Geriatric Dosage Handbook

— including —
Monitoring, Clinical Recommendations, and OBRA Guidelines

4th Edition   1998-99

D1809350

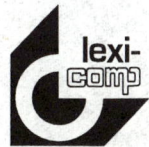

lexi-comp

APhA

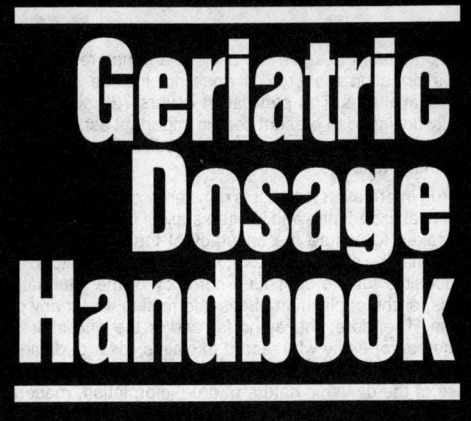

Geriatric Dosage Handbook

including

Monitoring, Clinical Recommendations, and OBRA Guidelines

4th Edition *1998-99*

Todd P. Semla, PharmD
Clinical Pharmacist
St Francis of Evanston
Evanston, Illinois
*Clinical Assistant Professor of Pharmacy Practice in
Medicine, Section of Geriatric Medicine*
University of Illinois at Chicago
Chicago, Illinois

Judith L. Beizer, PharmD
Associate Clinical Professor
College of Pharmacy and Allied Health Professions
St John's University
Jamaica, New York

Martin D. Higbee, PharmD
Associate Professor
Department of Pharmacy Practice and Science
The University of Arizona
Tucson, Arizona

NOTICE

This handbook is intended to serve the user as a handy reference and not as a complete drug information resource. It does not include information on every therapeutic agent available. The publication covers 735 commonly used drugs and is specifically designed to present certain important aspects of drug data in a more concise format than is typically found in medical literature or product material supplied by manufacturers.

The nature of drug information is that it is constantly evolving because of ongoing research and clinical experience and is often subject to interpretation. While great care has been taken to ensure the accuracy of the information presented, the reader is advised that the authors, editors, reviewers, contributors, and publishers cannot be responsible for the continued currency of the information or for any errors, omissions, or the application of this information, or for any consequences arising therefrom. Therefore, the author(s) and/or the publisher shall have no liability to any person or entity with regard to claims, loss, or damage caused, or alleged to be caused, directly or indirectly, by the use of information contained herein. Because of the dynamic nature of drug information, readers are advised that decisions regarding drug therapy must be based on the independent judgment of the clinician, changing information about a drug (eg, as reflected in the literature and manufacturer's most current product information), and changing medical practices. The editors are not responsible for any inaccuracy of quotation or for any false or misleading implication that may arise due to the text or formulas as used or due to the quotation of revisions no longer official.

The editors, authors, and contributors have written this book in their private capacities. No official support or endorsement by any federal or state agency or pharmaceutical company is intended or inferred.

The publishers have made every effort to trace the copyright holders for borrowed material. If they have inadvertently overlooked any, they will be pleased to make the necessary arrangements at the first opportunity.

If you have any suggestions or questions regarding any information presented in this handbook, please contact our drug information pharmacist at

1-800-837-LEXI

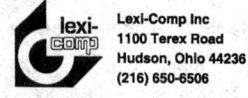

Lexi-Comp Inc
1100 Terex Road
Hudson, Ohio 44236
(216) 650-6506

ISBN 0-916589-65-X

TABLE OF CONTENTS

TABLE OF CONTENTS *(Continued)*

PREFACE

The *Geriatric Dosage Handbook* is designed to be a practical and convenient guide to the dosing and usage of medications in the elderly population. As the percentage of the population over the age of 65 increases, most healthcare professionals will be faced with the challenge of the appropriate use of medications in the elderly.

Many physiologic changes occur with aging, some of which affect the pharmacokinetics and/or pharmacodynamics of medications. For the majority of drugs, exact dosing guidelines for geriatric patients have not been established and most references do not specifically address the use of the medications in the elderly. For practical purposes, it has been recommended to "start low, go slow." Our objective in producing this handbook is to refine this recommendation and provide the reader with specific considerations when using medications in older adults. Information has been compiled from the current literature and our clinical experiences, emphasizing choice of medication, dosing, changes in pharmacokinetics or pharmacodynamics, monitoring parameters, and adverse effects. References are listed at the end of drug monographs to support this information when it exists. Additional clinical drug information which is relevant to the practice of geriatric pharmacotherapy is also included in each monograph and in the appendices.

This 4th edition of the handbook offers over 80 new and additional medications. Appendix information related to inhaled medications; depression scales; disease management (ie, asthma, osteoporosis, Parkinson's disease, constipation); new comparative drug charts; anticoagulant therapy guidelines; and various other useful tables and algorithms has been included.

We hope this reference proves to be a valuable and practical source of clinical drug information for healthcare professionals caring for the elderly. We welcome comments to improve future editions.

ACKNOWLEDGMENTS

The *Geriatric Dosage Handbook* exists in its present form as the result of the concerted efforts of the following individuals: the publisher and president of Lexi-Comp Inc, Robert D. Kerscher; Director of Books and Electronic Products, Julian I. Graubart, American Pharmaceutical Association (APhA); Lynn D. Coppinger, managing editor; and Barbara F. Kerscher, production manager.

Other members of the Lexi-Comp staff whose contributions deserve special mention include Diane Harbart, MT (ASCP), medical editor; Jeanne Wilson, Production/Systems Liason; Leslie Ruggles, Julie Katzen, Jennifer Rocky, and Stacey Hurd, project managers; Alexandra Hart, composition specialist; Jackie Mizer and Ginger Conner, production assistants; Tracey J. Reinecke, graphics designer; Jerry M. Reeves, Marc L. Long, and Patrick Grubb, sales managers; Jay L. Katzen and Brian B. Vossler, product managers; Kenneth J. Hughes, manager of authoring systems; Kristin M. Thompson, Matthew C. Kerscher, and Tina L. Collins, sales and marketing representatives; Edmund A. Harbart, vice-president, custom publishing division; Jack L. Stones, vice-president, reference publishing division; Dennis P. Smithers, David C. Marcus, and Sean Conrad, system analysts; Thury L. O'Connor, vice-president of technology; David J. Wasserbauer, vice-president, finance and administration; and Elizabeth M. Conlon and Rebecca A. Dryhurst, accounting.

Special thanks goes to Chris Lomax, PharmD, director of pharmacy, Children's Hospital, Los Angeles, who played a significant role in bringing APhA and Lexi-Comp together.

Much of the material contained in this book was a result of pharmacy contributors throughout the United States and Canada. Lexi-Comp has assisted many medical institutions to develop hospital-specific formulary manuals that contains clinical drug information as well as dosing. Working with these clinical pharmacists, hospital pharmacy and therapeutics committees, and hospital drug information centers, Lexi-Comp has developed an evolutionary drug database that reflects the practice of pharmacy in these major institutions.

In addition, the authors wish to thank their families, friends, and colleagues who supported them in their efforts to complete this handbook.

EDITORIAL ADVISORY PANEL

EDITORIAL ADVISORY PANEL *(Continued)*

Christopher J. Papasian, PhD
Director of Diagnostic Microbiology and Immunology Laboratories
Truman Medical Center
Kansas City, Missouri

Carol K. Taketomo, PharmD
Pharmacy Manager
Children's Hospital of Los Angeles
Los Angeles, California

Lowell L. Tilzer MD
Associate Medical Director
Community Blood Center of Greater Kansas City
Kansas City, Missouri

Richard L. Wynn, PhD
Professor and Chairman of Pharmacology
Baltimore College of Dental Surgery
Dental School
University of Maryland at Baltimore
Baltimore, Maryland

ABOUT THE AUTHORS

Todd P. Semla, MS, PharmD, BCPS, FCCP

Dr Semla received his Bachelor of Science in Pharmacy, his Master of Science in Clinical Pharmacy, and his Doctor of Pharmacy degrees from the University of Iowa. After earning his doctorate, Dr Semla was awarded the American Society of Health-System Pharmacists Fellowship in Geriatric Pharmacotherapy which he completed at the University of Iowa.

Dr Semla has more than 10 years experience in geriatric pharmacotherapy in a variety of clinical settings including ambulatory care, acute care and rehabilitation, and the nursing home. He is a Clinical Pharmacist at St Francis of Evanston with a practice in geriatric pharmacotherapy. Dr Semla is also a Clinical Assistant Professor of Pharmacy Practice in Medicine, Section of Geriatric Medicine, University of Illinois at Chicago College of Medicine. Prior to joining the staff at St Francis, Dr Semla was on the faculty of the University of Illinois at Chicago College of Pharmacy, the Pharmacotherapist for the Geriatric Assessment and Reactivation Unit and Geriatric Outpatient Assessment and Medicine Clinic at the University of Illinois and Clinics, and the Disciplinary Director for Pharmacy for the Illinois Geriatric Education Center.

Dr Semla's research interests include drug epidemiology in the elderly, Alzheimer's disease, and the effects of drugs on balance and postural control, and the role of the pharmacist in geriatric assessment. He has been an author of numerous publications in the geriatric, pharmacy, and medicine literature, and has presented original research at numerous professional meetings.

Dr Semla is an Associate Editor of the *Journal of Mental Health and Aging*, a member of the editorial board of the *Journal of the American Geriatrics Society*, and a member of the Geriatrics Editorial Panel for the *Annals of Pharmacotherapy*. He is an active member of several professional organizations, including the American Geriatrics Society (AGS) and the American College of Clinical Pharmacy (ACCP).

Judith L. Beizer, PharmD

Dr Beizer received her Bachelor of Science in Pharmacy from the St Louis College of Pharmacy and then earned a Doctor of Pharmacy degree from the University of Tennessee. After pursuing a residency in clinical pharmacy at the of the University of Pennsylvania, she completed a fellowship in geriatric pharmacy at Montefiore Medical Center, Bronx, NY. During her fellowship, Dr Beizer was involved in a National Institute on Aging (NIA) grant concerning medication use and pharmacist intervention in community-dwelling elderly.

Dr Beizer is currently an Associate Clinical Professor at St John's University College of Pharmacy and Allied Health Professions, Jamaica, NY. As part of her duties, she serves as Clinical Coordinator for Pharmacy at The Parker Jewish Institute for Healthcare and Rehabilitation, a long-term and sub-acute care facility in New Hyde Park, NY. At this facility she has expanded clinical pharmacy services and oversees students on rotation. Dr Beizer speaks regularly on the topic of medication use in the elderly and has published articles and abstracts on various issues in geriatric pharmacotherapy.

Dr Beizer is a member of numerous professional organizations, including the American Society of Health-System Pharmacists (ASHP), American Society of Consultant Pharmacists (ASCP), American College of Clinical Pharmacy (ACCP), the Gerontological Society of America (GSA), and the American Geriatric Society (AGS). She is a past chairperson of the ASHP Special Interest Group on Geriatric Pharmacy Practice. She currently serves on the Board of Commissioners for the Commission for Certification in Geriatric Pharmacy.

Martin D. Higbee, PharmD

Dr Higbee received his Bachelor of Science in Pharmacy from The University of Utah in 1973. After a year of pharmacy practice and clinical pharmacy experience received at The University of Utah, he entered the Doctor of Pharmacy degree program at The University of Texas at San Antonio. After graduation in 1977, he joined the University of Utah College of Pharmacy faculty. He became involved in the development of Salt Lake Veteran Administration Medical Center's Geriatric Treatment and Evaluation Unit. After the establishment of this unit, Dr Higbee created an ASHP accredited post-doctoral Geriatric Residency through the Veteran's Administration Medical Center and The University of Utah College of Pharmacy. Dr Higbee was also on the editorial staff for the Eli Lily - AACP

Geriatric Curriculum for Pharmacists project which created a geriatric textbook and curriculum for educators.

Dr Higbee joined the faculty at The University of Arizona in 1987. As part of his teaching responsibilities, he is a Clinical Pharmacist Consultant for the Hospital-Based Primary Care Team (division of Geriatric Care Center) at the Veterans Administration Medical Center in Tucson, Arizona, where he is preceptor for doctor of pharmacy students. Dr Higbee is also a nursing home consultant for local nursing homes in Arizona.

Dr Higbee regularly speaks locally and nationally on geriatric drug therapy topics and has published articles, chapters, and abstracts on various geriatric research and pharmacotherapy issues.

Dr Higbee is a member of numerous professional organizations, including American Society of Health-System Pharmacists (ASHP), American Pharmaceutical Association (APhA), American Society of Consultant Pharmacists (ASCP), American Association of Colleges of Pharmacy (AACP), and American College of Clinical Pharmacy (ACCP). He is a past chairman of the ASHP Special Interest Group on Geriatric Pharmacy Practice and past member of the AACP Task Force on Aging.

USE OF THE GERIATRIC DOSAGE HANDBOOK

The *Geriatric Dosage Handbook* is organized into a drug information section, an appendix, and a therapeutic category index.

The drug information section of the handbook, wherein all drugs are listed alphabetically, details information pertinent to each drug. Extensive cross referencing is provided by brand name and synonyms.

Drug information is presented in a consistent format and will provide the following:

Generic Name	U.S. Adopted Name
Pronunciation Guide	Phonetic pronunciation available by sound too
Related Information	Cross-reference to other pertinent drug information found in the Appendix
Brand Names	U.S. trade names (manufacturer specific)
Synonyms	Other names or accepted abbreviations of the generic name
Generic Available	Drugs available in generic form
Use	Information pertaining to appropriate indications of the drug. Includes both FDA approved and nonapproved indications.
Restrictions	The controlled substance classification from the Drug Enforcement Agency (DEA). U.S. schedules are I-V schedules vary by country and sometimes state (ie, Massachusetts uses I-VI).
Contraindications	Information pertaining to inappropriate use of the drug
Warnings	Hazardous conditions related to use of the drug and what to observe and parameters to monitor during therapy with the drug
Precautions	What to observe during therapy and disease states in which the drug should be cautiously used
Adverse Reactions	Side effects are grouped by body system (ie, dermatologic, gastrointestinal, etc)
Overdosage/	Signs or symptoms of excess drug
Toxicology	Suggested management of the patient with excess drug or overdose
Drug Interactions	Description of the interaction between the drug listed in the monograph and other drugs or drug classes. May include possible mechanisms and effect of combined therapy. May also include a strategy to manage the patient on combined therapy (ie, quinidine).
Drug/Food Interactions	Possible interactions between the drug listed in the monograph and certain foods and/or nutritional substances.
Stability	Information regarding storage of product or steps for reconstitution. Provides the time and conditions for which a solution or mixture will maintain full potency. For example, some solutions may require refrigeration after reconstitution while stored at room temperature prior to preparation.
Mechanism of Action	How drugs work in the body to elicit a response
Pharmacodynamics	Dose response relationships including onset of action, time of peak action, and duration of action

(continued)

Pharmacokinetics	Drug movement through the body over time. Pharmacokinetics deals with absorption, distribution, metabolism, half-life, bioavailability, protein binding, time to peak serum concentrations, and elimination of drugs. Pharmacokinetic parameters help predict drug concentration and dosage requirements.
Usual Dosage	The amount of the drug to be typically given or taken during therapy. Dosing information for geriatrics and adults as well as dosing adjustment information for renal failure or hepatic failure.
Administration	Information regarding the recommended final concentrations, rates of administration for parenteral drugs, or other guidelines when giving the medication.
Monitoring Parameters	Laboratory tests and patient physical parameters that should be monitored for safety and efficacy of drug therapy.
Reference Range	Therapeutic and toxic serum concentrations listed including peak and trough levels
Test Interactions	Listing of assay interference's when relevant (B = blood; S = serum; U = urine)
Patient Information	Advice, warnings, precautions, and other information of which the patient should be informed
Nursing Implications	Comments regarding nursing care of the patient. Includes additional instructions for the administration of the drug, also monitoring tips from the nursing perspective (ie, monitor for excessive sedation).
Additional Information	Information about sodium content and/or pertinent information about specific brands; dose equivalents (ie, metronidazole)
Special Geriatric Considerations	Pertinent information specific to the elderly
Dosage Forms	Information with regard to form, strength, and availability of the drug
References	Bibliographic information referring to specific geriatric literature findings

Appendix

The appendix offers a compilation of tables, guidelines, nomograms, and conversion information which can often be helpful when considering patient care.

Therapeutic Category Index

This index provides a useful listing of drugs by their therapeutic classification.

SAFE WRITING

Health professionals and their support personnel frequently produce handwritten copies of information they see in print; therefore, such information is subjected to even greater possibilities for error or misinterpretation on the part of others. Thus, particular care must be given to how drug names and strengths are expressed when creating written healthcare documents.

The following are a few examples of safe writing rules suggested by the Institute for Safe Medication Practices, Inc.*

1. There should be a space between a number and its units as it is easier to read. There should be no periods after the abbreviations mg or mL.

Correct	Incorrect
10 mg	10mg
100 mg	100mg

2. Never place a decimal and a zero after a whole number (2 mg is correct and 2.0 mg is incorrect). If the decimal point is not seen because it falls on a line or because individuals are working from copies where the decimal point is not seen, this causes a tenfold overdose.

3. Just the opposite is true for numbers less than 1. Always place a zero before a naked decimal (0.5 mL is correct, .5 mL is **in** correct).

4. Never abbreviate the word unit. The handwritten U or u, looks like a 0 (zero) and may cause a tenfold overdose error to be made.

5. Q.D. is not a safe abbreviation for once daily, as when the Q is followed by a sloppy dot, it looks like QID which means 4 times daily.

6. O.D. is not a safe abbreviation for once daily, as it is properly interpreted as meaning "right eye" and has caused liquid medications such as saturated solution of potassium iodide and Lugol's solution to be administered incorrectly. There is no safe abbreviation for once daily. It must be written out in full.

7. Do not use chemical names such as 6-mercaptopurine or 6-thioguanine, as sixfold overdoses have been given when these were not recognized as chemical names. The proper names of these drugs are mercaptopurine or thioguanine.

8. Do not abbreviate drug names (5FC, 6MP, 5-ASA, MTX, HCTZ CPZ, PBZ, etc) as they are misinterpreted and cause error.

9. Do not use the apothecary system or symbols.

10. When writing an outpatient prescription, write a complete prescription. A complete prescription can prevent the prescriber, the pharmacist, and/or the patient from making a mistake and can eliminate the need for further clarification.

    The legible prescriptions should contain:

    a. patient's full name

    b. for pediatric or geriatric patients: their age (or weight where applicable)

    c. drug name, dosage form and strength; if a drug is new or rarely prescribed, print this information

    d. number or amount to be dispensed

    e. complete patient instructions, including purpose of the medication

    f. when there are recognized contraindications for a prescribed drug, indicate to the pharmacist that you are aware of this fact (ie, when prescribing a potassium salt for a patient receiving an ACE inhibitor, write "K serum leveling being monitored")

*From "Safe Writing" by Davis NM, PharmD and Cohen MR, MS, Lecturers and Consultants for Safe Medication Practices, 1143 Wright Drive, Huntingdon Valley, PA 19006. Phone: (215) 947-7566.

ALPHABETICAL LISTING OF DRUGS

Abbokinase® *see* Urokinase *on page 974*

Abelcet™ Injection *see* Amphotericin B Lipid Complex *on page 72*

ABLC *see* Amphotericin B Lipid Complex *on page 72*

Absorbine® Antifungal [OTC] *see* Tolnaftate *on page 939*

Absorbine® Antifungal Foot Powder [OTC] *see* Miconazole *on page 625*

Absorbine® Jock Itch [OTC] *see* Tolnaftate *on page 939*

Absorbine Jr.® Antifungal [OTC] *see* Tolnaftate *on page 939*

Acarbose (AY car bose)

Brand Names Precose®

Therapeutic Category Alpha-Glucosidase Inhibitor

Use Treatment of type II diabetes mellitus (noninsulin-dependent diabetes mellitus); as monotherapy or in combination with a sulfonylurea when diet plus acarbose or a sulfonylurea does not result in adequate glycemic control

Contraindications Hypersensitivity to the drug; diabetic ketoacidosis, inflammatory bowel disease, colonic ulceration, partial intestinal obstruction, predisposition to intestinal obstruction, or chronic intestinal diseases associated with disorders of absorption or digestion, hernias, or other conditions which may be aggravated by increased gas

Warnings Not recommended for patients with significant renal impairment (S_{cr} >2 mg/dL)

Precautions See Overdosage

Adverse Reactions

Gastrointestinal: Flatulence, diarrhea, abdominal pain, dyspepsia, nausea, frequent or loose stools

Hepatic: Increased transaminase levels

Overdosage Hypoglycemia must be treated with oral or injectable glucose or injectable glucagon, but not sucrose (cane sugar)

Drug Interactions Insulin, oral hypoglycemics may increase risk of hypoglycemia; decreased bioavailability of metformin; charcoal and other intestinal adsorbents, digestive enzymes may decrease effectiveness of acarbose

Mechanism of Action Competitive inhibitor of pancreatic α-amylase and intestinal brush border α-glucosidases, resulting in delayed hydrolysis of ingested complex carbohydrates and disaccharides and absorption of glucose; dose-dependent reduction in postprandial serum insulin and glucose peaks; inhibits the metabolism of sucrose to glucose and fructose

Pharmacokinetics

Bioavailability: Systemic: 1% to 2%

Elimination: 51% unchanged in feces; degradation by gastrointestinal enzymes and microorganisms

Usual Dosage Geriatrics and Adults: Oral: Dosage must be individualized; initial dose: 25 mg 3 times/day just before meals or with first bite; increase at 4- to 8-week intervals; maximum dose: 100 mg 3 times/day for patients >60 kg body weight, 50 mg 3 times/day for patients <60 kg body weight

Administration See Usual Dosage

Monitoring Parameters Preprandial blood glucose, glycosylate hemoglobin A_{1c}, fructosamine, serum transaminase levels

Patient Information Must be taken at the start of a meal; review signs and symptoms of hypoglycemia and how to treat

Nursing Implications See Overdosage

Special Geriatric Considerations No specific trials in the elderly have been conducted; mean age in clinical trials has been <60 years; monitor change in preprandial blood glucose concentrations to account for potential age-related changes in postprandial glucose. Elderly, in clinical trials, had serum concentrations 1.5 times those of younger adults. Patients with creatinine clearance <25 mL/minute had serum concentrations 5 times those with normal renal clearance. No clinical significance can be attributed to this at this time. No adjustments in dose are recommended.

Dosage Forms Tablet: 50 mg, 100 mg

References

Balfour JA and McTavish D, "Acarbose: A Reappraisal," *Drugs*, 1993, 46(6):1025-54.

Bischoff H, "Pharmacology of α-Glucosidase Inhibition," *Eur J Clin Invest*, 1994, 24(Suppl 3):3-10.

Scheen AJ, de Magalhaes AC, Salvatore T, et al, "Reduction of the Acute Bioavailability of Metformin by the α-Glucosidase Inhibitor Acarbose in Normal Man," *Eur J Clin Invest*, 1994, 24(Suppl 3):50-4.

Accolate® *see* Zafirlukast *on page 993*

Accupril® *see* Quinapril *on page 813*

Acebutolol (a se BYOO toe lole)

Related Information
Beta-Blockers Comparison *on page 1026*

Brand Names Sectral®

Generic Available No

Therapeutic Category Antiarrhythmic Agent, Class II; Beta-Adrenergic Blocker

Use Treatment of hypertension; ventricular arrhythmias; although not an approved indication, beta-adrenergic blockers generally reduce angina

Contraindications Hypersensitivity to beta-blocking agents, uncompensated congestive heart failure; cardiogenic shock; bradycardia or heart block; sinus node dysfunction; A-V conduction abnormalities. Although acebutolol primarily blocks $beta_1$-receptors, high doses can result in $beta_2$-receptor blockage. Therefore, use with caution in elderly with bronchospastic lung disease and renal dysfunction. **Note:** Geriatric patients often have decreased renal function.

Warnings Abrupt withdrawal of beta-blockers may result in an exaggerated cardiac beta-adrenergic responsiveness. Symptomatology has included reports of tachycardia, hypertension, ischemia, angina, myocardial infarction, and sudden death. It is recommended that patients be tapered gradually off of beta-blockers over a 2-week period rather than via abrupt discontinuation.

Precautions Diabetes mellitus (may mask signs/symptoms of hypoglycemia), renal function decline, myasthenia gravis, and severe peripheral vascular disease; use with caution in patients with bronchospasm disease or congestive heart failure, patients undergoing anesthesia, and hyperthyroidism

Adverse Reactions

Cardiovascular: Persistent bradycardia, torsade de pointes, ventricular arrhythmias, shortness of breath, heart block, hypotension, chest pain, edema, heart failure, Raynaud's phenomena, facial edema

Central nervous system: Depression, confusion, dizziness, insomnia, lethargy, headache, nightmares, fatigue

Dermatologic: Rash, pruritus

Gastrointestinal: Constipation, diarrhea, nausea, xerostomia, gastritis, anorexia

Genitourinary: Impotence, decreased libido, urinary retention, polyuria

Neuromuscular & skeletal: Arthralgia, muscle cramps

Ocular: Blurred vision, visual disturbance

Miscellaneous: Cold extremities

Overdosage See Toxicology

Toxicology Sympathomimetics (eg, epinephrine or dopamine), glucagon or a pacemaker can be used to treat the toxic bradycardia, asystole, and/or hypotension. Initially, fluids may be the best treatment for toxic hypotension. Patients should remain supine; serum glucose and potassium should be measured. Use supportive measures: lavage, syrup of ipecac; atenolol may be removed by hemodialysis. I.V. glucose should be administered for hypoglycemia; seizures may be treated with phenytoin or diazepam intravenously; continuous monitoring of blood pressure and EKG is necessary. If PVCs occur, treat with lidocaine or phenytoin; avoid quinidine, procainamide, and disopyramide since these agents further depress myocardial function. Bronchospasm can be treated with theophylline on $beta_2$ agonists (epinephrine).

Drug Interactions

Pharmacologic action of beta antagonists may be decreased by aluminum compounds, calcium salts, barbiturates, cholestyramine, colestipol, NSAIDs, penicillins (ampicillin), rifampin, salicylates, sulfinpyrazone, thyroid hormones; hypoglycemic effect of sulfonylureas may be blunted

Pharmacologic effect of beta antagonists may be enhanced with concomitant use of calcium channel blockers, oral contraceptives, flecainide (bioavailability and effect of flecainide also enhanced), haloperidol (hypotensive effects of both drugs), H_2 antagonists (decreased metabolism), hydralazine (both drugs hypotensive effects increased), loop diuretics (increased serum concentration of beta-blockers except atenolol), MAO inhibitors, phenothiazines, propafenone, quinidine, quinolones, thioamines; beta-blockers may decrease clearance of acetaminophen; beta-blockers may increase anticoagulant effects of warfarin (propranolol); benzodiazepine effects enhanced by the lipophilic beta-blockers (atenolol does not interact); significant and fatal increases in blood pressure have occurred after decrease in dose or discontinuation of clonidine in patients receiving both clonidine and beta-blockers together (reduce doses of each cautiously with small decreases); peripheral ischemia of ergot alkaloids enhanced by beta-blockers; beta-

(Continued)

Acebutolol *(Continued)*

blockers increase serum concentration of lidocaine; beta-blockers increase hypotensive effect of prazosin

Mechanism of Action Competitively blocks $beta_1$-adrenergic receptors with little or no effect on $beta_2$-receptors except at high doses. Exhibits membrane stabilizing and intrinsic sympathomimetic activity; low lipid solubility, therefore, little crosses blood-brain barrier.

Pharmacokinetics

Absorption: Oral: Well absorbed, 90%

Protein binding: 25%

Metabolism: Undergoes extensive first-pass; substrate of CYP1A2 and 2E1

Half-life: 3-4 hours

Time to peak: 2-4 hours

Elimination: Primarily excreted by bile and intestinal wall 50% to 60%; renal excretion 30% to 40%; some hepatic elimination occurs

Usual Dosage Oral:

Geriatrics: Initial: 200-400 mg/day; dose reduction due to age-related decrease in Cl_{cr} will be necessary; do not exceed 800 mg/day

Adults: 400-800 mg/day in 2 divided doses; maximum: 1200 mg/day

Dosing adjustment in renal impairment:

Cl_{cr} 25-49 mL/minute/1.73 m^2: Reduce dose by 50%

Cl_{cr} <25 mL/minute/1.73 m^2: Reduce dose by 75%

Dosing adjustment in hepatic impairment: Use with caution

Monitoring Parameters Blood pressure, orthostatic hypotension, heart rate, CNS effects

Test Interactions Increased triglycerides, potassium, uric acid, cholesterol (S), glucose; decreased HDL

Patient Information Do not discontinue medication abruptly, sudden stopping of medication may precipitate or cause angina; consult pharmacist or physician before taking with other adrenergic drugs (eg, cold medications); notify physician if any of the following symptoms occur: difficult breathing, night cough, swelling of extremities, slow pulse, dizziness, lightheadedness, confusion, depression, skin rash, fever, sore throat, unusual bleeding or bruising; may produce drowsiness, dizziness, lightheadedness, blurred vision, confusion; use with caution while driving or performing tasks requiring alertness; may mask signs of hypoglycemia in diabetics; may be taken without regard to meals

Nursing Implications Advise against abrupt withdrawal (see Monitoring Parameters)

Special Geriatric Considerations Since bioavailability increased in elderly about twofold, geriatric patients may require lower maintenance doses, therefore, as serum and tissue concentrations increase $beta_1$ selectivity diminishes; due to alterations in the beta-adrenergic autonomic nervous system, beta-adrenergic blockade may result in less hemodynamic response than seen in younger adults. Studies indicate that despite decreased sensitivity to the chronotropic effects of beta blockade with age, there appears to be an increased myocardial sensitivity to the negative inotropic effect during stress (ie, exercise). Controlled trials have shown the overall response rate for propranolol to be only 20% to 50% in elderly populations. Therefore, all beta-adrenergic blocking drugs may result in a decreased response as compared to younger adults. Adjust dose for renal function in the elderly.

Dosage Forms Capsule, as hydrochloride: 200 mg, 400 mg

References

Kligman EW and Higbee MD, "Drug Therapy for Hypertension in the Elderly," *J Fam Pract*, 1989, 28(1):81-7.

Levison SP, "Treating Hypertension in the Elderly," *Clin Geriatr Med*, 1988, 4(1):1-12.

Vestal RE, Wood AJ, and Shand DG, "Reduced Beta-Adrenoceptor Sensitivity in the Elderly," *Clin Pharmacol Ther*, 1979, 26(2):181-6.

Yin FC, Raizes, GS, Guarnieri T, et al, "Age-Associated Decrease in Ventricular Response to Haemodynamic Stress During Beta-Adrenergic Blockade," *Br Heart J*, 1978, 40(12):1349-55.

ACE Inhibitors Comparison *see page 1019*

Acephen® [OTC] *see* Acetaminophen *on this page*

Aceta® [OTC] *see* Acetaminophen *on this page*

Acetaminophen *(a seet a MIN oh fen)*

Brand Names Acephen® [OTC]; Aceta® [OTC]; Apacet® [OTC]; Banesin® [OTC]; Dapa® [OTC]; Datril® [OTC]; Dorcol® [OTC]; Feverall™ [OTC]; Genapap® [OTC]; Halenol® [OTC]; Liquiprin® [OTC]; Mapap® [OTC]; Maranox® [OTC]; Panadol® [OTC]; Panex 500® [OTC]; Redutemp® [OTC];

Ridenol® [OTC]; Tempra® [OTC]; Tylenol® [OTC]; Tylenol® Extended Relief [OTC]; Uni Aco® [OTC]

Synonyms APAP; N-Acetyl-P-Aminophenol; Paracetamol

Generic Available Yes

Therapeutic Category Analgesic, Non-narcotic; Antipyretic

Use Treatment of mild to moderate pain and fever; does not have antirheumatic effects

Contraindications Hypersensitivity to acetaminophen, G-6-PD deficiency

Warnings May cause severe hepatic toxicity with overdose; chronic daily doses of 5-8 g over several weeks or 3-4 g/day for 1 year have resulted in liver damage; use with caution in patients with alcoholic liver disease

Adverse Reactions
Dermatologic: Rash
Renal: Renal injury with chronic use
Miscellaneous: Hypersensitivity reactions (rare)

Overdosage Symptoms of overdose include hepatic necrosis, transient azotemia, renal tubular necrosis with acute toxicity, anemia, and GI disturbances with chronic toxicity

Toxicology Acetylcysteine 140 mg/kg orally (loading) followed by 70 mg/kg every 4 hours for 17 doses; therapy should be initiated based upon laboratory analysis suggesting high probability of hepatotoxic potential. Activated charcoal is very effective at binding acetaminophen; however, the dose of acetylcysteine may need to be increased. Intravenous acetylcysteine should be reserved for patients unable to take oral forms.

Drug Interactions Potential hepatotoxicity of acetaminophen may be increased and the therapeutic effects may be decreased with the concomitant use of the following agents: barbiturates, carbamazepine, hydantoins, rifampin, sulfinpyrazone; increased toxicity with alcohol

Mechanism of Action Inhibits the synthesis of prostaglandins in the central nervous system and peripherally blocks pain impulse generation; produces antipyresis from inhibition of hypothalamic heat-regulating center

Pharmacokinetics
Protein binding: 20% to 50%
Metabolism: At normal therapeutic dosages the parent compound is metabolized in the liver to sulfate and glucuronide metabolites, while a small amount is metabolized by microsomal mixed function oxidases to a highly reactive intermediate (N-acetyl-imidoquinone) which is conjugated with glutathione and inactivated; at toxic doses (as little as 4 g in a single day) glutathione can become depleted, and conjugation becomes insufficient to meet the metabolic demand causing an increase in N-acetyl-imidoquinone concentration, which is thought to cause hepatic cell necrosis
Half-life: 1-3 hours; may be increased in the elderly, but this should not affect drug dosing
Time to peak serum concentration: Oral: 10-60 minutes after normal doses, but may be delayed in acute overdoses

Usual Dosage Geriatrics and Adults: Oral, rectal: 325-650 mg every 4-6 hours or 1000 mg 3-4 times/day; do **not** exceed 4 g/day

Dosing interval in renal impairment:
Cl_{cr} 10-50 mL/minute: Administer every 6 hours
Cl_{cr} <10 mL/minute: Administer every 8 hours (metabolites accumulate)
Moderately dialyzable (20% to 50%)
Dosing adjustment/comments in hepatic impairment: Appears to be well tolerated in cirrhosis; serum concentration may need monitoring with long-term use

Monitoring Parameters Relief of pain or fever

Reference Range Toxic concentration with probable hepatotoxicity: >200 μg/mL at 4 hours or 50 μg/mL at 12 hours

Test Interactions Increased chloride, bilirubin, uric acid, glucose, ammonia (B), chloride (S), uric acid (S), alkaline phosphatase (S), chloride (S); decreased sodium, bicarbonate, calcium (S)

Patient Information Do not exceed recommended dosage; check cough and cold preparations for acetaminophen content; avoid alcohol while taking acetaminophen

Nursing Implications Monitor patient for relief of pain and/or fever

Additional Information The American College of Rheumatology has recommended acetaminophen as the first-line drug in the treatment of osteoarthritis of the hip or knee

Special Geriatric Considerations See Warnings and Usual Dosage
(Continued)

Acetaminophen *(Continued)*

Dosage Forms
Caplet: 160 mg, 325 mg, 500 mg
Elixir: 120 mg/5 mL, 160 mg/5 mL, 167 mg/5 mL, 325 mg/5 mL
Liquid, oral: 160 mg/5 mL, 500 mg/15 mL
Suppository: 120 mg, 325 mg, 600 mg
Tablet: 80 mg, 325 mg, 500 mg, 650 mg

References
Hochberg MC, Altman RD, Brandt KD, et al, "Guidelines for the Medical Management of Osteoarthritis. Part I. Osteoarthritis of the Hip. American College of Rheumatology," *Arthritis Rheum*, 1995, 38(11):1535-40.

Hochberg MC, Altman RD, Brandt KD, et al, "Guidelines for the Medical Management of Osteoarthritis. Part II. Osteoarthritis of the Knee. American College of Rheumatology," *Arthritis Rheum*, 1995, 38(11):1541-6.

Acetaminophen and Codeine *(a seet a MIN oh fen & KOE deen)*

Brand Names Capital® and Codeine; Phenaphen® With Codeine; Tylenol® With Codeine

Synonyms Codeine and Acetaminophen

Generic Available Yes

Therapeutic Category Analgesic, Narcotic

Use Relief of mild to moderate pain

Restrictions C-III

Contraindications Hypersensitivity to acetaminophen or codeine phosphate

Warnings Tablets contain metabisulfite which may cause allergic reactions; acetaminophen may cause hepatic damage in overdose or with chronic use of high doses

Precautions Use with caution in patients with hypersensitivity reactions to other phenanthrene derivative opioid agonists (morphine, hydrocodone, hydromorphone, levorphanol, oxycodone, oxymorphone) or respiratory disease or compromise

Adverse Reactions
Cardiovascular: Palpitations, hypotension, bradycardia, peripheral vasodilation
Central nervous system: CNS depression, dizziness, drowsiness, sedation, increased intracranial pressure
Dermatologic: Pruritus
Endocrine & metabolic: Antidiuretic hormone release
Gastrointestinal: Nausea, vomiting, constipation
Ocular: Miosis
Respiratory: Respiratory depression
Miscellaneous: Physical and psychological dependence with prolonged use, biliary or urinary tract spasm, histamine release

Overdosage Symptoms of overdose include hepatic necrosis, blood dyscrasias, respiratory depression, transient azotemia, renal tubular necrosis with acute toxicity, anemia, and GI disturbances with chronic toxicity

Toxicology Acetylcysteine 140 mg/kg orally (loading) followed by 70 mg/kg every 4 hours for 17 doses; therapy should begin after availability of serum acetaminophen concentration. Naloxone (2 mg I.V.) can also be used to reverse the toxic effects of the opiate (see Naloxone monograph). Activated charcoal is effective at binding certain chemicals and this is especially true for acetaminophen; however, dose of acetylcysteine may need to be increased by 30% or charcoal should be removed first.

Drug Interactions Potential hepatotoxicity of acetaminophen may be increased and the therapeutic effects may be decreased with the concomitant use of the following agents: barbiturates, carbamazepine, hydantoins, rifampin, sulfinpyrazone; increased toxicity with alcohol; increased toxicity with CNS depressants, phenothiazines, tricyclic antidepressants, guanabenz, MAO inhibitors (may decrease blood pressure); codeine's conversion to morphine may be inhibited by SSRIs (CYP2D6)

Usual Dosage Doses should be titrated to appropriate analgesic effect
Geriatrics: 1 Tylenol® [#3] or 2 Tylenol® [#2] tablets every 4 hours; do not exceed 4 g/day acetaminophen
Adults: 1-2 tablets every 4 hours with a maximum of 12 tablets/24 hours

Monitoring Parameters Relief of pain, respiratory and mental status, blood pressure, bowel function

Patient Information May cause drowsiness; avoid alcoholic beverages; do not exceed recommended dose; check cough and cold preparations for acetaminophen content

Nursing Implications Observe patient for excessive sedation or confusion, respiratory depression, constipation

Special Geriatric Considerations The duration of action of codeine may be prolonged in the elderly; in addition, enhanced analgesia has been seen in elderly patients on therapeutic doses of narcotics; if 1 tablet/dose is used, it may be useful to add an additional 325 mg of acetaminophen to maximize analgesic effect

Dosage Forms
Capsule:
#2: Acetaminophen 325 mg and codeine phosphate 15 mg (C-III)
#3: Acetaminophen 325 mg and codeine phosphate 30 mg (C-III)
#4: Acetaminophen 325 mg and codeine phosphate 60 mg (C-III)
Elixir: Acetaminophen 120 mg and codeine phosphate 12 mg per 5 mL with alcohol 7% (C-V)
Suspension, oral, alcohol free: Acetaminophen 120 mg and codeine phosphate 12 mg per 5 mL (C-V)
Tablet: Acetaminophen 500 mg and codeine phosphate 30 mg (C-III); acetaminophen 650 mg and codeine phosphate 30 mg (C-III)
Tablet:
#1: Acetaminophen 300 mg and codeine phosphate 7.5 mg (C-III)
#2: Acetaminophen 300 mg and codeine phosphate 15 mg (C-III)
#3: Acetaminophen 300 mg and codeine phosphate 30 mg (C-III)
#4: Acetaminophen 300 mg and codeine phosphate 60 mg (C-III)

Acetaminophen and Hydrocodone *see* Hydrocodone and Acetaminophen *on page 461*

Acetaminophen and Oxycodone *see* Oxycodone and Acetaminophen *on page 705*

Acetazolamide (a set a ZOLE a mide)
Related Information
Glaucoma Drug Therapy Comparison *on page 1032*
I.V. Push Recommended Guidelines *on page 1083*
Brand Names Diamox®; Diamox Sequels®
Generic Available Yes
Therapeutic Category Anticonvulsant, Miscellaneous; Carbonic Anhydrase Inhibitor; Diuretic, Carbonic Anhydrase Inhibitor
Use Lower intraocular pressure to treat glaucoma; also used as a diuretic; adjunct treatment of refractory seizure disorders and acute altitude sickness
Contraindications Hypersensitivity to acetazolamide or other sulfonamides; patients with hepatic or significant renal insufficiency; patients with decreased serum sodium and/or potassium; patients with adrenocortical insufficiency; severe pulmonary obstruction; long-term use in noncongestive angle-closure glaucoma
Warnings I.M. administration is painful because of the alkaline pH of the drug
Precautions Use with caution in patients with respiratory acidosis and diabetes mellitus; impairment of mental alertness and/or physical coordination may occur; electrolyte balance should be monitored
Adverse Reactions
Central nervous system: Fever, drowsiness, fatigue, malaise, confusion, convulsions
Dermatologic: Rash (including Stevens-Johnson syndrome, erythema multiforme, toxic epidermal necrolysis)
Endocrine & metabolic: Hyperchloremic metabolic acidosis in up to 55% of older patients, hypokalemia, hyperglycemia
Gastrointestinal: GI irritation, anorexia, dryness of the mouth, vomiting, constipation
Genitourinary: Polyuria
Hematologic: Bone marrow suppression
Neuromuscular & skeletal: Muscular weakness, paresthesia
Ocular: Myopia
Renal: Dysuria, renal calculi, glycosuria, hematuria
Toxicology For decontamination, lavage/activated charcoal with cathartic; hemodialysis may remove as much as 30% of dose
Drug Interactions
Increased lithium excretion and decreased excretion of amphetamines, quinidine, procainamide, flecainide, phenobarbital, and salicylates by alkalinization of the urine
Salicylates may also increase risk of metabolic acidosis (see Additional Information)
Hypokalemia may be compounded with concurrent use of diuretics or steroids
(Continued)

Acetazolamide *(Continued)*

Primidone's absorption may be delayed

Digitalis toxicity may occur if hypokalemia is untreated

Stability Reconstituted solution may be stored under refrigeration (2°C to 8°C) for 24 hours (the product contains no preservative); discard unused solutions after 24 hours

Mechanism of Action Reversible inhibition of the enzyme carbonic anhydrase resulting in increased renal excretion of sodium, potassium, bicarbonate, and water; enzyme inhibition also decreases aqueous humor production, thus decreasing intraocular pressure

Pharmacodynamics

Onset of action: Lowering of intraocular pressure varies between 2 minutes with the I.V. form to 2 hours with the sustained release capsule

Peak effect:

I.V.: 15 minutes

Capsule, sustained release: 8-12 hours

Tablet: 1-4 hours

Duration:

I.V.: 4-5 hours

Capsule, sustained release: 18-24 hours

Tablet: 8-12 hours

Pharmacokinetics

Distribution: Into erythrocytes, kidneys and crosses the blood-brain barrier

Protein binding: 95% bound to serum proteins; may be lower in the elderly; increased plasma concentrations secondary to decreased clearance in older persons with decreased renal function; these changes increase the risk of hyperchloremic acidosis

Half-life: 2.4-5.8 hours

Elimination: 70% to 100% of the I.V. or tablet dose is excreted unchanged in the urine within 24 hours

Usual Dosage

Geriatrics: Oral: Initial: 250 mg once or twice daily; use lowest effective dose possible

Adults:

Glaucoma:

Oral: 250 mg 1-4 times/day or 500 mg sustained release capsule twice daily

I.M., I.V.: 250-500 mg, may repeat in 2-4 hours; standard doses may lead to excessive plasma concentrations

Edema: Oral, I.M., I.V.: 250-375 mg once daily

Epilepsy: Oral: 8-30 mg/kg/day in 1-4 divided doses

Altitude sickness: Oral: 250 mg every 6-12 hours

Dosing interval in renal impairment:

Cl_{cr} 10-50 mL/minute: Administer every 12 hours

Cl_{cr} <10 mL/minute: Avoid use; ineffective, may potentiate acidosis

Moderately dialyzable (20% to 50%)

Administration Reconstitute each 500 mg vial with 5 mL of sterile water for injection to yield a concentration of 100 mg/mL; may cause an alteration in taste, especially carbonated beverages; short-acting tablets may be crushed and suspended in cherry or chocolate syrup to disguise the bitter taste of the drug, do not use fruit juices, alternatively submerge tablet in 10 mL of hot water and add 10 mL honey or syrup

Monitoring Parameters Intraocular pressure, serum bicarbonate, sodium and potassium, periodic CBC with differential

Reference Range Total: 5-10 µg/mL; Free (unbound) 0.25-0.5 µg/mL

Test Interactions Increased chloride, bilirubin, uric acid, glucose, ammonia (B), chloride (S), uric acid (S), alkaline phosphatase (S), chloride (S); decreased sodium, bicarbonate, calcium (S)

Patient Information Report numbness or tingling of extremities to physician; do not crush, chew, or swallow contents of long-acting capsule, but may be opened and sprinkled on soft food; ability to perform tasks requiring mental alertness and/or physical coordination may be impaired; take with food

Additional Information Drug may cause substantial increase in blood glucose in some diabetic patients; sustained release capsule is not recommended for treatment of epilepsy; the use of analgesic doses of salicylates should be avoided in patients treated with acetazolamide, especially the elderly

Special Geriatric Considerations Malaise and complaints of tiredness and myalgia are signs of excessive dosing and acidosis in the elderly

Dosage Forms
Capsule, sustained release: 500 mg
Injection: 500 mg
Tablet: 125 mg, 250 mg

References
Chapron DJ, Gomolin IH, and Sweeney KR, "Acetazolamide Blood Concentrations are Excessive in the Elderly: Propensity for Acidosis and Relationship to Renal Function," *J Clin Pharmacol*, 1989, 29(4):348-53.

Chapron DJ, Sweeney KR, Feig PU, et al, "Influence of Advanced Age on the Disposition of Acetazolamide," *Br J Clin Pharmacol*, 1985, 19:363-71.

Heller I, Halevy J, Cohen S, et al, "Significant Metabolic Acidosis Induced by Acetazolamide," *Arch Intern Med*, 1985, 145:1815-7.

Reiss WG and Oles KS, "Acetazolamide in the Treatment of Seizures," *Ann Pharmacother*, 1996, 30(5):514-9.

Rousseau P and Fuentevilla-Clifton A, "Acetazolamide and Salicylate Interaction in the Elderly: A Case Report," *J Am Geriatr Soc*, 1993, 41(8):868-9.

Acetohexamide (a set oh HEKS a mide)

Related Information
Antacid Drug Interactions *on page 1096*

Brand Names Dymelor®

Generic Available Yes

Therapeutic Category Antidiabetic Agent; Hypoglycemic Agent, Oral; Sulfonylurea Agent

Use Adjunct to diet for the management of mild to moderately severe, stable noninsulin-dependent (type II) diabetes mellitus

Contraindications Diabetes complicated by ketoacidosis, therapy of type 1 diabetes, hypersensitivity to sulfonylureas

Precautions Avoid alcohol or products containing alcohol; patients with liver disease or reduced renal function may have increased risk for symptomatic hypoglycemia

Adverse Reactions
Central nervous system: Headache
Endocrine & metabolic: Severe hypoglycemia, hyponatremia, syndrome of inappropriate antidiuretic hormone
Gastrointestinal: Nausea, vomiting, epigastric fullness, heartburn, diarrhea

Overdosage Symptoms of overdose include low blood sugar, tingling of lips and tongue, nausea, yawning, confusion, agitation, tachycardia, sweating, convulsions, stupor, and coma

Toxicology Hypoglycemia should be managed with 50 mL I.V. dextrose 50% followed immediately with a continuous infusion of 10% dextrose in water (administer at a rate sufficient enough to approach a serum glucose level of 100 mg/dL). The use of corticosteroids to treat the hypoglycemia is controversial, however, the addition of 100 mg of hydrocortisone to the dextrose infusion may prove helpful.

Drug Interactions Monitor patient closely; large number of drugs interact with sulfonylureas to enhance their hypoglycemic effects including oral anticoagulants, salicylates, NSAIDs, sulfonamides, phenylbutazone, insulin, clofibrate, fenfluramine, fluconazole, gemfibrozil, H_2 antagonists, methyldopa, tricyclic antidepressants, urinary acidifiers; decreased hypoglycemic effects by beta-blockers, cholestyramine, diazoxide, hydantoins, rifampin, thiazides, urinary alkalinizers

Mechanism of Action Believed to cause hypoglycemia by stimulating insulin release from the pancreatic beta cells; reduces glucose output from the liver (decreases gluconeogenesis); insulin sensitivity is increased at peripheral target sites (alters receptor sensitivity/receptor density); potentiates effects of ADH; may produce mild diuresis and significant uricosuric activity

Pharmacodynamics
Peak hypoglycemic effect: Within 8-10 hours
Duration: 12-24 hours (prolonged with renal impairment)

Pharmacokinetics
Protein binding: ~90% (ionic/nonionic)
Metabolism: In the liver to potent active metabolite
Half-life: 5-6 hours (parent compound has half-life of 0.8-2.4 hours)
Elimination: Urinary excretion <40% as unchanged drug; metabolite, hydroxyhexamide is more potent and is excreted less rapidly; ~80% to 95% of dose excreted in urine within 24 hours; ~15% is excreted in bile

Usual Dosage Geriatrics and Adults: Oral: 250 mg to 1.5 g/day in 1-2 divided doses; if daily dose is ≤1 g it should be as a single daily dose

Dosing adjustment in renal impairment: Cl_{cr} <50 mL/minute: Avoid use; prolonged hypoglycemia occurs in azotemic patients
(Continued)

Acetohexamide *(Continued)*

Dosing adjustment in hepatic impairment: Initiate therapy at lower than recommended doses

Monitoring Parameters Fasting blood glucose, hemoglobin A_{1c} or fructosamine

Reference Range Fasting blood glucose: Geriatrics: 100-150 mg/dL; Adults: 80-140 mg/dL

Test Interactions Decreased glucose, uric acid, decreased prothrombin time, decreased sodium (S)

Patient Information If nausea or stomach upset occurs, may be taken with food; avoid hypoglycemia, eat regularly, do not skip meals; keep sugar source with you

Nursing Implications Blood (preferred) and urine glucose concentrations should be monitored when therapy is started; normally takes 7 days to determine therapeutic response; patients who are anorexic or NPO may need to have their dose held to avoid hypoglycemia

Additional Information Produces a diuretic effect and increases the urinary excretion of uric acid

Special Geriatric Considerations Not considered a drug of choice in the elderly because of the potentially prolonged half-life of the more active metabolite; has not been specifically studied in the elderly; how "tightly" a geriatric patient's blood sugar of <150 mg/dL is now an acceptable end point. Such a decision should be based on the patient's functional and cognitive status, how well they recognize hypoglycemic or hyperglycemic symptoms, and how to respond to them, and their other disease states.

Dosage Forms Tablet: 250 mg, 500 mg

Acetophenazine *(a set oh FEN a zeen)*

Related Information

Antacid Drug Interactions *on page 1096*
Antipsychotic Agents Comparison *on page 1023*
Antipsychotic Medication Guidelines *on page 1076*
Federal OBRA Regulations Recommended Maximum Doses - Antipsychotics *on page 1056*

Brand Names Tindal®

Generic Available No

Therapeutic Category Antipsychotic Agent; Neuroleptic Agent; Phenothiazine Derivative

Use Management of manifestations of psychotic disorders; treatment of depressive neurosis, alcohol withdrawal, nausea and vomiting, Tourette's syndrome, Huntington's chorea, spasmodic torticollis, and Reye's syndrome; treatment of nonpsychotic symptoms associated with dementia in elderly (see Special Geriatric Considerations)

Contraindications Known hypersensitivity to acetophenazine; severe CNS depression, cross-sensitivity to other phenothiazines may exist; avoid use in patients with narrow-angle glaucoma, blood dyscrasias, severe liver or cardiac disease; subcortical brain damage; circulatory collapse; severe hypotension or hypertension

Warnings

Tardive dyskinesia: Prevalence rate may be 40% in elderly; elderly women especially at risk; embarrassment from dyskinesias may lead to greater social isolation; development of the syndrome and the irreversible nature are proportional to duration and total cumulative dose over time. May be reversible if diagnosed early in therapy; intermittent use of antipsychotics (not proven to be clinically effective) helps decrease total cumulative dose.

EPS: Extrapyramidal reactions are more common in elderly with up to 50% developing these reactions after age 60. These reactions may be more common in dementia patients. Drug-induced **Parkinson's syndrome** occurs often. Discontinuation usually resolves symptoms but may take weeks to months (12+) to clear. **Akathisia** is the most common EPS reaction in elderly. The symptoms of motor restlessness are difficult to diagnose in demented elderly; increased nervousness, assertiveness, restlessness with constant movement may indicate this adverse event. Consider decreasing dose of antipsychotic to treat as well as diagnose problem; usually see this reaction within 2-3 months of initiating antipsychotic drug.

Anticholinergic effects: These side effects most common with low potency antipsychotics (eg, thioridazine, chlorpromazine). CNS toxicity occurs more frequently and severely in elderly; increased confusion, memory loss, psychotic behavior, and agitation frequently occur as a consequence of anticholinergic effects to antipsychotic agents. Peripheral anticholinergic action troublesome to elderly; most peripheral anticholinergic effects last only 2-3 weeks (see Adverse Reactions).

Orthostatic hypotension: More common with low potency agents (eg, thioridazine, chlorpromazine, and clozapine) but of concern with all antipsychotic agents; orthostasis due to alpha-receptor blockade by antipsychotic agents. Elderly present many risk factors for orthostatic hypotension: blunted baroreceptor reflexes, decreased vascular tone, decreased vascular volume, and possible presence of cardiac diseases which result in decreased cardiac output.

Sedation: Common side effect with antipsychotic therapy; should not be used as a hypnotic unless insomnia is associated with target behavior symptoms treated with antipsychotic medications (see Special Geriatric Considerations). Anecdotal reports suggesting antipsychotic sedation in nonpsychotic patients is extremely unpleasant due to feelings of depersonalization, derealization, and dysphoria. Due to the long duration of action with antipsychotic drugs, these reactions may last up to 24 hours and result in decreased daytime function.

Cardiac toxicity: Life-threatening arrhythmias have occurred at therapeutic doses of antipsychotics. Thioridazine more commonly demonstrates EKG changes than other antipsychotics; suggested to use high potency antipsychotic agents (ie, haloperidol) in patients with cardiac conduction defects.

Precautions Use with caution in patients with severe cardiovascular disorder, seizures, and Parkinson's disease; benefits of therapy must be weighed against risks

Adverse Reactions

Cardiovascular: EKG changes, hypotension (especially orthostatic), tachycardia, arrhythmias, abnormal T waves with prolonged ventricular repolarization

Central nervous system: Drowsiness, restlessness, anxiety, extrapyramidal reactions, dystonic reactions, pseudoparkinsonian signs and symptoms, tardive dyskinesia, neuroleptic malignant syndrome, seizures, altered central temperature regulation

Dermatologic: Hyperpigmentation, pruritus, rash, contact dermatitis, photosensitivity (rare)

Endocrine & metabolic: Amenorrhea, galactorrhea, gynecomastia

Gastrointestinal: Xerostomia (problem for denture user), constipation, adynamic ileus, GI upset, weight gain

Genitourinary: Overflow incontinence, urinary retention, priapism, sexual dysfunction (up to 60%)

Hematologic: Agranulocytosis, leukopenia

Hepatic: Cholestatic jaundice

Ocular: Retinal pigmentation (more common than with chlorpromazine), blurred vision, decreased visual acuity (may be irreversible)

Sedation and extrapyramidal effects are more pronounced than anticholinergic and orthostatic effects

Overdosage Symptoms of overdose include deep sleep, coma, extrapyramidal symptoms, abnormal involuntary muscle movements, hypotension or hypertension; agitation, restlessness, fever, hypothermia or hyperthermia, seizures, cardiac arrhythmias, EKG changes

Toxicology Following initiation of essential overdose management, toxic symptom treatment and supportive treatment should be initiated. Hypotension usually responds to I.V. fluids or Trendelenburg positioning. If unresponsive to these measures the use of a parenteral inotrope may be required (eg, norepinephrine 0.1-0.2 mcg/kg/minute titrated to response). Do not use epinephrine. Seizures commonly respond to diazepam (I.V. 5-10 mg bolus every 15 minutes if needed up to a total of 30 mg) or to phenytoin or phenobarbital. Also critical cardiac arrhythmias often respond to I.V. phenytoin (15 mg/kg up to 1 g), while other antiarrhythmics can be used. Neuroleptics often cause extrapyramidal symptoms (eg, dystonic reactions) requiring management with diphenhydramine 1-2 mg/kg up to a maximum of 50 mg I.M. or I.V. slow push followed by a maintenance dose for 48-72 hours. When these reactions are unresponsive to diphenhydramine, benztropine mesylate I.V. 1-2 mg may be effective. These agents are generally effective within 2-5 minutes.

Drug Interactions

Alcohol may increase CNS sedation

Anticholinergic agents may decrease pharmacologic effects; increase anticholinergic side effects; may enhance tardive dyskinesia

(Continued)

Acetophenazine *(Continued)*

Aluminum salts may decrease absorption of phenothiazines

Barbiturates may decrease phenothiazine serum concentrations

Bromocriptine may have decreased efficacy when administered with pheno-
. thiazines

Guanethidine's hypotensive effect is decreased by phenothiazines

Lithium administration with phenothiazines may increase disorientation

Meperidine and phenothiazine coadministration increases sedation and hypotension

Methyldopa administration with phenothiazine (trifluoperazine) may significantly increase blood pressure

Norepinephrine, epinephrine have decreased pressor effect when administered with chlorpromazine; therefore, be aware of possible decreased effectiveness or when any phenothiazine is used

Phenytoin serum concentrations may increase or decrease with phenothiazines; tricyclic antidepressants may have increased serum concentrations
with concomitant administration with phenothiazines

Propranolol administered with phenothiazines may increase serum concentrations of both drugs

Valproic acid may have increased half-life when administered with phenothiazines (chlorpromazine)

Stability Protect from light; dispense in amber or opaque vials

Mechanism of Action Blocks postsynaptic mesolimbic dopaminergic D_1 and
D_2 receptors in the brain; exhibits a strong alpha-adrenergic blocking and
anticholinergic effect, depresses the release of hypothalamic and hypophyseal hormones; believed to depress the reticular activating system thus
affecting basal metabolism, body temperature, wakefulness, vasomotor tone,
and emesis

Pharmacokinetics

Absorption: Absorption may be affected by the inherent anticholinergic action
on the gastrointestinal tissue causing variable absorption. Absorption from
tablets is erratic with less variation seen with solutions.

Distribution: Widely distributed in tissues with CNS concentrations exceeding
that of plasma due to their lipophilic characteristics

Protein binding: Antipsychotic agents are bound 90% to 99% to plasma or
proteins; highly bound to brain and lung tissue and other tissues with a high
blood perfusion

Time to peak: 2-4 hours

Elimination: Occurs through hepatic metabolism (oxidation) where numerous
active metabolites are produced; active metabolites excreted in urine; elimination half-lives of antipsychotics ranges from 20-40 hours which may be
extended in elderly due to decline in oxidative hepatic reactions (phase I)
with age. The biologic effect of a single dose persists for 24 hours. When
the patient has accommodated to initial side effects (sedation), once daily
dosing is possible due to the long half-life of antipsychotics.

Steady-state plasma levels are achieved in 4-7 days; therefore, if possible, do
not make dose adjustments more than once in a 7-day period. Due to the
long half-lives of antipsychotics, as needed (prn) use is ineffective since
repeated doses are necessary to achieve therapeutic tissue concentrations
in the CNS.

Usual Dosage Oral:

Geriatrics (nonpsychotic patients; dementia behavior): Initial: 20 mg once
daily; increase at 4- to 7-day intervals by 20 mg/day; increase dosing
intervals (bid, tid, etc) as necessary to control response or side effects. For
patients with sleep difficulty, administer 1 hour before bedtime; maximum
daily dose: 140 mg; gradual increases (titration) may prevent some side
effects or decrease their severity.

Adults: 20 mg 3 times/day up to 60-120 mg/day

Not dialyzable (0% to 5%)

Monitoring Parameters Orthostatic blood pressures; tremors, gait changes,
abnormal movement in trunk, neck, buccal area, or extremities; monitor target
behaviors for which the agent is given

Test Interactions Increased cholesterol (S), glucose; decreased uric acid (S)

Patient Information Do not take antacid within 1 hour of taking drug; may
cause drowsiness, avoid alcohol; avoid excess sun exposure (use sun block);
rise slowly from recumbent position; use of supportive stockings may help
prevent orthostatic hypotension

Nursing Implications Observe for tremor and abnormal movement or
posturing (extrapyramidal symptoms); increased confusion or psychotic
behavior, constipation, urinary retention, abnormal gait

Special Geriatric Considerations See Warnings.

Many elderly patients receive antipsychotic medications for inappropriate nonpsychotic behavior. Before initiating antipsychotic medication, the clinician should investigate any possible reversible cause; any stress or stress from any disease can cause acute "confusion" or worsening of baseline nonpsychotic behavior. Most commonly acute changes in behavior are due to increases in drug dose or addition of new drug to regimen; fluid electrolyte loss; infections; and changes in environment.

Any changes in disease status in any organ system can result in behavior changes.

In the treatment of agitated, demented, elderly patients, authors of metaanalysis of controlled trials of the response to the traditional antipsychotics (phenothiazines, butyrophenones) in controlling agitation have concluded that the use of neuroleptics results in a response rate of 18%. Clearly neuroleptic therapy for behavior control should be limited with frequent attempts to withdraw the agent given for behavior control.

Dosage Forms Tablet, as maleate: 20 mg

References

Peabody CA, Warner MD, Whiteford HA, et al, "Neuroleptics and the Elderly," *J Am Geriatr Soc*, 1987, 35(3):233-8.

Risse SC and Barnes R, "Pharmacologic Treatment of Agitation Associated With Dementia," *J Am Geriatr Soc*, 1986, 34(5):368-76.

Saltz BL, Woerner MG, Kane JM, et al, "Prospective Study of Tardive Dyskinesia Incidence in the Elderly," *JAMA*, 1991, 266(17):2402-6.

Seifert RD, "Therapeutic Drug Monitoring: Psychotropic Drugs," *J Pharm Pract*, 1984, 6:403-16.

Acetoxymethylprogesterone *see* Medroxyprogesterone Acetate *on page 578*

Acetylcholine (a se teel KOE leen)

Related Information

Glaucoma Drug Therapy Comparison *on page 1032*

Brand Names Miochol-E®

Generic Available No

Therapeutic Category Cholinergic Agent, Ophthalmic; Ophthalmic Agent, Miotic

Use Produce complete miosis in cataract surgery, keratoplasty, iridectomy, and other anterior segment surgery where rapid miosis is required

Contraindications Hypersensitivity to acetylcholine chloride; acute iritis and acute inflammatory disease of the anterior chamber

Warnings Open under aseptic conditions only

Precautions Systemic effects rarely occur, but can cause problems for patients with acute cardiac failure, bronchial asthma, peptic ulcer, hyperthyroidism, GI spasm, urinary trace obstruction, and Parkinson's disease. Retinal detachment may result in individuals with pre-existing retinal disease. An examination of the fundus is advised prior to treatment.

Adverse Reactions

Cardiovascular: Bradycardia, hypotension, flushing

Central nervous system: Headache

Ocular: Altered distance vision, decreased night vision, transient lenticular opacities

Respiratory: Dyspnea

Miscellaneous: Diaphoresis

Toxicology Treatment includes flushing eyes with water or normal saline and supportive measures; if accidentally ingested, induce emesis or perform gastric lavage

Drug Interactions

Decreased effect possible with flurbiprofen and suprofen, ophthalmic

Effects may be prolonged or enhanced in patients receiving tacrine

Stability Prepare solution immediately before use

Mechanism of Action Causes contraction of the sphincter muscles of the iris, resulting in miosis and contraction of the ciliary muscle, leading to accommodation

Pharmacodynamics

Onset of miosis: In seconds

Duration: ~10-20 minutes

Usual Dosage Geriatrics and Adults: Instill 0.5-2 mL of 1% injection (5-20 mg) instilled into anterior chamber before or after securing one or more sutures

Patient Information May sting on instillation; use caution while driving at night or performing hazardous tasks

(Continued)

Acetylcholine *(Continued)*

Nursing Implications Discard any solution that is not used; open under aseptic conditions only

Special Geriatric Considerations See Usual Dosage and Patient Information

Dosage Forms Powder, intraocular, as chloride: 1:100 [10 mg/mL] (2 mL, 15 mL)

Acetylsalicylic Acid *see Aspirin on page 84*
Aches-N-Pain® [OTC] *see Ibuprofen on page 475*
Achromycin® Ophthalmic *see Tetracycline on page 900*
Achromycin® Topical *see Tetracycline on page 900*
Achromycin® V Oral *see Tetracycline on page 900*
Aciclovir *see Acyclovir on this page*
Acidulated Phosphate Fluoride *see Fluoride on page 392*
Aclovate® *see Alclometasone on page 31*
ACT® [OTC] *see Fluoride on page 392*
Actagen® Syrup [OTC] *see Triprolidine and Pseudoephedrine on page 966*
Actagen® Tablet [OTC] *see Triprolidine and Pseudoephedrine on page 966*
Actifed® Allergy Tablet (Day) [OTC] *see Pseudoephedrine on page 802*
Actigall™ *see Ursodiol on page 975*
Activase® *see Alteplase on page 40*
Activated Dimethicone *see Simethicone on page 856*
Activated Ergosterol *see Ergocalciferol on page 340*
Activated Methylpolysiloxane *see Simethicone on page 856*
Actron® [OTC] *see Ketoprofen on page 515*
Acular® Ophthalmic *see Ketorolac Tromethamine on page 517*
Acutrim® Precision Release® [OTC] *see Phenylpropanolamine on page 741*
ACV *see Acyclovir on this page*
Acycloguanosine *see Acyclovir on this page*

Acyclovir *(ay SYE kloe veer)*

Related Information
   I.V. Medication Recommendations *on page 1080*
   Valacyclovir *on page 976*

Brand Names Zovirax®

Synonyms Aciclovir; ACV; Acycloguanosine

Generic Available Yes-Capsule

Therapeutic Category Antiviral Agent, Oral; Antiviral Agent, Parenteral; Antiviral Agent, Topical

Use Treatment of initial and prophylaxis of recurrent mucosal and cutaneous herpes simplex (HSV-1 and HSV-2) infections, herpes simplex encephalitis, herpes zoster (shingles), genital herpes infection, and varicella-zoster infections in immunocompromised patients

Contraindications Hypersensitivity to acyclovir

Precautions Use with caution in patients with pre-existing renal disease or in those receiving other nephrotoxic drugs concurrently; maintain adequate and urine output during the first 2 hours after I.V. infusion; use with caution in patients with underlying neurologic abnormalities and in patients with serious renal, hepatic, or electrolyte abnormalities or substantial hypoxia

Adverse Reactions
   Cardiovascular: Hypotension. tachycardia, vasodilation
   Central nervous system: Headache, delirium, dizziness, seizures, insomnia, fever, fatigue
   Dermatologic: Skin rash, pruritus
   Gastrointestinal: Nausea, vomiting, diarrhea, abdominal pain, sore throat
   Hematologic: Bone marrow suppression, anemia
   Hepatic: Elevation of liver enzymes
   Local: Phlebitis at injection site
   Neuromuscular & skeletal: Tremulousness, myalgia
   Ophthalmic: Eye pain, photophobia
   Renal: Nephrotoxicity, dysuria
   Miscellaneous: Diaphoresis, thirst

Overdosage Symptoms of overdose include elevated serum creatinine, renal failure

Toxicology In the event of an overdose, sufficient urine flow must be maintained to avoid drug precipitation within the renal tubules. Hemodialysis has resulted in up to 60% reductions in serum acyclovir concentrations.

Drug Interactions
Probenecid increases acyclovir bioavailability, terminal half-life may be increased and renal clearance may be decreased
Zidovudine increases drowsiness and lethargy

Stability Incompatible with blood products and protein-containing solutions; reconstituted 50 mg/mL solution should be used within 12 hours; do not refrigerate reconstituted solutions as they may precipitate

Mechanism of Action Inhibits DNA synthesis and viral replication by competing with deoxyguanosine triphosphate for viral DNA polymerase and being incorporated into viral DNA

Pharmacokinetics
Absorption: Oral: 15% to 30%; food does not appear to affect absorption
Distribution: Widely throughout the body including brain, kidney, lungs, liver, spleen, muscle, uterus, vagina, and the CSF
Protein binding: <30%
Half-life (adults): Inversely affected by renal function; see table.

Creatinine Clearance (mL/min/1.73 m²)	Half-life (h)
>80	2.5
50-80	3
15-50	3.5
0	19.5

Time to peak serum concentration: Within 1½ to 2 hours after an oral dose, and within 1 hour following intravenous administration
Elimination: Primary route of elimination is the kidney, following a small amount of hepatic metabolism; requires dosage adjustment with renal impairment, hemodialysis removes ~60% of the dose and to a much lesser extent by peritoneal dialysis

Usual Dosage Geriatrics and Adults:
Dosing weight should be based on the smaller of lean body weight or total body weight
Adult determination of lean body weight (LBW) in kg:
LBW males: 50 kg + (2.3 kg x inches >5 feet)
LBW females: 45 kg + (2.3 kg x inches >5 feet)
Treatment of herpes simplex virus infections:
Oral:
Treatment: 200 mg every 4 hours while awake (5 times/day)
Prophylaxis: 200 mg 3-4 times/day or 400 mg twice daily
Topical: ½" ribbon of ointment every 3 hours (6 times/day)
I.V.:
Mucocutaneous HSV infection: 5 mg/kg/dose every 8 hours for 5-10 days
HSV encephalitis: 10 mg/kg/dose every 8 hours for 10 days
Treatment of varicella-zoster virus infections:
Oral:
800 mg/dose every 4 hours while awake (5 times/day) for 7-10 days or 1000 mg every 6 hours for 5 days
I.V.: 10 mg/kg/dose every 8 hours for 5-10 days
Prophylaxis in immunocompromised patients:
Varicella or herpes zoster in HIV-positive patients: Oral: 400 mg 5 times/day
Bone marrow transplant recipients: I.V.:
Patients who are HSV seropositive: 5 mg/kg/dose divided every 8 hours
Patients who are CMV seropositive: 10 mg/kg/dose divided every 8 hours; for clinically significant CMV infections, ganciclovir should be used in place of acyclovir

Dosing interval in renal impairment: See tables.

Parenteral Acyclovir Dosage in Renal Function Impairment

Creatinine Clearance (mL/min/1.73 m²)	% of Recommended Dose	Dosing Interval (h)
>50	100%	8
25-50	100%	12
10-25	100%	24
0-10	50%	24

(Continued)

Acyclovir *(Continued)*

Oral Acyclovir Dosage in Renal Function Impairment

Normal Dosage Regimen (5 times/day)	Creatinine Clearance (mL/min/1.73 m²)	Dose (mg)	Dosing Interval
200 mg q4h	>10	200	q4h, 5 times/day
	0-10	200	q12h
400 mg q12h	>10	400	q12h
	0-10	200	q12h
800 mg q4h	>25	800	q4h, 5 times/day
	10-25	800	q8h
	0-10	800	q12h

Administration Infuse over at least 1 hour; wear gloves when applying ointment

Monitoring Parameters Urinalysis, BUN, serum creatinine, liver enzymes, CBC

Reference Range
Level guidelines:
Pre: 0.1-1.6 µg/mL
Post: 3-10 µg/mL
Panic value: >50 µg/mL
Infusion time: 1 hour

Test Interactions Increased BUN, creatinine

Patient Information Contagious only when viral shedding is occurring; avoid sexual intercourse when lesions are visible; recurrences tend to appear within 3 months of original infection; acyclovir is **not** a cure

Nursing Implications Maintain adequate hydration of patient; check infusion site for phlebitis, rotate site to prevent phlebitis

Additional Information Appears to reduce the length and severity of chickenpox, but should be used unless patient is immunosuppressed; oral doses of 800 mg 5 times/day have been associated with a lower incidence and shortened duration of postherpetic neuralgias

Special Geriatric Considerations For herpes zoster, acyclovir should be started within 72 hours of the appearance of the rash to be effective; calculate creatinine clearance (see renal impairment dosing in Usual Dosage)

Dosage Forms
Capsule: 200 mg
Powder for Injection: 500 mg (10 mL); 1000 mg (20 mL)
Ointment, topical: 5% [50 mg/g] (3 g, 15 g)
Suspension, oral (banana flavor): 200 mg/5 mL
Tablet: 400 mg, 800 mg

References
Dellamonica P, Carles M, Lokiec F, et al, "Preventing Recurrent Varicella and Herpes Zoster With Oral Acyclovir in HIV-Seropositive Patients," *Clin Pharm*, 1991, 10(4):301-2.

Huff JC, Bean B, Balfour HH Jr, et al, "Therapy of Herpes Zoster With Oral Acyclovir," *Am J Med*, 1988, 85(2A):84-9.

McKendrick MW, McGill JI, White JE, et al, "Oral Acyclovir in Acute Herpes Zoster," *Br Med J [Clin Res]*, 1986, 293:1529-32.

Morton P and Thomson AN, "Oral Acyclovir in the Treatment of Herpes Zoster in General Practice," *N Z Med J*, 1989, 102(863):93-5.

Wood MJ, Johnson RW, McKendrick MW, et al, "A Randomized Trial of Acyclovir for 7 Days or 21 Days With and Without Prednisolone for Treatment of Acute Herpes Zoster," *N Engl J Med*, 1994, 330(13):896-900.

Adalat® *see* Nifedipine *on page 671*

Adalat® CC *see* Nifedipine *on page 671*

Adamantanamine Hydrochloride *see* Amantadine *on page 49*

Adapin® Oral *see* Doxepin *on page 321*

Adenine Arabinoside *see* Vidarabine *on page 988*

ADH *see* Vasopressin *on page 983*

Adlone® Injection *see* Methylprednisolone *on page 611*

Adrenalin® *see* Epinephrine *on page 336*

Adrenaline *see* Epinephrine *on page 336*

Adsorbocarpine® Ophthalmic *see* Pilocarpine *on page 748*

Adsorbonac® Ophthalmic [OTC] *see* Sodium Chloride *on page 860*

Adsorbotear® Ophthalmic Solution [OTC] *see* Artificial Tears *on page 82*

Advil® [OTC] *see* Ibuprofen *on page 475*

AeroBid®-M Oral Aerosol Inhaler *see* Flunisolide *on page 390*

AeroBid® Oral Aerosol Inhaler *see* Flunisolide *on page 390*

Aerolate III® *see* Theophylline *on page 902*

Aerolate JR® *see* Theophylline *on page 902*

Aerolate SR® *see* Theophylline *on page 902*

Aeroseb-Dex® *see* Dexamethasone *on page 274*

Aeroseb-HC® *see* Hydrocortisone *on page 462*

Afrin® Children's Nose Drops [OTC] *see* Oxymetazoline *on page 706*

Afrin® Saline Mist [OTC] *see* Sodium Chloride *on page 860*

Afrin® Sinus [OTC] *see* Oxymetazoline *on page 706*

Afrin® Tablet [OTC] *see* Pseudoephedrine *on page 802*

Aftate® for Athlete's Foot [OTC] *see* Tolnaftate *on page 939*

Aftate® for Jock Itch [OTC] *see* Tolnaftate *on page 939*

Agoral® Plain [OTC] *see* Mineral Oil *on page 628*

A-hydroCort® *see* Hydrocortisone *on page 462*

Airet® *see* Albuterol *on this page*

Akarpine® Ophthalmic *see* Pilocarpine *on page 748*

AKBeta® *see* Levobunolol *on page 529*

AK-Chlor® Ophthalmic *see* Chloramphenicol *on page 203*

AK-Cide® Ophthalmic *see* Sulfacetamide Sodium and Prednisolone *on page 875*

AK-Con® Ophthalmic *see* Naphazoline *on page 653*

AK-Dex® Ophthalmic *see* Dexamethasone *on page 274*

AK-Dilate® Ophthalmic Solution *see* Phenylephrine *on page 740*

AK-Homatropine® Ophthalmic *see* Homatropine *on page 454*

Akineton® *see* Biperiden *on page 119*

AK-NaCl® [OTC] *see* Sodium Chloride *on page 860*

AK-Nefrin® Ophthalmic Solution *see* Phenylephrine *on page 740*

Akne-Mycin® Topical *see* Erythromycin, Topical *on page 347*

AK-Pred® Ophthalmic *see* Prednisolone *on page 774*

AKPro® Ophthalmic *see* Dipivefrin *on page 306*

AK-Sulf® Ophthalmic *see* Sulfacetamide Sodium *on page 874*

AKTob® Ophthalmic *see* Tobramycin *on page 929*

AK-Trol® *see* Neomycin, Polymyxin B, and Dexamethasone *on page 661*

Akwa Tears® Ophthalmic Ointment [OTC] *see* Ocular Lubricant *on page 688*

Akwa Tears® Solution [OTC] *see* Artificial Tears *on page 82*

Ala-Cort® *see* Hydrocortisone *on page 462*

Ala-Scalp® *see* Hydrocortisone *on page 462*

Alatrofloxacin/Trovafloxacin *see* Trovafloxacin/Alatrofloxacin *on page 969*

Alazide® *see* Hydrochlorothiazide and Spironolactone *on page 459*

Albalon-A® Ophthalmic *see* Naphazoline and Antazoline *on page 654*

Albalon® Liquifilm® Ophthalmic *see* Naphazoline *on page 653*

Albuterol (al BYOO ter ole)

Related Information

Asthma Guidelines *on page 1040*

Inhaled Medications Comparison *on page 1034*

Brand Names Airet®; Proventil®; Proventil® HFA; Ventolin®; Ventolin® Rotocaps®; Volmax®

Synonyms Salbutamol

Generic Available Yes

Therapeutic Category Adrenergic Agonist Agent; Beta$_2$-Adrenergic Agonist Agent; Bronchodilator

Use Bronchodilator in reversible airway obstruction due to asthma or COPD

Contraindications Hypersensitivity to albuterol, adrenergic amines, or any ingredients

Warnings Use with caution in patients with unstable vasomotor symptoms, diabetes, hyperthyroidism, prostatic hypertrophy, or a history of seizures; also use caution in the elderly and those patients with cardiovascular disorders such as coronary artery disease, arrhythmias, and hypertension

Precautions Excessive use may result in tolerance; deaths have been reported after excessive use; though the exact cause is unknown, cardiac arrest after a severe asthmatic crisis is suspected

(Continued)

Albuterol *(Continued)*

Adverse Reactions
Cardiovascular: Tachycardia, palpitations, elevation or depression of blood pressure

Central nervous system: Nervousness, CNS stimulation, hyperactivity, insomnia

Gastrointestinal: GI upset

Neuromuscular & skeletal: Tremors (may be more common in the elderly)

Overdosage
Symptoms of overdose include hypertension, tachycardia, seizures, angina, hypokalemia, and tachyarrhythmias

Toxicology
Prudent use of a cardioselective beta-adrenergic blocker (eg, atenolol or metoprolol); keep in mind the potential for induction of bronchoconstriction in an asthmatic. Dialysis has not been shown to be of value in the treatment of an overdose with this agent.

Drug Interactions
Decreased therapeutic effect: Beta-adrenergic blockers (eg, propranolol)

Increased therapeutic effect: Inhaled ipratropium may increase duration of bronchodilation, nifedipine may increase FEV-1

Increased toxicity (cardiovascular): MAO inhibitors, tricyclic antidepressants, sympathomimetic agents (eg, amphetamine, dopamine, dobutamine), inhaled anesthetics (eg, enflurane)

Mechanism of Action
Relaxes bronchial smooth muscle by action on beta$_2$-receptors with little effect on heart rate (minor beta$_1$ activity)

Pharmacodynamics
Peak bronchodilation effect: Within 0.5-2 hours

Duration: 3-4 hours

Pharmacokinetics
Metabolism: By the liver to an inactive sulfate, with 28% appearing in the urine as unchanged drug

Half-life:

Inhaled: 3.8 hours

Oral: 3.7-5 hours

Usual Dosage
Oral (see Special Geriatric Considerations):

Geriatrics: 2 mg 3-4 times/day; maximum: 8 mg 4 times/day

Adults: 2-4 mg 3-4 times/day; maximum: 8 mg 4 times/day; sustained release: 1-2 tablets every 12 hours

Inhalation: Geriatrics and Adults:

Nebulization: 2.5 mg 3-4 times/day (2.5 mg = 0.5 mL of the 0.5% inhalation solution) in 2.5 mL of normal saline; may be used more frequently in acute exacerbations

Metered dose inhaler: 2 puffs every 4-6 hours though some patients may be controlled on 1 puff every 4 hours; maximum: 12 puffs/day

Rotahaler®: 200 mcg inhaled every 4-6 hours using a Rotahaler® inhalation device

Monitoring Parameters
Pulmonary function, blood pressure, pulse

Patient Information
Do not exceed recommended dosage; rinse mouth with water following each inhalation to help with dry throat and mouth; follow specific instructions accompanying inhaler; if more than one inhalation is necessary, wait at least 1 full minute between inhalations. May cause nervousness, restlessness, insomnia - if these effects continue after dosage reduction, notify physician; also notify physician if palpitations, tachycardia, chest pain, muscle tremors, dizziness, headache, flushing, or if breathing difficulty persists.

Nursing Implications
Before using, the inhaler must be shaken well; assess lung sounds, pulse, and blood pressure before administration and during peak of medication; observe patient for wheezing after administration, if this occurs, call physician

Special Geriatric Considerations
Because of its minimal effect on beta$_1$-receptors and its relatively long duration of action, albuterol is a rational choice in the elderly when a beta agonist is indicated. Elderly patients may find it useful to utilize a spacer device when using a metered dose inhaler. The Ventolin® Rotahaler® is an alternative for patients who have difficulty using the metered dose inhaler. Oral use should be avoided due to adverse effects.

Dosage Forms
Aerosol: 90 mcg/dose (17 g)

Aerosol, chlorofluorocarbon free (Proventil® HFA): 90 mcg/dose (17 g)

Capsule, oral inhalation: 0.5% (20 mL)

Solution:
Inhalation: 0.5% (20 mL)
Concentrate for nebulization: 0.5%
Nebulization: 0.083% (3 mL)
Syrup, as sulfate (alcohol and sugar free): 2 mg/5 mL (480 mL)
Tablet, as sulfate: 2 mg, 4 mg
Tablet, extended release (Volmax®): 4 mg, 8 mg

Alclometasone (al kloe MET a sone)
Brand Names Aclovate®
Generic Available No
Therapeutic Category Anti-inflammatory Agent; Corticosteroid, Topical (Low Potency)
Use Relief of inflammatory and pruritic manifestations of corticosteroid-responsive dermatoses (low potency topical corticosteroid)
Contraindications Viral, fungal, or tubercular skin lesions, known hypersensitivity to alclometasone or any component
Precautions Systemic absorption of topical corticosteroids has produced reversible HPA axis suppression. This is more likely to occur when the preparation is used on large surfaces or denuded areas for prolonged periods of time or with an occlusive dressing.
Adverse Reactions
Dermatologic: Acne, hypopigmentation, allergic dermatitis, maceration of the skin, skin atrophy, striae, miliaria, telangiectasia
Endocrine & metabolic: HPA suppression, Cushing's syndrome, growth retardation
Local: Burning, itching, irritation, dryness, folliculitis, hypertrichosis
Systemic: HPA axis suppression, Cushing's syndrome, hyperglycemia; these reactions occur more frequently with occlusive dressings
Miscellaneous: Secondary infection
Mechanism of Action Topical corticosteroids have anti-inflammatory, antipruritic, vasoconstrictive, and antiproliferative actions
Usual Dosage Geriatrics and Adults: Topical: Apply a thin layer to the affected area 2-3 times/day
Monitoring Parameters Relief of symptoms
Patient Information Use only as prescribed and for no longer than the period prescribed; apply sparingly in a thin film and rub in lightly; avoid contact with eyes; notify physician if condition persists or worsens
Nursing Implications Use sparingly; should not be used on open or weeping lesions
Additional Information Considered a low potency steroid; avoid use on the face
Special Geriatric Considerations Due to age-related changes in skin, limit use of topical glucocorticosteroids (see Precautions)
Dosage Forms
Alclometasone dipropionate:
Cream: 0.05% (15 g, 45 g, 60 g)
Ointment, topical: 0.05% (15 g, 45 g, 60 g)

Alconefrin® Nasal Solution [OTC] *see* Phenylephrine *on page 740*
Aldactazide® *see* Hydrochlorothiazide and Spironolactone *on page 459*
Aldactone® *see* Spironolactone *on page 869*
Aldomet® *see* Methyldopa *on page 609*
Aldoril® *see* Methyldopa and Hydrochlorothiazide *on page 609*

Alendronate (a LEN droe nate)
Brand Names Fosamax®
Therapeutic Category Bisphosphonate Derivative
Use Nonhormonal prevention and treatment of osteoporosis; treatment of Paget's disease of bone
Contraindications Patients with hypocalcemia; hypersensitivity to bisphosphonates or hypersensitivity to any of the drug's components
Warnings Concomitant use of hormone replacement therapy is not recommended because of lack of clinical experience; since alendronate appears to be eliminated renally, caution in reduced renal function is advised; no dose reduction is recommended when creatinine clearance is >35 mL/minute. The use of alendronate in patients with creatinine clearances <35 mL/minute is not recommended.
Precautions Bisphosphonates should be used with caution in patients who have concomitant gastrointestinal disorders such as peptic ulcer disease, (Continued)

Alendronate *(Continued)*

gastritis, esophageal disease, or dysphagia; patients with hypocalcemia must have this abnormality corrected before initiating alendronate therapy. Additionally, patients who are hypomagnesemic or hypophosphatemic as well as vitamin D deficient, must be corrected prior to therapy; must assure adequate nutrition especially concerning vitamin D and calcium intake.

Adverse Reactions Incidence of adverse effects increases significantly in patients treated for Paget's disease at 40 mg/day, mostly GI adverse effects.

Central nervous system: Headache

Dermatologic: Rash

Gastrointestinal: Abdominal pain, flatulence, dyspepsia, dysphagia, gastritis, esophageal ulceration, abdominal distention

Neuromuscular & skeletal: Musculoskeletal pain

Overdosage Symptoms of overdose include heartburn, gastritis, abdominal pain, nausea, esophagitis, hypocalcemia, and hypophosphatemia

Toxicology Gastric lavage, treat hypocalcemia with I.V. calcium; may consider administering antacids or milk to bind alendronate; general supportive care

Drug Interactions Ranitidine (I.V.) increases bioavailability twofold; calcium products decrease absorption; aspirin-induced gastrointestinal adverse effects are increased when alendronate dose exceeds 10 mg/day; food/drug interaction (see Administration)

Drug/Food Interactions Due to significant inhibition to absorption, alendronate must not be taken with any other medication, food, or drink **other than plain water** (see Administration). When taken within or 2 hours before food, bioavailability is decreased up to 40%. When taken with liquids other than water, bioavailability is reduced 60%.

Mechanism of Action Decreases bone resorption by inhibiting osteocyte osteolysis; decreases mineral release and matrix or collagen breakdown in bone

Pharmacodynamics

Onset of action: Bone mineral density increases were noted at 3 months in trials

Duration of action: Trials noted continuous effect for the 3 years of study with daily use; upon discontinuation of daily use, no further increases in bone mass observed. Thus, it appears daily treatment is needed to maintain effect.

Pharmacokinetics

Absorption: Oral: Male: 0.6% given in a fasting state; Female: 0.7%

Protein binding: ~78%

Metabolism: Not metabolized

Bioavailability: Reduced up to 60% with food or drink

Half-life: Terminal: Exceeds 10 years; serum concentrations cleared >95% in 6 hours

Elimination: Renal with unabsorbed drug eliminated in feces

Usual Dosage Oral: Geriatrics and Adults: See Additional Information

Prevention of osteoporosis: 5 mg once daily

Osteoporosis: 10 mg once daily. **Note:** Safety studies beyond 4 years of treatment are in progress.

Paget's disease of bone: 40 mg once daily for 6 months; retreatment may be considered after a 6-month period post-treatment in those who relapse as demonstrated by an increase in alkaline phosphatase or in those who fail to decrease alkaline phosphatase to normal

Administration It is imperative to administer alendronate 30-60 minutes before the patient takes any food, drink, or other medications orally to avoid interference with absorption. The patient should take alendronate on an empty stomach with a full glass (8 oz) of **plain water** (not mineral water) and avoid lying down for 30 minutes after swallowing tablet to help delivery to stomach. Patient should have adequate calcium intake. Supplemental calcium is necessary for maximal effect.

Monitoring Parameters Alkaline phosphatase should be periodically measured; serum calcium, phosphate, and possibly potassium due to its drug class; use of absorptiometry may assist in noting benefit in osteoporosis; monitor pain and fracture rate

Reference Range Calcium (total): Adults: 9.0-11.0 mg/dL (2.05-2.54 mmol/L); may slightly decrease with aging; phosphorus: 2.5-4.5 mg/dL (0.81-1.45 mmol/L)

Patient Information Food, beverages (including mineral water), and other medications may significantly reduce the absorption and therefore the effectiveness; take with plain water (6-8 oz) at least 30 minutes before the first food, beverage, or medication of the day; must take supplemental calcium while treated with alendronate

Nursing Implications To facilitate the drug's delivery to the stomach, the patient should **not** lie down for at least 30 minutes after taking the medication; supplemental calcium is necessary to effect bone density; vitamin D should also be given if dietary intake is inadequate

Additional Information Esophageal irritation and gastric pain have been reported frequently. Proper administration may prevent or decrease this common adverse effect. Patients need to take supplemental calcium while treated with alendronate appropriate for age and hormonal status; vitamin D supplements suggested if patient is deficient in this vitamin. Patients treated with 10 mg of alendronate daily had significant increases in bone mineral density. Increases were absorbed as early as 3 months and continued throughout the 3 years of study. Mean bone mineral density increases at 3 years were: spine, trochanter 8%; femoral neck 6%; total body bone mineral density 2.5%.

Special Geriatric Considerations No dosage adjustment is needed in the elderly, however, alendronate is not recommended to be used in patients with Cl_{cr} <35 mL/minute until further data and experience are available. Since many elderly receive diuretics, evaluation of electrolyte status (calcium, phosphate, magnesium, potassium) may need to be done periodically due to the drug class (bisphosphonate). Should assure immobile patients are at least sitting up for 30 minutes after swallowing tablets.

Dosage Forms Tablet, as sodium: 5 mg, 10 mg, 40 mg

References

Chesnut CH 3rd, McClung MR, Ensrud KE, et al, "Alendronate Treatment of the Postmenopausal Osteoporatic Woman: Effect of Multiple Dosages on Bone Mass and Bone Remodeling," *Am J Med*, 1995, 99(2):144-52.

Watts NB, "Treatment of Osteoporosis With Bisphosphonates," *Rheum Dis Clin North Am*, 1994, 20(3):717-34.

Aleve® [OTC] *see* Naproxen *on page 655*

Alfenta® *see* Alfentanil *on this page*

Alfentanil (al FEN ta nil)

Brand Names Alfenta®

Generic Available No

Therapeutic Category Analgesic, Narcotic

Use Analgesic adjunct given by continuous infusion or in incremental doses in maintenance of anesthesia with barbiturate or N_2O or a primary anesthetic agent for the induction of anesthesia in patients undergoing general surgery in which endotracheal intubation and mechanical ventilation are required

Contraindications Hypersensitivity to alfentanil hydrochloride or narcotics; increased intracranial pressure, severe respiratory depression

Warnings Drug dependence, head injury, acute asthma and respiratory conditions; hypotension has occurred in neonates with respiratory distress syndrome; use caution when administering to patients with bradyarrhythmias and with supraventricular arrhythmias; rapid I.V. infusion may result in skeletal muscle and chest wall rigidity → impaired ventilation → respiratory distress/arrest; inject slowly over 3-5 minutes; nondepolarizing skeletal muscle relaxant may be required. Alfentanil may produce more hypotension compared to fentanyl, therefore, be sure to administer slowly and ensure patient has adequate hydration.

Precautions Sulfite sensitivity is found in some individuals, especially asthmatics in atopic patients; pulmonary disease; use caution postoperatively; supraventricular arrhythmias: the vagolytic action of narcotics may increase ventricular rate; use with caution in patients with seizures as narcotics lower seizure threshold with increased doses; abdominal disease may have altered presentation or have symptoms obscured with narcotics

Adverse Reactions

Cardiovascular: Bradycardia, tachycardia, peripheral vasodilation, cardiac arrhythmias, orthostatic hypotension, chest wall rigidity, facial flushing

Central nervous system: Drowsiness, sedation, increased intracranial pressure, lightheadedness, dizziness, dysphoria, delirium, agitation, lethargy, confusion, CNS depression, convulsions, mental depression, paradoxical CNS excitation or delirium, dysesthesia

Dermatologic: Rash, urticaria, itching

Endocrine & metabolic: Antidiuretic hormone release

(Continued)

Alfentanil *(Continued)*

Gastrointestinal: Nausea, vomiting, constipation, biliary tract spasm, abdominal pain, cramps

Genitourinary: Urinary tract spasm

Ocular: Miosis, diplopia, blurred vision

Respiratory: Respiratory depression, bronchospasm, laryngospasm

Miscellaneous: Physical and psychological dependence with prolonged use, cold, clammy skin, diaphoresis

Overdosage Symptoms of overdose include miosis, respiratory depression, seizures, CNS depression

Toxicology Naloxone 2 mg I.V. with repeat administration as necessary up to a total of 10 mg; may precipitate withdrawal

Drug Interactions Cytochrome P-450 3A enzyme substrate

Decreased effect: Phenothiazines may antagonize the analgesic effect of opiate agonists

Increased effect: Dextroamphetamine may enhance the analgesic effect of morphine and other opiate agonists; warfarin effect may be enhanced

Increased toxicity: CNS depressants (eg, benzodiazepines, barbiturates, phenothiazines, tricyclic antidepressants), erythromycin, reserpine, beta-blockers; increased respiratory effect with barbiturate anesthetics; diazepam may cause cardiovascular depression when given with high-dose alfentanil; nitrous oxide may cause cardiovascular depression with high-dose alfentanil

Drug/lab interactions: Increased biliary tract pressure may result in increased serum amylase or lipase

Stability Dilute in D_5W, NS, or LR

Mechanism of Action Binds with stereospecific receptors at many sites within the CNS, increases pain threshold, alters pain perception, inhibits ascending pain pathways; is an ultra short-acting narcotic

Pharmacokinetics

Distribution: V_d: 0.46 L/kg

Metabolism: Substrate CYP3A4

Half-life, elimination: 83-97 minutes

Usual Dosage Doses should be titrated to appropriate effects; wide range of doses is dependent upon desired degree of analgesia/anesthesia

Alfentanil

Indication	Approx Duration of Anesthesia (min)	Induction Period (Initial Dose) (mcg/kg)	Maintenance Period (Increments/ Infusion)	Total Dose (mcg/kg)	Effects
Incremental injection	≤30	8-20	3-5 mcg/kg or 0.5-1 mcg/kg/ min	8-40	Spontaneously breathing or assisted ventilation when required.
	30-60	20-50	5-15 mcg/kg	Up to 75	Assisted or controlled ventilation required. Attenuation of response to laryngoscopy and intubation.
Continuous infusion	>45	50-75	0.5-3 mcg/kg/ min average infusion rate 1-1.5 mcg/kg/ min	Dependent on duration of procedure	Assisted or controlled ventilation required. Some attenuation of response to intubation and incision, with intraoperative stability.
Anesthetic induction	>45	130-245	0.5-1.5 mcg/ kg/min or general anesthetic	Dependent on duration of procedure	Assisted or controlled ventilation required. Administer slowly (over 3 minutes). Concentration of inhalation agents reduced by 30% to 50% for initial hour.
MAC	≤30	3-8	3-5 mcg/kg every 5-20 min to 1 mcg/ kg/min	3-40 mcg/ kg	Assisted or controlled ventilation required.

Geriatrics (see Special Geriatric Considerations): It is recommended to reduce dose in elderly when initiating this drug; therefore, use dose at lowest recommended dose to initiate therapy; monitor closely

Adults: Dose should be based on ideal body weight; see table and Additional Information.

Monitoring Parameters Respiratory rate, blood pressure, heart rate

Reference Range 100-340 ng/mL (depending upon procedure)

Nursing Implications Monitor patient for CNS, respiratory depression, and urticaria

Additional Information Patients who are >20% above ideal body weight should have their doses calculated based on ideal body weight

Special Geriatric Considerations The elderly may be particularly susceptible to the CNS depressant and constipating effects of narcotics; use with caution and frequent monitoring in COPD patients since even moderate doses may compromise ventilation; best to use at lowest recommended doses initially

Dosage Forms Injection, preservative free, as hydrochloride: 500 mcg/mL (2 mL, 5 mL, 10 mL, 20 mL)

References

Bodenham A and Park GR, "Alfentanil Infusions in Patients Requiring Intensive Care," *Clin Pharmacokinet*, 1988, 15(4):216-26.

Kirkham SR and Pugh R, "Opioid Analgesia in Uraemic Patients," *Lancet*, 1995, 345(8958):1185.

Meistelman C, Saint-Maurice C, Lepaul M, et al, "A Comparison of Alfentanil Pharmacokinetics in Children and Adults," *Anesthesiology*, 1987, 66(1):13-6.

Pokela ML, Ryhanen PT, Koivisto ME, et al, "Alfentanil-Induced Rigidity in Newborn Infants," *Anesth Analg*, 1992, 75(2):252-7.

Alimenazine Tartrate see Trimeprazine on page 960

Alka-Mints® [OTC] see Calcium Salts (Oral) on page 152

Alkeran® see Melphalan on page 582

Allegra® see Fexofenadine on page 380

Aller-Chlor® [OTC] see Chlorpheniramine on page 208

Allercon® Tablet [OTC] see Triprolidine and Pseudoephedrine on page 966

Allerest® 12 Hour Nasal Solution [OTC] see Oxymetazoline on page 706

Allerest® Eye Drops [OTC] see Naphazoline on page 653

Allerfrin® Syrup [OTC] see Triprolidine and Pseudoephedrine on page 966

Allerfrin® Tablet [OTC] see Triprolidine and Pseudoephedrine on page 966

AllerMax® Oral [OTC] see Diphenhydramine on page 302

Allerphed Syrup [OTC] see Triprolidine and Pseudoephedrine on page 966

Allopurinol (al oh PURE i nole)

Related Information

Antacid Drug Interactions on page 1096

Brand Names Zyloprim®

Generic Available Yes

Therapeutic Category Uric Acid Lowering Agent; Xanthine Oxidase Inhibitor

Use Prevention of attack of gouty arthritis and nephropathy; treatment of secondary hyperuricemia which may occur during treatment of tumors or leukemia; prevent recurrent calcium oxalate calculi

Contraindications Do not use in patients with a previous severe allergy reaction

Precautions Reduce dosage in renal insufficiency, reinstate with caution in patients who have had a previous mild allergic reaction; monitor liver function and complete blood counts before initiating therapy and periodically during therapy

Adverse Reactions

Central nervous system: Neuritis, drowsiness, fever

Dermatologic: Pruritic maculopapular rash, exfoliative dermatitis

Gastrointestinal: GI irritation

Hematologic: Leukocytosis, leukopenia, thrombocytopenia, eosinophilia, bone marrow suppression

Hepatic: Hepatitis

Ocular: Cataracts

Renal: Renal impairment

Toxicology If significant amounts of allopurinol are thought to have been absorbed, it is a theoretical possibility that oxypurinol stones could be formed but no record of such occurrence in overdose exists. Alkalinization of the urine and forced diuresis can help prevent potential xanthine stone formation. (Continued)

Allopurinol (Continued)

Drug Interactions

Decreased effect: Alcohol decreases effectiveness

Increased toxicity: Inhibits metabolism of azathioprine and mercaptopurine; use with ampicillin or amoxicillin may increase the incidence of skin rash; doses of allopurinol >600 mg/day may decrease theophylline clearance to result in toxicity; use with ACE inhibitors may increase the risk of hypersensitivity reactions; thiazide diuretics increase the incidence of hypersensitivity reactions to allopurinol

Mechanism of Action Decreases the production of uric acid by inhibiting the action of xanthine oxidase, an enzyme that converts hypoxanthine to xanthine and xanthine to uric acid

Pharmacodynamics Decrease in serum uric acid occurs in 1-2 days with a nadir achieved in 1-3 weeks

Pharmacokinetics

Absorption: Oral: ~80% from GI tract

Protein binding: <1%

Metabolism: ~75% of the drug is metabolized to active metabolites, chiefly oxypurinol; allopurinol and oxypurinol are dialyzable

Half-life:

Parent: 1-3 hours

Oxypurinol: Normal renal function: 18-30 hours

Time to peak serum concentration: Within 2-4 hours

Usual Dosage Oral:

Geriatrics: Initial dose: 100 mg/day, increase until desired uric acid level is obtained

Adults: Daily doses >300 mg should be administered in divided doses

Gout: Average dose: 200-300 mg/day (mild); 400-600 mg/day (severe)

Maximum dose: 800 mg/day

Dosing interval in renal impairment: See table.

Adult Maintenance Doses of Allopurinol*

Creatinine Clearance (mL/min)	Maintenance Dose of Allopurinol (mg)
140	400 qd
120	350 qd
100	300 qd
80	250 qd
60	200 qd
40	150 qd
20	100 qd
10	100 q2d
0	100 q3d

*This table is based on a standard maintenance dose of 300 mg of allopurinol per day for a patient with a creatinine clearance of 100 mL/minute.

Myeloproliferative neoplastic disorders: 600-800 mg/day in 2-3 divided doses for prevention of acute uric acid nephropathy for 2-3 days starting 1-2 days before chemotherapy

Monitoring Parameters CBC, serum uric acid levels, I & O, hepatic and renal function, especially at start of therapy

Reference Range Uric acid, serum: Adults: Male: 3.4-7 mg/dL (SI: 202-416 μmol/L) or slightly more; Female: 2.4-6 mg/dL (SI: 143-357 μmol/L) or slightly more. Values >7 mg/dL (SI: 416 μmol/L) are sometimes arbitrarily regarded as hyperuricemia, but there is no sharp line between normals on the one hand, and the serum uric acid of those with clinical gout. Normal ranges cannot be adjusted for purine ingestion, but high purine diet increases uric acid. Uric acid may be increased with body size, exercise, and stress.

Test Interactions Increased alkaline phosphatase, AST, ALT; decreased uric acid (S)

Patient Information Take after meals with plenty of fluid; discontinue the drug and contact physician at first sign of rash, painful urination, blood in the urine, irritation of the eyes, or swelling of the lips or mouth; may cause drowsiness

Nursing Implications Administer after meals; encourage fluid intake

Additional Information Skin rash occurs most often in patients taking diuretics concurrently; may predispose patient to ampicillin-induced rash

Special Geriatric Considerations Adjust dose based on renal function (see Usual Dosage)

Dosage Forms Tablet: 100 mg, 300 mg

References

Emmerson BT, "The Management of Gout," *N Engl J Med*, 1996, 334(7):445-51.

Almora® [OTC] *see* Magnesium Salts (Various Salts) *on page 568*

Alomide® Ophthalmic *see* Lodoxamide Tromethamine *on page 547*

Alphamul® [OTC] *see* Castor Oil *on page 171*

Alphatrex® *see* Betamethasone *on page 114*

Alprazolam (al PRAY zoe lam)

Related Information

Antacid Drug Interactions *on page 1096*
Anxiolytic/Hypnotic Use in Long-Term Care Facilities *on page 1099*
Benzodiazepines Comparison *on page 1024*
Federal OBRA Regulations Recommended Maximum Doses - Anxiolytics *on page 1057*
Federal OBRA Regulations Recommended Maximum Doses - Hypnotics *on page 1057*

Brand Names Xanax®

Generic Available No

Therapeutic Category Antianxiety Agent; Benzodiazepine

Use Treatment of anxiety; adjunct in the treatment of depression; management of panic attacks

Restrictions C-IV

Contraindications Hypersensitivity to alprazolam or any component; there may be a cross-sensitivity with other benzodiazepines; severe uncontrolled pain, narrow-angle glaucoma, severe respiratory depression, pre-existing CNS depression

Warnings Withdrawal symptoms including seizures have occurred 18 hours to 3 days after abrupt discontinuation; when discontinuing therapy, decrease daily dose by no more than 0.5 mg every 3 days; reduce dose in patients with significant hepatic disease

Precautions Use with caution in patients with a history of drug dependence

Adverse Reactions

Central nervous system: Drowsiness, dizziness, confusion, sedation, ataxia, headache
Gastrointestinal: Xerostomia, constipation, diarrhea, nausea, vomiting
Neuromuscular & skeletal: Impaired coordination
Ocular: Blurred vision
Respiratory: Decreased respiratory rate, apnea, laryngospasm
Miscellaneous: Physical and psychological dependence with prolonged use

Overdosage Symptoms of overdose include somnolence, confusion, coma, and diminished reflexes

Toxicology Treatment for benzodiazepine overdose is supportive; rarely is mechanical ventilation required

Flumazenil has been shown to selectively block the binding of benzodiazepines to CNS receptors, resulting in a reversal of benzodiazepine-induced sedation; however, its use may not alter the course of overdose

Drug Interactions Benzodiazepines may decrease the effect of levodopa
Decreased metabolism: Cimetidine, fluoxetine
Increased metabolism: Rifampin
Increased toxicity: CNS depressants, alcohol

Mechanism of Action Benzodiazepines appear to potentiate the effects of GABA and other inhibitory neurotransmitters by binding to specific benzodiazepine-receptor sites in various areas of the CNS

Pharmacodynamics Studies have shown that the elderly are more sensitive to the effects of benzodiazepines as compared to younger adults

Pharmacokinetics

Absorption: Oral: Rapidly and well absorbed
Distribution: V_d: 0.9-1.2 L/kg
Protein binding: 80%
Metabolism: Extensive in the liver; major metabolite is inactive; alphahydroxy-alprazolam (active); substrate CYP3A4
Half-life: 12-15 hours
Time to peak serum concentration: Within 1-2 hours
Elimination: Metabolites and parent compound in the urine; elimination is prolonged in elderly men (half-life: 19.5 hours); elderly women had no significant change in alprazolam clearance

(Continued)

Alprazolam *(Continued)*

Usual Dosage Oral:
Geriatrics: Initial: 0.125-0.25 mg twice daily; increase by 0.125 mg/day as needed
Adults: 0.25-0.5 mg 2-3 times/day, titrate dose upward; maximum: 4 mg/day

Monitoring Parameters Respiratory and cardiovascular status, symptoms of anxiety, mental status

Test Interactions Increased alkaline phosphatase

Patient Information Avoid alcohol and other CNS depressants; may cause drowsiness; avoid activities needing good psychomotor coordination until CNS effects are known; may cause physical or psychological dependence; avoid abrupt discontinuation after prolonged use

Nursing Implications Assist with ambulation during initiation of therapy; monitor for alertness

Additional Information Not intended for management of anxieties and minor distresses associated with everyday life; treatment longer than 4 months should be re-evaluated to determine the patient's need for the drug; when decreasing the dose or discontinuing alprazolam, decrease by no more than 0.5 mg every 3 days

Special Geriatric Considerations Due to short duration of action, it is considered to be a benzodiazepine of choice in the elderly (see Pharmacodynamics, Pharmacokinetics, and Additional Information)

Dosage Forms Tablet: 0.25 mg, 0.5 mg, 1 mg, 2 mg

References
Greenblatt DJ, Divoll M, Abernethy DR, et al, "Alprazolam Kinetics in the Elderly: Relation to Antipyrine Disposition," *Arch Gen Psychiatry*, 1983, 40(3):287-90.
Reidenberg MM, Levy M, Warner H, et al, "Relationship Between Diazepam Dose, Plasma Level, Age, and Central Nervous System Depression," *Clin Pharmacol Ther*, 1978, 23(4):371-4.

Alprostadil *(al PROS ta dill)*

Brand Names Caverject® Injection; Edex® Injection; Muse® Pellet; Prostin VR Pediatric® Injection

Synonyms PGE_1; Prostaglandin E_1

Generic Available No

Therapeutic Category Prostaglandin

Use Diagnosis and treatment of erectile dysfunction of vasculogenic, psychogenic, or neurogenic etiology; adjunct in the diagnosis of erectile dysfunction

Contraindications Conditions predisposing patients to priapism (sickle cell anemia, multiple myeloma, leukemia); patients with anatomical deformation of the penis, penile implants; use in men for whom sexual activity is inadvisable or contraindicated

Warnings Priapism may occur; treat immediately to avoid penile tissue damage and permanent loss of potency; discontinue therapy if signs of penile fibrosis develop (penile angulation, cavernosal fibrosis, or Peyronie's disease)

Adverse Reactions
Cardiovascular: Flushing, bradycardia, hypotension, hypertension, tachycardia, cardiac arrest, edema, cerebral bleeding, congestive heart failure, second degree heart block, shock, supraventricular tachycardia, ventricular fibrillation, hyperemia
Central nervous system: Fever, seizures, headache, dizziness, hyperirritability, hypothermia, jitteriness, lethargy
Endocrine & metabolic: Hypokalemia, hypoglycemia, hyperkalemia
Gastrointestinal: Diarrhea, gastric regurgitation
Genitourinary: Penile pain, prolonged erection, penile fibrosis, penis disorder, penile rash, penile edema, anuria, balanitis, urethral bleeding, penile numbness, yeast infection, penile pruritus and erythema, abnormal ejaculation
Hematologic: Disseminated intravascular coagulation, anemia, bleeding, thrombocytopenia
Hepatic: Hyperbilirubinemia
Local: Injection site hematoma, injection site bruising
Neuromuscular & skeletal: Back pain, hyperextension of neck, stiffness
Renal: Hematuria
Respiratory: Apnea, upper respiratory infection, flu syndrome, sinusitis, nasal congestion, cough, bradypnea, bronchial wheezing
Miscellaneous: Sepsis, localized pain in structures other than the injection site, peritonitis

Toxicology If intracavernous overdose occurs, supervise until any systemic effects have resolved or until penile detumescence has occurred

Stability Erectile dysfunction: Refrigerate at 2°C to 8°C until dispensed; after dispensing, stable for up to 3 months at or below 25°C; do not freeze; use only the supplied diluent for reconstitution (ie, bacteriostatic/sterile water with benzyl alcohol 0.945%)

Mechanism of Action Relaxes trabecular smooth muscle by dilation of cavernosal arteries when injected along the penile shaft, allowing blood flow to and entrapment in the lacunar spaces of the penis (ie, corporeal veno-occlusive mechanism)

Pharmacokinetics

Distribution: Nonsignificant amounts distribute peripherally following penile injection

Protein binding, plasma: 81% to albumin

Metabolism: ~75% metabolized by oxidation in one pass through the lungs

Half-life: 5-10 minutes

Elimination: Metabolites excreted in urine (90% within 24 hours)

Usual Dosage Geriatrics and Adults: **Erectile dysfunction:**

Caverject®, Edex®:

Vasculogenic, psychogenic, or mixed etiology: Individualize dose by careful titration; usual dose: 2.5-60 mcg (doses >60 mcg are not recommended); initiate dosage titration at 2.5 mcg, increasing by 2.5 mcg to a dose of 5 mcg and then in increments of 5-10 mcg depending on the erectile response until the dose produces an erection suitable for intercourse, not lasting >1 hour; if there is absolutely no response to initial 2.5 mcg dose, the second dose may increased to 7.5 mcg, followed by increments of 5-10 mcg

Neurogenic etiology (eg, spinal cord injury): Initiate dosage titration at 1.25 mcg, increasing to a doses of 2.5 mcg and then 5 mcg; increase further in increments 5 mcg until the dose is reached that produces an erection suitable for intercourse, not lasting >1 hour

Note: Patient must stay in the physician's office until complete detumescence occurs; if there is no response, then the next higher dose may be given within 1 hour; if there is still no response, a 1-day interval before giving the next dose is recommended; increasing the dose or concentration in the treatment of impotence results in increasing pain and discomfort

Muse® Pellet: Intraurethral: Administer as needed to achieve an erection; duration of action is about 30-60 minutes; use only two systems per 24-hour period

Monitoring Parameters Degree of penile pain, length of erection, signs of infection

Patient Information Store in refrigerator; if self-injecting for the treatment of impotence, dilute with the supplied diluent and use immediately after diluting; see physician at least every 3 months to ensure proper technique and for dosage adjustment; alternate sides of the penis with each injection; do not inject more than 3 times/week, allowing at least 24 hours between each dose; dispose of the syringe, needle, and vial properly; discard single-use vials after each use; report moderate to severe penile pain or erections lasting >6 hours to a physician immediately; inform a physician as soon as possible if any new penile pain, nodules, hard tissue or signs of infection develop; the risk of transmission of blood-borne diseases is increased with use of alprostadil injections since a small amount of bleeding at the injection site is possible; do not share this medication or needles/syringes

Nursing Implications Erectile dysfunction: Use a ½", 27- to 30-gauge needle; inject into the dorsolateral aspect of the proximal third of the penis, avoiding visible veins; alternate side of the penis for injections; if the patient is going to be self-injecting at home, carefully assess their aseptic technique for injection and knowledge of proper disposal of the syringe, needle and vial; observe for signs of infection, penile fibrosis, and significant pain or priapism

Special Geriatric Considerations Elderly may have concomitant diseases which would contraindicate the use of alprostadil (see Adverse Reactions and Warnings). Other forms of attaining penile tumescence are recommended.

Dosage Forms

Injection:

Caverject®: 5 mcg, 10 mcg, 20 mcg

Edex® Injection: 5 mcg, 10 mcg, 20 mcg, 40 mcg

Pellet, urethral: 125 mcg, 250 mcg, 500 mcg, 1000 mcg

AL-R® [OTC] see Chlorpheniramine on page 208

Altace™ see Ramipril on page 821

Alteplase (AL te plase)

Brand Names Activase®

Synonyms Alteplase, Recombinant; Alteplase, Tissue Plasminogen Activator, Recombinant; t-PA

Generic Available No

Therapeutic Category Thrombolytic Agent

Use Management of acute myocardial infarction for the lysis of thrombi in coronary arteries; management of acute massive pulmonary embolism (PE) in adults

Acute myocardial infarction (AMI): Chest pain ≥20 minutes, ≤12-24 hours; S-T elevation ≥0.1 mV in at least two EKG leads

Acute pulmonary embolism (APE): Age ≤75 years: As soon as possible within 5 days of thrombotic event. Documented massive pulmonary embolism by pulmonary angiography or echocardiography or high probability lung scan with clinical shock.

Acute ischemic stroke (rule out hemorrhagic courses before administering)

Contraindications No central venous puncture (CVP line) or noncompressible arterial sticks. Blood pressure systolic ≥180, diastolic ≥110 unresponsive to nitrate or calcium antagonist; pregnancy; recent (within 1 month): cerebrovascular accident or transient ischemic attack, gastrointestinal bleeding, trauma or surgery, prolonged external cardiac massage; intracranial neoplasm, suspected aortic dissection, arteriovenous malformation or aneurysm, bleeding diathesis, severe hepatic or renal disease, hemostatic defects, severe uncontrolled hypertension

Warnings Doses >150 mg have been associated with an increase of intracranial hemorrhage

Adverse Reactions

Cardiovascular: Hypotension

Central nervous system: Fever

Dermatologic: Bruising

Gastrointestinal: GI hemorrhage, nausea, vomiting

Genitourinary: GU hemorrhage

Hematologic: Retroperitoneal hemorrhage, gingival hemorrhage, intracranial hemorrhage rapid lysis of coronary artery thrombi by thrombolytic agents may be associated with reperfusion-related atrial and/or ventricular arrhythmias

Respiratory: Epistaxis

Overdosage Increased incidence of intracranial bleeding

Drug Interactions Increased effect: Anticoagulants, aspirin, clopidogrel, ticlopidine, dipyridamole, and heparin are at least additive

Stability Refrigerate; must be used within 8 hours of reconstitution; alteplase is **incompatible** with dobutamine, dopamine, heparin, and nitroglycerin infusions; physically **compatible** with lidocaine, metoprolol, propranolol when administered via Y site; **compatible** with either D_5W or NS

Standard dose: 100 mg/100 mL 0.9% NaCl [total volume: 200 mL]

Mechanism of Action Initiates local fibrinolysis by binding to fibrin in a thrombus (clot) and converts entrapped plasminogen to plasmin

Pharmacokinetics Elimination: Cleared rapidly from circulating plasma at a rate of 550-650 mL/minute, primarily by the liver; >50% present in plasma is cleared within 5 minutes after the infusion has been terminated, and ~80% is cleared within 10 minutes

Usual Dosage

Coronary artery thrombi:

Patients >67 kg: I.V.: Front loading dose: Total dose is 100 mg over 1.5 hours. Add this dose to a 100 mL bag of 0.9% sodium chloride for a total volume of 200 mL. Infuse 15 mg (30 mL) over 1-2 minutes; infuse 50 mg (100 mL) over 30 minutes. (Begin heparin 5000-10,000 unit bolus followed by continuous infusion of 1000 units/hour.) Infuse 35 mg/hour (70 mL) for next 60 minutes.

Patients ≤67 kg: Administer 15 mg as an I.V. bolus, then 0.75 mg/kg over 30 minutes, not to exceed 50 mg, and then 0.5 mg/kg over the next 60 minutes not to exceed 35 mg

Acute pulmonary embolism: 100 mg over 2 hours

Acute ischemic stroke: Doses should be given within the first 3 hours of the onset of symptoms. Load with 0.09 mg/kg as a bolus, followed by 0.81 mg/kg as a continuous infusion over 60 minutes; maximum total dose should not exceed 90 mg

Administration Do not use bacteriostatic water for reconstitution

Reference Range

Not routinely measured; literature supports therapeutic levels of 0.52-1.8 µg/mL

Fibrinogen: 200-400 mg/dL

Activated partial thromboplastin time (APTT): 22.5-38.7 seconds

Prothrombin time (PT): 10.9-12.2 seconds

Nursing Implications Assess for hemorrhage during first hour of treatment (see Usual Dosage)

Special Geriatric Considerations No specific changes in use in elderly are necessary; use as indicated in Usual Dosage

Dosage Forms Powder for injection, lyophilized (recombinant): 20 mg [11.6 million units] (20 mL); 50 mg [29 million units] (50 mL); 100 mg [58 million units] (100 mL)

References

Meyer BJ and Chesebro JH, "New Accelerated rt-PA Strategy Has Sufficient Advantage Over Older Streptokinase Strategies That it Should Be the Thrombolytic Strategy of Choice in Anterior and Large Infarctions," *Am J Therapeut,* 1995, 2:123-7.

Alteplase, Recombinant *see* Alteplase *on previous page*

Alteplase, Tissue Plasminogen Activator, Recombinant *see* Alteplase *on previous page*

ALternaGEL® [OTC] *see* Aluminum Hydroxide *on this page*

Alu-Cap® [OTC] *see* Aluminum Hydroxide *on this page*

Aludrox® [OTC] *see* Aluminum Hydroxide and Magnesium Hydroxide *on page 43*

Aluminum Acetate and Calcium Acetate

(a LOO mi num AS e tate & KAL see um AS e tate)

Brand Names Bluboro® [OTC]; Boropak® [OTC]; Domeboro® Topical [OTC]; Pedi-Boro® [OTC]

Generic Available Yes

Therapeutic Category Topical Skin Product

Use Astringent wet dressing for relief of inflammatory conditions of the skin and to reduce weeping that may occur in dermatitis such as poison ivy and insect bites

Precautions Avoid contact with eyes; discontinue if irritation or extension of inflammatory condition occurs; if condition being treated lasts longer than 1 week, consult a physician

Drug Interactions Enzyme activity of collagenase used topically may be inhibited

Usual Dosage Topical: Soak affected area in the solution 2-4 times/day for 15-30 minutes or apply wet dressing soaked in the solution 2-4 times/day for 30-minute treatment periods; rewet dressing with solution every few minutes to keep it moist

Monitoring Parameters Monitor for decreasing inflammation and swelling

Nursing Implications Observe for response; report any increase in inflammation or swelling to physician

Special Geriatric Considerations No special considerations necessary

Dosage Forms

Powder, to make topical solution: 1 packet/pint of water [1:40 solution]

Tablet, effervescent: 1 tablet/pint [1:40 dilution]

Aluminum Hydroxide (a LOO mi num hye DROKS ide)

Brand Names ALternaGEL® [OTC]; Alu-Cap® [OTC]; Alu-Tab® [OTC]; Amphojel® [OTC]; Dialume® [OTC]; Nephrox Suspension [OTC]

Generic Available Yes

Therapeutic Category Antacid; Antidote, Hyperphosphatemia

Use Hyperacidity; hyperphosphatemia, treatment of GERD, hyperacidity associated with PUD

Contraindications Hypersensitivity to aluminum salts or dry components

Warnings Hypophosphatemia may occur with prolonged administration or large doses; aluminum intoxication and osteomalacia may occur in patients with uremia

Precautions Use with caution in patients with congestive heart failure, renal failure, edema, cirrhosis, low sodium diets, and patients who have recently suffered gastrointestinal hemorrhage; uremic patients not receiving dialysis may develop osteomalacia and osteoporosis due to phosphate depletion

Adverse Reactions

Central nervous system: Mental confusion, somnolence

(Continued)

Aluminum Hydroxide *(Continued)*

Endocrine & metabolic: Hypermagnesemia, aluminum toxicity, osteomalacia, hypophosphatemia, dehydration

Gastrointestinal: Constipation, decreased bowel motility, fecal impaction, diarrhea

Miscellaneous: Hemorrhoids

Overdosage Symptoms of overdose include bone pain, malaise, muscular weakness, encephalopathy

Toxicology Deferoxamine, traditionally used as an iron chelator, has been shown to increase urinary aluminum output. Deferoxamine chelation of aluminum has resulted in improvements of clinical symptoms and bone histology. Deferoxamine, however, remains an experimental treatment for aluminum poisoning and has a significant potential for adverse effects.

Drug Interactions

Aluminum compounds decrease the pharmacologic effect of allopurinol, chloroquine, corticosteroids, diflunisal, digoxin, ethambutol, H_2 antagonists, iron compounds, isoniazid, penicillamine, phenothiazines, tetracyclines, thyroid hormones, ticlopidine

Aluminum compounds increase the pharmacologic effect of benzodiazepines

Mechanism of Action Neutralize gastric acid and, therefore, increase pH of the stomach and duodenal bulb; with increased pH >4, the proteolytic activity of pepsin is diminished. Antacids also increase lower esophageal sphincter tone; aluminum ions inhibit gastric emptying by decreasing smooth muscle contraction; aluminum binds phosphate in the intestine to form insoluble aluminum phosphate which are then excreted in feces

Pharmacodynamics Acid-neutralizing capacity varies from product to product; antacids ingested in a fasting state give reduced acidity for 30 minutes; if ingested 1 hour after meals, reduced acidity may be extended for 3 hours

Usual Dosage Geriatrics and Adults (see Additional Information, Monitoring Parameters, and Neutralizing Capacity of Commonly Used Antacids table in the Appendix)

Oral: 500-1800 mg, 3-6 times/day, between meals and at bedtime

Suspension: 5-30 mL 3-6 times/day between meals and at bedtime

Monitoring Parameters Frequency of bowel movements, GI complaints (symptoms); phosphorous serum concentrations periodically when patient is on chronic therapy; when used as a phosphate binder, dose to achieve a serum phosphate concentration ≤4 mg/100 mL

Reference Range Aluminum normal range (serum): 0-6 ng/mL; dialysis patients may attain up to 40 ng/mL without symptoms of toxicity; >100 ng/mL possible CNS toxicity

Test Interactions Decreased phosphorus, inorganic (S)

Patient Information Dilute dose in water or juice, shake well; chew tablets thoroughly before swallowing with water; do not take oral drugs within 1-2 hours of administration; notify physician if relief is not obtained or if there are any signs to suggest bleeding from the GI tract

Nursing Implications Observe for constipation, fecal impaction, diarrhea, and hypophosphatemia

Additional Information When used primarily as a phosphate binder, dose should be followed with water; when used for peptic ulcer treatment, deliver 144 mEq neutralizing capacity 1 and 3 hours after meals as needed to control symptoms (see Neutralizing Capacity of Commonly Used Antacids table in the Appendix); often alternated with aluminum and magnesium combinations to decrease diarrhea

Special Geriatric Considerations Elderly, due to disease and/or drug therapy, may be predisposed to constipation and fecal impaction. Careful evaluation of possible drug interactions must be done. When used as an antacid in ulcer treatment, consider buffer capacity (mEq/mL) to calculate dose; consider renal insufficiency (<30 mL/minute) as predisposition to aluminum toxicity.

Dosage Forms

Capsule: 475 mg, 500 mg

Gel: 600 mg/5 mL (360 mL)

Suspension, oral: 320 mg/5 mL (500 mL), 675 mg/5 mL

Tablet: 300 mg, 500 mg, 600 mg

References

Bohannon AD and Lyles KW, "Drug-Induced Bone Disease," *Clin Geriatr Med*, 1994, 10(4):611-23.

Aluminum Hydroxide and Magnesium Hydroxide
(a LOO mi num hye DROKS ide & mag NEE zhum hye DROK side)

Brand Names Aludrox® [OTC]; Maalox® [OTC]; Maalox® Therapeutic Concentrate [OTC]

Synonyms Magnesium Hydroxide and Aluminum Hydroxide

Generic Available Yes

Therapeutic Category Antacid

Use Antacid, hyperphosphatemia in renal failure, GERD, hyperacidity associated with PUD

Contraindications Known hypersensitivity to aluminum hydroxide or magnesium hydroxide

Warnings Sodium content may be significant for patients with hypertension, renal failure, congestive heart failure; hypermagnesemia may result with renal insufficiency when >50 mEq of magnesium is administered daily; patients with Cl_{cr} <30 mL/minute are at risk for hypermagnesemia

Precautions Aluminum intoxication, osteomalacia, patients with GI hemorrhage; use with caution in patients on low sodium diets (patients with congestive heart failure, edema, hypertension), cirrhosis, and renal failure; magnesium intoxication may occur with renal insufficiency

Adverse Reactions
Central nervous system: Mental confusion

Endocrine & metabolic: Hypermagnesemia, aluminum intoxication, osteomalacia, hypophosphatemia, dehydration

Gastrointestinal: Constipation, diarrhea, fecal impaction

Overdosage
Aluminum: Osteomalacia (bone pain), malaise, weakness, and aluminum intoxication (encephalopathy) may occur in patients with renal insufficiency

Magnesium: CNS depression, confusion, hypotension, muscle weakness, blockage of peripheral neuromuscular transmission serum >4 mEq/L (4.8 mg/dL): deep tendon reflexes may be depressed; serum ≥10 mEq/L (12 mg/dL): deep tendon reflexes may disappear, respiratory paralysis may occur, heart block may occur

Toxicology Deferoxamine, traditionally used as an iron chelator, has been shown to increase urinary aluminum output. Deferoxamine chelation of aluminum has resulted in improvements of clinical symptoms and bone histology. Deferoxamine, however, remains an experimental treatment for aluminum poisoning and has a significant potential for adverse effects. Hypermagnesemia, toxic symptoms usually present with serum concentration >4 mEq/L; concurrent hypocalcemia, impaired clotting, somnolence, and disappearance of deep tendon reflexes. Serum concentration >12 mEq/L may be fatal, serum concentration ~10 mEq/L may cause complete heart block; I.V. calcium (5-10 mEq) will reverse respiratory depression or heart block; peritoneal dialysis or hemodialysis may be needed.

Drug Interactions
Magnesium and aluminum combination compounds decrease the pharmacologic effect of benzodiazepines, captopril, glucocorticosteroids, fluoroquinolones, H_2 antagonists, hydantoins, iron compounds, ketoconazole, penicillamine, phenothiazines, salicylates, tetracyclines, ticlopidine; concomitant use with sodium polystyrene sulfonate may cause metabolic alkalosis in patients with renal insufficiency

Magnesium and aluminum combination compounds increase the pharmacologic effect of levodopa, quinidine, sulfonylureas, valproic acid

Mechanism of Action Neutralize gastric acid and, therefore, increase pH of the stomach and duodenal bulb; with increased pH >4, the proteolytic activity of pepsin is diminished. Antacids also increase lower esophageal sphincter tone; aluminum ions inhibit gastric emptying by decreasing smooth muscle contraction. When used to treat hyperphosphatemia, aluminum binds phosphate in the intestine to form insoluble aluminum phosphate which is then excreted in feces.

Pharmacodynamics Acid-neutralizing capacity varies from product to product (see Appendix). Antacids ingested in a fasting state give reduced acidity for 30 minutes; if ingested 1 hour after meals, reduced acidity may be extended for 3 hours.

Usual Dosage Dosage depends upon disease condition being treated and specific agent used

Geriatrics and Adults: Oral:
Peptic ulcer disease: 144 mEq neutralizing capacity 1 and 3 hours after meals and as needed (see Neutralizing Capacity of Commonly Used Antacids table in the Appendix)
(Continued)

Aluminum Hydroxide and Magnesium Hydroxide
(Continued)

Reflux esophagitis: 15-30 mL 20-40 minutes after meals and at bedtime

Phosphate binding: Dose titrated to achieve high normal serum phosphate concentrations; doses administered with meals (see Monitoring Parameters)

Monitoring Parameters Frequency of bowel movements and GI complaints (symptoms)

Aluminum: Monitor phosphorous levels periodically when patient is on chronic therapy; when used as a phosphate binder, dose to achieve a serum phosphate concentration ≤4 mg/100 mL; observe for complaints or bone pain, malaise, and muscular weakness

Magnesium: See Overdosage; observe for signs of mental confusion and increased somnolence

Reference Range

Aluminum: Normal range (serum): 0-6 ng/mL; dialysis patients may attain up to 40 ng/mL without symptoms of toxicity; >100 ng/mL possible CNS toxicity

Magnesium: Normal range (serum): 1.5-2.3 mg/dL (1.25-1.9 mEq/L); toxicity occurs with serum concentration >4 mEq/L (4.8 mg/dL)

Test Interactions Decreased phosphorus, inorganic (S)

Patient Information Chew tablets thoroughly before swallowing with water; notify physician if relief is not obtained or if signs of bleeding from GI tract occur; if prescribed dose is exceeded in order to maintain symptom-free periods, advise physician

Nursing Implications Administer 1-2 hours apart from oral drugs; shake suspensions well; observe for constipation, fecal impaction, diarrhea, and hypophosphatemia (see Monitoring Parameters, Overdosage, and Reference Range)

Additional Information Sodium content varies with product; check for each product if important for patient

Special Geriatric Considerations Elderly, due to disease or drug therapy, may be predisposed to diarrhea or constipation. Diarrhea may result in electrolyte imbalance. Decreased renal function (Cl_{cr} <30 mL/minute) may result in toxicity of aluminum or magnesium. Drug interactions must be considered. If possible, administer antacid 1-2 hours apart from other drugs. When treating ulcers, consider buffer capacity (mEq/mL) to calculate dose of antacid (see Neutralizing Capacity of Commonly Used Antacids table in the Appendix).

Dosage Forms

Suspension:

Aludrox®: Aluminum hydroxide 307 mg and magnesium hydroxide 103 mg per 5 mL

Maalox®: Aluminum hydroxide 225 mg and magnesium hydroxide 200 mg per 5 mL

Maalox® TC (high potency): Aluminum hydroxide 600 mg and magnesium hydroxide 300 mg per 5 mL

Tablet, chewable (Maalox®): Aluminum hydroxide 600 mg and magnesium hydroxide 300 mg

Various other products available with various proportions of aluminum and magnesium

References

Bohannon AD and Lyles KW, "Drug-Induced Bone Disease," *Clin Geriatr Med*, 1994, 10(4):611-23.

Gams JG, "Clinical Significance of Magnesium: A Review," *Drug Intell Clin Pharm*, 1987, 21(3):240-6.

Peterson WL, Sturdevant RAL, Franki HD, et al, "Healing of Duodenal Ulcer With an Antacid Regimen," *N Engl J Med*, 1977, 297(7):341-5.

Aluminum Hydroxide, Magnesium Hydroxide, and Simethicone

(a LOO mi num hye DROKS ide, mag NEE zhum hye DROKS ide, & sye METH i kone)

Brand Names Di-Gel® [OTC]; Gas-Ban DS® [OTC]; Gelusil® [OTC]; Maalox® Plus [OTC]; Magalox Plus® [OTC]; Mylanta®-II [OTC]; Mylanta® [OTC]

Generic Available Yes

Therapeutic Category Antacid; Antiflatulent

Use Temporary relief of hyperacidity associated with gas; may also be used for indications associated with other antacids, such as hyperphosphatemia, prevention of stress ulcers, treatment of GERD

Contraindications Known hypersensitivity to aluminum hydroxide, magnesium hydroxide, or simethicone

Warnings Sodium content may be significant for patients with hypertension, renal failure, congestive heart failure; hypermagnesemia may result with renal insufficiency when >50 mEq of magnesium is administered daily; patients with Cl_{cr} <30 mL/minute are at risk for hypermagnesemia

Precautions Use with caution in patients with GI hemorrhage, patients on low sodium diets, patients with congestive heart failure, edema, hypertension, cirrhosis, and renal failure; magnesium intoxication may occur with renal insufficiency

Adverse Reactions

Central nervous system: Mental confusion, somnolence

Endocrine & metabolic: Dehydration or fluid restriction, hypermagnesemia, osteomalacia, hypophosphatemia

Gastrointestinal: Constipation, decreased bowel motility, fecal impaction, diarrhea

Overdosage

Aluminum: osteomalacia (bone pain), malaise, weakness, and aluminum intoxication (encephalopathy) may occur in patients with renal insufficiency

Magnesium: CNS depression, confusion, hypotension, muscle weakness, blockage of peripheral neuromuscular transmission serum >4 mEq/L (4.8 mg/dL): deep tendon reflexes may be depressed; serum ≥10 mEq/L (12 mg/dL): deep tendon reflexes may disappear, respiratory paralysis may occur, heart block may occur

Toxicology Deferoxamine, traditionally used as an iron chelator, has been shown to increase urinary aluminum output. Deferoxamine chelation of aluminum has resulted in improvements of clinical symptoms and bone histology. Deferoxamine, however, remains an experimental treatment for aluminum poisoning and has a significant potential for adverse effects. Hypermagnesemia, toxic symptoms usually present with serum concentration >4 mEq/L; concurrent hypocalcemia, impaired clotting, somnolence, and disappearance of deep tendon reflexes. Serum concentration >12 mEq/L may be fatal, serum concentration ~10 mEq/L may cause complete heart block; I.V. calcium (5-10 mEq) will reverse respiratory depression or heart block; peritoneal dialysis or hemodialysis may be needed.

Drug Interactions

Magnesium and aluminum combination compounds decrease the pharmacologic effect of benzodiazepines, captopril, glucocorticosteroids, fluoroquinolones, H_2 antagonists, hydantoins, iron compounds, ketoconazole, penicillamine, phenothiazines, salicylates, tetracyclines, ticlopidine; concomitant use with sodium polystyrene sulfonate may cause metabolic alkalosis in patients with renal insufficiency

Magnesium and aluminum combination compounds increase the pharmacologic effect of levodopa, quinidine, sulfonylureas, valproic acid

Mechanism of Action Neutralize gastric acid and, therefore, increase pH of the stomach and duodenal bulb; with increased pH >4, the proteolytic activity of pepsin is diminished. Antacids also increase lower esophageal sphincter tone; aluminum ions inhibit gastric emptying by decreasing smooth muscle contraction

Pharmacodynamics Acid-neutralizing capacity varies from product to product; antacids ingested in a fasting state give reduced acidity for 30 minutes; if ingested 1 hour after meals, reduced acidity may be extended for 3 hours

Usual Dosage Dosage depends upon disease condition being treated and specific agent used

Geriatrics and Adults: Oral:

Peptic ulcer disease: 144 mEq neutralizing capacity 1 and 3 hours after meals and as needed (see Neutralizing Capacity of Commonly Used Antacids table in the Appendix)

Reflux esophagitis: 15-30 mL 20-40 minutes after meals and at bedtime

Phosphate binding: Dose titrated to achieve high normal serum phosphate concentrations; doses administered with meals (see Monitoring Parameters)

Monitoring Parameters Frequency of bowel movements and GI complaints (symptoms)

Aluminum: Monitor phosphorous levels periodically when patient is on chronic therapy; when used as a phosphate binder, dose to achieve a serum phosphate concentration ≤4 mg/100 mL; observe for complaints or bone pain, malaise, and muscular weakness

(Continued)

Aluminum Hydroxide, Magnesium Hydroxide, and Simethicone *(Continued)*

Magnesium: Observe for signs of mental confusion and increased somnolence (see Overdosage)

Reference Range

Aluminum: Normal range (serum): 0-6 ng/mL; dialysis patients may attain up to 40 ng/mL without symptoms of toxicity; >100 ng/mL possible CNS toxicity

Magnesium: Normal range (serum): 1.5-2.3 mg/dL (1.25-1.9 mEq/L); toxicity occurs with serum concentration >4 mEq/L (4.8 mg/dL)

Test Interactions Decreased phosphorus, inorganic (S)

Patient Information Dilute dose in water or juice; chew tablets thoroughly before swallowing with water; shake well; notify physician if relief is not obtained or if signs of bleeding from GI tract occur

Nursing Implications Administer 1-2 hours apart from oral drugs (see Monitoring Parameters, Overdosage, and Reference Range)

Additional Information In order for simethicone to be effective, doses need to be 40-125 mg administered four times daily, not to exceed 500 mg daily; sodium content varies with product; check for each product if important for patient

Special Geriatric Considerations Elderly, due to disease or drug therapy, may be predisposed to diarrhea or constipation. Diarrhea may result in electrolyte imbalance. Decreased renal function (Cl_{cr} <30 mL/minute) may result in toxicity of aluminum or magnesium. Drug interactions must be considered. If possible, administer antacid 1-2 hours apart from other drugs. When treating ulcers, consider buffer capacity (mEq/mL) to calculate dose of antacid (see Neutralizing Capacity of Commonly Used Antacids table in the Appendix).

Dosage Forms

Liquid:

Gelusil®; Mylanta®: Aluminum hydroxide 200 mg, magnesium hydroxide 200 mg and simethicone 25 mg per 5 mL

Maalox® Plus: Aluminum hydroxide 225 mg, magnesium hydroxide 200 mg, and simethicone 25 mg per 5 mL (30 mL, 180 mL)

Mylanta®-II: Aluminum hydroxide 400 mg, magnesium hydroxide 400 mg, and simethicone 40 mg per 5 mL (150 mL, 360 mL)

Tablet, chewable:

Mylanta®: Aluminum hydroxide 200 mg, magnesium hydroxide 200 mg, and simethicone 20 mg

Mylanta®-II: Aluminum hydroxide 400 mg, magnesium hydroxide 400 mg, and simethicone 40 mg

Various other products available which contain various proportions of aluminum hydroxide, magnesium hydroxide, and simethicone

References

Bohannon AD and Lyles KW, "Drug-Induced Bone Disease," *Clin Geriatr Med*, 1994, 10(4):611-23.

Gams JG, "Clinical Significance of Magnesium: A Review," *Drug Intell Clin Pharm*, 1987, 21(3):240-6.

Peterson WL, Sturdevant RAL, Franki HD, et al, "Healing of Duodenal Ulcer With an Antacid Regimen," *N Engl J Med*, 1977, 297(7):341-5.

Aluminum Hydroxide, Magnesium Trisilicate, Sodium Bicarbonate, and Alginic Acid

(a LOO mi num hye DROK side, mag NEE zee um trye SIL eh kate, SOW dee um bye KAR bun ate, & al JIN ik AS id)

Brand Names Gaviscon®-2 [OTC]; Gaviscon® Extra Strength Relief Formula [OTC]

Generic Available No

Therapeutic Category Antacid

Use Temporary relief of hyperacidity

Unlabeled use: Gastroesophageal reflux

Contraindications Known hypersensitivity; not indicated for treatment of peptic ulcers

Warnings Sodium content may be significant for patients with hypertension, renal failure, congestive heart failure; hypermagnesemia may result with renal insufficiency when >50 mEq of magnesium is administered daily; patients with Cl_{cr} <30 mL/minute are at risk for hypermagnesemia

Precautions Aluminum intoxication, osteomalacia, patients with GI hemorrhage; use with caution in patients on low sodium diets (patients with congestive heart failure, edema, hypertension), cirrhosis, and renal failure; magnesium intoxication may occur with renal insufficiency

Adverse Reactions

Central nervous system: Mental confusion, somnolence

Endocrine & metabolic: Dehydration or fluid restriction, hypermagnesemia, osteomalacia, hypophosphatemia

Gastrointestinal: Constipation, decreased bowel motility, fecal impaction, diarrhea

Overdosage

Aluminum: osteomalacia (bone pain), malaise, weakness, and aluminum intoxication (encephalopathy) may occur in patients with renal insufficiency

Magnesium: CNS depression, confusion, hypotension, muscle weakness, blockage of peripheral neuromuscular transmission serum >4 mEq/L (4.8 mg/dL): deep tendon reflexes may be depressed; serum ≥10 mEq/L (12 mg/dL): deep tendon reflexes may disappear, respiratory paralysis may occur, heart block may occur; I.V. calcium (5-10 mEq) will reverse respiratory depression or heart block; in extreme cases, peritoneal dialysis or hemodialysis may be required

Drug Interactions

Magnesium and aluminum combination compounds decrease the pharmacologic effect of benzodiazepines, captopril, glucocorticosteroids, fluoroquinolones, H_2 antagonists, hydantoins, iron compounds, ketoconazole, penicillamine, phenothiazines, salicylates, tetracyclines, ticlopidine; concomitant use with sodium polystyrene sulfonate may cause metabolic alkalosis in patients with renal insufficiency

Magnesium and aluminum combination compounds increase the pharmacologic effect of levodopa, quinidine, sulfonylureas, valproic acid

Mechanism of Action Neutralize gastric acid and, therefore, increase pH of the stomach and duodenal bulb; with increased pH >4, the proteolytic activity of pepsin is diminished. Antacids also increase lower esophageal sphincter tone; aluminum ions inhibit gastric emptying by decreasing smooth muscle contraction

Pharmacodynamics Acid-neutralizing capacity varies from product to product; antacids ingested in a fasting state give reduced acidity for 30 minutes; if ingested 1 hour after meals, reduced acidity may be extended for 3 hours

Usual Dosage Geriatrics and Adults: Oral: Chew 2-4 tablets 4 times/day

Monitoring Parameters Frequency of bowel movements and GI complaints (symptoms)

Aluminum: Monitor phosphorous levels periodically when patient is on chronic therapy; observe for complaints or bone pain, malaise, and muscular weakness

Magnesium: Observe for signs of mental confusion and increased somnolence (see Overdosage)

Reference Range

Aluminum: Normal range (serum): 0-6 ng/mL; dialysis patients may attain up to 40 ng/mL without symptoms of toxicity; >100 ng/mL possible CNS toxicity

Magnesium: Normal range (serum): 1.5-2.3 mg/dL (1.25-1.9 mEq/L); toxicity occurs with serum concentration >4 mEq/L (4.8 mg/L)

Test Interactions Decreased phosphorus, inorganic (S)

Patient Information Chew tablets; do not swallow whole; can dilute liquid in water or juice; notify physician if relief is not obtained or if signs of bleeding from GI tract occur

Nursing Implications Administer 1-2 hours apart from oral drugs; observe for constipation, fecal impaction, diarrhea (see Monitoring Parameters, Overdosage, and References Range)

Additional Information Sodium content varies with product; check for each product if important for patient

Special Geriatric Considerations Elderly, due to disease or drug therapy, may be predisposed to diarrhea or constipation. Diarrhea may result in electrolyte imbalance. Decreased renal function (Cl_{cr} <30 mL/minute) may result in toxicity of aluminum or magnesium. Drug interactions must be considered. If possible, administer antacid 1-2 hours apart from other drugs. When treating ulcers, consider buffer capacity (mEq/mL) to calculate dose of antacid (see Neutralizing Capacity of Commonly Used Antacids table in the Appendix).

(Continued)

Aluminum Hydroxide, Magnesium Trisilicate, Sodium Bicarbonate, and Alginic Acid *(Continued)*

Dosage Forms
Liquid: Aluminum hydroxide 160 mg, magnesium trisilicate 40 mg, sodium alginate 400 mg, sodium bicarbonate 140 mg per 15 mL

Tablet, chewable: Aluminum hydroxide dried gel 80 mg, magnesium trisilicate 20 mg, sodium bicarbonate 70 mg, and alginic acid 200 mg

References
Bohannon AD and Lyles KW, "Drug-Induced Bone Disease," *Clin Geriatr Med*, 1994, 10(4):611-23.

Gams JG, "Clinical Significance of Magnesium: A Review," *Drug Intell Clin Pharm*, 1987, 21(3):240-6.

Peterson WL, Sturdevant RAL, Franki HD, et al, "Healing of Duodenal Ulcer With an Antacid Regimen," *N Engl J Med*, 1977, 297(7):341-5.

Aluminum Phosphate *(a LOO mi num FOS fate)*

Synonyms Aluminum Phosphate Gel

Generic Available No

Therapeutic Category Electrolyte Supplement, Oral

Use Increase fecal excretion of phosphates; no longer labeled for use as an antacid

Contraindications Known hypersensitivity to aluminum phosphate

Warnings Sodium content may be significant for patients with hypertension, renal failure, edema, cirrhosis, congestive heart failure, and those on low sodium diets

Precautions Aluminum intoxication, osteomalacia, patients with GI hemorrhage; caution in renal failure

Adverse Reactions
Endocrine & metabolic: Dehydration or fluid restriction
Gastrointestinal: Constipation, decreased bowel motility, fecal impaction
Miscellaneous: Hemorrhoids

Overdosage Symptoms of overdose include osteomalacia (bone pain), malaise, weakness, and in renal failure, encephalopathy

Toxicology Deferoxamine, traditionally used as an iron chelator, has been shown to increase urinary aluminum output. Deferoxamine chelation of aluminum has resulted in improvements of clinical symptoms and bone histology. Deferoxamine, however, remains an experimental treatment for aluminum poisoning and has a significant potential for adverse effects.

Drug Interactions
May decrease absorption of weak acidic drugs or increase absorption of weak basic drugs

Aluminum compounds decrease the pharmacologic effect of allopurinol, chloroquine, corticosteroids, diflunisal, digoxin, ethambutol, H_2 antagonists, iron compounds, isoniazid, penicillamine, phenothiazines, tetracyclines, thyroid hormones, triclodipine

Aluminum compounds increase the pharmacologic effect of benzodiazepines

Usual Dosage Geriatrics and Adults: Oral: 15-30 mL every 2 hours between meals (see Monitoring Parameters)

Monitoring Parameters Frequency of bowel movements and GI complaints (symptoms); observe for complaints of bone pain, malaise, and muscular weakness; phosphorous levels periodically when patient is on chronic therapy; when used as a phosphate binder, dose to achieve a serum phosphate concentration ≤4 mg/100 mL

Reference Range Normal range (serum): 0-6 ng/mL; dialysis patients may attain ≤40 ng/mL without symptoms of toxicity; >100 ng/mL possible CNS toxicity

Test Interactions Decreased phosphorus, inorganic (S)

Patient Information Dilute dose in water or juice, shake well; do not take within 1-2 hours of oral administration of other drugs unless instructed by physician, pharmacist, or nurse

Nursing Implications Observe for constipation, fecal impaction, and hypophosphatemia (see Monitoring Parameters)

Additional Information Used primarily as a phosphate binder; dose should be followed with water

Special Geriatric Considerations Elderly, due to disease and/or drug therapy, may be predisposed to constipation and fecal impaction. Must consider renal insufficiency (Cl_{cr} <30 mL/minute) as predisposition to aluminum toxicity.

Dosage Forms Suspension, oral: 233 mg/5 mL

References
Bohannon AD and Lyles KW, "Drug-Induced Bone Disease," *Clin Geriatr Med*, 1994, 10(4):611-23.

Aluminum Phosphate Gel *see* Aluminum Phosphate *on previous page*

Aluminum Sucrose Sulfate, Basic *see* Sucralfate *on page 873*

Alupent® *see* Metaproterenol *on page 596*

Alu-Tab® [OTC] *see* Aluminum Hydroxide *on page 41*

Amantadine (a MAN ta deen)
Brand Names Symadine®; Symmetrel®

Synonyms Adamantanamine Hydrochloride

Generic Available Yes

Therapeutic Category Anti-Parkinson's Agent; Antiviral Agent, Oral

Use Symptomatic and adjunct treatment of parkinsonism; also used in prophylaxis and treatment of influenza A viral infection; treatment of drug-induced extrapyramidal symptoms

Contraindications Hypersensitivity to amantadine hydrochloride or any component

Warnings Use with caution in patients with liver disease, a history of recurrent and eczematoid dermatitis, CHF, peripheral edema, uncontrolled psychosis or severe psychoneurosis, epilepsy or other seizures, and in those receiving CNS stimulant drugs

Precautions May cause CNS effects or blurred vision; when treating Parkinson's disease, do not discontinue abruptly

Adverse Reactions
Cardiovascular: Orthostatic hypotension, edema, congestive heart failure
Central nervous system: Dizziness, confusion, headache, insomnia, difficulty in concentrating, anxiety, restlessness, irritability, hallucinations, psychosis
Dermatologic: Livedo reticularis
Gastrointestinal: Nausea, constipation, xerostomia
Genitourinary: Urinary retention

Overdosage Symptoms of overdose include nausea, vomiting, slurred speech, blurred vision, lethargy, hallucinations, seizures, myoclonic jerking

Toxicology Treatment should be directed at reducing the CNS stimulation and at maintaining cardiovascular function. Seizures can be treated with diazepam 5-10 mg I.V. every 15 minutes as needed; up to a total of 30 mg in an adult, while a lidocaine infusion may be required for the cardiac dysrhythmias. CNS toxicity can be treated with physostigmine 1-2 mg slow I.V. every 1-2 hours.

Drug Interactions
Increased effect: Additive anticholinergic effects in patients receiving drugs with anticholinergic activity; additive CNS stimulant effect with CNS stimulants
Increased toxicity/levels with hydrochlorothiazide plus triamterene

Stability Protect from freezing

Mechanism of Action As an antiviral, blocks the uncoating of influenza A virus preventing penetration of virus into host; antiparkinsonian activity may be due to its blocking the reuptake of dopamine into presynaptic neurons and causing direct stimulation of postsynaptic receptors.

Pharmacodynamics Onset of action: Usually within 48 hours, antidyskinetic

Pharmacokinetics
Absorption: Well absorbed from GI tract
Distribution: Crosses the blood-brain barrier
Distribution: V_d:
Normal: 4.4±0.2 L/kg
Renal failure: 5.1±0.2 L/kg
Protein binding:
Normal renal function: ~67%
Hemodialysis patients: ~59%
Metabolism: Not appreciable, small amounts of an acetyl metabolite identified
Half-life:
Normal renal function: 2-7 hours
Elderly patients: 24-29 hours
Impaired renal function: 7-10 days
Hemodialysis patients: Usually within 8 days
Time to peak serum concentration: 1-4 hours
Elimination: 80% to 90% unchanged in urine by glomerular filtration and tubular secretion

(Continued)

Amantadine (Continued)

Usual Dosage

Geriatrics: Dose based on renal function; some patients tolerate the drug better when it is given in 2 divided daily doses; see table.

Amantadine Dosing Guidelines in Renal Impairment

Cl$_{cr}$ (mL/min/1.73 m^2)	Suggested Maintenance Regimen
>80	100 mg bid
60	200 mg/100 mg alternate days
50	100 mg/d
40	100 mg/d
30	200 mg 2 times/week*
20	100 mg 3 times/week
≤10	200 mg/100 mg alternating q7d†

*Loading dose of 200 mg recommended on the first day for Cl$_{cr}$ <30 mL/minute.

†Includes patients maintained on 3 times/week hemodialysis.

Adults:
  Parkinson's disease: 100 mg twice daily
  Influenza A viral infection: 200 mg/day in 1-2 divided doses, start as soon as possible after onset of symptoms, continue for 24-48 hours after symptoms disappear
  Prophylaxis: Minimum 10-day course of therapy following exposure or continue for 2-3 weeks after influenza A virus vaccine is given
Slightly dialyzable (5% to 20%)

Monitoring Parameters Renal function, Parkinson's symptoms, mental status, influenza symptoms, blood pressure

Patient Information Do not abruptly discontinue therapy, it may precipitate a parkinsonian crisis; may impair ability to perform activities requiring mental alertness or coordination; take second dose of the day in the early afternoon to decrease the incidence of insomnia

Nursing Implications If insomnia occurs, the last daily dose should be taken in the early afternoon; assess parkinsonian symptoms prior to and throughout course of therapy

Additional Information In many patients, the therapeutic benefits of amantadine are limited to a few months

Special Geriatric Considerations Elderly patients may be more susceptible to the CNS effects of amantadine; using 2 divided daily doses may minimize this effect. The syrup may be used to administer doses <100 mg; studies have demonstrated that young adults on 200 mg/day achieve a plasma concentration of 300 ng/mL. To achieve this concentration (for influenza prophylaxis) in older adults, studies have suggested a dose of 100 mg or 1.4 mg/kg/day.

Dosage Forms

Amantadine hydrochloride:
  Capsule: 100 mg
  Syrup: 50 mg/5 mL (480 mL)

References

Aoki FY and Sitar DS, "Amantadine Kinetics in Healthy Elderly Men: Implications for Influenza Prevention," *Clin Pharmacol Ther*, 1985, 37(2):137-44.

Aoki FY and Sitar DS, "Clinical Pharmacokinetics of Amantadine Hydrochloride," *Clin Pharmacokinet*, 1988, 14(1):35-51.

Koller WC, Silver DE, and Lieberman A, "An Algorithm for the Management of Parkinson's Disease," *Neurology*, 1994, 44(12 Suppl 10):S1-52.

Somani SK, Degelau J, Cooper SL, et al, "Comparison of Pharmacokinetic and Safety Profiles of Amantadine 50- and 100-mg Daily Doses in Elderly Nursing Home Residents," *Pharmacotherapy*, 1991, 11(6):460-6.

Stange KC, Little DW, and Blatnik B, "Adverse Reactions to Amantadine Prophylaxis of Influenza in a Retirement Home," *J Am Geriatr Soc*, 1991, 33(7):700-5.

Amaryl® see Glimepiride on page 425

Ambien™ see Zolpidem on page 996

AmBisome® see Amphotericin B Lipid Complex on page 72

Amcinonide (am SIN oh nide)

Brand Names Cyclocort®

Generic Available No

Therapeutic Category Anti-inflammatory Agent; Corticosteroid, Topical (Very High Potency)

Use Relief of the inflammatory and pruritic manifestations of corticosteroid-responsive dermatoses (very high potency corticosteroid)

Contraindications Viral, fungal, or tubercular skin lesions, known hypersensitivity to amcinonide or any component

Precautions Systemic absorption of topical corticosteroids has produced reversible HPA axis suppression. This is more likely to occur when the preparation is used on large surfaces or denuded areas for prolonged periods of time or with an occlusive dressing.

Adverse Reactions
Dermatologic: Acne, hypopigmentation, allergic dermatitis, maceration of the skin, skin atrophy, striae, miliaria, telangiectasia
Endocrine & metabolic: HPA suppression, Cushing's syndrome, growth retardation
Local: Burning, itching, irritation, dryness, folliculitis, hypertrichosis
Systemic: Suppression of HPA axis, Cushing's syndrome, hyperglycemia; these reactions occur more frequently with occlusive dressings
Miscellaneous: Secondary infection

Mechanism of Action Topical corticosteroids have anti-inflammatory, antipruritic, vasoconstrictive, and antiproliferative actions

Pharmacokinetics
Absorption: Adequate through intact skin; increases with skin inflammation or occlusion
Metabolism: In the liver
Elimination: By the kidney and in bile

Usual Dosage Geriatrics and Adults: Topical: Apply in a thin layer 2-3 times/day

Monitoring Parameters Relief of symptoms

Patient Information Use only as prescribed and for no longer than the period prescribed; apply sparingly in a thin film and rub in lightly; avoid contact with eyes; notify physician if condition persists or worsens

Nursing Implications Apply sparingly

Additional Information Considered a very high potency steroid; avoid use on the face

Special Geriatric Considerations Due to age-related changes in skin, limit use of topical glucocorticosteroids (see Precautions)

Dosage Forms
Cream: 0.1% (15 g, 30 g, 60 g)
Lotion: 0.1% (20 mL, 60 mL)
Ointment, topical: 0.1% (15 g, 30 g, 60 g)

Amcort® *see* Triamcinolone *on page 949*

Amen® Oral *see* Medroxyprogesterone Acetate *on page 578*

American Geriatrics Society Current Standards of Practice - Oral Anticoagulation for Older Adults *see page 1069*

A-methaPred® Injection *see* Methylprednisolone *on page 611*

Amethopterin *see* Methotrexate *on page 605*

Amfebutamone *see* Bupropion *on page 134*

Amikacin (am i KAY sin)
Related Information
Aminoglycoside Dosing Guidelines *on page 1009*
Cephalosporins, Aminoglycosides, Macrolides, & Quinolones *on page 1014*
I.V. Medication Recommendations *on page 1080*
Serum Drug Concentrations Commonly Monitored: Guidelines *on page 1114*

Brand Names Amikin®
Generic Available No
Therapeutic Category Antibiotic, Aminoglycoside

Use Treatment of documented gram-negative enteric infection resistant to gentamicin and tobramycin; documented infection of mycobacterial organisms susceptible to amikacin

Contraindications Hypersensitivity to amikacin sulfate or any component; cross-sensitivity may exist with other aminoglycosides

Warnings Aminoglycosides are associated with significant nephrotoxicity or ototoxicity; the ototoxicity is directly proportional to the amount of drug given and the duration of treatment; tinnitus or vertigo are indications of vestibular injury and impending bilateral irreversible damage; renal damage is usually reversible
(Continued)

Amikacin *(Continued)*

Precautions Dose and/or frequency of administration must be modified in patients with renal impairment and elderly

Adverse Reactions Risk of hypomagnesemia if decrease in magnesium intake

Central nervous system: Confusion, delirium

Dermatologic: Rash

Hepatic: Hepatotoxicity with elevated LFTs

Neuromuscular & skeletal: Neuromuscular blockade

Otic: Ototoxicity

Renal: Nephrotoxicity

Miscellaneous: Drug fever

Overdosage Symptoms of overdose include ototoxicity, nephrotoxicity, and neuromuscular toxicity

Toxicology Treatment of choice following a single acute overdose appears to be the maintenance of good urine output of at least 3 mL/kg/hour. Dialysis is of questionable value in the enhancement of aminoglycoside elimination. If required, hemodialysis is preferred over peritoneal dialysis in patients with normal renal function. Careful hydration may be all that is required to promote diuresis and, therefore, the enhancement of the drug's elimination.

Drug Interactions Synergy with penicillins and cephalosporins, penicillins may inactivate *in vitro*; loop diuretics may potentiate the ototoxicity of the aminoglycosides

Increased/prolonged effect: Depolarizing and nondepolarizing neuromuscular blocking agents

Increased toxicity: Concurrent use of amphotericin may increase nephrotoxicity

Stability Stable for 24 hours at room temperature when mixed in D_5W, $D_51/4NS$; $D_51/2NS$; NS; LR

Mechanism of Action Inhibits protein synthesis in susceptible bacteria by binding to ribosomal subunits

Pharmacokinetics

Absorption: I.M.: Aminoglycosides may be delayed in the bedridden patient

Half-life:

Adults: 2-3 hours

Anuria: 28-86 hours

Half-life and clearance are dependent on renal function primarily distributed into extracellular fluid (highly hydrophilic); penetrates the blood-brain barrier when meninges are inflamed

Time to peak serum concentration:

I.M.: Within 45-120 minutes

I.V.: Within 30 minutes

Elimination: 94% to 98% excreted unchanged in urine via glomerular filtration within 24 hours

Clearance (renal) may be reduced and half-life prolonged in geriatric patients

Usual Dosage

Geriatrics:

I.M., I.V.: Initial: 15-20 mg/kg/day divided every 12-24 hours; occasionally every 8- or 48-hour dosing may be required; dosage adjustments should be based on serum concentrations and calculated pharmacokinetic parameters

Once daily or extended interval: I.V.: 15-20 mg/kg/dose given every 24, 36, or 48 hours depending on Cl_{cr} (see below)

Adults: I.M., I.V.: 15-20 mg/kg/day divided every 8-12 hours

Dosing adjustment in renal impairment: Some patients may require larger or more frequent doses if serum concentrations document the need (ie, cystic fibrosis or febrile granulocytopenic patients). Administer a loading dose of 5-7.5 mg/kg; subsequent dosages and frequency of administration are best determined by measurement of serum concentration and assessment of renal insufficiency.

Cl_{cr} ≥60 mL/minute: Administer every 24 hours

Cl_{cr} 40-59 mL/minute: Administer every 36 hours

Cl_{cr} 20-39 mL/minute: Administer every 48 hours

Cl_{cr} <20 mL/minute: Individualize dose

Dialyzable (50% to 100%)

Administration Administer I.M. injection in large muscle mass

Monitoring Parameters BUN, serum creatinine, serum peak and trough concentrations, hydration and urine output. In cases where extended treatment is warranted (>10 days), audiology testing should be considered.

Reference Range
Therapeutic:
Peak: 25-30 µg/mL
Trough: 4-8 µg/mL
Toxic:
Peak: >35 µg/mL
Trough: >10 µg/mL
Once daily or extended interval dosing: Trough: <5 µg/mL

Test Interactions Increased BUN, AST, ALT, alkaline phosphatase, bilirubin, creatinine, LDH, protein; Decreased calcium, magnesium, potassium, sodium

Patient Information Report loss of hearing, ringing or roaring in the ears or feeling of fullness in head

Nursing Implications Aminoglycoside serum concentrations measured from blood taken from Silastic® central catheters can sometimes give falsely high readings; obtain culture for culture and sensitivity before first dose; weigh patient and obtain baseline renal function before therapy begins; monitor vital signs, serum concentrations are reportedly lower in patients with fever; administer around-the-clock rather than 3 times/day, to promote less variation in peak and trough serum concentrations

Additional Information Drug should be discontinued if signs of ototoxicity, nephrotoxicity, or hypersensitivity occurs; hearing should be tested before, during, and after treatment, when indicated; sodium content of 1 g: 29.9 mg (1.3 mEq)

Special Geriatric Considerations The aminoglycosides are important therapeutic interventions for infections due to susceptible organisms and as empiric therapy in seriously ill patients. Their use is not without risk of toxicity, however, these risks can be minimized if initial dosing is adjusted for estimated renal function and appropriate monitoring performed (see Warnings, Precautions, and Usual Dosage). High dose, once daily aminoglycosides have been advocated as an alternative to traditional dosing regimens. Once daily or extended interval dosing is as effective and may be safer than traditional dosing. Interval must be adjusted for renal function. See Pharmacokinetics and Usual Dosage.

Dosage Forms Injection, as sulfate: 50 mg/mL (2 mL, 4 mL); 250 mg/mL (2 mL, 4 mL)

References
Bauer LA and Blouin RA, "Influence of Age on Amikacin Pharmacokinetics in Patients Without Renal Disease. Comparison With Gentamicin and Tobramycin," *Eur J Clin Pharmacol*, 1983, 24(5):639-42.

Nicolau DP, Freeman CD, Belliveau PP, et al, "Experience With a Once-Daily Aminoglycoside Program Administered to 2184 Adult Patients," *Antimicrob Agents Chemother*, 1995, 39(3):650-5.

Preston SL and Briceland LL, "Single Daily Dosing of Aminoglycosides," *Pharmacotherapy*, 1995, 15(3):297-316.

Vanhaeverbeek M, Siska G, Douchamps J, et al, "Comparison of the Efficacy and Safety of Amikacin Once or Twice-a-Day in the Treatment of Severe Gram-Negative Infections in the Elderly," *Int J Clin Pharmacol Ther Toxicol*, 1993, 31(3):153-6.

Yasuhara H, Kobayashi S, Sakamoto K, et al, "Pharmacokinetics of Amikacin and Cephalothin in Bedridden Elderly Patients," *J Clin Pharmacol*, 1982, 22(8-9):403-9.

Amikin® *see* Amikacin *on page 51*

Amiloride (a MIL oh ride)

Brand Names Midamor®

Generic Available Yes

Therapeutic Category Diuretic, Potassium Sparing

Use Counteract potassium loss induced by other diuretics in the treatment of hypertension or edematous conditions including congestive heart failure, hepatic cirrhosis and hypoaldosteronism; usually used in conjunction with a more potent diuretic such as thiazides or loop diuretics

Contraindications Hyperkalemia, potassium supplementation and impaired renal function, hypersensitivity to amiloride or any component

Warnings May cause hyperkalemia (serum concentrations >5.5 mEq/L) which, if uncorrected, is potentially fatal

Precautions Potassium excretion may be decreased in the elderly increasing the risk of hyperkalemia with the use of amiloride

Adverse Reactions
Central nervous system: Headache, lethargy
Dermatological: Rash
Endocrine & metabolic: Hyperkalemia, gynecomastia, hyperchloremic metabolic acidosis, dehydration, hyponatremia
Gastrointestinal: Anorexia, nausea, vomiting, diarrhea
(Continued)

Amiloride *(Continued)*

Toxicology Clinical signs are consistent with dehydration and electrolyte disturbance; severe hyperkalemia (>6.5 mEq/L). Ingestion of large amounts of potassium-sparing diuretics may result in life-threatening hyperkalemia. This can be treated with I.V. insulin and glucose (dextrose 25% in water), with concurrent I.V. sodium bicarbonate (1 mEq/kg up to 44 mEq/dose). If needed, Kayexalate® oral or rectal solutions in sorbitol may also be useful.

Drug Interactions

NSAIDs may reduce the therapeutic effect of amiloride; amiloride may reduce the inotropic effects of digoxin

Increased risk of hyperkalemia if given with other potassium-sparing diuretics, potassium preparations, or ACE inhibitors

Mechanism of Action Interferes with potassium/sodium exchange in the distal tubule

Pharmacokinetics

Absorption: Oral: ~50%

Distribution: V_d: 350-380 L

Half-life: 6-9 hours

Elimination: Excreted unchanged equally in urine and feces; renal clearance of amiloride is decreased in elderly

Usual Dosage

Geriatrics: Initial: 5 mg once daily or every other day

Adults: 5-10 mg/day (up to 20 mg)

Monitoring Parameters Blood pressure (standing, sitting/supine), serum electrolytes, renal function, weight, I & O

Test Interactions Increased potassium (S); decreased magnesium; transient renal and hepatic function tests have been noted

Patient Information Take in the morning with food or milk; avoid excessive ingestion of foods high in potassium or use of salt substitutes; report any muscle cramps, weakness, nausea, or dizziness

Nursing Implications Monitor I & O ratios and daily weight throughout therapy

Additional Information Medication should be discontinued if potassium serum concentration exceeds 6.5 mEq/L; combined with hydrochlorothiazide as Moduretic®; amiloride is considered an alternative to triamterene or spironolactone

Special Geriatric Considerations See Precautions

Dosage Forms Tablet, as hydrochloride: 5 mg

Amiloride and Hydrochlorothiazide

(a MIL oh ride & hye droe klor oh THYE a zide)

Related Information

Amiloride *on previous page*

Hydrochlorothiazide *on page 458*

Brand Names Moduretic®

Synonyms Hydrochlorothiazide and Amiloride

Generic Available Yes

Therapeutic Category Diuretic, Combination

Use Antikaliuretic diuretic, antihypertensive

Contraindications Anuria, acute or chronic renal insufficiency; patients who are hypersensitive to this drug or to other sulfonamide-derived drugs

Precautions Should not be used in the presence of serum potassium concentrations >5.5 mEq/L

Adverse Reactions

Endocrine & metabolic: Hyperkalemia

Gastrointestinal: Nausea, diarrhea, GI pain

Usual Dosage Oral:

Geriatrics: Initial: 1/2 to 1 tablet daily

Adults: Start with 1 tablet daily, then may be increased to 2 tablets/day if needed; usually given in a single dose

Monitoring Parameters Blood pressure, serum electrolytes, renal function

Test Interactions Increased BUN, calcium, sodium, magnesium, chloride, uric acid

Patient Information Take with food in the morning

Special Geriatric Considerations Potassium excretion may be decreased in the elderly, increasing the risk of hyperkalemia with potassium-sparing diuretics such as amiloride.

Dosage Forms Tablet: Amiloride hydrochloride 5 mg and hydrochlorothiazide 50 mg

2-Amino-6-Trifluoromethoxy-benzothiazole *see* Riluzole *on page 831*

Aminobenzylpenicillin *see* Ampicillin *on page 73*

Aminoglycoside Dosing Guidelines *see page 1009*

Aminophyllin® *see* Aminophylline *on this page*

Aminophylline (am in OFF i lin)

Related Information

Asthma Guidelines *on page 1040*

I.V. Medication Recommendations *on page 1080*

I.V. Push Recommended Guidelines *on page 1083*

Serum Drug Concentrations Commonly Monitored: Guidelines *on page 1114*

Brand Names Aminophyllin®; Phyllocontin®; Somophyllin®; Truphylline®

Synonyms Theophylline Ethylenediamine

Generic Available Yes

Therapeutic Category Bronchodilator; Theophylline Derivative

Use Bronchodilator in reversible airway obstruction due to asthma or COPD

Contraindications Uncontrolled arrhythmias, untreated seizure disorders, and hypersensitivity to xanthine or ethylenediamine; infection or irritation of the rectum or large colon when using suppositories

Precautions Use with caution in patients with peptic ulcer, hyperthyroidism, hypertension, and patients with compromised cardiac function

Adverse Reactions

Cardiovascular: Palpitation, sinus tachycardia, extrasystoles, hypotension, ventricular arrhythmias, flushing

Central nervous system: Irritability, restlessness, headache, insomnia, seizures, fever

Endocrine & metabolic: Hyperglycemia

Gastrointestinal: Nausea, vomiting, esophageal reflux, diarrhea, hematemesis, rectal bleeding, epigastric pain

Neuromuscular & skeletal: Tremors, muscle twitching

Renal: Diuresis, proteinuria

Respiratory: Tachypnea, respiratory arrest

Adverse reactions are uncommon at serum theophylline concentrations <20 mcg/mL

Overdosage Symptoms of overdose include tachycardia, extrasystoles, nausea, vomiting, anorexia, tonic-clonic seizures, insomnia, circulatory failure; agitation, irritability, headache

Toxicology If seizures have not occurred, induce vomiting; ipecac syrup is preferred. Do not induce emesis in the presence of impaired consciousness. Repeated doses of charcoal have been shown to be effective in enhancing the total body clearance of theophylline. Do not repeat charcoal doses if an ileus is present. Charcoal hemoperfusion may be considered if the serum theophylline concentration exceeds 40 mcg/mL, the patient is unable to tolerate repeat oral charcoal administrations, or if severe toxic symptoms are present. Clearance with hemoperfusion is better than clearance from hemodialysis. Administer a cathartic, especially if sustained release agents were used. Phenobarbital administered prophylactically may prevent seizures.

Drug Interactions Changes in diet may affect the elimination of theophylline

Theophylline may decrease the effects of phenytoin, lithium, and neuromuscular blocking agents; theophylline increases the excretion of lithium; theophylline may have synergistic toxicity with sympathomimetics

Cimetidine, ranitidine, allopurinol, beta-blockers (nonspecific), erythromycin (macrolide antibiotics), calcium channel blockers, disulfiram, interferon, mexiletine, thiobendazole, influenza virus vaccine, corticosteroids, ephedrine, quinolones, thyroid hormones, oral contraceptives, amiodarone, troleandomycin, clindamycin, carbamazepine, isoniazid, loop diuretics, and lincomycin may increase theophylline concentrations

Cigarette and marijuana smoking, rifampin, barbiturates, hydantoins, ketoconazole, sulfinpyrazone, sympathomimetics, isoniazid, loop diuretics, charcoal, carbamazepine, and aminoglutethimide may decrease theophylline concentrations

Tetracyclines enhance toxicity and benzodiazepine's action may be antagonized

Stability Do not use solutions if discolored or if crystals are present

Mechanism of Action Causes bronchodilatation, diuresis, CNS and cardiac stimulation, and gastric acid secretion by blocking phosphodiesterase which (Continued)

Aminophylline *(Continued)*

increases tissue concentrations of cyclic adenine monophosphate (cAMP) which in turn promotes catecholamine stimulation of lipolysis, glycogenolysis, and gluconeogenesis and induces release of epinephrine from adrenal medulla cells. Other proposed mechanisms include inhibition of extracellular adenosine, stimulation of endogenous catecholamines, antagonism of PGE_2 and $PGE_{2\alpha}$, mobilization of intracellular calcium, and increased sensitivity of beta-adrenergic receptors in reactive airways.

Pharmacokinetics

Absorption: Oral: Depends upon dosage form; aminophylline is the ethylenediamine salt of theophylline, pharmacokinetic parameters are those of theophylline

Metabolism: Liver - extensive (85% to 90%)

Half-life: Highly variable and dependent upon age, liver function, cardiac function, lung disease, and smoking history

Elimination: In urine as metabolites; see tables.

Aminophylline

Patient Group	Approximate Half-Life (h)
Geriatrics and Adults	
Nonsmoker	4-16 (8.7 avg)
Smoker	4.4
Cardiac compromised, liver failure	20-30

Dosage Form	Time to Peak
Uncoated tablet	2 h
Enteric coated tablet	5 h
Chewable tablet	1-1.5 h
Extended release	4-7 h
Intravenous	<30 min

Usual Dosage Geriatrics and Adults (all dosages based upon **aminophylline**):

Treatment of acute bronchospasm:
Loading dose (in patients not currently receiving aminophylline or theophylline): 6 mg/kg (based on aminophylline) given I.V. over 20-30 minutes; administration rate should not exceed 25 mg/minute (aminophylline)

Approximate I.V. maintenance dosages are based upon **continuous infusions**; bolus dosing may be determined by multiplying the hourly infusion rate by 24 hours and dividing by the desired number of doses/day

Adults (healthy, nonsmoking): 0.7 mg/kg/hour

Older patients, patients with cor pulmonale, patients with congestive heart failure or liver failure: 0.25 mg/kg/hour

Oral:
Nonsustained release: 16-20 mg/kg/day in 4 divided doses
Sustained release: 9-13 mg/kg/day divided into 2-3 doses/day

Dosage should be adjusted according to serum concentration measurements during the first 12- to 24-hour period. Avoid using suppositories due to erratic, unreliable absorption. See table.

Guidelines for Obtaining Aminophylline Serum Concentrations

Dosage Form	Time to Draw Level
P.O. liquid, fast-release tab	Peak: 1 h post 4th dose
	Trough: Just before 4th dose
P.O. slow-release product	Peak: 4 h post 3rd dose
	Trough: Just before 3rd dose

Rectal: Geriatrics and Adults: 500 mg 3 times/day

Monitoring Parameters Heart rate, CNS effects (insomnia, irritability); respiratory rate (COPD patients often have resting controlled respiratory rates in low 20s)

Reference Range
Sample size: 0.5-1 mL serum (red top tube)

Therapeutic: 10-20 µg/mL; Toxic: >20 µg/mL some patients may have adequate clinical response with serum concentrations from 5-10 µg/mL

Timing of serum samples: If toxicity is suspected, draw serum concentration any time during a continuous I.V. infusion, or 2 hours after an oral dose; if lack of therapeutic is effected, draw a trough serum concentration immediately before the next oral dose or intermittent I.V. dose

Test Interactions May elevate uric acid serum concentrations

Patient Information Oral preparations should be taken with a full glass of water; avoid drinking or eating large quantities of caffeine-containing beverages or food; take at regular intervals; take sustained release tablets whole; do not chew beads; remain in bed for 15-20 minutes after inserting suppository; take with food if GI upset occurs; notify physician if nausea, vomiting, insomnia, nervousness, irritability, palpitations, seizures occur; do not change from one brand to another without consulting physician and pharmacist; do not change doses without consulting your physician

Nursing Implications Avoid I.M. injection, too painful; do not inject I.V. solution faster than 25 mg/minute; administer oral and I.V. administration around-the-clock rather than 4 times/day, 3 times/day, etc (ie, 12-6-12-6, not 9-1-5-9) to promote less variation in peak and trough serum concentrations; do not crush sustained release drug products; do not crush enteric coated drug product; monitor vital signs, serum concentrations, and CNS effects (insomnia, irritability); encourage patient to drink adequate fluids (2 L/day) to decrease mucous viscosity in airways

Additional Information Elderly, acutely ill, and patients with severe respiratory problems, pulmonary edema, or liver dysfunction are at greater risk of toxicity because of reduced drug clearance; 100 mg aminophylline = 79 mg theophylline

Special Geriatric Considerations Although there is a great intersubject variability for half-lives of methylxanthines (2-10 hours). The elderly, as a group, have slower hepatic clearance. Therefore, use lower initial doses and monitor closely for response and adverse reactions. Additionally, elderly are at greater risk for toxicity due to concomitant disease (eg, congestive heart failure, arrhythmias), and drug use (eg, cimetidine, ciprofloxacin, etc) (see Precautions and Drug Interactions).

Dosage Forms

Injection: 25 mg/mL (10 mL, 20 mL) - 250 mg (equivalent to 187 mg theophylline) per 10 mL; 500 mg (equivalent to 394 mg theophylline) per 20 mL

Liquid, oral (dye free): 105 mg (equivalent to 90 mg theophylline) per 5 mL (240 mL)

Suppository, rectal: 250 mg (equivalent to 198 mg theophylline) - 500 mg (equivalent to 395 mg theophylline)

Tablet: 100 mg (equivalent to 79 mg theophylline) - 200 mg (equivalent to 158 mg theophylline) - 500 mg (equivalent to 395 mg theophylline)

Tablet, controlled release: 225 mg (equivalent to 178 mg theophylline)

References

Kearney TE, Manoguerra AS, Curtis GP, et al, "Theophylline Toxicity and the Beta-Adrenergic System," *Ann Intern Med*, 1985, 102(6):766-9.

Mahler DA, Barlow PB, and Matthay RA, "Chronic Obstructive Pulmonary Disease," *Clin Geriatr Med*, 1986, 2(2):285-312.

Upton RA, "Pharmacokinetic Interactions Between Theophylline and Other Medication (Part II)," *Clin Pharmacokinet*, 1991, 20(2):135-50.

Aminosalicylic Acid (a mee noe sal i SIL ik AS id)

Brand Names Pamisyl®

Synonyms 4-Aminosalicylic Acid; PAS

Generic Available Yes

Therapeutic Category Anti-inflammatory Agent; Antipyretic; Antitubercular Agent; Nonsteroidal Anti-inflammatory Agent (NSAID), Oral

Use Treatment of tuberculosis with combination drugs

Unlabeled use: Lipid lowering agent

Contraindications Hypersensitivity to aminosalicylic acid or its components

Precautions Use with caution in persons with reduced renal or hepatic function; patients with gastric ulcer, CHF, or sodium restriction

Adverse Reactions

Cardiovascular: Vasculitis

Central nervous system: Fever, encephalopathy

Dermatologic: Skin eruptions

Endocrine & metabolic: Goiter

Gastrointestinal: Nausea, vomiting, diarrhea, abdominal pain

Hematologic: Leukopenia, agranulocytosis, thrombocytopenia, blood dyscrasias

(Continued)

Aminosalicylic Acid *(Continued)*

Hepatic: Jaundice, hepatitis

Miscellaneous: Infections, mononucleosis-like syndrome, hypersensitivity

Drug Interactions Decreased absorption of digoxin (oral dosing); vitamin B_{12} deficiency (administer I.M. if needed)

Mechanism of Action Bacteriostatic against *Mycobacterium tuberculosis*

Pharmacokinetics

Absorption: Sodium salt is readily absorbed in GI tract

Distribution: Wide with high concentrations in pleural and caseous tissue; CSF concentrations are low

Metabolism: Hepatic (>50% acetylation)

Half-life: 1 hour

Elimination: >80% excreted in urine as metabolites or free acid

Excretion may be reduced and half-life prolonged in persons with hepatic or renal impairment

Usual Dosage Geriatrics and Adults: Oral: 14-16 g/day in 2-3 divided doses

Monitoring Parameters Signs and symptoms of resolving infection

Test Interactions May decrease serum cholesterol concentrations; false-positive urine glucose with copper reduction methods

Patient Information Take with food; may discolor urine red; do not take tablet if brown or purple in color; do not store in bathroom or kitchen as tablets will deteriorate in high humidity environments; notify physician of sore throat, bruising, bleeding, or skin rash

Nursing Implications Store in dry place; do not administer tablets if discolored; administer with meals

Special Geriatric Considerations Elderly may require lower recommended dose (see Precautions)

Dosage Forms Tablet: 500 mg

4-Aminosalicylic Acid *see* Aminosalicylic Acid *on previous page*

5-Aminosalicylic Acid *see* Mesalamine *on page 591*

Amiodarone *(a MEE oh da rone)*

Brand Names Cordarone®

Generic Available No

Therapeutic Category Antiarrhythmic Agent, Class III

Use Management of resistant, life-threatening ventricular arrhythmias unresponsive to conventional therapy with less toxic agents; has also been used for treatment of supraventricular arrhythmias (atrial fibrillation, flutter, tachycardia) unresponsive to conventional therapy

Contraindications Hypersensitivity to amiodarone; severe sinus node dysfunction, marked sinus bradycardia; second and third degree A-V block; bradycardia-induced syncope, except if pacemaker is placed; thyroid disease

Warnings Not considered first-line antiarrhythmic due to high incidence of toxicity; 75% of patients experience adverse effects with large doses; exacerbation of arrhythmias (2% to 5%); discontinuation is required in 5% to 20% of patients; reserve for use in life-threatening arrhythmias refractory to other therapy; elevation of LFTs (AST/ALT), usually transient; discontinue if persistent

Precautions May be ineffective or cause arrhythmias in patients who have hypokalemia

Adverse Reactions Most patients develop adverse effects when administered chronically; gastrointestinal side effects are the most common

Patients ≥60 years of age may be at greater risk for adverse reactions

Cardiovascular: Atropine resistant bradycardia, heart block, sinus arrest, myocardial depression, congestive heart failure, paroxysmal ventricular tachycardia, hypotension; 10% to 20% of those who develop pulmonary toxicity die of cardiopulmonary adverse effects ammonia

Central nervous system: (5% to 14% incidence): Lack of coordination, fatigue, malaise, abnormal gait, ataxia, dizziness, headache, insomnia, nightmares, fever

Dermatologic: Slate blue discoloration of skin, photosensitivity (10%), rash

Endocrine & metabolic: Hypothyroidism (up to 11%) or less commonly hyperthyroidism; each 200 mg tablet contains 75 mg iodine; hyperglycemia, increased triglycerides; 49% of patients develop thyroid dysfunction, most have altered TFTs; amiodarone-induced hypothyroidism may be treated with thyroid supplement replacement; monitor serum T_4 and TSH with goal to achieve normal ranges of each

Gastrointestinal: Nausea, vomiting, anorexia, constipation

Hematologic: Coagulation abnormalities, thrombocytopenia

Hepatic: Increased liver enzymes, severe hepatic toxicity (potentially fatal), increased bilirubin, increased serum

Neuromuscular & skeletal: Tremors, paresthesia

Ocular: Corneal microdeposits (100% of patients), photophobia

Respiratory: Interstitial pneumonitis, hypersensitivity pneumonitis, pulmonary fibrosis (10% to 13% of patients); alveolar pneumonitis may present with cough, dyspnea, chest x-ray changes

Most patients develop adverse effects when administered chronically; gastrointestinal side effects are the most common

Patients ≥60 years of age may be at greater risk for adverse reactions

Overdosage Symptoms of overdose include sinus bradycardia and/or heart block, hypotension and Q-T prolongation; patients should be monitored for several days following ingestion; treat patient with general supportive measures

Toxicology Intoxication with amiodarone necessitates EKG monitoring. When bradycardia occurs, atropine may be given, however, atropine resistant bradycardia has been reported. In cases of difficult to treat amiodarone-induced bradycardia, injectable isoproterenol or a temporary pacemaker may be required; cholestyramine may enhance elimination

Drug Interactions

Amiodarone may increase plasma concentrations of digoxin and cardiac glycosides, flecainide, procainamide, quinidine, warfarin, theophylline, and phenytoin resulting in toxicities

Combined use with beta-blockers, digitalis, or calcium channel blockers may result in bradycardia, sinus arrest; use with class I antiarrhythmics may cause ventricular arrhythmias; amiodarone + general anesthetics may result in bradycardia, hypotension, heart block; cholestyramine may possibly decreased amiodarone serum concentration

Mechanism of Action A class III antiarrhythmic agent which inhibits adrenergic stimulation, prolongs the action potential and refractory period in myocardial tissue; decreases A-V conduction and sinus node function. These effects may be due to selective blockade of triiodothyronine (T_3) in myocardium; also has weak calcium channel blocking activity; noncompetitive alpha- and beta-receptor antagonist; exhibits some anticholinergic activity

Pharmacodynamics

Onset of effect: 3 days to 3 weeks after starting therapy

Peak effect: 1 week to 5 months

Duration of effects after discontinuation of therapy: 7-50 days

Pharmacokinetics

Distribution: V_d: 66 L/kg (range: 18-148 L/kg)

Protein binding: 96%

Metabolism: In the liver, major metabolite N-desethylamiodarone (active); eliminated via biliary excretion; possible enterohepatic recirculation; inhibits CYP2C9 and 2D6, substrate CYP3A4

Bioavailability: ~50% (range: 20% to 80%); maximum plasma concentration: 3-7 hours following oral administration

Half-life (oral chronic therapy): 40-55 days (range: 26-107 days)

Elimination: biphasic; 50% reduction of serum concentration in 2.5-10 days; slow terminal elimination 26-107 days; steady-state levels achieved between 130-535 days with 265 days average; <1% excreted unchanged in urine

Usual Dosage Geriatrics and Adults:

Oral: Ventricular arrhythmias: 800-1600 mg/day in 1-2 doses for 1-3 weeks, then 600-800 mg/day in 1-2 doses for 1 month; maintenance: 400-600 mg/day; lower doses are recommended for supraventricular arrhythmias. Administer with food if gastrointestinal side effects occur or when doses exceed 1000 mg/day; may be administered as a single daily dose once maintenance doses are achieved.

I.V.:

First 24 hours: 1000 mg according to following regimen

Step 1: 150 mg (10 mL) over first 10 minutes (mix 3 mL in 100 mL D_5W)

Step 2: 360 mg (200 mL) over next 6 hours (mix 18 mL in 500 mL D_5W)

Step 3: 540 mg (300 mL) over next 18 hours

After the first 24 hours: 0.5 mg/minute utilizing concentration of 1-6 mg/mL

Breakthrough VF or VT: 150 mg supplemental doses in 100 mL D_5W over 10 minutes

Note: When switching from I.V. to oral therapy, use the following as a guide:

<1-week I.V. infusion: 800-1600 mg/day

1- to 3-week I.V. infusion: 600-800 mg/day

(Continued)

Amiodarone *(Continued)*

>3-week I.V. infusion: 400 mg

Dosing adjustment in hepatic impairment: Probably necessary in substantial hepatic impairment

Hemodialysis effects: Not removed by hemodialysis or peritoneal dialysis (0% to 5%); no supplemental doses required

Monitoring Parameters Monitor heart rate and rhythm throughout therapy; monitor liver and thyroid function (particularly TSH)

Reference Range Therapeutic: 0.5-2.5 mg/L (SI: 1-4 µmol/L) (parent); desethyl metabolite is active and is present in equal concentration to parent drug

Test Interactions Thyroid function tests: Amiodarone partially inhibits the peripheral conversion of thyroxine (T_4) to triiodothyronine (T_3); serum T_4 and reverse triiodothyronine (RT_3) concentrations may be increased and serum T_3 may be decreased; most patients remain clinically euthyroid, however, clinical hypothyroidism or hyperthyroidism may occur

Patient Information Take with food; use sunscreen or stay out of sun to prevent burns; skin discoloration is reversible; photophobia may make sunglasses necessary

Nursing Implications Assess patient for signs of thyroid dysfunction, lethargy, edema of the hands, feet, weight loss, and pulmonary toxicity

Additional Information Onset of pharmacologic effects range from 5-30 days, full effect may take as long as 3 months; hospitalization required for initiation of therapy; response may require 1-2 weeks; CNS symptoms normally develops within 7 days, muscle weakness may present a great hazard for ambulation

Special Geriatric Considerations Information describing the clinical use and pharmacokinetics in elderly is lacking; however, elderly may be predisposed to toxicity (see Drug Interactions). Half-life may be prolonged due to decreased clearance; monitor closely.

Dosage Forms

Amiodarone hydrochloride:

Injection: 50 mg/mL with benzyl alcohol (3 mL)

Tablet, scored: 200 mg

References

Fenster PE and Nolan PE, "Antiarrhythmic Drugs," *Geriatric Pharmacology*, Bressler R and Katz MD, eds, New York, NY: McGraw-Hill, 1993, 6:105-49.

Amitone® [OTC] *see* Calcium Salts (Oral) *on page 152*

Amitriptyline *(a mee TRIP ti leen)*

Related Information

Antidepressant Agents Comparison *on page 1021*

Antidepressant Medication Guidelines *on page 1075*

Federal OBRA Regulations Recommended Maximum Doses - Antidepressants *on page 1056*

Serum Drug Concentrations Commonly Monitored: Guidelines *on page 1114*

Brand Names Elavil®; Endep®; Enovil®

Generic Available Yes

Therapeutic Category Antidepressant, Tricyclic

Use Treatment of various forms of depression, often in conjunction with psychotherapy; as an analgesic for certain chronic and neuropathic pain, migraine prophylaxis

Unlabeled use: Treatment of pathologic laughing or weeping associated with forebrain disease

Contraindications Hypersensitivity to amitriptyline (cross-sensitivity with other tricyclics may occur); narrow-angle glaucoma; patients receiving MAO inhibitor within past 14 days

Warnings To avoid cholinergic crisis, do not discontinue abruptly in patients receiving high doses chronically

Precautions Use with caution in patients with cardiac conduction disturbances, history of hyperthyroidism, renal or hepatic impairment, bipolar illness, benign prostatic hypertrophy; an EKG prior to initiation of therapy is advised

Adverse Reactions

Cardiovascular: Postural hypotension, arrhythmias, tachycardia, sudden death

Central nervous system: Sedation, fatigue, anxiety, confusion, insomnia, impaired cognitive function, seizures; extrapyramidal symptoms are possible, moderate to marked sedation can occur (tolerance to these effects usually occur)

Dermatologic: Photosensitivity

Endocrine and metabolic: Hypoglycemia, rarely SIADH

Gastrointestinal: Xerostomia, increased appetite, weight gain, constipation, decreased lower esophageal sphincter tone may cause GE reflux, paralytic ileus

Genitourinary: Urinary retention

Hematologic: Rarely agranulocytosis, leukopenia, eosinophilia

Hepatic: Increased liver enzymes, cholestatic jaundice

Neuromuscular & skeletal: Tremors, weakness

Ocular: Blurred vision, increased intraocular pressure

Miscellaneous: Allergic reactions

Anticholinergic effects may be pronounced; moderate to marked sedation can occur and is associated with falling

Overdosage Symptoms of overdose include agitation, confusion, hallucinations, urinary retention, hypothermia, hypotension, tachycardia

Toxicology Following initiation of essential overdose management, toxic symptoms should be treated. Ventricular arrhythmias often respond to phenytoin 15-20 mg/kg with concurrent systemic alkalinization (sodium bicarbonate 0.5-2 mEq/kg I.V.). Arrhythmias unresponsive to this therapy may respond to lidocaine 1 mg/kg I.V. followed by a titrated infusion. Physostigmine (1-2 mg I.V. slowly) may be indicated in reversing cardiac arrhythmias that are due to vagal blockade or for anticholinergic effects. Seizures usually respond to diazepam I.V. boluses (5-10 mg, up to 30 mg). If seizures are unresponsive or recur, phenytoin or phenobarbital may be required.

Drug Interactions

Amitriptyline may decrease the effects of guanethidine and may increase the effects of other CNS depressants, adrenergic agents (epinephrine, isoproterenol), anticholinergic agents and dicumarol

With MAO inhibitors, hyperpyrexia, tachycardia, hypertension, confusion, seizures, and death have been reported. Cimetidine, fluoxetine, methylphenidate, and haloperidol may decrease the metabolism and/or increase TCA levels and phenobarbital may increase the metabolism of amitriptyline; use with clonidine may result in hypertensive crisis.

Stability Keep oral solution in refrigerator, remains stable for 7 days after preparation; protect injection and Elavil® 10 mg tablets from light

Mechanism of Action Traditionally believed to increase the synaptic concentration of serotonin (5-HT) and or norepinephrine (NE) in the central nervous system by inhibition of their reuptake by the presynaptic neuronal membrane. However, additional receptor effects have been found including desensitization of adenyl cyclase, down regulation of beta-adrenergic receptors, and down regulation of serotonin receptors.

Pharmacodynamics Therapeutic effects begin in 7-21 days; NE <5-HT

Pharmacokinetics

Metabolism: In the liver to nortriptyline (active), hydroxy derivatives and conjugated derivatives; substrate CYP1A2, 2C9, 2D6

Half-life: Adults: 9-25 hours (15-hour average); half-life prolonged (mean: 21.7 hours)

Time to peak serum concentration: Within 4 hours

Elimination: Renal excretion of 18% as unchanged drug; small amounts eliminated in feces by bile

Plasma concentrations increase with age and steady-state plasma concentrations are significantly increased in older patients compared to younger patients after equal doses

Usual Dosage Oral:

Geriatrics: Initial: 10-25 mg at bedtime; dose should be increased in 10-25 mg increments every week if tolerated; dose range: 25-150 mg/day

Adults: 30-100 mg/day single dose at bedtime or in divided doses; dose may be gradually increased up to 300 mg/day; once symptoms are controlled, decrease gradually to lowest effective dose

Nondialyzable

Monitoring Parameters Blood pressure, pulse, EKG; target symptoms

Reference Range

Therapeutic:

Amitriptyline and nortriptyline 100-250 ng/mL (SI: 360-900 nmol/L)

Nortriptyline 50-150 ng/mL (SI: 190-570 nmol/L)

Toxic: >0.5 µg/mL

Test Interactions Elevated glucose

(Continued)

Amitriptyline *(Continued)*

Patient Information Avoid alcohol ingestion; do not discontinue medication abruptly; may cause urine to turn blue-green; may cause drowsiness, dry mouth, constipation, blurred vision; rise slowly to prevent dizziness

Nursing Implications Monitor blood pressure and pulse rate prior to and during initial therapy; evaluate mental status; monitor weight, may increase appetite and possibly a craving for sweets

Additional Information Plasma concentrations do not always correlate with clinical effectiveness; desired therapeutic effect (for depression) may take as long as 3-4 weeks, at that point dosage should be reduced to lowest effective level; when used for migraine headache prophylaxis, therapeutic effect may take as long as 6 weeks; a higher dosage may be required in a heavy smoker, because of increased metabolism

Special Geriatric Considerations The most anticholinergic and sedating of the antidepressants; pronounced effects on the cardiovascular system (hypotension), hence, many geropsychiatrists agree it is best to avoid in the elderly

Dosage Forms
Amitriptyline hydrochloride:
Injection: 10 mg/mL (10 mL)
Tablet: 10 mg, 25 mg, 50 mg, 75 mg, 100 mg, 150 mg

References
Nies A, Robinson DS, Friedman MJ, et al, "Relationship Between Age and Tricyclic Antidepressant Plasma Levels," *Am J Psychiatry*, 1977, 134:790-3.
Schulz P, Turner-Tamiyasu K, Smith G, et al, "Amitriptyline Disposition in Young and Elderly Normal Men," *Clin Pharmacol Ther*, 1983, 33(3):360-6.

Amitriptyline and Perphenazine
(a mee TRIP ti leen & per FEN a zeen)

Related Information
Amitriptyline *on page 60*
Perphenazine *on page 731*

Brand Names Etrafon®; Triavil®

Synonyms Perphenazine and Amitriptyline

Therapeutic Category Antidepressant, Tricyclic; Antipsychotic Agent; Neuroleptic Agent

Adverse Reactions See individual agents

Special Geriatric Considerations Avoid use of combination products; use of amitriptyline is not recommended in the elderly (see Amitriptyline monograph)

References
Peabody CA, Warner MD, Whiteford HA, et al, "Neuroleptics and the Elderly," *J Am Geriatr Soc*, 1987, 35(3):233-8.
Risse SC and Barnes R, "Pharmacologic Treatment of Agitation Associated With Dementia," *J Am Geriatr Soc*, 1986, 34(5):368-76.
Saltz BL, Woerner MG, Kane JM, et al, "Prospective Study of Tardive Dyskinesia Incidence in the Elderly," *JAMA*, 1991, 266(17):2402-6.
Seifert RD, "Therapeutic Drug Monitoring: Psychotropic Drugs," *J Pharm Pract*, 1984, 6:403-16.

Amlodipine (am LOE di peen)

Related Information
Calcium Channel Blocking Agents Comparison *on page 1027*

Brand Names Norvasc®

Generic Available No

Therapeutic Category Antianginal Agent; Calcium Channel Blocker

Use Treatment of hypertension alone or in combination with antihypertensives; chronic stable angina alone or with other antianginal agents; vasospastic angina alone or in combination with other agents

Contraindications Hypersensitivity to amlodipine or any component or other calcium channel blocker; severe hypotension or second or third degree heart block

Warnings Use with caution in titrating dosages for impaired renal or hepatic function patients; use with caution in patients with congestive heart failure; may increase frequency, severity, duration of angina during initiation of therapy; increased intracranial pressure, idiopathic hypertrophic subaortic stenosis; do not abruptly withdraw therapy; use with caution in elderly due to greater propensity to hypotension

The FDA's Cardiovascular and Renal Drug Advisory Committee reviewed current data regarding the risk of heart attacks in patients treated with calcium channel blockers and determined that as a class, the calcium channel antagonists are safe; however, they warned that short-acting nifedipine could increase the risk of myocardial infarction in some patients. The committee was in agreement with a statement issued September, 1995 by the National Heart Lung, and Blood Institute of the National Institute of Health, that warned that short-acting nifedipine should be used with great caution especially at higher doses.

Precautions Sick sinus syndrome, severe left ventricular dysfunction, congestive heart failure, hepatic or renal impairment, hypertrophic cardiomyopathy (especially obstructive), concomitant therapy with beta-blockers or digoxin, edema

Adverse Reactions

Cardiovascular: Reductions in systemic blood pressure, flushing, tachycardia, palpitations, chest pain, peripheral ischemia, irregular pulse, cardiac failure, migraine

Central nervous system: Dizziness, vertigo, rigors, ataxia, twitching, apathy, agitation, amnesia, depersonalization

Dermatologic: Acne, bruising

Gastrointestinal: Nausea, constipation, loose stools, increased appetite, taste changes

Genitourinary: Urinary incontinence

Hematologic: Petechiae, purpura, bruising

Miscellaneous: Abnormal vision, eye pain, conjunctivitis, abnormal visual accommodation, xerophthalmia, diplopia, gingival swelling and inflammation

Overdosage Symptoms of overdose include hypotension

Toxicology Ipecac-induced emesis can hypothetically worsen calcium antagonist toxicity, since it can produce vagal stimulation. Supportive and symptomatic treatment, including I.V. fluids and Trendelenburg positioning, should be initiated as intoxication may cause hypotension. Although calcium (calcium chloride I.V. 1-2 g in adults with repeats as needed) has been used as an "antidote" for acute intoxications, there is limited experience to support its routine use and should be reserved for those cases where definite signs of myocardial depression are evident. Heart block may respond to isoproterenol, glucagon, atropine and/or calcium, although a temporary pacemaker may be required.

Drug Interactions

Beta-blockers increased cardiac and A-V conduction depression

Fentanyl increased volume requirements and hypotension; although this drug is new, other drug interactions not reported to the same degree as older agents; however, should be suspect of any drug interaction reported with other calcium channel blockers

Amlodipine metabolism may be inhibited by erythromycin, ketoconazole, itraconazole, protease inhibitors; induced by rifampin, rifabutin

Mechanism of Action Inhibits calcium ion from entering "slow channels" or select voltage-sensitive areas of vascular smooth muscle and myocardium during depolarization, producing a relaxation of coronary vascular smooth muscle and coronary vasodilation; increases myocardial oxygen delivery in patients with vasospastic angina

Pharmacodynamics

Onset of action: 30-50 minutes

Peak effect: 6-12 hours

Duration: 24 hours

Pharmacokinetics

Absorption: Oral: Well absorbed; percent absorbed not determined to date

Protein binding: 93%

Metabolism: Hepatic, >90% to inactive compound; substrate CYP3A4

Bioavailability: 64% to 90%

Half-life: 30-50 hours

Elimination: Metabolite and parent drug excreted renally; 10% excreted unchanged in urine

Usual Dosage Oral:

Geriatrics: 2.5 mg once daily; increase by 2.5 mg increments at 7- to 14-day intervals; maximum recommended dose: 10 mg/day

Adults: 2.5-10 mg once daily

Monitoring Parameters Heart rate, blood pressure

Patient Information Do not discontinue abruptly; report any dizziness, shortness of breath, palpitations, or edema

Nursing Implications See Warnings, Precautions, Monitoring Parameters, Special Geriatric Considerations

Special Geriatric Considerations Elderly may experience a greater hypotensive response; constipation may be more of a problem in elderly; calcium channel blockers are no more effective in elderly than other therapies; (Continued)

Amlodipine *(Continued)*

however, they do not cause significant CNS effects which is an advantage over some antihypertensive agents.

Dosage Forms Tablet: 2.5 mg, 5 mg, 10 mg

Ammonium Chloride (a MOE nee um KLOR ide)

Generic Available Yes

Therapeutic Category Diuretic, Miscellaneous; Metabolic Alkalosis Agent; Urinary Acidifying Agent

Use Diuretic or systemic and urinary acidifying agent; treatment of hypochloremic states

Contraindications Severe hepatic and renal dysfunction; patients with primary respiratory acidosis; patients with metabolic alkalosis secondary to vomiting

Warnings Hepatic impairment: In severe liver disease (ie, cirrhosis, hepatitis), the liver may fail to convert the ammonia to urea with ammonia retention leading to hepatic coma

Precautions Observe patients for symptoms of toxicity (see Overdosage); administer slowly when giving by I.V. route to avoid pain, local irritation, and toxicity

Adverse Reactions
Cardiovascular: Bradycardia
Central nervous system: Mental confusion, coma, headache, febrile response
Dermatologic: Rash
Endocrine & metabolic: Metabolic acidosis secondary to hyperchloremia
Gastrointestinal: Gastric irritation, nausea, vomiting
Local: Pain at site of injection, venous thrombosis, phlebitis, extravasation
Respiratory: Hyperventilation

Overdosage Symptoms of overdose include acidosis, nausea, vomiting, thirst, headache, arrhythmias, drowsiness, confusion, hyperventilation, hypokalemia, pallor, sweating, retching, twitching, seizures, coma

Toxicology Administer sodium bicarbonate or lactate to treat acidosis; supplemental potassium for hypokalemia

Stability Avoid excessive heat; protect from freezing (will precipitate crystals); if crystals form, warm at room temperature in water bath; compatible with normal saline

Mechanism of Action Increases acidity by increasing free hydrogen ion concentration from conversion of ammonium to urea in the liver

Pharmacokinetics
Absorption: Rapid from GI tract, complete within 3-6 hours
Metabolism: In the liver
Elimination: In urine

Usual Dosage Metabolic alkalosis: The following equations represent different methods of correction utilizing either the serum HCO_3^-, the serum chloride, or the base excess

Equation 1: Dosing of mEq NH_4Cl via the chloride-deficit method (hypochloremia):
Dose of mEq NH_4Cl = [0.2 L/kg x body weight (kg)] x [103 - observed serum chloride]; administer 100% of dose over 12 hours, then re-evaluate
Note: 0.2 L/kg is the estimated chloride space and 103 is the average normal serum chloride concentration

Equation 2: Dosing of mEq NH_4Cl via the bicarbonate-excess method (refractory hypochloremic metabolic alkalosis):
Dose of NH_4Cl = [0.5 L/kg x body weight (kg) x (observed serum HCO_3^- ~24)]; administer 50% of dose over 12 hours, then re-evaluate
Note: 0.5 L/kg is the estimated bicarbonate space and 24 is the average normal serum bicarbonate concentration

Equation 3: Dosing of mEq NH_4Cl via the base-excess method:
Dose of NH_4Cl = [0.3 L/kg x body weight (kg) x measured base excess (mEq/L)]; administer 50% of dose over 12 hours, then re-evaluate
Note: 0.3 L/kg is the estimated extracellular bicarbonate and base excess is measured by the chemistry lab and reported with arterial blood gases

These equations will yield different requirements of ammonium chloride
Equation #1 is inappropriate to use if the patient has severe metabolic alkalosis without hypochloremia or if the patient has uremia
Equation #3 is the most useful for the first estimation of ammonium chloride dosage

Geriatrics and Adults: Urinary acidifying agent/diuretic:
Oral: 1-2 g every 4-6 hours

I.V.: 1.5 g/dose every 6 hours

Administration Rapid I.V. injection may increase the likelihood of ammonia toxicity; rate should not exceed 1 mEq/kg/hour; 26.75% solution must be diluted prior to administration

Monitoring Parameters Respiratory rate, signs of toxicity (see Overdosage)

Test Interactions ↑ ammonia (B); ↓ potassium (S), sodium (S)

Patient Information Take oral dose after meals

Additional Information Do not exceed a 1% to 2% concentration of ammonium chloride or an administration rate of more than 5 mL/minute; administer over approximately 3 hours for I.V. infusion

Special Geriatric Considerations No specific data available for elderly; monitor closely with hepatic disease for signs of toxicity

Dosage Forms
Injection: 26.75% [5 mEq/mL] (20 mL)
Tablet: 500 mg
Tablet, enteric coated: 486 mg

References
Bushinsky DA and Coe FL, "Hyperkalemia During Acute Ammonium Chloride Acidosis in Man," Nephron, 1985, 40(1):38-40.

Amobarbital (am oh BAR bi tal)

Related Information
Anxiolytic/Hypnotic Use in Long-Term Care Facilities on page 1099
Federal OBRA Regulations Recommended Maximum Doses - Hypnotics on page 1057

Brand Names Amytal®

Synonyms Amylobarbitone

Generic Available No

Therapeutic Category Barbiturate; Hypnotic; Sedative

Restrictions C-II

Special Geriatric Considerations Use of this agent in the elderly is not recommended

Amobarbital and Secobarbital
(am oh BAR bi tal & see koe BAR bi tal)

Related Information
Anxiolytic/Hypnotic Use in Long-Term Care Facilities on page 1099
Federal OBRA Regulations Recommended Maximum Doses - Hypnotics on page 1057

Brand Names Tuinal®

Synonyms Secobarbital and Amobarbital

Generic Available No

Therapeutic Category Barbiturate; Hypnotic

Restrictions C-II

Special Geriatric Considerations Use of this agent in the elderly is not recommended

Amoxapine (a MOKS a peen)

Related Information
Antidepressant Agents Comparison on page 1021
Antidepressant Medication Guidelines on page 1075
Federal OBRA Regulations Recommended Maximum Doses - Antidepressants on page 1056

Brand Names Asendin®

Generic Available Yes

Therapeutic Category Antidepressant

Use Treatment of neurotic and endogenous depression and mixed symptoms of anxiety and depression

Contraindications Hypersensitivity to amoxapine; cross-sensitivity with other tricyclics may occur; narrow-angle glaucoma; patients receiving MAO inhibitors within past 14 days

Warnings Do not discontinue abruptly in patients receiving high doses chronically

Precautions Use with caution in patients with seizures, bipolar illness, cardiac conduction disturbances, cardiovascular diseases, benign prostatic hypertrophy or urinary retention, hyperthyroidism, or those receiving thyroid replacement; an EKG prior to initiation is advised

Adverse Reactions Cardiac toxicities and risk of seizure are usually greater than anticholinergic effects
Cardiovascular: Cardiac toxicities, hypotension, arrhythmias
(Continued)

Amoxapine *(Continued)*

Central nervous system: Drowsiness, fever, dizziness, nervousness, insomnia, seizures, extrapyramidal effects, tardive dyskinesia, neuroleptic malignant syndrome

Dermatologic: Rash

Endocrine & metabolic: Amenorrhea, galactorrhea

Gastrointestinal: Constipation, xerostomia

Hematologic: Leukopenia

Ocular: Blurred vision

Overdosage Symptoms of overdose include grand mal convulsions, acidosis, coma, renal failure

Toxicology Following initiation of essential overdose management, toxic symptoms should be treated. Ventricular arrhythmias often respond to phenytoin 15-20 mg/kg with concurrent systemic alkalinization (sodium bicarbonate 0.5-2 mEq/kg I.V.). Arrhythmias unresponsive to this therapy may respond to lidocaine 1mg/kg I.V. followed by a titrated infusion. Physostigmine (1-2 mg I.V. slowly) may be indicated in reversing cardiac arrhythmias that are due to vagal blockade, or for anticholinergic effects. Seizures usually respond to diazepam I.V. boluses (5-10 mg, up to 30 mg). If seizures are unresponsive or recur, phenytoin or phenobarbital may be required.

Drug Interactions

May possibly decrease effects of clonidine and guanethidine

May increase effects of central nervous system depressants, adrenergic agents, anticholinergic agents; with monoamine oxidase inhibitors, hyperpyrexia, tachycardia, hypertension, seizures and death may occur

Fluoxetine may augment the effect of TCAs, delay starting TCA for 2-3 weeks after fluoxetine's discontinuation; similar interactions as with other tricyclics may occur

Mechanism of Action Traditionally believed to increase the synaptic concentration of serotonin and/or norepinephrine in the central nervous system by inhibition of their reuptake by the presynaptic neuronal membrane. However, additional receptor effects have been found including desensitization of adenyl cyclase, down regulation of beta-adrenergic receptors, and down regulation of serotonin receptors.

Pharmacodynamics Antidepressant effects usually occur after 1-3 weeks; NE >5-HT

Pharmacokinetics

Absorption: Oral: Rapidly and well absorbed

Distribution: V_d: 0.9-1.2 L/kg

Protein binding: 80%

Metabolism: Extensive in the liver

Half-life: 11-16 hours

Time to peak serum concentration: Within 1-2 hours

Elimination: Excretion of metabolites and parent compound in urine

8-hydroxy metabolite is active, with a half-life: 30 hours

Usual Dosage Oral (once symptoms are controlled, decrease gradually to lowest effective dose):

Geriatrics: Initial: 25 mg at bedtime increased by 25 mg weekly for outpatients and every 3 days for inpatients if tolerated; usual dose: 50-150 mg/day, but doses up to 300 mg may be necessary

Adults: Initial: 25 mg 2-3 times/day, if tolerated, dosage may be increased to 100 mg 2-3 times/day; may be given in a single bedtime dose when dosage <300 mg/day

Maximum daily dose:
Outpatient: 400 mg
Inpatient: 600 mg

Monitoring Parameters Blood pressure, pulse, EKG; target symptoms

Reference Range Therapeutic: Amoxapine 20-100 ng/mL (SI: 64-319 nmol/L); 8-OH amoxapine 150-400 ng/mL (SI: 478-1275 nmol/L); both 200-500 ng/mL (SI: 637-1594 nmol/L)

Test Interactions Elevated glucose

Patient Information Dry mouth may be helped by sips of water, sugarless gum or hard candy; avoid alcohol; very important to maintain established dosage regimen; photosensitivity to sunlight can occur; rise slowly to prevent dizziness

Nursing Implications Monitor blood pressure and pulse rate prior to and during initial therapy; evaluate mental status; monitor weight, may increase appetite and possibly a craving for sweets; recognize signs of neuroleptic malignant syndrome and tardive dyskinesia

Additional Information May take up to 2 weeks for full therapeutic effects to be apparent; maintenance dose is usually given at bedtime to reduce daytime sedation; tolerance develops in 1-3 months in some patients, close medical follow-up is essential

Special Geriatric Considerations Has not been studied exclusively in the elderly; because of the risk for tardive dyskinesia and extrapyramidal side effects, amoxapine is not a drug of choice in the elderly; significant anticholinergic and orthostatic effects

Dosage Forms Tablet: 25 mg, 50 mg, 100 mg, 150 mg

Amoxicillin (a moks i SIL in)

Related Information

Penicillins, Penicillin-Related Antibiotics, & Other Antibiotics *on page 1010*
Prevention of Bacterial Endocarditis *on page 1062*
Regimens Used to Treat *Helicobacter pylori* and Ulcers *on page 1033*

Brand Names Amoxil®; Biomox®; Polymox®; Trimox®; Wymox®

Synonyms Amoxycillin; *p*-Hydroxyampicillin

Generic Available Yes

Therapeutic Category Antibiotic, Penicillin

Use Treatment of otitis media, sinusitis, and infections caused by susceptible organisms involving the respiratory tract, skin, and urinary tract; prophylaxis of bacterial endocarditis

Contraindications Hypersensitivity to amoxicillin, penicillin, or any component

Precautions In patients with renal impairment, doses and/or frequency of administration should be modified in response to the degree of renal impairment; high percentage of patients with infectious mononucleosis have developed rash during therapy with amoxicillin; use with caution in patients with cephalosporin allergy (anaphylactic reaction)

Adverse Reactions

Central nervous system: Seizures, fever
Dermatologic: Rash (especially patients with mononucleosis)
Gastrointestinal: Diarrhea
Miscellaneous: Superinfection

Overdosage Symptoms of overdose include neuromuscular sensitivity, seizures

Toxicology Many beta-lactam-containing antibiotics have the potential to cause neuromuscular hyperirritability or convulsive seizures. Hemodialysis may be helpful to aid in the removal of the drug from the blood, otherwise most treatment is supportive or symptom directed.

Drug Interactions Probenecid increased amoxicillin levels, allopurinol theoretically increased risk for amoxicillin rash

Stability Oral suspension remains stable for 7 days at room temperature or 14 days if refrigerated

Mechanism of Action Interferes with bacterial cell wall synthesis during active multiplication causing cell death and resultant bactericidal activity against susceptible bacteria

Pharmacokinetics

Absorption: Oral: Rapid and nearly complete
Protein binding: 17% to 20%
Metabolism: Partial
Half-life (patients with Cl_{cr} <10 mL/minute): 7-21 hours
Time to peak:
  Capsule: Within 2 hours
  Suspension: 1 hour
Elimination: Renal excretion (80% as unchanged drug); ~30% removed by 3-hour hemodialysis

Usual Dosage Oral:

Geriatrics: Dosage may need to be adjusted based upon renal function
Adults: 250-500 mg every 8 hours; maximum dose: 2-3 g/day
  Uncomplicated gonorrhea: 3 g plus probenecid 1 g in a single dose
  Endocarditis prophylaxis: 3 g 1 hour before procedure and 1.5 g 6 hours later

Dosing interval in renal impairment:

Cl_{cr} 10-50 mL/minute: Administer every 12 hours
Cl_{cr} <10 mL/minute: Administer every 24 hours
Moderately dialyzable (20% to 50%)

Monitoring Parameters Signs and symptoms of infection (fever, urinary frequency or pain, etc) should begin to resolve after 1-2 days

Test Interactions Increased AST, ALT, protein

(Continued)

Amoxicillin *(Continued)*

Patient Information Report diarrhea promptly; entire course of medication (10-14 days) should be taken to ensure eradication of organism; should be taken in equal intervals around-the-clock to maintain adequate blood concentrations

Nursing Implications Assess patient at beginning and throughout therapy for infection; observe for signs and symptoms of anaphylaxis; obtain specimens for C&S before the first dose; administer around-the-clock rather than 3 times/day, etc (ie, 8-4-12, not 9-1-5) to promote less variation in peak and trough serum concentrations

Additional Information Food does not interfere with absorption; urticarial rash that appears after a few days of therapy may indicate hypersensitivity

Special Geriatric Considerations Resistance to amoxicillin has been a problem in patients on frequent antibiotics or in a nursing home. Alternative antibiotics may be necessary in these populations; consider renal function.

Dosage Forms

Capsule: 250 mg, 500 mg

Suspension, oral: 125 mg/5 mL (5 mL unit dose, 80 mL, 100 mL, 150 mL, 200 mL); 250 mg/5 mL (5 mL unit dose, 80 mL, 100 mL, 150 mL, 200 mL)

Tablet, chewable: 125 mg, 250 mg

References

Dajani AS, Bisno AL, Chung KJ, et al, "Prevention of Bacterial Endocarditis. Recommendations by the American Heart Association," *JAMA*, 1990, 264(22):2919-22.

Hill S, Yeates M, Pathy J, et al, "A Controlled Trial of Norfloxacin and Amoxicillin in the Treatment of Uncomplicated Urinary Tract Infection in the Elderly," *J Antimicrob Chemother*, 1985, 15(4):505-6.

Amoxicillin and Clavulanate Potassium

(a moks i SIL in & klav yoo LAN ate poe TASS ee um)

Related Information

Penicillins, Penicillin-Related Antibiotics, & Other Antibiotics *on page 1010*

Brand Names Augmentin®

Synonyms Amoxicillin and Clavulanic Acid

Generic Available No

Therapeutic Category Antibiotic, Penicillin

Use Treatment of otitis media, sinusitis, and infections caused by susceptible organisms involving the lower respiratory tract, skin and skin structure, and urinary tract

Contraindications Known hypersensitivity to amoxicillin, clavulanic acid, or penicillin

Precautions In patients with renal impairment, doses and/or frequency of administration should be modified in response to the degree of renal impairment; high percentage of patients with infectious mononucleosis have developed rash during therapy with amoxicillin; use with caution in patients who are allergic to cephalosporins (anaphylactic reactions)

Adverse Reactions

Central nervous system: Seizures, fever

Dermatologic: Rash, urticaria; urticarial rash that appears after a few days of therapy may indicate hypersensitivity

Gastrointestinal: Nausea, vomiting, incidence of diarrhea is higher than with amoxicillin alone

Genitourinary: Vaginitis

Toxicology Many beta-lactam-containing antibiotics have the potential to cause neuromuscular hyperirritability or convulsive seizures. Hemodialysis may be helpful to aid in the removal of the drug from the blood, otherwise most treatment is supportive or symptom directed.

Drug Interactions Probenecid increased amoxicillin levels, allopurinol theoretically increased risk for amoxicillin rash

Stability Reconstituted oral suspension should be kept in refrigerator; discard unused suspension after 10 days

Mechanism of Action Amoxicillin interferes with bacterial cell wall synthesis during active multiplication causing cell death and resultant bactericidal activity against susceptible bacteria; clavulanic acid binds and inhibits beta-lactamases that inactivate amoxicillin resulting in amoxicillin having an expanded spectrum of activity

Pharmacokinetics

Absorption: Oral: Both amoxicillin and clavulanate are well absorbed

Metabolism: Clavulanic acid is metabolized in the liver

Half-life: Adults with normal renal function: Both agents are ~1 hour; amoxicillin pharmacokinetics are not affected by clavulanic acid

Time to peak: Peak levels of each appearing within 2 hours

Elimination: Amoxicillin excreted primarily unchanged in urine

Usual Dosage Geriatrics and Adults: Oral (dose based on amoxicillin component - see Additional Information and Amoxicillin monograph):

500 mg every 12 hours or 250 mg every 8 hours

Respiratory tract infection, severe infection: 875 mg every 12 hours or 500 mg every 8 hours

Dosing interval in renal impairment (patients with severe renal impairment should not receive the 875 mg dose):

Cl_{cr} 10-30 mL/minute: Administer every 12 hours

Cl_{cr} <10 mL/minute: Administer every 24 hours

Moderately dialyzable (20% to 50%)

Test Interactions May interfere with urinary glucose determinations using Clinitest®

Patient Information Report diarrhea promptly; entire course of medication (10-14 days) should be taken to ensure eradication of organism; should be taken in equal intervals around-the-clock to maintain adequate blood concentrations; females should report onset of symptoms of candidal vaginitis

Nursing Implications Assess patient at beginning and throughout therapy for infection; observe for signs and symptoms of anaphylaxis; obtain specimens for C&S before the first dose; administer around-the-clock rather than 3 times/day to promote less variation in peak and trough serum concentrations; do not administer two 250 mg tablets as substitute for a 500 mg tablet (see Additional Information)

Additional Information Urticarial rash that appears after a few days of therapy may indicate hypersensitivity; incidence of diarrhea is higher than with amoxicillin alone; both '250' and '500' tablets contain the same amount of clavulanic acid, thus two '250' tablets are not equivalent to one '500' tablet; clavulanic acid inhibits beta-lactamase destruction of amoxicillin

Special Geriatric Considerations Expanded coverage of this combination makes it a useful alternative when amoxicillin resistance is present and patients cannot tolerate alternative treatments; consider renal function (Cl_{cr} estimation) in elderly. Considered one of the drugs of choice in the outpatient treatment of community-acquired pneumonia in older adults.

Dosage Forms

Suspension, oral:

125 (banana flavor): Amoxicillin trihydrate 125 mg and clavulanic acid 31.25 mg per 5 mL (75 mL, 150 mL)

200: Amoxicillin 200 mg and clavulanic acid 28.5 mg per 5 mL (50 mL, 75 mL, 100 mL)

250 (orange flavor): Amoxicillin trihydrate 250 mg and clavulanic acid 62.5 mg per 5 mL (75 mL, 150 mL)

400: Amoxicillin 400 mg and clavulanic acid 57 mg per 5 mL (50 mL, 75 mL, 100 mL)

Tablet:

250: Amoxicillin trihydrate 250 mg and clavulanic acid 125 mg

500: Amoxicillin trihydrate 500 mg and clavulanic acid 125 mg

875: Amoxicillin trihydrate 875 mg and clavulanic acid 125 mg

Tablet, chewable:

125: Amoxicillin trihydrate 125 mg and clavulanic acid 31.25 mg

250: Amoxicillin trihydrate 250 mg and clavulanic acid 62.5 mg

References

American Thoracic Society, "Guidelines for the Initial Management of Adults With Community-Acquired Pneumonia: Diagnosis, Assessment of Severity, and Initial Antimicrobial Therapy," *Am Rev Respir Dis*, 1993, 148(5):1418-26.

Ancill RJ, Ballard JH, and Capewell MA, "Urinary Tract Infections in Geriatric Inpatients: A Comparative Study of Amoxicillin-Clavulanic Acid and Co-trimoxazole," *Curr Ther Res*, 1987, 41(4):444-8.

Amoxicillin and Clavulanic Acid *see* Amoxicillin and Clavulanate Potassium *on previous page*

Amoxil® *see* Amoxicillin *on page 67*

Amoxycillin *see* Amoxicillin *on page 67*

Amphojel® [OTC] *see* Aluminum Hydroxide *on page 41*

Amphotec® *see* Amphotericin B Colloidal Dispersion *on page 71*

Amphotericin B (am foe TER i sin bee)

Related Information

I.V. Medication Recommendations *on page 1080*

Brand Names Fungizone®

Generic Available Yes

(Continued)

Amphotericin B *(Continued)*

Therapeutic Category Antifungal Agent, Systemic; Antifungal Agent, Topical

Use Treatment of severe systemic infections and meningitis caused by susceptible fungi; fungal peritonitis; irrigant for bladder fungal infections; and topically for cutaneous and mucocutaneous candidal infections

Contraindications Hypersensitivity to amphotericin or any component

Warnings I.V. amphotericin is used primarily for the treatment of patients with progressive and potentially fatal fungal infections; not to be used for common clinically inapparent forms of fungal disease

Precautions Because of the nephrotoxic potential of amphotericin, other nephrotoxic drugs should be avoided; BUN and serum creatinine concentrations should be determined every other day while therapy is increased and at least weekly thereafter

Adverse Reactions

Cardiovascular: Hypotension, hypertension, flushing
Central nervous system: Delirium, fever, headache, chills
Endocrine & metabolic: Hypokalemia, hypomagnesemia
Gastrointestinal: Nausea, vomiting
Hematologic: Bone marrow suppression
Local: Phlebitis
Renal: Renal failure, renal tubular acidosis
Miscellaneous: Generalized pain

Adverse effects due to intrathecal amphotericin:
Cardiovascular: Headache
Central nervous system: Arachnoiditis, pain along lumbar nerves
Gastrointestinal: Nausea, vomiting
Genitourinary: Urinary retention
Neuromuscular & skeletal: Paresthesia
Ocular: Vision changes

Overdosage Symptoms of overdose include renal dysfunction, anemia, thrombocytopenia, granulocytopenia, fever, nausea, and vomiting

Drug Interactions

Nephrotoxic effects of other drugs (cyclosporine, aminoglycosides) may be enhanced

Corticosteroids may increase potassium depletion caused by amphotericin

May predispose patients receiving cardiac glycosides or skeletal muscle relaxants to toxicity secondary to hypokalemia

Stability Reconstitute only with sterile water without preservatives, not bacteriostatic water; benzyl alcohol, sodium chloride, or other electrolyte solutions may cause precipitation; for I.V. infusion, an in-line filter (>1 micron mean pore diameter) may be used; short-term exposure (<24 hours) to light during I.V. infusion does **not** appreciably affect potency; lipid complex should be diluted in 5% dextrose to final concentration of 1 mg/mL

Mechanism of Action Binds to ergosterol altering cell membrane permeability in susceptible fungi and causing leakage of cell components with subsequent cell death

Pharmacokinetics

Distribution: Minimal amounts enter the aqueous humor, bile, CSF, amniotic fluid, pericardial fluid, pleural fluid and synovial fluid; poorly dialyzed
Protein binding: Plasma: 90%
Half-life:
Initial: 15-48 hours
Terminal phase: 15 days
Time to peak serum concentration: I.V.: During the first hour after a 4- to 6-hour infusion

Usual Dosage Minimum dilution for amphotericin B infusions: 0.1 mg/mL
Geriatrics and Adults:
Test dose: I.V.: 1 mg infused over 20-30 minutes. If the test dose is tolerated, the initial therapeutic dose is 0.25 mg/kg. The daily dose can then be gradually increased, usually in 0.25 mg/kg increments on each subsequent day until the desired daily dose is reached.
Maintenance dose: I.V.: 0.25-1 mg/kg/day or 1.5 mg/kg every other day; do not exceed 1.5 mg/kg/day.
Lipid complex: I.V.: 5 mg/kg as a single daily dose for aspergillosis infused at 2.5 mg/kg/hour; shake content in bag if infusion exceeds 2 hours
I.T.: 25-300 mcg every 48-72 hours; increase to 500 mcg as tolerated
Bladder irrigation: 50 mg/day in 1 L of sterile water irrigation solution instilled over 24 hours for 2-7 days or until cultures are clear

Dialysate: 1-2 mg/L of peritoneal dialysis fluid either with or without low-dose I.V. amphotericin B (a total dose of 2-10 mg/kg given over 7-14 days)

Topical: Apply to affected areas 2-4 times/day for 1-4 weeks depending on nature and severity of infection

Dosing adjustment in renal impairment: If renal dysfunction is due to the drug, the daily total can be decreased by 50% or the dose can be given every other day; I.V. therapy may take several months

Poorly dialyzed

Monitoring Parameters Monitor electrolytes, BUN, serum creatinine, LFTs, CBC regularly, I & O, signs of hypokalemia (muscle weakness, cramping, drowsiness, EKG changes, etc); if BUN exceeds 40 mg/dL or the serum creatinine exceeds 3 mg/dL, discontinue the drug or reduce the dose until renal function improves

Reference Range Therapeutic: 1-2 µg/mL (SI: 1-2.2 µmol/L)

Test Interactions Increased creatine phosphokinase [CPK] (S); decreased magnesium, potassium (S)

Patient Information Amphotericin cream may slightly discolor skin and stain clothing; personal hygiene is very important to help reduce the spread and recurrence of lesions; avoid covering topical applications with occlusive bandages; most skin lesions require 1-3 weeks of therapy

Nursing Implications May premedicate patients with acetaminophen and diphenhydramine 30 minutes prior to the amphotericin infusion. Meperidine (Demerol®) may help to reduce rigors. Dosage adjustments are not necessary with renal impairment. If renal dysfunction is due to the drug, the daily total can be decreased by 50% or the dose can be given every other day (see Stability and Usual Dosage).

Additional Information Lipid complex may be less nephrotoxic, but more expensive

Special Geriatric Considerations The pharmacokinetics and dosing of amphotericin have not been studied in the elderly. It appears that use is similar to young adults; caution should be exercised in renal function and desired effect monitored closely.

Dosage Forms
Cream: 3% (20 g)
Injection: 50 mg
Lotion: 3% (30 mL)
Ointment, topical: 3% (20 g)
Suspension, as lipid complex: 100 mg/20 mL

References
Gallis HA, Drew RH, and Pickard WW, "Amphotericin B: 30 Years of Clinical Experience," *Rev Infect Dis*, 1990, 12(2):308-29.

Wong-Beringer A, Beringer PM, and Rho JP, "Focus on Amphotericin B Lipid Complex," *Formulary*, 1996, 13(3):169-85.

Amphotericin B Colloidal Dispersion
(am foe TER i sin bee koe LOY dal dis PER shun)

Brand Names Amphotec®

Therapeutic Category Antifungal Agent, Systemic

Use Effective in the treatment of invasive mycoses in patient refractory to or intolerant of conventional amphotericin B

Contraindications Hypersensitivity to amphotericin B or its components

Warnings Anaphylaxis has been reported; facilities for cardiopulmonary resuscitation should be available; infusion reactions, sometimes, severe, usually subside with continued therapy

Adverse Reactions
Cardiovascular: Hypotension, tachycardia
Central nervous system: Headache, chills, fever
Dermatologic: Rash
Endocrine & metabolic: Hypokalemia, hypomagnesemia
Gastrointestinal: Nausea, diarrhea, abdominal pain
Hematologic: Thrombocytopenia
Hepatic: LFT change
Neuromuscular & skeletal: Rigors
Respiratory: Dyspnea

Note: Amphotericin B colloidal dispersion has an improved therapeutic index compared to conventional amphotericin B, and has been used safely in patients with amphotericin B-related nephrotoxicity; however, continued decline of renal function has occurred in some patients

(Continued)

Amphotericin B Colloidal Dispersion *(Continued)*

Overdosage Symptoms of overdose include renal dysfunction, anemia, thrombocytopenia, granulocytopenia, fever, nausea, vomiting

Toxicology Treatment is supportive

Drug Interactions Increased toxicity: Cyclosporine and aminoglycosides (nephrotoxicity), corticosteroids (hypokalemia)

Mechanism of Action Binds to ergosterol altering cell membrane permeability in susceptible fungi and causing leakage of cell components with subsequent cell death

Pharmacokinetics

Distribution: V_d: Total amphotericin B increases with increasing doses of total amphotericin B (with 4 mg/kg/day = 4 L/kg); predominantly distributed in the liver; concentrations in kidneys and other tissues are lower than observed with conventional amphotericin B

Half-life: 28-29 hours

Plasma concentration: Total amphotericin B remains between 1-3 mcg/mL

Elimination: Clearance: 0.1 L/hour/kg (with 4 mg/kg/day)

Usual Dosage Geriatrics and Adults: 3-4 mg/kg/day I.V. (infusion of 1 mg/kg/hour); maximum: 7.5 mg/kg/day; duration of therapy is often <6 weeks

Monitoring Parameters Liver function tests, electrolytes, BUN, creatinine clearance, temperature, CBC, I/O, signs of hypokalemia (muscle weakness, cramping, drowsiness, EKG changes)

Nursing Implications May premedicate with acetaminophen and diphenhydramine 30 minutes prior to infusion; meperidine may help reduce rigors; avoid injection faster than 1 mg/kg/hour

Special Geriatric Considerations The pharmacokinetics and dosing of amphotericin have not been studied in the elderly. It appears that use is similar to young adults; caution should be exercised and renal function and desired effect monitored closely.

Dosage Forms Suspension for injection: 5 mg/mL (20 mL)

Amphotericin B Lipid Complex
(am foe TER i sin bee LIP id KOM pleks)

Brand Names Abelcet™ Injection; AmBisome®

Synonyms ABLC

Generic Available No

Therapeutic Category Antifungal Agent, Systemic

Use Treatment of aspergillosis or any type of progressive fungal infection in patients who are refractory to or intolerant of conventional amphotericin B therapy; orphan drug status for cryptococcal meningitis

Contraindications Hypersensitivity to amphotericin or any component in the formulation

Warnings Anaphylaxis has been reported with amphotericin B desoxycholate and other amphotericin B-containing drugs. Facilities for cardiopulmonary resuscitation should be available during administration due to the possibility of anaphylactic reaction. If severe respiratory distress occurs, the infusion should be immediately discontinued and the patient should not receive further infusions. During the initial dosing, the drug should be administered intravenously and under close clinical observation by medically trained personnel. Acute reactions (including fever and chills) may occur 1-2 hours after starting an intravenous infusion. These reactions are usually more common with the first few doses and generally diminish with subsequent doses.

Adverse Reactions Reduced nephrotoxicity as well as frequent infusion related side effects have been reported with this formulation

Cardiovascular: Hypotension, cardiac arrest

Central nervous system: Chills, fever, headache, pain

Dermatologic: Rash

Endocrine & metabolic: Bilirubinemia, hypokalemia, acidosis

Gastrointestinal: Nausea, vomiting, diarrhea, gastrointestinal hemorrhage, abdominal pain

Renal: Increased serum creatinine, renal failure

Respiratory: Respiratory failure, dyspnea, pneumonia

Miscellaneous: Multiple organ failure

Drug Interactions Toxic effect of nephrotoxic drugs may be additive; corticosteroids may increase potassium depletion caused by amphotericin; may predispose patients receiving cardiac glycosides or skeletal muscle relaxants to toxicity secondary to hypokalemia

Mechanism of Action As a modification of dimyristoyl phosphatidylcholine:dimyristoyl phosphatidylglycerol 7:3 (DMPC:DMPG) liposome, amphotericin B lipid-complex has a higher drug to lipid ratio and the concentration of amphotericin B is 33 M; ABLC is a ribbon-like structure, not a liposome; mechanism is like amphotericin - includes binding to ergosterol altering cell membrane permeability in susceptible fungi and causing leakage of cell components with subsequent cell death

Usual Dosage Geriatrics and Adults: I.V.: 2.5-5 mg/kg/day as a single infusion
Note: Significantly higher dose of ABLC are tolerated; it appears that attaining higher doses with ABLC produce more rapid fungicidal activity *in vivo* than standard amphotericin B preparations

  Dosing adjustment in renal impairment: None necessary; effects of renal impairment are not currently known
  Hemodialysis: No supplemental dosage necessary
  Peritoneal dialysis: No supplemental dosage necessary
  Continuous arterio-venous or veno-venous hemofiltration (CAVH/CAVHD): No supplemental dosage necessary

Monitoring Parameters
  BUN and serum creatinine concentrations should be determined every other day while therapy is increased and at least weekly thereafter; monitor input and output
  Serum potassium and magnesium should be monitored closely; monitor for signs of hypokalemia (muscle weakness, cramping, drowsiness, EKG changes, etc)
  Monitor electrolytes, liver function, hematocrit, CBC, blood pressure, and temperature regularly

Patient Information I.V. therapy may take several months; personal hygiene is very important to help reduce the spread and recurrence of lesions; most skin lesions require 1-3 weeks of therapy; report any hearing loss

Special Geriatric Considerations The pharmacokinetics and dosing of amphotericin have not been studied in the elderly. It appears that use is similar to young adults; caution should be exercised and renal function and desired effect monitored closely.

Dosage Forms Injection: 50 mg; 5 mg/mL (20 mL)

Ampicillin (am pi SIL in)

Related Information
  I.V. Medication Recommendations *on page 1080*
  Penicillins, Penicillin-Related Antibiotics, & Other Antibiotics *on page 1010*
  Prevention of Bacterial Endocarditis *on page 1062*

Brand Names Marcillin®; Omnipen®; Omnipen®-N; Polycillin®; Polycillin-N®; Principen®; Totacillin®; Totacillin®-N

Synonyms Aminobenzylpenicillin

Generic Available Yes

Therapeutic Category Antibiotic, Penicillin

Use Treatment of susceptible bacterial infections

Contraindications Known hypersensitivity to ampicillin (penicillin)

Precautions Dosage adjustment may be necessary when Cl_{cr} <10-15 mL/minute; high percentage of patients with infectious mononucleosis have developed rash during therapy with ampicillin; use with caution in patients with cephalosporin allergy (anaphylactic reaction)

Adverse Reactions
  Central nervous system: Penicillin encephalopathy
  Dermatologic: Rash, itching
  Gastrointestinal: Diarrhea, nausea, vomiting, stomach cramps and pain, pseudomembranous colitis
  Miscellaneous: Superinfection

Overdosage Symptoms of overdose include neuromuscular sensitivity, seizures

Toxicology Many beta-lactam-containing antibiotics have the potential to cause neuromuscular hyperirritability or convulsive seizures. Hemodialysis may be helpful to aid in the removal of the drug from the blood, otherwise most treatment is supportive or symptom directed.

Drug Interactions Aminoglycosides (synergy possible), decreased elimination and increased serum concentrations with probenecid, allopurinol (rash)

Drug/Food Interactions Food decreases rate and extent of absorption; take on an empty stomach

Stability Oral suspension is stable for 14 days under refrigeration; solutions for I.M. or direct I.V. should be used within 1 hour; solutions for I.V. infusion will
(Continued)

Ampicillin *(Continued)*

be inactivated by dextrose at room temperature; if dextrose containing solutions are to be used, the resultant solution will only be stable for 2 hours versus 8 hours in the 0.9% sodium chloride injection.

Mechanism of Action Interferes with bacterial cell wall synthesis during active multiplication causing cell death and resultant bactericidal activity against susceptible bacteria

Pharmacokinetics

Absorption: Oral: 50%; not affected by age

Distribution: Into bile; penetration into CSF occurs with inflamed meninges only

Protein binding: 15% to 25%

Half-life:

Adults: 1-1.8 hours

Anuric patients: 8-20 hours

Time to peak serum concentration: Oral: Within 1-2 hours

Elimination: ~90% of drug excreted unchanged in urine within 24 hours, ~40% is removed by hemodialysis

Clearance has been reported to be decreased and half-life prolonged in older patients

Usual Dosage Geriatrics and Adults (for geriatric patients, administer usual adult dose unless renal function is markedly reduced):

I.M., I.V.: 8-12 g/day in 4-6 divided doses

Oral: 250-500 mg every 6 hours

Dosing interval in renal impairment:

Cl_{cr} 10-30 mL/minute: Administer every 6-12 hours

Cl_{cr} <10 mL/minute: Administer every 12 hours

Administration

Do not use D_5W as a diluent, D_5W has limited stability

Standard diluent: Dose/50 mL NS

Minimum volume: Concentration should not exceed 30 mg/mL; manufacturer may supply as either the anhydrous or the trihydrate form

Monitoring Parameters Signs and symptoms of infection (fever, urinary frequency or pain, etc) should begin to resolve after 1-2 days

Test Interactions Increased protein; urinary glucose (Benedict's solution, Clinitest®); increased AST, positive Coombs' [direct]

Patient Information Take on an empty stomach; complete full course of therapy; should be taken at equal intervals around-the-clock to maintain adequate blood concentrations; women should report onset of symptoms of candidal vaginitis

Nursing Implications Ampicillin and gentamicin should not be mixed in the same I.V. tubing or administered concurrently; do C&S before starting therapy; observe patient for signs and symptoms of hypersensitivity; keep resuscitation equipment, epinephrine, and antihistamine close by in the event of an anaphylactic reaction. Administer on an empty stomach (ie, 1 hour prior to, or 2 hours after meals) to increase total absorption. Administer around-the-clock rather than 4 times/day (ie, 12-6-12-6, not 9-1-5-9) to promote less variation in peak and trough serum concentrations. Dosage adjustment may be necessary when Cl_{cr} <10-15 mL/minute.

Additional Information Appearance of a rash should be carefully evaluated to differentiate a nonallergic ampicillin rash from a hypersensitivity reaction; ampicillin rash is dull red, macular or maculopapular, and only mildly pruritic; normally appears on pressure areas like knees, elbows, palms, or soles, and may spread in symmetric pattern over most of the body; incidence of ampicillin rash is higher in patients with viral infections, *Salmonella* infections, lymphocytic leukemia, or patients that have hyperuricemia

Sodium content of suspension (250 mg/5 mL, 5 mL): 10 mg (0.4 mEq)

Sodium content of 1 g: 66.7 mg (3 mEq)

Special Geriatric Considerations Adjust dose for renal function (see Pharmacokinetics and Usual Dosage)

Dosage Forms

Ampicillin trihydrate:

Capsule, as trihydrate: 250 mg, 500 mg

Suspension, oral, as trihydrate: 125 mg/5 mL (5 mL unit dose, 80 mL, 100 mL, 150 mL, 200 mL); 250 mg/5 mL (5 mL unit dose, 80 mL, 100 mL, 150 mL, 200 mL); 500 mg/5 mL (5 mL unit dose, 100 mL)

Capsule, as anhydrous: 250 mg, 500 mg

Injection, as sodium: 125 mg, 250 mg, 500 mg, 1 g, 2 g, 10 g

References
Triggs EJ, Johnson JM, and Learoyd B, "Absorption and Disposition of Ampicillin in the Elderly," *Eur J Clin Pharmacol*, 1980, 18(2):195-8.

Ampicillin and Sulbactam (am pi SIL in & SUL bak tam)

Related Information
I.V. Medication Recommendations *on page 1080*
Penicillins, Penicillin-Related Antibiotics, & Other Antibiotics *on page 1010*
Brand Names Unasyn®
Synonyms Sulbactam and Ampicillin
Generic Available No
Therapeutic Category Antibiotic, Penicillin
Use Treatment of susceptible bacterial infections involved with skin and skin structure, intra-abdominal infections, gynecological infections; spectrum is that of ampicillin plus organisms producing beta-lactamases such as *S. aureus*, *H. influenzae*, *E. coli*, *Klebsiella*, *Acinetobacter*, *Enterobacter*, and anaerobes
Contraindications Hypersensitivity to ampicillin, sulbactam or any component, or penicillins
Warnings Should not be administered to patients with mononucleosis
Precautions Use with caution in patients allergic to cephalosporins; a high percentage of patients with infectious mononucleosis have developed rash during therapy with ampicillin; modify dosage in patients with renal impairment whose Cl_{cr} is <10-15 mL/minute
Adverse Reactions
Cardiovascular: Chest pain
Central nervous system: Fatigue, malaise, headache, chills
Dermatologic: Rash, itching
Gastrointestinal: Diarrhea, nausea, vomiting, enterocolitis, pseudomembranous colitis, hairy tongue
Genitourinary: Dysuria
Hematologic: Decreased WBC, neutrophils, platelets, hemoglobin, and hematocrit
Hepatic: Increased liver enzymes
Local: Pain at injection site (I.M.: 16%, I.V.: 3%), thrombophlebitis
Renal: Increased BUN and creatinine
Miscellaneous: Candidiasis, hypersensitivity reactions
Toxicology Many beta-lactam-containing antibiotics have the potential to cause neuromuscular hyperirritability or convulsive seizures. Hemodialysis may be helpful to aid in the removal of the drug from the blood, otherwise most treatment is supportive or symptom directed.
Drug Interactions Aminoglycosides, bacteriostatic agents, uricosuric agents (probenecid, indomethacin, sulfinpyrazone, and high-dose aspirin >3-4 g/day), chlorpropamide, diuretics, pyrazinamide, diazoxide, alcohol, mecamylamine
Stability I.M. and direct I.V. administration: used within 1 hour after preparation; reconstitute with sterile water for injection or 0.5% or 2% lidocaine hydrochloride injection (I.M.); sodium chloride 0.9% (NS) is the diluent of choice for I.V. piggyback use, solutions made in NS are stable up to 72 hours when refrigerated whereas dextrose solutions (same concentration) are stable for only 4 hours
Mechanism of Action The addition of sulbactam, a beta-lactamase inhibitor, to ampicillin extends the spectrum of ampicillin to include beta-lactamase producing organisms; ampicillin acts by inhibiting bacterial cell wall synthesis during the stage of active multiplication
Pharmacokinetics
Protein binding:
Ampicillin: 28%
Sulbactam: 38%
Half-life: Ampicillin and sulbactam are similar: 1-1.8 hours and 1-1.3 hours, respectively
Time to peak serum concentration: Immediate
Elimination: ~75% to 85% of both drugs are excreted unchanged in the urine within 8 hours following administration
Reduced clearance and prolonged half-life in the elderly have been found for both compounds; age and renal function were negatively correlated with clearance
Usual Dosage Unasyn® (ampicillin/sulbactam) is a combination product; each 3 g vial contains 2 g of ampicillin and 1 g of sulbactam. Sulbactam has very little antibacterial activity by itself, but effectively extends the spectrum of
(Continued)

Ampicillin and Sulbactam *(Continued)*

ampicillin to include beta-lactamase producing strains that are resistant to ampicillin alone. Therefore, dosage recommendations for Unasyn® are based on the ampicillin component.

Geriatrics and Adults: I.M., I.V.: 1-2 g ampicillin every 6-8 hours; maximum: 8 g ampicillin/day, 4 g sulbactam/day

Dosing interval in renal impairment:
Cl$_{cr}$ 15-29 mL/minute: Administer every 12 hours
Cl$_{cr}$ 5-14 mL/minute: Administer every 24 hours

Monitoring Parameters Signs and symptoms of infection (fever, urinary frequency or pain, etc) should begin to resolve after 1-2 days; with prolonged therapy, monitor hematologic, renal, and hepatic function

Test Interactions False-positive urinary glucose levels (Benedict's solution, Clinitest®)

Patient Information Report sore throat, fever, fatigue, or diarrhea

Nursing Implications Do C&S before starting therapy; observe patient for signs and symptoms of hypersensitivity; keep resuscitation equipment, epinephrine, and antihistamine close by in the event of an anaphylactic reaction; observe for superinfection; for I.M. injection reconstitute with sterile water or 0.5% or 2% lidocaine hydrochloride. Reduce dose with decreased renal function.

Additional Information Appearance of a rash should be carefully evaluated to differentiate a nonallergic ampicillin rash from a hypersensitivity reaction; ampicillin rash is dull red, macular or maculopapular, and only mildly pruritic; normally appears on pressure areas like knees, elbows, palms, or soles, and may spread in symmetric pattern over most of the body; incidence of ampicillin rash is higher in patients with viral infections, *Salmonella* infections, lymphocytic leukemia, or patients that have hyperuricemia

Special Geriatric Considerations Adjust dose for renal function (see Pharmacokinetics and Usual Dosage)

Dosage Forms
Powder for injection:
1.5 g: Ampicillin sodium 1 g and sulbactam sodium 0.5 g
3 g: Ampicillin sodium 2 g and sulbactam sodium 1 g

References
Meyers BR, Wilkinson P, Mendelson MH,. et al, "Pharmacokinetics of Ampicillin-Sulbactam in Healthy Elderly and Young Volunteers," *Antimicrob Agents Chemother*, 1991, 35(10):2098-101.
Rho SP, Jones A, Woo M, et al, "Single Dose Pharmacokinetics of Intravenous Ampicillin plus Sulbactam in Healthy Elderly and Young Subjects," *J Antimicrob Chemother*, 1989, 24(4):573-80.

Amrinone *(AM ri none)*

Brand Names Inocor®

Generic Available No

Therapeutic Category Adrenergic Agonist Agent

Use Treatment of low cardiac output states (sepsis, congestive heart failure); adjunctive therapy of pulmonary hypertension

Contraindications Hypersensitivity to amrinone lactate or sulfites (contains 0.25 mg sodium metabisulfite)

Warnings Inotropic effects additive to other inotropic agents (digitalis, theophylline); use cautiously in patients with atrial and ventricular arrhythmias; may increase ventricular response since amrinone increases slightly atrioventricular condition; hypersensitivity may occur rapidly, within a few weeks of continued therapy

Precautions Monitor fluids and electrolytes; diuresis may result from improvement in cardiac output and may require dosage reduction of diuretics; do not use in valvular disease, idiopathic subaortic stenosis, or myocardial infarction; may cause arrhythmias; thrombocytopenia with continuous therapy; hepatotoxicity, hypovolemic patients (dehydrated diuresis) may have inadequate filling pressure

Adverse Reactions
Cardiovascular: Hypotension (1.3%), ventricular and supraventricular arrhythmias (3%) (may be related to infusion rate), chest pain (0.2%), pericarditis, vasculitis
Central nervous system: Fever (0.9%)
Gastrointestinal: Nausea, vomiting, abdominal pain, and anorexia
Hematologic: Thrombocytopenia (2.4% incidence) may be dose related; may be reversed with dose reduction within 4 weeks

Hepatic: Hepatotoxicity (0.2% incidence) discontinue amrinone if significant increase in liver enzymes with symptoms of idiosyncratic hypersensitivity reaction, ascites

Local: Burning at injection site

Neuromuscular & skeletal: Myositis

Respiratory: Pleuritis

Overdosage Symptoms of overdose include hypotension

Toxicology There is no specific antidote for amrinone intoxication. Overdosage with amrinone has caused severe hypotension by vasodilation, if this occurs general measures for circulatory support should be taken; decrease dose.

Drug Interactions When furosemide is admixed with amrinone, a precipitate immediately forms; diuretics may cause significant hypovolemia and decrease filling pressure

Stability May be administered undiluted for I.V. bolus doses. For continuous infusion, dilute with 0.45% or 0.9% sodium chloride to final concentration of 1-3 mg/mL; use within 24 hours; do not directly dilute with dextrose-containing solutions, chemical interaction occurs; may be administered I.V. into running dextrose infusions. Furosemide forms a precipitate when injected in I.V. lines containing amrinone.

Mechanism of Action Inhibits myocardial cyclic adenosine monophosphate (cAMP) phosphodiesterase activity and increases cellular levels of cAMP resulting in a positive inotropic effect and increased cardiac output; also possesses systemic and pulmonary vasodilator effects resulting in pre- and afterload reduction; slightly increases atrioventricular conduction

Pharmacodynamics

Onset of action: I.V.: Following administration, hemodynamic actions occur within 2-5 minutes

Peak effects: Within 10 minutes

Duration: Dose dependent with low doses lasting ~30 minutes and higher doses lasting ~2 hours

Pharmacokinetics

Distribution: V_d: 1.2 L/kg

Protein binding: 10% to 49%

Metabolism: In the liver

Half-life:

Normal adult volunteers: 3.6 hours

Congestive heart failure: 5.8 hours, range: 3-15 hours

Elimination: Excreted (60% to 90% as metabolites) in urine within 24 hours; 10% to 40% excreted unchanged in urine

Usual Dosage Note: Dose should not exceed 10 mg/kg/24 hours

Geriatrics and Adults: 0.75 mg/kg I.V. bolus over 2-3 minutes followed by maintenance infusion of 5-10 mcg/kg/minute

Monitoring Parameters Thrombocytopenia, hepatotoxicity, GI effects, blood pressure and heart rate every 5 minutes during infusion, CVP, PCWP, respiratory rate; monitor renal function and fluid electrolyte status (particularly potassium)

Reference Range 0.5-7 µg/mL

Patient Information Change position slowly because of postural hypotension

Nursing Implications Should be administered solely via an I.V. pump; patients should be carefully monitored for hemodynamic response (hypotension) and potential adverse effects (ie, thrombocytopenia, hepatotoxicity, and GI effects)

Additional Information Normally prescribed for patients who have not responded well to therapy with digitalis, diuretics, and vasodilators; dosage is based on clinical response

Special Geriatric Considerations While amrinone is not specifically arrhythmogenic, elderly may be at high risk for ventricular and particularly atrial arrhythmias due to high incidence of arrhythmias in this population; also, elderly are often hypovolemic due to dehydration; therefore, monitor fluid status carefully (CVP line) in order to have effective falling pressure for maximal response; found to be as effective as dobutamine in elderly with heart failure in one study despite the decline in beta-adrenergic response with age

Dosage Forms Injection, as lactate: 5 mg/mL (20 mL)

References

Rich MW, Woods WL, Davila-Roman VG, et al, "A Randomized Comparison of Intravenous Amrinone Versus Dobutamine in Older Patients With Decompensated Congestive Heart Failure," *J Am Geriatr Soc*, 1995, 43(3):271-4.

Amylobarbitone see Amobarbital *on page 65*

Amytal® see Amobarbital on page 65

Anacin® [OTC] see Aspirin on page 84

Anafranil® see Clomipramine on page 236

Anaprox® see Naproxen on page 655

Anaspaz® see Hyoscyamine on page 471

Ancef® see Cefazolin on page 175

Ancobon® see Flucytosine on page 388

Androderm® Transdermal System see Testosterone on page 895

Android® see Methyltestosterone on page 613

Andro-L.A.® Injection see Testosterone on page 895

Andropository® Injection see Testosterone on page 895

Anergan® see Promethazine on page 791

Anestacon® see Lidocaine on page 537

Aneurine Hydrochloride see Thiamine on page 906

Anexsia® see Hydrocodone and Acetaminophen on page 461

Anodynos-DHC® see Hydrocodone and Acetaminophen on page 461

Ansaid® Oral see Flurbiprofen on page 400

Ansamycin see Rifabutin on page 829

Antacid Drug Interactions see page 1096

Antazoline-V® Ophthalmic see Naphazoline and Antazoline on page 654

Anticoagulant Therapy Guidelines see page 1069

Antidepressant Agents Comparison see page 1021

Antidepressant Medication Guidelines see page 1075

Antidiuretic Hormone see Vasopressin on page 983

Antidotes see page 1097

Antiepileptic Drug Interactions Comparison see page 1022

Antihist-1® [OTC] see Clemastine on page 231

Antilirium® see Physostigmine on page 745

Antipsychotic Agents Comparison see page 1023

Antipsychotic Medication Guidelines see page 1076

Antispas® Injection see Dicyclomine on page 285

Anti-Tuss® Expectorant [OTC] see Guaifenesin on page 437

Antivert® see Meclizine on page 574

Antrizine® see Meclizine on page 574

Anturane® see Sulfinpyrazone on page 879

Anucort-HC® Suppository see Hydrocortisone on page 462

Anuprep HC® Suppository see Hydrocortisone on page 462

Anusol® HC-1 [OTC] see Hydrocortisone on page 462

Anusol® HC-2.5% [OTC] see Hydrocortisone on page 462

Anusol-HC® Suppository see Hydrocortisone on page 462

Anxanil® see Hydroxyzine on page 470

Anxiolytic/Hypnotic Use in Long-Term Care Facilities see page 1099

Anzemet® see Dolasetron on page 314

Apacet® [OTC] see Acetaminophen on page 16

APAP see Acetaminophen on page 16

Aplisol® see Tuberculin Purified Protein Derivative on page 971

Aplitest® see Tuberculin Purified Protein Derivative on page 971

Aplonidine see Apraclonidine on this page

APPG see Penicillin G Procaine on page 723

Apraclonidine (a pra KLOE ni deen)

Brand Names Iopidine®

Synonyms Aplonidine; p-Aminoclonidine

Generic Available Yes

Therapeutic Category Adrenergic Agonist Agent, Ophthalmic; Alpha$_2$-Adrenergic Agonist Agent, Ophthalmic

Use

0.5% solution: Short-term adjunctive therapy in patients on maximally tolerated medical therapy who require additional intraocular pressure (IOP) reduction

1% solution: Prevention and treatment of postsurgical intraocular pressure elevation

Contraindications Known hypersensitivity to apraclonidine or clonidine; concurrent use of a monoamine oxidase inhibitor

Warnings Closely monitor patients who develop exaggerated reductions in intraocular pressure; use with caution in patients with cardiovascular disease and in patients with a history of vasovagal reactions

Precautions Efficacy as an adjunctive therapy may be limited in patients already using two aqueous suppressing drugs

Adverse Reactions
Cardiovascular: Arrhythmias, peripheral edema
Central nervous system: Dizziness, depression, insomnia, lethargy, nervousness, somnolence
Dermatologic: Dermatitis
Gastrointestinal: Xerostomia, nausea, constipation
Neuromuscular & skeletal: Paresthesia
Ocular: Conjunctival blanching, mydriasis, upper lid elevation, burning, discomfort, itching, conjunctival microhemorrhage, blurred vision
Respiratory: Dyspnea, rhinitis
Miscellaneous: Allergic response

Overdosage No cases of human ingestion reported; supportive treatment is indicated

Drug Interactions Increased effect: Topical beta-blockers, pilocarpine may cause additive decreased intraocular pressure; monoamine oxidase inhibitors (see Contraindications); may exacerbate effects of CNS depressants; tricyclic antidepressants have competitive effects (theoretical); additive effects possible with cardiovascular and other agents with hypotensive effects

Stability Store in tight, light-resistant containers

Mechanism of Action Apraclonidine is a potent alpha-adrenergic agent similar to clonidine; relatively selective for alpha$_2$-receptors but does retain some binding to alpha$_1$-receptors; appears to result in reduction of aqueous humor formation; more polar than clonidine which reduces its penetration through the blood-brain barrier and suggests that its pharmacological profile is characterized by peripheral rather than central effects

Pharmacodynamics
Onset of action: 1 hour
Maximum IOP: 3-5 hours

Pharmacokinetics Half-life: 8 hours

Usual Dosage Geriatrics and Adults: Ophthalmic:
0.5% solution: Instill 1-2 drops in the affected eye(s) 3 times/day
1% solution: Instill 1 drop in operative eye 1 hour prior to laser surgery, second drop in eye upon completion of procedure

Administration Wait 5 minutes between instillation of other ophthalmic agents to avoid washout of previous dose; after topical instillation, finger pressure should be applied to lacrimal sac to decrease drainage into the nose and throat and minimize possible systemic absorption

Monitoring Parameters Intraocular pressure, fundoscopic exam, visual field testing

Reference Range Steady-state concentration: Peak: 0.9 ng/mL; trough: 0.5 ng/mL

Patient Information May sting on instillation, do not touch dropper to eye; visual acuity may be decreased after administration; night vision may be decreased; distance vision may be altered; read package instructions for insertion

Nursing Implications See Administration and Patient Information

Special Geriatric Considerations Determine that the patient or caregiver can adequately administer ophthalmic medication dosage form

Dosage Forms Solution, ophthalmic, as hydrochloride: 0.5% (5 mL); 1% (0.1 mL, 0.25 mL)

Apresazide® *see* Hydralazine and Hydrochlorothiazide *on page 457*

Apresoline® *see* Hydralazine *on page 456*

Aprodine® Syrup [OTC] *see* Triprolidine and Pseudoephedrine *on page 966*

Aprodine® Tablet [OTC] *see* Triprolidine and Pseudoephedrine *on page 966*

Aquachloral® Supprettes® *see* Chloral Hydrate *on page 200*

AquaMEPHYTON® *see* Phytonadione *on page 747*

Aquaphyllin® *see* Theophylline *on page 902*

AquaSite® Ophthalmic Solution [OTC] *see* Artificial Tears *on page 82*

Aqueous Procaine Penicillin G *see* Penicillin G Procaine *on page 723*

Aqueous Testosterone *see* Testosterone *on page 895*

Ara-A *see* Vidarabine *on page 988*

Arabinofuranosyladenine *see* Vidarabine *on page 988*

Ardeparin (ar dee PA rin)

Brand Names Normiflo®

Therapeutic Category Anticoagulant

Use Prevention of deep vein thrombosis (DVT) which may lead to pulmonary embolism following knee replacement surgery

Contraindications Hypersensitivity to ardeparin, pork products, or other low-molecular weight heparins; cerebrovascular disease or other active hemorrhage; cerebral aneurysm; severe uncontrolled hypertension; thrombocytopenia associated with a positive *in vitro* test for antiplatelet antibodies in the presence of ardeparin

Warnings Not intended for I.M. or I.V. use; use with extreme caution in patients with history of heparin-induced thrombocytopenia; may cause allergic-type reaction including anaphylactic symptoms and life-threatening or less severe asthmatic episodes in certain susceptible individuals; sulfite sensitivity more likely in asthmatics than nonasthmatics; watch for fall in Hct, blood pressure, or other unexplained symptom which may indicate bleeding event; use with extreme caution in patients with conditions having increased risk of hemorrhage (ie, bacterial endocarditis, congenital or acquired bleeding disorders, active ulcerative or angiodysplastic gastrointestinal disease, severe uncontrolled hypertension, hemorrhagic stroke, or shortly after brain, spinal, or ophthalmologic surgery) or in patients treated concomitantly with platelet inhibitors; equivalent postoperative incidence of thrombocytopenia in patients who received ardeparin and patients receiving either warfarin, aspirin, or placebo; use with caution in patients with hypersensitivity to methylparaben or propylparaben; do not mix with other injections or infusions; use with caution in patients with bleeding diathesis, recent GI bleeding, thrombocytopenia or platelet defects, severe liver disease, hypertensive or diabetic retinopathy, or if undergoing invasive procedure especially if receiving other drugs known to interfere with hemostasis

Adverse Reactions

Central nervous system: Fever, confusion

Dermatologic: Pruritus, rash

Gastrointestinal: Nausea, constipation, vomiting

Hematologic: Hemorrhage, thrombocytopenia, anemia

Overdosage Main symptom of overdose is bleeding which may first be indicated with bleeding at the surgical site or at the venipuncture site; other symptoms include epistaxis, hematuria, or blood in stool; easy bruising or petechiae may precede frank bleeding

Toxicology Treatment includes discontinuing the drug and applying pressure to the site, if possible, and replacing volume and hemostatic blood elements (eg, fresh frozen plasma, platelets) as necessary. 1 mg protamine sulfate neutralizes approximately 100 anti-Xa units of aldeparin. Anti-IIa activity of I.V. aldeparin is completely neutralized within 10 minutes following I.V. infusion dose of equal weight protamine sulfate (about 1 mg protamine sulfate for each 100 anti-Xa units of aldeparin). The anti-Xa and Heptest® activities of ardeparin are reduced by about 75% within 10 minutes and are almost completely neutralized within 30 minutes after protamine sulfate administration. Protamine sulfate may cause anaphylactoid reactions that can be life-threatening, it should be given only when resuscitation techniques and treatment of anaphylactic shock are available.

Drug Interactions Use with anticoagulants or platelet inhibitors, including aspirin and NSAIDs may induce or augment bleeding

Stability Store at room temperature 15°C to 25°C (59°F to 77°F)

Mechanism of Action A low molecular weight heparin with antithrombotic properties; a partially depolymerized porcine mucosal heparin that has the same molecular subunits as heparin sodium, USP; acts at multiple sites in the normal coagulation system; binds to and accelerates the activity of antithrombin III, thereby inhibiting thrombosis by inactivating factor Xa and thrombin; inhibits thrombin by binding to heparin cofactor II

Pharmacokinetics

Absorption: Well absorbed

Bioavailability:

Anti-Xa: 92% ± 16%

Anti-IIa: 63% ± 19%

Peak plasma concentrations:

Peak anti-Xa: 0.09 ± 0.03 to 0.32 ± 0.05 units/mL after 30-100 anti-Xa units/kg single doses reached in 2.7 ± 0.6 hours

Mean anti-IIa: 0.07 ± 0.02 units/mL after 100 anti-Xa units/kg single doses reached in 3 ± 1 hours

Half-life: Anti-Xa: Longer than heparin sodium, USP

Note: Mean plasma clearances of ardeparin anti-Xa and anti-IIa activities in normal volunteers following a single 90 anti-Xa units/kg I.V. bolus dose are 30 ± 7 and 46 ± 16 mL/hour/kg respectively, and the mean disposition half-lives are 3.3 ± 2.4 and 1.2 ± 0.3 hours respectively

Usual Dosage Geriatrics and Adults: Subcutaneous: 50 anti-Xa units every 12 hours

Volume of Normiflo® to Be Administered by Patient Weight

Patient Weight in Pounds	Patient Weight in Kilograms	Volume of Normiflo (mL)	
		5000 anti-Xa units/0.5 mL	10,000 anti-Xa units/0.5 mL
44-54	20-24	0.10	
55-76	25-34	0.15	
77-98	35-44	0.20	
99-120	45-54	0.25	
121-142	55-64	0.30	
143-164	65-74	0.35	
165-186	75-84	0.40	
187-208	85-94	0.45	
209-230	95-104	0.50	0.25
231-285	105-129		0.30
286-329	130-149		0.35
330-373	150-169		0.40
374-417	170-189		0.45
418-440	190-200		0.50

Dosage adjustment in renal impairment: No adjustment necessary Not dialyzable

Administration Administer by deep subcutaneous injection; do not administer I.M.; patient should be sitting or lying down. May be injected into abdomen (avoid the navel), the anterior aspect of the thighs, or the outer aspect of the upper arms. Vary site with each injection. A skinfold held between the thumb and forefinger must be lifted. Entire length of the needle is inserted into the fold at a 45° to 90° angle. Before injecting, draw back on the plunger to ensure the needle is not in the intravascular space. Do not rub injection site after completing injection. Treatment should begin the evening of the day of surgery or the following morning and is continued for up to 14 days or until patient is fully ambulatory.

Monitoring Parameters Monitor CBC including platelet counts, urinalysis, and occult blood in stool

Test Interactions At recommended doses, ardeparin has no effect on PT; APTT may show no change or be prolonged; asymptomatic increases in AST and ALT levels >3 times the upper limit of normal have been reported in 20 of 16 and 4 of 16 normal subjects; because aminotransferase determinations are important in the differential diagnosis of myocardial infarction, liver disease, and pulmonary embolism, elevations that might be caused by drugs like ardeparin should be interpreted with caution; ardeparin may increase activity of lipoprotein lipase; paradoxical elevations in serum triglyceride levels have been seen in clinical trails

Additional Information Peak anti-Xa plasma concentrations produced by ardeparin were about twice as high as those produced by heparin sodium, and ardeparin anti-Xa half-life in plasma was longer than that for heparin sodium.

Special Geriatric Considerations No significant differences in safety in patients >65 years of age vs those <65 years of age

Dosage Forms Injection, as sodium: Anti-Xa units 5000 (0.5 mL); Anti-Xa units 10,000 (0.5 mL)

Aristospan® **Intralesional** see Triamcinolone on page 949
Arm-a-Med® **Isoetharine** see Isoetharine on page 499
Arm-a-Med® **Isoproterenol** see Isoproterenol on page 501
Arm-a-Med® **Metaproterenol** see Metaproterenol on page 596
Armour® **Thyroid** see Thyroid on page 917
Arrestin® see Trimethobenzamide on page 961
Artane® see Trihexyphenidyl on page 958
Artha-G® see Salsalate on page 847
Arthritis Foundation® **Pain Reliever [OTC]** see Aspirin on page 84
Arthropan® see Salicylates (Various Salts) on page 842
Articulose-50® **Injection** see Prednisolone on page 774

Artificial Tears (ar ti FISH il tears)

Brand Names Adsorbotear® Ophthalmic Solution [OTC]; Akwa Tears® Solution [OTC]; AquaSite® Ophthalmic Solution [OTC]; Bion® Tears Solution [OTC]; Comfort® Tears Solution [OTC]; Dakrina® Ophthalmic Solution [OTC]; Dry Eye® Therapy Solution [OTC]; Dry Eyes® Solution [OTC]; Dwelle® Ophthalmic Solution [OTC]; Eye-Lube-A® Solution [OTC]; HypoTears PF Solution [OTC]; HypoTears Solution [OTC]; Isopto® Plain Solution [OTC]; Isopto® Tears Solution [OTC]; Just Tears® Solution [OTC]; Lacril® Ophthalmic Solution [OTC]; Liquifilm® Tears Solution [OTC]; Liquifilm® Forte Solution [OTC]; LubriTears® Solution [OTC]; Moisture® Ophthalmic Drops [OTC]; Murine® Solution [OTC]; Murocel® Ophthalmic Solution [OTC]; Nature's Tears® Solution [OTC]; Nu-Tears® Solution [OTC]; Nu-Tears® II Solution [OTC]; OcuCoat® Ophthalmic Solution [OTC]; OcuCoat® PF Ophthalmic Solution [OTC]; Puralube® Tears Solution [OTC]; Refresh® Ophthalmic Solution [OTC]; Refresh® Plus Ophthalmic Solution [OTC]; Tear Drop® Solution [OTC]; TearGard® Ophthalmic Solution [OTC]; Teargen® Ophthalmic Solution [OTC]; Tearisol® Solution [OTC]; Tears Naturale® Free Solution [OTC]; Tears Naturale® II Solution [OTC]; Tears Naturale® Solution [OTC]; Tears Plus® Solution [OTC]; Tears Renewed® Solution [OTC]; Ultra Tears® Solution [OTC]; Viva-Drops® Solution [OTC]
Synonyms Hydroxyethylcellulose; Polyvinyl Alcohol
Generic Available Yes
Therapeutic Category Opiate Partial Agonist
Use Ophthalmic lubricant; for relief of dry eyes and eye irritation
Contraindications Hypersensitivity to any component
Warnings Not for use with soft contact lenses
Adverse Reactions Ocular: Mild stinging, temporary blurred vision
Usual Dosage Use as needed to relieve symptoms, 1-2 drops into eye(s) 3-4 times/day
Patient Information Wash hands thoroughly; if irritation or condition worsens or persists for longer than 3 days, discontinue use; do not touch tip of container to any surface; close immediately after use
Nursing Implications Not for use with soft contact lenses
Special Geriatric Considerations Assure the patient or caregiver can adequately administer ophthalmic medication
Dosage Forms Solution, ophthalmic: 15 mL and 30 mL with dropper

ASA see Aspirin on page 84
A.S.A. [OTC] see Aspirin on page 84
5-ASA see Mesalamine on page 591
Asacol® **Oral** see Mesalamine on page 591

Ascorbic Acid (a SKOR bik AS id)

Brand Names Ascorbicap® [OTC]; C-Crystals® [OTC]; Cebid® Timecelles® [OTC]; Cecon® [OTC]; Cevalin® [OTC]; Cevi-Bid® [OTC]; Ce-Vi-Sol® [OTC]; Dull-C® [OTC]; Flavorcee® [OTC]; N'ice® Vitamin C Drops [OTC]; Vita-C® [OTC]
Synonyms Vitamin C
Generic Available Yes
Therapeutic Category Urinary Acidifying Agent; Vitamin, Water Soluble
Use Prevention and treatment of scurvy; urinary acidification; dietary supplementation; has been promoted in prevention and decreasing the severity of colds, wounds; urinary acidifier (4-12 g/day); idiopathic methemoglobinemia
Warnings Diabetics and patients prone to recurrent renal calculi should not take excessive doses for extended periods of time
Precautions Some products contain tartrazine and sulfites; avoid in sensitive patients

Adverse Reactions
Cardiovascular: Flushing
Central nervous system: Faintness, dizziness, headache, fatigue
Gastrointestinal: Nausea, vomiting, heartburn, diarrhea
Renal: Hyperoxaluria, large doses precipitate cystine, oxalate and urate renal stones

Overdosage Symptoms of overdose include renal calculi, nausea, gastritis, diarrhea

Toxicology Diuresis with forced fluids may be useful following a massive ingestion

Drug Interactions Iron, aspirin, estrogens, warfarin
Drug-lab tests: False-negative urine glucose determinations with doses >500 mg/day; occult blood tests may be falsely negative if vitamin C ingested within 48-72 hours of test

Stability Injectable form should be stored under refrigeration (2°C to 8°C); protect oral dosage forms from light; is rapidly oxidized when in solution in air and alkaline media

Mechanism of Action Vitamin C's biologic functions are not fully understood; it is necessary for collagen formation and tissue repair in the body; involved in some oxidation-reduction reactions as well as other metabolic reactions, such as synthesis of carnitine, steroids, and catecholamines; conversion of folic acid to folinic acid

Pharmacokinetics
Absorption: Oral: Readily absorbed with a wide distribution; absorption is an active process and is thought to be dose-dependent
Metabolism: In the liver by oxidation and sulfation
Elimination: In urine; there is an individual specific renal threshold for ascorbic acid; when blood levels are high, ascorbic acid is excreted in urine, whereas when the levels are subthreshold very little if any ascorbic acid is cleared into urine

Usual Dosage Geriatrics and Adults: Oral, I.M., I.V., S.C.:
Scurvy: 500-1000 mg/day for at least 2 weeks
Urinary acidification: 4-12 g/day in 3-4 divided doses
RDA dietary supplement: 60 mg/day
Wound healing: 300-500 mg/day; larger amounts have been also recommended; maximum 7-10 days pre- and postoperatively
Burns: 1-2 g/day
Prevention and treatment of cold: 1-3 g/day

Monitoring Parameters Monitor for renal calculi; monitor pH of urine when acidifying

Reference Range None

Test Interactions False-positive urinary glucose with cupric sulfate reagent, false-negative urinary glucose with glucose oxidase method

Patient Information Do not use in large doses if diabetic or have a history of renal stones; do not exceed 3 g/day without physician's advice

Nursing Implications Avoid rapid I.V. injection; monitor urine pH when using as an acidifying agent

Additional Information Sodium content of 1 g of sodium ascorbate: ~5 mEq

Special Geriatric Considerations Minimum RDA for elderly is not established; vitamin C is provided mainly in citrus fruits and tomatoes; the elderly, however, avoid citrus fruits due to cost and difficulty preparing (peeling); daily replacement through a single multiple vitamins recommended; use of natural vitamin C or rose hips offers no advantages; acidity may produce GI complaints

Dosage Forms
Capsule, timed release: 500 mg
Crystals: 4 g/teaspoonful (1000 g)
Drops: 100 mg/mL (50 mL)
Injection: 100 mg/mL (2 mL, 10 mL); 250 mg/mL (30 mL, 50 mL)
Liquid: 35 mg/0.6 mL (50 mL)
Powder: 4 g/teaspoonful (1000 g)
Syrup: 500 mg/5 mL (5 mL, 10 mL, 120 mL, 480 mL)
Tablet: 50 mg, 100 mg, 250 mg, 500 mg, 1000 mg
Tablet:
  Chewable: 100 mg, 250 mg, 500 mg
  Timed release: 500 mg, 1500 mg

References
Myrianthopoulos M, "Dietary Treatment of Hyperlipidemia in the Elderly," *Clin Geriatr Med*, 1987, 3(2):343-59.

Ascorbicap® [OTC] *see* Ascorbic Acid *on previous page*

Ascriptin® [OTC] *see* Aspirin *on this page*

Asendin® *see* Amoxapine *on page 65*

Asmalix® *see* Theophylline *on page 902*

A-Spas® S/L *see* Hyoscyamine *on page 471*

Aspergum® [OTC] *see* Aspirin *on this page*

Aspirin (AS pir in)

Brand Names Anacin® [OTC]; Arthritis Foundation® Pain Reliever [OTC]; A.S.A. [OTC]; Ascriptin® [OTC]; Aspergum® [OTC]; Asprimox® [OTC]; Bayer® Aspirin [OTC]; Bayer® Buffered Aspirin [OTC]; Bayer® Low Adult Strength [OTC]; Bufferin® [OTC]; Buffex® [OTC]; Cama® Arthritis Pain Reliever [OTC]; Easprin®; Ecotrin® [OTC]; Ecotrin® Low Adult Strength [OTC]; Empirin® [OTC]; Extra Strength Adprin-B® [OTC]; Extra Strength Bayer® Enteric 500 Aspirin [OTC]; Extra Strength Bayer® Plus [OTC]; Halfprin® 81® [OTC]; Measurin® [OTC]; Regular Strength Bayer® Enteric 500 Aspirin [OTC]; St Joseph® Adult Chewable Aspirin [OTC]; Synalgos® [OTC]; ZORprin®

Synonyms Acetylsalicylic Acid; ASA

Generic Available Yes

Therapeutic Category Analgesic, Non-narcotic; Anti-inflammatory Agent; Antiplatelet Agent; Antipyretic; Nonsteroidal Anti-inflammatory Agent (NSAID), Oral; Salicylate

Use Treatment of mild to moderate pain, inflammation and fever; management of rheumatoid arthritis, rheumatic fever, osteoarthritis, and gout (high dose); may be used as a prophylaxis of myocardial infarction and transient ischemic attacks (TIA)

Unlabeled use: Stroke prevention in patients with atrial fibrillation who are not good candidates for warfarin therapy; stent implantation

Contraindications Bleeding disorders (factor VII or IX deficiencies), hypersensitivity to salicylates or other nonsteroidal anti-inflammatory drugs (NSAIDs); tartrazine dye and asthma

Warnings Tinnitus or impaired hearing may indicate toxicity; discontinue use 1 week prior to surgical procedures

Precautions Use with caution in patients with platelet and bleeding disorders, renal dysfunction, hepatic disease, history of salicylate-induced gastric irritation, peptic ulcer disease, erosive gastritis, bleeding disorders, hypoprothrombinemia, and vitamin K deficiency; use cautiously in asthmatics, especially those with aspirin intolerance and nasal polyps

Adverse Reactions

Central nervous system: Dizziness, mental confusion, CNS depression, fever, headache, lassitude

Dermatologic: Rash, urticaria, angioedema

Gastrointestinal: Nausea, vomiting, dyspepsia, epigastric discomfort, GI distress, ulcers, thirst

Hematologic: Occult bleeding, prolongation of bleeding time, leukopenia, thrombocytopenia, inhibition of platelet aggregation

Hepatic: Hepatotoxicity

Otic: Tinnitus

Respiratory: Bronchospasm, hyperventilation

Miscellaneous: Diaphoresis

Overdosage 10-30 g; symptoms of overdose include tinnitus, headache, dizziness, confusion, metabolic acidosis, hyperpyrexia, hyperpnea, tachypnea, nausea, vomiting, irritability, disorientation, hallucinations, lethargy, stupor, dehydration, hyperventilation, hyperthermia, hyperactivity, depression leading to coma, respiratory failure, and collapse; laboratory abnormalities include hypokalemia, hypoglycemia or hyperglycemia with alterations in pH

Aspirin or Other Salicylate Toxicity

Toxic Symptoms	Treatment
Overdose	Induce emesis with ipecac, and/or lavage with saline, followed with activated charcoal
Dehydration	I.V. fluids with KCl (no D$_5$W only)
Metabolic acidosis (must be treated)	Sodium bicarbonate
Hyperthermia	Cooling blankets or sponge baths
Coagulopathy/hemorrhage	Vitamin K I.V.
Hypoglycemia (with coma, seizures, or change in mental status)	Dextrose 25 g I.V.
Seizures	Diazepam 5-10 mg I.V.

Toxicology The "Done" nomogram is very helpful for estimating the severity of aspirin poisoning and directing treatment using serum salicylate concentration. Treatment can also be based upon symptomatology; see table.

Drug Interactions

Aspirin may increase methotrexate serum concentration and may displace valproic acid from binding sites which can result in toxicity; warfarin and aspirin may increase bleeding

NSAIDs and aspirin may increase GI adverse effects, possible decreased serum concentration of NSAIDs

Aspirin may antagonize effects of probenecid and sulfinpyrazone since salicylates in low dose (<2.4 g/day) antagonize uricosuric effect

Corticosteroids increased salicylate serum concentration

Nizatidine increased serum salicylate concentration

ACE inhibitors, anticoagulants, beta-blockers, heparin, loop diuretics, nitroglycerin, sulfinpyrazone, spironolactone, sulfonylureas, insulin, valproic acid

Stability Keep suppositories in refrigerator, do not freeze; hydrolysis of aspirin occurs upon exposure to water or moist air, resulting in salicylate and acetate, which possess a vinegar-like odor; do not use if a strong odor is present

Mechanism of Action Inhibits prostaglandin synthesis, acts on the hypothalamus heat-regulating center to reduce fever, blocks prostaglandin synthetase action which prevents formation of the platelet-aggregating substance thromboxane A_2; decreases pain receptor sensitivity. Other proposed mechanisms of action for salicylate anti-inflammatory action are lysosomal stabilization, inhibition of kinin and leukotriene production, alteration of chemotactic factors, and inhibition of neutrophil activation. This latter mechanism may be the most significant pharmacologic action to reduce inflammation.

Pharmacokinetics

Absorption: From the stomach and small intestine

Distribution: Readily into most body fluids and tissues; aspirin is hydrolyzed to salicylate (active) by esterases in the GI mucosa, red blood cells, synovial fluid and blood

Protein binding: Plasma protein bound (albumin) >90% at low concentrations and 76% at high concentrations (400 mcg/mL)

Metabolism: Metabolism of salicylate occurs primarily by hepatic microsomal enzymes

Half-life, aspirin: 15-20 minutes

Metabolic pathways are saturable such that salicylates half-life is dose-dependent ranging from 3 hours at lower doses (300-600 mg), 5-6 hours (after 1 g) and 15-30 hours with higher doses; in therapeutic anti-inflammatory doses, half-lives generally range from 6-12 hours

Time to peak plasma concentrations: ~1-2 hours

Usual Dosage Geriatrics and Adults:

Analgesic and antipyretic: Oral, rectal: 325-1000 mg every 4-6 hours up to 4 g/day

Anti-inflammatory: Oral: Initial: 2.4-3.6 g/day in divided doses; usual maintenance: 3.6-5.4 g/day, monitor serum concentrations

Stent implantation: Oral: 325 mg 2 hours prior to implantation and 160-325 mg daily thereafter

TIA: Oral: 1.3 g/day in 2-4 divided doses; other studies have demonstrated equal efficacy with fewer side effects at a dose of 300 mg/day

Myocardial infarction, stroke, and atrial fibrillation prophylaxis: 81-325 mg/day

Dialyzable (50% to 100%)

Monitoring Parameters Serum concentrations, renal function; hearing changes or tinnitus; monitor for response (ie, pain, inflammation, range of motion, grip strength); observe for abnormal bleeding, bruising, weight gain

Reference Range

Sample size: 1.5-2 mL blood (purple top tube)

Timing of serum samples: Peak concentration usually occurs 2 hours after ingestion; the half-life increases with the dosage (eg, the half-life after 300 mg is 3 hours, and after 1 g is 5-6 hours, and after 8-10 g is 10-15 hours). Salicylate serum concentrations correlate with the pharmacological actions and adverse effects observed. Anti-inflammatory therapeutic serum concentrations 150-300 mcg/mL. See table on following page.

Test Interactions False-negative results for glucose oxidase urinary glucose tests (Clinistix®); false-positives using the cupric sulfate method (Clinitest®); also, interferes with Gerhardt test (urinary ketone analysis), VMA determination; 5-HIAA, xylose tolerance test, and T_3 and T_4; increased PBI; increased uric acid

(Continued)

Aspirin *(Continued)*

Serum Salicylate: Clinical Correlations

Serum Salicylate Concentration (mcg/mL)	Desired Effects	Adverse Effects/Intoxication
~100	Antiplatelet Antipyresis Analgesia	GI intolerance and bleeding, hypersensitivity, hemostatic defects
150-300	Anti-inflammatory	Mild salicylism
250-400	Treatment of rheumatic fever	Nausea/vomiting, hyperventilation, salicylism, flushing, sweating, thirst, headache, diarrhea, and tachycardia
>400-500		Respiratory alkalosis, hemorrhage, excitement, confusion, asterixis, pulmonary edema, convulsions, tetany, metabolic acidosis, fever, coma, cardiovascular collapse, renal and respiratory failure

Patient Information Watch for bleeding gums or any signs of GI bleeding; take with food or milk to minimize GI distress, notify physician if ringing in ears or persistent GI pain occurs; do not crush or chew sustained release or enteric coated preparation; avoid other aspirin or salicylate containing products

Nursing Implications Administer with food or a full glass of water to minimize GI distress; do not crush sustained release tablets or enteric coated tablets; monitor for bleeding, bruising, tinnitus

Special Geriatric Considerations Elderly are a high-risk population for adverse effects from nonsteroidal anti-inflammatory agents. As much as 60% of elderly with GI complications to NSAIDs can develop peptic ulceration and/or hemorrhage asymptomatically. The concomitant use of H_2 blockers, omeprazole, and sucralfate is not effective as prophylaxis with the exception of NSAID-induced duodenal ulcers which may be prevented by the use of ranitidine. Misoprostol and proton pump inhibitors are the only agents proven to help prevent the development of NSAID-induced ulcers. Also, concomitant disease and drug use contribute to the risk for GI adverse effects. Use lowest effective dose for shortest period possible. Consider renal function decline with age. Use of NSAIDs can compromise existing renal function especially when Cl_{cr} is ≤30 mL/minute. Tinnitus may be a difficult and unreliable indication of toxicity due to age-related hearing loss or eighth cranial nerve damage. CNS adverse effects such as confusion, agitation, and hallucination are generally seen in overdose or high dose situations, but elderly may demonstrate these adverse effects at lower doses than younger adults.

Dosage Forms

Capsule: 356.4 mg with caffeine 30 mg
Suppository, rectal: 120 mg, 200 mg, 300 mg, 600 mg
Tablet: 81 mg, 325 mg, 500 mg
Tablet:
  With caffeine: 400 mg with caffeine 32 mg
  Buffered: 325 mg with magnesium-aluminum hydroxide 150 mg
  Chewable: 81 mg
  Coated: 325 mg
  Effervescent: 325 mg, 500 mg
  Enteric coated: 81 mg, 325 mg, 500 mg
  Sustained release: 650 mg, 800 mg

References

Albers GW, "Atrial Fibrillation and Stroke", *Arch Intern Med*, 1994, 154(13):1443-8.

Clinch D, Banerjee AK, Ostrik G, "Absence of Abdominal Pain in Elderly Patients With Peptic Ulcer," *Age Ageing*, 1984, 13:120-3.

Clive DM and Stoff JS, "Renal Syndromes Associated With Nonsteroidal Anti-inflammatory Drugs," *N Engl J Med*, 1984, 310(9):563-72.

Hawkey CJ, Karrasch JA, Szczepaski L, et al, "Omeprazole Compared With Misoprostrol for Ulcers Associated With Nonsteroidal Anti-inflammatory Drugs," *N Engl J Med*, 1998, 338(11):727-34.

Knodel LC, "Preventing NSAID-Induced Ulcers: The Role of Misoprostol," *Consult Pharm*, 1989, 4:37-41.

Schömig A, Neumann, FJ, Kastrati A, et al, "A Randomized Comparison of Antiplatelet and Anticoagulant Therapy After the Placement of Coronary-Artery Stents," *N Engl J Med*, 1996, 334(17):1084-9.

Weissmann G, "Aspirin," *Sci Am*, 1991, 264(1):84-90.

Yeomans ND, Tulassay Z, Juhasz L, et al, "A Comparison of Omeprazole With Ranitidine for Ulcers Associated With Nonsteroidal Anti-inflammatory Drugs," *N Engl J Med*, 1998, 338:719-26.

Aspirin and Codeine (AS pir in & KOE deen)

Related Information
Aspirin *on page 84*
Codeine *on page 246*

Brand Names Empirin® With Codeine

Synonyms Codeine and Aspirin

Generic Available Yes

Therapeutic Category Analgesic, Narcotic

Use Relief of mild to moderate pain

Restrictions C-III

Contraindications Hypersensitivity to aspirin, codeine or any component

Precautions Use with caution in patients with impaired renal function, erosive gastritis, or peptic ulcer

Adverse Reactions
Cardiovascular: Palpitations, hypotension, bradycardia, peripheral vasodilation
Central nervous system: CNS depression, increased intracranial pressure
Dermatologic: Pruritus, rash, urticaria
Endocrine & metabolic: Antidiuretic hormone release
Gastrointestinal: Nausea, vomiting, constipation
Hematologic: Occult bleeding
Hepatic: Hepatotoxicity
Respiratory: Respiratory depression, bronchospasm
Ocular: Miosis
Miscellaneous: Physical and psychological dependence, biliary or urinary tract spasm, histamine release

Drug Interactions Refer to individual monographs for Aspirin and Codeine

Usual Dosage
Geriatrics: One #3 tablet (30 mg codeine) or two #2 tablets (15 mg codeine/each) every 4-6 hours as needed for pain
Adults: 1-2 tablets every 4-6 hours as needed for pain

Monitoring Parameters Pain relief, respiratory status, blood pressure, mental status

Test Interactions Urine glucose, urinary 5-HIAA, serum uric acid

Patient Information May cause drowsiness, avoid alcoholic beverages; check cough and cold preparations for aspirin content

Nursing Implications Observe patient for excessive sedation or confusion, respiratory depression, constipation

Special Geriatric Considerations The duration of action of codeine may be prolonged in the elderly; in addition, enhanced analgesia has been seen in elderly patients on therapeutic doses of narcotics; if one tablet/dose is used, it may be useful to add an additional 325 mg of aspirin to maximize analgesic effect

Dosage Forms
Tablet:
#2: Aspirin 325 mg and codeine phosphate 15 mg
#3: Aspirin 325 mg and codeine phosphate 30 mg
#4: Aspirin 325 mg and codeine phosphate 60 mg

Aspirin and Oxycodone *see* Oxycodone and Aspirin *on page 706*

Asprimox® [OTC] *see* Aspirin *on page 84*

Asproject® *see* Salicylates (Various Salts) *on page 842*

Astelin® *see* Azelastine *on page 100*

Astemizole (a STEM mi zole)

Brand Names Hismanal®

Generic Available No

Therapeutic Category Antihistamine

Use Perennial and seasonal allergic rhinitis and other allergic symptoms including urticaria

Contraindications Hypersensitivity to astemizole or any component

Warnings Rare cases of severe cardiovascular events (cardiac arrest, arrhythmias) have been reported in the following situations: overdose (even as low
(Continued)

Astemizole *(Continued)*

as 20-30 mg/day), significant hepatic dysfunction, when used in combination with erythromycin, ketoconazole, or itraconazole

Adverse Reactions

Central nervous system: Not likely to cause drowsiness, dizziness, nervousness, headache. **Note:** Minimal sedation and anticholinergic effects are seen as compared to older antihistamines.

Gastrointestinal: Appetite increase, xerostomia, weight gain

Overdosage Symptoms of overdose include sedation, apnea, diminished mental alertness, ventricular tachycardia, torsade de pointes

Toxicology There is no specific treatment for an antihistamine overdose, however most of its clinical toxicity is due to anticholinergic effects. Acetylcholinesterase inhibitors including physostigmine, neostigmine, pyridostigmine, and edrophonium may be useful for the overdose with severe life-threatening symptoms. Physostigmine 1-2 mg I.V., slowly may be given to reverse the anticholinergic effects. Cases of ventricular arrhythmias following dosages >200 mg have been reported, however, overdoses of up to 500 mg have been reported without ill effect. Patients should be carefully observed with EKG monitoring in cases of suspected overdose. Magnesium may be helpful for torsade de pointes or a lidocaine bolus followed by a titrated infusion.

Drug Interactions Increased toxicity: Erythromycin, other macrolide antibiotics, itraconazole, ketoconazole, nefazodone

Mechanism of Action Competes with histamine for H_1-receptor sites on effector cells in the gastrointestinal tract, blood vessels, and respiratory tract; binds to lung receptors significantly greater than it binds to cerebellar receptors, resulting in a reduced sedative potential

Pharmacokinetics

Distribution: Nonsedating action reportedly due to the drugs low lipid solubility and poor penetration through the blood-brain barrier

Protein binding: 97%

Metabolism: Undergoes exclusive first-pass metabolism

Half-life: 20 hours

Time to peak serum concentration: Oral: Long-acting, with steady-state plasma levels of parent compound and metabolites seen within 4-8 weeks following initiation of chronic therapy peak plasma levels appear in 1-4 hours following administration

Elimination: Eliminated by metabolism in the liver to active and inactive metabolites, which are thereby excreted in the feces and to a lesser degree in the urine

Usual Dosage Oral:

Geriatrics: 10 mg/day

Adults: 10 mg/day; to decrease time to steady-state, administer 30 mg on first day, 20 mg on second day, then 10 mg/day in a single dose

Monitoring Parameters Relief of symptoms

Patient Information Take on an empty stomach, at least 2 hours after a meal or 1 hour before a meal. Because of its delayed onset, astemizole is useful for prophylaxis of allergic symptoms, rather than for acute relief. Do not exceed recommended doses.

Nursing Implications Administer on an empty stomach

Additional Information Not likely to cause drowsiness

Special Geriatric Considerations Because of its low incidence of sedation and anticholinergic effects, astemizole would be a rational choice in the elderly when an antihistamine is indicated

Dosage Forms Tablet: 10 mg

Asthma Guidelines *see page 1040*

AsthmaHaler® *see* Epinephrine *on page 336*

AsthmaNefrin® [OTC] *see* Epinephrine *on page 336*

Astramorph™ PF Injection *see* Morphine Sulfate *on page 640*

Atarax® *see* Hydroxyzine *on page 470*

Atenolol *(a TEN oh lole)*

Related Information

Beta-Blockers Comparison *on page 1026*

Brand Names Tenormin®

Generic Available Yes

Therapeutic Category Antianginal Agent; Beta-Adrenergic Blocker

Use Treatment of hypertension, alone or in combination with other agents; also used in management of angina pectoris; selective inhibitor of beta$_1$-adrenergic receptors; postmyocardial infarction patients

Unlabeled use: Acute alcohol withdrawal, supraventricular and ventricular arrhythmias, and migraine headache prophylaxis; diastolic congestive heart failure

Contraindications Hypersensitivity to beta-blocking agents, pulmonary edema, cardiogenic shock, bradycardia, heart block, uncompensated congestive heart failure, sinus node dysfunction, A-V conduction abnormalities, diabetes mellitus. Although atenolol primarily blocks beta$_1$-receptors, high doses can result in beta$_2$-receptor blockade. Use with caution in elderly with bronchospastic lung disease and renal dysfunction. Geriatric patients often have decreased renal function (see Usual Dosage).

Warnings Abrupt withdrawal of beta-blockers may result in an exaggerated cardiac beta-adrenergic responsiveness. Symptomatology has included reports of tachycardia, hypertension, ischemia, angina, myocardial infarction, and sudden death. It is recommended that patients be tapered gradually off of beta-blockers over a 2-week period rather than via abrupt discontinuation.

Precautions Administer to congestive heart failure patients with caution; administer with caution to patients with bronchospastic disease, diabetes mellitus, hyperthyroidism, myasthenia gravis and renal function decline and severe peripheral vascular disease.

Adverse Reactions

Cardiovascular: Persistent bradycardia, hypotension, chest pain, edema, heart failure, second or third degree A-V block, Raynaud's phenomena

Central nervous system: Dizziness, fatigue, insomnia, lethargy, confusion, mental depression, headache, nightmares

Gastrointestinal: Constipation, diarrhea, nausea

Genitourinary: Impotence

Respiratory: Dyspnea has occurred when daily dosage exceeds 100 mg/day, wheezing

Miscellaneous: Cold extremities

Overdosage Symptoms of overdose include bradycardia, congestive heart failure, hypotension, bronchospasm, hypoglycemia (see Toxicology)

Toxicology Sympathomimetics (eg, epinephrine or dopamine), glucagon or a pacemaker can be used to treat the toxic bradycardia, asystole, and/or hypotension. Initially, fluids may be the best treatment for toxic hypotension. Patients should remain supine; serum glucose and potassium should be measured. Use supportive measures: lavage, syrup of ipecac; atenolol may be removed by hemodialysis. I.V. glucose should be administered for hypoglycemia; seizures may be treated with phenytoin or diazepam intravenously; continuous monitoring of blood pressure and EKG is necessary. If PVCs occur, treat with lidocaine or phenytoin; avoid quinidine, procainamide, and disopyramide since these agents further depress myocardial function. Bronchospasm can be treated with theophylline on beta$_2$ agonists (epinephrine).

Drug Interactions

Pharmacologic action of beta antagonists may be decreased by aluminum compounds, calcium salts, barbiturates, cholestyramine, colestipol, NSAIDs, penicillins (ampicillin), rifampin, salicylates, sulfinpyrazone, thyroid hormones; hypoglycemic effect of sulfonylureas may be blunted

Pharmacologic effect of beta antagonists may be enhanced with concomitant use of calcium channel blockers, oral contraceptives, flecainide (bioavailability and effect of flecainide also enhanced), haloperidol (hypotensive effects of both drugs), H$_2$ antagonists (decreased metabolism), hydralazine (both drugs' hypotensive effects increased), loop diuretics (increased serum concentration of beta-blockers except atenolol), MAO inhibitors, phenothiazines, propafenone, quinidine, quinolones, thioamines; beta-blockers may decrease clearance of acetaminophen; beta-blockers may increase anticoagulant effects of warfarin (propranolol); benzodiazepine effects enhanced by the lipophilic beta-blockers (atenolol does not interact)

Significant and fatal increases in blood pressure have occurred after decrease in dose or discontinuation of clonidine in patients receiving both clonidine and beta-blockers together (reduce doses of each cautiously with small decreases); peripheral ischemia of ergot alkaloids enhanced by beta-blockers; beta-blockers increase serum concentration of lidocaine; beta-blockers increase hypotensive effect of prazosin

Stability Dilutions in dextrose, sodium chloride, and sodium chloride and dextrose stable for 48 hours

Mechanism of Action Competitively blocks response to beta$_1$-adrenergic receptors with little or no effect on beta$_2$-receptors except at high doses; (Continued)

Atenolol *(Continued)*

consider renal function (see Usual Dosage). Does not exhibit membrane stabilizing or intrinsic sympathomimetic activity; low lipid solubility, therefore, little crosses blood-brain barrier.

Pharmacokinetics

Absorption: Incompletely from GI tract (50%)

Distribution: Does **not** cross the blood-brain barrier

Protein binding: Low (3% to 15%)

Half-life: 6-9 hours (longer in patients with reduced renal function; 16-27 hours with Cl_{cr} 15-35 mL/minute and >27 hours in Cl_{cr} <15 mL/minute)

Time to peak serum concentrations: Oral: Within 2-4 hours

Elimination: 40% excreted as unchanged drug in urine, 50% in feces

Usual Dosage Geriatrics and Adults:

Oral: 50-100 mg/dose given daily; doses >100 mg/day are unlikely to produce further response for blood pressure control, however, some patients with angina may require 200 mg/day to achieve control of symptoms; **geriatrics initial dose: 25 mg/day**

I.V.: For early treatment of myocardial infarction: 5 mg slow I.V. over 5 minutes; may repeat in 10 minutes; if both doses are tolerated, may start oral atenolol 50 mg every 12 hours

Dosing interval in renal impairment:

Cl_{cr} 15-35 mL/minute: Administer 50 mg/day maximum

Cl_{cr} <15 mL/minute: Administer 50 mg every other day maximum

Postmyocardial infarction:

I.V.: Administer as soon as possible 5 mg over 5 minutes; follow with 5 mg I.V. 10 minutes later

Oral: Follow with 100 mg/day or 50 mg twice daily for 6-9 days postmyocardial infarction

Moderately dialyzable (20% to 50%)

Monitoring Parameters
Blood pressure, orthostatic hypotension, heart rate, CNS effects, EKG

Test Interactions
Increased triglycerides, potassium, uric acid, cholesterol (S), glucose; decreased HDL

Patient Information
Adhere to dosage regimen; watch for postural hypotension; do not discontinue medication abruptly, sudden stopping of medication may precipitate or cause angina; consult pharmacist or physician before taking with other adrenergic drugs (eg, cold medications); notify physician if any of the following symptoms occur: difficult breathing, night cough, swelling of extremities, slow pulse, dizziness, lightheadedness, confusion, depression, skin rash, fever, sore throat, unusual bleeding or bruising; may produce drowsiness, dizziness, lightheadedness, blurred vision, confusion; use with caution while driving or performing tasks requiring alertness; may mask signs of hypoglycemia in diabetics; may be taken without regard to meals

Nursing Implications
Patient's therapeutic response may be evaluated by looking at blood pressure, apical and radial pulses, fluid I & O, daily weight, respirations, and circulation in extremities before and during therapy; monitor for CNS side effects; modify dosage in patients with renal insufficiency

Additional Information
May potentiate hypoglycemia in a diabetic patient and mask signs and symptoms; patients who receive hemodialysis should receive 50 mg oral dose after each dialysis

Special Geriatric Considerations
Due to alterations in the beta-adrenergic autonomic nervous system, beta-adrenergic blockade may result in less hemodynamic response than seen in younger adults. Studies indicate that despite decreased sensitivity to the chronotropic effects of beta blockade with age, there appears to be an increased myocardial sensitivity to the negative inotropic effect during stress (ie, exercise). Controlled trials have shown the overall response rate for propranolol to be only 20% to 50% in elderly populations. Therefore, all beta-adrenergic blocking drugs may result in a decreased response as compared to younger adults.

Dosage Forms

Injection: 0.5 mg/mL (10 mL)

Tablet: 25 mg, 50 mg, 100 mg

References

Aagaard GN, "Treatment of Hypertension in The Elderly," *Drug Treatment in the Elderly*, Vestal RE, ed, Boston, MA: ADIS Health Science Press, 1984, 77.

Ativan® see Lorazepam *on page 551*

Atolone® see Triamcinolone *on page 949*

Atorvastatin (a TORE va sta tin)

Related Information
Antacid Drug Interactions *on page 1096*

Brand Names Lipitor®

Therapeutic Category Antilipemic Agent; HMG-CoA Reductase Inhibitor

Use Adjunct to diet for the primary reduction of elevated total, LDL-cholesterol, apolipoprotein B, and triglyceride levels in patients with primary hypercholesterolemia or mixed dyslipidemia; used in hypercholesterolemic patients without clinically evident heart disease to reduce the risk of myocardial infarction, to reduce the risk for revascularization, and reduce the risk of death due to cardiovascular causes

Contraindications Hypersensitivity to atorvastatin or its components (may have cross-sensitivity with other HMG-CoA reductase inhibitors); patients with active liver disease

Warnings Discontinue therapy if symptoms of myopathy or renal failure due to rhabdomyolysis develop

Precautions Use with caution in patients with history of liver disease or who consume excessive amounts of alcohol

Adverse Reactions
Central nervous system: Headache, giddiness, euphoria, mild confusion, impaired short-term memory
Gastrointestinal: Diarrhea, flatulence, abdominal pain
Hepatic: Mild LFT increases
Neuromuscular & skeletal: Myalgia
Respiratory: Pharyngitis, rhinitis

Overdosage Few symptoms anticipated

Toxicology Treatment is supportive

Drug Interactions
Increased toxicity: Gemfibrozil (musculoskeletal effects such as myopathy, myalgia and/or muscle weakness accompanied by markedly elevated CK concentrations, rash and/or pruritus); clofibrate, niacin (myopathy), erythromycin, clarithromycin, cyclosporine, itraconazole, protease inhibitors, oral anticoagulants (elevated PT)
Increased effect/toxicity of levothyroxine
Concurrent use of erythromycin and atorvastatin may result in rhabdomyolysis

Mechanism of Action Inhibitor of 3-hydroxy-3-methylglutaryl coenzyme A (HMG-CoA) reductase, the rate limiting enzyme in cholesterol synthesis (reduces the production of mevalonic acid from HMG-CoA); this then results in a compensatory increase in the expression of LDL receptors on hepatocyte membranes and a stimulation of LDL catabolism

Pharmacokinetics
Absorption: Rapid
Protein binding: 98%
Metabolism: Undergoes enterohepatic recycling; not a prodrug; metabolized to active ortho- and parahydroxylated derivates and an inactive beta-oxidation product; substrate for CYP3A4
Half-life: 14 hours (parent)
Time to peak serum concentration: 1-2 hours (maximal reduction in plasma cholesterol and triglycerides in 2 weeks)
Elimination: 2% excreted as unchanged drug in the urine
Note: In the elderly, C_{max} (42.5%) and AUC (27%) were increased; since activity does not correlate with plasma concentration, it is unknown if these changes are clinically significant

Usual Dosage Geriatrics and Adults: Oral: Initial: 10 mg once daily, titrate up to 80 mg/day if needed

Dosing adjustment in renal impairment: No dosage adjustment necessary
Dosing adjustment in hepatic impairment: Decrease dosage with severe disease (eg, chronic alcoholic liver disease)

Monitoring Parameters Lipid serum concentrations after 2-4 weeks; LFTs, CPK

Patient Information May take with food if desired; may take without regard to time of day

Nursing Implications The best effect is seen when administered at night; monitor for symptoms of adverse effects (See Adverse Reactions and Special Geriatric Considerations)

Special Geriatric Considerations Effective and well tolerated in the elderly. The definition of and, therefore, when to treat hyperlipidemia in the elderly is a
(Continued)

Atorvastatin *(Continued)*

controversial issue. The National Cholesterol Education Program recommends that all adults 20 years of age and older maintain a plasma cholesterol <200 mg/dL. By this definition, 60% of all elderly would be considered to have a borderline high (200-239 mg/dL) or high (≥240 mg/dL) plasma cholesterol. However, plasma cholesterol has been shown to be a less reliable predictor of coronary heart disease in the elderly. Therefore, it is the authors' belief that pharmacologic treatment be reserved for those who are unable to obtain a desirable plasma cholesterol concentration by diet alone and for whom the benefits of treatment are believed to outweigh the potential adverse effects, drug interactions, and cost of treatment.

Dosage Forms Tablet: 10 mg, 20 mg, 40 mg

References

Gibson DM, Bron NJ, Richens A, et al, "Effect of Age and Gender on Pharmacokinetics of Atorvastatin in Humans," *J Clin Pharmacol*, 1996, 36(3):242-6.

"Summary of the Second Report of the National Cholesterol Education Program (NCEP) Expert Panel on Detection, Evaluation, and Treatment of High Blood Cholesterol in Adults (Adult Treatment Panel II)," *JAMA*, 1993, 269(23):3015-23.

Atovaquone *(a TOE va kwone)*

Brand Names Mepron™

Therapeutic Category Antiprotozoal

Use Acute oral treatment of mild to moderate *Pneumocystis carinii* pneumonia (PCP) in patients who are intolerant to co-trimoxazole

Contraindications Life-threatening allergic reaction to the drug or formulation

Warnings Has only been used in mild to moderate PCP; use with caution in elderly patients because of potentially impaired renal, hepatic, and cardiac function

Adverse Reactions

Central nervous system: Fever, insomnia, headache, anxiety, dizziness

Dermatologic: Rash, pruritus

Endocrine & metabolic: Hypoglycemia, amylase, hyponatremia

Gastrointestinal: Nausea, diarrhea, vomiting, abdominal pain, anorexia, dyspepsia, oral *Monilia*, constipation

Hematologic: Leukopenia, neutropenia, anemia

Hepatic: Elevated liver enzymes (ALT, AST, alkaline phosphatase)

Neuromuscular & skeletal: Weakness

Renal: Elevated BUN and creatinine

Respiratory: Cough

Drug Interactions Possible increased toxicity with other highly protein bound drugs; however, serum concentrations of 15 mcg/mL of phenytoin failed to cause an interaction

Mechanism of Action Mechanism has not been fully elucidated; may inhibit electron transport in mitochondria inhibiting metabolic enzymes

Pharmacokinetics

Absorption: Decreased significantly in single doses >750 mg; increased threefold when administered with a high fat meal

Distribution: Enterohepatically recirculated

Protein binding: >99.9%

Bioavailability: ~30%

Half-life: 2.9 days

Elimination: In feces

Usual Dosage Geriatrics and Adults: Oral: 750 mg twice daily with food for 21 days

Patient Information Take only prescribed dose; take each dose with a meal, preferably one with high fat content

Nursing Implications Notify physician if patient is unable to eat significant amounts of food on an ongoing basis

Special Geriatric Considerations Has not been extensively evaluated in patients >65 years of age (see Warnings)

Dosage Forms Suspension, oral (citrus flavor): 750 mg/5 mL (210 mL)

Atozine® *see* Hydroxyzine *on page 470*

Atretol® *see* Carbamazepine *on page 160*

Atromid-S® *see* Clofibrate *on page 235*

Atropair® *see* Atropine *on this page*

Atropine *(A troe peen)*

Related Information

Antidotes *on page 1097*

Asthma Guidelines *on page 1040*
I.V. Push Recommended Guidelines *on page 1083*

Brand Names Atropair®; Atropine-Care®; Atropisol®; Isopto® Atropine; I-Tropine®; Ocu-Tropine®

Generic Available Yes

Therapeutic Category Anticholinergic Agent; Anticholinergic Agent, Ophthalmic; Antidote, Organophosphate Poisoning; Antispasmodic Agent, Gastrointestinal; Bronchodilator; Ophthalmic Agent, Mydriatic

Use Preoperative medication to inhibit salivation and secretions; treatment of sinus bradycardia; management of peptic ulcer; treatment of exercise-induced bronchospasm; urinary incontinence; antidote for organophosphate pesticide poisoning; used to produce mydriasis and cycloplegia for examination of the retina and optic disk and accurate measurement of refractive errors; uveitis

Contraindications Hypersensitivity to atropine sulfate or any component; narrow-angle glaucoma; tachycardia; thyrotoxicosis; obstructive disease of the GI tract; obstructive uropathy, asthma

Precautions Use with caution in geriatric patients since they may be more sensitive to its effects. Low doses cause a paradoxical decrease in heart rate. Some commercial products contain sodium metabisulfite, which can cause allergic-type reactions. Heat prostration may occur in hot weather. Use with caution in patients with autonomic neuropathy, prostatic hypertrophy, hyperthyroidism, congestive heart failure, cardiac arrhythmias, chronic lung disease, biliary tract disease.

Adverse Reactions
Cardiovascular: Tachycardia, palpitations
Central nervous system: Fatigue, ataxia, delirium, headache, restlessness, ataxia. **Note: The elderly may be at increased risk for confusion and hallucinations**.
Dermatologic: Dry hot skin
Gastrointestinal: Impaired GI motility, xerostomia
Genitourinary: Dysuria
Neuromuscular & skeletal: Tremors
Ocular: Mydriasis, blurred vision
Miscellaneous: Heat intolerance

Toxicology Anticholinergic toxicity is caused by strong binding of the drug to cholinergic receptors. Cholinesterase inhibitors reduce acetylcholinesterase, the enzyme that breaks down acetylcholine and thereby allows acetylcholine to accumulate and compete for receptor binding with the offending anticholinergic. For anticholinergic overdose with severe life-threatening symptoms, physostigmine 1-2 mg S.C. or I.V., slowly may be given to reverse these effects.

Drug Interactions
Decreased effect of phenothiazines, levodopa, metoclopramide, cisapride
Increased toxicity: Amantadine, tricyclic antidepressants, some antihistamines
Antagonistic effect: Tacrine, donepezil

Stability Store injection below 40°C, avoid freezing

Mechanism of Action Blocks the action of acetylcholine at parasympathetic sites in smooth muscle, secretory glands and the CNS; increases cardiac output, dries secretions, antagonizes histamine and serotonin

Pharmacokinetics
Absorption: Well absorbed from all dosage forms
Distribution: Wide throughout the body; crosses the blood-brain barrier
Metabolism: In the liver
Half-life: 2-3 hours
Elimination: Into urine of both metabolites and unchanged drug (30% to 50%)

Usual Dosage Geriatrics and Adults:
Preanesthetic: I.M., I.V., S.C.: 0.4-0.6 mg 30-60 minutes preop
Bradycardia: I.V.: 0.5-1 mg every 5 minutes, not to exceed a total of 2 mg
Ophthalmic, 1% solution: 1-2 drops before the procedure
Uveitis: 1-2 drops 4 times/day

Monitoring Parameters Blood pressure, pulse, mental status, anticholinergic effects

Patient Information Maintain good oral hygiene habits, because lack of saliva may increase chance of cavities. Observe caution while driving or performing other tasks requiring alertness, as may cause drowsiness, dizziness, or blurred vision. Notify physician if skin rash, flushing or eye pain occurs, or if difficulty in urinating, constipation, or sensitivity to light becomes severe or persists.

(Continued)

Atropine (Continued)

Nursing Implications Observe for tachycardia if patient has cardiac problems; lack of saliva may increase chance of cavities, therefore, good oral hygiene should be promoted

Additional Information Because of its bothersome and potentially dangerous side effects, atropine is rarely used except as a preoperative agent or in the acute treatment of bradyarrhythmias

Special Geriatric Considerations Anticholinergic agents are generally not well tolerated in the elderly and their use should be avoided when possible (see Precautions, Adverse Reactions). In the elderly, anticholinergic agents should not be used as prophylaxis against extrapyramidal symptoms.

Dosage Forms

Atropine sulfate:

Injection: 0.1 mg/mL (5 mL, 10 mL); 0.3 mg/mL (1 mL, 30 mL); 0.4 mg/mL (1 mL, 20 mL, 30 mL); 0.5 mg/mL (1 mL, 5 mL, 30 mL); 0.8 mg/mL (0.5 mL, 1 mL); 1 mg/mL (1 mL, 10 mL)

Ophthalmic:

Ointment: 0.5%, 1% (3.5 g)

Solution: 0.5% (5 mL); 1% (2 mL); 2% (1 mL, 2 mL); 3% (5 mL)

Tablet: 0.4 mg

Tablet, soluble: 0.4 mg, 0.6 mg

References

Feinberg M, "The Problems of Anticholinergic Adverse Effects in Older Patients," *Drugs Aging,* 1993, 3(4):335-48.

Atropine and Diphenoxylate *see* Diphenoxylate and Atropine *on page 303*

Atropine-Care® *see* Atropine *on page 92*

Atropisol® *see* Atropine *on page 92*

Atrovent® *see* Ipratropium *on page 495*

A/T/S® Topical *see* Erythromycin, Topical *on page 347*

Attapulgite (at a PULL gite)

Brand Names Children's Kaopectate® [OTC]; Diasorb® [OTC]; Kaopectate® Advanced Formula [OTC]; Kaopectate® Maximum Strength Caplets; Rheaban® [OTC]

Generic Available Yes

Therapeutic Category Antidiarrheal

Use Symptomatic treatment of diarrhea

Restrictions See Warnings and Precautions

Contraindications Fecal impaction; constipation, ileus

Warnings Do not use with diarrhea associated with toxigenic bacteria or pseudomembranous colitis

Precautions Use with caution in patients >60 years of age due to fecal impaction potential; presence of high fever; do not use in patients predisposed to fecal impaction

Adverse Reactions Gastrointestinal: Constipation, fecal impaction

Overdosage May cause bowel impaction and intestinal obstruction

Drug Interactions Digoxin absorption may be decreased due to adsorbent action of attapulgite; caution should be used with concomitant administration of any drug due to attapulgite's adsorbent action

Mechanism of Action Controls diarrhea because of its adsorbent action

Pharmacokinetics Absorption: Not absorbed from GI tract

Usual Dosage Geriatrics and Adults: Oral: 1200-1500 mg after each loose bowel movement or every 2 hours; 15-30 mL up to 8 times/day, or up to 9000 mg/24 hours

Monitoring Parameters Monitor for reduction of stools per day and increased consistency; monitor for signs of fluid and electrolyte loss

Patient Information If diarrhea is not controlled in 48 hours, contact a physician

Nursing Implications Shake well before giving; re-evaluate cause of diarrhea if not controlled in 48 hours; diarrhea should also be treated by diet (ie, clear liquids, bland foods, and no dairy products for first 24-48 hours); monitor for signs of fluid and electrolyte loss

Special Geriatric Considerations Elderly often present bowel impaction with diarrhea. The use of adsorbents in the face of fecal impaction could aggravate this serious condition. Also, diarrhea causes fluid/electrolyte loss which elderly do not tolerate well. Use of adsorbents can cause further loss of fluid/electrolytes.

Dosage Forms
Liquid, oral concentrate: 600 mg/15 mL (180 mL, 240 mL, 360 mL, 480 mL); 750 mg/15 mL (120 mL)
Tablet: 750 mg
Tablet, chewable: 300 mg, 600 mg

Attenuvax® see Measles Virus Vaccine, Live on page 574

Augmentin® see Amoxicillin and Clavulanate Potassium on page 68

Auranofin (au RANE oh fin)

Brand Names Ridaura®

Generic Available No

Therapeutic Category Gold Compound

Use Management of active stage of classic or definite rheumatoid arthritis in patients that do not respond to or tolerate other agents; psoriatic arthritis; adjunctive or alternative therapy for pemphigus

Contraindications Renal disease, history of blood dyscrasias, congestive heart failure, exfoliative dermatitis, necrotizing enterocolitis, history of anaphylactic reactions

Warnings Therapy should be discontinued if platelet count falls to <100,000/mm³, WBC to <4000, or <1500 granulocytes/mm³; explain the possibility of adverse reactions before initiating therapy; signs of gold toxicity include decrease in hemoglobin, leukopenia, granulocytes and platelets; proteinuria, hematuria, pruritus, stomatitis, persistent diarrhea, rash, metallic taste; diabetes mellitus and congestive heart failure should be in control before initiating therapy; use cautiously in patients with a history of blood dyscrasias, bone marrow suppression, inflammatory bowel disease, allergic hemolytic anemias, drug allergy, or hypersensitivity, skin rash, history of renal or liver disease, uncontrolled hypertension, or compromised cerebral or cardiovascular circulation.

Precautions Use with caution in patients with impaired renal or hepatic function; NSAIDs and corticosteroids may be discontinued over time after initiating gold therapy; do not use with penicillamine, antimalarials, immunosuppressives, other than corticosteroids; for mild or minor adverse reactions, hold therapy until reaction resolves then may resume therapy at reduced doses; moderate to severe reaction requires discontinuation of gold therapy

Adverse Reactions
Central nervous system: Confusion, hallucination, seizures, fever, headache
Dermatologic: Dermatitis, pruritus, alopecia, gray-to-blue pigmentation
Gastrointestinal: Diarrhea (50%), loose stools, stomatitis, abdominal cramping, constipation, flatulence, dyspepsia, melena, GI bleeding, mouth ulcers, dysgeusia, dysphagia, metallic taste
Genitourinary: Vaginitis
Hematologic: Thrombocytopenia, aplastic anemia, eosinophilia
Hepatic: Hepatitis, increased LFTs, jaundice
Ocular: Iritis, corneal ulcers
Renal: Proteinuria, hematuria, nephrotic syndrome, glomerulitis
Respiratory: Bronchitis, interstitial pneumonitis, fibrosis
Miscellaneous: "Nitritoid" reactions include flushing, syncope, dizziness, diaphoresis, nausea, vomiting, weakness

Overdosage Symptoms of overdose include hematuria, proteinuria, fever, nausea, vomiting, diarrhea

Toxicology For mild gold poisoning, dimercaprol 2.5 mg/kg 4 times/day for 2 days or for more severe forms of gold intoxication, dimercaprol 3 mg/kg every 4 hours for 2 days, should be initiated; then after 2 days, the initial dose should be repeated twice daily on the third day, and once daily thereafter for 10 days. Other chelating agents have been used with some success.

Drug Interactions Penicillamine, antimalarials, phenytoin, cytotoxic drugs, or immunosuppressive agents

Mechanism of Action The exact mechanism of action of gold is unknown; gold is taken up by macrophages which results in inhibition of phagocytosis and lysosomal membrane stabilization; other actions observed are decreased serum rheumatoid factor and alterations in immunoglobulins. Additionally, complement activation is decreased, prostaglandin synthesis is inhibited, and lysosomal enzyme activity is decreased.

Pharmacodynamics Therapeutic response may not be seen for 3-4 months after start of therapy

Pharmacokinetics
Absorption: Oral: ~15% to 33% (25% average) of gold in a dose
(Continued)

Auranofin (Continued)

Protein binding: 60%

Half-life: 21-31 days (half-life dependent upon single or multiple dosing)

Time to peak: Peak blood gold concentrations are seen within 2 hours; peak serum concentration: 1-2 hours

Elimination: 60% of absorbed gold is eliminated in urine while the remainder is eliminated in feces

Usual Dosage Geriatrics and Adults: Oral: 6 mg/day in 1-2 divided doses; after 6 months may be increased to 9 mg/day in 3 divided doses; if still no response after 3 months at 9 mg/day, discontinue drug; to start oral therapy after gold injections, discontinue parenteral gold and start oral gold at 6 mg/day either in divided doses or single daily dose

Monitoring Parameters Urinalysis, CBC with platelets done monthly; monitor for other side effects (see Adverse Reactions)

Reference Range Gold: Normal: 0-0.1 µg/mL (SI: 0-0.0064 µmol/L); Therapeutic: 1-3 µg/mL (SI: 0.06-0.18 µmol/L); urine <0.1 µg/24 hours

Test Interactions May enhance the response to a tuberculin skin test

Patient Information Minimize exposure to sunlight; report any signs of toxicity to physician (ie, pruritus, rash, sore mouth, indigestion, metallic taste); joint pain may take 1-2 months to start to subside

Nursing Implications Monitor urine for protein; CBC and platelets; monitor for mouth ulcers and skin reactions; may monitor serum concentration

Additional Information Metallic taste may indicate stomatitis

Special Geriatric Considerations Tolerance to gold decreases with advanced age; use cautiously only after traditional therapy and other disease modifying antirheumatic drugs (DMARDs) have been attempted

Dosage Forms Capsule: 3 mg = 29% gold

Auro® Ear Drops [OTC] see Carbamide Peroxide on page 162

Aurolate® see Gold Sodium Thiomalate on page 432

Aurothioglucose (aur oh thye oh GLOO kose)

Brand Names Solganal®

Generic Available No

Therapeutic Category Gold Compound

Use Adjunctive treatment in adult active rheumatoid arthritis; alternative or adjunct in treatment of pemphigus; treatment for psoriatic patients who do not respond to NSAIDs

Contraindications Renal disease, history of blood dyscrasias, congestive heart failure, exfoliative dermatitis, hepatic disease, SLE, history of hypersensitivity to gold or any component

Warnings Explain the possibility of adverse reactions before initiating therapy; signs of gold toxicity include decrease in hemoglobin, leukopenia, granulocytes and platelets; proteinuria, hematuria, pruritus, stomatitis, persistent diarrhea, rash, metallic taste; diabetes mellitus and congestive heart failure should be in control before initiating therapy; use cautiously in patients with a history of blood dyscrasias, bone marrow suppression, inflammatory bowel disease, allergic hemolytic anemias, drug allergy, or hypersensitivity, skin rash, history of renal or liver disease, uncontrolled hypertension, or compromised cerebral or cardiovascular circulation. Therapy should be discontinued if platelet count falls to <100,000/mm³, WBC to <4000, or <1500 granulocytes/mm³.

Precautions Use with caution in patients with impaired renal or hepatic function; NSAIDs and corticosteroids may be discontinued over time after initiating gold therapy; do not use with penicillamine, antimalarials, immunosuppressives, other than corticosteroids; for mild or minor adverse reactions, hold therapy until reaction resolves then may resume therapy at reduced doses; moderate to severe reaction requires discontinuation of gold therapy

Adverse Reactions

Central nervous system: Confusion, hallucinations, seizures, fever, headache

Dermatologic: Dermatitis, pruritus, alopecia, gray-to-blue pigmentation

Gastrointestinal: Stomatitis, flatulence, dyspepsia, melena, GI bleeding, mouth ulcers, dysgeusia, dysphagia, metallic taste

Genitourinary: Vaginitis

Hematologic: Thrombocytopenia, aplastic anemia, eosinophilia

Hepatic: Hepatitis, increased LFTs, jaundice

Ocular: Iritis, corneal ulcers

Renal: Proteinuria, hematuria, nephrotic syndrome, glomerulitis

Respiratory: Bronchitis, interstitial pneumonitis, fibrosis

Miscellaneous: "Nitritoid" reactions include flushing, syncope, dizziness, diaphoresis, nausea, vomiting, weakness

Overdosage Symptoms of overdose include hematuria, proteinuria, fever, nausea, vomiting, diarrhea, thrombocytopenia, agranulocytopenia, skin reaction (papulovesicular lesions, urticaria, pruritus, exfoliative dermatitis)

Toxicology For mild gold poisoning, dimercaprol 2.5 mg/kg 4 times/day for 2 days or for more severe forms of gold intoxication, dimercaprol 3-5 mg/kg every 4 hours for 2 days, should be initiated. Then after 2 days, the initial dose should be repeated twice daily on the third day, and once daily thereafter for 10 days. Other chelating agents have been used with some success.

Drug Interactions One report of increased phenytoin serum concentration with auranofin

Stability Protect from light and store at 15°C to 30°C

Mechanism of Action The exact mechanism of action of gold is unknown; gold is taken up by macrophages which results in inhibition of phagocytosis and lysosomal membrane stabilization; other actions observed are decreased serum rheumatoid factor and alterations in immunoglobulins. Additionally, complement activation is decreased, prostaglandin synthesis is inhibited, and lysosomal enzyme activity is decreased.

Pharmacodynamics Gold injections may result in decreased morning stiffness in 1-2 months; significant benefit may not be noted for 3-6 months

Pharmacokinetics
Absorption: I.M.: Erratic and slow
Protein binding: 95% to 99%
Metabolism: Unknown
Half-life: 3-27 days (single dose); 14-40 days (third dose); up to 168 days (11th dose)
Mean steady-state plasma concentration: 1-5 mcg/mL
Time to peak serum concentration: Within 4-6 hours
Elimination: Majority ultimately eliminated in urine and the remainder in feces; 70% renal excretion, 30% fecal

Usual Dosage Doses should initially be given at weekly intervals
Geriatrics and Adults: I.M.: 10 mg first week; 25 mg second and third week; then 50 mg/week until 800 mg to 1 g cumulative dose has been given; if improvement occurs without adverse reactions, administer 25-50 mg every 2-3 weeks for 2-20 weeks; then every 3-4 weeks if patient remains stable; if no response after cumulative dose of 1 g, discontinue therapy

Monitoring Parameters Each visit, the patient should have urinalysis, CBC with platelets initially; then every 6 months on maintenance therapy; monitor for other adverse reactions (see Adverse Reactions)

Reference Range Gold: Normal: 0-0.1 μg/mL (SI: 0-0.0064 μmol/L); Therapeutic: 1-3 μg/mL (SI: 0.06-0.18 μmol/L); urine <0.1 μg/24 hours

Patient Information Minimize exposure to sunlight; report any signs of toxicity to physician (ie, pruritus, rash, sore mouth, indigestion, metallic taste); joint pain may take 1-2 months to start to subside

Nursing Implications Deep I.M. injection into the upper outer quadrant of the gluteal region; addition of 0.1 mL of 1% lidocaine to each injection may reduce the discomfort with injection; vial should be thoroughly shaken before withdrawing a dose; explain the possibility of adverse reactions before initiating therapy; advise patients to report any symptoms of toxicity; monitor serum concentration, CBC, platelets, urine protein (see Adverse Reactions, Warnings, Patient Information)

Additional Information Patients with HLA-D locus histocompatibility antigens DRw2 and DRw3 may have genetic predisposition to toxic reactions

Special Geriatric Considerations Elderly have decreased tolerance to gold with age and may experience increased adverse effects; use cautiously only after traditional therapy and other disease modifying antirheumatic drugs (DMARDs) have been attempted

Dosage Forms Injection, suspension: 50 mg/mL [gold 50%] (10 mL)

Avapro® see Irbesartan on page 496

Aventyl® Hydrochloride see Nortriptyline on page 684

Axid® see Nizatidine on page 681

Axid® AR [OTC] see Nizatidine on page 681

Ayr® Saline [OTC] see Sodium Chloride on page 860

Azactam® see Aztreonam on page 102

Azatadine (a ZA ta deen)

Brand Names Optimine®
Generic Available No
(Continued)

Azatadine *(Continued)*

Therapeutic Category Antihistamine

Use Treatment of perennial and seasonal allergic rhinitis and chronic urticaria

Contraindications Hypersensitivity to azatadine or other components; patients receiving MAO inhibitors. Antihistamines should not be used to treat lower respiratory tract symptoms.

Warnings Use with caution in patient with narrow-angle glaucoma, stenosing peptic ulcer, urinary bladder obstruction, prostatic hypertrophy, asthmatic attacks. Antihistamines are more likely to cause dizziness, excessive sedation, syncope, toxic confusion states, and hypotension in the elderly.

Adverse Reactions
Central nervous system: Slight to moderate drowsiness, dizziness
Gastrointestinal: Nausea, vomiting, xerostomia
Ocular: Blurred vision
Respiratory: Thickening of bronchial secretions

Overdosage Symptoms of overdose include CNS depression or stimulation, dry mouth, flushed skin, fixed and dilated pupils, apnea

Toxicology There is no specific treatment for an antihistamine overdose, however, most of its clinical toxicity is due to anticholinergic effects. Cholinesterase inhibitors may be useful by reducing acetylcholinesterase. Acetylcholinesterase inhibitors include physostigmine, neostigmine, pyridostigmine, and edrophonium. For anticholinergic overdose with severe life-threatening symptoms, physostigmine 1-2 mg I.V., slowly may be given to reverse these effects.

Drug Interactions Increased effect/toxicity: Procarbazine, CNS depressants, tricyclic antidepressants, alcohol, MAO inhibitors

Mechanism of Action Azatadine is a piperidine-derivative antihistamine; has both anticholinergic and antiserotonin activity; has been demonstrated to inhibit mediator release from human mast cells *in vitro*; mechanism of this action is suggested to prevent calcium entry into the mast cell through voltage-dependent calcium channels

Pharmacokinetics
Absorption: Oral: 90%
Distribution: Crosses the blood-brain barrier
Protein binding: Minimally bound to plasma protein
Metabolism: Extensively conjugated in the liver
Half-life: 9 hours
Time to peak serum concentration: 4 hours after the dose
Elimination: 20% excreted unchanged in urine

Usual Dosage Oral:
Geriatrics: 1 mg once or twice daily
Adults: 1-2 mg twice daily

Monitoring Parameters Relief of symptoms, mental status

Patient Information May cause drowsiness; avoid CNS depressants and alcohol

Nursing Implications See Monitoring Parameters

Additional Information Azatadine offers no significant advantage over other antihistamines

Special Geriatric Considerations Anticholinergic effects are not well tolerated in elderly and frequently result in bowel, bladder, and mental adverse effects (ie, constipation, confusion, and urinary retention); see Warnings and Additional Information

Dosage Forms Tablet, as maleate: 1 mg

Azathioprine *(ay za THYE oh preen)*

Brand Names Imuran®

Generic Available No

Therapeutic Category Immunosuppressant Agent

Use Adjunct with other agents in prevention of rejection of renal transplants; also used in severe rheumatoid arthritis unresponsive to other agents; Crohn's disease, ulcerative colitis, multiple sclerosis

Contraindications Hypersensitivity to azathioprine or any component; patients with rheumatoid arthritis treated previously with alkylating agents may be at risk for secondary neoplasia

Warnings Chronic immunosuppression increases the risk of neoplasia; mutagenic potential; possible hematologic toxicities (leukopenia, thrombocytopenia); severe infections (fungal, bacterial, viral)

Precautions Use with caution in patients with liver disease, renal impairment, and those with cadaveric kidneys; reduce usual dosage 25% to 33% in patients receiving both allopurinol and azathioprine

Adverse Reactions
Cardiovascular: Hypotension
Central nervous system: Fever
Dermatologic: Alopecia, rash, maculopapular rash
Gastrointestinal: Nausea, vomiting, anorexia, diarrhea, aphthous stomatitis
Hematologic: Leukopenia, thrombocytopenia, bone marrow suppression
Hepatic: Hepatotoxicity
Neuromuscular & skeletal: Arthralgias, which include myalgias, rigors
Ocular: Retinopathy
Respiratory: Dyspnea
Miscellaneous: Rare hypersensitivity reactions

Overdosage Symptoms of overdose include nausea, vomiting, diarrhea

Toxicology Following initiation of essential overdose management, symptomatic and supportive treatment should be instituted. Dialysis has been reported to remove significant amounts of the drug and its metabolites, and should be considered as a treatment option in those patients who deteriorate despite established forms of therapy.

Drug Interactions Allopurinol; reduce dose to $1/4$ to $1/3$ of usual dosage if allopurinol is given concurrently

Stability
Stability of parenteral admixture at room temperature (25°C) and refrigeration (4°C): 24 hours
Stable in neutral or acid solutions, but is hydrolyzed to mercaptopurine in alkaline solutions

Mechanism of Action Antagonizes purine metabolism and may inhibit synthesis of DNA, RNA, and proteins; may also interfere with cellular metabolism and inhibit mitosis

Pharmacokinetics
Protein binding: ~30%
Metabolism: Extensive by hepatic xanthine oxidase to 6-mercaptopurine (active)
Half-life:
Parent: 12 minutes
6-mercaptopurine: 0.7-3 hours
Elimination: Small amounts excreted as unchanged drug; metabolites eliminated eventually in urine

Usual Dosage
Rheumatoid arthritis: Oral:
Geriatrics: 1 mg/kg/day (50-100 mg); titrate gradually by 25 mg/day until response or toxicity (see dose adjustment for renal function)
Adults: 1 mg/kg/day for 6-8 weeks; increase by 0.5 mg/kg every 4 weeks until response or up to 2.5 mg/kg/day I.V. dose is equivalent to oral dose
Renal transplantation: Geriatrics and Adults: Oral, I.V.: Initial: 3-5 mg/kg/day; maintenance: 1-3 mg/kg/day
Dosing adjustment in renal impairment:
Cl_{cr} 10-50 mL/minute: Administer 75% of dose
Cl_{cr} <10 mL/minute: Administer 50% of dose
Slightly dialyzable (5% to 20%)

Monitoring Parameters Perform CBC with platelets weekly for first month, twice monthly for second and third months, then monthly. Dose increases will require more frequent monitoring; early sign of toxicity is WBC count dropping to <3000-4000/mm³

Test Interactions Increased AST, ALT, bilirubin, alkaline phosphatase, amylase (S), prothrombin time; decreased uric acid, albumin

Patient Information Response in rheumatoid arthritis may not occur for up to 3 months; do not stop taking without the physician's approval, do not have any vaccinations before checking with your physician; check with your physician if you have a persistent sore throat, unusual bleeding or bruising, fatigue, abdominal pain, pale stools, darkened urine. May cause nausea, vomiting, fever, joint pain, and diarrhea; notify physician if persistent.

Nursing Implications Hematologic status should be monitored during therapy (see Monitoring Parameters)

Additional Information Azathioprine is an imidazolyl derivative of 6-mercaptopurine. If infection occurs, drug dosage should be reduced; NSAID therapy should be continued when beginning initial therapy with azathioprine in the treatment of rheumatoid arthritis

(Continued)

Azathioprine *(Continued)*

Special Geriatric Considerations Toxicity to immunosuppressives is increased in elderly. Start with lowest recommended adult doses. Signs of infection, such as fever and WBC rise, may not occur. Lethargy and confusion may be more prominent signs of infection. Adjust dose for renal function in elderly.

Dosage Forms
Injection, as sodium: 5 mg/mL (20 mL)
Tablet, scored: 50 mg

References
Hutchins LF and Lipschitz DA, "Cancer, Clinical Pharmacology, and Aging," *Clin Geriatr Med*, 1987, 3(3):483-503.
Kaplan HG, "Use of Cancer Chemotherapy in the Elderly," *Drug Treatment in the Elderly*, Vestal RE, ed, Boston, MA: ADIS Health Science Press, 1984, 338-49.

Azelastine *(a ZEL as teen)*

Brand Names Astelin®

Therapeutic Category Antihistamine, Intranasal

Use Treatment of symptoms of seasonal allergic rhinitis (ie, rhinorrhea, sneezing, nasal pruritus)

Contraindications Patients with a known hypersensitivity to azelastine or any of its components

Precautions Azelastine may cause somnolence; caution should be exercised when performing activities that require mental alertness. Concurrent use of alcohol or other CNS depressants with azelastine should be avoided. Avoid use of azelastine with other antihistamines unless advised by a physician; avoid spraying into eyes.

Adverse Reactions
Cardiovascular: Flushing, hypertension, tachycardia
Central nervous system: Headache (14.8%), somnolence (11.5%), fatigue, dizziness, hypoesthesia, vertigo, anxiety, depersonalization, depression, nervousness, sleep disorder, abnormal thinking
Dermatological: Contact dermatitis, eczema, hair and follicle infection, furunculosis
Endocrine & metabolic: Amenorrhea, breast pain
Gastrointestinal: Bitter taste (19.7%), dry mouth, nausea, weight increase, constipation, gastroenteritis, glossitis, increased appetite, ulcerative stomatitis, vomiting, increased ALT, aphthous stomatitis, taste loss
Neuromuscular & skeletal: Myalgia, temporomandibular dislocation, hyperkinesia
Ocular: Conjunctivitis, eye abnormality, eye pain, watery eyes
Renal: Albuminuria, hematuria, increased urinary frequency
Respiratory: Nasal burning, pharyngitis, paroxysmal sneezing, rhinitis, epistaxis, bronchospasm, coughing, throat burning, laryngitis
Body as a whole: Allergic reaction, back pain, herpes simplex, viral infection, malaise, pain in extremities, abdominal pain

Toxicology There have been no reported overdoses with azelastine; increased somnolence is likely to occur; supportive measures should be employed

Drug Interactions Increased effect: Alcohol and CNS depressants cause additive somnolence and CNS impairment. Cimetidine 400 mg twice daily increases the AUC and C_{max} of azelastine by 65%. (Ranitidine, erythromycin, and ketoconazole have shown no effect on azelastine pharmacokinetics.)

Mechanism of Action Azelastine competes with histamine for histamine$_1$-receptor sites on effector cells in the GI tract, blood vessels, and respiratory tract. This action inhibits the symptoms associated with seasonal allergic rhinitis (ie, sneezing, pruritus, increased mucus production).

Pharmacokinetics
Distribution: 14.5 L/kg
Protein binding: 88%, 97% for active metabolite, desmethylazelastine
Metabolism: Hepatic
Bioavailability: 40%
Half-life: Azelastine 22 hours, desmethylazelastine 54 hours
Time to peak: 2-3 hours
Elimination: 75% feces

Usual Dosage Geriatrics and Adults: 2 sprays (137 mcg/spray) per nostril twice daily. Before initial use, the delivery system should be primed with 4 sprays or until a fine mist appears. If 3 or more days have elapsed since last use, the delivery system should be reprimed.

Monitoring Parameters Relief of symptoms

Patient Information Avoid spraying in eyes; store bottle in upright position with pump tightly closed. Before initial use, prime the pump with 4 sprays or until a fine mist appears. If not used for 3 or more days, prime the pump with 2 sprays. Do not take other antihistamines without telling your physician.

Nursing Implications Instruct patient in appropriate technique (see Patient Information)

Additional Information Azelastine is absorbed systemically; will cause sedation in some patients. Although this agent is clinically effective, the side effects of sedation, bitter taste, and high cost will limit its use in many patients.

Special Geriatric Considerations Only a small number of older subjects were included in premarketing trials. In those patients, side effects were no different than in younger patients (see Adverse Effects, Additional Information, and Patient Information).

Dosage Forms Spray, nasal, as hydrochloride: 137 mcg/actuation [100 actuations/bottle]

Azithromycin (az ith roe MYE sin)

Related Information

Cephalosporins, Aminoglycosides, Macrolides, & Quinolones *on page 1014*

Prevention of Bacterial Endocarditis *on page 1062*

Brand Names Zithromax™

Generic Available No

Therapeutic Category Antibiotic, Macrolide

Use Treatment of adult patients (>16 years of age) with mild to moderate infections of susceptible strains in upper and lower respiratory tract, skin and skin structure, and sexually transmitted diseases due to nongonococcal urethritis and cervicitis due to *Chlamydia trachomatis*; prevention of *Mycobacterium avium* complex (MAC) in patients with advanced HIV infection

Contraindications Hypersensitivity to azithromycin, erythromycin, or other macrolide antibiotics; use with pimozide

Warnings Patients with a community-acquired pneumonia due to *S. pneumoniae* or *H. influenzae* should be stable enough for outpatient oral treatment. Patients who are dehydrated, not eating, have respiratory, cardiac, or other chronic illnesses that may be exacerbated by pneumonia should be hospitalized. Not for nosocomial pneumonia, patients with documented or suspected bacteremia, or in patients who are immunocompromised. Pseudomembranous colitis is possible with any broad spectrum antibiotic, if suspected, stop the drug and pursue appropriate diagnostic work-up and treatment. Patients treated for nongonococcal urethritis or cervicitis should have a serological test for syphilis and gonococcal culture taken. Use caution in patients with impaired hepatic or renal function. Cardiac effects have been reported with other macrolides, but not with azithromycin.

Adverse Reactions All adverse reactions are reportedly reversible after discontinuation of the drug

Cardiovascular: Palpitations, chest pain

Central nervous system: Dizziness, headache, fatigue

Dermatologic: Allergy and rash, photosensitivity, angioedema

Gastrointestinal: Diarrhea (5%), nausea (3%), and abdominal pain (3%), dyspepsia, flatulence, vomiting, melena

Genitourinary: Vaginitis, *Monilia*

Hematologic: Leukopenia, neutropenia, decreased platelet count, alkaline bilirubin, blood glucose, LDH and phosphate; increased phosphokinase, potassium, ALT, GGT, and AST

Hepatic: Cholestatic jaundice

Renal: Nephritis, elevated BUN, serum creatinine

Overdosage Information is limited, GI symptoms such as nausea, vomiting

Toxicology Evacuation of unabsorbed drug when possible and other general supportive measures

Drug Interactions Aluminum- and magnesium-containing antacids will decrease peak serum concentrations, but not the extent of absorption; other macrolide antibiotics such as erythromycin, have been shown to increase theophylline serum concentrations and enhance warfarin's anticoagulant effect. These findings have not been identified with azithromycin, still careful monitoring is advised.

Drug/Food Interactions Food decreases C_{max} and bioavailability by 52% and 43% respectively (see Usual Dosage)

(Continued)

Azithromycin (Continued)

Mechanism of Action Inhibits microbial protein synthesis by binding to the 50S ribosomal subunit

Pharmacokinetics

Absorption: Oral: Rapidly absorbed from the GI tract

Distribution: Rapidly and widely distributed to body tissues and fluids; CSF concentrations are minimal in the presence of noninflamed meninges; tissue concentrations, particularly in fibroblasts and phagocytes, are greater than those in plasma or serum; steady-state volume of distribution: 31.1 L/kg

Protein binding: Serum protein binding appears to be concentration-dependent, ranging from 51% at 0.02 mcg/mL to 7% at 2 mcg/mL

Half-life, terminal: Averages 68 hours in healthy young adults

Elimination: Biliary excretion of unchanged drug is the primary route of elimination, with ~6% of unchanged drug eliminated in the urine over a 1-week period

The long half-life and large volume of distribution are believed to be secondary to the high affinity for tissues. In elderly women, but not in elderly men, peak serum concentrations were 30% to 50% greater compared to young adults; however, no significant accumulation was noted.

Usual Dosage Geriatrics and Adults:

Oral: 500 mg as a single loading dose on day 1 followed by 250 mg/day on days 2-5 (1.5 g total); the recommended dose for nongonococcal urethritis and cervicitis due to *C. trachomatis* is a single 1 g dose; take 1 hour before or 2 hours after meals

Mycobacterium avium prevention: Oral: 1200 mg once weekly

I.V.:

Community-acquired pneumonia: 500 mg as a single dose for at least 2 days, follow I.V. therapy by the oral route with a single daily dose of 500 mg to complete a 7- to 10-day course of therapy

Pelvic inflammatory disease (PID): 500 mg as a single dose for 1-2 days, follow I.V. therapy by the oral route with a single daily dose of 250 mg to complete a 7-day course of therapy

Monitoring Parameters Signs and symptoms of infection, mental status, appetite; hydration; cultures and sensitivity, if appropriate

Patient Information Complete full course of therapy; take on an empty stomach (1 hour before or 2 hours after meals); do not take with aluminum- or magnesium-containing antacids; notify physician if sore throat, unusual bleeding, or other infections occur

Nursing Implications Monitor tolerance to medication; do not administer concurrently with aluminum or magnesium antacids (see Drug Interactions); monitor respiratory, cardiac, and fluid status of nursing home patients being treated for pneumonia

Special Geriatric Considerations Dosage adjustment does not appear to be necessary in the elderly (see Usual Dosage and Pharmacokinetics); considered one of the drugs of choice in the treatment of outpatient treatment of community-acquired pneumonia in older adults (see Warnings)

Dosage Forms

Azithromycin dihydrate:

Capsule: 250 mg

Powder for injection: 500 mg

Powder for oral suspension: 100 mg/5 mL (15 mL); 200 mg/5 mL (15 mL, 22.5 mL); 1 g (single-dose packet)

Tablet: 250 mg, 600 mg

References

American Thoracic Society, "Guidelines for the Initial Management of Adults With Community-Acquired Pneumonia: Diagnosis, Assessment of Severity, and Initial Antimicrobial Therapy," *Am Rev Respir Dis*, 1993, 148(5):1418-26.

Coates P, Daniel R, Houston AC, et al, "An Open Study to Compare the Pharmacokinetics, Safety, and Tolerability of a Multiple-Dose Regimen of Azithromycin in Young and Elderly Volunteers," *Eur J Clin Microbiol Infect Dis*, 1991, 10(10):850-2.

Peters DH, Friedel HA, and McTavish D, "Azithromycin: A Review of Its Antimicrobial Activity, Pharmacokinetic Properties and Clinical Efficacy," *Drugs*, 1992, 44(5):750-99.

Azmacort™ see Triamcinolone *on page 949*

Azo-Standard® [OTC] see Phenazopyridine *on page 734*

Azthreonam see Aztreonam *on this page*

Aztreonam (AZ tree oh nam)

Related Information

I.V. Medication Recommendations *on page 1080*

Penicillins, Penicillin-Related Antibiotics, & Other Antibiotics *on page 1010*

Brand Names Azactam®

Synonyms Azthreonam

Generic Available No

Therapeutic Category Antibiotic, Miscellaneous

Use Treatment of patients with documented multidrug-resistant aerobic gram-negative infection in which beta-lactam therapy is contraindicated; used for urinary tract infection, lower respiratory tract infections, septicemia, skin/skin structure infections, intra-abdominal infections, and gynecological infections

Contraindications Hypersensitivity to aztreonam or any component

Warnings Check hypersensitivity to other beta-lactams; may have cross-allergenicity to penicillins and cephalosporins

Precautions Requires dosage reduction in renal impairment

Adverse Reactions
  Cardiovascular: Hypotension, transient EKG changes
  Central nervous system: Seizures, confusion, insomnia, dizziness
  Dermatologic: Rash, purpura, erythema multiforme, urticaria, petechiae, exfoliative dermatitis
  Gastrointestinal: Diarrhea, nausea, vomiting, pseudomembranous colitis
  Hematologic: Thrombocytopenia, eosinophilia, leukopenia, neutropenia
  Hepatic: Elevation of liver enzymes, jaundice
  Local: Pain at injection site, thrombophlebitis

Toxicology If necessary, dialysis can reduce the drug concentration in the blood

Drug Interactions Avoid antibiotics that induce beta-lactamase production (cefoxitin, imipenem); probenecid and furosemide significantly increase aztreonam serum concentrations

Stability Reconstituted solutions are colorless to light yellow straw colored and may turn pink upon standing without affecting potency; use reconstituted solutions and I.V. solutions (in NS and D₅W) within 48 hours if kept at room temperature or 7 days if kept in refrigerator; reconstituted solutions are **not** for multiple-dose use; incompatible when mixed with nafcillin, metronidazole

Mechanism of Action Inhibits bacterial cell wall synthesis during active multiplication causing cell wall destruction

Pharmacokinetics
  Absorption: I.M.: Well absorbed
  Distribution: V_d (adults): 0.2 L/kg
  Protein binding: 56%
  Half-life: 1.3-2.2 hours (half-life prolonged in renal failure)
  Time to peak serum concentration: Within 60 minutes following a dose
  Elimination: 60% to 70% excreted unchanged in urine and partially excreted in feces
  In healthy older adults with normal renal function (mean Cl_{cr}: 99 mL/minute), there were no significant changes in pharmacokinetic parameters. However, in older adults with impaired renal function (mean Cl_{cr}: 24 mL/minute) serum concentrations were inversely related to Cl_{cr}

Usual Dosage
  Geriatrics: Similar to adult dosing with appropriate adjustments for renal function (see below):
  Adults:
    Urinary tract infection: I.M., I.V.: 500 mg to 1 g every 8-12 hours
    Moderately severe systemic infections: 1 g I.V. or I.M. or 2 g I.V. every 8-12 hours
    Severe systemic or life-threatening infections (especially caused by *Pseudomonas aeruginosa*): I.V.: 2 g every 6-8 hours; maximum: 8 g/day
  Dosing interval in renal impairment:
    Cl_{cr} 10-30 mL/minute: Initial dose of 500 mg, 1 g, or 2 g, then reduce dose 50% given at the usual interval
    Cl_{cr} <10 mL/minute: Initial dose of 500 mg, 1 g, or 2 g, then reduce dose 75% given at the usual interval
  Moderately dialyzable (20% to 50%)

Administration I.V. route preferred for single doses >1 g or in patients with severe life-threatening infections; administer by IVP over 3-5 minutes or by intermittent infusion over 20-60 minutes at a final concentration not to exceed 20 mg/mL

Monitoring Parameters Resolution of signs and symptoms of infection, periodic liver function tests

Test Interactions Urine glucose (Clinitest®)

Nursing Implications See Administration
(Continued)

Aztreonam (Continued)

Additional Information Normally used with other antibiotics in life-threatening situations; member of new class of antibiotics called monobactams, with excellent gram-negative bacteria effectiveness, without ototoxicity or nephrotoxicity

Special Geriatric Considerations Adjust dose to renal function (see Pharmacokinetics and Usual Dosage)

Dosage Forms Injection: 500 mg (15 mL, 100 mL); 1 g (15 mL, 100 mL); 2 g (15 mL, 100 mL)

References

Creasey WA, Platt TB, Frantz M, et al, "Pharmacokinetics of Aztreonam in Elderly Male Volunteers," Br J Clin Pharmacol, 1985, 19:233-7.

Settler FR, Schramm M, Swabb EA, "Safety of Aztreonam and SQ 26,992 in Elderly Patients With Renal Insufficiency," Rev Infect Dis, 1985, (Suppl 4):5622.

Azulfidine® see Sulfasalazine on page 877

Azulfidine® EN-tabs® see Sulfasalazine on page 877

Bacid® [OTC] see Lactobacillus acidophilus and Lactobacillus bulgaricus on page 522

Baclofen (BAK loe fen)

Brand Names Lioresal®

Generic Available No

Therapeutic Category Skeletal Muscle Relaxant

Use Treatment of reversible spasticity associated with multiple sclerosis or spinal cord lesions

Unlabeled use: Trigeminal neuralgia, tardive dyskinesia, restless legs syndrome

Contraindications Hypersensitivity to baclofen or any component

Warnings Avoid abrupt withdrawal of the drug

Precautions Use with caution in patients with seizure disorder, impaired renal function

Adverse Reactions

Cardiovascular: Hypotension

Central nervous system: Drowsiness, fatigue, vertigo, dizziness, psychiatric disturbances, insomnia, slurred speech, headache, ataxia, hypotonia

Dermatologic: Rash

Gastrointestinal: Nausea, constipation, anorexia

Genitourinary: Polyuria, impotence

Overdosage Symptoms of overdose include vomiting, muscle hypotonia, salivation, drowsiness, coma, seizures, respiratory depression

Toxicology Following initiation of essential overdose management, symptomatic and supportive treatment should be instituted; atropine has been used to improve ventilation, heart rate, blood pressure, and core body temperature

Drug Interactions

Increased effect of opiate analgesics, benzodiazepines, hypertensive agents

Increased toxicity: CNS depressants (sedation), tricyclic antidepressants (short-term memory loss), clindamycin (neuromuscular blockade), guanabenz (sedation), MAO inhibitors (decreased blood pressure, CNS, and respiratory effects)

Mechanism of Action Inhibits the transmission of both monosynaptic and polysynaptic reflexes at the spinal cord level, possibly by hyperpolarization of primary afferent fiber terminals, with resultant relief of muscle spasticity

Pharmacodynamics

Onset of muscle relaxation effects: 3-4 days

Maximum clinical effects: Not seen for 5-10 days

Pharmacokinetics

Absorption: Oral: Rapid; absorption from the GI tract is thought to be dose dependent

Protein binding: 30%

Metabolized: Minimally in the liver

Half-life: 3.5 hours

Time to peak serum concentration: Within 2-3 hours

Elimination: 85% of oral dose excreted in urine and feces as unchanged drug

Usual Dosage Oral (the lowest effective dose is recommended; if benefits are not seen, withdraw the drug slowly):

Geriatrics: Initial: 5 mg 2-3 times/day, increasing gradually as needed

Adults: 5 mg 3 times/day, may increase 5 mg/dose every 3 days to a maximum of 80 mg/day

Intrathecal:

Test dose: 50-100 mcg, doses >50 mcg should be given in 25 mcg increments, separated by 24 hours

Maintenance: After positive response to test dose, a maintenance intrathecal infusion can be administered via an implanted intrathecal pump. Initial dose via pump: Infusion at a 24-hourly rate dosed at twice the test dose.

Dosing adjustment in renal impairment: May be necessary to reduce dosage

Monitoring Parameters Symptoms, blood pressure, mental status

Test Interactions Increased alkaline phosphatase, AST, glucose, ammonia (B); decreased bilirubin (S)

Patient Information Take with food or milk; abrupt withdrawal after prolonged use may cause anxiety, hallucinations, tachycardia or spasticity. Avoid alcohol and other CNS depressants. May cause drowsiness, dizziness, and fatigue.

Nursing Implications Epileptic patients should be closely monitored; supervise ambulation; avoid abrupt withdrawal of the drug

Additional Information Not indicated for muscle spasm associated with rheumatic disorders; not recommended in Parkinson's disease or stroke since the efficacy has not been established

Special Geriatric Considerations The elderly are more sensitive to the effects of baclofen and are more likely to experience adverse CNS effects at higher doses. Two cases of encephalopathy were reported after inadvertent high doses (50 mg/day and 90 mg/day) were given to elderly patients.

Dosage Forms

Injection, intrathecal, preservative free: 500 mcg/mL (20 mL); 2000 mcg/mL (5 mL)

Tablet: 10 mg, 20 mg

References

Abarbanel J, Herishanu Y, Frisher S, "Encephalopathy Associated With Baclofen," *Ann Neurol*, 1985, 17(6):617-8.

Tan AK and Tan CB, "The Syndrome of Painful Legs and Moving Toes...A Case Report," *Singapore Med J*, 1996, 37(4):446-7.

Bactocill® see Oxacillin *on page 698*

BactoShield® Topical [OTC] see Chlorhexidine Gluconate *on page 206*

Bactrim™ see Co-Trimoxazole *on page 253*

Bactrim™ DS see Co-Trimoxazole *on page 253*

Bactroban® see Mupirocin *on page 643*

Bactroban® Nasal see Mupirocin *on page 643*

Baking Soda see Sodium Bicarbonate *on page 858*

Baldex® see Dexamethasone *on page 274*

Bancap HC® see Hydrocodone and Acetaminophen *on page 461*

Banesin® [OTC] see Acetaminophen *on page 16*

Banophen® Oral [OTC] see Diphenhydramine *on page 302*

Barbidonna® see Hyoscyamine, Atropine, Scopolamine, and Phenobarbital *on page 472*

Barbita® see Phenobarbital *on page 737*

Baridium® [OTC] see Phenazopyridine *on page 734*

Barophen® see Hyoscyamine, Atropine, Scopolamine, and Phenobarbital *on page 472*

Baycol® see Cerivastatin *on page 199*

Bayer® Aspirin [OTC] see Aspirin *on page 84*

Bayer® Buffered Aspirin [OTC] see Aspirin *on page 84*

Bayer® Low Adult Strength [OTC] see Aspirin *on page 84*

Beclomethasone (be kloe METH a sone)

Related Information

Asthma Guidelines *on page 1040*

Estimated Comparative Daily Dosages for Inhaled Corticosteroids *on page 1045*

Inhaled Medications Comparison *on page 1034*

Brand Names Beclovent® Oral Inhaler; Beconase AQ® Nasal Inhaler; Beconase® Nasal Inhaler; Vancenase® AQ Inhaler; Vancenase® Nasal Inhaler; Vanceril® Oral Inhaler

Generic Available No

Therapeutic Category Anti-inflammatory Agent; Corticosteroid, Inhalant

(Continued)

Beclomethasone (Continued)

Use
Oral inhalation: Treatment of bronchial asthma in patients who require chronic administration of corticosteroids

Nasal aerosol: Symptomatic treatment of seasonal or perennial rhinitis and nasal polyposis

Contraindications Status asthmaticus; hypersensitivity to the drug or fluorocarbons, oleic acid in the formulation

Warnings Not to be used in status asthmaticus

Precautions Avoid using higher than recommended dosages since suppression of hypothalamic, pituitary, or adrenal function may occur

Adverse Reactions
Central nervous system: Headache

Gastrointestinal: Xerostomia

Local: Growth of *Candida* in the mouth

Respiratory: Cough, sneezing, pulmonary infiltrates, hoarseness, rhinorrhea, nasal congestion, irritation and burning of the nasal mucosa, nasal ulceration

Miscellaneous: Epistaxis

Overdosage Nasal: Irritation and burning of the nasal mucosa, sneezing, intranasal and pharyngeal *Candida* infections, nasal ulceration, epistaxis, rhinorrhea, nasal stuffiness, headache

Toxicology When consumed in excessive quantities for prolonged periods, systemic hypercorticism and adrenal suppression may occur; in those cases, discontinuation and withdrawal of the corticosteroid should be done judiciously.

Stability Do not store near heat or open flame

Mechanism of Action Controls the rate of protein synthesis, depresses the migration of polymorphonuclear leukocytes, fibroblasts, reverses capillary permeability, and lysosomal stabilization at the cellular level to prevent or control inflammation

Pharmacokinetics
Absorption:

Oral: 90%

Inhalation: Readily, ~10% to 25% of an inhaled dose reaches the respiratory tract

Protein binding: 87%

Metabolism: Oral: Hepatic

Half-life: 15 hours (biphasic decay terminal decay is 15 hours, initial phase half-life: 3 hours); after inhalation, it is quickly hydrolyzed by pulmonary esterases prior to absorption

Elimination: Renal excretion with oral administration

Usual Dosage
Inhalation: Geriatrics and Adults: 2 inhalations 3 or 4 times/day or 4 inhalations twice daily, not to exceed 20 inhalations/day

Aerosol inhalation (nasal): Adults: 1 spray in each nostril 2-4 times/day

Aqueous inhalation (nasal): 1 spray in each nostril 2-4 times/day; once daily (84 mcg)

Patient Information Follow instructions that accompany product; inhaled beclomethasone makes many asthmatics cough, to reduce chance, inhale drug slowly or use prescribed inhaled bronchodilator 5 minutes before beclomethasone is used; keep inhaler clean and unobstructed, wash in warm water and dry thoroughly; notify physician if sore throat or sore mouth occurs; do not stop abruptly

Nursing Implications Take drug history of patients with perennial rhinitis, may be drug related; check mucous membranes for signs of fungal infection

Additional Information Not used in status asthmaticus; shake thoroughly before using; nasal inhalation and oral inhalation dosage forms are **not** to be used interchangeably

Special Geriatric Considerations Older patients may have difficulty with oral metered dose inhalers and may benefit from the use of a spacer or chamber device

Dosage Forms
Beclomethasone dipropionate:

Nasal:

Inhalation: (Beconase®, Vancenase®): 42 mcg/inhalation [200 metered doses] (16.8 g)

Spray (Vancenase® AQ Nasal): 0.084% [120 actuations] (19 g)

Spray, aqueous (Beconase AQ®, Vancenase® AQ): 42 mcg/inhalation [≥200 metered doses] (25 g); 84 mcg/inhalation [≥200 metered doses] (25 g)

Oral: Inhalation:
Beclovent®, Vanceril®: 42 mcg/inhalation [200 metered doses] (16.8 g)
Vanceril® Double Strength: 84 mcg/inhalation (5.4 g - 40 metered doses, 12.2 g - 120 metered doses)

Beclovent® Oral Inhaler *see* Beclomethasone *on page 105*

Beconase AQ® Nasal Inhaler *see* Beclomethasone *on page 105*

Beconase® Nasal Inhaler *see* Beclomethasone *on page 105*

Beepen-VK® *see* Penicillin V Potassium *on page 725*

Belix® Oral [OTC] *see* Diphenhydramine *on page 302*

Bellergal-S® *see* Ergotamine *on page 343*

Benadryl® Injection *see* Diphenhydramine *on page 302*

Benadryl® Oral [OTC] *see* Diphenhydramine *on page 302*

Benadryl® Topical *see* Diphenhydramine *on page 302*

Ben-Allergin-50® Injection *see* Diphenhydramine *on page 302*

Benazepril (ben AY ze pril)
Related Information
ACE Inhibitors Comparison *on page 1019*
Brand Names Lotensin®
Generic Available No
Therapeutic Category Angiotensin-Converting Enzyme (ACE) Inhibitors
Use Treatment of hypertension, either alone or in combination with other antihypertensive agents, particularly diuretics
Unlabeled use: Although there are no data for its use, ACE inhibitors as a class are indicated in the treatment of systolic congestive heart failure
Contraindications Hypersensitivity to benazepril or any component or any other angiotensin-converting enzyme inhibitor
Warnings ACE inhibitors prevent potassium excretion, approximately as much as amiloride or spironolactone; may cause neutropenia, agranulocytosis, angioedema, hepatic dysfunction, first-dose hypotension, proteinuria; use cautiously in elderly, may see exaggerated response
Precautions Use with caution and modify dosage in patients with renal impairment; use with caution in patients with collagen vascular disease, congestive heart failure, hypovolemia, valvular stenosis, hyperkalemia (>5.7 mEq/L), anesthesia
Adverse Reactions
Cardiovascular: Orthostatic blood pressure changes, angina, palpitations, chest pain, hypotension, syncope, flushing
Central nervous system: Nervousness, depression, anxiety, somnolence, fatigue, dizziness, headache, insomnia
Dermatologic: Rash, pruritus, angioedema
Endocrine & metabolic: Hyperkalemia, hyponatremia
Gastrointestinal: Ageusia, pancreatitis, xerostomia, constipation, nausea, vomiting, abdominal pain
Genitourinary: Impotence, decreased libido
Hematologic: Neutropenia, eosinophilia
Hepatic: Hepatitis
Neuromuscular & skeletal: Myalgia, arthralgia, arthritis, paresthesia, weakness
Ocular: Blurred vision
Renal: Proteinuria, oliguria, increased BUN, serum creatinine
Respiratory: Chronic cough (nonproductive, persistent; more often in women and seen in 5% to 29% of patients), asthma, bronchitis, bronchospasm, dyspnea, sinusitis
Miscellaneous: Diaphoresis
Overdosage Symptoms of overdose include severe hypotension; supportive measures only (see Toxicology)
Toxicology Following initiation of essential overdose management, toxic symptom treatment and supportive treatment should be initiated. Hypotension usually responds to I.V. fluids or Trendelenburg positioning. If unresponsive to these measures, the use of a parenteral inotrope may be required (eg, norepinephrine 0.1-0.2 mcg/kg/minute titrated to response). Seizures commonly respond to diazepam (I.V. 5-10 mg bolus every 15 minutes if needed up to a total of 30 mg) or to phenytoin or phenobarbital.
(Continued)

Benazepril (Continued)

Drug Interactions

Benazepril and potassium-sparing diuretics may cause additive hyperkalemic effect

Benazepril and indomethacin or nonsteroidal anti-inflammatory agents may cause reduced antihypertensive response to benazepril

Allopurinol and benazepril may cause neutropenia

Antacids and ACE inhibitors may decrease absorption of ACE inhibitors

Phenothiazines and ACE inhibitors may increase ACE inhibitor effect

Probenecid and ACE inhibitors (benazepril) may increase ACE inhibitors (benazepril) levels

Rifampin and ACE inhibitors (benazepril) may decrease ACE inhibitor effect

Digoxin and ACE inhibitors may increase serum digoxin concentration

Lithium and ACE inhibitors may increase lithium serum concentration

Tetracycline and ACE inhibitors (benazepril) may decrease tetracycline absorption (up to 37%)

Mechanism of Action Competitive inhibitor of angiotensin-converting enzyme (ACE); prevents conversion of angiotensin I to angiotensin II, a potent vasoconstrictor; results in lower levels of angiotensin II which causes an increase in plasma renin activity and a reduction in aldosterone secretion; a CNS mechanism may also be involved in hypotensive effect as angiotensin II increases adrenergic outflow from CNS; vasoactive kallikreins may be decreased in conversion to active hormones by ACE inhibitors, thus reducing blood pressure

Pharmacodynamics

Reduction in plasma angiotensin-converting enzyme activity:

Peak effect: 1-2 hours after oral administration of 2-20 mg dose

Duration of action: >90% inhibition for 24 hours has been observed after 5-20 mg oral dose

Reduction in blood pressure:

Single oral dose: Peak effect: 2-6 hours

With continuous therapy:

Maximum response: 2 weeks

Duration: 2 years

Pharmacokinetics

Absorption: Oral: Rapid, 37%; food does not alter significantly; metabolite (benazeprilat) itself unsuitable for oral administration due to poor absorption

Distribution: V_d: ~8.7 L

Protein binding: 96.7%; benazeprilat: 95.3%

Metabolism: Rapid and extensive in the liver to its active metabolite, benazeprilat, via enzymatic hydrolysis; undergoes significant first-pass metabolism and is completely eliminated from plasma in 4 hours

Half-life: Prolonged with renal impairment

Parent drug: 0.6 hours; prolonged with renal impairment

Metabolite elimination: 22 hours (from 24 hours after dosing onward) (average 10-11 hours with multiple dosing for benazeprilat the active metabolite)

Time to peak serum concentration:

Unchanged parent: 1-1.5 hours

Metabolite: 1.5-2 hours after fasting or 2-4 hours after a meal

Elimination: Nonrenal clearance (ie, biliary, metabolic) appears to contribute to the elimination of benazeprilat (11% to 12%), particularly in patients with severe renal impairment; hepatic clearance is the main elimination route of unchanged benazepril

Dialyzable: ~6% of metabolite removed by 4 hours of dialysis following 10 mg of benazepril administered 2 hours prior to procedure; parent compound was not found in the dialysate

Usual Dosage Patients taking diuretics should have them discontinued 2-3 days prior to starting benazepril; if they cannot be discontinued, then initial dose should be 5 mg; restart after blood pressure is stabilized if needed

Geriatrics: Oral: Initial: 5-10 mg/day in single or divided doses; usual range: 20-40 mg/day; adjust for renal function

Adults: Oral: 20-40 mg/day as a single dose or 2 divided doses

Unlabeled use: Congestive heart failure: Since ACE inhibitors are indicated as a class for treatment of congestive heart failure, patients receiving benazepril should be slowly titrated to a "target dose" of 20 mg/day; maximum dose should be limited to 40 mg/day; no data available to date for this drug and dose in congestive heart failure

Dosing interval in renal impairment: Cl_{cr} <30 mL/minute: Administer 5 mg/ day initially; titrate to response or maximum dose of 40 mg/day

Monitoring Parameters Serum potassium concentration, BUN, serum creatinine, renal function, WBC

Patient Information Notify physician of persistent cough; do not stop therapy except under prescriber advice; notify physician if you develop sore throat, fever, swelling of hands, feet, face, eyes, lips, and tongue; difficult breathing, irregular heartbeats, chest pains, or cough. May cause dizziness, fainting, and lightheadedness, especially in first week of therapy, sit and stand up slowly; may cause changes in taste or rash; do not add a salt substitute (potassium) without advice of physician.

Nursing Implications May cause depression in some patients; discontinue if angioedema of the face, extremities, lips, tongue, or glottis occurs; watch for hypotensive effect within 1-3 hours of first dose or new higher dose (see Precautions, Warnings, Monitoring Parameters, and Special Geriatric Considerations)

Special Geriatric Considerations Due to frequent decreases in glomerular filtration (also creatinine clearance) with aging, elderly patients may have exaggerated responses to ACE inhibitors; differences in clinical response due to hepatic changes are not observed. ACE inhibitors may be preferred agents in elderly patients with congestive heart failure and diabetes mellitus. Diabetic proteinuria is reduced and insulin sensitivity is enhanced. In general, the side effect profile is favorable in elderly and causes little or no CNS confusion; use lowest dose recommendations initially.

Dosage Forms Tablet, as hydrochloride: 5 mg, 10 mg, 20 mg, 40 mg

References

Konstam MA, Drakup K, Baker DW, et al, "Heart Failure: Evaluation and Care of Patients With Left Ventricular Systolic Dysfunction," *Clinical Practice Guideline No 11*, Rockville, MD: Agency for Health Care Policy and Research, Public Health Service, U.S. Department of Health and Human Services, 1994.

McAreavey D and Robertson JIS, "Angiotensin Converting Enzyme Inhibitors and Moderate Hypertension," *Drugs*, 1990, 40(3):326-45.

Williams JF, Bristow MR, Fowler MB, et al, "Guidelines for the Evaluation and Management of Heart Failure: Report of the American College of Cardiology/American Heart Association Task Force on Practice Guidelines (Committee on Evaluation and Management of Heart Failure)," *J Am Coll Cardiol*, 1995, 26:1376-8.

Benazepril and Hydrochlorothiazide
(ben AY ze pril & hye droe klor oh THYE a zide)

Related Information
Benazepril *on page 107*
Hydrochlorothiazide *on page 458*

Brand Names Lotensin HCT®

Generic Available No

Therapeutic Category Antihypertensive, Combination

Use Treatment of hypertension

Usual Dosage Dose is individualized

Dosage Forms Tablet: Benazepril 5 mg and hydrochlorothiazide 6.25 mg; benazepril 10 mg and hydrochlorothiazide 12.5 mg; benazepril 20 mg and hydrochlorothiazide 12.5 mg; benazepril 20 mg and hydrochlorothiazide 25 mg

Benemid® *see* Probenecid *on page 779*

Bentyl® Hydrochloride Injection *see* Dicyclomine *on page 285*

Bentyl® Hydrochloride Oral *see* Dicyclomine *on page 285*

Benylin® Cough Syrup [OTC] *see* Diphenhydramine *on page 302*

Benylin DM® [OTC] *see* Dextromethorphan *on page 278*

Benylin® Expectorant [OTC] *see* Guaifenesin and Dextromethorphan *on page 439*

Benylin® Pediatric [OTC] *see* Dextromethorphan *on page 278*

Benzathine Benzylpenicillin *see* Penicillin G Benzathine *on page 720*

Benzathine Penicillin G *see* Penicillin G Benzathine *on page 720*

Benzene Hexachloride *see* Lindane *on page 538*

Benzhexol Hydrochloride *see* Trihexyphenidyl *on page 958*

Benzodiazepines Comparison *see page 1024*

Benzonatate (ben ZOE na tate)

Brand Names Tessalon® Perles

Generic Available No

Therapeutic Category Antitussive; Cough Preparation; Local Anesthetic, Oral

(Continued)

Benzonatate *(Continued)*

Use Symptomatic relief of nonproductive cough

Contraindications Known hypersensitivity to benzonatate or related compounds

Precautions Release of benzonatate in the mouth can cause a temporary local anesthesia of the oral mucosa; capsules should be swallowed whole

Adverse Reactions

Central nervous system: Sedation, headache, dizziness

Gastrointestinal: GI upset, constipation, nausea

Ocular: Sensation of burning in the eyes

Respiratory: Nasal congestion

Overdosage Symptoms of overdose include restlessness, tremor, CNS stimulation

Toxicology The drug's local anesthetic activity can reduce the patient's gag reflex and, therefore, may contradict the use of ipecac following ingestion, this is especially true when the capsules are chewed. Gastric lavage may be indicated if initiated early on following an acute ingestion or in comatose patients. The remaining treatment is supportive and symptomatic. Treat convulsions with an I.V. short-acting barbiturate.

Mechanism of Action Tetracaine congener with antitussive properties; suppresses cough by topical anesthetic action on the respiratory stretch receptors

Pharmacodynamics

Onset of action: Therapeutic: Within 15-20 minutes

Duration: 3-8 hours

Usual Dosage Geriatrics and Adults: Oral: 100 mg 3 times/day, up to 600 mg/day

Monitoring Parameters Patient's chest sounds and respiratory pattern, mental status

Patient Information Swallow capsule whole; use of hard candy may increase saliva flow to aid in protecting pharyngeal mucosa

Nursing Implications Monitor patient's chest sounds and respiratory pattern; change patient position every 2 hours to prevent pooling of secretions in lung; capsules are not to be crushed

Special Geriatric Considerations No specific geriatric information is available about benzonatate; avoid use in patients with impaired gag reflex or who cannot swallow the capsule whole

Dosage Forms Capsule: 100 mg

Benzquinamide Hydrochloride

(benz KWIN a mide hye droe KLOR ide)

Brand Names Emete-Con®

Generic Available No

Therapeutic Category Antiemetic

Use Antiemetic associated with anesthesia and surgery

Contraindications Hypersensitivity to benzquinamide hydrochloride or any component

Warnings May mask signs of intestinal obstruction and brain tumor

Precautions I.V. administration has been associated with hypertension and transient arrhythmias. I.M. is the preferred route

Adverse Reactions

Cardiovascular: Hypertension hypotension, cardiac arrhythmias, PVCs, PACF, atrial fibrillation

Central nervous system: Drowsiness (most common), insomnia, restlessness, headache, chills, shivering

Dermatologic: Urticaria, rash

Gastrointestinal: Anorexia, nausea, xerostomia

Neuromuscular & skeletal: Weakness, twitching, shaking, tremors

Ocular: Blurred vision

Miscellaneous: Diaphoresis

Very large doses have produced extrapyramidal symptoms; hyperthermia, hiccups, flushing, salivation

Overdosage No specific antidote/supportive measures; see CNS stimulation and depressant symptoms in combination

Toxicology General supportive measures; no specific antidote. Not dialyzable since benzquinamide is moderately protein bound.

Drug Interactions May increase action of pressor drugs

Stability Protect from light; do not reconstitute with NS, as a precipitate will result; when reconstituted as directed remains stable for 14 days at room temperature

Mechanism of Action Mechanism is unknown, but probably acts directly on the chemoreceptor trigger zone; has antiemetic, antihistaminic, anticholinergic, and mild sedative action

Pharmacodynamics
Onset of action: ~15 minutes
Duration: 3-4 hours

Pharmacokinetics
Absorption: I.M.: Rapid
Protein binding: 58%
Metabolism: Mainly by the liver
Time to peak blood concentration: 30 minutes after administration
Elimination: In urine, feces, and bile

Usual Dosage Geriatrics and Adults:
I.M.: 50 mg (0.5-1 mg/kg) may be repeated in 1 hour, then every 3-4 hours as needed
I.V.: 25 mg (0.2-0.4 mg/kg); not recommended route; restrict I.V. route to patients without any cardiovascular disease (see Precautions)

Monitoring Parameters Monitor emetic episodes, monitor blood pressure, heart rate

Patient Information May cause drowsiness and dry mouth

Nursing Implications Reconstitute with 2.2 mL of sterile water; potent for 14 days at room temperature; do **not** reconstitute with normal saline (precipitate may develop); administer either deep I.M. or by slow I.V. no faster than 25 mg/minute

Special Geriatric Considerations Due to higher incidence of cardiovascular disease in elderly, it would be best to avoid use if possible (see Precautions); since this agent has anticholinergic action (mild), be aware of possibility of CNS effects including confusion and delirium

Dosage Forms Injection: 50 mg

Benztropine (BENZ troe peen)

Related Information
I.V. Push Recommended Guidelines *on page 1083*

Brand Names Cogentin®

Generic Available Yes: Tablet

Therapeutic Category Anticholinergic Agent; Anti-Parkinson's Agent

Use Adjunctive treatment of all forms of parkinsonism; also used in treatment of drug-induced extrapyramidal effects (except tardive dyskinesia) and acute dystonic reactions

Contraindications Patients with narrow-angle glaucoma; hypersensitivity to any component; pyloric or duodenal obstruction, stenosing peptic ulcers; bladder neck obstructions; achalasia; myasthenia gravis

Precautions Use with caution in hot weather or during exercise. Elderly patients frequently develop increased sensitivity and require strict dosage regulation - side effects may be more severe in elderly patients with atherosclerotic changes. Use with caution in patients with tachycardia, cardiac arrhythmias, hypertension, hypotension, prostatic hypertrophy (especially in the elderly) or any tendency toward urinary retention, liver or kidney disorders and obstructive disease of the GI or GU tract. May exacerbate mental symptoms and precipitate a toxic psychosis when used to treat extrapyramidal reactions resulting from phenothiazines. When given in large doses or to susceptible patients, may cause weakness and inability to move particular muscle groups. Anticholinergic agents can aggravate tardive dyskinesia caused by neuroleptic agents.

Adverse Reactions
Cardiovascular: Tachycardia
Central nervous system: Drowsiness, nervousness, hallucinations, memory loss, coma (**the elderly may be at increased risk for confusion and hallucinations**)
Gastrointestinal: Nausea, vomiting, constipation, dryness of mouth
Genitourinary: Urinary hesitancy or retention
Ocular: Blurred vision, mydriasis
Miscellaneous: Heat intolerance

Overdosage Symptoms of overdose include CNS depression, confusion, nervousness, hallucinations, dizziness, blurred vision, nausea, vomiting, hyperthermia
(Continued)

Benztropine *(Continued)*

Toxicology Anticholinergic toxicity is caused by strong binding of the drug to cholinergic receptors. Cholinesterase inhibitors reduce acetylcholinesterase, the enzyme that breaks down acetylcholine and thereby allows acetylcholine to accumulate and compete for receptor binding with the offending anticholinergic. For anticholinergic overdose with severe life-threatening symptoms, physostigmine 1-2 mg S.C. or I.V., slowly may be given to reverse these effects.

Drug Interactions
Decreased effect of levodopa (decreased absorption), metoclopramide, cisapride
Increased toxicity (central anticholinergic syndrome): Narcotic analgesics, phenothiazines, and other antipsychotics, tricyclic antidepressants, some antihistamines, quinidine, disopyramide
Antagonistic effect: Tacrine, donepezil

Mechanism of Action Thought to partially block striatal cholinergic receptors to help balance cholinergic and dopaminergic activity

Pharmacodynamics
Onset of action:
Parenteral dose: Within 15 minutes
Oral: Within 60 minutes
Duration: Activity can last from as little as 6 hours to as long as 48 hours

Usual Dosage Titrate dose in 0.5 mg increments at 5- to 6-day intervals
Geriatrics: Initial: 0.5 mg once or twice daily; increase by 0.5 mg as needed every 5-6 days; maximum: 6 mg/day
Adults:
Drug-induced extrapyramidal reaction: Oral, I.M., I.V.: 1-4 mg/dose 1-2 times/day
Acute dystonia: I.M., I.V.: 1-2 mg
Parkinsonism: Oral: 0.5-6 mg/day in 1-2 divided doses; if one dose is greater, administer at bedtime

Monitoring Parameters Symptoms of EPS or Parkinson's, pulse, anticholinergic effects (ie, CNS, bowel, and bladder function)

Patient Information Take after meals or with food if GI upset occurs; do not discontinue drug abruptly; notify physician if adverse GI effects, rapid or pounding heartbeat, confusion, eye pain, rash, fever or heat intolerance occurs. Observe caution when performing hazardous tasks or those that require alertness such as driving, as may cause drowsiness. Avoid alcohol and other CNS depressants. May cause dry mouth - adequate fluid intake or hard sugar-free candy may relieve. Difficult urination or constipation may occur - notify physician if effects persist; may increase susceptibility to heat stroke.

Nursing Implications No significant difference in onset of I.M. or I.V. injection, therefore, there is usually no need to use the I.V. route. Improvement is sometimes noticeable a few minutes after injection. Do not discontinue drug abruptly.

Special Geriatric Considerations Anticholinergic agents are generally not well tolerated in the elderly (often results in bowel, bladder, and CNS adverse effects) and their use should be avoided when possible (see Precautions and Adverse Reactions). In the elderly, anticholinergic agents should not be used as prophylaxis against extrapyramidal symptoms.

Dosage Forms
Benztropine mesylate:
Injection: 1 mg/mL (2 mL)
Tablet: 0.5 mg, 1 mg, 2 mg

References
Feinberg M, "The Problems of Anticholinergic Adverse Effects in Older Patients," *Drugs Aging*, 1993, 3(4):335-48.

Benzylpenicillin Benzathine *see* Penicillin G Benzathine *on page 720*

Benzylpenicillin Potassium *see* Penicillin G, Parenteral, Aqueous *on page 722*

Benzylpenicillin Sodium *see* Penicillin G, Parenteral, Aqueous *on page 722*

Bepridil *(BE pri dil)*
Related Information
Calcium Channel Blocking Agents Comparison *on page 1027*
Brand Names Vascor®
Generic Available No
Therapeutic Category Antianginal Agent; Calcium Channel Blocker

Use Treatment of chronic stable angina; primarily due to ventricular arrhythmias and agranulocytosis, this drug should be reserved for patients who have been intolerant of other antianginal therapy; bepridil may be used alone or in combination with nitrates or beta-blockers (see Adverse Reactions)

Contraindications Sinus bradycardia; advanced heart block; ventricular tachycardia; cardiogenic shock, hypotension, congestive heart failure; hypersensitivity to verapamil or any component, hypersensitivity to calcium channel blockers and adenosine; atrial fibrillation or flutter associated with accessory conduction pathways; not to be given within a few hours of I.V. beta-blocking agents

Warnings Hypotension, congestive heart failure; cardiac conduction defects, PVCs, idiopathic hypertrophic subaortic stenosis; may cause platelet aggregation inhibition; do not abruptly withdraw (chest pain); hepatic dysfunction, renal function impairment, increased angina, increased intracranial pressure with cranial tumors; elderly may have greater hypotensive effect

The FDA's Cardiovascular and Renal Drug Advisory Committee reviewed current data regarding the risk of heart attacks in patients treated with calcium channel blockers and determined that as a class, the calcium channel antagonists are safe; however, they warned that short-acting nifedipine could increase the risk of myocardial infarction in some patients. The committee was in agreement with a statement issued September, 1995 by the National Heart Lung, and Blood Institute of the National Institute of Health, that warned that short-acting nifedipine should be used with great caution especially at higher doses.

Precautions Sick sinus syndrome, severe left ventricular dysfunction, congestive heart failure, hepatic or renal impairment, hypertrophic cardiomyopathy (especially obstructive), concomitant therapy with beta-blockers or digoxin, edema

Adverse Reactions

Cardiovascular: Hypertension, PVC (VT/VF), prolonged Q-T intervals, torsade de pointes, palpitations, bradycardia, tachycardia, syncope, peripheral edema

Central nervous system: Fever, psychotic behavior, akathisia, dizziness, lightheadedness, drowsiness, nervousness, equilibrium disturbances, headache, insomnia, tinnitus, anxiety

Dermatologic: Skin rash and irritation

Gastrointestinal: GI upset, pharyngitis, gastritis, increased appetite, nausea, diarrhea, constipation, abdominal pain, xerostomia, flatulence, dysgeusia

Genitourinary: Impotence, urinary incontinence

Hematologic: Agranulocytosis

Neuromuscular & skeletal: Pain, muscle weakness, arthritis, hand tremor, paresthesia

Ocular: Blurred vision

Respiratory: Shortness of breath, wheezing, cough, respiratory infection, nasal congestion

Miscellaneous: Superinfection, flu syndrome, diaphoresis, gingival swelling and inflammation

Overdosage Symptoms of overdose include heartblock, hypotension, asystole, nausea, weakness, dizziness, drowsiness, confusion, and slurred speech; profound bradycardia and occasionally hyperglycemia; monitor potassium

Toxicology Ipecac-induced emesis can hypothetically worsen calcium antagonist toxicity, since it can produce vagal stimulation. The potential for seizures precipitously following acute ingestion of large doses of a calcium antagonist may also contraindicate the use of ipecac. Supportive and symptomatic treatment, including I.V. fluids and Trendelenburg positioning, should be initiated as intoxication may cause hypotension. Although calcium (calcium chloride I.V. 1-2 g in adults over 5-10 minutes with repeats as needed) has been used as an "antidote" for acute intoxications, there is limited experience to support its routine use and should be reserved for those cases where definite signs of myocardial depression are evident. Heart block may respond to isoproterenol, glucagon, atropine and/or calcium although a temporary pacemaker may be required.

Drug Interactions Beta-blockers (increased cardiac and A-V conduction depression); fentanyl (increased volume requirements and hypotension); although this drug is new, other drug interactions not reported to the same degree as older agents; however, should be suspect of any drug interaction reported with other calcium channel blockers

Mechanism of Action Inhibits calcium ion from entering the "slow channels" or select voltage-sensitive areas of vascular smooth muscle and myocardium (Continued)

Bepridil *(Continued)*

during depolarization; produces a relaxation of coronary vascular smooth muscle and coronary vasodilation; increases myocardial oxygen delivery in patients with vasospastic angina; this agent also inhibits fast sodium channels (inward) which may account for some of its side effects (eg, arrhythmias)

Pharmacodynamics Onset of action: Within 1 hour

Pharmacokinetics

Absorption: Oral: 95% to 100%

Metabolism/Bioavailability: Due to first-pass elimination, absolute bioavailability is ~60%

Half-life: ~24 hours

Time to peak: Within 2-3 hours

Elimination: Primarily by hepatic metabolism

Usual Dosage Geriatrics and Adults: Initial: 200 mg/day; adjust dosage after 10 days of administration; maximum daily dose: 400 mg; elderly require frequent monitoring due to side effect profile (cardiac) (see Special Geriatric Considerations and Additional Information)

Monitoring Parameters Heart rate, blood pressure, signs and symptoms of congestive heart failure

Reference Range Therapeutic: 1-2 ng/mL

Nursing Implications May cause cardiac arrhythmias if potassium is low

Additional Information This agent is not considered the drug of first choice, but is used for cases refractory to other calcium channel blockers

Special Geriatric Considerations Elderly may experience a greater hypotensive response; constipation may be more of a problem in elderly; calcium channel blockers are no more effective in elderly than other therapies, however, they do not cause significant CNS effects which is an advantage over some antihypertensive agents (see Additional Information)

Dosage Forms Tablet, as hydrochloride: 200 mg, 300 mg, 400 mg

Berubigen® *see* Cyanocobalamin *on page 257*

Beta-2® *see* Isoetharine *on page 499*

Beta-Blockers Comparison *see page 1026*

Betachron E-R® **Capsule** *see* Propranolol *on page 797*

Betagan® **Liquifilm®** *see* Levobunolol *on page 529*

Betamethasone *(bay ta METH a sone)*

Related Information

Antacid Drug Interactions *on page 1096*

Corticosteroids Comparison, Topical *on page 1030*

Brand Names Alphatrex®; Betatrex®; Beta-Val®; Celestone®; Celestone® Soluspan®; Cel-U-Jec®; Diprolene®; Diprolene® AF; Diprosone®; Maxivate®; Psorion® Cream; Selestoject®; Teladar®; Valisone®

Synonyms Flubenisolone

Generic Available Yes: Dipropionate, sodium phosphate, sodium phosphate and acetate, valerate

Therapeutic Category Adrenal Corticosteroid; Anti-inflammatory Agent; Corticosteroid, Systemic; Corticosteroid, Topical (Medium Potency); Corticosteroid, Topical (Medium/High Potency)

Use Inflammatory dermatoses such as seborrheic or atopic dermatitis, neurodermatitis, anogenital pruritus, psoriasis, inflammatory phase of xerosis, late phase of allergic dermatitis or irritant dermatitis

Contraindications Systemic fungal infections; hypersensitivity to betamethasone or any component

Precautions Use with caution in patients with hypothyroidism, cirrhosis, nonspecific ulcerative colitis and patients at increased risk for peptic ulcer disease; do not use occlusive dressings on weeping or exudative lesions and general caution with occlusive dressings should be observed; discontinue if skin irritation or contact dermatitis should occur; do not use in patients with decreased skin circulation; avoid the use of high potency steroids on the face

Adverse Reactions

Cardiovascular: Hypertension, edema

Central nervous system: Convulsions, vertigo, confusion, headache, seizures, psychoses, pseudotumor cerebri

Dermatologic: Acne, hypopigmentation, skin atrophy, impaired wound healing, striae, miliaria, telangiectasia

Endocrine & metabolic: Cushing's syndrome, pituitary-adrenal axis suppression, glucose intolerance, hypokalemia, alkalosis, postmenopausal bleeding, hot flashes

Gastrointestinal: Peptic ulcer, nausea, vomiting, pancreatitis

Local: Burning, itching, acne

Neuromuscular & skeletal: Muscle weakness, osteoporosis, fractures, aseptic necrosis of femoral and humeral heads, steroid myopathy

Ocular: Cataracts, glaucoma

Miscellaneous: Accelerated atherogenesis, sodium retention

Toxicology When consumed in excessive quantities, systemic hypercorticism and adrenal suppression may occur; in those cases, discontinuation and withdrawal of the corticosteroid should be done judiciously

Drug Interactions

Decreased effect with barbiturates, phenytoin, rifampin; decreased effect of salicylates, vaccines, toxoids, insulin, and oral hypoglycemics

Increased effect with estrogens

Increased hypokalemia when given with diuretics; could increase risk of digoxin toxicity

Mechanism of Action Controls the rate of protein synthesis, depresses the migration of polymorphonuclear leukocytes, fibroblasts, reverses capillary permeability, and lysosomal stabilization at the cellular level to prevent or control inflammation

Pharmacokinetics

Protein binding: 64%

Metabolism: Extensive in the liver

Half-life: 6.5 hours

Time to peak serum concentration: I.V.: Within 10-36 minutes

Elimination: <5% of dose excreted renally as unchanged drug

Usual Dosage

Geriatrics: Use the lowest effective dose

Adults:

Oral: 0.6-7.2 mg/day

I.M., I.V.: Betamethasone sodium phosphate: 0.6-9 mg/day divided every 12-24 hours

I.M.: Betamethasone sodium phosphate and betamethasone acetate: 0.5-9 mg/day ($^1/_3$ to $^1/_2$ of oral dose)

Intrabursal, intra-articular: 0.5-2 mL

Topical: Apply thin film 2-4 times/day

Monitoring Parameters Blood pressure, blood glucose, electrolytes

Test Interactions Increased amylase (S), chloride (S), cholesterol (S), glucose, protein, sodium (S); decreased calcium (S), chloride (S), potassium (S), thyroxine (S)

Patient Information Take with food or milk; take single daily dose in the morning; do not stop oral products abruptly; if taking oral product, carry an identification card or bracelet advising that you are on steroids; apply topical preparations in a thin layer

Nursing Implications Apply sparingly to areas; not for alternate day therapy; once daily doses should be given in the morning; not for use on broken skin or in areas of infection; do not apply to wet skin unless directed; do not apply to face or inguinal area; do not administer injectable suspension I.V.

Additional Information

Alphatrex® = betamethasone dipropionate

Betatrex® = betamethasone valerate

Beta-Val® = betamethasone valerate

B-S-P® = betamethasone sodium phosphate

Celestone® = betamethasone

Celestone® Soluspan® = betamethasone sodium phosphate/betamethasone acetate

Diprolene® = betamethasone dipropionate

Diprosone® = betamethasone dipropionate

Maxivate® = betamethasone dipropionate

Selestoject® = betamethasone sodium phosphate

Uticort® = betamethasone benzoate

Valisone® = betamethasone valerate

Special Geriatric Considerations Because of the risk of adverse effects, systemic corticosteroids should be used cautiously in the elderly, in the smallest possible dose, and for the shortest possible time.

Dosage Forms

Betamethasone dipropionate salt (Diprosone®)

Aerosol: 0.1% (85 g)

Cream: 0.05% (15 g, 45 g)

Lotion: 0.05% (20 mL, 30 mL, 60 mL)

Ointment: 0.05% (15 g, 45 g)

(Continued)

Betamethasone *(Continued)*

Base (Celestone®)
  Tablet: 0.6 mg
  Syrup: 0.6 mg/5 mL (118 mL)
Benzoate salt (Uticort®)
  Cream: 0.025% (60 g)
  Gel: 0.025% (15 g, 60 g)
  Lotion: 0.025% (60 mL)
Dipropionate salt, augmented (Diprolene®)
  Cream: 0.05% (15 g, 45 g)
  Gel: 0.05% (15 g, 45 g)
  Lotion: 0.05% (30 mL, 60 mL)
  Ointment, topical: 0.05% (15 g, 45 g)
Valerate salt (Betatrex®, Beta-Val®, Valisone®)
  Cream: 0.1% (15 g, 45 g, 110 g, 430 g); 0.01% (15 g, 60 g)
  Lotion: 0.1% (20 mL, 60 mL)
  Ointment, topical: 0.1% (15 g, 45 g)
Sodium phosphate salt (Selestoject®)
  Injection: 4 mg/mL (equivalent to 3 mg/mL) (5 mL)
Sodium phosphate and acetate salt (Celestone® Soluspan®)
  Injection, suspension: 6 mg/mL (3 mg of betamethasone sodium phosphate
    and 3 mg of betamethasone acetate per mL) (5 mL)

Betapace® *see Sotalol on page 866*

Betapen®-VK *see Penicillin V Potassium on page 725*

Betasept® [OTC] *see Chlorhexidine Gluconate on page 206*

Betaseron® *see Interferon Beta-1b on page 493*

Betatrex® *see Betamethasone on page 114*

Beta-Val® *see Betamethasone on page 114*

Betaxolol *(be TAKS oh lol)*

Related Information
  Beta-Blockers Comparison *on page 1026*
  Glaucoma Drug Therapy Comparison *on page 1032*

Brand Names Betoptic® Ophthalmic; Betoptic® S Ophthalmic; Kerlone® Oral

Generic Available No

Therapeutic Category Beta-Adrenergic Blocker; Beta-Adrenergic Blocker, Ophthalmic

Use Treatment of chronic open-angle glaucoma, ocular hypertension; management of hypertension

Contraindications Bronchial asthma, sinus bradycardia, second and third degree A-V block, cardiac failure, cardiogenic shock, hypersensitivity to betaxolol or any component

Precautions Use with caution in patients with cardiac failure or diabetes mellitus

Adverse Reactions
  Cardiovascular: Bradycardia, palpitations, edema, congestive heart failure
  Central nervous system: Headache, dizziness, fatigue, lethargy
  Neuromuscular & skeletal: Exacerbation of myasthenia gravis
  Ocular: Mild ocular stinging and discomfort, tearing, erythema, itching, keratitis, photophobia, decreased corneal sensitivity
  Miscellaneous: Cold extremities

Overdosage Symptoms of overdose include bradycardia, hypotension, A-V block, CHF, bronchospasm, hypoglycemia

Toxicology Sympathomimetics (eg, epinephrine or dopamine), glucagon or a pacemaker can be used to treat the toxic bradycardia, asystole, and/or hypotension; initially, fluids may be the best treatment for toxic hypotension

Drug Interactions Increased toxicity (hypotension): Ophthalmic: Systemic beta-blockers, reserpine, carbonic anhydrase inhibitors

Stability Avoid freezing

Mechanism of Action Competitively blocks beta$_1$-receptors, with little or no effect on beta$_2$-receptors resulting in the inhibition of the chronotropic, inotropic, and vasodilator effects of beta-adrenergic stimulation. Ophthalmic reduces intraocular pressure by reducing the production of aqueous humor.

Pharmacodynamics
  Onset of action:
    Ophthalmic instillation: Within 30-60 minutes with maximal effects occurring within 2 hours
    Oral: Blood pressure significantly decreases within 3 hours

Duration of action:
　Ophthalmic instillation: 12 hours or longer
　Oral: 25 hours

Pharmacokinetics
Absorption: Systemically absorbed from the eye
Metabolism: To multiple metabolites
Half-life: 12-22 hours
Elimination: Renal

Usual Dosage
Oral:
　Geriatrics: Initial: 5 mg/day
　Adults: 10 mg/day; may increase dose to 20 mg/day after 7-14 days if desired response is not achieved
Ophthalmic: Geriatrics and Adults: Instill 1 drop twice daily

Monitoring Parameters
Ophthalmic: Intraocular pressure
Systemic: Blood pressure, pulse

Patient Information May sting on instillation; do not touch dropper to eye; visual acuity may be decreased after administration; distance vision may be altered; assess patient's or caregiver's ability to administer; apply gentle pressure to lacrimal sac during and immediately following instillation (1 minute) to avoid systemic absorption; stop drug if breathing difficulty occurs

Nursing Implications Monitor for signs of congestive heart failure, hypotension, respiratory difficulty (bronchospasm); use cautiously in diabetics receiving hypoglycemic agents; teach proper instillation of eye drops; monitor blood pressure and heart rate

Additional Information Because of betaxolol's low lipid solubility, it is less likely to enter the CNS, decreasing the likelihood of CNS side effects

Special Geriatric Considerations Due to alterations in the beta-adrenergic autonomic nervous system, beta-adrenergic blockade may result in less hemodynamic response than seen in younger adults. Studies indicate that despite decreased sensitivity to the chronotropic effects of beta blockade with age, there appears to be an increased myocardial sensitivity to the negative inotropic effect during stress (ie, exercise). Controlled trials have shown the overall response rate for propranolol to be only 20% to 50% in elderly populations. Therefore, all beta-adrenergic blocking drugs may result in a decreased response as compared to younger adults.

Dosage Forms
Betaxolol hydrochloride:
　Solution, ophthalmic (Betoptic®): 0.5% (2.5 mL, 5 mL, 10 mL)
　Suspension, ophthalmic (Betoptic® S): 0.25% (2.5 mL, 10 mL, 15 mL)
　Tablet (Kerlone®): 10 mg, 20 mg

Bethanechol (be THAN e kole)
Brand Names Duvoid®; Myotonachol™; Urabeth®; Urecholine®
Generic Available Yes: Tablet
Therapeutic Category Cholinergic Agent
Use Nonobstructive urinary retention and retention due to neurogenic bladder; treatment and prevention of bladder dysfunction caused by phenothiazines and tricyclic antidepressants; diagnosis of flaccid or atonic neurogenic bladder

Contraindications Hypersensitivity to bethanechol; do not use in patients with mechanical obstruction of the GI or GU tract or when the strength or integrity of the GI or bladder wall is in question. It is also contraindicated in patients with hyperthyroidism, peptic ulcer disease, latent or active asthma, epilepsy, parkinsonism, obstructive pulmonary disease, bradycardia, vasomotor instability, atrioventricular conduction defects, or hypotension

Warnings For S.C. injection only; do not administer I.M. or I.V. since it may cause a severe cholinergic reaction

Precautions Potential for reflux infection if the sphincter fails to relax as bethanechol contracts the bladder; Myotonachol™ contains tartrazine

Adverse Reactions
Cardiovascular: Hypotension, cardiac arrest, flushed skin
Gastrointestinal: Abdominal cramps, diarrhea, nausea, vomiting, salivation
Respiratory: Bronchial constriction
Miscellaneous: Diaphoresis, vasomotor response

Overdosage Symptoms of overdose include nausea, vomiting, abdominal cramps, diarrhea, involuntary defecation, flushed skin, hypotension, bronchospasm

(Continued)

Bethanechol *(Continued)*

Toxicology Atropine is the treatment of choice for intoxications manifesting with significant muscarinic symptoms. Atropine I.V. 0.6 mg every 3-60 minutes should be repeated to control symptoms and then continued as needed for 1-2 days following the acute ingestion. Epinephrine 0.1-1 mg S.C. may be useful in reversing severe cardiovascular or pulmonary sequels.

Drug Interactions
Decreased effect: Procainamide, quinidine
Increased toxicity: Ganglionic blockers (critical decrease in blood pressure)
Increased cholinergic effects: Anticholinesterase agents, tacrine, donepezil

Mechanism of Action Stimulates cholinergic receptors in the smooth muscle of the urinary bladder and gastrointestinal tract resulting in increased peristalsis, increased GI and pancreatic secretions, bladder muscle contraction, and increased ureteral peristaltic waves

Pharmacodynamics
Onset of action:
Oral 30-90 minutes
S.C.: 5-15 minutes
Duration: Usually 1 hour

Pharmacokinetics Absorption: Oral: Variable

Usual Dosage Geriatrics (use lowest recommended dose) and Adults:
Oral: 10-50 mg 2-4 times/day
S.C.: 2.5-5 mg 3-4 times/day, up to 7.5-10 mg every 4 hours for neurogenic bladder

Monitoring Parameters Urinary output, blood pressure, pulse

Test Interactions Increased lipase, amylase (S), bilirubin, aminotransferase [ALT (SGPT)/AST (SGOT)] (S)

Patient Information Oral should be taken 1 hour before meals or 2 hours after meals to avoid nausea or vomiting; may cause abdominal discomfort, salivation, sweating or flushing - notify physician if these symptoms become pronounced. Rise slowly from sitting/lying down.

Nursing Implications Contraindicated for I.M. or I.V. use due to a likely severe cholinergic reaction; for S.C. injection only; observe closely for side effects; have bedpan readily available if administered for urinary retention

Additional Information Syringe containing atropine should be readily available for treatment of serious side effects

Special Geriatric Considerations Urinary incontinence in an elderly patient should be investigated. Bethanechol may be used for overflow incontinence (dribbling) caused by an atonic or hypotonic bladder, but clinical efficacy is variable (see Contraindications, Precautions, and Adverse Reactions).

Dosage Forms
Bethanechol chloride:
Injection: 5 mg/mL (1 mL)
Tablet: 5 mg, 10 mg, 25 mg, 50 mg

References
Romanowski GL, Shimp LA, Balson AB, et al, "Urinary Incontinence in the Elderly: Etiology and Treatment," *Drug Intell Clin Pharm*, 1988, 22(7-8):525-33.

Betimol® Ophthalmic *see* Timolol *on page 925*

Betoptic® Ophthalmic *see* Betaxolol *on page 116*

Betoptic® S Ophthalmic *see* Betaxolol *on page 116*

Biavax®ᵢᵢ *see* Rubella and Mumps Vaccines, Combined *on page 840*

Biaxin™ *see* Clarithromycin *on page 229*

Bicalutamide *(bye ka LOO ta mide)*

Brand Names Casodex®

Generic Available No

Therapeutic Category Androgen; Antiandrogen; Antineoplastic Agent, Hormone

Use Combination therapy with a luteinizing hormone-releasing hormone (LHRH) analog for the treatment of advanced prostate cancer

Contraindications Known hypersensitivity to bicalutamide or any of its components

Warnings Hypersensitivity or adverse reactions to flutamide or nilutamide; patients with liver disease

Adverse Reactions
Cardiovascular: Peripheral edema
Central nervous system: Dizziness, headache, fatigue
Dermatologic: Skin rash, pruritus

Endocrine & metabolic: Breast tenderness, gynecomastia, hot flashes, loss of libido

Gastrointestinal: Nausea, vomiting, diarrhea, constipation

Genitourinary: Impotence, Leydig cell tumors

Hematologic: Anemia

Hepatic: Enzyme elevation

Neuromuscular & skeletal: Pelvic or back pain

Ophthalmic: Visual disturbances

Mechanism of Action Pure nonsteroidal antiandrogen that binds to androgen receptors; specifically a competitive inhibitor for the binding of dihydrotestosterone and testosterone; prevents testosterone stimulation of cell growth in prostate cancer

Pharmacokinetics

Protein binding: 96%

Metabolism: Not yet studied

Half-life: Up to 10 days

Elimination: Not yet studied

Usual Dosage Geriatrics and Adults: Oral: 50 mg once daily (morning or evening), with or without food, in combination with a LHRH analog

Monitoring Parameters Serum prostate-specific antigen, alkaline phosphatase, acid phosphatase, or prostatic acid phosphatase; prostate gland dimensions; skeletal survey; liver scans; chest x-rays; physical exam every 3 months; bone scan every 3-6 months; CBC, LFTs, EKG, echocardiograms, and serum testosterone and luteinizing hormone (periodically)

Patient Information Take at the same time as treatment with LHRH analog; advise of potential side effects; notify the physician if any visual disturbances or yellow discoloration of the skin or eyes

Nursing Implications See Usual Dosage

Special Geriatric Considerations Renal impairment has no clinically significant changes in elimination of the parent compound or active metabolite; therefore, no dosage adjustment is needed in the elderly. In dosage studies, no difference was found between young adults and elderly with regard to steady-state serum concentrations for bicalutamide and its active R-enantiomer metabolite.

Dosage Forms Tablet: 50 mg

Bicillin® C-R 900/300 Injection *see* Penicillin G Benzathine and Procaine Combined *on page 721*

Bicillin® C-R Injection *see* Penicillin G Benzathine and Procaine Combined *on page 721*

Bicillin® L-A *see* Penicillin G Benzathine *on page 720*

Bicitra® *see* Sodium Citrate and Citric Acid *on page 861*

Biocef *see* Cephalexin *on page 194*

Biohist-LA® *see* Carbinoxamine and Pseudoephedrine *on page 164*

Biomox® *see* Amoxicillin *on page 67*

Bion® Tears Solution [OTC] *see* Artificial Tears *on page 82*

Bio-Tab® Oral *see* Doxycycline *on page 322*

Biozyme-C® *see* Collagenase *on page 251*

Biperiden (bye PER i den)

Brand Names Akineton®

Generic Available No

Therapeutic Category Anticholinergic Agent; Anti-Parkinson's Agent

Use Treatment of all forms of parkinsonism including drug-induced type (extrapyramidal symptoms); principally affects tremor

Contraindications Hypersensitivity to any component; narrow-angle glaucoma, pyloric or duodenal obstruction; stenosing peptic ulcers; bladder neck obstructions; achalasia; myasthenia gravis

Precautions Use with caution in hot weather or during exercise. Elderly patients frequently develop increased sensitivity and require strict dosage regulation - side effects may be more severe in elderly patients with atherosclerotic changes. Use with caution in patients with tachycardia, cardiac arrhythmias, hypertension, hypotension, prostatic hypertrophy (especially in the elderly) or any tendency toward urinary retention, liver or kidney disorders and obstructive disease of the GI or GU tract. May exacerbate mental symptoms and precipitate a toxic psychosis when used to treat extrapyramidal reactions resulting from phenothiazines. When given in large doses or to susceptible patients, may cause weakness and inability to move particular muscle groups. Anticholinergic agents can aggravate tardive dyskinesia caused by neuroleptic agents.

(Continued)

Biperiden *(Continued)*

Adverse Reactions
Cardiovascular: Tachycardia

Central nervous system: Coma, nervousness, memory loss, drowsiness; the elderly may be at increased risk for confusion and hallucinations

Gastrointestinal: Nausea, vomiting, constipation, dryness of mouth

Genitourinary: Urinary retention

Ocular: Blurred vision, mydriasis

Miscellaneous: Heat intolerance

Overdosage Symptoms of overdose include CNS depression, confusion, nervousness, hallucinations, dizziness, blurred vision, nausea, vomiting, hyperthermia

Toxicology Anticholinergic toxicity is caused by strong binding of the drug to cholinergic receptors; cholinesterase inhibitors reduce acetylcholinesterase, the enzyme that breaks down acetylcholine and thereby allows acetylcholine to accumulate and compete for receptor binding with the offending anticholinergic. For anticholinergic overdose with severe life-threatening symptoms, physostigmine 1-2 mg S.C. or I.V., slowly may be given to reverse these effects.

Drug Interactions
Decreased effect of levodopa (decreased absorption)

Increased toxicity (central anticholinergic syndrome): Narcotic analgesics, phenothiazines, and other antipsychotics, tricyclic antidepressants, some antihistamines, quinidine, disopyramide

Antagonistic effect: Tacrine, donepezil

Mechanism of Action Thought to partially block striatal cholinergic receptors to help balance cholinergic and dopaminergic activity

Pharmacokinetics
Bioavailability: 29%

Half-life: 18.4-24.3 hours

Time to peak serum concentration: 1-1.5 hours

Usual Dosage
Geriatrics: Oral: Initial: 2 mg 1-2 times/day

Adults:

Parkinsonism: Oral: 2 mg 3-4 times/day; maximum: 16 mg/day

Drug-induced extrapyramidal reaction:

Oral: 2 mg 1-3 times/day

I.M., I.V.: 2 mg every 30 minutes until symptoms resolved; maximum: 8 mg/day

Monitoring Parameters Symptoms of EPS or Parkinson's, pulse, anticholinergic effects (ie, CNS, bowel, and bladder function)

Patient Information Take after meals or with food if GI upset occurs; do not discontinue drug abruptly; notify physician if adverse GI effects, rapid or pounding heartbeat, confusion, eye pain, rash, fever or heat intolerance occurs. Observe caution when performing hazardous tasks or those that require alertness such as driving, as may cause drowsiness. Avoid alcohol and other CNS depressants. May cause dry mouth - adequate fluid intake or hard sugar-free candy may relieve. Difficult urination or constipation may occur - notify physician if effects persist; may increase susceptibility to heat stroke.

Nursing Implications No significant difference in onset of I.M. or I.V. injection, therefore, there is usually no need to use the I.V. route. Improvement is sometimes noticeable a few minutes after injection. Do not discontinue drug abruptly.

Special Geriatric Considerations Anticholinergic agents are generally not well tolerated in the elderly (often results in bowel, bladder, and CNS adverse reactions) and their use should be avoided when possible (see Precautions, Adverse Reactions). In the elderly, anticholinergic agents should not be used as prophylaxis against extrapyramidal symptoms.

Dosage Forms
Injection, as lactate: 5 mg/mL (1 mL)

Tablet, as hydrochloride: 2 mg

References
Feinberg M, "The Problems of Anticholinergic Adverse Effects in Older Patients," *Drugs Aging*, 1993, 3(4):335-48.

Bisac-Evac® [OTC] *see* Bisacodyl *on next page*

Bisacodyl (bis a KOE dil)

Brand Names Bisac-Evac® [OTC]; Bisacodyl Uniserts®; Bisco-Lax® [OTC]; Carter's Little Pills® [OTC]; Clysodrast®; Dacodyl® [OTC]; Deficol® [OTC]; Dulcolax® [OTC]; Fleet® Laxative [OTC]; Theralax® [OTC]

Generic Available Yes

Therapeutic Category Laxative, Stimulant

Use Treatment of constipation; colonic evacuation prior to procedures or examination

Contraindications Do not use in patients with abdominal pain, obstruction, nausea, or vomiting; appendicitis, acute surgical abdomen

Warnings Excessive use may lead to fluid and electrolyte imbalance

Precautions Drug is habit-forming and may result in laxative dependence and loss of normal bowel function with prolonged use; rectal bleeding and failure to respond to therapy may require further evaluation; discoloration of urine may occur

Adverse Reactions
Endocrine & metabolic: Electrolyte and fluid imbalance (metabolic acidosis or alkalosis, hypocalcemia)
Gastrointestinal: Abdominal cramps, nausea, vomiting, diarrhea, griping, bloating
Miscellaneous: Rectal burning, diaphoresis

Overdosage Symptoms of overdose include diarrhea, abdominal pain, nausea, vomiting, fluid/electrolyte loss, hypotension, lethargy, fatigue

Drug Interactions Milk and antacids will cause early release of drug in stomach rather than in small intestine

Mechanism of Action Stimulates peristalsis by directly irritating the smooth muscle of the intestine, possibly the colonic intramural plexus; alters water and electrolyte secretion producing net intestinal fluid accumulation and laxation

Pharmacodynamics Onset of action:
Oral: Within 6-10 hours
Rectal: 15-60 minutes

Pharmacokinetics
Absorption: Oral, rectal: <5% absorbed systemically
Metabolism: In the liver with conjugated metabolites
Elimination: Excreted in bile and urine

Usual Dosage
Geriatrics:
Oral: Initial: 5 mg/day
Rectal: 5-10 mg/day
Adults:
Oral: 10-15 mg/day as a single dose
Rectal: 10 mg/day as a single dose

Monitoring Parameters Monitor stools daily or weekly; fluid/electrolyte status

Patient Information Swallow tablets whole, do **not** crush or chew; do not take antacid or milk within 2 hours of taking drug; patients should assure proper dietary fiber and fluid intake with adequate exercise if medically appropriate; do not use if abdominal pain, nausea, or vomiting are present; laxative use should be used for a short period of time (<1 week); prolonged use may result in abuse, dependence, as well as fluid and electrolyte loss; notify physician if bleeding occurs or if constipation is not relieved

Nursing Implications Administer tablets 2 hours prior to or 4 hours after antacids; increased pH may dissolve the enteric coating leading to GI distress; do not crush enteric coated drug product

Special Geriatric Considerations The chronic use of stimulant cathartics is inappropriate and should be avoided; although constipation is a common complaint from elderly, such complaints require evaluation; elderly are often predisposed to constipation due to disease, drugs, immobility, and a decreased fluid intake, partially because they have a blunted "thirst reflex" with aging; short-term use of stimulants is best; if prophylaxis is desired, this can be accomplished with bulk agents (psyllium), stool softeners, and hyperosmotic agents (sorbitol 70%); stool softeners are unnecessary if stools are well hydrated, soft, or "mushy"

Dosage Forms
Enema: 10 mg/30 mL
Powder, as tannex: 2.5 g
Suppository, rectal: 5 mg, 10 mg
Tablet, enteric coated: 5 mg

Bisacodyl Uniserts® *see* Bisacodyl *on this page*

Bisco-Lax® [OTC] *see* Bisacodyl *on previous page*
Bismatrol® [OTC] *see* Bismuth *on this page*

Bismuth (BIZ muth)
Related Information
Regimens Used to Treat *Helicobacter pylori* and Ulcers *on page 1033*
Brand Names Bismatrol® [OTC]; Devrom® [OTC]; Pepto-Bismol® [OTC]; Pink Bismuth® [OTC]
Generic Available Yes
Therapeutic Category Antidiarrheal
Use Symptomatic treatment of mild, nonspecific diarrhea; indigestion, nausea; control of traveler's diarrhea (enterotoxigenic *Escherichia coli*); as an adjunct in the treatment of *Helicobacter pylori*-associated peptic ulcer disease
Contraindications Do not use subsalicylate in patients with influenza or chickenpox because of risk of Reye's syndrome; do not use in patients with known hypersensitivity to salicylates; history of severe GI bleeding; history of coagulopathy
Warnings Do not use prior to radiologic examinations of GI tract; bismuth is radiopaque (see Precautions)
Precautions Subsalicylate should be used with caution if patient is taking aspirin, additive toxicity; use with caution in anticoagulated patients; use in debilitated, immobile patients may lead to bowel impaction
Adverse Reactions Gastrointestinal: Impaction may occur in debilitated patients
Overdosage Symptoms of overdose include tinnitus (subsalicylate), fever
Toxicology It is unusual to develop toxicity from short-term administrations of bismuth salts, and most toxic symptoms occur following subacute or chronic intoxications. Chelation with dimercaprol in doses of 3 mg/kg or penicillamine 100 mg/kg/day for 5 days can hasten recovery from bismuth-induced encephalopathy. When associated with methemoglobinemia, bismuth intoxications should be treated with methylene blue 1-2 mg/kg in a 1% sterile aqueous solution I.V. push over 4-6 minutes. This may be repeated within 60 minutes if necessary, up to a total dose of 7 mg/kg. Seizures usually respond to I.V. diazepam.
Drug Interactions
Decreased effect: Tetracyclines and uricosurics
Increased toxicity: Aspirin, warfarin, hypoglycemics
Mechanism of Action Bismuth subsalicylate exhibits both antisecretory and antimicrobial action. This agent may provide some anti-inflammatory action as well. The salicylate moiety provides antisecretory effect and the bismuth exhibits antimicrobial directly against bacterial and viral gastrointestinal pathogens. Bismuth has some antacid properties.
Pharmacokinetics
Absorption: Minimally absorbed across the GI tract while the salt (eg, salicylate) may be readily absorbed
Metabolism: Undergoes chemical dissociation to various bismuth salts after oral administration
Usual Dosage Geriatrics and Adults: Oral:
Nonspecific diarrhea: Subsalicylate: 2 tablets or 30 mL every 30 minutes to 1 hour as needed up to 8 doses/24 hours
Prevention of traveler's diarrhea: 2.1 g/day or 2 tablets 4 times/day before meals and at bedtime
Subgallate: 1-2 tablets 3 times/day with meals
H. pylori: 2 tablets 4 times/day as part of a 3- or 4-drug regimen (see Appendix for Regimens Used to Treat *Helicobacter pylori* and Ulcers)
Dosing adjustment in renal impairment: Should probably be avoided in patients with renal failure
Monitoring Parameters Signs/symptoms of nausea, diarrhea, tinnitus, CNS toxic effects, GI bleeding
Reference Range Mild toxicity, serum concentration ≥30 mg/dL; severe, >50 mg/dL
Test Interactions Increased uric acid
Patient Information Chew tablet well or shake suspension well before using; may darken stools; if diarrhea persists for more than 2 days, consult a physician; tinnitus may indicate toxicity and use should be discontinued
Nursing Implications Seek causes for diarrhea; monitor for tinnitus; may aggravate or cause gout attack; may enhance bleeding if used with anticoagulants

Additional Information Pepto-Bismol® contains bismuth 58% and salicylate 42%; do not exceed 4.2 g/day dosage; bismuth is radiopaque; 2 tablets yield 204 mg salicylate; 30 mL of suspension yields 258 mg

Special Geriatric Considerations Tinnitus and CNS side effects (confusion, dizziness, high tone deafness, delirium, psychosis) may be difficult to assess in some elderly. Limit use of this agent in elderly.

Dosage Forms
Bismuth subsalicylate:
  Suspension: 262 mg/15 mL (240 mL)
  Tablet, chewable: 262 mg
Tablet, chewable, as subgallate: 200 mg

Bisoprolol (bis OH proe lol)

Related Information
Beta-Blockers Comparison *on page 1026*

Brand Names Zebeta®

Therapeutic Category Antianginal Agent; Beta-Adrenergic Blocker

Use Treatment of hypertension, alone or in combination with other agents
  Unlabeled use: Angina pectoris, supraventricular arrhythmias, PVCs

Contraindications Hypersensitivity to beta-blocking agents, uncompensated congestive heart failure; cardiogenic shock; bradycardia or heart block; sinus node dysfunction; A-V conduction abnormalities. Although bisoprolol primarily blocks beta$_1$-receptors, high doses can result in beta$_2$-receptor blockage. Therefore, use with caution in elderly with bronchospastic lung disease and renal dysfunction. **Note:** Geriatric patients often have decreased renal function.

Warnings Use with caution in patients with inadequate myocardial function; abrupt withdrawal of beta-blockers may result in an exaggerated cardiac beta-adrenergic responsiveness. Symptomatology has included reports of tachycardia, hypertension, ischemia, angina, myocardial infarction, and sudden death. It is recommended that patients be tapered gradually off of beta-blockers over a 2-week period rather than via abrupt discontinuation.

Precautions Diabetes mellitus (may mask signs/symptoms of hypoglycemia), renal function decline, myasthenia gravis, and severe peripheral vascular disease; use with caution in patients with bronchospasm disease or congestive heart failure, patients undergoing anesthesia, and hyperthyroidism

Adverse Reactions
Cardiovascular: Persistent bradycardia, hypotension, chest pain, edema, heart failure, Raynaud's phenomena, heart block, facial edema
Central nervous system: Fatigue, dizziness, insomnia, lethargy, nightmares, depression, confusion, headache
Dermatologic: Rash, pruritus
Gastrointestinal: Constipation, diarrhea, nausea, xerostomia, anorexia
Genitourinary: Impotence, urinary retention
Neuromuscular & skeletal: Muscle cramps
Ocular: Blurred vision
Respiratory: Shortness of breath
Miscellaneous: Cold extremities

Overdosage Symptoms of overdose include severe hypotension, bradycardia, heart failure and bronchospasm, hypoglycemia

Toxicology Sympathomimetics (eg, epinephrine or dopamine), glucagon or a pacemaker can be used to treat the toxic bradycardia, asystole, and/or hypotension. Initially, fluids may be the best treatment for toxic hypotension. Patients should remain supine; serum glucose and potassium should be measured. Use supportive measures: lavage, syrup of ipecac; not significantly dialyzable. I.V. glucose should be administered for hypoglycemia; seizures may be treated with phenytoin or diazepam intravenously; continuous monitoring of blood pressure and EKG is necessary. If PVCs occur, treat with lidocaine or phenytoin; avoid quinidine, procainamide, and disopyramide since these agents further depress myocardial function. Bronchospasm can be treated with theophylline on beta$_2$ agonists (epinephrine).

Drug Interactions
Pharmacologic action of beta antagonists may be decreased by aluminum compounds, calcium salts, barbiturates, cholestyramine, colestipol, NSAIDs, penicillins (ampicillin), rifampin, salicylates, sulfinpyrazone, thyroid hormones; hypoglycemic effect of sulfonylureas may be blunted
Pharmacologic effect of beta antagonists may be enhanced with concomitant use of calcium channel blockers, oral contraceptives, flecainide (bioavailability and effect of flecainide also enhanced), haloperidol (hypotensive effects of both drugs), H$_2$ antagonists (decreased metabolism), hydralazine
(Continued)

Bisoprolol *(Continued)*

(both drugs hypotensive effects increased), loop diuretics (increased serum concentration of beta-blockers except atenolol), MAO inhibitors, phenothiazines, propafenone, quinidine, quinolones, thioamines; beta-blockers may decrease clearance of acetaminophen; beta-blockers may increase anticoagulant effects of warfarin (propranolol); benzodiazepine effects enhanced by the lipophilic beta-blockers (atenolol does not interact)

Significant and fatal increases in blood pressure have occurred after decrease in dose or discontinuation of clonidine in patients receiving both clonidine and beta-blockers together (reduce doses of each cautiously with small decreases); peripheral ischemia of ergot alkaloids enhanced by beta-blockers; beta-blockers increase serum concentration of lidocaine; beta-blockers increase hypotensive effect of prazosin

Mechanism of Action Selective inhibitor of beta$_1$-adrenergic receptors; competitively blocks beta$_1$-receptors, with little or no effect on beta$_2$-receptors at doses <10 mg; low lipid solubility, therefore, little crosses the blood-brain barrier

Pharmacokinetics

Absorption: Rapid and almost complete from GI tract (≥90%)

Distribution: Wide to body tissues; highest concentrations in heart, liver, lungs, and saliva; crosses the blood-brain barrier to a limited extent

Protein binding: 26% to 33%

Metabolism: Significant first-pass metabolism; metabolized in the liver

Half-life: 9-12 hours

Time to peak serum concentration: 1.7-3 hours

Elimination: ~50% unchanged in urine, <2% excreted in feces

Usual Dosage Oral:

Geriatrics: Initial dose: 2.5-5 mg/day; may be increased by 2.5-5 mg/day; maximum recommended dose: 20 mg/day

Adults: 5 mg once daily, may be increased to 10 mg, and then up to 20 mg once daily, if necessary; may be given without regard to meals

Dosing adjustment in renal/hepatic impairment: Cl$_{cr}$ <40 mL/minute: Initial: 2.5 mg/day; increase cautiously

Not dialyzable

Monitoring Parameters Blood pressure, EKG, orthostatic hypotension, heart rate, CNS effects

Test Interactions Increased thyroxine (S), cholesterol (S), glucose; increased triglycerides, uric acid; decreased HDL

Patient Information Adhere to dosage regimen; watch for postural hypotension; do not discontinue medication abruptly, sudden stopping of medication may precipitate or cause angina; consult pharmacist or physician before taking with other adrenergic drugs (eg, cold medications); notify physician if any of the following symptoms occur: difficult breathing, night cough, swelling of extremities, slow pulse, dizziness, lightheadedness, confusion, depression, skin rash, fever, sore throat, unusual bleeding or bruising; may produce drowsiness, dizziness, lightheadedness, blurred vision, confusion; use with caution while driving or performing tasks requiring alertness; may mask signs of hypoglycemia in diabetics; may be taken without regard to meals

Nursing Implications Patient's therapeutic response may be evaluated by looking at blood pressure, apical and radial pulses, fluid I & O, daily weight, respirations, and circulation in extremities before and during therapy; monitor for CNS side effects; modify dosage in patients with renal insufficiency

Additional Information May potentiate hypoglycemia in a diabetic patient and mask signs and symptoms

Special Geriatric Considerations Due to alterations in the beta-adrenergic autonomic nervous system, beta-adrenergic blockade may result in less hemodynamic response than seen in younger adults. Studies indicate that despite decreased sensitivity to the chronotropic effects of beta blockade with age, there appears to be an increased myocardial sensitivity to the negative inotropic effect during stress (ie, exercise). Controlled trials have shown the overall response rate for propranolol to be only 20% to 50% in elderly populations. Therefore, all beta-adrenergic blocking drugs may result in a decreased response as compared to younger adults.

Dosage Forms Tablet, as fumarate: 5 mg, 10 mg

References

Aagaard GN, "Treatment of Hypertension in The Elderly," *Drug Treatment in the Elderly*, Vestal RE, ed, Boston, MA: ADIS Health Science Press, 1984, 77.

Bitolterol (bye TOLE ter ole)

Related Information
Asthma Guidelines *on page 1040*
Inhaled Medications Comparison *on page 1034*

Brand Names Tornalate®

Generic Available No

Therapeutic Category Adrenergic Agonist Agent; Beta$_2$-Adrenergic Agonist Agent; Bronchodilator

Use Prevent and treat bronchial asthma and bronchospasm

Contraindications Known hypersensitivity to bitolterol

Warnings Use with caution in patients with unstable vasomotor symptoms, diabetes, hyperthyroidism, prostatic hypertrophy or a history of seizures; also use caution in the elderly and those patients with cardiovascular disorders such as coronary artery disease, arrhythmias, and hypertension

Precautions Excessive use may result in tolerance; deaths have been reported after excessive use; though the exact cause is unknown, cardiac arrest after a severe asthmatic crisis is suspected

Adverse Reactions
Cardiovascular: Tachycardia, palpitations, hypertension
Central nervous system: CNS stimulation, nervousness, hyperactivity, insomnia, dizziness, headache
Gastrointestinal: Nausea, vomiting, GI upset, dysgeusia
Neuromuscular & skeletal: Tremors (may be more common in the elderly)

Overdosage Symptoms of overdose include tremor, dizziness, nervousness, headache, nausea, coughing, seizures, angina, hypertension

Toxicology In cases of overdose, supportive therapy should be instituted, and prudent use of a cardioselective beta-adrenergic blocker (eg, atenolol or metoprolol) should be considered, keeping in mind the potential for induction of bronchoconstriction in an asthmatic individual. Dialysis has not been shown to be of value in the treatment of an overdose with this agent.

Drug Interactions
Decreased therapeutic effect: Beta-adrenergic blockers (eg, propranolol)
Increased therapeutic effect: Inhaled ipratropium may increase duration of bronchodilation, nifedipine may increase FEV-1
Increased toxicity (cardiovascular): MAO inhibitors, tricyclic antidepressants, sympathomimetic agents (eg, amphetamine, dopamine, dobutamine), inhaled anesthetics (eg, enflurane)

Mechanism of Action Selectively stimulates beta$_2$-adrenergic receptors in the lungs producing bronchial smooth muscle relaxation; minor beta$_1$ activity

Pharmacodynamics
Onset of action: 3-4 minutes
Duration: 4-8 hours

Pharmacokinetics
Metabolism: Bitolterol, a prodrug, is hydrolyzed to colterol (active) following inhalation
Half-life: 3 hours
Time to peak plasma colterol concentration: Inhalation: Within 1 hour
Elimination: In urine and feces

Usual Dosage Geriatrics and Adults:
Bronchospasm: 2 inhalations at an interval of at least 1-3 minutes, followed by a third inhalation if needed
Prevention of bronchospasm: 2 inhalations every 8 hours; do not exceed 3 inhalations every 6 hours or 2 inhalations every 4 hours

Monitoring Parameters Pulmonary function, blood pressure, pulse

Patient Information Do not exceed recommended dosage; rinse mouth with water following each inhalation to help with dry throat and mouth. Follow specific instructions accompanying inhaler; if more than one inhalation is necessary, wait at least 1 full minute between inhalations. May cause nervousness, restlessness, insomnia - if these effects continue after dosage reduction, notify physician. Also notify physician if palpitations, tachycardia, chest pain, muscle tremors, dizziness, headache, flushing or if breathing difficulty persists.

Nursing Implications Before using, the inhaler must be shaken well; assess lung sounds, pulse, and blood pressure before administration and during peak of medication; observe patient for wheezing after administration, if this occurs, call physician

Special Geriatric Considerations Elderly patients may find it useful to utilize a spacer device when using a metered dose inhaler; difficulty in using the inhaler often limits its effectiveness (see Adverse Reactions)

(Continued)

Bitolterol (Continued)

Dosage Forms
Bitolterol mesylate:
Aerosol, oral: 0.8% [370 mcg/metered spray, 300 inhalations] (15 mL)
Solution, inhalation: 0.2% (10 mL, 30 mL, 60 mL)

Black Draught® [OTC] *see* Senna *on page 853*

Bleph®-10 Ophthalmic *see* Sulfacetamide Sodium *on page 874*

Blephamide® Ophthalmic *see* Sulfacetamide Sodium and Prednisolone *on page 875*

Blis-To-Sol® [OTC] *see* Tolnaftate *on page 939*

Blocadren® Oral *see* Timolol *on page 925*

Bluboro® [OTC] *see* Aluminum Acetate and Calcium Acetate *on page 41*

Bonine® [OTC] *see* Meclizine *on page 574*

Boropak® [OTC] *see* Aluminum Acetate and Calcium Acetate *on page 41*

Breathe Free® [OTC] *see* Sodium Chloride *on page 860*

Breezee® Mist Antifungal [OTC] *see* Miconazole *on page 625*

Breezee® Mist Antifungal [OTC] *see* Tolnaftate *on page 939*

Breonesin® [OTC] *see* Guaifenesin *on page 437*

Brethaire® *see* Terbutaline *on page 893*

Brethine® *see* Terbutaline *on page 893*

Bretylium (bre TIL ee um)

Related Information
I.V. Push Recommended Guidelines *on page 1083*

Brand Names Bretylol®

Generic Available Yes

Therapeutic Category Antiarrhythmic Agent, Class III

Use Treatment and prophylaxis of ventricular tachycardia and fibrillation which have failed to respond to traditional first-line therapies; also used in the treatment of other serious ventricular arrhythmias resistant to lidocaine

Contraindications Digitalis intoxication-induced arrhythmias

Warnings Hypotension to which tolerance develops over days of use; transient hypertension; transient aggravation of existing arrhythmia; use caution or avoid use in patients with fixed cardiac output, aortic stenosis, pulmonary hypertension (see Precautions and Adverse Reactions)

Precautions Hypotension (50% in supine position), patients with fixed cardiac output (severe pulmonary hypertension or aortic stenosis) may experience severe hypotension due to decrease in peripheral resistance without ability to increase cardiac output; reduce dose in renal failure patients

Adverse Reactions
Cardiovascular: Hypotension (incidence 50% to 75%), transient initial hypertension, increase in PVCs, bradycardia, flushing, syncope
Central nervous system: Vertigo, confusion, anxiety, paranoid reactions, lethargy, emotional lability, hyperthermia
Dermatologic: Rash
Gastrointestinal: Nausea, vomiting, rarely diarrhea, abdominal pain
Local: Muscle atrophy and necrosis with repeated I.M. injections at same site
Ocular: Conjunctivitis
Renal: Renal impairment
Respiratory: Nasal congestion, shortness of breath
Miscellaneous: Hiccups, diaphoresis

Overdosage Underdosing occurs more frequently than overdose; overdose results in significant hypertension followed by severe hypotension (see Toxicology)

Toxicology Administration of short-acting hypotensive agent, nitroprusside (Nipride®), should be used for the hypertensive response; do not use long-acting hypotensive agents which may enhance hypotensive action of bretylium; hypotension should be treated with fluid administration and pressor agents such as dopamine or norepinephrine

Drug Interactions
Other antiarrhythmic agents may potentiate or antagonize cardiac effects, toxic effects may be additive
Pressor effects of catecholamines may be enhanced by bretylium
May potentiate digitalis toxicity due to initial release of norepinephrine

Stability The premix infusion should be stored at room temperature and protected from freezing; compatible solutions for dilution: D_5W for injection, D_5W in 0.45% NS; D_5W in 0.9% NS; 5% D_5W in lactated Ringer's, 0.9% NS;

5% sodium bicarbonate; 20% mannitol; lactated Ringer's; D_5W with potassium chloride 40 mEq/L; calcium chloride 54.4 mEq/L in D_5W

Mechanism of Action Class II antiarrhythmic; after an initial release of norepinephrine at the peripheral adrenergic nerve terminals, inhibits further release by postganglionic nerve endings in response to sympathetic nerve stimulation and inhibits reuptake into postganglionic adrenergic neurons; this action apparently increases ventricular fibrillation threshold, increases refractory period and action potential duration, and increases pacemaker tissue firing rate and ventricular conduction velocity

Pharmacodynamics
Onset of action:
I.M.: May require 2 hours following administration
I.V.: Antiarrhythmic effects seen within 6-20 minutes following administration
Peak effects: Within 6-9 hours
Duration: 6-24 hours

Pharmacokinetics
Absorption: I.M.: Well absorbed; suppression of ventricular fibrillation and tachycardia may not begin for 20 minutes to 2 hours
Protein binding: 1% to 6%
Metabolism: Not metabolized
Half-life: 7-8 hours; will increase 2-4 times with renal impairment/failure
Elimination: 70% to 80% (of I.M. dose) unchanged in urine over the first 24 hours with 10% over following 3 days

Usual Dosage Geriatrics and Adults (intended for short-term use only):
Immediate life-threatening ventricular arrhythmias; ventricular fibrillation; unstable ventricular tachycardia. **Note:** Patients should undergo defibrillation/cardioversion before and after bretylium doses as necessary. Adjust dose for renal function in elderly.
Initial dose: I.V.: 5 mg/kg (undiluted) over 1 minute; if arrhythmias persist, administer 10 mg/kg (undiluted) over 1 minute and repeat as necessary (usually at 15- to 30-minute intervals) up to a total dose of 30 mg/kg
Other life-threatening ventricular arrhythmias:
Initial dose: I.M., I.V.: 5-10 mg/kg, may repeat every 1-2 hours if arrhythmias persist; administer I.V. dose (diluted) over 10-30 minutes
Maintenance dose:
I.M.: 5-10 mg/kg every 6-8 hours
I.V. (diluted): 5-10 mg/kg every 6 hours
I.V. infusion (diluted): 1-2 mg/minute (little experience with doses >40 mg/kg/day)

Dosing adjustment in renal impairment:
Cl_{cr} 10-50 mL/minute: Administer 25% to 50% of dose
Cl_{cr} <10 mL/minute: Avoid use
Moderately dialyzable (20% to 50%)

Monitoring Parameters EKG and blood pressure throughout therapy is absolutely essential

Reference Range None clearly established

Patient Information Anticipate vomiting

Nursing Implications I.M. injection should not exceed 5 mL volume in any one site; administer around-the-clock rather than 4 times/day, 3 times/day, etc (ie, 12-6-12-6, not 9-1-5-9) to promote less variation in peak and trough serum concentration

Additional Information Subtherapeutic doses may cause hypotension

Special Geriatric Considerations Since renal function may be decreased, calculate or measure Cl_{cr} to guide dosing (see Usual Dosage); may have prolonged half-life with aging; adjust dose for renal function in elderly (see Precautions and Adverse Reactions)

Dosage Forms
Bretylium tosylate:
Injection: 50 mg/mL (10 mL, 20 mL)
Injection, premixed, in D_5W: 1 mg/mL (500 mL); 2 mg/mL (250 mL); 4 mg/mL (250 mL, 500 mL)

References
Fenster PE and Nolan PE, "Antiarrhythmic Drugs," *Geriatric Pharmacology*, Bressler R and Katz MD, eds, New York, NY: McGraw-Hill, 1993, 6:105-49.

Bretylol® *see Bretylium on previous page*

Brevibloc® *see Esmolol on page 348*

Bricanyl® *see Terbutaline on page 893*

Bromaline® Elixir [OTC] *see Brompheniramine and Phenylpropanolamine on page 130*

Bromanate® Elixir [OTC] *see* Brompheniramine and Phenylpropanolamine *on page 130*

Bromarest® [OTC] *see* Brompheniramine *on next page*

Bromatapp® [OTC] *see* Brompheniramine and Phenylpropanolamine *on page 130*

Brombay® [OTC] *see* Brompheniramine *on next page*

Bromocriptine (broe moe KRIP teen)

Brand Names Parlodel®

Generic Available No

Therapeutic Category Anti-Parkinson's Agent; Ergot Alkaloid

Use Treatment of parkinsonism in patients unresponsive or allergic to levodopa; also used in conditions associated with hyperprolactinemia and acromegaly

Contraindications Hypersensitivity to bromocriptine or any component, severe ischemic heart disease or peripheral vascular disorders

Precautions Use with caution in impaired renal or hepatic function

Adverse Reactions

Cardiovascular: Hypotension, hypertension, syncope, exacerbation of Raynaud's syndrome

Central nervous system: Dizziness, drowsiness, fatigue, insomnia, headache, hallucinations, nightmares, psychosis, lightheadedness, confusion, "on-off" phenomena, ataxia, depression, vertigo, anxiety, nervousness, nightmares

Dermatologic: Skin rash

Gastrointestinal: Nausea, vomiting, anorexia, abdominal cramps, constipation

Genitourinary: Urinary incontinence, urinary retention

Neuromuscular & skeletal: Paresthesia (fingers), numbness, muscle cramps (legs and feet), weakness

Ocular: Visual disturbances, blepharospasm

Respiratory: Nasal congestion, shortness of breath

Miscellaneous: Cold extremities

Note: Incidence of adverse effects is high, especially at beginning of treatment and with dosages >20 mg/day; adverse reactions may be relieved by reducing dose temporarily

Overdosage Symptoms of overdose include nausea, vomiting, hypotension

Toxicology When unresponsive to I.V. fluids or Trendelenburg positioning, patient often responds to norepinephrine infusions started at 0.1-0.2 mcg/kg/minute followed by a titrated infusion

Drug Interactions

Decreased effect: Phenothiazines, haloperidol, reserpine, metoclopramide, methyldopa

Increased toxicity: Ergot alkaloids, hypotensive agents

Mechanism of Action Semisynthetic ergot alkaloid derivative with dopaminergic properties; inhibits prolactin secretion; can improve symptoms of Parkinson's disease by directly stimulating dopamine receptors in the corpus striatum

Pharmacokinetics

Protein binding: 90% to 96%

Metabolism: Majority metabolized in the liver; substrate CYP3A4

Half-life:

Biphasic: 6-8 hours

Terminal phase: 50 hours

Time to peak serum concentration: Oral: Within 1-2 hours

Elimination: In bile, with only 2% to 6% being excreted unchanged in urine

Usual Dosage Geriatrics and Adults: Oral:

Parkinsonism: 1.25 mg twice daily, increase by 1.25-2.5 mg/day in 2- to 4-week intervals; usual dose range: 30-90 mg/day in 3 divided doses, though elderly patients can usually be managed on lower doses

Hyperprolactinemia: 2.5 mg 2-3 times/day

Acromegaly: Initial: 1.25-2.5 mg, increasing as necessary every 3-7 days; usual dose: 20-30 mg/day

Monitoring Parameters Monitor blood pressure closely as well as hepatic, hematopoietic, and cardiovascular function

Test Interactions Increased BUN, AST, ALT, CPK, alkaline phosphatase, uric acid; usually these laboratory test abnormalities are transient and not clinically significant; if they occur, monitor for resolution

Patient Information Take with food or milk to minimize nausea; drowsiness commonly occurs upon initiation of therapy; limit use of alcohol; avoid exposure to cold; rise slowly from sitting or lying position

Nursing Implications Raise bed rails and institute safety measures; aid patient with ambulation; may cause postural hypotension and drowsiness; incidence of side effects is high (68%) with nausea the most common

Additional Information Usually used with levodopa or levodopa/carbidopa to treat Parkinson's disease; when adding bromocriptine, the dose of levodopa/carbidopa can usually and should be decreased

Special Geriatric Considerations No special considerations are recommended since drug is dosed to response; however, elderly may have concomitant diseases or drug therapy which may complicate therapy; see Adverse Reactions, Drug Interactions, and Usual Dosage

Dosage Forms
Bromocriptine mesylate:
Capsule: 5 mg
Tablet: 2.5 mg

References
Koller WC, Silver DE, and Lieberman A, "An Algorithm for the Management of Parkinson's Disease," *Neurology*, 1994, 44(12 Suppl 10):S1-52.
Stern MB, "Contemporary Approaches to the Pharmacotherapeutic Management of Parkinson's Disease: An Overview," *Neurology*, 1997, 49(1 Suppl 1):S2-9.
Watts RL, "The Role of Dopamine Agonists in Early Parkinson's Disease," *Neurology*, 1997, 49(1 Suppl 1):S34-48.

Bromphen® [OTC] *see* Brompheniramine *on this page*

Brompheniramine (brome fen IR a meen)

Brand Names Bromarest® [OTC]; Brombay® [OTC]; Bromphen® [OTC]; Brotane® [OTC]; Chlorphed® [OTC]; Cophene-B®; Diamine T.D.® [OTC]; Dimetane® Extentabs® [OTC]; Nasahist B®; ND-Stat®; Oraminic® II; Sinusol-B®; Veltane®

Synonyms Parabromdylamine

Generic Available Yes

Therapeutic Category Antihistamine

Use Perennial and seasonal allergic rhinitis and other allergic symptoms including urticaria

Contraindications Narrow-angle glaucoma, bladder neck obstruction, symptomatic prostatic hypertrophy, asthmatic attacks, and stenosing peptic ulcer, hypersensitivity to brompheniramine or any component

Warnings Antihistamines are more likely to cause dizziness, excessive sedation, syncope, toxic confusional states, and hypotension in the elderly.

Precautions Use with caution in patients with heart disease, hypertension, thyroid disease, and asthma

Adverse Reactions
Central nervous system: Paradoxical excitability, drowsiness, dizziness, confusion
Dermatologic: Rash
Gastrointestinal: Nausea, anorexia, xerostomia
Note: Compared with other first generation antihistamines, brompheniramine is relatively nonsedating.

Overdosage Symptoms of overdose include dry mouth, flushed skin, dilated pupils, CNS depression

Toxicology There is no specific treatment for an antihistamine overdose, however, most of its clinical toxicity is due to anticholinergic effects. Cholinesterase inhibitors may be useful by reducing acetylcholinesterase. Acetylcholinesterase inhibitors include physostigmine, neostigmine, pyridostigmine, and edrophonium. For anticholinergic overdose with severe life-threatening symptoms, physostigmine 1-2 mg I.V., slowly may be given to reverse these effects.

Drug Interactions Increased toxicity: CNS depressants, MAO inhibitors, alcohol, tricyclic antidepressants

Stability Solutions may crystallize if stored below 0°C, crystals will dissolve when warmed

Mechanism of Action Competes with histamine for H_1-receptor sites on effector cells in the gastrointestinal tract, blood vessels, and respiratory tract

Pharmacodynamics
Onset of action: Maximal clinical effects seen within 3-9 hours
Duration of action varies with formulation

Pharmacokinetics
Metabolism: Extensive by the liver
Half-life: 12-34 hours
Time to peak serum concentration: Oral: Within 2-5 hours
Elimination: In urine as inactive metabolites; 2% fecal elimination
(Continued)

Brompheniramine *(Continued)*

Usual Dosage
Oral:

Geriatrics: Initial: 4 mg once or twice daily. **Note:** Duration of action may be 36 hours or more, even when serum concentrations are low.

Adults: 4 mg every 4-6 hours or 8 mg of sustained release form every 8-12 hours or 12 mg of sustained release every 12 hours; maximum: 24 mg/day

I.M., I.V., S.C.: Adults: 5-20 mg every 4-12 hours; maximum: 40 mg/24 hours

Monitoring Parameters Relief of symptoms

Patient Information May cause drowsiness; avoid alcohol; take with food or milk; swallow whole; do not crush or chew sustained release products

Nursing Implications Raise bed rails and institute safety measures; aid patient with ambulation

Additional Information Causes less drowsiness than some conventional antihistamines

Special Geriatric Considerations Anticholinergic action may cause significant confusional symptoms; constipation and problems with voiding urine (see Contraindications, Warnings, and Usual Dosage)

Dosage Forms
Brompheniramine maleate:

Elixir: 2 mg/5 mL with 3% alcohol (120 mL, 480 mL, 4000 mL)

Injection: 10 mg/mL (10 mL)

Tablet: 4 mg, 8 mg

Tablet, sustained release: 8 mg, 12 mg

Brompheniramine and Phenylpropanolamine
(brome fen IR a meen & fen il proe pa NOLE a meen)

Related Information

Brompheniramine *on previous page*

Phenylpropanolamine *on page 741*

Brand Names Bromaline® Elixir [OTC]; Bromanate® Elixir [OTC]; Bromatapp® [OTC]; Bromphen® Tablet [OTC]; Cold & Allergy® Elixir [OTC]; Dimaphen® Elixir [OTC]; Dimaphen® Tablets [OTC]; Dimetapp® 4-Hour Liqui-Gel Capsule [OTC]; Dimetapp® Elixir [OTC]; Dimetapp® Tablet [OTC]; Dimetapp® Extentabs® [OTC]; Genatap® Elixir [OTC]; Myphetapp® [OTC]; Tamine® [OTC]; Vicks® DayQuil® Allergy Relief 4 Hour Tablet [OTC]

Synonyms Phenylpropanolamine and Brompheniramine

Generic Available Yes

Therapeutic Category Antihistamine/Decongestant Combination

Adverse Reactions

Cardiovascular: Palpitations

Central nervous system: Excitability, drowsiness, dizziness, headache

Dermatologic: Rash

Gastrointestinal: Anorexia, nausea, xerostomia

Hematologic: Leukopenia

Usual Dosage Geriatrics and Adults: Oral:

Elixir: 10 mL

Tablet: 1 tablet every 4-6 hours

Sustained release: 1 tablet every 12 hours

Special Geriatric Considerations Anticholinergic action may cause significant confusional symptoms; constipation and problems with voiding urine. Use cautiously in patients with cardiovascular disease (see Warnings and Precautions for individual agents).

Dosage Forms

Elixir: Brompheniramine maleate 2 mg and phenylpropanolamine hydrochloride 12.5 mg per 5 mL with 2.3% alcohol (120 mL)

Tablet, immediate release: Brompheniramine maleate 4 mg and phenylpropanolamine hydrochloride 25 mg

Tablet, sustained release: Brompheniramine maleate 12 mg and phenylpropanolamine hydrochloride 75 mg

Bromphen® Tablet [OTC] *see* Brompheniramine and Phenylpropanolamine *on this page*

Bronitin® *see* Epinephrine *on page 336*

Bronkaid® Mist [OTC] *see* Epinephrine *on page 336*

Bronkodyl® *see* Theophylline *on page 902*

Bronkometer® *see* Isoetharine *on page 499*

Bronkosol® *see* Isoetharine *on page 499*

Brontex® Liquid *see* Guaifenesin and Codeine *on page 438*
Brontex® Tablet *see* Guaifenesin and Codeine *on page 438*
Brotane® [OTC] *see* Brompheniramine *on page 129*
Bucladin®-S Softab® *see* Buclizine *on this page*

Buclizine (BYOO kli zeen)

Brand Names Bucladin®-S Softab®
Generic Available Yes
Therapeutic Category Antiemetic; Antihistamine, H_1 Blocker
Use Prevention and treatment of motion sickness; symptomatic treatment of vertigo
Contraindications Known hypersensitivity to buclizine
Warnings Severe emesis should be evaluated as to etiology before drug treatment is initiated; such treatment may obscure serious disease (ie, intestinal obstruction, appendicitis, brain tumors, and drug overdoses)
Precautions Product contains tartrazine; use with caution in patients with angle-closure glaucoma, peptic ulcer, urinary tract obstruction, hyperthyroidism; some preparations contain sodium bisulfite; syrup contains alcohol
Adverse Reactions
Cardiovascular: Hypotension, palpitations
Central nervous system: Drowsiness, sedation, dizziness, paradoxical excitement, fatigue, insomnia and confusion in elderly
Gastrointestinal: Nausea, vomiting, constipation, GI blockage in elderly
Genitourinary: Urinary retention
Neuromuscular & skeletal: Tremor
Ocular: Blurred vision
Overdosage CNS stimulation or depression; overdose may result in death in infants and children
Toxicology There is no specific treatment for an antihistamine overdose, however, most of its clinical toxicity is due to anticholinergic effects; anticholinesterase inhibitors including physostigmine, neostigmine, pyridostigmine, and edrophonium may be useful by reducing acetylcholinesterase; for anticholinergic overdose with severe life-threatening symptoms, physostigmine 1-2 mg I.V., slowly may be given to reverse these effects
Drug Interactions Increased toxicity: CNS depressants, MAO inhibitors, tricyclic antidepressants
Mechanism of Action Buclizine acts centrally by blocking chemoreceptor trigger zone to suppress nausea and vomiting. It is a piperazine antihistamine closely related to cyclizine and meclizine. It also has CNS depressant, anticholinergic, antispasmodic, and local anesthetic effects, and suppresses labyrinthine activity and conduction in vestibular-cerebellar nerve pathways.
Pharmacodynamics
Onset of action: 30-60 minutes
Duration: 8-12 hours
Pharmacokinetics Metabolism: In the liver
Usual Dosage Geriatrics and Adults: Oral:
Motion sickness (prophylaxis): 50 mg 30 minutes prior to traveling; may repeat 50 mg after 4-6 hours
Vertigo: 50 mg twice daily, up to 150 mg/day
Administration May be chewed, swallowed whole, or dissolved in mouth
Monitoring Parameters Monitor for CNS, urinary, and gastrointestinal effects in elderly
Patient Information May cause drowsiness; caution should be exercised when performing mechanical functions; avoid alcohol and other CNS depressants; may cause dry mouth, constipation, and difficulty urinating
Nursing Implications Bucladin®-S Softab® may be chewed, swallowed whole, or allowed to dissolve in mouth; monitor for CNS side effects (ie, confusion), urinary retention, and constipation
Special Geriatric Considerations Due to anticholinergic action, use lowest dose in divided doses to avoid side effects and their inconvenience; limit use if possible; may cause confusion or aggravate symptoms of confusion in those with dementia; constipation and difficulty voiding urine may occur
Dosage Forms Tablet, chewable, as hydrochloride: 50 mg
References
Atkinson R and Appenzeller O, "Headache," *Postgrad Med J*, 1984, 60(710):841-6.

Budesonide (byoo DES oh nide)

Related Information
Asthma Guidelines *on page 1040*
(Continued)

Budesonide *(Continued)*

Estimated Comparative Daily Dosages for Inhaled Corticosteroids *on page 1045*

Brand Names Rhinocort™

Generic Available No

Therapeutic Category Corticosteroid, Nasal; Corticosteroid, Topical (Medium Potency)

Use Management of symptoms of seasonal or perennial rhinitis and nonallergic perennial rhinitis

Contraindications Hypersensitivity to budesonide or any components

Warnings Use with caution in patients receiving systemic or other inhaled corticosteroids

Precautions Use with caution, if at all, in patients with active or quiescent tuberculosis, untreated fungal, bacterial, or systemic viral infections, or ocular herpes simplex

Adverse Reactions

Cardiovascular: Pounding heartbeat (>10%)

Central nervous system: Nervousness (>10%), headache (>10%), dizziness (>10%)

Dermatologic: Itching (>10%), rash (>10%)

Gastrointestinal: GI irritation (>10%), bitter taste (>10%), oral candidiasis (>10%), xerostomia, dry throat, loss of taste perception

Respiratory: Coughing (>10%), upper respiratory tract infection (>10%), bronchitis (>10%), hoarseness (>10%), epistaxis, bronchospasm, shortness of breath

Miscellaneous: Increased susceptibility to infections (>10%), diaphoresis (>10%), loss of smell

Drug Interactions Although there have been no reported drug interactions to date, one would expect budesonide could potentially interact with drugs known to interact with other corticosteroids

Mechanism of Action Inhibits cells and mediators involved in allergic and nonallergic/irritant-mediated inflammation

Pharmacokinetics

Absorption: ~20% is systemically absorbed from intranasal dose

Metabolism: Liver

Usual Dosage Geriatrics and Adults: Aerosol inhalation: Nasal: Initial: 8 sprays (4 sprays/nostril) per day (256 mcg/day), given as either 2 sprays in each nostril in the morning and evening or as 4 sprays in each nostril in the morning; after symptoms decrease (usually by 3-7 days), reduce dose slowly every 2-4 weeks to the smallest amount needed to control symptoms

Monitoring Parameters Relief of symptoms

Patient Information For intranasal use only; inhaler should be shaken well immediately prior to use; clear nasal passage by blowing nose prior to use; keep inhaler clean and unobstructed; wash in warm water and dry thoroughly; contact physician if symptoms are not improved by 3 weeks of treatment, if condition worsens, or if nasal irritation or burning persists

Nursing Implications Follow instructions which accompany product; for nasal use only

Special Geriatric Considerations Ensure that patients can correctly use nasal inhaler

Dosage Forms Aerosol: 50 mcg released per actuation to deliver ~32 mcg to patient via nasal adapter [200 metered doses] (7 g)

Bufferin® [OTC] *see* Aspirin *on page 84*

Buffex® [OTC] *see* Aspirin *on page 84*

Bumetanide *(byoo MET a nide)*

Related Information

I.V. Push Recommended Guidelines *on page 1083*

Brand Names Bumex®

Generic Available No

Therapeutic Category Diuretic, Loop

Use Management of edema associated with congestive heart failure or hepatic or renal disease including nephrotic syndrome; used alone or in combination with antihypertensives in the treatment of hypertension

Contraindications Hypersensitivity to bumetanide or any component; allergy to sulfonamides may result in cross-hypersensitivity to bumetanide; anuria or increasing azotemia

Warnings Loop diuretics are potent diuretics; excess amounts can lead to profound diuresis with fluid and electrolyte loss; close medical supervision and dose evaluation is required, particularly in the elderly

Adverse Reactions
Cardiovascular: Hypotension
Central nervous system: Dizziness, headache, encephalopathy
Dermatologic: Rash, photosensitivity
Endocrine & metabolic: Hyperglycemia, hypokalemia, hypochloremia, hyponatremia
Gastrointestinal: Cramps, nausea, vomiting
Genitourinary: Azotemia
Hepatic: Alteration of liver function test results
Neuromuscular & skeletal: Weakness
Otic: Impaired hearing
Renal: Decreased uric acid excretion, increased serum creatinine

Overdosage Symptoms of overdose include electrolyte depletion, volume depletion

Toxicology Treatment is primarily symptomatic and supportive; hypotension responds to fluids and Trendelenburg position; replace electrolytes as necessary

Drug Interactions
Decreased effect: Indomethacin, other NSAIDs
Increased hypotensive effect: Other antihypertensives
Increased level of lithium
Increased risk of ototoxicity: Aminoglycosides, other loop diuretics, vancomycin
When given with digoxin, diuretic-induced hypokalemia increases the risk of digoxin toxicity

Stability I.V. infusion solutions should be used within 24 hours after preparation

Mechanism of Action Inhibits reabsorption of sodium and chloride in the ascending loop of Henle and distal renal tubule, interfering with the chloride-binding cotransport system, thus causing increased excretion of water, sodium, chloride, magnesium, and calcium

Pharmacodynamics
Onset of action:
Oral, I.M.: 30-60 minutes
I.V.: Within a few minutes
Duration: 6 hours

Pharmacokinetics
Distribution: V_d: 13-25 L/kg
Protein binding: 95%
Metabolism: Partial in the liver
Half-life: 1-1.5 hours
Elimination: Majority of unchanged drug and metabolites excreted in urine

Usual Dosage
Geriatrics: Initial: Oral: 0.5 mg once daily, increase as necessary
Adults:
Oral: 0.5-2 mg/dose (maximum: 10 mg/day) 1-2 times/day
I.M., I.V.: 0.5-1 mg/dose (maximum: 10 mg/day)

Monitoring Parameters Blood pressure (standing and sitting/supine), serum electrolytes, renal function; in high doses, monitor auditory function, I & O, weight

Test Interactions Increased BUN, creatinine, ammonia (B), amylase (S), glucose, uric acid (S); decreased sodium, calcium, chloride, potassium

Patient Information May be taken with food or milk; get up slowly from a lying or sitting position to minimize dizziness, lightheadedness or fainting; also use extra care when exercising, standing for long periods of time and during hot weather; take in the morning; may cause increased sensitivity to sunlight

Nursing Implications Administer I.V. slowly, over 1-2 minutes; be alert to complaints about hearing difficulty; check patient for orthostasis (see Monitoring Parameters)

Additional Information Can be used in furosemide-allergic patients; 1 mg = 40 mg furosemide

Special Geriatric Considerations Severe loss of sodium and/or increases in BUN can cause confusion; for any change in mental status in patients on bumetanide, monitor electrolytes and renal function (see Warnings)

Dosage Forms
Injection: 0.25 mg/mL (2 mL, 4 mL, 10 mL)
Tablet: 0.5 mg, 1 mg, 2 mg

Bumex® *see Bumetanide on page 132*
Buprenex® *see Buprenorphine on this page*

Buprenorphine (byoo pre NOR feen)
Related Information
Pharmacokinetics of Narcotic Agonist Analgesics *on page 1037*
Brand Names Buprenex®
Generic Available No
Therapeutic Category Analgesic, Narcotic
Use Management of moderate to severe pain
Restrictions C-V
Contraindications Hypersensitivity to buprenorphine or any component
Warnings If used in narcotic-dependent patients, may cause withdrawal effects
Precautions Use with caution in severe impairment of hepatic, pulmonary, or renal function
Adverse Reactions
Cardiovascular: Hypotension
Central nervous system: Vertigo, confusion, sedation, dizziness, headache
Gastrointestinal: Nausea
Respiratory: Respiratory depression
Overdosage Symptoms of overdose include CNS depression, pinpoint pupils, hypotension, bradycardia
Toxicology Treatment of an overdose includes support of the patient's airway, establishment of an I.V. line, and administration of naloxone 2 mg I.V. with repeat administration as necessary up to a total of 10 mg
Drug Interactions Increased toxicity: CNS depressants, barbiturate anesthetics, benzodiazepines
Stability Protect from excessive heat or light
Mechanism of Action Opiate agonist/antagonist that produces analgesia by binding to kappa and mu opiate receptors in the CNS
Pharmacodynamics Onset of analgesia: Within 10-30 minutes
Pharmacokinetics
Absorption: I.M.: 30% to 40%
Distribution: V_d: 97-187 L/kg
Protein binding: Highly protein bound
Metabolism: Mainly in the liver; undergoes extensive first-pass metabolism
Half-life: 2.2-3 hours
Elimination: 70% in feces via bile and 20% in urine as unchanged drug
Usual Dosage I.M., slow I.V.:
Geriatrics: 0.15 mg every 6 hours
Adults: 0.3-0.6 mg every 6 hours as needed
Monitoring Parameters Pain relief, respiratory and mental status, blood pressure
Test Interactions Increased amylase, lipase
Patient Information May cause drowsiness and/or dizziness
Nursing Implications Monitor respiratory status during therapy; gradual withdrawal of drug is necessary to avoid withdrawal symptoms
Additional Information 0.3 mg = 10 mg morphine or 75 mg meperidine, has longer duration of action than either; may precipitate abstinence syndrome in narcotic-dependent patients; therefore, use buprenorphine before starting a patient on a narcotic. Long-term use is not recommended.
Special Geriatric Considerations One postmarketing study found that elderly patients were more likely to suffer from confusion and drowsiness after buprenorphine as compared to younger patients
Dosage Forms Injection, as hydrochloride: 0.3 mg/mL (1 mL)
References
Harcus AH, Ward AE, and Smith DW, "Buprenorphine: Experience in an Elderly Population of 975 Patients During a Year's Monitored Release," *Br J Clin Pract*, 1980, 34(5):144-6.

Bupropion (byoo PROE pee on)
Related Information
Antidepressant Agents Comparison *on page 1021*
Antidepressant Medication Guidelines *on page 1075*
Brand Names Wellbutrin®; Wellbutrin® SR; Zyban®
Synonyms Amfebutamone
Generic Available No
Therapeutic Category Antidepressant
Use Treatment of depression; as an aid to smoking cessation treatment

Contraindications Seizure disorder, prior diagnosis of bulimia or anorexia nervosa, known hypersensitivity to bupropion, concurrent use of a mono-amine oxidase (MAO) inhibitor

Precautions Estimated seizure potential is increased many fold in doses in the 450-600 mg/day dosage; giving a single dose of 150 mg or less will lessen the seizure potential; recent myocardial infarction or unstable heart disease

Adverse Reactions
Central nervous system: Agitation, insomnia, fever, headache, psychosis, confusion, anxiety, restlessness, seizures, chills, akathisia
Gastrointestinal: Nausea, vomiting, weight loss
Genitourinary: Impotence
Neuromuscular & skeletal: Tremors
Ocular: Blurred vision

Overdosage Symptoms of overdose include labored breathing, salivation, arched back, ataxia, convulsions

Toxicology Hospitalize patient if still conscious, induce vomiting, administer activated charcoal every 6 hours for two times and obtain baseline labs, obtain EKG and EEG over the next 48 hours; maintain hydration. In patients who are comatose, stuporous, or seizing, perform gastric lavage after adequate airway has been established via intubation. Treat seizures with I.V. benzodiazepines and supportive therapies; dialysis may be of limited value after drug absorption because of slow tissue to plasma diffusion.

Drug Interactions Carbamazepine, phenytoin, cimetidine, phenobarbital (bupropion may enhance metabolism), enhanced acute toxicity with phenelzine; levodopa increases nausea and agitation; risk of seizure activity following abrupt withdrawal of benzodiazepines; MAO inhibitors separate by at least 14 days (see Contraindications)

Mechanism of Action Bupropion is an antidepressant structurally different from all other previously marketed antidepressants; like other antidepressants the mechanism of bupropion's activity is not fully understood; the drug is a weak blocker of serotonin and norepinephrine reuptake, inhibits neuronal dopamine reuptake and is not a monoamine oxidase A or B inhibitor

Pharmacodynamics May take up to 4 weeks or longer until full effect is seen

Pharmacokinetics
Absorption: Rapidly from the GI tract
Distribution: V_d: 1.4-3.2 L/kg
Protein binding: 82% to 88%; has not been studied in the elderly
Metabolism: Extensive in the liver to multiple metabolites (whose elimination may be decreased by liver or renal dysfunction)
Bioavailability, oral: 5%
Half-life: 14 hours
Time to peak plasma concentration: Oral: Within 2 hours

Usual Dosage Oral:
Geriatrics: Initial: 50-100 mg/day, increase by 50-100 mg every 3-4 days as tolerated; there is evidence that the elderly respond at 150 mg/day in divided doses, but some may require a higher dose
Adults: 100 mg 3 times/day; begin at 100 mg twice daily; increase after days if tolerated; may increase to a maximum dose of 450 mg/day
Smoking cessation: Initiate with 150 mg once daily for 3 days; increase to 150 mg twice daily; treatment should continue for 7-12 weeks

Monitoring Parameters Signs and symptoms of depression; mood; weight; blood pressure

Patient Information Take in equally divided doses 3-4 times/day to minimize the risk of seizures; avoid alcohol; may impair driving or other motor or cognitive skills and judgment

Nursing Implications Monitor body weight; be aware that drug may cause seizures

Additional Information Use in patients with renal or hepatic impairment increases the possibilities of possible toxic effects

Special Geriatric Considerations Limited data available about the use of bupropion in the elderly; two studies have found it equally effective when compared to imipramine. Its side effect profile (minimal anticholinergic and blood pressure effects) may make it useful in persons who do not tolerate traditional cyclic antidepressants (see Usual Dosage).

Dosage Forms
Tablet (Wellbutrin®): 75 mg, 100 mg
Tablet, sustained release (Wellbutrin® SR, Zyban®): 100 mg, 150 mg
(Continued)

Bupropion *(Continued)*

References

Branconnier RJ, Cole JO, Ghazvinian S, et al, "Clinical Pharmacology of Bupropion and Imipramine in Elderly Depressives," *J Clin Psychiatry*, 1983, 44(5 Pt 2):130-3.

Hayes PE and Kristoff CA, "Adverse Reactions to Five New Antidepressants," *Clin Pharm*, 1986, 5:471-80.

Kane JM, Cole K, Sarantakos S, et al, "Safety and Efficacy of Bupropion in Elderly Patients: Preliminary Observations," *J Clin Psychiatry*, 1983, 44(5 Pt 2):134-6.

BuSpar® *see Buspirone on this page*

Buspirone *(byoo SPYE rone)*

Brand Names BuSpar®

Generic Available No

Therapeutic Category Antianxiety Agent

Use Management of anxiety

    Unlabeled use: Panic attacks

Contraindications Hypersensitivity to buspirone or any component

Warnings Use in hepatic or renal impairment is not recommended

Precautions Causes less sedation than other anxiolytics, but patients should be cautioned about driving until they are certain buspirone does not affect them adversely; avoid alcoholic beverages

Adverse Reactions

    Central nervous system: Sedation, disorientation, excitement, dizziness, fever, headache, encephalopathy, ataxia

    Dermatologic: Rash, urticaria

    Gastrointestinal: Nausea, vomiting, diarrhea, flatulence

    Hematologic: Leukopenia, eosinophilia

Overdosage Symptoms of overdose include dizziness, drowsiness, pinpoint pupils, nausea, vomiting

Toxicology There is no known antidote for buspirone and most therapies are supportive and symptomatic in nature

Drug Interactions

    Increased effect: Cimetidine

    Increased toxicity: MAO inhibitors, CNS depressants, alcohol, increased haloperidol concentrations

Drug/Food Interactions Food may decrease the absorption of buspirone, but it may also decrease the first-pass metabolism, thereby increasing the bioavailability of buspirone

Mechanism of Action Selectively antagonizes CNS serotonin 5-HT$_1$A receptors without affecting benzodiazepine-GABA receptors; may down-regulate postsynaptic 5-HT$_2$ receptors as do antidepressants

Pharmacodynamics Onset of action: Decrease in anxiety is seen after 1 week of therapy, but it may take several weeks for the full effects to be seen

Pharmacokinetics Studies in the elderly found no significant changes in pharmacokinetic parameters

    Protein binding: 95%

    Metabolism: In the liver by oxidation and undergoes extensive first-pass metabolism

    Half-life: 2-3 hours; range: 2-11 hours

    Time to peak serum concentration: Within 40-60 minutes

Usual Dosage Oral:

    Geriatrics: Initial: 5 mg twice daily, increase by 5 mg/day every 2-3 days as needed up to 20-30 mg/day; maximum daily dose: 60 mg/day (see Additional Information)

    Adults: 15 mg/day (5 mg 3 times/day); increase by 5 mg/day every 2-3 days, as needed to a maximum of 60 mg/day (see Additional Information)

    Dosage adjustment in hepatic impairment: Dose should be decreased with severe hepatic insufficiency; anuric patients should be dosed at 25% to 50% of the usual dose

Monitoring Parameters Mental status, symptoms of anxiety

Test Interactions Increased AST, ALT

Patient Information May cause drowsiness or dizziness; take with food; report any change in senses (ie, smelling, hearing, vision); cautious use with alcohol is recommended; takes 2-3 weeks to see the full effect of this medication

Nursing Implications See Monitoring Parameters

Additional Information Has shown little potential for abuse; not effective when used prn; maximal effect may not be achieved until 3-4 weeks after adequate dose is achieved. Some response may be seen in 1-2 weeks after initiation of therapy. Buspirone, in the treatment of agitation, has been shown to be effective in elderly at an average daily dose of 30-35 mg; slow titration, as described in Usual Dosage, is necessary to avoid side effects and achieve maximum tolerable doses for individual patients.

Special Geriatric Considerations Because buspirone is less sedating than other anxiolytics, it may be a useful agent in geriatric patients when an anxiolytic is indicated

Dosage Forms Tablet, as hydrochloride: 5 mg, 10 mg

References

Gammans RE, Westrick ML, Shea JP, et al, "Pharmacokinetics of Buspirone in Elderly Subjects," *J Clin Pharmacol*, 1989, 29(1):72-8.

Kunik ME, Yudofsky SC, Silver JM, et al, "Pharmacologic Approach to Management of Agitation Associated With Dementia," *J Clin Psychiatry*, 1994, 55(Suppl 2):13-7.

Weis KJ, "Management of Anxiety and Depression Syndromes in Elderly," *J Clin Psychiatry*, 1994, 55(Suppl 2):5-12.

Busulfan (byoo SUL fan)

Brand Names Myleran®

Generic Available No

Therapeutic Category Antineoplastic Agent, Alkylating Agent

Use Chronic myelogenous leukemia and marrow-ablative conditioning regimens prior to bone marrow transplantation

Contraindications Hypersensitivity to busulfan or any component; failure to respond to previous courses

Warnings The U.S. Food and Drug Administration (FDA) currently recommends that procedures for proper handling and disposal of antineoplastic agents be considered. May cause severe and serious bone marrow suppression (pancytopenia) that may be more prolonged than that produced by other alkylating agents. May take 1 month to 2 years to recover bone marrow function after discontinuing therapy; bronchopulmonary dysplasia (busulfan lung) with fibrosis occurs rarely; carcinogenic potential has been described as with other alkylating agents.

Precautions May induce severe bone marrow hypoplasia; reduce or discontinue dosage at first sign, as reflected by an abnormal decrease in any of the formed elements of the blood; use with caution in patients recently given other myelosuppressive drugs or radiation treatment

Adverse Reactions

Central nervous system: Dizziness, seizures
Dermatologic: Hyperpigmentation
Endocrine & metabolic: Addison-like syndrome, hyperuricemia
Gastrointestinal: Nausea, vomiting
Hematologic: Leukopenia, thrombocytopenia, anemia
Hepatic: Hepatic dysfunction, increased LFTs
Ocular: Blurred vision
Renal: Hemorrhagic cystitis
Respiratory: Pulmonary fibrosis

Overdosage Symptoms of overdose include leukopenia, thrombocytopenia, pancytopenia (rare)

Toxicology Initiate general supportive measures; monitor hematologic status closely; transfusions as needed

Drug Interactions Thioguanine (esophageal varices formed with long-term use); increased myelosuppression when used concomitantly with other immunosuppressives

Mechanism of Action Interferes with the normal function of DNA by alkylation and cross-linking the strands of DNA

Pharmacokinetics

Absorption: Oral: Rapidly and well absorbed
Metabolism: Extensive in the liver 10% to 50%
Time to peak:
I.V.: Peak plasma concentration occurs within 5 minutes
Oral: Within 4 hours
Elimination: In urine as metabolites within 24 hours

Usual Dosage Oral (refer to individual protocols):

Geriatrics: Start with lowest recommended doses for adults
Adults: 4-8 mg/day for remission induction of CML
Maintenance dose: Controversial, range from 1-4 mg/day to 2 mg/week

Monitoring Parameters Decrease in leukocytes not seen in first 10-15 days of therapy. Leukocyte count may increase during initiation of therapy and does not reflect resistance to therapy. Do not increase dose if WBC count increases during initiation of therapy. Monitor CBC and platelets weekly. Once remission is achieved, monitoring intervals may be increased according

(Continued)

Busulfan *(Continued)*

to protocol with physician discretion. Observe for signs of bleeding, bruising, infection, or pulmonary disease (see Additional Information).

Test Interactions Increased potassium (S)

Patient Information Watch for signs of bleeding, bruising, coughing, difficulty breathing, fever, joint pain, or flank pain. May cause darkening of skin, dizziness, fatigue, mental confusion, nausea, vomiting, anorexia. Take medication the same time each day. Excellent oral hygiene is needed to minimize oral discomfort.

Nursing Implications Avoid I.M. injection if platelet count falls to <100,000/mm^3 (see Monitoring Parameters)

Additional Information Use with caution in patients recently given other myelosuppressive drugs or radiation treatment

Myelosuppressive effects:
WBC: Moderate
Platelets: Moderate
Onset (days): 7
Nadir (days): 14-21
Recovery (days): 28

Special Geriatric Considerations Toxicity to immunosuppressives is increased in elderly. Start with lowest recommended adult doses (see Usual Dosage). Signs of infection, such as fever and rise in WBCs, may not occur. Lethargy and confusion may be more prominent signs of infection.

Dosage Forms Tablet: 2 mg

References

Heard BE and Cooke RA, "Busulphan Lung," *Thorax*, 1968, 23(2):187-93.

Hutchins LF and Lipschitz DA, "Cancer, Clinical Pharmacology, and Aging," *Clin Geriatr Med*, 1987, 3(3):483-503.

Kaplan HG, "Use of Cancer Chemotherapy in the Elderly," *Drug Treatment in the Elderly*, Vestal RE, ed, Boston, MA: ADIS Health Science Press, 1984, 338-49.

Butabarbital Sodium (byoo ta BAR bi tal SOW dee um)

Related Information

Anxiolytic/Hypnotic Use in Long-Term Care Facilities *on page 1099*
Federal OBRA Regulations Recommended Maximum Doses - Hypnotics *on page 1057*

Brand Names Butalan®; Buticaps®; Butisol Sodium®

Generic Available Yes

Therapeutic Category Barbiturate; Hypnotic; Sedative

Restrictions C-III

Special Geriatric Considerations Use of this agent in the elderly is not recommended

Butalan® *see Butabarbital Sodium on this page*

Buticaps® *see Butabarbital Sodium on this page*

Butisol Sodium® *see Butabarbital Sodium on this page*

Butorphanol (byoo TOR fa nole)

Related Information

I.V. Push Recommended Guidelines *on page 1083*
Pharmacokinetics of Narcotic Agonist Analgesics *on page 1037*

Brand Names Stadol®; Stadol® NS

Generic Available No

Therapeutic Category Analgesic, Narcotic

Use Management of moderate to severe pain; nasal butorphanol has been found useful in the treatment of migraine headache pain

Contraindications Hypersensitivity to butorphanol or any component; avoid use in opiate-dependent patients who have not been detoxified, may precipitate opiate withdrawal

Warnings Use with caution in hepatic or renal disease, may elevate CSF pressure, may increase cardiac workload

Precautions May cause CNS effects, such as drowsiness

Adverse Reactions

Cardiovascular: Hypotension
Central nervous system: CNS depression, headache
Gastrointestinal: Anorexia, nausea, vomiting, constipation, xerostomia
Respiratory: Respiratory depression

Overdosage Symptoms of overdose include respiratory depression, cardiac and CNS depression

Toxicology Treatment of an overdose includes support of the patient's airway, establishment of an I.V. line and administration of naloxone 2 mg I.V. with repeat administration as necessary up to a total of 10 mg.

Drug Interactions Increased toxicity: CNS depressants, barbiturate anesthetics

Stability Store at room temperature, protect from freezing

Mechanism of Action Mixed narcotic agonist-antagonist with central analgesic actions; binds to opiate receptors in the CNS, causing inhibition of ascending pain pathways, altering the perception of and response to pain; produces generalized CNS depression

Pharmacodynamics Peak effect:
I.M.: Within 30-60 minutes
I.V.: Within 4-5 minutes
Nasal: 1-2 hours

Pharmacokinetics Plasma concentrations after a single dose were not significantly different between elderly and young subjects
Absorption: I.M.: Rapidly and well absorbed
Protein binding: 80%
Metabolism: In the liver
Half-life:
Geriatrics: 5.5 hours
Adults: 2.5-4 hours
Elimination: Primarily in urine

Usual Dosage
Geriatrics:
I.M., I.V.: 0.5-2 mg every 6-8 hours, increase as necessary
Nasal: 1 mg (1 spray in one nostril); after 90-120 minutes, assess whether a second dose is needed; may repeat in 3-4 hours
Adults:
I.M.: 1-4 mg every 3-4 hours as needed
I.V.: 0.5-2 mg every 3-4 hours as needed
Nasal: 1 mg (1 spray in one nostril); after 60-90 minutes, assess whether a second dose is needed; may repeat in 3-4 hours
Dosing adjustment in renal impairment:
Cl_{cr} 10-50 mL/minute: Administer 75% of dose
Cl_{cr} <10 mL/minute: Administer 50% of dose

Monitoring Parameters Pain relief, respiratory and mental status, blood pressure

Patient Information May cause drowsiness, avoid alcohol; follow instructions for use of nasal spray

Nursing Implications Observe for excessive sedation or confusion, respiratory depression; raise bed rails; aid with ambulation

Special Geriatric Considerations Adjust dose for renal function in elderly (see Pharmacokinetics and Usual Dosage)

Dosage Forms
Butorphanol tartrate:
Injection: 1 mg/mL (1 mL); 2 mg/mL (1 mL, 2 mL, 10 mL)
Spray, nasal: 10 mg/mL [14-15 doses] (2.5 mL)

References
Ramsey R, Higbee M, Maesner J, et al, "Influence of Age on the Pharmacokinetics of Butorphanol," *Acute Care*, 1986, 12(Suppl 1):8-16.

BW-430C *see* Lamotrigine *on page 524*

Byclomine® Injection *see* Dicyclomine *on page 285*

Bydramine® Cough Syrup [OTC] *see* Diphenhydramine *on page 302*

Cafatine® *see* Ergotamine *on page 343*

Cafatine-PB® *see* Ergotamine *on page 343*

Cafergot® *see* Ergotamine *on page 343*

Cafetrate® *see* Ergotamine *on page 343*

Calan® *see* Verapamil *on page 986*

Calan® SR *see* Verapamil *on page 986*

Cal Carb-HD® [OTC] *see* Calcium Salts (Oral) *on page 152*

Calci-Chew™ [OTC] *see* Calcium Salts (Oral) *on page 152*

Calciday-667® [OTC] *see* Calcium Salts (Oral) *on page 152*

Calcifediol (kal si fe DYE ole)
Brand Names Calderol®
Synonyms 25-HCC; 25-Hydroxycholecalciferol; 25-Hydroxyvitamin D_3
Generic Available No
(Continued)

Calcifediol *(Continued)*

Therapeutic Category Vitamin D Analog

Use Treatment and management of metabolic bone disease associated with chronic renal failure

Contraindications Hypercalcemia, known hypersensitivity to calcifediol, vitamin D toxicity, malabsorption syndrome, hypervitaminosis D, decreased renal function

Warnings Must administer concomitant calcium supplementation; maintain adequate fluid intake; calcium-phosphate product (serum calcium times phosphorus) must not exceed 70; avoid hypercalcemia; renal function impairment with secondary hyperparathyroidism

Precautions Use with caution in coronary artery disease, decreased renal function, renal stones, and elderly

Adverse Reactions
Cardiovascular: Hypotension, cardiac arrhythmias
Central nervous system: Irritability, headache, somnolence, convulsions
Dermatologic: Pruritus
Endocrine & metabolic: Metastatic calcification, polydipsia
Gastrointestinal: Anorexia, weight loss, pancreatitis, nausea, vomiting, xerostomia, constipation, metallic taste
Hematologic: Anemia
Hepatic: Elevated AST/ALT
Neuromuscular & skeletal: Myalgia, bone pain, weakness
Ocular: Conjunctivitis, photophobia
Renal: Polyuria, renal damage

Overdosage Symptoms of overdose include hypercalcemia, hypercalciuria

Toxicology Following withdrawal of the drug, treatment consists of bed rest, liberal intake of fluids, reduced calcium intake, and cathartic administration. Severe hypercalcemia requires I.V. hydration and forced diuresis with I.V. furosemide (20-40 mg I.V. every 4-6 hours for adults). Urine output should be monitored and maintained at >3 mL/kg/hour. I.V. saline can quickly and significantly increase excretion of calcium into the urine. Calcitonin, cholestyramine, prednisone, sodium EDTA and mithramycin have all been used successfully to treat the more resistant cases of vitamin D-induced hypercalcemia.

Drug Interactions
Vitamin D may increase absorption of magnesium from magnesium compounds; hypercalcemia may be precipitated by vitamin D and, therefore, may increase cardiac arrhythmias in patients taking digitalis glycosides and verapamil; hypoparathyroid patients may develop hypercalcemia when using thiazide diuretics
Phenytoin and barbiturates decrease half-life of vitamin D; mineral oil with prolonged use decreases vitamin D absorption; cholestyramine reduces absorption of vitamin D

Stability Store in light-resistant container

Mechanism of Action Vitamin D analog that (along with calcitonin and parathyroid hormone) regulates serum calcium homeostasis by promoting absorption of calcium and phosphorus in the small intestine; promotes renal tubule resorption of phosphate; increases rate of accretion and resorption in bone minerals

Pharmacodynamics Maximal calcemic effects: Seen in 4 weeks with daily administration

Pharmacokinetics
Absorption: Rapid from the small intestine
Half-life: 12-22 days
Time to peak serum concentration: Oral: Within 4 hours
Elimination: In bile and feces, stored in liver and fat depots, muscle, skin, and bones

Usual Dosage Daily supplement for elderly (800 IU): 20 mcg
Geriatrics and Adults: Hepatic osteodystrophy: 20-100 mcg/day or every other day; titrate to obtain normal serum calcium/phosphate concentration; increase dose at 4-week intervals (see Additional Information)

Monitoring Parameters Urine output; obtain serum calcium concentration twice weekly during titration phase; if hypercalcemia is encountered, discontinue agent until calcium concentrations return to normal

Reference Range Calcium (serum) 9-10 mg/dL (4.5-5 mEq/L); phosphate 2.5-5 mg/dL

Test Interactions Increased calcium (S), cholesterol (S)

Patient Information Do not take more than the recommended amount. While taking this medication, your physician may want you to follow a special diet or take a calcium supplement. Follow this diet closely. Avoid taking magnesium supplements or magnesium containing antacids. Early symptoms of hypercalcemia include weakness, fatigue, somnolence, headache, anorexia, dry mouth, metallic taste, nausea, vomiting, cramps, diarrhea, muscle pain, bone pain, and irritability.

Nursing Implications Monitor calcium and phosphate levels closely; monitor symptoms of hypercalcemia (see Adverse Reactions)

Additional Information 1000 mcg = 40,000 units of vitamin D activity; this product not generally recommended for daily supplementation due to dosage forms, strengths, and cost

Special Geriatric Considerations Recommended daily allowances (RDA) have not been developed for persons >65 years of age; vitamin D, folate, and B_{12} (cyanocobalamin) have decreased absorption with age, but the clinical significance is yet unknown. Calorie requirements decrease with age and therefore, nutrient density must be increased to ensure adequate nutrient intake, including vitamins and minerals. Therefore, the use of a daily supplement with a multiple vitamin with minerals is recommended. Elderly consume less vitamin D, absorption may be decreased, and many elderly have decreased sun exposure; therefore, elderly should receive supplementation with 800 units (20 mcg)/day. This is a recommendation of particular need to those with high risk for osteoporosis.

Dosage Forms Capsule: 20 mcg, 50 mcg

References

Letsou AP and Price LS, "Health Aging and Nutrition: An Overview," *Clin Geriatr Med*, 1987, 3(2):253-60.

Myrianthopoulos M, "Dietary Treatment of Hyperlipidemia in the Elderly," *Clin Geriatr Med*, 1987, 3(2):343-59.

Riggs BL and Melton LJ, "The Prevention and Treatment of Osteoporosis," *N Engl J Med*, 1992, 327(9):620-7.

Calciferol™ Injection *see* Ergocalciferol *on page 340*

Calciferol™ Oral *see* Ergocalciferol *on page 340*

Calcijex™ *see* Calcitriol *on page 143*

Calcimar® Injection *see* Calcitonin *on next page*

Calci-Mix™ [OTC] *see* Calcium Salts (Oral) *on page 152*

Calcipotriene (kal si POE try een)

Brand Names Dovonex®

Generic Available No

Therapeutic Category Antipsoriatic Agent, Topical

Use Treatment of moderate plaque psoriasis

Contraindications Hypersensitivity to any of the components; hypercalcemia or evidence of vitamin D toxicity; do not use on the face

Warnings Apply directly to skin lesions; warn patient not to exceed the prescribed dose. In clinical studies, skin-related adverse effects were more severe in the elderly compared to younger adults.

Precautions May cause irritation of lesions and surrounding uninvolved skin; transient, reversible hypercalcemia has occurred with the use of calcipotriene

Adverse Reactions

Dermatologic: Burning, stinging, pruritus, erythema, facial dermatitis, worsening of psoriasis, skin atrophy, hyperpigmentation

Endocrine & metabolic: Hypercalcemia

Toxicology Topically applied calcipotriene can be absorbed in sufficient amounts to produce systemic effects

Mechanism of Action Synthetic vitamin D_3 analog which regulates skin cell production and proliferation

Pharmacokinetics

Absorption: ~6% when applied to psoriasis plaque

Metabolism: Within 24 hours most of the drug is converted to inactive metabolites by the liver

Usual Dosage Geriatrics and Adults: Apply to skin lesions twice daily; rub in gently and completely

Monitoring Parameters Healing of lesions, serum calcium concentration

Patient Information Apply only to affected areas; do not exceed the prescribed dose; avoid contact with face or eyes; wash hands after application; report any local adverse effects

Special Geriatric Considerations See Warnings

Dosage Forms

Cream: 0.005% (30 g, 60 g, 100 g)

(Continued)

Calcipotriene *(Continued)*
Ointment, topical: 0.005% (30 g, 60 g, 100 g)

Calcitonin (kal si TOE nin)
Brand Names Calcimar® Injection; Cibacalcin® Injection; Miacalcin® Injection; Miacalcin® Nasal Spray; Osteocalcin® Injection; Salmonine® Injection

Synonyms Calcitonin (Human); Calcitonin (Salmon)

Generic Available No

Therapeutic Category Antidote, Hypercalcemia

Use
Calcitonin (salmon): Treatment of Paget's disease of bone and as adjunctive therapy for hypercalcemia; also used in postmenopausal osteoporosis
Calcitonin (human): Treatment of Paget's disease of bone (orphan drug status)

Contraindications Hypersensitivity to salmon protein or gelatin diluent

Precautions A skin test should be performed prior to initiating therapy with salmon calcitonin; the skin test is 0.1 mL of 10 IU dilution of calcitonin (must be prepared) injected intradermally; observe injection site for 15 minutes for wheal or significant erythema

Adverse Reactions
Cardiovascular: Flushing of the face, edema, local edema
Central nervous system: Dizziness, headache, parasthesia, chills
Dermatologic: Rash, urticaria
Gastrointestinal: Nausea, vomiting, diarrhea, anorexia
Local: Pain at the injection site
Neuromuscular & skeletal: Weakness
Renal: Diuresis
Respiratory: Shortness of breath, nasal congestion

Overdosage Symptoms of overdose include hypocalcemia, hypocalcemic tetany

Stability Refrigeration is recommended for salmon calcitonin, stable for up to 2 weeks at room temperature; normal saline has been recommended for the dilution to prepare a skin test; protect from light; calcitonin human may be stored at room temperature

Mechanism of Action Structurally similar to human calcitonin; regulates serum calcium concentration along with vitamin D and parathyroid hormone; acts on bone to decrease osteoclast activity, in the kidney to decrease tubular reabsorption of sodium and calcium, and in the GI tract to increase the absorption of calcium

Pharmacokinetics
Metabolism: Rapidly by the kidneys
Half-life: S.C.: 1.2 hours
Elimination: As inactive metabolites in urine

Usual Dosage Geriatrics and Adults:
Hepatic osteodystrophy: 20-100 mcg/kg/day or every other day, titrate to obtain normal serum calcium/phosphate levels
Calcitonin salmon:
Skin test: 1 unit/0.1 mL intracutaneously
Paget's disease: I.M., S.C.: 100 units/day
Postmenopausal osteoporosis:
I.M., S.C.: 100 units/day
Nasal: 200 IU/day, alternating nostrils daily
Hypercalcemia: I.M., S.C.: 4 units/kg every 12 hours, may increase to maximum of 8 units/kg every 6 hours
Analgesic effects related to bone pain:
I.M., S.C.: 50-100 IU/day
Nasal: 200 IU/day
Calcitonin human: Paget's disease: I.M., S.C.: 0.5 mg/day; some patients require as little as 0.25 mg or 0.5 mg 2-3 times/week; severe cases may require 0.5 mg twice daily

Administration I.M. route is preferred

Monitoring Parameters Serum alkaline phosphatase, 24-hour urinary hydroxyproline before and every 3 months; symptom response (pain, fracture); serum calcium and electrolytes

Reference Range Therapeutic: <19 pg/mL (SI: 19 ng/L) basal, depending on the assay

Test Interactions Decreased calcium (S)

Patient Information Keep in refrigerator; take at bedtime to minimize nausea and flushing; follow instructions accompanying nasal product

Nursing Implications Keep in refrigerator when volume exceeds 2 mL; skin test should be performed prior to administration of salmon calcitonin

Special Geriatric Considerations Studies have shown calcitonin's effects on bone density and fracture rates are beneficial particularly in women unable to tolerate estrogens; calcium and vitamin D supplements should also be given. Calcitonin may also be effective in steroid-induced osteoporosis and other states associated with high bone turnover. Nasal spray may provide faster onset of analgesic effects than I.M.

Dosage Forms

Injection:

Human (Cibacalcin®): 0.5 mg/vial

Salmon: 200 units/mL (2 mL)

Spray, nasal: 200 units/activation (0.09 mL/dose) (2 mL glass bottle with pump)

References

Lyritis GP, Tsakalakos N, Magiasis B, et al, "Analgesic Effect of Salmon Calcitonin in Osteoporotic Vertebral Fractures: A Double-Blind, Placebo-Controlled Clinical Study," *Calcif Tissue Int*, 1991, 49(6):369-72.

Pontiroli AE, Pajetta E, Scaglia L, et al, "Analgesic Effect of Intranasal and Intramuscular Salmon Calcitonin in Post-Menopausal Osteoporosis: A Double-Blind, Double-Placebo Study," *Aging*, 1994, 6(6):459-63.

Reginster JY, "Calcitonin for Prevention and Treatment of Osteoporosis," *Am J Med*, 1993, 95(5A):44S-47S.

Reginster JY, Deroisy R, Lecart MP, et al, "A Double-Blind, Placebo-Controlled, Dose-Finding Trial of Intermittent Nasal Salmon Calcitonin for Prevention of Postmenopausal Lumbar Spine Bone Loss," *Am J Med*, 1995, 98(5):452-8.

Calcitonin (Human) *see* Calcitonin *on previous page*

Calcitonin (Salmon) *see* Calcitonin *on previous page*

Calcitriol (kal si TRYE ole)

Related Information

Antacid Drug Interactions *on page 1096*

Brand Names Calcijex™; Rocaltrol®

Synonyms 1,25 Dihydroxycholecalciferol

Generic Available No

Therapeutic Category Vitamin D Analog

Use Management of hypocalcemia in patients on chronic renal dialysis; reduce elevated parathyroid hormone levels; decrease severity of psoriatic lesions in psoriatic vulgaris

Contraindications Hypercalcemia; vitamin D toxicity; abnormal sensitivity to the effects of vitamin D; malabsorption syndrome; decreased function

Warnings Must administer concomitant calcium supplementation; maintain adequate fluid intake; calcium-phosphate product (serum calcium times phosphorus) must not exceed 70; avoid hypercalcemia; renal function impairment with secondary hyperparathyroidism

Precautions Use with caution in coronary artery disease, decreased renal function, renal stones, and elderly

Adverse Reactions

Cardiovascular: Increased blood pressure, cardiac arrhythmias

Central nervous system: Somnolence, headache, hyperthermia

Dermatologic: Pruritus

Endocrine & metabolic: Hypercholesterolemia, hypercalcemia

Gastrointestinal: Nausea, vomiting, constipation, anorexia, weight loss, xerostomia, pancreatitis, metallic taste

Genitourinary: Nocturia, uremia

Hepatic: Increased liver enzymes

Neuromuscular & skeletal: Myalgia, bone pain, weakness

Ocular: Calcific conjunctivitis, photophobia

Renal: Polyuria, polydipsia, albuminuria

Respiratory: Rhinorrhea

Overdosage Symptoms of overdose include hypercalcemia, hypercalciuria

Toxicology Following withdrawal of the drug, treatment consists of bedrest, liberal intake of fluids, reduced calcium intake, and cathartic administration. Severe hypercalcemia requires I.V. hydration and forced diuresis with I.V. furosemide (20-40 mg I.V. every 4-6 hours for adults). Urine output should be monitored and maintained at >3 mL/kg/hour. I.V. saline can quickly and significantly increase excretion of calcium into the urine. Calcitonin, cholestyramine, prednisone, sodium EDTA, and mithramycin have all been used successfully to treat the more resistant cases of vitamin D-induced hypercalcemia.

(Continued)

Calcitriol *(Continued)*

Drug Interactions
Vitamin D may increase absorption of magnesium from magnesium compounds; hypercalcemia may be precipitated by vitamin D and, therefore, may increase cardiac arrhythmias in patients taking digitalis glycosides and verapamil; hypoparathyroid patients may develop hypercalcemia when using thiazide diuretics

Phenytoin and barbiturates decrease half-life of vitamin D; mineral oil with prolonged use decreases vitamin D absorption; cholestyramine reduces absorption of vitamin D

Stability Store in tight, light-resistant container

Mechanism of Action Promotes absorption of calcium in the intestines and retention at the kidneys thereby increasing calcium levels in the serum; decreases excessive serum phosphatase levels, parathyroid hormone levels, and decreases bone resorption; increases renal tubule phosphate resorption

Pharmacodynamics
Onset of action: ~2-6 hours
Duration: 3-5 days
Maximum calcemic effects: 2-4 weeks after daily administration

Pharmacokinetics
Absorption: Oral: Rapid
Metabolism: Primarily to 1,24,25-trihydroxycholecalciferol and 1,24,25-trihydroxy ergocalciferol
Half-life: 1.5 days
Elimination: Principally in bile and feces, and 4% to 6% excreted in urine; stored primarily in liver but also in skin, fat, bone, and muscle

Usual Dosage Geriatrics and Adults: Individualize dosage to maintain calcium levels of 9-10 mg/dL (adjust for low albumin)

Renal failure: Oral: 0.25 mcg/day or every other day (may require 0.5-1 mcg/day); increase doses by 0.25 mcg/day at 4- to 8-week intervals; obtain serum calcium concentrations twice weekly during titration phase (see Additional Information)

Unlabeled use:
Renal failure: I.V.: 0.5 mcg (0.01 mcg/kg) 3 times/week; most doses in the range of 0.5-3 mcg (0.01-0.05 mcg/kg) 3 times/week
Hypoparathyroidism/pseudohypoparathyroidism: Oral: 0.5-2 mcg/day, administer in the morning (see Additional Information)

Monitoring Parameters Monitor renal function, serum calcium and phosphate concentrations; if hypercalcemia is encountered, discontinue agent until serum calcium returns to normal

Reference Range Calcium (serum) 9-10 mg/dL (4.5-5 mEq/L) but do not include the I.V. dosages; phosphate 2.5-5 mg/dL

Test Interactions Increased calcium, cholesterol, magnesium, BUN, AST, ALT, calcium (S), cholesterol (S); decreased alkaline phosphatase

Patient Information Do not take more than the recommended amount. While taking this medication, your physician may want you to follow a special diet or take a calcium supplement. Follow this diet closely. Avoid taking magnesium supplements or magnesium containing antacids. Early symptoms of hypercalcemia include weakness, fatigue, somnolence, headache, anorexia, dry mouth, metallic taste, nausea, vomiting, cramps, diarrhea, muscle pain, bone pain, and irritability.

Nursing Implications Monitor calcium and phosphate levels closely; monitor symptoms of hypercalcemia (see Adverse Reactions)

Additional Information Calcitriol degrades upon prolonged exposure to light; not used as a daily supplement due to dosage forms, strengths, and cost (1 mcg = 40,000 units)

Special Geriatric Considerations Recommended daily allowances (RDA) have not been developed for persons >65 years of age; vitamin D, folate, and B_{12} (cyanocobalamin) have decreased absorption with age, but the clinical significance is yet unknown. Calorie requirements decrease with age and therefore, nutrient density must be increased to ensure adequate nutrient intake, including vitamins and minerals. Therefore, the use of a daily supplement with a multiple vitamin with minerals is recommended. Elderly consume less vitamin D, absorption may be decreased, and many elderly have decreased sun exposure; therefore, elderly should receive supplementation with 800 units of vitamin D (20 mcg)/day. This is a recommendation of particular need to those with high risk for osteoporosis.

Dosage Forms
Capsule: 0.25 mcg, 0.5 mcg

Injection: 1 mcg/mL, 2 mcg/mL

References

Letsou AP and Price LS, "Health Aging and Nutrition: An Overview," *Clin Geriatr Med*, 1987, 3(2):253-60.

Myrianthopoulos M, "Dietary Treatment of Hyperlipidemia in the Elderly," *Clin Geriatr Med*, 1987, 3(2):343-59.

Riggs BL and Melton LJ, "The Prevention and Treatment of Osteoporosis," *N Engl J Med*, 1992, 327(9):620-7.

Calcium Acetate (KAL see um AS e tate)

Brand Names Calphron®; Phos-Ex®; PhosLo®

Generic Available No

Therapeutic Category Calcium Salt

Use Control of hyperphosphatemia in end stage renal failure and does not promote aluminum absorption; calcium acetate binds phosphorus in the GI tract better than other calcium salts due to its lower solubility and subsequent reduction in calcium or phosphorus absorption

Contraindications Hypercalcemia, renal calculi, hypophosphatemia, ventricular fibrillation, and patients with risk of digitalis toxicity

Warnings Use with caution in patients on digitalis, because hypercalcemia may precipitate cardiac arrhythmias. Always start at low-dose and do not increase without careful monitoring of serum calcium; estimate of daily dietary calcium intake should be made initially and the intake adjusted as needed. Use with caution in patients with CHF, renal failure. No other calcium supplements should be given concurrently; progressive hypercalcemia due to overdose may be severe as to require emergency measures; chronic hypercalcemia may lead to vascular calcification, and other soft tissue calcification. The serum calcium level should be monitored twice weekly during the early dose adjustment period.

Precautions Use caution when administering to patients with renal failure; hypercalcemia and hypercalciuria may develop at therapeutic doses over long periods of time; hypoparathyroidism may induce hypercalcemia and hypercalciuria, especially when patients receive high doses of vitamin D; administer cautiously to a digitalized patient, may precipitate arrhythmias

Adverse Reactions

Central nervous system: Mood and mental changes

Endocrine & metabolic: Metastatic calcinosis, milk-alkali syndrome

Gastrointestinal: Constipation, flatulence, laxative effect, acid rebound, dyspepsia, nausea, vomiting, GI hemorrhage, fecal impaction

Hematologic: Hypophosphatemia, hypercalcemia (with prolonged use), hypomagnesemia

Renal: Renal calculi, renal dysfunction, polyuria, hypercalciuria

Overdosage Symptoms of overdose include lethargy, nausea, vomiting, anorexia, constipation, abdominal pain, dry mouth, thirst, polyuria; severe hypercalcemia: Confusion, delirium, stupor, coma

Toxicology Following withdrawal of the drug, treatment consists of bed rest, liberal intake of fluids, reduced calcium intake, and cathartic administration. Severe hypercalcemia requires I.V. hydration and forced diuresis with I.V. furosemide (20-40 mg I.V. every 4-6 hours for adults). Urine output should be monitored and maintained at >3 mL/kg/hour. I.V. saline can quickly and significantly increase excretion of calcium into urine. Calcitonin, cholestyramine, prednisone, sodium EDTA, biphosphonates, and mithramycin have all been used successfully to treat the more resistant cases of vitamin D-induced hypercalcemia

Drug Interactions

Calcium may antagonize the effects of verapamil; renders tetracycline antibiotics inactive (orally)

Thiazide diuretics may induce hypercalcemia

Decreased atenolol absorption

Iron salts, quinolones have decreased absorption

Polystyrene sulfonate has decreased binding of potassium and may precipitate metabolic alkalosis

Stability Admixture incompatibilities: Carbonates, phosphates, sulfates, tartrates

Mechanism of Action Moderates nerve and muscle performance via action potential excitation threshold regulation; combines with dietary phosphate to form insoluble calcium phosphate which is excreted in feces

Pharmacokinetics Calcium is absorbed in soluble, ionized form; solubility of calcium is increased in an acid environment (except calcium lactate); therefore, administer with meals to maximize acidity and solubility to enhance absorption

(Continued)

Calcium Acetate *(Continued)*

Absorption: From the GI tract, requires vitamin D

Elimination: Mainly in feces as unabsorbed calcium with 20% eliminated by the kidneys

Usual Dosage Geriatrics and Adults: Oral: 2 tablets with each meal; dosage may be increased to bring serum phosphate value to <6 mg/dL; most patients require 3-4 tablets with each meal

Administration Tablets must be taken with meals to be effective

Monitoring Parameters Plasma and urine concentrations; plasma phosphate, EKG in hyperkalemic states

Reference Range Serum calcium: 9-10.4 mg/dL; due to a poor correlation between the serum ionized calcium (free) and total serum calcium, particularly in states of low albumin or acid/base imbalances, direct measurement of ionized calcium is recommended. In low albumin states, the corrected **total** serum calcium may be estimated by this equation (assuming a normal albumin of 4 g/dL); corrected total calcium = total serum calcium + 0.8 (4 - measured serum albumin)

Test Interactions Increased calcium (S); decreased magnesium; decreased phosphorus

Patient Information Take with food; do not take calcium supplements within 1-2 hours of taking other medicine by mouth or eating large amounts of fiber-rich foods; do not drink large amounts of alcohol or caffeine-containing beverages or use tobacco if calcium causes dyspepsia

Nursing Implications See Adverse Reactions, Additional Information, Overdosage, and Special Geriatric Considerations

Additional Information

Doses for calcium supplementation are given in elemental calcium; calcium salts vary in their amount of elemental calcium

Calcium carbonate (40% elemental calcium)

Calcium gluconate (9% elemental calcium)

Calcium lactate (13% elemental calcium)

Calcium citrate (21% elemental calcium)

Dibasic calcium phosphate (23% elemental calcium)

Calcium acetate (25% elemental calcium)

Tricalcium phosphate (39% elemental calcium)

All calcium preparations should be administered in divided doses to maximize calcium absorption; no more than 300-350 mg of elemental calcium should be given at a time. Women receiving estrogen therapy require 900-1000 mg total daily elemental calcium intake. Women not receiving estrogens require 1500 mg elemental calcium daily to maintain calcium balance.

12.7 mEq/g; 250 mg/g elemental calcium (25% elemental calcium)

Special Geriatric Considerations Constipation and gas can be significant in elderly, but are usually mild (see Warnings)

Dosage Forms Elemental calcium listed in brackets

Capsule (Phos-Ex® 125): 500 mg [125 mg]

Tablet:

Phos-Ex® 62.5: 250 mg [62.5 mg]

Phos-Ex® 167: 668 mg [167 mg]

Phos-Ex® 250: 1000 mg [250 mg]

PhosLo®: 667 mg [169 mg]

Calcium Channel Blocking Agents Comparison *see page 1027*

Calcium Chloride *(KAL see um KLOR ide)*

Generic Available Yes

Therapeutic Category Calcium Salt; Electrolyte Supplement, Parenteral

Use Cardiac resuscitation when epinephrine fails to improve myocardial contractions, cardiac disturbances of hyperkalemia, hypocalcemia, or calcium channel blocking agent toxicity; emergent treatment of hypocalcemic tetany, treatment of hypermagnesemia

Contraindications In ventricular fibrillation during cardiac resuscitation, hypercalcemia, and in patients with risk of digitalis toxicity, renal or cardiac disease

Warnings Avoid too rapid I.V. administration (<1 mL/minute) and extravasation; may cause hypotension, peripheral vasodilitation I.V.; use with caution in digitalized patients, respiratory failure, or acidosis; hypercalcemia may occur in patients with renal failure, and frequent determination of serum calcium is necessary; avoid metabolic acidosis (ie, administer only 2-3 days then change to another calcium salt); extravasation may cause tissue necrosis, tissue sloughing, abscess (see Nursing Implications for treatment)

Precautions Rapid I.V. may cause bradycardia, feeling of "heat waves", metallic or chalky taste, tingling, or sense of oppression; high doses reaching the heart may cause cardiac syncope

Adverse Reactions

Cardiovascular: Vasodilation, hypotension, bradycardia, cardiac arrhythmias, ventricular fibrillation, syncope

Central nervous system: Lethargy, coma, mania

Dermatologic: Erythema

Endocrine & metabolic: Decreased serum magnesium, hypercalcemia

Gastrointestinal: Elevated serum amylase

Local: Tissue necrosis, local burning sensation (I.V.)

Neuromuscular & skeletal: Muscle weakness

Renal: Hypercalciuria

Overdosage Symptoms of overdose include lethargy, nausea, vomiting, coma

Toxicology Following withdrawal of the drug, treatment consists of bed rest, liberal intake of fluids, reduced calcium intake, and cathartic administration. Severe hypercalcemia requires I.V. hydration and forced diuresis. Urine output should be monitored and maintained at >3 mL/kg/hour. I.V. saline can quickly and significantly increase excretion of calcium into urine.

Drug Interactions

Decreased effect: Calcium may antagonize the effects of calcium channel blockers

Increased toxicity: Administer cautiously to a digitalized patient, may precipitate arrhythmias

Stability

Do not refrigerate solutions; IVPB solutions/I.V. infusion solutions are stable for 24 hours at room temperature

Maximum concentration in parenteral nutrition solutions: 15 mEq/L of calcium and 30 mmol/L of phosphate

Incompatibilities include sodium bicarbonate, carbonates, phosphates, sulfates, and tartrates

Mechanism of Action Moderates nerve and muscle performance via action potential excitation threshold regulation

Pharmacokinetics

Absorption: I.V. calcium salts are absorbed directly into the circulation

Elimination: Mainly in feces as unabsorbed calcium with 20% eliminated by the kidneys

Usual Dosage Geriatrics and Adults: I.V.: **Note:** Calcium chloride is 3 times as potent as calcium gluconate

Cardiac arrest in the presence of hyperkalemia or hypocalcemia, magnesium toxicity, or calcium antagonist toxicity: 2-4 mg/kg (10% solution), repeated every 10 minutes

Hypocalcemia: 500 mg to 1 g (7-14 mEq), repeated at 1- to 3-day intervals if necessary

Hypocalcemic tetany: 4.5-16 mEq may be administered until response occurs

Hypocalcemia secondary to citrated blood transfusion: Administer 0.45 mEq **elemental** calcium for each 100 mL citrated blood infused

Administration See Warnings and Precautions

Monitoring Parameters Serum calcium and magnesium, blood pressure, heart rate, EKG, signs of extravasation and muscle weakness

Reference Range

Serum calcium: 8.4-10.2 mg/dL

Due to a poor correlation between the serum ionized calcium (free) and total serum calcium, particularly in states of low albumin or acid/base imbalances, direct measurement of ionized calcium is recommended

In low albumin states, the corrected **total** serum calcium may be estimated by this equation (assuming a normal albumin of 4 g/dL)

Corrected total calcium = total serum calcium + 0.8 (4.0 - measured serum albumin)

or

Corrected calcium = measured calcium - measured albumin + 4.0

Serum/plasma chloride: 95-108 mEq/L

Test Interactions ↑ calcium (S); ↓ magnesium

Nursing Implications Do not inject calcium chloride I.M. or administer S.C. or use scalp, small hand or foot veins for I.V. administration since severe necrosis and sloughing may occur. Monitor EKG if calcium is infused faster than 2.5 mEq/minute; usual: 0.7-1.5 mEq/minute (0.5-1 mL/minute); **stop the**

(Continued)

Calcium Chloride *(Continued)*

infusion if the patient complains of pain or discomfort. Warm to body temperature; administer slowly, do not exceed 1 mL/minute (inject into ventricular cavity - not myocardium); **do not infuse calcium chloride in the same I.V. line as phosphate-containing solutions.**

Extravasation treatment:
Hyaluronidase: Add 1 mL NS to 150 unit vial to make 150 units/mL of concentration; mix 0.1 mL of above with 0.9 mL NS in 1 mL syringe to make final concentration = 15 units/mL

Additional Information 14 mEq/g/10 mL; 270 mg elemental calcium/g (27% elemental calcium)

Special Geriatric Considerations When using in elderly, check albumin status and make appropriate decisions concerning reference serum concentrations; elderly, especially the ill, often have low albumin due to malnutrition

Dosage Forms Elemental calcium listed in brackets
Injection: 10% = 100 mg/mL [27.2 mg/mL] (10 mL)

References

Bilezikian JP, "Management of Acute Hypercalcemia," *N Engl J Med*, 1992, 326(18):1196-215.

Binder LS, "Acute Arthropod Envenomation: Incidence, Clinical Features, and Management," *Med Toxicol Adverse Drug Exp*, 1989, 4(3):163-73.

Chin RL, Garmel GM, and Harter PM, "Development of Ventricular Fibrillation After Intravenous Calcium Chloride Administration in a Patient With Supraventricular Tachycardia," *Ann Emerg Med*, 1995, 25(3):416-9.

McIvor ME, "Acute Fluoride Toxicity. Pathophysiology and Management," *Drug Saf*, 1990, 5(2):79-84.

Pearigen PD and Benowitz NL, "Poisoning Due to Calcium Antagonists. Experience With Verapamil, Diltiazem, and Nifedipine," *Drug Saf*, 1991, 6(6):408-30.

Slattery A, King WD, Nichols M, et al, "Hypercalcemia Following Damp-Rid™ Ingestion," *Clin Toxicol*, 1995, 33(5):487.

Worthley LI and Phillips PJ, "Intravenous Calcium Salts," *Lancet*, 1980, 2(8186):149.

Calcium Gluceptate *(KAL see um gloo SEP tate)*

Generic Available Yes

Therapeutic Category Calcium Salt; Electrolyte Supplement, Parenteral

Use Treatment of cardiac disturbances of hyperkalemia, hypocalcemia, or calcium channel blocker toxicity; cardiac resuscitation when epinephrine fails to improve myocardial contractions; treatment of hypermagnesemia and hypocalcemia

Contraindications In ventricular fibrillation during cardiac resuscitation; patients with risk of digitalis toxicity, renal or cardiac disease; hypercalcemia; may cause hypotension and peripheral vasodilation I.V.

Warnings Avoid too rapid I.V. administration; avoid extravasation; use with caution in digitalized patients, respiratory failure or acidosis; metabolic acidosis (administer for only 2-3 days then change to another calcium salt)

Precautions Rapid I.V. may cause bradycardia, feeling of "heat waves", metallic or chalky taste, tingling, or sense of oppression; high doses reaching the heart may cause cardiac syncope

Adverse Reactions
Cardiovascular: Vasodilation, hypotension, bradycardia, cardiac arrhythmias, ventricular fibrillation, syncope
Central nervous system: Lethargy, mania, coma
Dermatologic: Erythema
Endocrine & metabolic: Hypomagnesemia, hypercalcemia
Gastrointestinal: Elevated serum amylase
Local: Tissue necrosis, local burning sensation (I.V.)
Neuromuscular & skeletal: Muscle weakness
Renal: Hypercalciuria

Overdosage Symptoms of overdose include lethargy, nausea, vomiting, coma

Toxicology Following withdrawal of the drug, treatment consists of bed rest, liberal intake of fluids, reduced calcium intake, and cathartic administration. Severe hypercalcemia requires I.V. hydration and forced diuresis with I.V. furosemide (20-40 mg I.V. every 4-6 hours for adults). Urine output should be monitored and maintained at >3 mL/kg/hour. I.V. saline can quickly and significantly increase excretion of calcium into urine. Calcitonin, cholestyramine, prednisone, sodium EDTA, biphosphonates, and mithramycin have all been used successfully to treat the more resistant cases of vitamin D-induced hypercalcemia.

Drug Interactions Administer cautiously to digitalized patients, may precipitate arrhythmias; calcium may antagonize effects of calcium channel blockers

Stability Admixture **incompatibilities** include carbonates, phosphates, sulfates, tartrates

Mechanism of Action Moderates nerve and muscle performance via action potential excitation threshold regulation

Pharmacokinetics

Absorption: I.M. and I.V. calcium salts are absorbed directly into the bloodstream

Elimination: Mainly in feces as unabsorbed calcium with 20% eliminated by the kidneys

Usual Dosage Geriatrics and Adults: I.V. (dose expressed in mg of calcium glucptate):

Cardiac resuscitation in the presence of hypocalcemia, hyperkalemia, magnesium toxicity, or calcium channel blocker toxicity: 1.1-1.5 g (5-7 mL)

Hypocalcemia: 500 mg to 1.1 g/dose as needed

After citrated blood administration: 0.4 mEq/100 mL blood infused

Administration See Warnings and Precautions

Monitoring Parameters Serum calcium and magnesium, EKG, blood pressure, heart rate, signs of extravasation and muscle weakness

Reference Range

Serum calcium: 8.4-10.2 mg/dL

Due to a poor correlation between the serum ionized calcium (free) and total serum calcium, particularly in states of low albumin or acid/base imbalances, direct measurement of ionized calcium is recommended

In low albumin states, the corrected **total** serum calcium may be estimated by this equation (assuming a normal albumin of 4 g/dL)

Corrected total calcium = total serum calcium + 0.8 (4.0 - measured serum albumin)

or

Corrected calcium = measured calcium - measured albumin + 4.0

Test Interactions ↑ calcium (S); ↓ magnesium

Nursing Implications Warm to body temperature; administer slowly, do not exceed 1 mL/minute (inject into ventricular cavity - not myocardium).

Do not inject calcium glucptate I.M. or administer S.C. or use scalp, small hand or foot veins for I.V. administration since severe necrosis and sloughing may occur. Monitor EKG if calcium is infused faster than 2.5 mEq/minute; usual: 0.7-1.5 mEq/minute (0.5-1 mL/minute); **stop the infusion if the patient complains of pain or discomfort.** Warm to body temperature; administer slowly, do not exceed 1 mL/minute (inject into ventricular cavity - not myocardium); **do not infuse calcium glucptate in the same I.V. line as phosphate-containing solutions.**

Extravasation treatment:

Hyaluronidase: Add 1 mL NS to 150 unit vial to make 150 units/mL of concentration; mix 0.1 mL of above with 0.9 mL NS in 1 mL syringe to make final concentration = 15 units/mL

Additional Information 4.1 mEq/g; 82 mg elemental calcium/g (8% elemental calcium)

Special Geriatric Considerations When using in elderly, check albumin status and make appropriate decisions concerning reference serum concentrations; elderly, especially the ill, often have low albumin due to malnutrition

Dosage Forms Elemental calcium listed in brackets

Injection: 220 mg/mL [18 mg/mL] (5 mL, 50 mL)

Calcium Gluconate (Parenteral)

(KAL see um GLOO koe nate pa REN ter al)

Related Information

Antidotes *on page 1097*

I.V. Push Recommended Guidelines *on page 1083*

Brand Names Kalcinate®

Generic Available Yes

Therapeutic Category Calcium Salt

Use Treatment and prevention of hypocalcemia, treatment of tetany, cardiac disturbances of hyperkalemia, cardiac resuscitation when epinephrine fails to improve myocardial contractions, or calcium channel blocker toxicity

Contraindications In ventricular fibrillation during cardiac resuscitation, and in patients with risk of digitalis toxicity, renal or cardiac disease; hypercalcemia, renal calculi, hypophosphatemia

Warnings May produce cardiac arrest

Precautions Use caution when administering to patients with renal failure; avoid too rapid I.V. administration; use with caution in digitalized patients, (Continued)

Calcium Gluconate (Parenteral) *(Continued)*

respiratory failure or acidosis; avoid extravasation; hypercalcemia and hyper-calciuria may develop at therapeutic doses over long periods of time; hypo-parathyroidism may induce hypercalcemia and hypercalciuria, especially when patients receive high doses of vitamin D; administer cautiously to a digitalized patient, may precipitate arrhythmias

Adverse Reactions

Cardiovascular: Vasodilatation, hypotension, bradycardia, cardiac arrhyth-mias, ventricular fibrillation

Central nervous system: Lethargy, mental confusion, coma, mania, headache

Dermatologic: Erythema, tissue necrosis, sloughing, abscess formation

Endocrine & metabolic: Decrease serum magnesium, hypercalcemia, hypo-phosphatemia

Gastrointestinal: Vomiting, constipation (not proven), dyspepsia, flatulence

Hepatic: Elevated serum amylase

Neuromuscular & skeletal: Muscle weakness

Renal: Hypercalciuria

Overdosage Symptoms of overdose include hypercalcemia, mild hypercal-cemia: Lethargy, nausea, vomiting, anorexia, constipation, abdominal pain, dry mouth, thirst, polyuria; severe hypercalcemia: Confusion, delirium, stupor, coma

Drug Interactions

Calcium may antagonize the effects of verapamil; renders tetracycline antibi-otics inactive (orally)

Thiazide diuretics may induce hypercalcemia

Decreased atenolol absorption

Iron salts, quinolone have decreased absorption

Polystyrene sulfonate has decreased binding of potassium and may precipi-tate metabolic alkalosis

Stability Admixture incompatibilities: carbonates, phosphates, sulfates, tartrates; store at room temperature; do not use if precipitate occurs

Mechanism of Action Moderates nerve and muscle performance via action potential excitation threshold regulation; may prevent negative calcium balance when used as a supplement orally

Usual Dosage Geriatrics and Adults (dosage is in terms of elemental calcium): I.V.:

Hypocalcemia: 2-15 g/24 hours as a continuous infusion or in divided doses

Hypocalcemia secondary to citrated blood infusion; administer 0.45 mEq **elemental** calcium for each 100 mL citrated blood infused

Calcium antagonist toxicity, magnesium intoxication; cardiac arrest in the presence of hyperkalemia or hypocalcemia: 1-3 g

Tetany: 1-3 g may be administered until therapeutic response occurs

Cardiac resuscitation: 500-800 mg/dose (5-8 mL) every 10 minutes

Exchange transfusion: 300 mg/100 mL of citrated blood exchanged

Monitoring Parameters EKG, plasma and urine calcium concentrations

Reference Range Mild hypercalcemia: >10.5 mg/dL; severe hypercalcemia: >12 mg/dL; serum calcium: 9-10.4 mg/dL; due to a poor correlation between the serum ionized calcium (free) and total serum calcium, particularly in states of low albumin or acid/base imbalances, direct measurement of ionized calcium is recommended. In low albumin states, the corrected **total** serum calcium may be estimated by this equation (assuming a normal albumin of 4 g/dL); corrected total calcium = total serum calcium + 0.8 (4 - measured serum albumin).

Test Interactions Increased calcium (S); decreased magnesium; decreased phosphorus

Nursing Implications I.M. injections should be administered in the gluteal region in adults, usually in volumes <5 mL; do not use scalp veins or small hand or foot veins for I.V. administration; generally, I.V. infusion rates should not exceed 0.7-1.5 mEq/minute (1.5-3.3 mL/minute); stop the infusion if the patient complains of pain or discomfort. Warm to body temperature; admin-ister slowly, usually no faster than 1.5-3.3 mL/minute, do not inject directly into the myocardium when using calcium during advanced cardiac life support (see Adverse Reactions, Overdosage, Additional Information, and Special Geriatric Considerations).

Extravasation treatment:

Hyaluronidase: Add 1 mL NS to 150 unit vial to make 150 units/mL of concentration; mix 0.1 mL of above with 0.9 mL NS in 1 mL syringe to make final concentration = 15 units/mL

Additional Information 1 g calcium gluconate = 90 mg elemental calcium = 4.8 mEq calcium;

Doses for calcium supplementation are given in elemental calcium; calcium salts vary in their amount of elemental calcium

Calcium carbonate (40% elemental calcium)
Calcium gluconate (9% elemental calcium)
Calcium lactate (13% elemental calcium)
Calcium citrate (21% elemental calcium)
Dibasic calcium phosphate (23% elemental calcium)
Calcium acetate (25% elemental calcium)
Tricalcium phosphate (39% elemental calcium)

All calcium preparations should be administered in divided doses to maximize calcium absorption; no more than 300-350 mg of elemental calcium should be given at a time. Women receiving estrogen therapy require 900-1000 mg total daily elemental calcium intake. Women not receiving estrogens require 1500 mg elemental calcium daily to maintain calcium balance.

Special Geriatric Considerations Constipation and gas can be significant in elderly, but are usually mild (see Warnings and Nursing Implications)

Dosage Forms Injection: 100 mg/mL (10 mL)

Calcium Polycarbophil (KAL see um pol i KAR boe fil)

Brand Names Equalactin® Chewable Tablet [OTC]; Fiberall® Chewable Tablet [OTC]; FiberCon® Tablet [OTC]; Fiber-Lax® Tablet [OTC]; Mitrolan® Chewable Tablet [OTC]

Generic Available Yes

Therapeutic Category Antidiarrheal; Laxative, Bulk-Producing

Use Treatment of constipation or acute nonspecific diarrhea by restoring a more normal moisture level and providing bulk in the patient's intestinal tract; polycarbophil is indicated for constipation in diarrhea associated with irritable bowel syndrome and diverticulosis; calcium polycarbophil is supplied as the approved substitute whenever a bulk-forming laxative is ordered in a tablet, capsule, wafer, or other oral solid dosage form

Contraindications Hypersensitivity to any component; do not use if patient is experiencing nausea, vomiting, appendicitis, fecal impaction, acute surgical abdomen, intestinal obstruction, undiagnosed abdominal pain

Warnings Laxatives used excessively may lead to fluid/electrolyte imbalance; stimulant cathartics may lead to abuse or dependency with chronic use (laxative abuse syndrome); cathartic colon, which may present as ulcerative colitis, occurs with chronic use of stimulant cathartics; melanosis coli is a dark pigmentation of the colonic mucosa from chronic use of anthraquinone derivatives

Precautions Habit-forming and may result in laxative dependence and loss of normal bowel function with prolonged use; rectal bleeding or failure to respond requires further evaluation for possibly serious medical problems

Adverse Reactions
Cardiovascular: Palpitations
Central nervous system: Dizziness, faintness
Gastrointestinal: Nausea, vomiting, diarrhea, abdominal cramps, bloating, flatulence, perianal irritation
Neuromuscular & skeletal: Weakness
Miscellaneous: Diaphoresis

Overdosage Symptoms of overdose include abdominal pain, diarrhea, flatulence, possible impaction

Drug Interactions Decreased effect of oral anticoagulants, digoxin, potassium-sparing diuretics, salicylates, tetracyclines

Mechanism of Action Calcium polycarbophil is a hydrophilic agent which retains free water within the intestinal lumen and indirectly opposes dehydrating forces of the bowel, promoting formed stools; in diarrhea, it absorbs free fecal water, forming a gel and produces formed stools

Pharmacodynamics
Onset of action: 12-24 hours; can be up to 72 hours
Site of action: Small and large intestines

Usual Dosage Geriatrics and Adults: Oral: 1 g 4 times/day, up to 6 g/day; for severe diarrhea, repeat doses every 30 minutes; do not exceed 6 g/day

Administration When using as a laxative, patient should drink with adequate fluids (8 oz of water or other fluids) with each dose

Monitoring Parameters Monitor for diarrhea, abdominal pain, bowel obstruction, or impaction

Test Interactions Decreased potassium (S)

(Continued)

Calcium Polycarbophil *(Continued)*

Patient Information Drink a full glass of liquid with each dose; must drink fluids throughout the day to be effective and avoid impaction; report bleeding or failure to respond to physician, pharmacist, or nurse; do not use for acute constipation

Nursing Implications Bulk laxatives increase stool frequency; watch for signs of fluid/electrolyte loss (see Warnings and Contraindications)

Additional Information Each calcium polycarbophil tablet contains ~100 mg of absorbable elemental calcium; chewable tablets are available

Special Geriatric Considerations Elderly may have insufficient fluid intake which may predispose them to fecal impaction and bowel obstruction; bloating and flatulence may be a problem when used short-term; use cautiously in patients with a history of bowel impaction/obstruction

Dosage Forms
Tablet:
  Chewable:
    Equalactin®, Mitrolan®: 500 mg
    Fiberall®: 1250 mg
  Sodium free:
    FiberCon®: 500 mg
    Fiber-Lax®, FiberNorm®: 625 mg

Calcium Salts (Oral) (KAL see um salts OR al)

Brand Names Alka-Mints® [OTC]; Amitone® [OTC]; Cal Carb-HD® [OTC]; Calci-Chew™ [OTC]; Calciday-667® [OTC]; Calci-Mix™ [OTC]; Cal-Plus® [OTC]; Caltrate® 600 [OTC]; Caltrate, Jr.® [OTC]; Chooz® [OTC]; Citracal® [OTC]; Dicarbosil® [OTC]; Equilet® [OTC]; Florical® [OTC]; Gencalc® 600 [OTC]; Mallamint® [OTC]; Mylanta® Soothing Antacids [OTC]; Neo-Calglucon® [OTC]; Nephro-Calci® [OTC]; Os-Cal® 500 [OTC]; Oyst-Cal 500 [OTC]; Oystercal® 500; Posture® [OTC]; Rolaids® Calcium Rich [OTC]; Titralac® Plus Liquid [OTC]; Tums® [OTC]; Tums® E-X Extra Strength Tablet [OTC]; Tums® Extra Strength Liquid [OTC]; Tums® Ultra [OTC]

Generic Available Yes

Therapeutic Category Antacid; Antidote, Hyperphosphatemia; Calcium Salt

Use Antacid and calcium supplement

Contraindications Hypercalcemia, renal calculi, hypophosphatemia, ventricular fibrillation. In ventricular fibrillation during cardiac resuscitation, and in patients with risk of digitalis toxicity, renal or cardiac disease

Precautions Use caution when administering to patients with renal failure; hypercalcemia and hypercalciuria may develop at therapeutic doses over long periods of time; hypoparathyroidism may induce hypercalcemia and hypercalciuria, especially when patients receive high doses of vitamin D; administer cautiously to a digitalized patient, may precipitate arrhythmias

Adverse Reactions
Central nervous system: Mental confusion, headache, mood changes
Endocrine & metabolic: Hypercalcemia, milk-alkali syndrome (doses >2 g/day), hypophosphatemia, hypercalcinosis, hypomagnesemia
Gastrointestinal: Constipation (not proven), nausea, vomiting, dyspepsia, flatulence, laxative effect, acid rebound, fecal impaction, GI hemorrhage
Renal: Hypercalciuria, renal calculi, renal dysfunction, polyuria

Overdosage Symptoms of overdose include hypercalcemia, lethargy, nausea, vomiting, coma; following withdrawal of the drug, treatment consists of bed rest, liberal intake of fluids, reduced calcium intake, and cathartic administration.

Toxicology Severe hypercalcemia requires I.V. hydration and forced diuresis with I.V. furosemide (20-40 mg I.V. every 4-6 hours for adults). Urine output should be monitored and maintained at >3 mL/kg/hour. I.V. saline can quickly and significantly increase excretion of calcium into urine. Calcitonin, cholestyramine, prednisone, sodium EDTA, biphosphonates, and mithramycin have all been used successfully to treat the more resistant cases of vitamin D-induced hypercalcemia.

Drug Interactions
Calcium may antagonize the effects of verapamil; renders tetracycline antibiotics inactive (orally)
Thiazide diuretics may induce hypercalcemia
Decreased atenolol absorption
Iron salts, quinolones have decreased absorption

Stability Admixture incompatibilities: carbonates, phosphates, sulfates, tartrates

Mechanism of Action Moderates nerve and muscle performance via action potential excitation threshold regulation; may prevent negative calcium balance when used as dietary supplement as treatment or for osteoporosis; calcium carbonate is used as an antacid for acute dyspepsia

Pharmacokinetics Calcium is absorbed in soluble, ionized form; solubility of calcium is increased in an acid environment (except calcium lactate); therefore, administer with meals to maximize acidity and solubility to enhance absorption

Usual Dosage Geriatrics and Adults: Oral (dosage in terms of elemental calcium):

Dietary supplement: 500 mg to 2 g, 2-4 times/day (see Additional Information)

Osteoporosis/bone loss: 1000-1500 mg in divided doses/day (see Additional Information)

Antacid: Calcium carbonate: 0.5-2 g divided in 2-6 doses/day

Recommended daily allowance: 800 mg/day

Monitoring Parameters Plasma and urine calcium concentrations; EKG if hypercalcemic

Reference Range Mild hypercalcemia: >10.5 mg/dL; severe hypercalcemia: >12 mg/dL; serum calcium: 9-10.4 mg/dL; due to a poor correlation between the serum ionized calcium (free) and total serum calcium, particularly in states of low albumin or acid/base imbalances, direct measurement of ionized calcium is recommended. In low albumin states, the corrected **total** serum calcium may be estimated by this equation (assuming a normal albumin of 4 g/dL); corrected total calcium = total serum calcium + 0.8 (4 - measured serum albumin).

Test Interactions Increased calcium (S); decreased magnesium; decreased phosphorus

Patient Information Do not take calcium supplements within 1-2 hours of taking other medicine by mouth or eating large amounts of fiber-rich foods; do not drink large amounts of alcohol or caffeine-containing beverages or use tobacco; take with meals

Nursing Implications See Adverse Reactions, Additional Information, Overdosage, and Special Geriatric Considerations

Additional Information Doses for calcium supplementation are given in elemental calcium; calcium salts vary in their amount of elemental calcium

Calcium glubionate (6.5% elemental calcium)
Calcium carbonate (40% elemental calcium)
Calcium gluconate (9% elemental calcium)
Calcium lactate (13% elemental calcium)
Calcium citrate (21% elemental calcium)
Dibasic calcium phosphate (23% elemental calcium)
Calcium acetate (25% elemental calcium)
Tricalcium phosphate (39% elemental calcium)

All calcium preparations should be administered in divided doses to maximize calcium absorption; no more than 300-350 mg of elemental calcium should be given at a time. Women receiving estrogen therapy require 900-1000 mg total daily elemental calcium intake. Women not receiving estrogens require 1500 mg elemental calcium daily to maintain calcium balance.

Special Geriatric Considerations Constipation and gas can be significant in elderly but are usually mild and may be eliminated by switching to another salt form. Calcium carbonate has been associated with the highest incidence of side effects, probably due to its high calcium content. Calcium carbonate absorption is impaired in achlorhydria. Since achlorhydria is common in elderly, calcium carbonate may not be the ideal calcium supplement for dietary or treatment use. Administration with food helps this problem.

Dosage Forms Elemental calcium listed in brackets

Calcium carbonate:

Capsule: 1500 mg [600 mg]
Calci-Mix™: 1250 mg [500 mg]
Florical®: 364 mg [145.6 mg] with sodium fluoride 8.3 mg
Liquid (Tums® Extra Strength): 1000 mg/5 mL (360 mL)
Lozenge (Mylanta® Soothing Antacids): 600 mg [240 mg]
Powder (Cal Carb-HD®): 6.5 g/packet [2.6 g]
Suspension, oral: 1250 mg/5 mL [500 mg]
Tablet: 650 mg [260 mg], 1500 mg [600 mg]
Calciday-667®: 667 mg [267 mg]
Os-Cal® 500, Oyst-Cal 500, Oystercal® 500: 1250 mg [500 mg]
Cal-Plus®, Caltrate® 600, Gencalc® 600, Nephro-Calci®: 1500 mg [600 mg]

(Continued)

Calcium Salts (Oral) (Continued)

Chewable:
Alka-Mints®: 850 mg [340 mg]
Amitone®: 350 mg [140 mg]
Caltrate, Jr.®: 750 mg [300 mg]
Calci-Chew™, Os-Cal®: 750 mg [300 mg]
Chooz®, Dicarbosil®, Equilet®, Tums®: 500 mg [200 mg]
Mallamint®: 420 mg [168 mg]
Rolaids® Calcium Rich: 550 mg [220 mg]
Tums® E-X Extra Strength: 750 mg [300 mg]
Tums® Ultra®: 1000 mg [400 mg]
Florical®: 364 mg [145.6 mg] with sodium fluoride 8.3 mg

Calcium carbonate and simethicone (Titralac® Plus Liquid):
Liquid: Calcium carbonate 500 mg [200 mg] and simethicone 20 mg per 5 mL

Calcium citrate (Citracal®):
Tablet: 950 mg [200 mg]
Tablet, effervescent: 2376 mg [500 mg]

Calcium glubionate (Neo-Calglucon®):
Syrup: 1.8 g/5 mL [115 mg/5 mL] (480 mL)

Calcium gluconate:
Tablet: 500 mg [45 mg], 650 mg [58.5 mg], 975 mg [87.75 mg], 1 g [90 mg]

Calcium lactate:
Tablet: 325 mg [42.25 mg], 650 mg [84.5 mg]

Calcium phosphate, tribasic (Posture®):
Tablet, sugar free: 1565.2 mg [600 mg]

References

Bauwens SF, Drinka PJ, and Boh LE, "Pathogenesis and Management of Primary Osteoporosis," Clin Pharm, 1986, 5(8):639-59.
Heaney RP, Recker RR, and Saville PD, "Menopausal Changes in Calcium Balance Performance," J Lab Clin Med, 1978, 92(6):953-63.
Recker RR, "Calcium Absorption and Achlorhydria," N Engl J Med, 1985, 313(2):70-3.
Sagraves R, "Prevention and Treatment of Osteoporosis in Women," U.S. Pharmacist, 1994, 19(9 Suppl):3-16.

Caldecort® see Hydrocortisone on page 462

Caldecort® Anti-Itch Spray see Hydrocortisone on page 462

Calderol® see Calcifediol on page 139

Calm-X® Oral [OTC] see Dimenhydrinate on page 300

Calphron® see Calcium Acetate on page 145

Cal-Plus® [OTC] see Calcium Salts (Oral) on page 152

Caltrate® 600 [OTC] see Calcium Salts (Oral) on page 152

Caltrate, Jr.® [OTC] see Calcium Salts (Oral) on page 152

Cama® Arthritis Pain Reliever [OTC] see Aspirin on page 84

Capastat® Sulfate see Capreomycin on this page

Capital® and Codeine see Acetaminophen and Codeine on page 18

Capoten® see Captopril on page 156

Capozide® see Captopril and Hydrochlorothiazide on page 159

Capreomycin (kap ree oh MYE sin)

Brand Names Capastat® Sulfate

Generic Available No

Therapeutic Category Antibiotic, Miscellaneous; Antitubercular Agent

Use In conjunction with at least one other antituberculosis agent in the treatment of tuberculosis

Contraindications Known hypersensitivity to capreomycin sulfate

Warnings The use of capreomycin in patients with renal insufficiency or preexisting auditory impairment must be undertaken with great caution, and the risk of additional eighth nerve impairment or renal injury should be weighed against the benefits to be derived from therapy. Since other parenteral antituberculous agents (eg, streptomycin) also have similar and sometimes irreversible toxic effects, particularly on eighth cranial nerve and renal function, simultaneous administration of these agents with capreomycin is not recommended. Use with nonantituberculous drugs (ie, aminoglycoside antibiotics) having ototoxic or nephrotoxic potential should be undertaken only with great caution.

Adverse Reactions
Dermatologic: Rash
Hematologic: Eosinophilia, leukocytosis, thrombocytopenia

Local: Pain induration, bleeding at injection site
Otic: Ototoxicity, tinnitus
Renal: Nephrotoxicity

Overdosage Symptoms of overdose include renal failure, ototoxicity, thrombocytopenia; treatment is supportive

Drug Interactions Aminoglycosides increased risk for nephrotoxicity or respiratory paralysis; increased effect/duration of nondepolarizing neuromuscular blocking agents

Mechanism of Action Capreomycin is a cyclic polypeptide antimicrobial. It is administered as a mixture of capreomycin IA and capreomycin IB. The mechanism of action of capreomycin is not well understood. Mycobacterial species that have become resistant to other agents are usually still sensitive to the action of capreomycin. However, significant cross-resistance with viomycin, kanamycin, and neomycin occurs.

Pharmacokinetics
Absorption: Oral: Poor absorption necessitates parenteral administration
Half-life: Dependent upon renal function and varies with creatinine clearance; 4-6 hours
Time to peak serum concentration: I.M.: 1 hour
Elimination: Essentially excreted unchanged in the urine; no significant accumulation after ≥30 day of 1 g/day dosing in patients with normal renal function

Usual Dosage I.M.:
Geriatrics: Usual adult dose with adjustments for dosing in renal impairment; see table.

Capreomycin Sulfate

Cl$_{cr}$ (mL/min)	Dose (mg/kg) for each dosing interval		
	24 h	48 h	72 h
0	1.29	2.58	3.87
10	2.43	4.87	7.3
20	3.58	7.16	10.7
30	4.72	9.45	14.2
40	5.87	11.7	
50	7.01	14	
60	8.16		
80	10.4		
100	12.7		
110	13.9		

Adults: 1 g/day (not to exceed 20 mg/kg/day) for 60-120 days, followed by 1 g 2-3 times/week for a total of 12-24 months

Administration Administer by deep I.M. injection into large muscle mass

Monitoring Parameters Check hearing with audiometry and assess vestibular function regularly. Monitor BUN, creatinine, and potassium throughout the course of treatment.

Test Interactions Decreased potassium (S), increased BUN, leukocytosis, decreased platelets

Patient Information Report hearing loss to physician immediately; do not discontinue without notifying physician

Nursing Implications See Administration

Special Geriatric Considerations Has not been studied in the elderly. I.M. administration may limit use due to painful injection or lack of sites in patients with decreased muscle mass; adjust dose for renal function

Dosage Forms Injection, as sulfate: 100 mg/mL (10 mL)

Capsaicin (kap SAY sin)

Brand Names Capsin® [OTC]; Capzasin-P® [OTC]; No Pain-HP® [OTC]; R-Gel® [OTC]; Zostrix® [OTC]; Zostrix-® HP [OTC]

Generic Available No

Therapeutic Category Analgesic, Topical; Topical Skin Product

Use
Zostrix®: Temporary relief of pain (neuralgia) following herpes zoster infections
Zostrix®-HP: Relief of neuralgias such as diabetic neuropathy and postsurgical pain

(Continued)

Capsaicin *(Continued)*

Unlabeled use: Psoriasis, vitiligo, intractable pruritus, phantom limb pain, osteoarthritis of the knee, migraine headaches (intranasally)

Adverse Reactions Local: Transient burning on application

Mechanism of Action Renders the skin insensitive to pain by depleting and preventing reaccumulation of substance P in peripheral sensory neurons. Substance P is thought to be the primary chemomediator of pain impulses from the periphery to the central nervous system.

Usual Dosage Geriatrics and Adults: Apply to affected area up to 3-4 times/ day

Monitoring Parameters Relief of pain

Patient Information Wash hands immediately after application; for external use only; avoid contact with eyes; do not use on broken or irritated skin; transient burning may occur upon application but should disappear after a few days; if symptoms get worse or persist longer than 28 days, or clear up and recur, discontinue use and consult physician

Nursing Implications Wash hands immediately after application

Additional Information If used less than 3 times/day, this product may not be effective

Special Geriatric Considerations Capsaicin products are available over-the-counter. Counsel patients about the appropriate use of these products. The American College of Rheumatology recommends capsaicin for the symptomatic treatment of osteoarthritis of the knee.

Dosage Forms
Cream:
Capzasin-P®, Zostrix®: 0.025% (45 g, 90 g)
Zostrix®-HP: 0.075% (30 g, 60 g)
Gel (R-Gel®): 0.025% (15 g, 30 g)
Lotion (Capsin®): 0.025% (59 mL); 0.075% (59 mL)
Roll-on (No Pain-HP®): 0.075% (60 mL)

References
Cordell GA and Araujo OE, "Capsaicin: Identification, Nomenclature, and Pharmacotherapy," *Ann Pharmacother*, 1993, 27(3):330-6.
Hochberg MC, Altman RD, Brandt KD, et al, "Guidelines for the Medical Management of Osteoarthritis. Part II. Osteoarthritis of the Knee. American College of Rheumatology," *Arthritis Rheum*, 1995, 38(11):1541-6.

Capsin® [OTC] *see* Capsaicin *on previous page*

Captopril *(KAP toe pril)*
Related Information
ACE Inhibitors Comparison *on page 1019*
Antacid Drug Interactions *on page 1096*

Brand Names Capoten®

Generic Available Yes

Therapeutic Category Angiotensin-Converting Enzyme (ACE) Inhibitors

Use Management of hypertension and treatment of systolic congestive heart failure; increase circulation in Raynaud's phenomenon; idiopathic edema; diabetic nephropathy; postmyocardial infarction for prevention of ventricular failure

Unlabeled use: Hypertensive crisis, diabetic nephropathy, rheumatoid arthritis, diagnosis of anatomic renal artery stenosis, hypertension secondary to scleroderma renal crisis, diagnosis of aldosteronism, idiopathic edema, Bartter's syndrome

Contraindications Hypersensitivity to captopril or any component or any ACE inhibitor

Warnings Neutropenia, agranulocytosis, angioedema, decreased renal function (hypertension, renal artery stenosis, congestive heart failure), hepatic dysfunction (elimination, activation), proteinuria, first-dose hypotension (hypovolemia, CHF, dehydrated patients at risk, eg, diuretic use, elderly), elderly (due to renal function changes)

Precautions Use with caution and modify dosage in patients with renal impairment; use with caution in patients with collagen vascular disease, congestive heart failure, hypovolemia, valvular stenosis, hyperkalemia (>5.7 mEq/L), anesthesia

Adverse Reactions
Cardiovascular: Hypotension, tachycardia, arrhythmias, orthostatic blood pressure, angina, palpitations, chest pain, syncope, congestive heart failure, Raynaud's syndrome, flushing, vasculitis

Central nervous system: Nervousness, depression, confusion, somnolence, fatigue, dizziness, headache, insomnia

Dermatologic: Rash, photosensitivity, pruritus, angioedema

Endocrine & metabolic: Hyperkalemia, hyponatremia

Gastrointestinal: Pancreatitis, constipation, anorexia, nausea, gastritis, dysgeusia, xerostomia, peptic ulcer, weight loss, vomiting, diarrhea, abdominal pain, ageusia

Genitourinary: Impotence, polyuria

Hematologic: Neutropenia, agranulocytosis, pancytopenia, thrombocytopenia

Hepatic: Hepatitis

Neuromuscular & skeletal: Myalgia, arthralgia, arthritis, paresthesia

Ocular: Blurred vision

Renal: Proteinuria, oliguria, renal insufficiency, nephrotic syndrome, interstitial nephritis, increased BUN, serum creatinine

Respiratory: Chronic cough (nonproductive, persistent; more often in women and seen in 15% to 30% of patients), bronchospasm, dyspnea

Miscellaneous: Diaphoresis

Overdosage Symptoms of overdose include severe hypotension

Toxicology Following initiation of essential overdose management, toxic symptom treatment and supportive treatment should be initiated. Hypotension usually responds to I.V. fluids or Trendelenburg positioning. If unresponsive to these measures, the use of a parenteral inotrope may be required (eg, norepinephrine 0.1-0.2 mcg/kg/minute titrated to response). Seizures commonly respond to diazepam (I.V. 5-10 mg bolus in adults every 15 minutes if needed up to a total of 30 mg) or to phenytoin or phenobarbital.

Drug Interactions

Captopril and potassium-sparing diuretics may cause additive hyperkalemic effect

Captopril and indomethacin or nonsteroidal anti-inflammatory agents may cause reduced antihypertensive response to captopril

Allopurinol and captopril may cause neutropenia

Antacids and ACE inhibitors may decrease absorption of ACE inhibitors

Phenothiazines and ACE inhibitors may increase ACE inhibitor effect

Probenecid and ACE inhibitors (captopril) may increase ACE inhibitors (captopril) levels

Rifampin and ACE inhibitors (captopril) may decrease ACE inhibitor effect

Digoxin and ACE inhibitors may increase serum digoxin concentrations

Lithium and ACE inhibitors may increase lithium serum concentration

Tetracycline and ACE inhibitors (captopril) may decrease tetracycline absorption (up to 37%)

Capsaicin may cause or exacerbate coughing with ACE inhibitors

Food decreases captopril absorption (see Additional Information)

Stability All solutions made must be stored in glass bottles; syrup is stable for 7 days at 4°C and 22°C; distilled water is stable at 7 days at 22°C and 14 days at 4°C; distilled water with sodium ascorbate is stable 14 days at 22°C and 56 days at 4°C

Stability in aqueous solution is temperature dependent and related to geographical source and chemical (metal) content of tap water used. A 1 mg/mL solution (made by crushing a 25 mg tablet and adding it to 25 mL of tap water from Edmonton, Alberta, Canada) has been found to be stable for 27 days at 5°C, 11.8 days at 25°C, 3.6 days at 50°C, and 2.1 days at 75°C. However, captopril 1 mg/mL in tap water from Rochester, New York was extremely unstable. Captopril 1 mg/mL in sterile water for irrigation was stable for at least 3 days when kept refrigerated. Other factors not yet identified may influence captopril oxidation in aqueous solution. Powder papers can be made; powder papers are stable for 12 weeks when stored at room temperature.

Anaizi NH and Swenson C, "Instability of Aqueous Captopril Solutions," *Am J Hosp Pharm*, 1993, 50:486-8.

Pereira CM and Tam YK, "Stability of Captopril in Tap Water," *Am J Hosp Pharm*, 1992, 49(3):612-5.

Taketomo CK, Chu SA, Cheng MH, et al, "Stability of Captopril in Powder Papers Under Three Storage Conditions," *Am J Hosp Pharm*, 1990, 47(8):1799-801.

Mechanism of Action Competitive inhibitor of angiotensin-converting enzyme (ACE); prevents conversion of angiotensin I to angiotensin II, a potent vasoconstrictor; results in lower levels of angiotensin II which causes an increase in plasma renin activity and a reduction in aldosterone secretion; a CNS mechanism may also be involved in hypotensive effect as angiotensin II increases adrenergic outflow from CNS; vasoactive kallikreins may be
(Continued)

Captopril *(Continued)*

decreased in conversion to active hormones by ACE inhibitors, thus reducing blood pressure

Pharmacodynamics
Onset of action: Oral: Maximal decrease in blood pressure in 60-90 minutes after dose
Duration: Dose related; may require several weeks of therapy before full hypotensive effect is seen

Pharmacokinetics
Absorption: Oral: 60% to 75%
Distribution: V_d: 7 L/kg
Protein binding: 25% to 30%
Metabolism: 50%
Half-life:
    Normal adults: Dependent upon renal and cardiac function: 1.9 hours
    Impaired renal function: 3.5-32 hours
    Anuria: 20-40 hours
Time to peak serum concentrations: Within 1-2 hours
Elimination: 95% excreted in urine in 24 hours; 40% to 50% excreted unchanged urine

Usual Dosage Note: Dosage must be titrated according to patient's response; use lowest effective dose (see Additional Information, Administration, and Stability)

Geriatrics and Adults: Oral: Initial: 12.5-25 mg/dose given every 8-12 hours; increase by 12.5-25 mg/dose to maximum of 450 mg/day; increase doses at 1- to 2-week intervals
    Congestive heart failure: Initial: 6.25-12.5 mg 3 times/day; titrate to 25 mg 3 times/day over several days; titrate slowly over several weeks to "target dosage" of 50 mg 3 times/day. Maximum dose may be attained at 100 mg 3 times/day; do not exceed a daily dose of 450 mg.
    Diabetic nephropathy: 25 mg 3 times/day
    Left ventricular dysfunction following myocardial infarction: Initiate doses at 6.25-12.5 mg 3 times/day; increase to 25 mg 3 times/day over several days with the intent of achieving the "target dosage" of 50 mg 3 times/day over several weeks of slow titration

Note: Smaller dosages (6.25-12.5 mg) given every 8-12 hours are indicated in patients with renal dysfunction; renal function and leukocyte count should be carefully monitored during therapy; increase at intervals of 1-2 weeks
Moderately dialyzable (20% to 50%)

Administration Tablets may be used to make a solution of captopril (see Stability)

Monitoring Parameters Serum potassium concentrations, BUN, serum creatinine, renal function, WBC, CBC with platelets

Test Interactions Increased BUN, creatinine, potassium, positive Coombs' [direct]; decreased cholesterol (S); may cause false-positive results in urine acetone determinations using sodium nitroprusside reagent

Patient Information Administer 1 hour before meals; do not stop therapy except under prescriber advice; notify physician if you develop sore throat, fever, swelling of hands, feet, face, eyes, lips, and tongue; difficult breathing, irregular heartbeats, chest pains, or cough. May cause dizziness, fainting, and lightheadedness, especially in first week of therapy, sit and stand up slowly; may cause changes in taste or rash; do not add a salt substitute (potassium) without advice of physician.

Nursing Implications Watch for hypotensive effect within 1-3 hours of first dose or new higher dose (see Precautions, Warnings, Monitoring Parameters, and Special Geriatric Considerations)

Additional Information Many patients complain of transient cough during early therapy; food decreases absorption of captopril 30% to 40%; administer captopril 1 hour before meals; clinical significance not known; therefore, observe for loss of effect. Newer data demonstrate that lower doses of ACE inhibitors are effective and toxic reactions are decreased.

Special Geriatric Considerations Due to frequent decreases in glomerular filtration (also creatinine clearance) with aging, elderly patients may have exaggerated responses to ACE inhibitors; differences in clinical response due to hepatic changes are not observed. ACE inhibitors may be preferred agents in elderly patients with congestive heart failure and diabetes mellitus. Diabetic proteinuria is reduced and insulin sensitivity is enhanced. In general, the side effect profile is favorable in elderly and causes little or no CNS confusion; use lowest dose recommendations initially.

Dosage Forms Tablet: 12.5 mg, 25 mg, 50 mg, 100 mg

References

Anaizi NH and Swenson C, "Instability of Aqueous Captopril Solutions," *Am J Hosp Pharm*, 1993, 50(3):486-8.

Konstam MA, Drakup K, Baker DW, et al, "Heart Failure: Evaluation and Care of Patients With Left Ventricular Systolic Dysfunction," *Clinical Practice Guideline No 11*, Rockville, MD: Agency for Health Care Policy and Research, Public Health Service, U.S. Department of Health and Human Services, 1994.

Lewis EJ, Hunsicker LG, Bain RP, et al, "The Effect of Angiotensin-Converting Enzyme Inhibition on Diabetic Nephropathy," *N Engl J Med*, 1993, 329(20):1456-62.

McAreavey D and Robertson JIS, "Angiotensin Converting Enzyme Inhibitors and Moderate Hypertension," *Drugs*, 1990, 40(3):326-45.

Pereira CM and Tam YK, "Stability of Captopril in Tap Water," *Am J Hosp Pharm*, 1992, 49(3):612-5.

Taketomo CK, Chu SA, Cheng MH, et al, "Stability of Captopril in Powder Papers Under Three Storage Conditions," *Am J Hosp Pharm*, 1990, 47(8):1799-801.

Williams JF, Bristow MR, Fowler MB, et al, "Guidelines for the Evaluation and Management of Heart Failure: Report of the American College of Cardiology/American Heart Association Task Force on Practice Guidelines (Committee on Evaluation and Management of Heart Failure)," *J Am Coll Cardiol*, 1995, 26:1376-8.

Captopril and Hydrochlorothiazide
(KAP toe pril & hye droe klor oh THYE a zide)

Related Information
Captopril *on page 156*
Hydrochlorothiazide *on page 458*

Brand Names Capozide®

Generic Available No

Therapeutic Category Antihypertensive, Combination

Special Geriatric Considerations Combination products are not recommended for first-line treatment and divided doses of diuretics may increase the incidence of nocturia in the elderly

Dosage Forms
Tablet:
25/15: Captopril 25 mg and hydrochlorothiazide 15 mg
25/25: Captopril 25 mg and hydrochlorothiazide 25 mg
50/15: Captopril 50 mg and hydrochlorothiazide 15 mg
50/25: Captopril 50 mg and hydrochlorothiazide 25 mg

Capzasin-P® [OTC] *see* Capsaicin *on page 155*

Carafate® *see* Sucralfate *on page 873*

Carbachol (KAR ba kole)

Related Information
Glaucoma Drug Therapy Comparison *on page 1032*

Brand Names Carbastat® Ophthalmic; Carboptic® Ophthalmic; Isopto® Carbachol Ophthalmic; Miostat® Intraocular

Synonyms Carbacholine; Carbamylcholine Chloride

Generic Available No

Therapeutic Category Cholinergic Agent, Ophthalmic; Ophthalmic Agent, Miotic

Use Lower intraocular pressure in the treatment of glaucoma; to cause miosis during surgery

Contraindications Acute iritis, acute inflammatory disease of the anterior chamber, hypersensitivity to carbachol or any component

Precautions Use with caution in patients undergoing general anesthesia and in presence of corneal abrasion

Adverse Reactions
Cardiovascular: Syncope, arrhythmias, flushing
Central nervous system: Headache
Gastrointestinal: Salivation, GI cramps, vomiting, diarrhea
Genitourinary: Increased bladder tone
Local: Ciliary spasm with temporary decrease of visual acuity
Ocular: Corneal clouding, persistent bullous keratopathy, postoperative keratitis, retinal detachment, transient ciliary and conjunctival injection
Respiratory: Asthma
Miscellaneous: Diaphoresis

Overdosage Symptoms of overdose include miosis, flushing, vomiting, bradycardia, bronchospasm, involuntary urination; flush eyes with water or normal saline; if accidentally ingested, induce emesis or perform gastric lavage

Toxicology Atropine is the treatment of choice for intoxications manifesting with significant muscarinic symptoms. Atropine I.V. 2-4 mg every 3-60 minutes should be repeated to control symptoms and then continued as (Continued)

Carbachol *(Continued)*

needed for 1-2 days following the acute ingestion. Epinephrine 0.1-1 mg S.C. may be useful in reversing severe cardiovascular or pulmonary sequel.

Mechanism of Action Synthetic direct-acting cholinergic agent that causes miosis by stimulating muscarinic receptors in the eye

Pharmacodynamics
Onset of miosis:
Ophthalmic: Within 10-20 minutes
Intraocular: Within 2-5 minutes
Duration of action:
Ophthalmic: Reductions in intraocular pressure persist for 4-8 hours
Intraocular: Lasts 24 hours

Usual Dosage Geriatrics and Adults:
Intraocular: 0.5 mL instilled in anterior chamber before or after securing sutures
Ophthalmic: Instill 1-2 drops up to 4 times/day

Administration Finger pressure should be applied on the lacrimal sac for 1-2 minutes following topical instillation; remove excess around the eye with a tissue

Patient Information May sting on instillation; may cause headache, altered distance vision, and decreased night vision; do not touch dropper to eye

Nursing Implications Instillation for miosis prior to eye surgery should be gentle and parallel to the iris face and tangential to the pupil border; discard unused portion (see Administration)

Special Geriatric Considerations Assess patient's ability to self-administer (see Usual Dosage)

Dosage Forms
Solution:
Intraocular: 0.01% (1.5 mL)
Ophthalmic: 0.75% (15 mL, 30 mL); 1.5% (15 mL, 30 mL); 2.25% (15 mL); 3% (15 mL, 30 mL)

Carbacholine *see Carbachol on previous page*

Carbamazepine *(kar ba MAZ e peen)*

Related Information
Antiepileptic Drug Interactions Comparison *on page 1022*
Serum Drug Concentrations Commonly Monitored: Guidelines *on page 1114*

Brand Names Atretol®; Depitol®; Epitol®; Tegretol®; Tegretol-XR®

Generic Available Yes: Tablet

Therapeutic Category Anticonvulsant, Miscellaneous

Use Prophylaxis of generalized tonic-clonic, partial (especially complex partial), and mixed partial (treatment of choice) or generalized seizure disorder; may be used to relieve pain in trigeminal neuralgia or diabetic neuropathy

Unlabeled use: Has been used to treat bipolar disorders and other schizoaffective disorders; resistant schizophrenia, alcohol withdrawal, post-traumatic stress syndrome, atypical psychosis, unipolar depression; restless leg syndrome, and psychotic behavior associated with dementia

Contraindications Hypersensitivity to carbamazepine or any component; may have cross-sensitivity with tricyclic antidepressants; should not be used in any patient with bone marrow suppression, MAO inhibitor use, or history of bone marrow suppression

Warnings Potentially fatal blood cell abnormalities have been reported following treatment; early detection of hematologic change is important; advise patients of early signs and symptoms which are fever, sore throat, mouth ulcers, infections, easy bruising, petechial or purpuric hemorrhage; use with caution in glaucoma due to mild anticholinergic action; may cause confusion or activate latent psychosis; elderly at risk for confusion or agitation

Precautions MAO inhibitors should be discontinued for a minimum of 14 days before carbamazepine is begun; administer with caution to patients with history of cardiac damage or hepatic disease; may cause drowsiness, dizziness, or blurred vision

Adverse Reactions
Cardiovascular: Edema, congestive heart failure, syncope, hypertension, hypotension, arrhythmias
Central nervous system: Sedation, dizziness, slurred speech, difficulty concentrating, fatigue, ataxia

Dermatologic: Rash (but does not necessarily mean the drug should not be stopped), pruritus, alopecia, urticaria, Stevens-Johnson syndrome, exfoliative dermatitis, toxic epidermal necrolysis

Endocrine & metabolic: Hyponatremia, SIADH

Gastrointestinal: Nausea, gastric distress, abdominal pain, diarrhea, constipation, anorexia, xerostomia, glossitis, stomatitis

Genitourinary: Urinary retention

Hematologic: Neutropenia (can be transient), aplastic anemia (1 in 200,000 patients), agranulocytosis, thrombocytopenia; leukopenia is the most frequent hematologic effect

Hepatic: Hepatitis

Local: Thrombophlebitis

Neuromuscular & skeletal: Arthralgias, leg cramps

Ocular: Nystagmus, diplopia

Respiratory: Dyspnea

Overdosage Symptoms of overdose include dizziness, ataxia, drowsiness, nausea, vomiting, tremor, agitation, nystagmus, urinary retention, tachycardia, hypotension, hypertension, shock, dysrhythmias, coma, seizures, twitches, respiratory depression, neuromuscular disturbances

Toxicology Activated charcoal (50-100 g initially; ≥12 g/hour with nasogastric tube) is effective at binding carbamazepine; monitor EKG, blood pressure, body temperature, pupillary reflexes, bladder function for several days following ingestion; provide general supportive care

Drug Interactions

Erythromycin, clarithromycin, isoniazid, propoxyphene, verapamil, danazol, nicotinamide, diltiazem, and cimetidine may inhibit hepatic metabolism of carbamazepine with resultant increase of carbamazepine serum concentrations and toxicity

Carbamazepine may induce the metabolism of warfarin, doxycycline, oral contraceptives, phenytoin, theophylline, benzodiazepines, ethosuximide, lamotrigine, valproic acid, corticosteroids, and thyroid hormones

May increase metabolism of acetaminophen increasing the possibility of hepatotoxicity and decreasing its analgesic/antipyretic activity

Barbiturates and primidone may decrease serum concentrations of carbamazepine

Lithium may have increased CNS toxicity; valproic acid levels may decrease

Mechanism of Action May depress activity in the nucleus ventralis of the thalamus or decrease synaptic transmission or to decrease summation of temporal stimulation leading to neural discharge by limiting influx of sodium ions across cell membrane or other unknown mechanisms; stimulates the release of ADH and potentiates its action in promoting reabsorption of water; chemically related to tricyclic antidepressants; in addition to anticonvulsant effects, carbamazepine has anticholinergic, antineuralgic, antidiuretic, muscle relaxant, and antiarrhythmic properties

Pharmacokinetics

Absorption: Slow from GI tract

Distribution: V_d (adults): 0.59-2 L/kg

Protein binding 75% to 90%

Metabolism: Induces liver enzymes to increase its own metabolism and shortens half-life over time; metabolized in liver to active epoxide metabolite; substrated inducer of CYP3A4

Bioavailability: 85% oral

Half-life:
Initial: 18-55 hours
Multiple dosing: 12-17 hours

Time to peak: Unpredictable peak concentrations occur within 4-8 hours

Elimination: 1% to 3% excreted unchanged in urine

Usual Dosage Oral (dosage must be adjusted according to patient's response and serum concentrations):

Geriatrics and Adults: 200 mg twice daily to start, increase by 200 mg/day at 2- to 3-week intervals until therapeutic levels achieved and autoinduction adjustment of its own metabolism; usual dose: 800-1200 mg/day in 2-4 divided doses; some patients have required up to 1.6-2.4 g/day; most common chronic dose range: 7-15 mg/kg/day; must administer at least twice daily due to autoinduction

Monitoring Parameters CBC, serum concentrations, and response; select "target symptoms" for behavior monitoring

Reference Range Therapeutic: 6-12 μg/mL (SI: 25-51 μmol/L). Patients who require higher concentrations (8-12 μg/mL (SI: 34-51 μmol/L)) should be watched closely; trough concentrations >4 μg/mL are often needed. Side (Continued)

Carbamazepine *(Continued)*

effects including CNS effects occur commonly at higher dosage levels. If other anticonvulsants are given therapeutic range is 4-8 µg/mL (SI: 17-34 µmol/L).

Test Interactions Increased BUN, AST, ALT, bilirubin, alkaline phosphatase (S); decreased calcium, T_3, T_4, sodium (S)

Patient Information Take with food, may cause drowsiness, periodic blood test monitoring required; notify physician if you observe bleeding, bruising, jaundice, abdominal pain, pale stools, mental disturbances, fever, chills, sore throat, or mouth ulcers

Nursing Implications Observe patient for excessive sedation

Additional Information Suspension dosage form must be given on a 3-4 times/day schedule versus tablets which can be given 2-4 times/day; may cause a rash, but does not necessarily mean the drug should be stopped

Special Geriatric Considerations Elderly may have increased risk of SIADH-like syndrome (see Adverse Reactions)

Dosage Forms
Suspension, oral (citrus-vanilla flavor): 100 mg/5 mL (450 mL)
Tablet: 200 mg
Tablet, chewable: 100 mg
Tablet, extended release: 100 mg, 200 mg, 400 mg

Carbamide Peroxide *(KAR ba mide per OKS ide)*

Brand Names Auro® Ear Drops [OTC]; Debrox® Otic [OTC]; E•R•O Ear [OTC]; Gly-Oxide® Oral [OTC]; Mollifene® Ear Wax Removing Formula [OTC]; Murine® Ear Drops [OTC]; Orajel® Perioseptic [OTC]; Proxigel® Oral [OTC]

Synonyms Urea Peroxide

Generic Available Yes

Therapeutic Category Anti-infective Agent, Oral; Otic Agent, Cerumenolytic

Use
Oral: Relief of minor inflammation of gums, oral mucosal surfaces and lips including canker sores and dental irritation
Otic: Emulsify and disperse ear wax

Contraindications Otic preparation should not be used in patients with a perforated tympanic membrane; ear drainage, ear pain, or rash in the ear; dizziness

Warnings With prolonged use of oral carbamide peroxide, there is a potential for overgrowth of opportunistic organisms; damage to periodontal tissues; delayed wound healing

Adverse Reactions
Central nervous system: Dizziness
Dermatologic: Rash
Local: Irritation, tenderness, pain, redness

Stability Store in tight, light-resistant containers; oral gel should be stored under refrigeration

Mechanism of Action Carbamide peroxide releases hydrogen peroxide which serves as a source of nascent oxygen upon contact with catalase; deodorant action is probably due to inhibition of odor-causing bacteria; softens impacted cerumen due to its foaming action

Usual Dosage Geriatrics and Adults:
Oral (should not be used for >7 days):
Gel: Massage on affected area 4 times/day
Solution: Apply several drops undiluted to affected area of the mouth 4 times/day and at bedtime for up to 7 days, expectorate after 2-3 minutes; as an adjunct to oral hygiene after brushing, swish 10 drops for 2-3 minutes, then expectorate
Otic (should not be used for longer than 4 days): Instill 5-10 drops twice daily for up to 4 days; keep drops in ear for several minutes by keeping head tilted or placing cotton in ear

Administration See Usual Dosage

Patient Information Contact physician if dizziness or otic redness, rash, irritation, tenderness, pain, drainage, or discharge develop; do not drink or rinse mouth for 5 minutes after oral use of gel

Nursing Implications Patient may complain of foaming

Additional Information Otic preparation should not be used for >4 days; oral preparation should not be used for longer than 7 days

Special Geriatric Considerations Avoid contact with hearing aids

Dosage Forms
Gel, oral (Proxigel®): 11% (36 g)
Solution:
Oral (Cankaid®, Gly-Oxide®, Orajel® Brace-Aid Rinse): 10% in glycerin (15 mL, 22.5 mL, 30 mL, 60 mL)
Otic (Auro® Ear Drops, Debrox®, Murine® Ear Drops): 6.5% in glycerin (15 mL, 30 mL)

Carbamylcholine Chloride *see Carbachol on page 159*

Carbastat® Ophthalmic *see Carbachol on page 159*

Carbenicillin (kar ben i SIL in)

Brand Names Geocillin®
Synonyms Carindacillin
Generic Available No
Therapeutic Category Antibiotic, Penicillin
Use Treatment of serious infections caused by susceptible gram-negative aerobic bacilli or mixed aerobic-anaerobic bacterial infections and/or urinary tract infections excluding those secondary to *Klebsiella* sp and *Serratia marcescens*
Contraindications Hypersensitivity to carbenicillin or any component or penicillins
Warnings Oral carbenicillin should be limited to treatment of urinary tract infections and prostatitis
Precautions Do not use in patients with severe renal impairment (Cl$_{cr}$ <10 mL/ minute); use with caution in patients with history of cephalosporin allergy; dosage modification required in patients with impaired renal and/or hepatic function; because of its high sodium content (5 mEq/g), use with caution in patients with hypertension, congestive heart failure, or cephalosporin allergy
Adverse Reactions
Dermatologic: Rash, urticaria, pruritus
Endocrine & metabolic: Hypokalemia
Gastrointestinal: Nausea, vomiting, diarrhea, abdominal cramps
Hematologic: Eosinophilia, hemolytic anemia, neutropenia, thrombocytopenia
Hepatic: Elevation in liver enzymes
Miscellaneous: Furry tongue
Overdosage Symptoms of overdose include neuromuscular hypersensitivity, convulsions
Toxicology Many beta-lactam-containing antibiotics have the potential to cause neuromuscular hyperirritability or convulsive seizures. Hemodialysis may be helpful to aid in the removal of the drug from the blood, otherwise most treatment is supportive or symptom directed.
Drug Interactions Probenecid significantly prolongs half-life; decreased effect with administration of aminoglycosides within 1 hour, may inactivate both drugs
Mechanism of Action Interferes with bacterial cell wall synthesis during active multiplication
Pharmacokinetics
Absorption: Oral: 30% to 40%
Distribution: Into bile, low concentrations attained in CSF
Protein binding: 50%
Half-life: 60-90 minutes and is prolonged to 10-20 hours with renal insufficiency
Time to peak: Within 30-120 minutes; in patients with normal renal function, serum concentrations of carbenicillin following oral absorption are inadequate for the treatment of systemic infections
Elimination: ~80% to 99% of dose excreted unchanged in urine
Usual Dosage Geriatrics and Adults:
Oral: 1-2 tablets (382-764 mg) every 6 hours
Prostatitis: 2 tablets every 6 hours
Dosing interval in renal impairment:
Cl$_{cr}$ 10-50 mL/minute: Administer every 12-24 hours
Cl$_{cr}$ <10 mL/minute: Administer every 24-48 hours
Moderately dialyzable (20% to 50%)
Monitoring Parameters Signs and symptoms of infection (fever, urinary frequency, dysuria, etc)
Reference Range Therapeutic: Not established; Toxic: >250 µg/mL (SI: >660 µmol/L)
Test Interactions False-positive urine or serum proteins; false-positive urine glucose (Clinitest®)
(Continued)

Carbenicillin *(Continued)*

Patient Information Tablets have a bitter taste, can be taken with food; complete full course of treatment; notify physician of edema, difficulty breathing, bruising, or bleeding

Nursing Implications Watch for increased edema, rales, or signs of congestion, bruising, or bleeding; administer around-the-clock to promote less variation in peak and trough serum concentrations

Special Geriatric Considerations Has not been studied in the elderly (see Usual Dosage); adjust dose for renal function in the elderly

Dosage Forms Tablet, as indanyl sodium: 382 mg

Carbidopa *(kar bi DOE pa)*

Brand Names Lodosyn®

Generic Available No

Therapeutic Category Anti-Parkinson's Agent

Additional Information Usually used in combination with levodopa (Sinemet®); plain carbidopa tablets are available from Merck & Co to physicians for use in patients requiring individual titration of carbidopa and levodopa (see Levodopa and Carbidopa monograph)

Dosage Forms Tablet: 25 mg

Carbidopa and Levodopa *see* Levodopa and Carbidopa *on page 530*

Carbinoxamine and Pseudoephedrine

(kar bi NOKS a meen & soo doe e FED rin)

Brand Names Biohist-LA®; Carbiset® Tablet; Carbiset-TR® Tablet; Carbodec® Syrup; Carbodec® Tablet; Carbodec TR® Tablet; Cardec-S® Syrup; Rondec® Drops; Rondec® Filmtab®; Rondec® Syrup; Rondec-TR®

Generic Available Yes

Therapeutic Category Adrenergic Agonist Agent; Antihistamine, H_1 Blocker; Decongestant

Use Temporary relief of nasal congestion, running nose, sneezing, itching of nose or throat, and itchy, watery eyes due to the common cold, hay fever, or other respiratory allergies

Contraindications Hypersensitivity to carbinoxamine or pseudoephedrine or any component; severe hypertension or coronary artery disease, MAO inhibitor therapy, GI or GU obstruction, narrow-angle glaucoma; avoid use in premature or term infants due to a possible association with SIDS

Warnings Narrow-angle glaucoma, bladder neck obstruction, symptomatic prostatic hypertrophy, asthmatic attack, and stenosing peptic ulcer

Precautions Use with caution in patients with hyperthyroidism, diabetes mellitus, cardiovascular disease (ie, CAD, ischemic disease)

Adverse Reactions

Cardiovascular: Edema, palpitations, pallor

Central nervous system: Slight to moderate drowsiness or stimulation, headache, fatigue, nervousness, dizziness, fear, tenseness, restlessness, insomnia, depression, hallucinations, psychological symptoms

Dermatologic: Angioedema, photosensitivity, rash

Gastrointestinal: Appetite increase, weight gain, nausea, vomiting, diarrhea, abdominal pain, xerostomia

Genitourinary: Dysuria

Hepatic: Hepatitis

Neuromuscular & skeletal: Arthralgia, myalgia, paresthesia, tremor

Ocular: Blepharospasm, occular photosensitivity

Respiratory: Thickening of bronchial secretions, pharyngitis, bronchospasm, epistaxis

Miscellaneous: Diaphoresis

Overdosage Symptoms of overdose include dry mouth, flushed skin, dilated pupils, CNS depression

Toxicology There is no specific treatment for an antihistamine overdose, however, most of its clinical toxicity is due to anticholinergic effects. Anticholinesterase inhibitors including physostigmine, neostigmine, pyridostigmine, and edrophonium may be useful by reducing acetylcholinesterase; for anticholinergic overdose with severe life-threatening symptoms, physostigmine 1-2 mg (0.5 or 0.02 mg/kg for children) I.V., slowly may be given to reverse these effects.

Drug Interactions

Increased toxicity/adverse effect: Barbiturates, TCAs, MAO inhibitors, ethanolamine antihistamines, beta-blockers, methyldopa, bromocriptine, caffeine

Decreased effect: Phenothiazines, insulin, oral decongestants

Mechanism of Action Carbinoxamine competes with histamine for H_1-receptor sites on effector cells in the gastrointestinal tract, blood vessels, and respiratory tract

Pseudoephedrine: Pseudoephedrine has beta-adrenergic properties and alpha-adrenergic action; stimulates alpha-adrenergic receptors of the vascular smooth muscle, thus constricting dilated arterioles within the nasal mucosa and reducing blood flow to the engaged area; increases urethral sphincter tone due to alpha-adrenergic actions

Usual Dosage Geriatrics and Adults: Oral:
Liquid: 5 mL 4 times/day
Tablets: 1 tablet 4 times/day

Monitoring Parameters Monitor pulse, blood pressure; monitor for tremor, insomnia, and changes in mental function

Patient Information May cause drowsiness, impaired coordination, or judgment; may cause blurred vision; may also cause CNS excitation and difficulty sleeping

Nursing Implications Raise bed rails; institute safety measures; assist with ambulation

Special Geriatric Considerations Elderly are more predisposed to adverse effects of sympathomimetics since they frequently have cardiovascular diseases and diabetes mellitus as well as multiple drug therapies. It may be advisable to treat with a short-acting/immediate-release formulation before initiating sustained-release/long-acting formulations. Carbinoxamine exhibits anticholinergic action which may cause constipation, urinary retention and mental confusion in elderly.

Dosage Forms
Drops: Carbinoxamine maleate 2 mg and pseudoephedrine hydrochloride 25 mg per mL (30 mL with dropper)
Syrup: Carbinoxamine maleate 4 mg and pseudoephedrine hydrochloride 60 mg per 5 mL (120 mL, 480 mL)
Tablet:
Film-coated: Carbinoxamine maleate 4 mg and pseudoephedrine hydrochloride 60 mg
Sustained release: Carbinoxamine maleate 8 mg and pseudoephedrine hydrochloride 120 mg

Carbiset® Tablet *see* Carbinoxamine and Pseudoephedrine *on previous page*

Carbiset-TR® Tablet *see* Carbinoxamine and Pseudoephedrine *on previous page*

Carbodec® Syrup *see* Carbinoxamine and Pseudoephedrine *on previous page*

Carbodec® Tablet *see* Carbinoxamine and Pseudoephedrine *on previous page*

Carbodec TR® Tablet *see* Carbinoxamine and Pseudoephedrine *on previous page*

Carboptic® Ophthalmic *see* Carbachol *on page 159*

Cardec-S® Syrup *see* Carbinoxamine and Pseudoephedrine *on previous page*

Cardene® *see* Nicardipine *on page 667*

Cardene® SR *see* Nicardipine *on page 667*

Cardioquin® *see* Quinidine *on page 815*

Cardizem® CD *see* Diltiazem *on page 298*

Cardizem® Injectable *see* Diltiazem *on page 298*

Cardizem® SR *see* Diltiazem *on page 298*

Cardizem® Tablet *see* Diltiazem *on page 298*

Cardura® *see* Doxazosin *on page 320*

Carindacillin *see* Carbenicillin *on page 163*

Carisoprodate *see* Carisoprodol *on this page*

Carisoprodol (kar i soe PROE dole)

Brand Names Rela®; Sodol®; Soma®; Soma® Compound; Soma® Compound with Codeine; Soprodol®; Soridol®

Synonyms Carisoprodate; Isobamate

Generic Available Yes

Therapeutic Category Skeletal Muscle Relaxant

Use Relief of discomfort associated with acute, painful musculoskeletal conditions

Contraindications Acute intermittent porphyria, hypersensitivity to carisoprodol, meprobamate or any component

Warnings Use with caution in addiction-prone individuals; abrupt withdrawal has caused mild symptoms in some patients and psychological dependence has been reported, though rare. Idiosyncratic reactions may occur rarely
(Continued)

Carisoprodol *(Continued)*

within minutes or hours of the first dose; symptoms include weakness, transient quadriplegia, dizziness, ataxia, temporary loss of vision, diplopia, agitation, euphoria, disorientation; symptoms subside in a few hours; use with caution in renal and hepatic dysfunction

Adverse Reactions

Cardiovascular: Tachycardia, orthostatic hypotension, facial flushing, syncope

Central nervous system: Sedation, dizziness, fatigue, vertigo, agitation, headache, insomnia, ataxia

Gastrointestinal: Nausea, vomiting

Neuromuscular & skeletal: Tremors

Miscellaneous: Cross-hypersensitivity with meprobamate has been reported

Overdosage Symptoms of overdose include CNS depression, stupor, coma, shock, respiratory depression

Toxicology Treatment is supportive following attempts to enhance drug elimination; hypotension should be treated with I.V. fluids and/or Trendelenburg positioning; carisoprodol is dialyzable

Drug Interactions Increased toxicity: Alcohol, CNS depressants, phenothiazines, clindamycin, MAO inhibitors

Mechanism of Action Precise mechanism is not yet clear, but many effects have been ascribed to its central depressant actions

Pharmacodynamics

Onset of action: Within 30 minutes

Duration: 4-6 hours

Pharmacokinetics

Metabolism: By the liver

Half-life: 8 hours

Elimination: Excreted by kidneys

Usual Dosage

Geriatrics: See Special Geriatric Considerations

Adults: Oral: 350 mg 3-4 times/day; take last dose at bedtime; compound: 1-2 tablets 4 times/day

Dosing adjustment in hepatic impairment: Dosage may need to be decreased in patients with severe hepatic dysfunction

Monitoring Parameters Relief of pain and/or muscle spasm, mental status

Patient Information May cause drowsiness or dizziness; avoid alcohol and other CNS depressants; because of the risk of postural hypotension, rise slowly from sitting or lying down

Nursing Implications Raise bed rails and institute safety measures; assist with ambulation

Special Geriatric Considerations No data available on the use of skeletal muscle relaxants in the elderly; because of the risk of orthostatic hypotension and CNS depression, avoid or use with caution in the elderly; not considered a drug of choice in the elderly

Dosage Forms

Tablet:

Sodol®, Soma®, Soprodol®; 350 mg

Soma® Compound: Carisoprodol 200 mg and aspirin 325 mg

Soma® Compound with codeine: Carisoprodol 200 mg, aspirin 325 mg, and codeine phosphate 16 mg

Carteolol *(KAR tee oh lole)*

Related Information

Beta-Blockers Comparison *on page 1026*

Brand Names Cartrol® Oral; Ocupress® Ophthalmic

Generic Available No

Therapeutic Category Antianginal Agent; Beta-Adrenergic Blocker; Beta-Adrenergic Blocker, Ophthalmic

Use Management of hypertension; treatment of chronic open-angle glaucoma and intraocular hypertension

Contraindications Uncompensated congestive heart failure, cardiogenic shock, bradycardia or heart block, asthma or any other bronchospastic disorder; diabetes mellitus, or hypersensitivity to beta-blocking agents

Warnings Abrupt withdrawal of beta-blockers may result in an exaggerated cardiac beta-adrenergic responsiveness. Symptomatology has included reports of tachycardia, hypertension, ischemia, angina, myocardial infarction, and sudden death. It is recommended that patients be tapered gradually off of beta-blockers over a 2-week period rather than via abrupt discontinuation.

Precautions Administer to congestive heart failure patients with caution; administer with caution to patients with bronchospastic disease, diabetes mellitus, hyperthyroidism, myasthenia gravis and renal function decline and severe peripheral vascular disease. Abrupt withdrawal of the drug should be avoided, drug should be discontinued over 2 weeks.

Adverse Reactions

Cardiovascular: Mesenteric arterial thrombosis, A-V block, persistent bradycardia, hypotension, chest pain, edema, heart failure, Raynaud's phenomena

Central nervous system: Fatigue, dizziness, headache, insomnia, lethargy, nightmares, depression, confusion

Dermatologic: Purpura

Gastrointestinal: Ischemic colitis, constipation, nausea, diarrhea

Genitourinary: Impotence

Hematologic: Thrombocytopenia

Respiratory: Bronchospasm

Miscellaneous: Cold extremities

Overdosage Symptoms of overdose include bradycardia, congestive heart failure, hypotension, bronchospasm, hypoglycemia (see Toxicology)

Toxicology Sympathomimetics (eg, epinephrine or dopamine), glucagon or a pacemaker can be used to treat the toxic bradycardia, asystole, and/or hypotension. Initially, fluids may be the best treatment for toxic hypotension. Patients should remain supine; serum glucose and potassium should be measured. Use supportive measures: lavage, syrup of ipecac; I.V. glucose should be administered for hypoglycemia; seizures may be treated with phenytoin or diazepam intravenously; continuous monitoring of blood pressure and EKG is necessary. If PVCs occur, treat with lidocaine or phenytoin; avoid quinidine, procainamide, and disopyramide since these agents further depress myocardial function. Bronchospasm can be treated with theophylline on beta$_2$ agonists (epinephrine).

Drug Interactions

Phenobarbital, rifampin may decrease beta-blocker bioavailability and may decrease its activity

Cimetidine may reduce beta-blocker clearance and increase its effects

Aluminum-containing antacid may reduce GI absorption of beta-blockers; nonsteroidal anti-inflammatory agents, sulfinpyrazone, flecainide, MAO inhibitors, phenothiazines, aluminum compounds, calcium, cholestyramine, colestipol, haloperidol, H$_2$ blockers, loop diuretics, ciprofloxacin, quinidine, ergot alkaloids, salicylates, sympathomimetics, thyroid hormones, insulins, lidocaine, calcium channel blockers, catecholamine depleting drugs, clonidine, disopyramide, prazosin, theophylline

Mechanism of Action Blocks both beta$_1$- and beta$_2$-receptors and has mild intrinsic sympathomimetic activity; has negative inotropic and chronotropic effects and can significantly slow A-V nodal conduction; low lipid solubility will decrease CNS side effects

Pharmacodynamics Ophthalmic: 22% to 25% reduction of IOP given twice daily

Onset: Not known

Maximum effect: Not described

Duration: 12 hours

Pharmacokinetics

Absorption: Well absorbed, 80%

Protein binding: 25% to 30%

Bioavailability: Oral: 85%

Half-life: 6 hours

Elimination: 50% to 70% excreted unchanged in urine

Usual Dosage Geriatrics and Adults:

Oral: 2.5 mg as a single daily dose, with a maintenance dose normally 2.5-5 mg once daily; maximum daily dose: 10 mg; doses >10 mg do not increase response and may in fact decrease effect

Ophthalmic: Instill 1 drop in affected eye(s) twice daily (see Additional Information)

Dosing interval in renal impairment:

Cl$_{cr}$ >60 mL/minute/1.73 m^2: Administer every 24 hours

Cl$_{cr}$ 20-60 mL/minute/1.73 m^2: Administer every 48 hours

Cl$_{cr}$ <20 mL/minute/1.73 m^2: Administer every 72 hours

Monitoring Parameters Blood pressure, orthostatic hypotension, heart rate, CNS effects

(Continued)

Carteolol *(Continued)*

Patient Information Do not discontinue medication abruptly, sudden stopping of medication may precipitate or cause angina; consult pharmacist or physician before taking with other adrenergic drugs (eg, cold medications); notify physician if any of the following symptoms occur: difficult breathing, night cough, swelling of extremities, slow pulse, dizziness, lightheadedness, confusion, depression, skin rash, fever, sore throat, unusual bleeding or bruising; may produce drowsiness, dizziness, lightheadedness, blurred vision, confusion; use with caution while driving or performing tasks requiring alertness; may mask signs of hypoglycemia in diabetics; may be taken without regard to meals

Nursing Implications Advise against abrupt withdrawal; monitor orthostatic blood pressures, apical and peripheral pulse and mental status changes (ie, confusion, depression)

Additional Information Since bioavailability increased in elderly about twofold, geriatric patients may require lower maintenance doses, therefore, as serum and tissue concentrations increase beta$_1$ selectivity diminishes; when treating glaucoma/intraocular hypertension, if the desired IOP is not achieved, consider adding concomitant therapy with pilocarpine, dipivefrin, etc

Special Geriatric Considerations Due to alterations in the beta-adrenergic autonomic nervous system, beta-adrenergic blockade may result in less hemodynamic response than seen in younger adults. Studies indicate that despite decreased sensitivity to the chronotropic effects of beta blockade with age, there appears to be an increased myocardial sensitivity to the negative inotropic effect during stress (ie, exercise). Controlled trials have shown the overall response rate for propranolol to be only 20% to 50% in elderly populations. Therefore, all beta-adrenergic blocking drugs may result in a decreased response as compared to younger adults; adjust dose for renal function in elderly.

Dosage Forms

Carteolol hydrochloride:
Solution, ophthalmic (Ocupress®): 1% (5 mL, 10 mL)
Tablet (Cartrol®): 2.5 mg, 5 mg

Carter's Little Pills® [OTC] *see* Bisacodyl *on page 121*
Cartrol® Oral *see* Carteolol *on page 166*

Carvedilol *(KAR ve dil ole)*

Related Information

Beta-Blockers Comparison *on page 1026*

Brand Names Coreg®

Therapeutic Category Alpha-/Beta- Adrenergic Blocker

Use Management of hypertension; can be used alone or in combination with other antihypertensive agents; mild or moderate NYHA class II or III heart failure of ischemic or cardiomyopathic origin (in conjunction with digoxin, diuretics, and ACE inhibitors)

Unlabeled use: Angina pectoris; idiopathic cardiomyopathy

Contraindications Uncompensated congestive heart failure (NYHA class IV), cardiogenic shock, bradycardia or heart block, asthma, COPD; hypersensitivity to carvedilol or to any component

Warnings Acute withdrawal may exacerbate symptoms; use with caution in patients undergoing anesthesia with agents that depress myocardial function (eg, trichloroethylene, cyclopropane). Use with caution in bronchospastic disease, those with hyperthyroidism may have symptomatic signs masked due to beta-blockade, impaired hepatic function, or diabetes mellitus. Abrupt withdrawal of the drug should be avoided, drug should be discontinued over 1-2 weeks; may potentiate hypoglycemia in a diabetic patient and mask signs and symptoms; sweating will continue; patients with peripheral vascular disease may have symptoms aggravated by carvedilol. Worsening cardiac failure or fluid retention may occur during up-titration of carvedilol (in that case, increase diuretics and do not increase dose of carvedilol until stable).

Precautions Since carvedilol exhibits beta-blocking activity, bradycardia may occur; dose should be reduced if heart rate is <55 beats/minute; postural hypotension may be encountered upon initiation of therapy or following dose increases; avoid abrupt discontinuation, especially in patients with ischemic heart disease. Discontinue over a 1- to 2-week period; use with caution in patients with a history of anaphylactic reactions to allergens since the use of beta-blockers may block effective treatment with epinephrine. Use of beta-blockers is generally contraindicated in patients with reactive airway disease. Use with caution in patients who require beta-blockade for concomitant disease; liver dysfunction may be precipitated by carvedilol. Monitor for subjective signs and symptoms (jaundice, dark urine, pruritus, etc).

Adverse Reactions

Cardiovascular: Bradycardia, bundle branch block, congestive heart failure, arrhythmia, A-V block, extrasystoles, hypertension, reduced peripheral circulation, hypotension, dependent edema, peripheral edema, palpitations, angina, atrial fibrillation, myocardial infarction, chest pain, syncope

Central nervous system: Anxiety, dizziness, insomnia, somnolence, hallucinations, nightmares, vivid dreams, ataxia, amnesia, paresis, vertigo, migraine, depression, fatigue, nervousness

Dermatologic: Skin rash, itching, alopecia

Endocrine & metabolic: Decreased libido, hyperkalemia, hypokalemia, hot flashes

Gastrointestinal: Diarrhea, abdominal pain, nausea, stomach discomfort, constipation, flatulence, xerostomia, vomiting

Genitourinary: Impotence, increased polyuria

Hematologic: Thrombocytopenia, anemia, eosinophilia, leukopenia

Hepatic: Bilirubinemia, hypertriglyceridemia, increased LFTs, increased alkaline phosphatase, increased BUN, decreased HDL

Neuromuscular & skeletal: Back pain, arthralgia, weakness, numbness of extremities, neuralgia, leg cramps, myalgia

Ocular: Dry eyes, abnormal vision

Otic: Tinnitus, decreased hearing

Renal: Hematuria, albuminuria

Respiratory: Dyspnea, rhinitis, dyspnea, asthma, bronchospasms, respiratory alkalosis, cough

Miscellaneous: Diaphoresis

Overdosage Symptoms include hypotension, bradycardia, cardiac insufficiency, cardiogenic shock, cardiac arrest, bronchospasm, vomiting, delirium, and generalized seizure

Toxicology Gastric lavage or induced emesis if short time has elapsed since ingestion; where possible, observe in intensive care; administer general supportive care; bradycardia may be treated with atropine 2 mg I.V.; to support cardiovascular function, glucagon 5-10 mg I.V. followed by continuous infusion at 5 mg/hour; sympathomimetics for pressor effect; bronchospasm is treated with beta-sympathomimetics as aerosol or I.V. infusion. Aminophylline I.V. may be effective for bronchospasm; for seizures, I.V. diazepam or clonazepam is recommended; treatment for toxicity may require a long period due to carvedilol's long half-life.

Drug Interactions Carvedilol with antidiabetic agent may **enhance** hypoglycemia; carvedilol with calcium channel blockers **increases** conduction disturbances; carvedilol with clonidine **increases** blood pressure and heart rate lowering effects; carvedilol **increases** digoxin concentrations (15%); rifampin **decreases** serum concentrations of carvedilol (70%); cimetidine increases carvedilol AUC by 30%

Mechanism of Action Carvedilol blocks alpha, beta$_1$, and beta$_2$-adrenergic receptors; carvedilol exhibits no intrinsic sympathomimetic activity; its pharmacologic actions result in reduced cardiac output, reduced exercise-induced tachycardia, and reduced reflex orthostatic tachycardia. Carvedilol reduces plasma renin and increases atrial natriuretic peptide.

Pharmacodynamics

Onset of action: Within 1 hour of oral administration and blood pressure lowering effect is seen within 30 minutes of ingestion

Pharmacokinetics

Absorption: Rapidly and extensively absorbed

Protein binding: >98% bound to plasma proteins, mostly albumin

Metabolism: Significant first-pass metabolism in liver; three active metabolites are generated with beta-blockade activity. These metabolites, however, have weak antihypertensive action. Substrate CYP2D6.

Bioavailability: 25% to 35%

Half-life: 7-10 hours; elderly have serum concentrations 50% higher than young adults

Usual Dosage Geriatrics and Adults: Oral:

Hypertension: 6.25 mg twice daily, if tolerated, should be maintained for 1-2 weeks, then increased to 12.5 mg twice daily; dosage may be increased to a maximum of 25 mg twice daily; if pulse rate drops below 55 beats/minute, the dosage should be reduced; total daily dose should not exceed 50 mg (see Additional Information and Special Geriatric Considerations)

(Continued)

Carvedilol *(Continued)*

Congestive heart failure: 3.125 mg twice daily for 2 weeks; if this dose is tolerated, may increase to 6.25 mg twice daily. Double the dose every 2 weeks to the highest dose tolerated by patient.

Maximum recommended dose:
  <85 kg: 25 mg twice daily
  >85 kg: 50 mg twice daily

Administration Should be taken with food to slow the rate of absorption which will reduce the possibility of orthostatic hypotension

Monitoring Parameters Monitor blood pressure standing and sitting/supine, pulse, mental status; if used in diabetic patients, monitor fasting blood glucose closely; if used in patients with COPD, monitor respiratory rate and function; monitor for signs and symptoms of liver dysfunction

Patient Information Should be taken with food to minimize the risk of hypotension; do not stop or interrupt use without a physician's advice; if dizziness and fainting occur, contact physician; avoid driving or hazardous work if experiencing dizziness or fainting; patients with contact lenses may experience decreased lacrimation

Nursing Implications At initiation of each new dose, observe patient for signs of dizziness or lightheadedness for at least 1 hour (see Monitoring Parameters, Usual Dosage, and Administration)

Additional Information Carvedilol should not be given to patients with severe hepatic failure; addition of a diuretic or adding carvedilol to diuretic therapy can result in exaggerated hypotension. Monitor closely upon initiation. Some studies have demonstrated a reduced risk of death, hospitalization in patients with CHF treated with digoxin, diuretics, and ACEI therapy.

Special Geriatric Considerations Due to alterations in the beta-adrenergic autonomic nervous system, beta-adrenergic blockade may result in less hemodynamic response than seen in younger adults. Studies indicate that despite decreased sensitivity to the chronotropic effects of beta blockade with age, there appears to be an increased myocardial sensitivity to the negative inotropic effect during stress (ie, exercise). Carvedilol serum concentrations are 50% higher in elderly than in young adults; however, no dose changes are recommended for elderly. The authors would suggest that doses of 6.25 mg/day for hypertension or 3.125 mg/day for congestive heart failure be initiated for elderly who may be at risk for orthostatic hypotension (volume depleted, receives diuretics or other antihypertensives). If tolerated, then dose increases can continue at 1- to 2-week intervals.

Dosage Forms Tablet: 3.125 mg, 6.25 mg, 12.5 mg, 25 mg

References
Packer M, Bristow MR, Cohn JN, et al, "The Effect of Carvedilol on Morbidity and Mortality in Patients With Chronic Heart Failure," *N Engl J Med*, 1996, 334(21):1349-55.

Casanthranol and Docusate *see* Docusate and Casanthranol *on page 313*

Cascara Sagrada (kas KAR a sah GRAH dah)

Generic Available Yes

Therapeutic Category Laxative, Stimulant

Use Temporary relief of constipation; sometimes used with milk of magnesia ("black and white" mixture)

Contraindications Nausea, vomiting, abdominal pain, fecal impaction, intestinal obstruction, GI bleeding, appendicitis, congestive heart failure; hypersensitivity to cascara sagrada or any component

Warnings Laxatives used excessively may lead to fluid/electrolyte imbalance; stimulant cathartics may lead to abuse or dependency with chronic use (laxative abuse syndrome); cathartic colon, which may present as ulcerative colitis, occurs with chronic use of stimulant cathartics; melanosis coli is a dark pigmentation of the colonic mucosa from chronic use of anthraquinone derivatives

Precautions Habit-forming and may result in laxative dependence and loss of normal bowel function with prolonged use; rectal bleeding or failure to respond requires further evaluation for possibly serious medical problems

Adverse Reactions

Central nervous system: Faintness

Endocrine & metabolic: Electrolyte and fluid imbalance

Genitourinary: Urine discoloration (reddish pink or brown)

Gastrointestinal: Abdominal cramps, nausea, diarrhea, bloating, flatulence

Miscellaneous: Diaphoresis, perianal irritation

Overdosage Symptoms of overdose include hypokalemia, hypocalcemia, metabolic acidosis or alkalosis, abdominal pain, diarrhea, malabsorption, weight loss and protein-losing enteropathy

Stability Protect from light and heat

Mechanism of Action Direct chemical irritation of the intestinal mucosa resulting in an increased rate of colonic motility; stimulation of the myenteric plexus and change in fluid and electrolyte secretion of the gastrointestinal mucosa

Pharmacodynamics Onset of action: 6-10 hours

Pharmacokinetics
  Absorption: Oral: Small amount from small intestine
  Metabolism: In the liver

Usual Dosage Geriatrics and Adults: Oral:
  Aromatic fluid extract: 5 mL/day (range 2-6 mL) as needed at bedtime
  Tablet: 1 tablet (325 mg) at bedtime as needed; avoid chronic use
  Black and white cocktail (M.O.M./cascara): 5 mL cascara sagrada fluid extract with 25 mL milk of magnesia (total 30 mL) at bedtime as needed

Monitoring Parameters Monitor stools per day, consistency, occult or gross blood; also with chronic use, monitor serum electrolytes; monitor for dehydration and hypotension

Test Interactions Decreased calcium (S), decreased potassium (S)

Patient Information Should not be used regularly for more than 1 week; may discolor urine or feces (yellow-brown); do not use in presence of nausea, vomiting, or abdominal pain; stimulant laxative use should be limited; notify physician if unrelieved by laxative, rectal bleeding occurs, or signs of electrolyte imbalance develop (dizziness, weakness, muscle cramps); take with a full glass of water

Nursing Implications See Warnings, Precautions, Monitoring Parameters, Additional Information, and Special Geriatric Considerations

Additional Information Cascara sagrada fluid extract is five times more potent than cascara sagrada aromatic fluid extract and contains 18% alcohol

Special Geriatric Considerations Elderly are often predisposed to constipation due to disease, immobility, drugs, low residue diets, and a decreased fluid intake usually due to a decreased "thirst reflex" with age. Avoid stimulant cathartic use on a chronic basis if possible. Use osmotic, lubricant, stool softeners, and bulk agents as prophylaxis. Patients should be instructed for proper dietary fiber and fluid intake as well as regular exercise. Monitor closely for fluid/electrolyte imbalance, CNS signs of fluid/electrolyte loss, and hypotension.

Dosage Forms
  Aromatic fluid extract: 120 mL, 473 mL (contains 18% alcohol)
  Tablet: 325 mg

Casodex® *see Bicalutamide on page 118*

Castor Oil (KAS tor oyl)

Brand Names Alphamul® [OTC]; Emulsoil® [OTC]; Fleet® Flavored Castor Oil [OTC]; Neoloid® [OTC]; Purge® [OTC]

Synonyms Oleum Ricini

Generic Available Yes

Therapeutic Category Laxative, Stimulant

Use Preparation for rectal or bowel examination or surgery; occasionally used to relieve constipation; also applied to skin as emollient and protectant

Contraindications Known hypersensitivity to castor oil; nausea, vomiting, abdominal pain, fecal impaction, GI bleeding, appendicitis, congestive heart failure, dehydration

Warnings Castor oil induces a strong purgative action and therefore should not be used for routine treatment of constipation

Precautions Use only when a prompt and thorough catharsis is desired

Adverse Reactions
  Cardiovascular: Hypotension
  Central nervous system: Dizziness
  Endocrine & metabolic: Electrolyte disturbance
  Gastrointestinal: Abdominal cramps, nausea, diarrhea

Overdosage Symptoms of overdose include diarrhea, abdominal cramps, nausea, vomiting, hypotension, dizziness

Stability Protect from heat (castor oil emulsion should be protected from freezing)

Mechanism of Action Acts primarily in the small intestine; hydrolyzed to ricinoleic acid which stimulates secretory processes, decreases glucose
(Continued)

Castor Oil (Continued)

absorption, therefore, reduces net absorption of fluid and electrolytes and stimulates peristalsis

Pharmacodynamics Onset of action: Oral: 2-6 hours after dose

Usual Dosage
Geriatrics and Adults: 15-60 mL as a single dose
Adults: Emulsified castor oil: 30-60 mL/dose

Monitoring Parameters Monitor number of stools per day; consistency, fluid status, and blood pressure if fluid loss is excessive

Patient Information Laxative use should be short-term (< 7 days); discontinue use when bowel regularity returns; notify physician if constipation is unrelieved, blood appears in stool, or if dizziness, muscle weakness, or cramping is experienced; take with full glass of water or juice; maintain adequate fluid intake

Nursing Implications Do not administer at bedtime because of rapid onset of action (see Monitoring Parameters)

Additional Information Chill or give with juice or carbonated beverage to improve palatability

Special Geriatric Considerations Elderly are often predisposed to constipation due to disease, immobility, drugs, low residue diets, and a decreased fluid intake usually due to a decreased "thirst reflex" with age. Avoid stimulant cathartic use on a chronic basis if possible. Use osmotic, lubricant, stool softeners, and bulk agents as prophylaxis. Patients should be instructed for proper dietary fiber and fluid intake as well as regular exercise. Monitor closely for fluid/electrolyte imbalance, CNS signs of fluid/electrolyte loss, and hypotension. Strong and chronic purging may cause severe fluid and electrolyte loss which may affect mental function (CNS) (see Warnings); not a drug of first choice for constipation in elderly

Dosage Forms
Emulsion, castor oil: 36.4%, 60%, 67%, 95%
Liquid, castor oil: 95%, 100%

Cataflam® Oral see Diclofenac on page 281

Catapres® Oral see Clonidine on page 238

Catapres-TTS® Transdermal see Clonidine on page 238

Caverject® Injection see Alprostadil on page 38

C-Crystals® [OTC] see Ascorbic Acid on page 82

Cebid® Timecelles® [OTC] see Ascorbic Acid on page 82

Cecon® [OTC] see Ascorbic Acid on page 82

Cedax® see Ceftibuten on page 190

Cefaclor (SEF a klor)

Related Information
Cephalosporins, Aminoglycosides, Macrolides, & Quinolones on page 1014

Brand Names Ceclor®; Ceclor® CD

Generic Available No

Therapeutic Category Antibiotic, Cephalosporin (Second Generation)

Use Treatment of otitis media, sinusitis, and infections caused by susceptible organisms involving the respiratory tract, skin and skin structure, bone and joint, and urinary tract and gynecologic as well as septicemia

Contraindications Hypersensitivity to cefaclor or any component or cephalosporins

Warnings Prolonged use may result in superinfection

Precautions Use with caution in patients with impaired renal function and a history of colitis; modify dosage in patients with severe renal impairment; use with caution in patients with penicillin allergy (anaphylactic reactions, pruritic rash)

Adverse Reactions
Dermatologic: Rash, urticaria, pruritus, Stevens-Johnson syndrome
Gastrointestinal: Nausea, vomiting, diarrhea, pseudomembranous colitis
Hematologic: Eosinophilia, hemolytic anemia, neutropenia
Hepatic: Cholestatic jaundice, slight elevation of AST, ALT
Neuromuscular & skeletal: Arthralgia

Overdosage Symptoms of overdose include neuromuscular hypersensitivity, convulsions

Toxicology Many beta-lactam-containing antibiotics have the potential to cause neuromuscular hyperirritability or convulsive seizures. Hemodialysis may be helpful to aid in the removal of the drug from the blood, otherwise most treatment is supportive or symptom directed.

Drug Interactions Probenecid prolongs half-life and decreases clearance

Stability Refrigerate suspension after reconstitution; discard after 14 days

Mechanism of Action Interferes with bacterial cell wall synthesis during active multiplication causing cell death and resultant bactericidal activity against susceptible bacteria

Pharmacokinetics
Absorption: Oral: Acid stable, well absorbed
Half-life: 30-60 minutes (prolonged with renal impairment)
Time to peak serum concentration: Within 30-60 minutes
Elimination: Most of a dose (80%) is excreted unchanged in urine

Usual Dosage Geriatrics and Adults: Oral: 250-500 mg every 8 hours or daily dose can be given in 2 divided doses
Dosing adjustment in renal impairment: Cl_{cr} <50 mL/minute: Administer 50% of dose in 2 divided doses
Moderately dialyzable (20% to 50%)

Monitoring Parameters Signs and symptoms of infections, including mental status

Test Interactions Positive Coombs' [direct], false-positive urine glucose (Clinitest®), false increase in serum or urine creatinine

Patient Information Complete full course of therapy; may take with food or milk

Nursing Implications Monitor patient for rash and pruritus which are common adverse effects; monitor for resolution of infection

Special Geriatric Considerations Has not been studied in the elderly (see Usual Dosage); adjust dose for renal function in elderly; considered one of the drugs of choice in the outpatient treatment of community-acquired pneumonia in older adults

Dosage Forms
Capsule: 250 mg, 500 mg
Powder for oral suspension (strawberry flavor): 125 mg/5 mL (75 mL, 150 mL); 187 mg/5 mL (50 mL, 100 mL); 250 mg/5 mL (75 mL, 150 mL); 375 mg/5 mL (50 mL, 100 mL)
Tablet, extended release: 375 mg, 500 mg

References
American Thoracic Society, "Guidelines for the Initial Management of Adults With Community-Acquired Pneumonia: Diagnosis, Assessment of Severity, and Initial Antimicrobial Therapy," *Am Rev Respir Dis*, 1993, 148(5):1418-26.

Cefadroxil (sef a DROKS il)
Related Information
Cephalosporins, Aminoglycosides, Macrolides, & Quinolones *on page 1014*
Prevention of Bacterial Endocarditis *on page 1062*
Brand Names Duricef®; Ultracef®
Generic Available No
Therapeutic Category Antibiotic, Cephalosporin (First Generation)
Use Treatment of susceptible bacterial infections, including those caused by group A beta-hemolytic *Streptococcus*
Contraindications Hypersensitivity to cefadroxil and/or cephalosporins
Precautions Use with caution in patients allergic to penicillin; reduce dose for decreased renal function; prolonged use may result in superinfection
Adverse Reactions
Dermatologic: Maculopapular and erythematous rash
Gastrointestinal: Dyspepsia, diarrhea, pseudomembranous colitis, nausea, vomiting
Hematologic: Neutropenia
Miscellaneous: Superinfection
Overdosage Symptoms of overdose include neuromuscular hypersensitivity, convulsions
Drug Interactions Increased serum concentrations with probenecid
Stability Refrigerate suspension after reconstitution; discard after 14 days
Mechanism of Action Interferes with bacterial cell wall synthesis during active multiplication causing cell death and resultant bactericidal activity against susceptible bacteria
Pharmacokinetics
Absorption: Oral: Rapidly and well absorbed from GI tract
(Continued)

173

Cefadroxil *(Continued)*

Distribution: V_d: 0.31 L/kg
Protein binding: 20%
Half-life: 1-2 hours; in renal failure, the half-life increases to 20-24 hours
Time to peak serum concentration: Within 70-90 minutes
Elimination: >90% of dose excreted unchanged in urine within 8 hours
Effects of aging on the pharmacokinetics of cefadroxil are not well studied; only older patients with impaired renal function have been studied

Usual Dosage Oral:
Geriatrics: Usual adult dosage with adjustments for patients with renal impairment
Adults: 1-2 g/day in 2 divided doses

Dosing interval (for 500 mg dose) in renal impairment (following an initial 1 g dose):
Cl_{cr} >50 mL/minute: No adjustment necessary
Cl_{cr} 25-50 mL/minute: Administer every 12 hours
Cl_{cr} 10-25 mL/minute: Administer every 24 hours
Cl_{cr} 0-10 mL/minute: Administer every 36 hours

Monitoring Parameters Signs and symptoms of infection, including mental status

Test Interactions Positive Coombs' [direct], glucose, protein; decreased glucose

Patient Information Complete full course of therapy; can be taken with food or milk; report persistent diarrhea to physician

Nursing Implications Administer around-the-clock to promote less variation in peak and trough serum concentrations

Special Geriatric Considerations Adjust dose for renal function in elderly (see Pharmacokinetics and Usual Dosage)

Dosage Forms
Cefadroxil monohydrate:
Capsule: 500 mg
Suspension, oral: 125 mg/5 mL, 250 mg/5 mL, 500 mg/5 mL (50 mL, 100 mL)
Tablet: 1 g

References
Cutler RE, Blair AD, and Kelly MR, "Cefadroxil Kinetics in Patients With Renal Insufficiency," *Clin Pharmacol Ther*, 1979, 25(5 Pt 1):514-21.

Cefadyl® *see Cephapirin on page 197*

Cefamandole *(sef a MAN dole)*

Related Information
Cephalosporins, Aminoglycosides, Macrolides, & Quinolones *on page 1014*
I.V. Medication Recommendations *on page 1080*

Brand Names Mandol®

Generic Available No

Therapeutic Category Antibiotic, Cephalosporin (Second Generation)

Use Treatment of susceptible bacterial infection; mainly respiratory tract, skin and skin structure, bone and joint, urinary tract and gynecologic as well as septicemia

Contraindications Hypersensitivity to cefamandole nafate or any component and cephalosporins

Precautions Use with caution in patients allergic to penicillins; reduce dose for decreased renal function; increased tendency for bleeding

Adverse Reactions
Central nervous system: CNS irritation, seizures, fever
Dermatologic: Rash, urticaria
Gastrointestinal: Diarrhea, abdominal cramps, pseudomembranous colitis
Hematologic: Leukopenia, thrombocytopenia, positive Coombs' test, eosinophilia, hypoprothrombinemia
Hepatic: Transient elevation of liver enzymes, cholestatic jaundice
Local: Pain at injection site
Miscellaneous: Superinfection

Overdosage Symptoms of overdose include neuromuscular hypersensitivity, convulsions

Toxicology Many beta-lactam-containing antibiotics have the potential to cause neuromuscular hyperirritability or convulsive seizures. Hemodialysis may be helpful to aid in the removal of the drug from the blood, otherwise most treatment is supportive or symptom directed.

Drug Interactions

Disulfiram-like reaction has been reported when taken within 72 hours of alcohol consumption

The hypoprothrombinemic effects of anticoagulants and heparin may be increased

Probenecid will increase and prolong cefamandole plasma concentrations

May potentiate aminoglycoside nephrotoxicity

Stability After reconstitution CO_2 gas is liberated which allows solution to be withdrawn without injecting air; solution is stable for 24 hours at room temperature and 96 hours when refrigerated; for I.V. infusion in NS and D_5W is stable for 24 hours at room temperature; 1 week when refrigerated or 26 weeks when frozen

Mechanism of Action Interferes with bacterial cell wall synthesis during active multiplication causing cell death and resultant bactericidal activity against susceptible bacteria

Pharmacokinetics

Distribution: Well throughout the body, except the CSF poor penetration even with inflamed meninges; extensive enterohepatic circulation; high concentrations in the bile

Protein binding: 56% to 78%

Half-life: 30-60 minutes

Time to peak serum concentration:

I.M.: Within 1-2 hours

I.V.: Within 10 minutes

Elimination: Majority of drug excreted unchanged in urine

Cefamandole's pharmacokinetics were not altered in older men with "normal" renal function (S_{cr} ≤1.5 mg/dL)

Usual Dosage I.M., I.V.:

Geriatrics: Usual adult dose with adjustments for renal impairment when appropriate

Adults: 4-12 g/24 hours divided every 4-6 hours

Dosing interval in renal impairment:

Cl_{cr} 50-80 mL/minute: 1-2 g every 6 hours

Cl_{cr} 25-50 mL/minute: 1-2 g every 8 hours

Cl_{cr} 10-25 mL/minute: 1 g every 8 hours

Cl_{cr} 2-10 mL/minute: 1 g every 12 hours

Cl_{cr} <2 mL/minute: 0.5-0.75 g every 12 hours

Moderately dialyzable (20% to 50%)

Monitoring Parameters Signs and symptoms of infection, including mental status

Test Interactions Increased alkaline phosphatase, AST, ALT, BUN, creatinine, prothrombin time, glucose, protein; decreased glucose; positive Coombs' [direct]

Patient Information Avoid alcoholic beverages; report signs of bleeding, bruising, or superinfection

Nursing Implications Watch for signs of bruising or bleeding

Additional Information Sodium content of 1 g: 3.3 mEq

Special Geriatric Considerations The risk of coagulation abnormalities (increased PT) limits the use of cefamandole in the elderly; adjust dose for renal function in elderly (see Pharmacokinetics and Usual Dosage)

Dosage Forms Injection, as nafate: 500 mg, 1 g, 2 g, 10 g

References

Mellin HE, Welling PG, and Madsen PO, "Pharmacokinetics of Cefamandole in Patients With Normal and Impaired Renal Function," *Antimicrob Agents Chemother*, 1977, 11:262-6.

Cefazolin (sef A zoe lin)

Related Information

Cephalosporins, Aminoglycosides, Macrolides, & Quinolones *on page 1014*

I.V. Medication Recommendations *on page 1080*

Prevention of Bacterial Endocarditis *on page 1062*

Brand Names Ancef®; Kefzol®; Zolicef®

Generic Available Yes

Therapeutic Category Antibiotic, Cephalosporin (First Generation)

Use Treatment of gram-positive bacilli and cocci (except enterococcus); some gram-negative bacilli including *E. coli*, *Proteus*, and *Klebsiella* may be susceptible

Contraindications Hypersensitivity to cefazolin sodium or any component, cephalosporins

(Continued)

Cefazolin *(Continued)*

Precautions Modify dosage in patients with renal impairment; use with caution in patients with penicillin allergy

Adverse Reactions

Central nervous system: CNS irritation, seizures, confusion, fever

Dermatologic: Rash, urticaria

Gastrointestinal: Diarrhea

Hematologic: Leukopenia, thrombocytopenia, neutropenia

Hepatic: Transient elevation of liver enzymes, cholestatic jaundice

Overdosage Symptoms of overdose include neuromuscular hypersensitivity, convulsions

Toxicology Many beta-lactam-containing antibiotics have the potential to cause neuromuscular hyperirritability or convulsive seizures. Hemodialysis may be helpful to aid in the removal of the drug from the blood, otherwise most treatment is supportive or symptom directed.

Drug Interactions

Furosemide may be a possible additive to nephrotoxicity

Probenecid may decrease cephalosporin elimination

May potentiate aminoglycoside-induced nephrotoxicity

Stability Reconstituted solution is stable for 24 hours at room temperature and 96 hours when refrigerated; for I.V. infusion in NS or D_5W solution is stable for 24 hours at room temperature, 96 hours when refrigerated or 12 weeks when frozen; after freezing, thawed solution is stable for 48 hours at room temperature or 10 days when refrigerated

Mechanism of Action Interferes with bacterial cell wall synthesis during active multiplication causing cell death and resultant bactericidal activity against susceptible bacteria

Pharmacokinetics

Distribution: V_d: No change

Protein binding: 74% to 86%

Metabolism: Hepatic metabolism is minimal

Half-life: 90-150 minutes (prolonged with renal impairment); mean half-life was twice as long, 3.5 hours, and mean total clearance was reduced by 50% in older adults compared to younger adults

CSF penetration is poor

Time to peak serum concentration:

I.M.: Within 30 minutes to 2 hours

I.V.: Within 5 minutes

Elimination: 80% to 100% excreted unchanged in urine

Usual Dosage I.M., I.V.:

Geriatrics: Usual adult dose with adjustments for renal function when appropriate

Adults: 1-2 g every 8 hours

Dosing interval in renal impairment:

Cefazolin Sodium

Cl_{cr} (mL/min)	Dose (mg) for Each Dosing Interval
≥55	250-1000 q8h
35-54	250-1000 q12h
11-34	125-500 q12h
≤10	125-500 q24h

Moderately dialyzable (20% to 50%)

Monitoring Parameters Signs and symptoms of infection; WBC, mental status

Test Interactions False-positive urine glucose using Clinitest®, positive Coombs' [direct], false increase in serum or urine creatinine

Nursing Implications Administer around-the-clock rather than 3 times/day (ie, 8-4-12) to promote less variation in peak and trough serum concentrations; dosage modification required in renal insufficiency

Additional Information Sodium content of 1 g: 47 mg (2 mEq)

Special Geriatric Considerations Adjust dose for renal function (see Pharmacokinetics and Usual Dosage)

Dosage Forms

Cefazolin sodium:

Infusion, premixed, in D_5W (frozen) (Ancef®): 500 mg (50 mL); 1 g (50 mL)

Injection (Kefzol®): 500 mg, 1 g

Powder for injection (Ancef®, Zolicef®): 250 mg, 500 mg, 1 g, 5 g, 10 g, 20 g

References
Simon VC, Malerczyk V, Tenschert B, et al, "Die Geriatrische Pharmakologie von Cefazolin, Cefradin, und Sulfisomidin," *Arzneim Forsch*, 1976, 26(7):1377-82.

Cefepime (SEF e pim)

Related Information
Cephalosporins, Aminoglycosides, Macrolides, & Quinolones *on page 1014*
I.V. Medication Recommendations *on page 1080*

Brand Names Maxipime®

Therapeutic Category Antibiotic, Cephalosporin (Fourth Generation)

Use Treatment of respiratory tract infections (including bronchitis and pneumonia), cellulitis and other skin and soft tissue infections, and urinary tract infections; considered a fourth generation cephalosporin because it has gram-negative coverage similar to ceftazidime and gram-positive coverage similar to cefotaxime

Contraindications Hypersensitivity to cefepime or its components, or other cephalosporins

Precautions Modify dosage in patients with severe renal impairment; prolonged use may result in superinfection; a low incidence of cross-hypersensitivity to penicillins exists

Adverse Reactions
Central nervous system: Headache, lightheadedness
Dermatologic: Rash
Gastrointestinal: Dyspepsia, antibiotic-associated diarrhea, nausea
Hepatic: Transient elevations in LFTs
Local: Phlebitis
Ocular: Blurred vision

Overdosage Symptoms of overdose include neuromuscular hypersensitivity, convulsions

Toxicology Hemodialysis may be helpful to aid in the removal of the drug from the blood; however, most often treatment is supportive and symptom directed

Drug Interactions
Increased effect: High-dose probenecid decreases clearance
Increased toxicity: Aminoglycosides increase nephrotoxic potential

Mechanism of Action Inhibits bacterial cell wall synthesis by binding to one or more of the penicillin-binding proteins (PBPs) which in turn inhibits the final transpeptidation step of peptidoglycan synthesis in bacterial cell walls, thus inhibiting cell wall biosynthesis. Bacterial eventually lyse due to ongoing activity of cell wall autolytic enzymes (autolysis and murein hydrolases) while cell wall assembly is arrested. Cefepime has greater resistance to beta-lactamases than other cephalosporins.

Pharmacokinetics Note: A longer half-life (mean 3 hours) and reduced renal and total clearances have been reported in the elderly compared to younger subjects
Absorption: I.M.: Rapid and complete; T_{max}: 0.5-1.5 hours
Distribution: V_d: Adults: 14-20 L; penetrates into inflammatory fluid at concentrations ~80% of serum concentrations and into bronchial mucosa at concentrations ~60% of those reached in the plasma
Protein binding, plasma: 16% to 19%
Metabolism: ≤15% hydrolyzed to inactive metabolites
Half-life: 2 hours
Elimination: ≥85% as unchanged drug in urine

Usual Dosage Geriatrics: I.M., I.V.: Should be based on renal function and severity of infection

Dosing adjustment in renal impairment: See table.

Cefepime

Cl_{cr} (mL/min)	Infection		
	Mild to Moderate	**Moderate to Severe**	**Severe***
>60	0.5-1 g q12h	1-2 g q12h	2 g q12h
30-60	0.5-1 g q24h	1-2 g q24h	2 g q24h
11-29	0.5 g q24h	0.5-1 g q24h	1 g q24h
≤10	0.25 g q24h	0.25-0.5 g q24h	0.5 g q24h

*Severe infections should only be treated with I.V. infusion.

(Continued)

Cefepime *(Continued)*

Hemodialysis effects: Removed by dialysis; administer supplemental dose of 250 mg after each dialysis session

Peritoneal dialysis effects: Removed to a lesser extent than hemodialysis; administer 1-2 g every 48 hours

Monitoring Parameters Obtain specimen for culture and sensitivity prior to the first dose; signs and symptoms of infection; mental status

Test Interactions As with other cephalosporins; false-positive Coombs' test; may falsely elevate creatinine values when Jaffé reaction is used; may cause false-positive results in urine glucose tests when using cupric sulfate (Benedict's solution, Clinitest®), false-positive urinary proteins and steroids

Patient Information Report side effects such as diarrhea, dyspepsia, headache, blurred vision, and lightheadedness to your physician

Nursing Implications Do not admix with aminoglycosides in the same bottle/bag; observe for signs and symptoms of bacterial infection, including defervescence; observe for anaphylaxis during first dose

Special Geriatric Considerations See Pharmacokinetics and Usual Dosage

Dosage Forms
Cefepime hydrochloride:
Infusion: 1.2 g
Infusion (Addvantage®): 1 g
Injection: 1 g, 2 g

References
Barbhaiya RH, Knupp CA, and Pittman KA, "Effects of Age and Gender on Pharmacokinetics of Cefepime," *J Antimicrob Chemother*, 1992, 36(6):1181-5.
Wynd MA and Paladino JA, "Cefepime: A Fourth-Generation Parenteral Cephalosporin," *Ann Pharmacother*, 1997, 30(12):1414-24.

Cefixime (sef IKS eem)

Related Information
Cephalosporins, Aminoglycosides, Macrolides, & Quinolones *on page 1014*

Brand Names Suprax®

Generic Available No

Therapeutic Category Antibiotic, Cephalosporin (Third Generation)

Use Treatment of urinary tract infections, otitis media, respiratory infections due to susceptible organisms; documented poor compliance with other oral antimicrobials; outpatient therapy of serious soft tissue or skeletal infections due to susceptible organisms; single dose for *N. gonorrhoeae*

Contraindications Hypersensitivity to cefixime or cephalosporins

Warnings Prolonged use may result in superinfection

Precautions Modify dosage in patients with renal impairment; use with caution in patients hypersensitive to penicillin, and patients with a history of colitis

Adverse Reactions
Central nervous system: Fever, headache, dizziness, malaise, somnolence
Dermatologic: Skin rash
Gastrointestinal: Nausea, diarrhea, abdominal pain, flatulence, dyspepsia, pseudomembranous colitis
Hematologic: Transient thrombocytopenia, leukopenia, eosinophilia, and decreased hemoglobin and hematocrit
Hepatic: Transient elevation of liver enzymes
Renal: Transient elevation of BUN or creatinine

Overdosage Symptoms of overdose include neuromuscular hypersensitivity, convulsions

Drug Interactions
Probenecid may prolong cefixime's half-life and increase serum concentration
Salicylates may decrease peak serum concentrations and AUC

Stability Reconstituted oral solution may be kept at room temperature without potency loss for 14 days; **do not refrigerate**

Mechanism of Action Interferes with bacterial cell wall synthesis during active multiplication causing cell death and resultant bactericidal activity against susceptible bacteria

Pharmacokinetics
Absorption: Oral: 40% to 50%
Protein binding: 65%
Half-life:
Normal renal function: 3-4 hours
Renal failure: Up to 11.5 hours
Time to peak serum concentration: Within 2-6 hours

Elimination: 50% of absorbed dose is excreted as active drug in urine and 10% in bile

Decreased clearance and prolonged half-life have been reported in older adults

Usual Dosage Oral:

Geriatrics: Usual adult dose with adjustments for renal function when appropriate

Adults: 400 mg/day in 1-2 divided doses

N. gonorrhoeae: Single 400 mg dose followed with doxycycline is recommended

Dosing adjustment in renal impairment:

Cl_{cr} 21-60 mL/minute or renal hemodialysis: Administer 75% of the standard dose

Cl_{cr} ≤20 mL/minute or continuous ambulatory peritoneal dialysis: Administer 50% of the standard dose

10% removed by hemodialysis

Monitoring Parameters With prolonged therapy, monitor renal and hepatic function periodically; signs and symptoms of infection

Test Interactions False-positive reaction for urine glucose using Clinitest®

Patient Information Complete full course of therapy; can be taken with food or milk; report persistent diarrhea

Nursing Implications Modify dosage in patients with renal impairment

Additional Information Otitis media should be treated with the suspension since it results in higher peak blood levels than the tablet

Special Geriatric Considerations Adjust dose for renal impairment (see Pharmacokinetics and Usual Dosage)

Dosage Forms

Suspension, oral: 100 mg/5 mL (50 mL, 100 mL)

Tablet: 200 mg, 400 mg

References

Faulkner RD, Bohaycheck W, Lanc RA, et al, "Pharmacokinetic of Cefixime in Young and Elderly," *J Antimicrob Chemother*, 1988, 21(6):787-94.

Cefizox® *see* Ceftizoxime *on page 190*

Cefmetazole (sef MET a zole)

Related Information

Cephalosporins, Aminoglycosides, Macrolides, & Quinolones *on page 1014*

Brand Names Zefazone®

Generic Available No

Therapeutic Category Antibiotic, Cephalosporin (Second Generation)

Use Second generation cephalosporin with an antibacterial spectrum similar to cefoxitin, useful on many aerobic and anaerobic gram-positive and gram-negative bacteria; prophylaxis for vaginal or abdominal hysterectomy, cesarean section, colorectal surgery, cholecystectomy (high-risk patients)

Contraindications Hypersensitivity to cefmetazole or any component, cephalosporins

Precautions Use with caution in patients with impaired renal or impaired function; patients with a history of gastrointestinal disease (colitis) or penicillin allergy

Adverse Reactions

Cardiovascular: Hypotension, shock

Central nervous system: Fever, headache

Dermatologic: Rash

Endocrine & metabolic: Hot flashes

Gastrointestinal: Diarrhea, nausea, vomiting, epigastric pain, pseudomembranous colitis

Genitourinary: Vaginitis

Hematologic: Bleeding

Local: Pain at injection site, phlebitis

Respiratory: Dyspnea, respiratory distress

Miscellaneous: candidiasis, epistaxis

Overdosage Symptoms of overdose include neuromuscular hypersensitivity, convulsions

Toxicology Many beta-lactam-containing antibiotics have the potential to cause neuromuscular hyperirritability or convulsive seizures. Hemodialysis may be helpful to aid in the removal of the drug from the blood, otherwise most treatment is supportive or symptom directed.

Drug Interactions

Probenecid may prolong cephalosporin half-life

(Continued)

Cefmetazole *(Continued)*

May potentiate aminoglycoside nephrotoxicity

Stability Reconstituted solution and I.V. infusion in NS or D_5W solution are stable for 24 hours at room temperature, 7 days when refrigerated, or 6 weeks when frozen; after freezing, thawed solution is stable for 24 hours at room temperature or 7 days when refrigerated

Mechanism of Action Interferes with bacterial cell wall synthesis during active multiplication causing cell death and resultant bactericidal activity against susceptible bacteria

Pharmacokinetics

Protein binding: 65%
Metabolism: <15%
Half-life: 72 minutes
Elimination: Renal

Usual Dosage Geriatrics and Adults: I.V.:

Infections: 2 g every 6-12 hours for 5-14 days
Prophylaxis: 1-2 g 30-90 minutes before surgery
Dosing interval in renal impairment: See table.

Cefmetazole Sodium

Cl_{cr} (mL/min/1.73 m²)	Dose (g) for Each Dosing Interval
50-90	1-2 q12h
30-49	1-2 q16h
10-29	1-2 q24h
<10	1-2 q48h

Monitoring Parameters Signs and symptoms of infection including mental status and prothrombin times

Test Interactions Positive Coombs' [direct], falsely elevated urinary 17-ketosteroid values

Patient Information Do not drink alcohol for at least 24 hours after receiving dose; report persistent diarrhea; females should report symptoms of vaginitis

Nursing Implications Do not admix with aminoglycosides in same bottle/bag

Additional Information Sodium content of 1 g: 2 mEq

Special Geriatric Considerations Cefmetazole has not been studied in the elderly (see Usual Dosage); adjust dose for renal function

Dosage Forms Powder for injection, as sodium: 1 g, 2 g

References

Donowitz GR and Mandell GL, "Beta-Lactam Antibiotics," *N Engl J Med*, 1988, 318(7):419-26.

Cefobid® *see Cefoperazone on next page*

Cefonicid *(se FON i sid)*

Related Information

Cephalosporins, Aminoglycosides, Macrolides, & Quinolones *on page 1014*
I.V. Medication Recommendations *on page 1080*

Brand Names Monocid®

Generic Available No

Therapeutic Category Antibiotic, Cephalosporin (Second Generation)

Use Treatment of susceptible bacterial infection; mainly respiratory tract, skin and skin structure, bone and joint, urinary tract and gynecologic as well as septicemia; second generation cephalosporin

Contraindications Hypersensitivity to cefonicid sodium or any component and cephalosporins

Precautions Use with caution in patients allergic to penicillin; reduce dose for decreased renal function

Adverse Reactions

Central nervous system: Fever, headache
Dermatologic: Skin rash
Gastrointestinal: Nausea, diarrhea, abdominal pain, pseudomembranous colitis
Hematologic: Increased platelets and eosinophils
Hepatic: Transient elevations in liver enzymes
Local: Pain at injection site
Renal: Transient increase in BUN or creatinine

Overdosage Symptoms of overdose include neuromuscular hypersensitivity, convulsions

Toxicology Many beta-lactam-containing antibiotics have the potential to cause neuromuscular hyperirritability or convulsive seizures. Hemodialysis may be helpful to aid in the removal of the drug from the blood, otherwise most treatment is supportive or symptom directed.

Drug Interactions
Probenecid may prolong half-life and increase serum concentration
May potentiate aminoglycoside nephrotoxicity

Stability Reconstituted solution and I.V. infusion in NS or D_5W solution are stable for 24 hours at room temperature or 72 hours if refrigerated

Mechanism of Action Interferes with bacterial cell wall synthesis during active multiplication causing cell death and resultant bactericidal activity against susceptible bacteria

Usual Dosage Geriatrics and Adults: I.M., I.V.: 1 g every 24 hours
Prophylaxis: Preop: 1 g 1 hour prior to procedure
Dosing interval in renal impairment: See table.

Cefonicid Sodium

Cl_{cr} (mL/min/1.73 m²)	Dose (mg/kg) for each dosing interval
60-79	10-24 q24h
40-59	8-20 q24h
20-39	4-15 q24h
10-19	4-15 q48h
5-9	4-15 q3-5d
<5	3-4 q3-5d

Administration I.M. injection into relatively large muscle and aspirate; dose of 2 g should be divided in half and given into two separate sites

Monitoring Parameters Signs and symptoms of infection including mental status

Test Interactions False-positive urine glucose using Clinitest®, positive Coombs' [direct], false elevation of serum or urine creatinine

Nursing Implications See Administration

Special Geriatric Considerations Adjust dose for renal function (estimated Cl_{cr}) (see Usual Dosage). I.M. administration should be avoided in patients with limited muscle mass.

Dosage Forms Powder for injection, as sodium: 500 mg, 1 g, 10 g

Cefoperazone (sef oh PER a zone)

Related Information
Cephalosporins, Aminoglycosides, Macrolides, & Quinolones *on page 1014*
I.V. Medication Recommendations *on page 1080*

Brand Names Cefobid®

Generic Available No

Therapeutic Category Antibiotic, Cephalosporin (Third Generation)

Use Treatment of susceptible bacterial infection; mainly respiratory tract, skin and skin structure, bone and joint, urinary tract and gynecologic as well as septicemia

Contraindications Hypersensitivity to cefoperazone or any component, cephalosporins

Precautions Use with caution in patients allergic to penicillin, increased tendency for bleeding

Adverse Reactions
Dermatologic: Maculopapular and erythematous rash
Gastrointestinal: Dyspepsia, diarrhea, pseudomembranous colitis, nausea
Hematologic: Increased risk of bleeding
Local: Bleeding (increased PT), pain, and induration at injection site

Overdosage Symptoms of overdose include neuromuscular hypersensitivity, convulsions

Toxicology Many beta-lactam-containing antibiotics have the potential to cause neuromuscular hyperirritability or convulsive seizures. Hemodialysis may be helpful to aid in the removal of the drug from the blood, otherwise most treatment is supportive or symptom directed.

Drug Interactions May have synergy with aminoglycosides and theoretically increase risk of nephrotoxicity; disulfiram-like reactions have been reported when alcohol was ingested within 72 hours after administration
(Continued)

Cefoperazone (Continued)

Stability Reconstituted solution and I.V. infusion in NS or D_5W solution is stable for 24 hours at room temperature, 5 days when refrigerated or 3 weeks when frozen; after freezing, thawed solution is stable for 48 hours at room temperature or 10 days when refrigerated

Mechanism of Action Interferes with bacterial cell wall synthesis during active multiplication causing cell death and resultant bactericidal activity against susceptible bacteria

Pharmacokinetics

Half-life: 2 hours (half-life higher with hepatic disease or biliary obstruction); mean half-life in the elderly has been reported to be as long as 10.5 hours and appears to be affected by both renal dysfunction and nonrenal clearance

Time to peak serum concentration:
I.M.: Within 1-2 hours
I.V.: Within 15-20 minutes

Serum concentrations following I.V. administration are 2-3 times serum concentrations following I.M. administration

Elimination: Primarily via hepatobiliary pathway, 25% is eliminated renally

Usual Dosage Geriatrics and Adults: I.M., I.V.: 2-4 g/day in divided doses every 12 hours (up to 12 g/day)

Dosing adjustment in biliary or hepatic impairment: Reduce dose 50% in patients with advanced cirrhosis; total daily doses >4 g should not be necessary

Monitoring Parameters Signs and symptoms of infection including mental status

Test Interactions Prothrombin time, false-positive urine glucose with cupric sulfate solution (Clinitest®), positive Coombs' [direct]

Patient Information Report bleeding or bruising; avoid alcoholic beverages during and 72 hours after completion of therapy

Nursing Implications Monitor for coagulation abnormalities; may need to reduce dose in hepatic disease or biliary obstruction

Additional Information Sodium content of 1 g: 1.5 mEq

Special Geriatric Considerations See Pharmacokinetics and Usual Dosage

Dosage Forms

Cefoperazone sodium:
Injection, premixed (frozen): 1 g (50 mL); 2 g (50 mL)
Powder for injection: 1 g, 2 g

References

Deeter RG, Weinstein MP, Swanson KA, et al, "Crossover Assessment of Serum Bactericidal Activity and Pharmacokinetics of Five Broad-Spectrum Cephalosporins in the Elderly," *Antimicrob Agents Chemother*, 1990, 34(6):1007-13.

Meyers BR, Mendelson MN, Deeter RG, et al, "Pharmacokinetics of Cefoperazone in Ambulatory Elderly Volunteers Compared With Young Adults," *Antimicrob Agents Chemother*, 1987, 31(6):925-9.

Naber K, Adam D, Schalkhauser K, et al, "Pharmacokinetics of Cefoperazone in Geriatric Patients and Concentrations in Different Tissues of the Urinary Tract," *Excerpta Medica*, 1982, 114.

Cefotan® see Cefotetan on next page

Cefotaxime (sef oh TAKS eem)

Related Information

Cephalosporins, Aminoglycosides, Macrolides, & Quinolones on page 1014

I.V. Medication Recommendations on page 1080

Brand Names Claforan®

Generic Available No

Therapeutic Category Antibiotic, Cephalosporin (Third Generation)

Use Treatment of documented or suspected infections including *N. gonorrhoeae* and meningitis due to susceptible organisms

Contraindications Hypersensitivity to cefotaxime or any component, cephalosporins

Warnings Prolonged use may result in superinfection

Precautions Use with caution in patients with impaired renal function or history of colitis; modify dosage in patients with renal impairment; use with caution in patients with penicillin allergy

Adverse Reactions

Central nervous system: Fever, headache, agitation, confusion
Dermatologic: Rash, pruritus
Gastrointestinal: Pseudomembranous colitis, diarrhea, nausea, vomiting

Hematologic: Transient neutropenia, thrombocytopenia

Hepatic: Transient elevation of liver enzymes

Local: Phlebitis, pain at injection site

Renal: Transient elevations of BUN or creatinine

Overdosage Symptoms of overdose include neuromuscular hypersensitivity, convulsions

Toxicology Many beta-lactam-containing antibiotics have the potential to cause neuromuscular hyperirritability or convulsive seizures. Hemodialysis may be helpful to aid in the removal of the drug from the blood, otherwise most treatment is supportive or symptom directed.

Drug Interactions

Probenecid may prolong cephalosporin half-life

May have synergy with aminoglycosides and theoretically increase risk of nephrotoxicity

Stability Reconstituted solution is stable for 24 hours at room temperature and 10 days when refrigerated; for I.V. infusion in NS or D_5W solution is stable for 24 hours at room temperature, 5 days when refrigerated or 13 weeks when frozen; after freezing, thawed solution is stable for 24 hours at room temperature or 10 days when refrigerated

Mechanism of Action Interferes with bacterial cell wall synthesis during active multiplication by binding to penicillin binding proteins, causing cell death and resultant bactericidal activity against susceptible bacteria

Pharmacokinetics

Protein binding: 31% to 50%

Metabolism: Partially in the liver to active metabolite, desacetylcefotaxime

Half-life:

Cefotaxime: 1-1.5 hours (prolonged with renal and/or hepatic impairment)

Desacetylcefotaxime: 1.5-1.9 hours (prolonged with renal impairment)

Time to peak serum concentration:

I.M.: Within 30 minutes

I.V.: Within ~5 minutes

In patients 60-80 years of age, the serum half-life was prolonged, the clearance decreased, and AUC increased for cefotaxime and less so for its desacetyl metabolite. A significantly greater increase in half-life and decrease in clearance in patients >80 years of age has been reported.

Usual Dosage Geriatrics and Adults: I.M., I.V.:

Uncomplicated gonorrhea: I.M.: Single 1 g dose

Uncomplicated infection: 1 g every 12 hours

Moderate to severe infection: 1-2 g every 6-8 hours

Life-threatening infection: 2 g/dose every 4 hours; maximum dose: 12 g/day

Dosing adjustment in renal impairment: Cl_{cr} <20 mL/minute: Reduce dose 50%

Moderately dialyzable (20% to 50%)

Administration Cefotaxime can be administered IVP over 3-5 minutes, or I.V. retrograde or I.V. intermittent infusion over 15-30 minutes; final concentration for I.V. administration should not exceed 100 mg/mL; I.M. dosing should be in a large muscle mass (ie, gluteus maximus)

Monitoring Parameters Signs and symptoms of infection including mental status

Test Interactions Positive Coombs' [direct]

Nursing Implications See Administration

Special Geriatric Considerations Adjust dose for renal impairment (see Pharmacokinetics and Usual Dosage)

Dosage Forms

Cefotaxime sodium:

Infusion, premixed, in D_5W (frozen): 1 g (50 mL); 2 g (50 mL)

Powder for injection: 500 mg, 1 g, 2 g, 10 g

References

Deeter RG, Weinstein MP, Swanson KA, et al,"Crossover Assessment of Serum Bactericidal Activity and Pharmacokinetics of Five Broad-Spectrum Cephalosporins in the Elderly," *Antimicrob Agents Chemother*, 1990, 34(6):1007-13.

Ludwig E, Székely É, Csiba A, et al,"Pharmacokinetics of Cefotaxime and Desacetylcefotaxime in Elderly Patients," *Drugs*, 1988, 35(Suppl 2):51-6.

Cefotetan (SEF oh tee tan)

Related Information

Cephalosporins, Aminoglycosides, Macrolides, & Quinolones *on page 1014*

I.V. Medication Recommendations *on page 1080*

Brand Names Cefotan®

Generic Available No

(Continued)

Cefotetan *(Continued)*

Therapeutic Category Antibiotic, Cephalosporin (Second Generation)

Use Treatment of susceptible bacterial infection; mainly respiratory tract, skin and skin structure, bone and joint, urinary tract and gynecologic as well as septicemia

Contraindications Hypersensitivity to cefotetan or any component, cephalosporins

Precautions Use with caution in patients with a history of penicillin allergy

Adverse Reactions

Central nervous system: Fever

Dermatologic: Rash, pruritus, urticaria

Gastrointestinal: Diarrhea, nausea, vomiting, pseudomembranous colitis, abdominal pain

Hematologic: Prolongation of bleeding time or prothrombin time, neutropenia, thrombocytopenia, eosinophilia, agranulocytosis, hemolytic anemia

Local: Phlebitis

Miscellaneous: Super infection

Overdosage Symptoms of overdose include neuromuscular hypersensitivity, convulsions

Toxicology Many beta-lactam-containing antibiotics have the potential to cause neuromuscular hyperirritability or convulsive seizures. Hemodialysis may be helpful to aid in the removal of the drug from the blood, otherwise most treatment is supportive or symptom directed.

Drug Interactions

Probenecid may prolong cephalosporin half-life

Alcohol (disulfiram-like reaction)

May have synergy with aminoglycosides and theoretically increase risk of nephrotoxicity

Stability Reconstituted solution is stable for 24 hours at room temperature and 96 hours when refrigerated; for I.V. infusion in NS or D_5W solution and after freezing, thawed solution is stable for 24 hours at room temperature or 96 hours when refrigerated; frozen solution is stable for 12 weeks

Mechanism of Action Interferes with bacterial cell wall synthesis during active multiplication causing cell death and resultant bactericidal activity against susceptible bacteria

Pharmacokinetics

Protein binding: 76% to 90%

Half-life: 3-5 hours

Time to peak plasma concentration: I.M.: Within 1.5-3 hours

Elimination: Primarily excreted unchanged in urine with 20% excreted in bile

Usual Dosage I.M., I.V.:

Geriatrics: Usual adult dose adjusted for renal function

Adults: 1-6 g/day in divided doses every 12 hours, 1-2 g may be given every 24 hours for urinary tract infection

Dosing interval in renal impairment:

Cl_{cr} 10-30 mL/minute: Administer every 24 hours

Cl_{cr} <10 mL/minute: Administer every 48 hours

Slightly dialyzable (5% to 20%)

Administration I.M. doses should be given in a large muscle mass (ie, gluteus maximus)

Monitoring Parameters Signs and symptoms of infection including mental status

Test Interactions Increased alkaline phosphatase, AST, ALT, BUN, creatinine, glucose, protein; decreased glucose; positive Coombs' test

Patient Information Avoid alcoholic beverages during and for 72 hours after completion of therapy

Nursing Implications Administer around-the-clock to promote less variation in peak and trough serum concentrations; reduce dose in patients with impaired renal function (see Administration)

Additional Information Sodium content of 1 g: 3.5 mEq

Special Geriatric Considerations Cefotetan has not been studied in the elderly (see Usual Dosage); adjust dose for renal function in elderly

Dosage Forms Powder for injection, as disodium: 1 g (10 mL, 100 mL); 2 g (20 mL, 100 mL); 10 g (100 mL)

Cefoxitin *(se FOKS i tin)*

Related Information

Cephalosporins, Aminoglycosides, Macrolides, & Quinolones *on page 1014*

I.V. Medication Recommendations *on page 1080*

Brand Names Mefoxin®

Generic Available No

Therapeutic Category Antibiotic, Cephalosporin (Second Generation)

Use Less active against staphylococci and streptococci than first generation cephalosporins, but active against anaerobes including *Bacteroides fragilis*; active against gram-negative enteric bacilli including *E. coli*, *Klebsiella*, and *Proteus*

Contraindications Hypersensitivity to cefoxitin or any component, cephalosporins

Warnings Prolonged use may result in superinfection

Precautions Use with caution in patients with history of colitis; cefoxitin may increase resistance of organisms by inducing beta-lactamase; use with caution and modify dosage in patients with renal impairment; use with caution in patients with a history of penicillin allergy

Adverse Reactions
Central nervous system: Fever
Dermatologic: Rash, exfoliative dermatitis
Gastrointestinal: Nausea, vomiting, pseudomembranous colitis, diarrhea
Hematologic: Transient leukopenia, thrombocytopenia, anemia, eosinophilia
Hepatic: Transient elevation in serum AST concentration
Local: Pain at injection site, thrombophlebitis
Renal: Elevations in BUN or serum creatinine

Overdosage Symptoms of overdose include neuromuscular hypersensitivity, convulsions

Toxicology Many beta-lactam-containing antibiotics have the potential to cause neuromuscular hyperirritability or convulsive seizures. Hemodialysis may be helpful to aid in the removal of the drug from the blood, otherwise most treatment is supportive or symptom directed.

Drug Interactions
Probenecid prolongs half-life and elevates serum concentrations
Theoretically increases risk of nephrotoxicity with other nephrotoxic drugs

Stability Reconstituted solution is stable for 24 hours at room temperature and 48 hours when refrigerated; for I.V. infusion in NS or D_5W solution is stable for 24 hours at room temperature, 1 week when refrigerated or 26 weeks when frozen; after freezing, thawed solution is stable for 24 hours at room temperature or 5 days when refrigerated

Mechanism of Action Interferes with bacterial cell wall synthesis during active multiplication causing cell death and resultant bactericidal activity against susceptible bacteria

Pharmacokinetics
Protein binding: 65% to 79%
Half-life: 45-60 minutes, increases significantly with renal insufficiency
Time to peak serum concentration:
 I.M.: Within 20-30 minutes
 I.V.: Within 5 minutes
Elimination: Rapidly excreted as unchanged drug (85%) in urine; poorly penetrates into CSF even with inflammation of the meninges
Compared to younger patients (<55 years), older patients (66-94 years) have been reported to have a reduced total body clearance, prolonged half-life, increased volume of distribution, and reduced protein binding

Usual Dosage I.M., I.V.:
Geriatrics: Usual adult dose adjusted for estimated Cl_{cr}
Adults: 1-2 g every 6-8 hours (I.M. injection is painful)
 Dosing interval in renal impairment:
 Cl_{cr} 30-50 mL/minute: Administer every 8-12 hours
 Cl_{cr} 10-29 mL/minute: Administer every 12-24 hours
 Cl_{cr} 5-9 mL/minute: Administer 500 mg every 12-24 hours
 Cl_{cr} <5 mL/minute: Administer 500 mg every 24-48 hours
Moderately dialyzable (20% to 50%)

Administration I.M. dose should be administered in a large muscle mass (ie, gluteus maximus)

Monitoring Parameters Monitor renal function periodically when used in combination with other nephrotoxic drugs

Test Interactions Positive Coombs' [direct]; false-positive urine glucose (Clinitest®), false increase in serum or urine creatinine

Nursing Implications Administer around-the-clock rather than 4 times/day, 3 times/day, etc (ie, 12-6-12-6, not 9-1-5-9) to promote less variation in peak and trough serum concentrations; modify dosage in patients with renal insufficiency (see Usual Dosage and Administration)
(Continued)

Cefoxitin *(Continued)*

Additional Information Sodium content of 1 g: 53 mg (2.3 mEq)

Special Geriatric Considerations Adjust dose for renal function in elderly (see Pharmacokinetics and Usual Dosage)

Dosage Forms
Cefoxitin sodium:
Infusion, premixed, in D_5W (frozen): 1 g (50 mL); 2 g (50 mL)
Powder for injection: 1 g, 2 g, 10 g

References
Garcia MJ, Garcia A, Nieto MJ, et al, "Disposition of Cefoxitin in the Elderly," *Int J Clin Pharmacol Ther Toxicol*, 1980, 18(11):503-9.

Cefpodoxime *(sef pode OKS eem)*

Related Information
Cephalosporins, Aminoglycosides, Macrolides, & Quinolones *on page 1014*

Brand Names Vantin®

Generic Available No

Therapeutic Category Antibiotic, Cephalosporin (Second Generation)

Use Treatment of susceptible acute, community-acquired pneumonia caused by *S. pneumoniae* or nonbeta-lactamase producing *H. influenzae*; acute uncomplicated gonorrhea caused by *N. gonorrhoeae*; uncomplicated skin and skin structure infections caused by *S. aureus* or *S. pyogenes*; acute otitis media caused by *S. pneumoniae*, *H. influenzae*, or *M. catarrhalis*; pharyngitis or tonsillitis; and uncomplicated urinary tract infections caused by *E. coli*, *Klebsiella*, and *Proteus*

Contraindications Hypersensitivity to cefpodoxime or cephalosporins

Warnings Modify dosage in patients with severe renal impairment; prolonged use may result in superinfection; hypersensitivity to penicillins

Adverse Reactions
Central nervous system: Headache
Dermatologic: Rash
Gastrointestinal: Nausea (3.8%), vomiting, abdominal pain, diarrhea (7.1%), pseudomembranous colitis
Genitourinary: Vaginal fungal infections (3.3%)
Hematologic: Eosinophilia; leukocytosis; thrombocytosis; decrease in hemoglobin, hematocrit; leukopenia; prolonged PT and PTT
Hepatic: Transient elevation in AST, ALT, bilirubin
Renal: Increase in BUN and creatinine

Overdosage Symptoms of overdose include neuromuscular hypersensitivity, convulsions

Toxicology Many beta-lactam-containing antibiotics have the potential to cause neuromuscular hyperirritability or convulsive seizures. Hemodialysis may be helpful to aid in the removal of the drug from the blood, otherwise most treatment is supportive or symptom directed.

Drug Interactions
Antacids and H_2-receptor antagonists (reduce absorption and serum concentration of cefpodoxime)
Probenecid (inhibits renal excretion of cefpodoxime)

Stability After mixing, keep suspension in refrigerator, shake well before using; discard unused portion after 14 days

Mechanism of Action Interferes with bacterial cell wall synthesis during active multiplication, causing cell wall death and resultant bactericidal activity against susceptible bacteria

Pharmacokinetics
Absorption: Oral: Rapidly and well absorbed, acid stable; enhanced in the presence of food or low gastric pH
Distribution: Good tissue penetration, including lung and tonsils; penetrates into pleural fluid
Protein binding: 18% to 23%
Metabolism: Oral: De-esterified in the GI tract to the active metabolite, cefpodoxime
Bioavailability: Oral: 50%
Half-life: 2.2 hours (prolonged with renal impairment); elderly: 3.65 hours
Peak concentrations: Within 2-3 hours
Elimination: Plasma clearance: ~200-300 mL/minute; primarily eliminated by the kidney with 80% of dose excreted unchanged in urine in 24 hours

Usual Dosage Geriatrics and Adults: Oral: 100-400 mg every 12 hours for 7-14 days

Uncomplicated gonorrhea: 200 mg as a single dose

Dosing adjustment in renal impairment: Cl_{cr} <30 mL/minute: Administer every 24 hours

Hemodialysis patients: Dose 3 times/week following dialysis

Monitoring Parameters Signs and symptoms of infection

Test Interactions Positive Coombs' [direct]

Patient Information Take with food; chilling improves flavor (do not freeze); report persistent diarrhea; entire course of medication (10-14 days) should be taken to ensure eradication of organism; should be taken in equal intervals around-the-clock to maintain adequate blood levels; females should report symptoms of vaginitis

Nursing Implications Assess patient at beginning and throughout therapy for infection; administer around-the-clock to promote less variation in peak and trough serum concentrations

Additional Information Dose adjustment is not necessary in patients with cirrhosis

Special Geriatric Considerations Considered one of the drugs of choice for outpatient treatment of community-acquired pneumonia in older adults; dosage adjustment is not necessary unless renal impairment (see Usual Dosage and Pharmacokinetics)

Dosage Forms

Cefpodoxime proxetil:

Granules for oral suspension (lemon creme flavor): 50 mg/5 mL (100 mL); 100 mg/5 mL (100 mL)

Tablet, film coated: 100 mg, 200 mg

References

American Thoracic Society, "Guidelines for the Initial Management of Adults With Community-Acquired Pneumonia: Diagnosis, Assessment of Severity, and Initial Antimicrobial Therapy," *Am Rev Respir Dis*, 1993, 148(5):1418-26.

Backhouse C, Wade A, Williamson P, et al, "Multiple Dose Pharmacokinetics of Cefpodoxime in Young Adult and Elderly Patients," *J Antimicrob Chemother*, 1990, 26(Supp E):29-34.

Cefprozil (sef PROE zil)

Related Information

Cephalosporins, Aminoglycosides, Macrolides, & Quinolones *on page 1014*

Brand Names Cefzil®

Generic Available No

Therapeutic Category Antibiotic, Cephalosporin (Second Generation)

Use Treatment of otitis media, sinusitis, and infections caused by susceptible organisms involving the respiratory tract, skin and skin structure

Contraindications Known hypersensitivity to cefprozil or any cephalosporin

Warnings Cross-allergenicity with penicillin 5% to 16%; serum sickness-like reactions and seizures (in patients with severe renal impairment) have been reported with some cephalosporins

Precautions Dose adjustment required in patients with impaired renal function; pseudomembranous colitis, superinfection

Adverse Reactions

Central nervous system: Dizziness, fatigue, confusion, tonic-clonic seizures, headache

Dermatologic: Stevens-Johnson syndrome, erythema multiforme, toxic epidermal necrolysis

Gastrointestinal: Cholestasis, nausea, vomiting, diarrhea

Hematologic: Anemia (hemolytic, aplastic), hemorrhage, hematological disorders

Hepatic: Elevated liver enzymes, total bilirubin, alkaline phosphatase, hepatic dysfunction

Renal: Renal dysfunction

Miscellaneous: Hypersensitivity reactions

Toxicology Many beta-lactam-containing antibiotics have the potential to cause neuromuscular hyperirritability or seizures. Hemodialysis may be helpful in the removal of the drug from the blood, otherwise most treatment should be supportive or symptom directed; seizures should be treated with anticonvulsant therapy such as 5-10 mg I.V. diazepam.

Drug Interactions Probenecid (elevated plasma concentrations and risk of toxicity)

Stability Reconstituted suspension should be refrigerated and any unused portion discarded after 14 days

(Continued)

Cefprozil *(Continued)*

Mechanism of Action Interferes with bacterial cell wall synthesis during active multiplication causing cell death and resultant bactericidal activity against susceptible bacteria

Pharmacokinetics A mixture of cis- (90%) and trans- (10%) isomers; well absorbed from the GI tract (90%); food does not delay or reduce absorption; distribution is to most body tissues including the aqueous humor, bone, soft tissues, and the CSF. Elimination is primarily renal with 60% to 70% of the drug excreted in the urine in 24 hours; hepatic dysfunction does not appear to significantly alter elimination. Significantly greater peak concentrations and area under the curve is found in patients with Cl_{cr} <30 mL/minute; also, the half-life is prolonged 1.7 vs 5.9 hours and renal clearance reduced 198 mL/minute vs 18.8 mL/minute compared to patients with normal renal function.

Usual Dosage

Geriatrics and Adults: Duration of treatment ≥10 days:

Upper respiratory tract infections: 500 mg every 24 hours

Lower respiratory tract infections: 500 mg every 12 hours

Uncomplicated skin and skin structure infections: 250-500 mg every 12 hours or 500 mg every 24 hours

Adults: 250-500 mg every 12-24 hours for 10 days

Dosing adjustment in renal impairment: Cl_{cr} 0-30 mL/minute: Administer 50% of standard dose at the standard interval

Hemodialysis patients: Administer dose at the completion of hemodialysis

Monitoring Parameters Culture and sensitivity; response to treatment (fever, WBC, mental status, appetite)

Test Interactions Positive Coombs' (direct), false-positive urine glucose therapy with Clinitest® tablets, Benedict's or Fehling's solution; false-positive test for proteinuria; false-elevated urinary 17-ketosteroid values

Patient Information Complete full course of therapy; take at regular intervals; may take with food or milk; report persistent diarrhea; chilling suspension improves flavor (do not freeze)

Nursing Implications Observe patient for signs of infection resolution; monitor for rash, pruritus, and confusion (see Special Geriatric Considerations)

Special Geriatric Considerations Has not been studied exclusively in the elderly; adjust dose for estimated renal function (see Usual Dosage)

Dosage Forms

Powder for oral suspension: 125 mg/5 mL (50 mL, 100 mL); 250 mg/5 mL (50 mL, 100 mL)

Tablet: 250 mg, 500 mg

References

Shukla UA, Pittman KA, and Barbhaiya RH, "Pharmacokinetic Interactions of Cefprozil With Food, Propantheline, Metoclopramide, and Probenecid in Healthy Volunteers," *J Clin Pharmacol*, 1992, 32(8):725-31.

Shyu WC, Pittman KA, Wilber RB, et al, "Pharmacokinetics of Cefprozil in Healthy Subjects and Patients With Hepatic Impairment," *J Clin Pharmacol*, 1991, 31(4):372-6.

Ceftazidime *(SEF tay zi deem)*

Related Information

Cephalosporins, Aminoglycosides, Macrolides, & Quinolones *on page 1014*

I.V. Medication Recommendations *on page 1080*

Brand Names Ceptaz™; Fortaz®; Tazicef®; Tazidime®

Generic Available No

Therapeutic Category Antibiotic, Cephalosporin (Third Generation)

Use Treatment of documented susceptible *Pseudomonas aeruginosa* infection; *Pseudomonas* infection in patient at risk of developing aminoglycoside-induced nephrotoxicity and/or ototoxicity; empiric therapy of a febrile, granulocytopenic patient

Contraindications Hypersensitivity to ceftazidime or any component, cephalosporins

Warnings Prolonged use may result in superinfection

Precautions Use with caution and modify dosage in patients with impaired renal function; use with caution in patients with history of colitis or penicillin allergy

Adverse Reactions

Central nervous system: Fever, headache

Dermatologic: Rash

Gastrointestinal: Nausea, vomiting, pseudomembranous colitis

Hematologic: Eosinophilia, thrombocytosis, transient leukopenia, hemolytic anemia
Hepatic: Transient elevation in liver enzymes
Local: Phlebitis
Renal: BUN and creatinine increases
Miscellaneous: Candidiasis

Overdosage Symptoms of overdose include neuromuscular hypersensitivity, convulsions

Toxicology Many beta-lactam-containing antibiotics have the potential to cause neuromuscular hyperirritability or convulsive seizures. Hemodialysis may be helpful to aid in the removal of the drug from the blood, otherwise most treatment is supportive or symptom directed.

Drug Interactions Aminoglycosides: *in vitro* studies indicate additive or synergistic effect against some strains of *Enterobacteriaceae* and *Pseudomonas aeruginosa*, and theoretically may increase risk of nephrotoxicity; increased levels with probenecid

Stability Reconstituted solution and I.V. infusion in NS or D_5W solution is stable for 24 hours at room temperature, 10 days when refrigerated or 12 weeks when frozen; after freezing, thawed solution is stable for 24 hours at room temperature or 4 days when refrigerated; 96 hours under refrigeration, after mixing

Mechanism of Action Interferes with bacterial cell wall synthesis during active multiplication causing cell death and resultant bactericidal activity against susceptible bacteria

Pharmacokinetics
Distribution: Widely throughout the body including bone, bile, skin, CSF (diffuses into CSF with higher concentrations when the meninges are inflamed) endometrium, heart, pleural and lymphatic fluids
Protein binding: 17%, <10% protein binding in the elderly; in the elderly half-life increased, volume of distribution decreased, and AUC increased
Half-life: 1-2 hours (prolonged with renal impairment)
Time to peak serum concentration: I.M.: Within 60 minutes
Elimination: By glomerular filtration with 80% to 90% of the dose excreted as unchanged drug within 24 hours

Usual Dosage I.M., I.V.:
Geriatrics: Dosage should be based on renal function with a dosing interval not more frequent then every 12 hours
Adults: 1-2 g every 8-12 hours (250-500 mg every 8-12 hours for urinary tract infections)
Dosing interval in renal impairment:
Cl_{cr} 30-50 mL/minute: Administer every 12 hours
Cl_{cr} 10-30 mL/minute: Administer every 24 hours
Cl_{cr} <10 mL/minute: Administer every 48 hours
Dialyzable (50% to 100%)
Dosing in hemodialysis: 1 g loading dose, then 1 g after each dialysis session. Neurotoxicity and convulsions have been reported in dialysis patients receiving 2-3 g every 12 hours.

Administration Any carbon dioxide bubbles that may be present in the withdrawn solution should be expelled prior to injection. Ceftazidime can be administered IVP over 3-5 minutes, or I.V. retrograde or I.V. intermittent infusion over 15-30 minutes; final concentration for I.V. administration should not exceed 100 mg/mL; can be reconstituted for I.M. administration with 0.5% or 1% lidocaine if volume tolerated.

Monitoring Parameters Serum creatinine with concurrent use of an aminoglycoside; a change in renal function necessitates a change in dose; signs of infection such as fever, WBC, mental status

Test Interactions Positive Coombs' [direct], false-positive urine glucose (Clinitest®)

Nursing Implications Observe patient for signs of infection resolution; monitor for rash, pruritus, and confusion (see Special Geriatric Considerations)

Additional Information Sodium content of 1 g: 54 mg (2.3 mEq). For most elderly; weak third generation cephalosporin strongest against anaerobes and gram-positive bacteria; *Pseudomonas* sp.

Special Geriatric Considerations Changes in renal function associated with aging and corresponding alterations in pharmacokinetics result in every 12-hour dosing being an adequate dosing interval

Dosage Forms
Infusion, premixed (frozen): 500 mg in D_5W (50 mL); 1 g in $D_{1.4}W$ (50 mL); 2 g in $D_{3.2}W$ (50 mL); 1 g in NS (50 mL); 2 g in NS (100 mL)
(Continued)

Ceftazidime *(Continued)*

Injection: 500 mg, 1 g, 2 g, 6 g, 10 g

References

Sirgo MA and Norris S, "Ceftazidime in the Elderly: Appropriateness of Twice-Daily Dosing," *DICP Ann Pharmacother*, 1991, 25(3):284-8.

Slaker RA and Danielson B, "Neurotoxicity Associated With Ceftazidime Therapy in Geriatric Patients With Renal Dysfunction," *Pharmacotherapy*, 1991, 11(4):351-2.

Ceftibuten (sef TYE byoo ten)

Related Information

Cephalosporins, Aminoglycosides, Macrolides, & Quinolones *on page 1014*

Brand Names Cedax®

Therapeutic Category Antibiotic, Cephalosporin (Third Generation)

Use Treatment of acute bacterial exacerbations of chronic bronchitis; treatment of acute bacterial otitis media due to *H. influenzae*, *Moraxella catarrhalis*, or *Streptococcus pyogenes* but not when due to *Streptococcus pneumoniae*; treatment of pharyngitis or tonsillitis due to *S. pyogenes*

Contraindications Hypersensitivity to ceftibuten or cephalosporins

Warnings Prolonged use may result in superinfection

Precautions Use with caution in patients hypersensitive to penicillin

Adverse Reactions

Gastrointestinal: Diarrhea, nausea, vomiting, heartburn, epigastralgia

Hematologic: Eosinophilia

Hepatic: Increased LFTs

Overdosage Symptoms of overdose include neuromuscular hypersensitivity, convulsions

Toxicology Many beta-lactam-containing antibiotics have the potential to cause neuromuscular hyperirritability or convulsive seizures. Hemodialysis may be helpful to aid in the removal of the drug from the blood, otherwise most treatment is supportive or symptom directed.

Drug Interactions Increased effect of oral anticoagulants (theoretical)

Drug/Food Interactions Administer suspension at least 2 hours before or 1 hour after a meal

Mechanism of Action Interferes with bacterial cell wall synthesis during active multiplication causing cell death and resultant bactericidal activity against susceptible bacteria

Pharmacokinetics

Absorption: T_{max}: 2-3 hours; F = 80%

Protein binding: 65% to 77%

Metabolism: 7% to 10% to weakly active olefinic isomer

Half-life: 1.5-2.5 hours

Elimination: 67% to 75% recovered unchanged in the urine after 24 hours

Usual Dosage Geriatrics and Adults: Oral: 400 mg once daily

Dosage adjustment in renal impairment:

Cl_{cr} 30-49 mL/minute: Administer 200 mg every 24 hours

Cl_{cr} 5-20 mL/minute: Administer 100 mg every 24 hours

Monitoring Parameters Signs and symptoms of infection including mental status

Patient Information Complete full course of therapy; report persistent diarrhea; capsules can be taken with food

Nursing Implications See Food/Drug Interactions

Special Geriatric Considerations Has not been studied specifically in the elderly; adjust dose for renal function (see Usual Dosage)

Dosage Forms

Capsule: 400 mg

Powder for oral suspension (cherry flavor): 90 mg/5 mL (30 mL, 60 mL, 120 mL); 180 mg/5 mL (30 mL, 60 mL, 120 mL)

Ceftin® Oral *see* Cefuroxime *on page 193*

Ceftizoxime (sef ti ZOKS eem)

Related Information

Cephalosporins, Aminoglycosides, Macrolides, & Quinolones *on page 1014*

I.V. Medication Recommendations *on page 1080*

Brand Names Cefizox®

Generic Available No

Therapeutic Category Antibiotic, Cephalosporin (Third Generation)

Use Treatment of susceptible bacterial infection; mainly respiratory tract, skin and skin structure, bone and joint, urinary tract and gynecologic as well as septicemia

Contraindications Hypersensitivity to ceftizoxime or any component, cephalosporins

Precautions Use with caution in patients allergic to penicillin; reduce dosage in patients with decreased renal function

Adverse Reactions

Central nervous system: Fever, headache

Dermatologic: Rash, pruritus

Gastrointestinal: Pseudomembranous colitis, diarrhea, nausea, vomiting

Hematologic: Transient neutropenia, thrombocytopenia

Hepatic: Transient elevation of liver enzymes

Local: Burning at the injection site, phlebitis

Renal: Transient elevations in BUN or serum creatinine

Overdosage Symptoms of overdose include neuromuscular hypersensitivity, convulsions

Toxicology Many beta-lactam-containing antibiotics have the potential to cause neuromuscular hyperirritability or convulsive seizures. Hemodialysis may be helpful to aid in the removal of the drug from the blood, otherwise most treatment is supportive or symptom directed.

Drug Interactions Increased levels with probenecid; concurrent use with an aminoglycoside may increase risk of nephrotoxicity

Stability Reconstituted solution is stable for 24 hours at room temperature and 96 hours when refrigerated; for I.V. infusion in NS or D_5W solution is stable for 24 hours at room temperature, 96 hours when refrigerated or 12 weeks when frozen; after freezing, thawed solution is stable for 24 hours at room temperature or 10 days when refrigerated

Mechanism of Action Interferes with bacterial cell wall synthesis during active multiplication causing cell death and resultant bactericidal activity against susceptible bacteria

Pharmacokinetics

Distribution: V_d: 0.35-0.5 L/kg

Protein binding: 30%

Half-life: 1.6 hours (half-life increases to 25 hours when Cl_{cr} fall <10 mL/minute)

Time to peak serum concentration: I.M.: Within 30-60 minutes

Elimination: Excreted unchanged in urine

One study has reported the pharmacokinetics of ceftizoxime in the elderly. Following a single 2 g I.V. dose the mean serum half-life was 3.5 hours; mean V_{dss}: 14.2 L/1.73 m²; mean clearance: 62.5 mL/minute/1.73 m²

Usual Dosage Geriatrics and Adults: I.M., I.V.: 0.5-2 g every 8-12 hours, up to 2 g every 4 hours or 4 g every 8 hours for life-threatening infections

Dosing interval in renal impairment:

Cl_{cr} 50-79 mL/minute: Administer 500-1500 mg every 8 hours

Cl_{cr} 5-49 mL/minute: Administer 250-1000 mg every 12 hours

Cl_{cr} 0-4 mL/minute (dialysis): Administer 250-1000 mg every 24-48 hours
Moderately dialyzable (20% to 50%)

Administration Administer I.M. injections in a large muscle mass (ie, gluteus maximus)

Monitoring Parameters Signs and symptoms of infection including mental status

Test Interactions Increased alkaline phosphatase, AST, ALT, BUN, creatinine, glucose, protein, positive Coombs' reaction [direct]; decreased glucose; tests have been reported, false-positive urinary glucose determinations

Nursing Implications Administer around-the-clock to promote less variation in peak and trough serum concentrations (see Administration)

Additional Information Sodium content of 1 g: 60 mg (2.6 mEq)

Special Geriatric Considerations Adjust dose for renal function in elderly (see Pharmacokinetics and Usual Dosage)

Dosage Forms

Ceftizoxime sodium:

Injection, in D_5W (frozen): 1 g (50 mL); 2 g (50 mL)

Powder for injection: 500 mg, 1 g, 2 g, 10 g

References

Deeter RG, Weinstein MP, Swanson KA, et al, "Crossover Assessment of Serum Bactericidal Activity and Pharmacokinetics of Five Broad-Spectrum Cephalosporins in the Elderly," *Antimicrob Agents Chemother*, 1990, 34(6):1007-13.

Ceftriaxone (sef trye AKS one)

Related Information
Cephalosporins, Aminoglycosides, Macrolides, & Quinolones *on page 1014*
I.V. Medication Recommendations *on page 1080*

Brand Names Rocephin®

Generic Available No

Therapeutic Category Antibiotic, Cephalosporin (Third Generation)

Use Treatment of documented infection due to susceptible organisms including the lower respiratory tract, skin and skin structure, bone and joint, intra-abdominal, urinary tract, meningitis, septicemia, and gonorrhea

Contraindications Hypersensitivity to ceftriaxone sodium or any component, cephalosporins

Warnings Prolonged use may result in superinfection

Precautions Use with caution in patients with gallbladder, biliary tract, liver, pancreatic disease, or history of colitis; use with caution in patients allergic to penicillin

Adverse Reactions
Dermatologic: Rash
Gastrointestinal: Diarrhea, nausea, vomiting, colitis, sludging in the gallbladder
Hematologic: Eosinophilia, thrombocytosis, leukopenia, anemia, increased prothrombin time
Hepatic: Jaundice, transient elevation in liver enzymes, cholelithiasis
Local: Pain at injection site
Renal: Increased BUN

Overdosage Symptoms of overdose include neuromuscular hypersensitivity, convulsions

Toxicology Many beta-lactam-containing antibiotics have the potential to cause neuromuscular hyperirritability or convulsive seizures. Hemodialysis may be helpful to aid in the removal of the drug from the blood, otherwise most treatment is supportive or symptom directed.

Drug Interactions Increased levels with probenecid; may have synergy with the aminoglycosides and theoretically increase the risk of nephrotoxicity; alcohol (disulfiram-like reaction)

Stability Reconstituted solution (100 mg/mL) is stable for 3 days at room temperature and 3 days when refrigerated; for I.V. infusion in NS or D$_5$W solution is stable for 3 days at room temperature, 10 days when refrigerated or 26 weeks when frozen; after freezing, thawed solution is stable for 3 days at room temperature or 10 days when refrigerated

Mechanism of Action Interferes with bacterial cell wall synthesis during active multiplication causing cell death and resultant bactericidal activity against susceptible bacteria

Pharmacokinetics
Distribution: Widely throughout the body including gallbladder, lungs, bone, bile, CSF (diffuses into the CSF at higher concentrations when the meninges are inflamed)
Protein binding: 85% to 95%
Half-life: 5-9 hours (with normal renal and hepatic function)
Time to peak serum concentration:
I.M.: Within 1-2 hours
I.V.: Within minutes
Elimination: Excreted unchanged in urine (33% to 65%) by glomerular filtration and in feces
Studies of ceftriaxone in the elderly have found a prolonged serum half-life (15 hours) and a reduced total clearance with or without a change in the volume of distribution. The change in renal clearance has been correlated to a reduction in Cl$_{cr}$. An increased free fraction was also found in one study suggesting a reduction in protein binding.

Usual Dosage Geriatrics and Adults: I.M., I.V.: 1-2 g every 12-24 hours depending on the type and severity of the infection; usual dose: 1-2 g every 24 hours; maximum dose: 4 g/day

Dosing adjustment in renal or hepatic impairment: Not necessary
Uncomplicated gonorrhea: I.M.: 250 mg as a single dose

Administration Administer I.M. doses in a large muscle mass (ie, maximus gluteus)

Monitoring Parameters Signs and symptoms of infection including mental status

Test Interactions False-positive urine glucose with Clinitest®

Nursing Implications Administer around-the-clock to promote less variation in peak and trough serum concentrations (see Administration)

Additional Information Sodium content of 1 g: 2.6 mEq

Special Geriatric Considerations No adjustment for renal function necessary (see Pharmacokinetics and Usual Dosage)

Dosage Forms

Ceftriaxone sodium:

Infusion, premixed (frozen): 1 g in $D_{3.8}W$ (50 mL); 2 g in $D_{2.4}W$ (50 mL)

Injection: 350 mg/mL

Powder for injection: 250 mg, 500 mg, 1 g, 2 g, 10 g

References

Deeter RG, Weinstein MP, Swanson KA, et al, "Crossover Assessment of Serum Bactericidal Activity and Pharmacokinetics of Five Broad-Spectrum Cephalosporins in the Elderly," *Antimicrob Agents Chemother*, 1990, 34(6):1007-13.

Hayton WL and Stoeckel K, "Age-Associated Changes in Ceftriaxone Pharmacokinetics," *Clin Pharmacokinet*, 1986, 11(1):76-82.

Luderer JR, Patel IH, Durkin J, et al, "Age and Ceftriaxone Kinetics," *Clin Pharmacol Ther*, 1984, 35(1):19-25.

Richards DM, Heel RC, Brogden RN, et al, "Ceftriaxone: A Review of Its Antibacterial Activity, Pharmacological Properties and Therapeutic Use," *Drugs*, 1984, 27(6):469-527.

Cefuroxime (se fyoor OKS eem)

Related Information

Cephalosporins, Aminoglycosides, Macrolides, & Quinolones *on page 1014*

I.V. Medication Recommendations *on page 1080*

Brand Names Ceftin® Oral; Kefurox® Injection; Zinacef® Injection

Generic Available No

Therapeutic Category Antibiotic, Cephalosporin (Second Generation)

Use Infections caused by staphylococci, group B streptococci, *H. influenzae* (type A and B), *E. coli*, *Enterobacter*, *Salmonella*, and *Klebsiella*; treatment of susceptible infections of the lower respiratory tract, otitis media, urinary tract, skin and soft tissue, bone and joint, sepsis, and gonorrhea

Contraindications Hypersensitivity to cefuroxime or any component, cephalosporins

Warnings Prolonged use may result in superinfection

Precautions Use with caution and modify dosage in patients with renal impairment; use with caution in patients with history of colitis; use with caution in patients allergic to penicillin

Adverse Reactions

Central nervous system: Dizziness, fever, headache

Dermatologic: Rash

Gastrointestinal: Nausea, vomiting, diarrhea, stomach cramps, GI bleeding, pseudomembranous colitis

Genitourinary: Vaginitis

Hematologic: Transient neutropenia and leukopenia, decreased hemoglobin and hematocrit, eosinophilia

Hepatic: Transient increase in liver enzymes

Local: Pain at the injection site, thrombophlebitis

Renal: Transient elevation in creatinine or BUN

Overdosage Symptoms of overdose include neuromuscular hypersensitivity, convulsions

Toxicology Many beta-lactam-containing antibiotics have the potential to cause neuromuscular hyperirritability or convulsive seizures. Hemodialysis may be helpful to aid in the removal of the drug from the blood, otherwise most treatment is supportive or symptom directed.

Drug Interactions Concomitant administration with an aminoglycoside may result in synergy and theoretically increase the risk of nephrotoxicity; probenecid increases serum concentrations of cefuroxime

Stability Reconstituted solution is stable for 24 hours at room temperature and 48 hours when refrigerated; for I.V. infusion in NS or D_5W solution is stable for 24 hours at room temperature, 7 days when refrigerated or 26 weeks when frozen; after freezing, thawed solution is stable for 24 hours at room temperature or 21 days when refrigerated

Mechanism of Action Interferes with bacterial cell wall synthesis during active multiplication causing cell death and resultant bactericidal activity against susceptible bacteria

Pharmacokinetics

Absorption: Increased when given with or shortly after food

Protein binding: 33% to 50%

Bioavailability: Oral cefuroxime axetil: 37% to 52%

(Continued)

Cefuroxime (Continued)

Half-life (adults): 1-2 hours (prolonged in renal impairment)
The serum half-life of cefuroxime is prolonged in the elderly due to decreased renal function; mean half-life: 2-4 hours
Time to peak plasma concentration:
    I.M.: Within 15-60 minutes
    I.V.: 2-3 minutes
Elimination: Primarily excreted 66% to 100% as unchanged drug in urine by both glomerular filtration and tubular secretion; can be removed by dialysis

Usual Dosage Geriatrics and Adults:
Oral: 125-500 mg twice daily, depending on severity of infection
I.M., I.V.: 750-1.5 g every 6 hours; maximum: 6 g/24 hours

Dosing interval in renal impairment:
Cl_{cr} >20 mL/minute: Administer 750-1500 mg every 8 hours
Cl_{cr} 10-20 mL/minute: Administer 750 mg every 12 hours
Cl_{cr} <10 mL/minute: Administer 750 mg every 24 hours
Hemodialysis patients: Administer doses following dialysis

Administration Tablets can be crushed and given with soft foods to mask the bitter taste; I.M. doses should be given deep into a large muscle (ie, gluteus maximus)

Monitoring Parameters Signs and symptoms of infection including mental status

Test Interactions Positive Coombs' [direct]; false-positive urine glucose with Clinitest®

Patient Information Complete full course of therapy, do not skip doses; can be taken with food or milk; notify physician if severe diarrhea occurs

Nursing Implications Administer around-the-clock to promote less variation in peak and trough serum concentrations (see Administration)

Additional Information Sodium content of 1 g: 54.2 mg (2.4 mEq)

Special Geriatric Considerations Adjust dose for renal function in elderly; consider one of the drugs of choice for outpatient treatment of community-acquired pneumonia in the older adult (see Pharmacokinetics and Usual Dosage)

Dosage Forms
Cefuroxime sodium:
    Infusion, premixed (frozen) (Zinacef®): 750 mg (50 mL); 1.5 g (50 mL)
    Powder for injection: 750 mg, 1.5 g, 7.5 g
    Powder for injection (Kefurox®, Zinacef®): 750 mg, 1.5 g, 7.5 g
Cefuroxime axetil:
    Powder for oral suspension (tutti-frutti flavor) (Ceftin®): 125 mg/5 mL (50 mL, 100 mL, 200 mL)
    Tablet (Ceftin®): 125 mg, 250 mg, 500 mg

References

American Thoracic Society, "Guidelines for the Initial Management of Adults With Community-Acquired Pneumonia: Diagnosis Assessment of Severity and Initial Antimicrobial Therapy," *Am Rev Respir Dis*, 1993, 148(5):1418-26.
Broekhuysen J, Deger F, Douchamps J, et al, "Pharmacokinetic Study of Cefuroxime in the Elderly," *Br J Clin Pharmacol*, 1981, 21(6):801-5.
Douglas JG, Bax RP, and Munro JF, "The Pharmacokinetics of Cefuroxime in the Elderly," *J Antimicrob Chemother*, 1980, 6(4):543-9.

Cefzil® see Cefprozil on page 187

Celestone® see Betamethasone on page 114

Celestone® Soluspan® see Betamethasone on page 114

Celontin® see Methsuximide on page 607

Cel-U-Jec® see Betamethasone on page 114

Cenafed® [OTC] see Pseudoephedrine on page 802

Cenafed® Plus Tablet [OTC] see Triprolidine and Pseudoephedrine on page 966

Cena-K® see Potassium Chloride on page 763

Centrax® see Prazepam on page 771

Cephalexin (sef a LEKS in)

Related Information
Cephalosporins, Aminoglycosides, Macrolides, & Quinolones on page 1014
Prevention of Bacterial Endocarditis on page 1062

Brand Names Biocef; Keflex®; Keftab®

Generic Available Yes

Therapeutic Category Antibiotic, Cephalosporin (First Generation)

Use Treatment of susceptible bacterial infections, including those caused by group A beta-hemolytic *Streptococcus*, *Staphylococcus*, *Klebsiella pneumoniae*, *E. coli*, *Proteus mirabilis*, and *Shigella*

Contraindications Hypersensitivity to cephalexin or any component, cephalosporins

Warnings Prolonged use may result in superinfection

Precautions Use with caution and modify dosage in patients with renal impairment; use with caution in patients with history of colitis; use with caution in patients with penicillin allergy

Adverse Reactions
Central nervous system: Dizziness, fatigue, headache
Dermatologic: Rash
Gastrointestinal: Nausea, vomiting, pseudomembranous colitis, abdominal cramps
Hematologic: Transient neutropenia, anemia, positive Coombs' test
Hepatic: Transient elevation in liver enzymes

Overdosage Symptoms of overdose include neuromuscular hypersensitivity, convulsions

Toxicology Many beta-lactam-containing antibiotics have the potential to cause neuromuscular hyperirritability or convulsive seizures. Hemodialysis may be helpful to aid in the removal of the drug from the blood, otherwise most treatment is supportive or symptom directed.

Drug Interactions Increased levels with probenecid; theoretical synergy and increased risk of nephrotoxicity with aminoglycosides

Stability Refrigerate suspension after reconstitution; discard after 14 days

Mechanism of Action Interferes with bacterial cell wall synthesis during active multiplication causing cell death and resultant bactericidal activity against susceptible bacteria

Pharmacokinetics
Half-life: 0.5-1.2 hours (prolonged with renal impairment)
Protein binding: 6% to 15%
Time to peak serum concentration: Oral: Within 60 minutes
Elimination: 80% to 100% of dose excreted as unchanged drug in urine within 8 hours

Usual Dosage Geriatrics and Adults: Oral: 250-1000 mg every 6 hours
Dosing interval in renal impairment:
Cl_{cr} 10-40 mL/minute: Administer every 8-12 hours
Cl_{cr} 5-10 mL/minute: Administer every 12 hours
Cl_{cr} <5 mL/minute: Administer every 12-24 hours
Moderately dialyzable (20% to 50%)

Monitoring Parameters Signs and symptoms of infection

Test Interactions False-positive urine glucose with Clinitest®; positive Coombs' test [direct]; false increase in serum or urine creatinine

Patient Information Complete full course of therapy; may take with food or milk if GI upset occurs; notify physician if severe diarrhea occurs

Nursing Implications Administer on an empty stomach (ie, 1 hour prior to, or 2 hours after meals) to increase total absorption; administer around-the-clock rather than 4 times/day to promote less variation in peak and trough serum concentrations

Special Geriatric Considerations Adjust dose for renal function (see Usual Dosage)

Dosage Forms
Cephalexin monohydrate:
Capsule: 250 mg, 500 mg
Powder for oral suspension: 125 mg/5 mL (5 mL unit dose, 60 mL, 100 mL, 200 mL); 250 mg/5 mL (5 mL unit dose, 100 mL, 200 mL)
Suspension, oral: pediatric: 100 mg/mL [5 mg/drop] (10 mL)
Tablet: 250 mg, 500 mg, 1 g
Tablet, as hydrochloride: 500 mg

Cephalosporins, Aminoglycosides, Macrolides, & Quinolones *see page 1014*

Cephalothin (sef A loe thin)
Related Information
Cephalosporins, Aminoglycosides, Macrolides, & Quinolones *on page 1014*

Brand Names Keflin®

Generic Available Yes

Therapeutic Category Antibiotic, Cephalosporin (First Generation)

(Continued)

Cephalothin *(Continued)*

Use Treatment of susceptible bacterial infections, including those caused by group A beta-hemolytic *Streptococcus*

Contraindications Hypersensitivity to cephalothin, cephalosporins

Warnings Prolonged use might result in superinfection

Precautions Modify dosage according to renal function; use with caution in patients with penicillin allergy

Adverse Reactions

Dermatologic: Maculopapular and erythematous rash

Gastrointestinal: Dyspepsia, diarrhea, pseudomembranous colitis, nausea, vomiting

Local: Bleeding, pain, and induration at injection site

Overdosage Symptoms of overdose include neuromuscular hypersensitivity, convulsions

Toxicology Many beta-lactam-containing antibiotics have the potential to cause neuromuscular hyperirritability or convulsive seizures. Hemodialysis may be helpful to aid in the removal of the drug from the blood, otherwise most treatment is supportive or symptom directed.

Drug Interactions Increased levels with probenecid; concomitant administration with an aminoglycoside may result in synergy and theoretically increase the risk of nephrotoxicity

Stability Reconstituted solution is stable for 12-24 hours at room temperature and 96 hours when refrigerated; for I.V. infusion in NS or D_5W solution is stable for 24 hours at room temperature, 96 hours when refrigerated or 12 weeks when frozen; after freezing, thawed solution is stable for 24 hours at room temperature or 96 hours when refrigerated

Mechanism of Action Interferes with bacterial cell wall synthesis during active multiplication causing cell death and resultant bactericidal activity against susceptible bacteria

Pharmacokinetics

Protein binding: 65% to 80%; does not penetrate the CSF unless the meninges are inflamed

Metabolism: Partially deacetylated in the liver and kidney

Half-life: 30-60 minutes

Time to peak serum concentration:

I.M.: Within 30 minutes

I.V.: Within 15 minutes

Elimination: 50% to 75% of dose appears as unchanged drug in urine

In a small number (4) of bedridden elderly, the half-life and volume of distribution were increased and the total clearance decreased compared to younger healthy volunteers

Usual Dosage Geriatrics and Adults: I.M., I.V.: 500 mg to 2 g every 4-6 hours

Dosing interval in renal impairment: See table.

Cephalothin Sodium

Cl_{cr} (mL/min)	Maximum dose (g) for Each Dosing Interval
50-80	2 q6h
25-50	1.5 q6h
10-25	1 q6h
2-10	0.5 q6h
<2	0.5 q8h

Monitoring Parameters Signs and symptoms of infection including mental status

Test Interactions Increased creatinine (S), prothrombin time, glucose; positive Coombs' [direct], increased protein; decreased glucose

Nursing Implications Administer I.M. dose deep into large muscle mass (ie, gluteus maximus) to decrease pain and induration

Additional Information Sodium content of 1 g: 2.8 mEq

Special Geriatric Considerations Adjust dose for renal function in elderly (see Pharmacokinetics and Usual Dosage)

Dosage Forms

Cephalothin sodium:

Infusion, in D_5W (frozen): 1 g (50 mL); 2 g (50 mL)

Powder for injection: 1 g, 2 g, 20 g

References

Yasuhara H, Kobayashi S, Sakamoto K, et al, "Pharmacokinetics of Amikacin and Cephalothin in Bedridden Elderly Patients," *J Clin Pharmacol*, 1982, 22(8-9):403-9.

Cephapirin (sef a PYE rin)

Related Information

Cephalosporins, Aminoglycosides, Macrolides, & Quinolones *on page 1014*

Brand Names Cefadyl®

Generic Available No

Therapeutic Category Antibiotic, Cephalosporin (First Generation)

Use Treatment of infections when caused by susceptible strains in serious respiratory, genitourinary, gastrointestinal, skin and soft-tissue, bone and joint infections; septicemia; endocarditis

Contraindications Hypersensitivity to cephapirin or any component, cephalosporins

Warnings Prolonged use might result in superinfection

Precautions Modify dose according to renal function; use with caution in patients with penicillin allergy

Adverse Reactions

Central nervous system: CNS irritation, seizures, fever

Dermatologic: Rash, urticaria

Gastrointestinal: Diarrhea, pseudomembranous colitis

Hematologic: Leukopenia, thrombocytopenia, positive Coombs' test

Hepatic: Transient elevation of liver enzymes

Overdosage Symptoms of overdose include neuromuscular hypersensitivity, convulsions

Toxicology Many beta-lactam-containing antibiotics have the potential to cause neuromuscular hyperirritability or convulsive seizures. Hemodialysis may be helpful to aid in the removal of the drug from the blood, otherwise most treatment is supportive or symptom directed.

Drug Interactions Decreased elimination and increased serum concentration with probenecid; theoretic synergy and increased risk for nephrotoxicity with aminoglycosides

Stability Reconstituted solution is stable for 24 hours at room temperature and 10 days when refrigerated; for I.V. infusion in NS or D_5W solution is stable for 24 hours at room temperature, 10 days when refrigerated or 14 days when frozen; after freezing, thawed solution is stable for 12 hours at room temperature or 10 days when refrigerated

Mechanism of Action Interferes with bacterial cell wall synthesis during active multiplication causing cell death and resultant bactericidal activity against susceptible bacteria

Pharmacokinetics

Protein binding: 22% to 25%

Metabolism: Partially in the liver, kidney and plasma

Half-life: 36-60 minutes

Time to peak serum concentration:

I.M.: Within 30 minutes

I.V.: Within 5 minutes

Elimination: Metabolites (50% active) excreted in urine; 60% to 85% is excreted as unchanged drug in urine

Usual Dosage Geriatrics and Adults: I.M., I.V.: 1 g every 6 hours up to 12 g/day

Dosing interval in renal impairment: Cl_{cr} <10 mL/minute: Administer every 12 hours

Hemodialysis patients: 7.5-15 mg/kg just prior to dialysis and every 12 hours thereafter

Administration Administer I.M. doses deep into a large muscle mass (ie, gluteus maximus)

Monitoring Parameters Signs and symptoms of infection including mental status

Test Interactions Positive Coombs' [direct]; increased glucose, protein; decreased glucose

Nursing Implications See Administration

Special Geriatric Considerations Cephapirin has not been studied in the elderly (see Usual Dosage); adjust dose for renal function

Dosage Forms Powder for injection, as sodium: 500 mg, 1 g, 2 g, 4 g, 20 g

Cephradine (SEF ra deen)

Related Information
  Cephalosporins, Aminoglycosides, Macrolides, & Quinolones *on page 1014*

Brand Names Velosef®

Generic Available Yes

Therapeutic Category Antibiotic, Cephalosporin (First Generation)

Use Treatment of susceptible bacterial infections, including those caused by group A beta-hemolytic *Streptococcus*

Contraindications Hypersensitivity to cephradine or any component, cephalosporins

Warnings Prolonged use may result in superinfection

Precautions Modify dose according to renal function; use with caution in patients with penicillin allergy

Adverse Reactions
  Dermatologic: Rash
  Gastrointestinal: Nausea, vomiting, diarrhea, pseudomembranous colitis
  Renal: Increased BUN and creatinine

Overdosage Symptoms of overdose include neuromuscular hypersensitivity, convulsions

Toxicology Many beta-lactam-containing antibiotics have the potential to cause neuromuscular hyperirritability or convulsive seizures. Hemodialysis may be helpful to aid in the removal of the drug from the blood, otherwise most treatment is supportive or symptom directed.

Drug Interactions Decreased elimination and increased serum concentrations with probenecid; theoretical synergy and increased risk of nephrotoxicity with aminoglycosides

Stability Reconstituted solution is stable for 2 hours at room temperature and 24 hours when refrigerated; for I.V. infusion in NS or D_5W solution is stable for 10 hours at room temperature, 48 hours when refrigerated or 6 weeks when frozen; after freezing, thawed solution is stable for 10 hours at room temperature or 48 hours when refrigerated

Mechanism of Action Interferes with bacterial cell wall synthesis during active multiplication causing cell death and resultant bactericidal activity against susceptible bacteria

Pharmacokinetics
  Absorption: Oral: Faster than I.M. absorption, yet well absorbed from all routes
  Protein binding: 18% to 20%
  Half-life: 1-2 hours
  Time to peak serum concentration: Oral, I.M.: Within 1-2 hours
  Elimination: ~80% to 90% of drug recovered in urine as unchanged drug within 6 hours

Usual Dosage Geriatrics and Adults: Oral, I.M., I.V.: 2-4 g/day in 4 equally divided doses up to 8 g/day

  Dosing adjustment in renal impairment:
  Cl_{cr} >20 mL/minute: Administer 500 mg every 6 hours
  Cl_{cr} 5-20 mL/minute: Administer 250 mg every 6 hours
  Cl_{cr} <5 mL/minute: Administer 250 mg every 12 hours
  Hemodialysis patients: 250 mg at the start of dialysis, then 250 mg at 12 and 36-48 hours later

Administration I.M. doses should be given deep into a large muscle mass (ie, gluteus maximus)

Monitoring Parameters Signs and symptoms of infection including mental status

Test Interactions Positive Coombs' [direct]; increased glucose, protein; decreased glucose

Patient Information Complete full course of therapy, do not miss doses; may be taken with food or milk; call physician if severe diarrhea occurs

Nursing Implications See Administration

Special Geriatric Considerations Cephradine has not been studied in the elderly (see Usual Dosage); adjust dose for renal function in elderly

Dosage Forms
  Capsule: 250 mg, 500 mg
  Powder for injection: 250 mg, 500 mg, 1 g, 2 g vials
  Suspension, oral: 125 mg/5 mL (100 mL); 250 mg/5 mL (200 mL)
  Tablet: 1 g

Cephulac® *see Lactulose on page 523*

Ceptaz™ *see* Ceftazidime *on page 188*
Cerebyx® *see* Fosphenytoin *on page 412*

Cerivastatin (se ree va STAT in)
Brand Names Baycol®
Therapeutic Category Antilipemic Agent; HMG-CoA Reductase Inhibitor
Use Adjunct to dietary therapy to for the reduction of elevated total and LDL cholesterol levels in patients with primary hypercholesterolemia and mixed dyslipidemia when the response to dietary restriction of saturated fat and cholesterol and other nonpharmacological measures alone has been inadequate
Contraindications Hypersensitivity to cerivastatin
Adverse Reactions
Hepatic: Increased LFTs
Neuromuscular & skeletal: Increased creatinine kinase, myalgia, muscle weakness; rhabdomyolysis, myoglobinemia, and acute renal failure have been reported with other statins
Drug Interactions Decreased absorption with cholestyramine; possible increased risk of myopathy when used concurrently with CYP3A4 inhibitors as has been reported with other statins; erythromycin increases cerivastatin concentrations in the plasma
Usual Dosage Geriatrics and Adults: Oral: 0.3 mg once daily in the evening; may be taken with or without food

Dosage adjustment with moderate to severe renal impairment: Start at 0.2 mg once daily in the evening
Monitoring Parameters Serum cholesterol, LFTs, CPK
Patient Information Promptly report any unexplained muscle pain, tenderness, or weakness, especially if accompanied by malaise or fever; follow prescribed diet
Nursing Implications The best effect is seen when administered at night; monitor for symptoms of adverse effects (see Adverse Reactions and Special Geriatric Considerations)
Special Geriatric Considerations The definition of and, therefore, when to treat hyperlipidemia in the elderly is a controversial issue. The National Cholesterol Education Program recommends that all adults 20 years of age and older maintain a plasma cholesterol <200 mg/dL. By this definition, 60% of all elderly would be considered to have a borderline high (200-239 mg/dL) or high (≥240 mg/dL) cholesterol. However, plasma cholesterol has been shown to be a less reliable predictor of coronary heart disease in the elderly. Therefore, it is the authors' belief that pharmacologic treatment be reserved for those who are unable to obtain a desirable plasma cholesterol concentration by diet alone and for whom the benefits of treatment are believed to outweigh the potential adverse effects, drug interactions, and cost of treatment.
Dosage Forms Tablet, as sodium: 0.2 mg, 0.3 mg
References
"Summary of the Second Report of the National Cholesterol Education Program (NCEP) Expert Panel on Detection, Evaluation, and Treatment of High Blood Cholesterol in Adults (Adult Treatment Panel II)," *JAMA*, 1993, 269(23):3015-23.

Cerumenex® Otic *see* Triethanolamine Polypeptide Oleate-Condensate *on page 954*
C.E.S. *see* Estrogens, Conjugated *on page 353*
Cetamide® Ophthalmic *see* Sulfacetamide Sodium *on page 874*
Cetapred® Ophthalmic *see* Sulfacetamide Sodium and Prednisolone *on page 875*

Cetirizine (se TI ra zeen)
Brand Names Zyrtec™
Synonyms P-071; UCB-P071
Generic Available No
Therapeutic Category Antihistamine
Use Perennial and seasonal allergic rhinitis and other allergic symptoms including chronic urticaria
Contraindications Contraindicated in patients who are hypersensitive to cetirizine or hydroxyzine, any of its constituents, or to any other antihistamine with a similar chemical structure
Precautions May cause drowsiness or sedation in doses >10 mg/day; dosage should be reduced in the elderly, patients with renal insufficiency, hepatic dysfunction, or who are on hemodialysis
(Continued)

Cetirizine *(Continued)*

Adverse Reactions
Central nervous system: Somnolence, fatigue, dizziness
Gastrointestinal: Xerostomia, pharyngitis

Overdosage Symptoms of overdose include somnolence

Toxicology No specific antidote; treatment should be symptomatic or supportive

Drug Interactions
Large doses of theophylline cause a small decrease in cetirizine clearance
Increased CNS effect with alcohol, other CNS depressants

Mechanism of Action Selective inhibition of peripheral H_1 receptors; cetirizine is a metabolite of hydroxyzine

Pharmacodynamics
Onset of action: Within 1 hour
Duration of action: 24 hours

Pharmacokinetics
Distribution: Minimal penetration into central nervous system
Protein binding: 93%
Metabolism: Not extensively metabolized by the liver
Half-life: 7.4-9 hours; in mild-moderate renal failure the half-life is increased to 19-21 hours
Time to peak: 0.5-1 hour; food may delay time to peak and decrease C_{max}
Elimination: 60% of dose is excreted unchanged in urine within 24 hours
Note: In the elderly, there was a 50% increase in half-life and a 40% decrease in clearance, most likely due to change in renal function; not removed by hemodialysis

Usual Dosage Oral:
Geriatrics: Initial: 5 mg once daily; may increase to 10 mg/day
Adults: 5-10 mg once daily
Dosage adjustment in renal/hepatic impairment: Cl_{cr} 11-31 mL/minute: Administer 5 mg once daily
Hemodialysis: Administer 5 mg once daily

Monitoring Parameters Relief of symptoms

Patient Information May be taken at any time during the day, with or without food

Nursing Implications Monitor for effectiveness

Additional Information Unlike other second generation antihistamines, cetirizine has not been associated with torsade de pointes and does **not** interact with macrolide antibiotics or ketoconazole

Special Geriatric Considerations Adjust dose for renal function (see Usual Dosage and Pharmacokinetics)

Dosage Forms
Cetirizine hydrochloride:
Syrup: 5 mg/5 mL (120 mL)
Tablet: 5 mg, 10 mg

Cevalin® [OTC] *see Ascorbic Acid on page 82*

Cevi-Bid® [OTC] *see Ascorbic Acid on page 82*

Ce-Vi-Sol® [OTC] *see Ascorbic Acid on page 82*

Cheracol® *see Guaifenesin and Codeine on page 438*

Cheracol® D [OTC] *see Guaifenesin and Dextromethorphan on page 439*

Chibroxin™ Ophthalmic *see Norfloxacin on page 683*

Children's Advil® Oral Suspension [OTC] *see Ibuprofen on page 475*

Children's Hold® [OTC] *see Dextromethorphan on page 278*

Children's Kaopectate® [OTC] *see Attapulgite on page 94*

Children's Motrin® Oral Suspension [OTC] *see Ibuprofen on page 475*

Children's Silfedrine® [OTC] *see Pseudoephedrine on page 802*

Chlo-Amine® [OTC] *see Chlorpheniramine on page 208*

Chloral *see Chloral Hydrate on this page*

Chloral Hydrate *(KLOR al HYE drate)*

Related Information
Anxiolytic/Hypnotic Use in Long-Term Care Facilities *on page 1099*
Federal OBRA Regulations Recommended Maximum Doses - Hypnotics *on page 1057*

Brand Names Aquachloral® Supprettes®

Synonyms Chloral; Trichloroacetaldehyde Monohydrate

Generic Available Yes

Therapeutic Category Hypnotic; Sedative

Use Short-term sedative and hypnotic (<2 weeks), sedative/hypnotic for dental and diagnostic procedures; sedative prior to EEG evaluations

Restrictions C-IV

Contraindications Hypersensitivity to chloral hydrate or any component; hepatic or renal impairment; gastritis or ulcers; severe cardiac disease

Warnings Trichloroethanol (TCE), a metabolite of chloral hydrate, is a carcinogen in mice; no data available in humans

Precautions Use with caution in patients with porphyria

Adverse Reactions

Central nervous system: Disorientation, sedation, ataxia, excitement (paradoxical), dizziness, fever, headache, "hangover" effect

Dermatologic: Rash, urticaria

Gastrointestinal: Gastric irritation, nausea, vomiting, diarrhea, flatulence

Hematologic: Leukopenia, eosinophilia

Miscellaneous: Physical and psychological dependence may occur with prolonged use of large doses

Overdosage Symptoms of overdose include hypotension, respiratory depression, coma, hypothermia, cardiac arrhythmias

Toxicology Treatment is supportive and symptomatic; lidocaine or propranolol may be used for ventricular dysrhythmias, while isoproterenol or atropine may be required for torsade de pointes; activated charcoal may prevent drug absorption

Drug Interactions

Increased effect of warfarin, CNS depressants, alcohol

Increased toxicity with alcohol (flushing, tachycardia, etc), furosemide, intravenous (flushing, diaphoresis, and blood pressure changes)

Stability Sensitive to light; exposure to air causes volatilization; store in light-resistant, airtight container

Mechanism of Action Central nervous system depressant effects are due to its active metabolite trichloroethanol, mechanism unknown

Pharmacodynamics

Peak effect: Within 30-60 minutes

Duration: 4-8 hours

Pharmacokinetics

Absorption: Oral, rectal: Well absorbed

Protein binding: Trichloroacetic acid is highly protein bound and displaces other acidic drugs

Metabolism: Rapid to trichloroethanol; variable amounts metabolized in liver and kidney to trichloroacetic acid (inactive)

Half-life: Trichloroethanol: 8-11 hours

Elimination: Metabolites excreted in urine; small amounts excreted in feces via bile

Usual Dosage

Geriatrics: Hypnotic: Initial: Oral: 250 mg at bedtime

Adults:

Sedation, anxiety: Oral, rectal: 250 mg 3 times/day

Hypnotic: Oral, rectal: 500-1000 mg at bedtime or 30 minutes prior to procedure, not to exceed 2 g/24 hours

Dosing adjustment/comments in renal impairment: Cl_{cr} <50 mL/minute: Avoid use

Dialyzable (50% to 100%)

Dosing adjustment/comments in hepatic impairment: Avoid use in patients with severe hepatic impairment

Administration Do not crush capsule; contains drug in liquid form

Monitoring Parameters Mental status, vital signs

Test Interactions False-positive urine glucose using Clinitest® method; may interfere with fluorometric urine catecholamine and urinary 17-hydroxycorticosteroid tests

Patient Information Take capsule with a full glass of water or fruit juice; swallow capsules whole, do not chew; avoid alcohol and other CNS depressants; avoid activities needing good psychomotor coordination until CNS effects are known; drug may cause physical or psychological dependence; avoid abrupt discontinuation after prolonged use; if taking at home prior to a diagnostic procedure, have someone else transport you

Nursing Implications Gastric irritation may be minimized by diluting dose in water or other oral liquid

(Continued)

Chloral Hydrate *(Continued)*

Additional Information Tolerance to hypnotic effect develops, therefore, not recommended for use >2 weeks; taper dosage to avoid withdrawal with prolonged use

Special Geriatric Considerations Chloral hydrate is considered a second or third line hypnotic agent in the elderly; interpretive guidelines from the Health Care Financing Administration (HCFA) discourage the use of chloral hydrate in residents of long-term care facilities

Dosage Forms

Capsule: 250 mg, 500 mg

Suppository: 324 mg, 500 mg, 648 mg

Syrup: 250 mg/5 mL, 500 mg/5 mL

Chlorambucil *(klor AM byoo sil)*

Brand Names Leukeran®

Generic Available No

Therapeutic Category Antineoplastic Agent, Alkylating Agent (Nitrogen Mustard)

Use Management of chronic lymphocytic leukemia (CLL), Hodgkin's and non-Hodgkin's lymphoma; management of nephrotic syndrome unresponsive to conventional therapy; breast and ovarian carcinoma; Waldenström macroglobulinemia, testicular carcinoma, thrombocythemia, choriocarcinoma; rheumatoid arthritis; idiopathic membranous nephropathy

Contraindications Hypersensitivity to chlorambucil or any component, or previous resistance, severe bone marrow suppression; cross-hypersensitivity with other alkylating agents may occur

Warnings The U.S. Food and Drug Administration (FDA) currently recommends that procedures for proper handling and disposal of antineoplastic agents be considered. Can severely suppress bone marrow function; affects human fertility; carcinogenic in humans and probably mutagenic and teratogenic as well; chromosomal damage has been documented; secondary AML may be associated with chronic therapy.

Precautions Use with caution in patients with seizure disorder and bone marrow suppression; reduce initial dosage if patient has received radiation therapy, myelosuppressive drugs or has a depressed baseline leukocyte or platelet count within the previous 4 weeks

Adverse Reactions

Central nervous system: Confusion, ataxia, seizures

Dermatologic: Rash

Endocrine & metabolic: Hyperuricemia

Gastrointestinal: Nausea, vomiting, oral ulcers

Genitourinary: Oligospermia

Hematologic: Leukopenia, thrombocytopenia, anemia

Hepatic: Hepatotoxicity with jaundice

Neuromuscular & skeletal: Peripheral neuropathy, tremors, muscle twitching, weakness

Respiratory: Pulmonary fibrosis

Miscellaneous: Drug fever

Overdosage Symptoms of overdose include vomiting, ataxia, coma, seizures, agitation, tremor, confusion, pancytopenia

Toxicology There are no known antidotes for chlorambucil intoxication, and treatment is mainly supportive, directed at decontaminating the GI tract and controlling symptoms; blood products may be used to treat the hematologic toxicity

Drug Interactions Bone marrow suppression may be enhanced with other antineoplastic agents

Stability Protect from light

Mechanism of Action Interferes with DNA replication and RNA transcription by alkylation and cross-linking the strands of DNA (bifunctional alkylating agent)

Pharmacokinetics

Absorption: Oral: Well absorbed

Protein binding (mostly albumin): ~99%

Metabolism: In the liver to an active metabolite

Half-life: 6 minutes

Time to peak plasma concentrations: Within 1 hour

Elimination: 60% excreted in urine within 24 hours principally as metabolites

Usual Dosage Oral (refer to individual protocols):

Geriatrics: Use lowest recommended doses for adults; usual dose for elderly is 2-4 mg/day, particularly for use in treatment of rheumatoid arthritis

Adults: General short courses: 0.1-0.2 mg/kg/day or 4-8 mg/m²/day for 2-3 weeks for remission induction, then adjust dose on basis of blood counts; maintenance therapy: 0.03-0.1 mg/kg/day

Nephrotic syndrome: 0.1-0.2 mg/kg/day every day for 5-15 weeks with low dose prednisone

CLL: Biweekly regimen: Initial: 0.4 mg/kg dose is increased by 0.1 mg/kg every 2 weeks until a response occurs and/or myelosuppression occurs; monthly regimen: Initial: 0.4 mg/kg, increase dose by 0.2 mg/kg every 4 weeks until a response occurs and/or myelosuppression occurs

Malignant lymphomas: Non-Hodgkin's lymphoma: 0.1 mg/kg/day; Hodgkin's: 0.2 mg/kg/day

Not dialyzable

Monitoring Parameters Monitor WBC and platelet counts closely (weekly); observe for CNS side effects/toxicity

Test Interactions Increased potassium (S)

Patient Information Any signs of infection (fever, chills, sore throat), easy bruising or bleeding, shortness of breath, black tarry stools, yellow discoloration of skin or eyes, bloody or dark urine, joint pain, swelling, or painful or burning urination should be brought to physician's attention. Nausea, vomiting or hair loss sometimes occurs. Food may delay absorption; take on empty stomach; avoid alcohol, prolonged sun exposure. May cause loss of appetite.

Nursing Implications See Monitoring Parameters, Patient Information, and Additional Information

Additional Information

Myelosuppressive effects:

WBC: Moderate

Platelets: Moderate

Onset (days): 7

Nadir (days): 10-14

Recovery (days): 28

Special Geriatric Considerations Toxicity to immunosuppressives is increased in elderly. Start with lowest recommended adult doses (see Usual Dosage). Signs of infection, such as fever and rise in WBCs, may not occur. Lethargy and confusion may be more prominent signs of infection.

Dosage Forms Tablet, sugar coated: 2 mg

References

Hutchins LF and Lipschitz DA, "Cancer, Clinical Pharmacology, and Aging," *Clin Geriatr Med*, 1987, 3(3):483-503.

Kaplan HG, "Use of Cancer Chemotherapy in the Elderly," *Drug Treatment in the Elderly*, Vestal RE, ed, Boston, MA: ADIS Health Science Press, 1984, 338-49.

Chloramphenicol (klor am FEN i kole)

Related Information

Penicillins, Penicillin-Related Antibiotics, & Other Antibiotics *on page 1010*

Brand Names AK-Chlor® Ophthalmic; Chloromycetin®; Chloroptic® Ophthalmic

Generic Available Yes

Therapeutic Category Antibacterial, Topical; Antibiotic, Ophthalmic; Antibiotic, Otic; Antibiotic, Miscellaneous

Use Treatment of serious infections due to organisms resistant to other less toxic antibiotics or when its penetrability into the site of infection is clinically superior to other antibiotics to which the organism is sensitive; useful in infections caused by *Bacteroides*, *H. influenzae*, *Neisseria meningitidis*, *Salmonella*, and *Rickettsia*

Contraindications Hypersensitivity to chloramphenicol or any component

Warnings Serious and fatal blood dyscrasias have occurred after both short-term and prolonged therapy; should not be used when less potentially toxic agents are effective; prolonged use may result in superinfection; use with care in patients with glucose 6-phosphate dehydrogenase deficiency

Precautions Reduce dose with impaired liver function

Adverse Reactions

Central nervous system: Nightmares, headache, mental depression, confusion, delirium

Dermatologic: Rash

Gastrointestinal: Diarrhea, stomatitis, enterocolitis, dysgeusia, nausea, vomiting

Hematologic: Bone marrow suppression, aplastic anemia

(Continued)

Chloramphenicol *(Continued)*

Neuromuscular & skeletal: Peripheral neuropathy
Ocular: Optic neuritis

Overdosage Symptoms of overdose include anemia, metabolic acidosis, hypotension, hypothermia

Drug Interactions
Chloramphenicol inhibits the metabolism and may increase the effects of chlorpropamide, tolbutamide, phenytoin, phenobarbital, oral anticoagulants, cyclophosphamide
Phenobarbital and rifampin may decrease concentration of chloramphenicol
Acetaminophen may increase chloramphenicol serum concentrations
Response to iron and vitamin B_{12} may be decreased; avoid concomitant use with other drugs that may cause bone marrow suppression

Stability Refrigerate ophthalmic solution; constituted solutions remain stable for 30 days; use only clear solutions; frozen solutions remain stable for 6 months

Mechanism of Action Reversibly binds to 50S ribosomal subunits of susceptible organisms preventing amino acids from being transferred to growing peptide chains thus inhibiting protein synthesis

Pharmacokinetics
Absorption: Oral: 75% to 100%
Chloramphenicol palmitate is hydrolyzed in the GI tract to the base; chloramphenicol sodium succinate must be hydrolyzed by esterases to active base
Protein binding: 60%
Metabolism: Extensive metabolism in the liver (90%) to inactive metabolites, principally by glucuronidation
Half-life: 1.6-3.3 hours (increased with hepatic insufficiency)
Time to peak serum concentration: Oral: Within 0.5-3 hours
Elimination: 5% to 15% excreted as unchanged drug in urine and 4% excreted in bile

Usual Dosage Geriatrics and Adults:
Ophthalmic: Apply 1-2 drops or small amount of ointment every 3-6 hours; increase interval between applications after 48 hours
Topical: Gently rub into the affected area 3-4 times/day
Meningitis: Oral, I.V.: 50 mg/kg/day in divided doses every 6 hours; maximum daily dose: 4 g/day
Slightly dialyzable (5% to 20%)

Monitoring Parameters Complete blood count with reticulocyte count should be done before therapy and then weekly; periodic liver and renal function (see Reference Levels)

Reference Range
Sample size: 0.5-2 mL blood (red top tube) or 0.1-1 mL serum (separated)
Therapeutic: 15-20 µg/mL; Toxic: >40 µg/mL
Timing of serum samples: Draw levels 1.5 hours and 3 hours after I.V. dose or oral dose

Test Interactions Increased iron (B), prothrombin time; decreased urea nitrogen (B)

Patient Information Take on empty stomach; take with food if GI upset, at evenly spaced intervals (every 6 hours around-the-clock); notify physician if fever, sore throat, unusual bruising or bleeding, or decreased energy are experienced

Nursing Implications Administer around-the-clock rather than 4 times/day to promote less variation in peak and trough serum concentration (see Monitoring Parameters)

Additional Information Sodium content of 1 g (injection): 51.8 mg (2.25 mEq)

Special Geriatric Considerations Chloramphenicol has not been studied in the elderly; it is not necessary to adjust the dose based upon the decrease in renal function associated with age. Chloramphenicol should be reserved for serious infections and the oral form avoided.

Dosage Forms
Capsule: 250 mg
Cream: 1% (30 g)
Injection, as sodium succinate: 100 mg/mL
Ointment, ophthalmic: 1% (3.5 g)
Powder for solution, ophthalmic: 25 mg/vial
Solution:
Ophthalmic: 0.5% (7.5 mL)
Otic: 0.5% (15 mL)

References
Nahata MC and Powell DA, "Bioavailability and Clearance of Chloramphenicol After Intravenous Chloramphenicol Succinate," *Clin Pharmacol Ther*, 1981, 30(3):368-72.

Yoshikawa TT, "Antimicrobial Therapy for the Elderly Patient," *J Am Geriatr Soc*, 1990, 38(12):1353-72.

Chlorate® [OTC] *see* Chlorpheniramine *on page 208*

Chlordiazepoxide (klor dye az e POKS ide)

Related Information
Antacid Drug Interactions *on page 1096*
Anxiolytic/Hypnotic Use in Long-Term Care Facilities *on page 1099*
Benzodiazepines Comparison *on page 1024*
Federal OBRA Regulations Recommended Maximum Doses - Anxiolytics *on page 1057*
I.V. Push Recommended Guidelines *on page 1083*

Brand Names Libritabs®; Librium®; Mitran® Oral; Reposans-10® Oral

Synonyms Methaminodiazepoxide Hydrochloride

Generic Available Yes

Therapeutic Category Antianxiety Agent; Benzodiazepine; Hypnotic; Sedative

Use Management of anxiety and as a preoperative sedative, symptoms of alcohol withdrawal

Restrictions C-IV

Contraindications Hypersensitivity to chlordiazepoxide or any component, may be cross-sensitive with other benzodiazepines; pre-existing CNS depression, severe uncontrolled pain, narrow-angle glaucoma, severe respiratory depression

Precautions Use with caution in patients with liver dysfunction or a history of drug dependence

Adverse Reactions
Cardiovascular: Hypotension, tachycardia, edema
Central nervous system: Drowsiness, ataxia, confusion, mental impairment
Dermatologic: Skin eruptions
Gastrointestinal: Nausea, constipation
Hematologic: Blood dyscrasias
Neuromuscular & skeletal: Reflex slowing
Miscellaneous: Drug dependence, **falls in the elderly**

Overdosage Symptoms of overdose include hypotension, respiratory depression, coma, hypothermia, cardiac arrhythmias

Toxicology Treatment for benzodiazepine overdose is supportive; rarely is mechanical ventilation required; flumazenil has been shown to selectively block the binding of benzodiazepines to CNS receptors, resulting in a reversal of benzodiazepine-induced CNS depression; respiratory depression may not be reversed

Drug Interactions Benzodiazepines may decrease the effect of levodopa
Decreased metabolism: Cimetidine, fluoxetine
Increased metabolism: Rifampin
Increased toxicity: CNS depressants, alcohol

Stability Refrigerate injection; protect from light

Mechanism of Action Benzodiazepines appear to potentiate the effects of GABA and other inhibitory neurotransmitters by binding to specific benzodiazepine-receptor sites in various areas of the CNS

Pharmacodynamics Studies have shown that the elderly are more sensitive to the effects of benzodiazepines as compared to younger adults

Pharmacokinetics
Absorption: I.M.: Slow and erratic
Distribution: V_d: 3.3 L/kg
Protein binding: 90% to 98%
Metabolism: Extensive in the liver to desmethyldiazepam (active and long-acting)
Half-life: 6.6-25 hours; increased in elderly and in severe liver disease
Time to peak serum concentration:
Oral: Within 2 hours
I.M.: Results in lower peak plasma concentrations than oral administration
Elimination: Very little excreted in urine as unchanged drug

Usual Dosage
Geriatrics: Anxiety: Oral: 5 mg 2-4 times/day
Adults:
Anxiety: Oral: 15-100 mg divided 3-4 times/day
(Continued)

Chlordiazepoxide (Continued)

Alcohol withdrawal symptoms: Oral, I.V.: 50-100 mg to start, dose may be repeated in 2-4 hours as necessary to a maximum of 300 mg/24 hours

Dosing adjustment in renal impairment: Cl_{cr} <10 mL/minute: 50% of dose
Not dialyzable (0% to 5%)

Administration I.V. form is a powder and should be reconstituted with 5 mL of sterile water or saline prior to administration; do not use diluent provided with ampul for I.V. administration

Monitoring Parameters Respiratory, cardiovascular and mental status; check for orthostasis

Reference Range Therapeutic: 0.1-3 µg/mL (SI: 0-10 µmol/L); Toxic: >23 µg/mL (SI: >77 µmol/L)

Patient Information Avoid alcohol and other CNS depressants; may cause drowsiness; avoid activities needing good psychomotor coordination until CNS effects are known; may cause physical or psychological dependence; avoid abrupt discontinuation after prolonged use

Nursing Implications Up to 300 mg may be given I.M. or I.V. during a 6-hour period, but not more than this in any 24-hour period (see Administration); assist patient with ambulation during initiation of therapy

Special Geriatric Considerations Due to its long-acting metabolite, chlordiazepoxide is not considered a drug of choice in the elderly (see Pharmacodynamics and Pharmacokinetics); long-acting benzodiazepines have been associated with falls in the elderly; interpretive guidelines from the Health Care Financing Administration (HCFA) discourage the use of this agent in residents of long-term care facilities

Dosage Forms

Capsule, as hydrochloride: 5 mg, 10 mg, 25 mg
Powder for injection, as hydrochloride: 100 mg
Tablet: 5 mg, 10 mg, 25 mg

References

Hicks R, Dysken MW, Davis JM, et al, "The Pharmacokinetics of Psychotropic Medication in the Elderly: A Review," *J Clin Psychiatry*, 1981, 42(10):374-85.
Reidenberg MM, Levy M, Warner H, et al, "Relationship Between Diazepam Dose, Plasma Level, Age, and Central Nervous System Depression," *Clin Pharmacol Ther*, 1978, 23(4):371-4.

Chlordiazepoxide and Clidinium see Clidinium and Chlordiazepoxide on page 231

Chlorhexidine Gluconate (klor HEKS i deen GLOO koe nate)

Brand Names BactoShield® Topical [OTC]; Betasept® [OTC]; Dyna-Hex® Topical [OTC]; Exidine® Scrub [OTC]; Hibiclens® Topical [OTC]; Hibistat® Topical [OTC]; Peridex® Oral Rinse; PerioGard®

Generic Available No

Therapeutic Category Antibiotic, Oral Rinse; Antibiotic, Topical

Use Skin cleanser for surgical scrub, cleanser for skin wounds, germicidal hand rinse, and as antibacterial dental rinse; chlorhexidine is active against gram-positive and gram-negative organisms, facultative anaerobes, aerobes, and yeast

Contraindications Known hypersensitivity to chlorhexidine gluconate

Adverse Reactions Staining of oral surfaces (mucosa, teeth, dorsum of tongue) may be visible as soon as one week after therapy begins and is more pronounced when there is a heavy accumulation of unremoved plaque and when teeth fillings have rough surfaces. Stain does not have a clinically adverse effect but because removal may not be possible, patient with frontal restoration should be advised of the potential permanency of the stain. Inform patient that reduced taste perception during treatment is reversible with discontinuation of chlorhexidine.

Usual Dosage

Geriatrics and Adults:

Oral rinse (Peridex®):

Precede use of solution by flossing and brushing teeth, completely rinse toothpaste from mouth; swish 15 mL undiluted oral rinse around in mouth for 30 seconds, then expectorate. Caution patient not to swallow the medicine; avoid eating for 2-3 hours after treatment. (The cap on bottle of oral rinse is a measure for 15 mL.)

When used as a treatment of gingivitis, the regimen begins with oral prophylaxis. Patient treats mouth with 15 mL chlorhexidine; swish for 30 seconds, then expectorate. This is repeated twice daily (morning and evening). Patient should have a re-evaluation followed by a dental prophylaxis every 6 months.

Cleanser:
   Surgical scrub: Scrub 3 minutes and rinse thoroughly, wash for an additional 3 minutes
   Hand wash: Wash for 15 seconds and rinse
   Hand rinse: Rub 15 seconds and rinse
Patient Information Do not swallow, do not rinse after use; may cause reduced taste perception which is reversible; keep out of eyes and ears; may discolor teeth
Nursing Implications See Usual Dosage
Special Geriatric Considerations See Usual Dosage
Dosage Forms
Liquid, topical, with isopropyl alcohol 4%:
   Dyna-Hex® Skin Cleanser: 2% (120 mL, 240 mL, 480 mL, 960 mL, 4000 mL); 4% (120 mL, 240 mL, 480 mL, 4000 mL)
   Exidine® skin cleanser, Hibiclens® skin cleanser: 4% (15 mL, 120 mL, 240 mL, 480 mL, 960 mL, 4000 mL)
Rinse:
   Oral (mint flavor) (Peridex®): 0.12% with alcohol 11.6% (480 mL)
   Topical (Hibistat® hand rinse): 0.5% with isopropyl alcohol 70% (120 mL, 240 mL)
Sponge/Brush (Hibiclens®): 4% with isopropyl alcohol 4% (22 mL)
Wipes (Hibistat®): 0.5% (50s)

Chloromycetin® see Chloramphenicol on page 203
Chloroptic® Ophthalmic see Chloramphenicol on page 203

Chlorothiazide (klor oh THYE a zide)
Brand Names Diurigen®; Diuril®
Generic Available Yes: Tablet
Therapeutic Category Diuretic, Thiazide
Use Management of mild to moderate hypertension, or edema associated with congestive heart failure, or nephrotic syndrome in patients unable to take oral hydrochlorothiazide, when a thiazide is the diuretic of choice
Contraindications Hypersensitivity to chlorothiazide or any component; cross-sensitivity with other thiazides or sulfonamides; do not use in anuric patients.
Warnings The injection must not be administered S.C. or I.M.; I.V. chlorothiazide should only be used in emergency situations or when the patient is unable to take the oral form
Precautions May cause hyperbilirubinemia, fluid and electrolyte imbalance, hyperglycemia, hyperuricemia
Adverse Reactions
Cardiovascular: Hypotension
Dermatologic: Rash, photosensitivity
Endocrine & metabolic: Hypokalemia, hypochloremic alkalosis, hyperglycemia, hyperlipidemia, hyponatremia, hyperuricemia
Genitourinary: Prerenal azotemia
Hematologic: Rarely blood dyscrasias
Overdosage Symptoms of overdose include electrolyte depletion, volume depletion
Toxicology Treatment is primarily symptomatic and supportive; hypotension responds to fluids and Trendelenburg position; replace electrolytes as necessary
Drug Interactions
Decreased effect: NSAIDs
Decreased effect of oral hypoglycemics; decreased absorption with cholestyramine and colestipol
Increased effect with furosemide and other loop diuretics
Increased toxicity/levels of lithium; when given with digoxin, diuretic-induced hypokalemia increases the risk of digoxin toxicity
Stability Reconstituted solution is stable for 24 hours at room temperature; precipitation will occur in <24 hours in pH is <7.4
Mechanism of Action Inhibits sodium reabsorption in the distal tubules causing increased excretion of sodium and water as well as potassium and hydrogen ions
Pharmacodynamics
Onset of action: Oral: Diuresis: 2 hours
Duration:
   Oral: 6-12 hours
   I.V.: Diuretic action: ~2 hours
(Continued)

Chlorothiazide *(Continued)*

Pharmacokinetics
Absorption: Oral: Poor
Half-life: 1-2 hours
Time to peak serum concentration: Within 4 hours

Usual Dosage
Geriatrics: Oral: 500 mg once daily or 1 g 3 times/week
Adults: Oral, I.V.: 500 mg to 2 g/day divided in 1-2 doses

Administration I.V. must be prepared with at least 15 mL of diluent

Monitoring Parameters Blood pressure (standing and sitting/supine), serum electrolytes, renal function, I & O, weight

Test Interactions Increased ammonia (B), amylase (S), calcium (S), chloride (S), cholesterol (S), glucose, uric acid (S); decreased chloride (S), magnesium, potassium (S), sodium (S)

Patient Information Take in the morning; may cause increased sensitivity to sunlight; rise slowly from lying down or sitting

Nursing Implications Injection must **not** be administered S.C. or I.M. (see Monitoring Parameters); check patient for orthostasis

Additional Information Sodium content of 500 mg injection: 57.5 mg (2 mEq)

Special Geriatric Considerations Chlorothiazide is minimally effective in patients with a Cl_{cr} <30 mL/minute; this may limit the usefulness of chlorothiazide in the elderly

Dosage Forms
Injection, as sodium: 25 mg/mL (20 mL)
Suspension: 250 mg/5 mL (237 mL)
Tablet: 250 mg, 500 mg

Chlorphed® [OTC] *see* Brompheniramine *on page 129*
Chlorphed®-LA Nasal Solution [OTC] *see* Oxymetazoline *on page 706*

Chlorpheniramine *(klor fen IR a meen)*

Brand Names Aller-Chlor® [OTC]; AL-R® [OTC]; Chlo-Amine® [OTC]; Chlorate® [OTC]; Chlor-Pro® [OTC]; Chlor-Trimeton® [OTC]; Kloromin® [OTC]; Phenetron®; Telachlor®; Teldrin® [OTC]

Synonyms CTM

Generic Available Yes

Therapeutic Category Antihistamine

Use Perennial and seasonal allergic rhinitis and other allergic symptoms including urticaria

Contraindications Hypersensitivity to chlorpheniramine maleate or any component; narrow-angle glaucoma, bladder neck obstruction, symptomatic prostate hypertrophy, asthmatic attacks, and stenosing peptic ulcer

Warnings Antihistamines are more likely to cause dizziness, excessive sedation, syncope, toxic confusional states, and hypotension in the elderly

Precautions Use with caution in patients with heart disease, hypertension, thyroid disease, and asthma

Adverse Reactions
Central nervous system: Drowsiness, headache, paradoxical excitability
Dermatologic: Dermatitis
Gastrointestinal: Nausea, xerostomia
Ocular: Diplopia
Genitourinary: Polyuria, urinary retention
Neuromuscular & skeletal: Weakness
Respiratory: Thick bronchial secretions

Overdosage Symptoms of overdose include dry mouth, flushed skin, dilated pupils, CNS depression

Toxicology There is no specific treatment for an antihistamine overdose, however, most of its clinical toxicity is due to anticholinergic effects. Cholinesterase inhibitors may be useful by reducing acetylcholinesterase. Acetylcholinesterase inhibitors include physostigmine, neostigmine, pyridostigmine, and edrophonium. For anticholinergic overdose with severe life-threatening symptoms, physostigmine 1-2 mg I.V., slowly may be given to reverse these effects.

Drug Interactions Increased toxicity (CNS depression): CNS depressants, monoamine oxidase inhibitors, alcohol, tricyclic antidepressants, phenothiazines

Mechanism of Action Competes with histamine for H_1-receptor sites on effector cells in the gastrointestinal tract, blood vessels, and respiratory tract

Pharmacokinetics
Protein binding: 69% to 72%
Metabolism: In the liver
Half-life: 20-24 hours; one study found no significant difference in the half-life in elderly subjects though there was wide interindividual variation
Elimination: Metabolites and parent drug (3% to 4%) excreted in urine; 35% of total within 48 hours

Usual Dosage Oral:
Geriatrics: 4 mg once or twice daily or 8 mg sustained release at bedtime. **Note:** Duration of action may be 36 hours or more even when serum concentrations are low.
Adults: 4 mg every 4-6 hours, not to exceed 24 mg/day or sustained release 8-12 mg every 12 hours

Administration Do not crush sustained release tablet

Monitoring Parameters Relief of symptoms

Patient Information May cause drowsiness; avoid CNS depressants and alcohol; swallow whole, do not crush or chew

Nursing Implications Raise bed rails and institute safety measures; assist with ambulation

Additional Information Chlorpheniramine is available in various combinations. These include acetaminophen; phenylephrine; phenylpropanolamine; pseudoephedrine; phenylephrine and phenyltoloxamine; phenylpropanolamine and acetaminophen; pseudoephedrine and iodine; phenyltoloxamine, phenylpropanolamine, and phenylephrine.

Special Geriatric Considerations Anticholinergic action may cause significant confusional symptoms, constipation, or problems voiding urine (see Contraindications, Warnings, and Usual Dosage)

Dosage Forms
Chlorpheniramine maleate:
Capsule: 12 mg
Capsule, timed release: 8 mg, 12 g
Syrup: 2 mg/5 mL (120 mL, 473 mL)
Tablet: 4 mg, 8 mg, 12 mg
Tablet:
Chewable: 2 mg
Timed release: 8 mg, 12 mg

References
Simons KJ, Martin TJ, Watson WT, et al, "Pharmacokinetics and Pharmacodynamics of Terfenadine and Chlorpheniramine in the Elderly," *J Allergy Clin Immunol*, 1990, 85(3):540-7.

Chlor-Pro® [OTC] *see Chlorpheniramine on previous page*

Chlorpromazine (klor PROE ma zeen)
Related Information
Antacid Drug Interactions *on page 1096*
Antipsychotic Agents Comparison *on page 1023*
Antipsychotic Medication Guidelines *on page 1076*
Federal OBRA Regulations Recommended Maximum Doses - Antipsychotics *on page 1056*
I.V. Push Recommended Guidelines *on page 1083*

Brand Names Ormazine; Thorazine®

Generic Available Yes

Therapeutic Category Antiemetic; Antipsychotic Agent; Neuroleptic Agent; Phenothiazine Derivative

Use Treatment of nausea and vomiting; psychoses; Tourette's syndrome; mania; intractable hiccups (adults); behavioral problems in nonpsychotic symptoms associated with dementia in elderly; Huntington's chorea; spasmodic torticollis (see Special Geriatric Considerations)

Contraindications Hypersensitivity to chlorpromazine hydrochloride or any component; cross-sensitivity with other phenothiazines may exist; avoid use in patients with narrow-angle glaucoma, bone marrow suppression, severe liver or cardiac disease; subcortical brain damage; circulatory collapse; severe hypotension or hypertension

Warnings Significant hypotension may occur, especially when the drug is administered parenterally; extended release capsules and injection contain benzyl alcohol; injection also contains sulfites which may cause allergic reaction

Tardive dyskinesia: Prevalence rate may be 40% in elderly; elderly women especially at risk; embarrassment from dyskinesias may lead to greater social isolation; development of the syndrome and the irreversible nature
(Continued)

Chlorpromazine *(Continued)*

are proportional to duration and total cumulative dose over time. May be reversible if diagnosed early in therapy; intermittent use of antipsychotics (not proven use) helps decrease total cumulative dose.

EPS: Extrapyramidal reactions are more common in elderly with up to 50% developing these reactions after age 60. These reactions may be more common in dementia patients. Drug-induced **Parkinson's syndrome** occurs often. Discontinuation usually resolves symptoms but may take weeks to months (12+) to clear. **Akathisia** is the most common EPS reaction in elderly. The symptoms of motor restlessness are difficult to diagnose in demented elderly; increased nervousness, assertiveness, restlessness with constant movement may indicate this adverse event. Consider decreasing dose if antipsychotic to treat as well as diagnose problem; usually see this reaction within 2-3 months of initiating antipsychotic drug.

Anticholinergic effects: These side effects most common with low potency antipsychotics (eg, thioridazine, chlorpromazine). CNS toxicity occurs more frequently and severely in elderly; increased confusion, memory loss, psychotic behavior, and agitation frequently occur as a consequence of anticholinergic effects to antipsychotic agents. Peripheral anticholinergic action troublesome to elderly; most peripheral anticholinergic effects last only 2-3 weeks (see Adverse Reactions).

Orthostatic hypotension: More common with low potency agents (eg, thioridazine, chlorpromazine, and clozapine) but of concern with all antipsychotic agents; orthostasis due to alpha-receptor blockade by antipsychotic agents. Elderly present many risk factors for orthostatic hypotension: blunted baroreceptor reflexes, decreased vascular tone, decreased vascular volume, and possible presence of cardiac diseases which result in decreased cardiac output.

Sedation: Common side effect with antipsychotic therapy; should not be used as a hypnotic unless insomnia is associated with target behavior symptoms treated with antipsychotic medications (see Special Geriatric Considerations). Anecdotal reports suggesting antipsychotic sedation in nonpsychotic patients is extremely unpleasant due to feelings of depersonalization, derealization, and dysphoria. Due to the long duration of action with antipsychotic drugs, these reactions may last up to 24 hours and result in decreased daytime function.

Cardiac toxicity: Life-threatening arrhythmias have occurred at therapeutic doses of antipsychotics. Thioridazine more commonly demonstrates EKG changes than other antipsychotics; suggested to use high potency antipsychotic agents (ie, haloperidol) in patients with cardiac conduction defects.

Precautions Use with caution in patients with cardiovascular disease, seizures, and Parkinson's disease; benefits of therapy must be weighed against risks

Adverse Reactions

Cardiovascular: Hypotension (especially with I.V. use), orthostatic hypotension, tachycardia, arrhythmias, abnormal T waves with prolonged ventricular repolarization

Central nervous system: Sedation, drowsiness, restlessness, anxiety, extrapyramidal reactions, pseudoparkinsonian signs and symptoms, tardive dyskinesia, neuroleptic malignant syndrome, seizures, altered central temperature regulation

Dermatologic: Hyperpigmentation, pruritus, rash, photosensitivity

Endocrine & metabolic: Amenorrhea, galactorrhea, gynecomastia

Gastrointestinal: GI upset, xerostomia (problem for denture users), constipation, adynamic ileus, weight gain

Genitourinary: Urinary retention, overflow incontinence, priapism, sexual dysfunction (up to 60%), impotence

Hematologic: Agranulocytosis, leukopenia (usually in patients with large doses for prolonged periods), thrombocytopenia, hemolytic anemia, eosinophilia

Hepatic: Cholestatic jaundice (rare)

Ocular: Retinal pigmentation, blurred vision

Miscellaneous: Anaphylactoid reactions

Overdosage Symptoms of overdose include deep sleep, coma, extrapyramidal symptoms, abnormal involuntary muscle movements, hypotension or hypertension; agitation, restlessness, fever, hypothermia or hyperthermia, seizures, cardiac arrhythmias, EKG changes

Toxicology Following initiation of essential overdose management, toxic symptom treatment and supportive treatment should be initiated. Hypotension usually responds to I.V. fluids or Trendelenburg positioning. If unresponsive to these measures the use of a parenteral inotrope may be required (eg, norepinephrine 0.1-0.2 mcg/kg/minute titrated to response). Do not use epinephrine. Seizures commonly respond to diazepam (I.V. 5-10 mg bolus every 15 minutes if needed up to a total of 30 mg) or to phenytoin or phenobarbital. Also critical cardiac arrhythmias often respond to I.V. phenytoin (15 mg/kg up to 1 g), while other antiarrhythmics can be used. Neuroleptics often cause extrapyramidal symptoms (eg, dystonic reactions) requiring management with diphenhydramine 1-2 mg/kg up to a maximum of 50 mg I.V. slow push followed by a maintenance dose for 48-72 hours. When these reactions are unresponsive to diphenhydramine, benztropine mesylate I.V. 1-2 mg may be effective. These agents are generally effective within 2-5 minutes.

Drug Interactions

Alcohol may increase CNS sedation

Anticholinergic agents may decrease pharmacologic effects; increase anticholinergic side effects; may enhance tardive dyskinesia

Aluminum salts may decrease absorption of phenothiazines

Anorexiants with phenothiazines may decrease the effects of amphetamines and their congenes

Barbiturates may decrease phenothiazine serum concentrations

Bromocriptine may have decreased efficacy when administered with phenothiazines

Guanethidine's hypotensive effect is decreased by phenothiazines

Lithium administration with phenothiazines may increase disorientation

Meperidine and phenothiazine coadministration increases sedation and hypotension

Methyldopa administration with phenothiazine (trifluoperazine) may significantly increase blood pressure

Norepinephrine, epinephrine have decreased pressor effect when administered with chlorpromazine; therefore, be aware of possible decreased effectiveness or when any phenothiazine is used

Phenytoin serum concentrations may increase or decrease with phenothiazines; tricyclic antidepressants may have increased serum concentrations with concomitant administration with phenothiazines

Propranolol administered with phenothiazines may increase serum concentrations of both drugs

Tricyclic antidepressants may have serum concentrations increased by phenothiazines

Valproic acid may have increased half-life when administered with phenothiazines (chlorpromazine)

Stability Slightly yellowed solution does not indicate potency loss, but a markedly discolored solution should be discarded; diluted injection (1 mg/mL) with NS and stored in 5 mL vials remain stable for 30 days; protect all dosage forms from light, clear or slightly yellow solutions may be used; should be dispensed in amber or opaque vials/bottles. Solutions may be diluted or mixed with fruit juices or other liquids but must be administered immediately after mixing; do not prepare bulk dilutions or store bulk dilutions.

Mechanism of Action Blocks postsynaptic mesolimbic dopaminergic D_1 and D_2 receptors in the brain; exhibits a strong alpha-adrenergic blocking and anticholinergic effect, depresses the release of hypothalamic and hypophyseal hormones; believed to depress the reticular activating system thus affecting basal metabolism, body temperature, wakefulness, vasomotor tone, and emesis

Pharmacokinetics

Metabolism: Extensive in the liver to active and inactive metabolites; substrate CYP2D6 and 3A4

Half-life:

Biphasic: 30 hours

Phase 1 half-life: 2 hours

Elimination: <1% excreted as unchanged drug in urine within 24 hours

Usual Dosage

Geriatrics (nonpsychotic patient; dementia behavior): Oral: Initial: 10-25 mg 1-2 times/day; increase at 4- to 7-day intervals by 10-25 mg/day. Increase dose intervals (bid, tid, etc) as necessary to control behavior response or side effects; maximum daily dose: 800 mg; gradual increases (titration) may prevent some side effects or decrease their severity.

(Continued)

Chlorpromazine *(Continued)*

Adults:
  Psychosis:
    Oral: Range: 30-800 mg/day in 1-4 divided doses, initiate at lower doses and titrate as needed; usual dose is 200 mg/day; some patients may require 1-2 g/day
    I.M., I.V.: Initial: 25 mg, may repeat (25-50 mg) in 1-4 hours, gradually increase to a maximum of 400 mg/dose every 4-6 hours until patient controlled; usual dose 300-800 mg/day
  Nausea and vomiting:
    Oral: 10-25 mg every 4-6 hours
    I.M., I.V.: 25-50 mg every 4-6 hours
    Rectal: 25-100 mg every 6-8 hours
  Not dialyzable (0% to 5%)

Monitoring Parameters Orthostatic blood pressures; tremors, gait changes, abnormal movement in trunk, neck, buccal area, or extremities; monitor target behaviors for which the agent is given

Reference Range Therapeutic: 30-300 ng/mL (SI: 157-942 nmol/L); Toxic: >750 ng/mL (SI: >2355 nmol/L); serum concentrations not often obtained since dose is titrated to best response, also correlation to response is controversial

Test Interactions False-positives for phenylketonuria, amylase, uroporphyrins, urobilinogen; possible false-negative pregnancy urinary test

Patient Information Oral concentrate must be diluted in 2-4 oz of liquid (water, fruit juice, carbonated drinks, milk, or pudding); do not take antacid within 1 hour of taking drug; avoid alcohol; avoid excess sun exposure (use sun block); may cause drowsiness, rise slowly from recumbent position; use of supportive stockings may help prevent orthostatic hypotension

Nursing Implications Dilute oral concentrate with water or juice before administration; avoid skin contact with oral suspension or solution; may cause contact dermatitis; monitor orthostatic blood pressures 3-5 days after initiation of therapy or a dose increase; observe for tremor and abnormal movement or posturing (extrapyramidal symptoms); watch for hypotension when administering I.M. or I.V.

Special Geriatric Considerations See Warnings.

Many elderly patients receive antipsychotic medications for inappropriate nonpsychotic behavior. Before initiating antipsychotic medication, the clinician should investigate any possible reversible cause; any stress or stress from any disease can cause acute "confusion" or worsening of baseline nonpsychotic behavior. Most commonly acute changes in behavior are due to increases in drug dose or addition of new drug to regimen; fluid electrolyte loss; infections; and changes in environment.

Any changes in disease status in any organ system can result in behavior changes.

In the treatment of agitated, demented, elderly patients, authors of meta-analysis of controlled trials of the response to the traditional antipsychotics (phenothiazines, butyrophenones) in controlling agitation have concluded that the use of neuroleptics results in a response rate of 18%. Clearly neuroleptic therapy for behavior control should be limited with frequent attempts to withdraw the agent given for behavior control.

Dosage Forms

Chlorpromazine hydrochloride:
    Capsule, sustained action: 30 mg, 75 mg, 150 mg, 200 mg, 300 mg
    Concentrate, oral: 30 mg/mL (120 mL); 100 mg/mL (60 mL, 240 mL)
    Injection: 25 mg/mL (1 mL, 2 mL, 10 mL)
    Syrup: 10 mg/5 mL (120 mL)
    Tablet: 10 mg, 25 mg, 50 mg, 100 mg, 200 mg
  Suppository, rectal, as base: 25 mg, 100 mg

References

Peabody CA, Warner MD, Whiteford HA, et al, "Neuroleptics and the Elderly," *J Am Geriatr Soc*, 1987, 35(3):233-8.

Risse SC and Barnes R, "Pharmacologic Treatment of Agitation Associated With Dementia," *J Am Geriatr Soc*, 1986, 34(5):368-76.

Saltz BL, Woerner MG, Kane JM, et al, "Prospective Study of Tardive Dyskinesia Incidence in the Elderly," *JAMA*, 1991, 266(17):2402-6.

Seifert RD, "Therapeutic Drug Monitoring: Psychotropic Drugs," *J Pharm Pract*, 1984, 6:403-16.

Chlorpropamide *(klor PROE pa mide)*

Related Information

Antacid Drug Interactions *on page 1096*

Brand Names Diabinese®

Generic Available Yes

Therapeutic Category Antidiabetic Agent; Hypoglycemic Agent, Oral; Sulfonylurea Agent

Use Adjunct to diet for the management of mild to moderately severe, stable noninsulin-dependent (type II) diabetes mellitus

Unlabeled use: Neurogenic diabetes insipidus

Contraindications Cross-sensitivity may exist with other hypoglycemics or sulfonamides; do not use with type 1 diabetes, or with severe renal, hepatic, thyroid, or other endocrine disease, diabetes complicated by ketoacidosis; patients with reduced renal function, dietary noncompliance or irregular meals, alcohol abusers

Precautions Patients should be properly instructed in the early detection and treatment of hypoglycemia

Adverse Reactions

Cardiovascular: Edema

Central nervous system: Headache, dizziness

Dermatologic: Rash, urticaria, photosensitivity

Endocrine & metabolic: Hypoglycemia, hyponatremia, SIADH

Gastrointestinal: Anorexia, nausea, vomiting, diarrhea, constipation, heartburn, epigastric fullness

Hematologic: Aplastic anemia, hemolytic anemia, bone marrow suppression, agranulocytosis

Hepatic: Jaundice

Overdosage Symptoms of overdose include low blood glucose levels, tingling of lips and tongue, tachycardia, convulsions, stupor, coma

Toxicology Intoxications with sulfonylureas can cause hypoglycemia and are best managed with glucose administration (oral for milder hypoglycemia or by injection in more severe forms)

Drug Interactions

Decreased chlorpropamide effectiveness with thiazides, hydantoins (eg, phenytoin), and beta-adrenergic blockers

Increased toxicity: Increased alcohol-associated disulfiram reactions; increased oral anticoagulant effect; salicylates can increase chlorpropamide effect and can decrease blood glucose; MAO inhibitors increased hypoglycemic response; sulfonamides can decrease sulfonylureas clearance

Mechanism of Action Stimulates insulin release from the pancreatic beta cells; reduces glucose output from the liver; insulin sensitivity is increased at peripheral target sites

Pharmacodynamics

Peak clinical effect: Oral: Within 6-8 hours

Duration: May exceed 60 hours in the elderly

Pharmacokinetics

Distribution: V_d: 0.13-0.23 L/kg, increased in older diabetics

Protein binding: 88% to 99%

Metabolism: Extensive (~80%) in the liver; clearance decreased in older patients with diabetes

Half-life: 30-42 hours, prolonged in the elderly or with renal disease; in older diabetics: 99 hours

Time to peak serum concentration: Within 3-4 hours

Elimination: 10% to 30% excreted in urine as unchanged drug

Usual Dosage Oral (dosage is variable and should be individualized based upon the patient's response):

Geriatrics: Initial: 100 mg once daily; increase by 50-125 mg/day at 3- to 5-day intervals; maximum daily dose: 750 mg

Adults: 250 mg once daily; subsequent dosages may be increased or decreased by 50-125 mg/day at 3- to 5-day intervals; maximum daily dose: 750 mg

Monitoring Parameters Fasting blood glucose, Hgb A_{1c} or fructosamine levels

Reference Range Glucose: Adults: 60-115 mg/dL; elderly fasting blood glucose: 100-150 mg/dL

Test Interactions Positive Coombs' [direct]; decreased cholesterol (S), decreased prothrombin time, decreased sodium (S)

Patient Information Avoid hypoglycemia, eat regularly, do not skip meals; carry a quick source of sugar with you

Nursing Implications Patients who are anorexic or NPO may need to hold the dose to avoid hypoglycemia

(Continued)

Chlorpropamide *(Continued)*

Additional Information Long half-life may complicate recovery from excess effects

Special Geriatric Considerations Because of chlorpropamide's long half-life, duration of action, drug interactions, and the increased risk for hypoglycemia, it is not considered a hypoglycemic agent of choice in the elderly (see Pharmacokinetics and Pharmacodynamics). How "tightly" a geriatric patient's blood glucose should be controlled is controversial; however, a fasting blood sugar of <150 mg/dL is now an acceptable end point. Such a decision should be based on the patient's functional and cognitive status, how well they recognize hypoglycemic or hyperglycemic symptoms, and how to respond to them, and their other disease states.

Dosage Forms Tablet: 100 mg, 250 mg

References
Arrigoni L, Fundak G, Horn J, et al, "Chlorpropamide Pharmacokinetics in Young Healthy Adults and Older Diabetic Patients," *Clin Pharm*, 1987, 6(2):162-4.

Chlorprothixene *(klor proe THIKS een)*

Related Information

Antacid Drug Interactions *on page 1096*
Antipsychotic Agents Comparison *on page 1023*
Antipsychotic Medication Guidelines *on page 1076*
Federal OBRA Regulations Recommended Maximum Doses - Antipsychotics *on page 1056*

Brand Names Taractan®

Generic Available No

Therapeutic Category Antipsychotic Agent; Neuroleptic Agent; Phenothiazine Derivative; Thioxanthene Derivative

Use Management of manifestations of psychotic disorders; depressive neurosis; alcohol withdrawal; nausea and vomiting; nonpsychotic symptoms associated with dementia in elderly, Tourette's syndrome; Huntington's chorea; spasmodic torticollis and Reye's syndrome (see Special Geriatric Considerations)

Contraindications Circulatory collapse, hypersensitivity to chlorprothixene or any component; may cross react with thiothixene; comatose states due to central depressant drugs; severe CNS depression; subcortical brain damage; severe hypotension or hypertension; avoid use in patients with narrow-angle glaucoma, blood dyscrasias, severe liver or cardiac disease

Warnings

Tardive dyskinesia: Prevalence rate may be 40% in elderly; elderly women especially at risk; embarrassment from dyskinesias may lead to greater social isolation; development of the syndrome and the irreversible nature are proportional to duration and total cumulative dose over time. May be reversible if diagnosed early in therapy; intermittent use of antipsychotics (not proven use) helps decrease total cumulative dose.

EPS: Extrapyramidal reactions are more common in elderly with up to 50% developing these reactions after age 60. These reactions may be more common in dementia patients. Drug-induced **Parkinson's syndrome** occurs often. Discontinuation usually resolves symptoms but may take weeks to months (12+) to clear. **Akathisia** is the most common EPS reaction in elderly. The symptoms of motor restlessness are difficult to diagnose in demented elderly; increased nervousness, assertiveness, restlessness with constant movement may indicate this adverse event. Consider decreasing dose if antipsychotic to treat as well as diagnose problem; usually see this reaction within 2-3 months of initiating antipsychotic drug.

Anticholinergic effects: These side effects most common with low potency antipsychotics (eg, thioridazine, chlorpromazine). CNS toxicity occurs more frequently and severely in elderly; increased confusion, memory loss, psychotic behavior, and agitation frequently occur as a consequence of anticholinergic effects to antipsychotic agents. Peripheral anticholinergic action troublesome to elderly; most peripheral anticholinergic effects last only 2-3 weeks (see Adverse Reactions).

Orthostatic hypotension: More common with low potency agents (eg, thioridazine, chlorpromazine, and clozapine) but of concern with all antipsychotic agents; orthostasis due to alpha-receptor blockade by antipsychotic agents. Elderly present many risk factors for orthostatic hypotension: blunted baroreceptor reflexes, decreased vascular tone, decreased vascular volume, and possible presence of cardiac diseases which result in decreased cardiac output.

Sedation: Common side effect with antipsychotic therapy; should not be used as a hypnotic unless insomnia is associated with target behavior symptoms treated with antipsychotic medications (see Special Geriatric Considerations). Anecdotal reports suggesting antipsychotic sedation in nonpsychotic patients is extremely unpleasant due to feelings of depersonalization, derealization, and dysphoria. Due to the long duration of action with antipsychotic drugs, these reactions may last up to 24 hours and result in decreased daytime function.

Cardiac toxicity: Life-threatening arrhythmias have occurred at therapeutic doses of antipsychotics. Thioridazine more commonly demonstrates EKG changes than other antipsychotics; suggested to use high potency antipsychotic agents (ie, haloperidol) in patients with cardiac conduction defects.

Adverse Reactions

Cardiovascular: EKG changes, hypotension (especially orthostatic), tachycardia, arrhythmias, abnormal T waves with prolonged ventricular repolarization

Central nervous system: Drowsiness, restlessness, anxiety, extrapyramidal reactions, dystonic reactions, pseudoparkinsonian signs and symptoms, tardive dyskinesia, neuroleptic malignant syndrome, seizures, altered central temperature regulation

Dermatologic: Hyperpigmentation, pruritus, rash, contact dermatitis, photosensitivity (rare)

Endocrine & metabolic: Amenorrhea, galactorrhea, gynecomastia

Gastrointestinal: Xerostomia (problem for denture user), constipation, adynamic ileus, GI upset, weight gain

Genitourinary: Urinary retention, overflow incontinence, priapism, sexual dysfunction (up to 60%)

Hematologic: Agranulocytosis, leukopenia (usually in patients with large doses for prolonged periods)

Hepatic: Cholestatic jaundice

Ocular: Retinal pigmentation (more common than with chlorpromazine), blurred vision, decreased visual acuity (may be irreversible)

Sedation and anticholinergic effects are more pronounced than extrapyramidal effects

Overdosage Symptoms of overdose include deep sleep, coma, extrapyramidal symptoms, abnormal involuntary muscle movements, hypotension or hypertension; agitation, restlessness, fever, hypothermia or hyperthermia, seizures, cardiac arrhythmias, EKG changes

Toxicology Following initiation of essential overdose management, toxic symptom treatment and supportive treatment should be initiated. Hypotension usually responds to I.V. fluids or Trendelenburg positioning. If unresponsive to these measures the use of a parenteral inotrope may be required (eg, norepinephrine 0.1-0.2 mcg/kg/minute titrated to response). Do not use epinephrine. Seizures commonly respond to diazepam (I.V. 5-10 mg bolus in adults every 15 minutes if needed up to a total of 30 mg) or to phenytoin or phenobarbital. Also critical cardiac arrhythmias often respond to I.V. phenytoin (15 mg/kg up to 1 g), while other antiarrhythmics can be used. Neuroleptics often cause extrapyramidal symptoms (eg, dystonic reactions) requiring management with diphenhydramine 1-2 mg/kg up to a maximum of 50 mg I.M. or I.V. slow push followed by a maintenance dose for 48-72 hours. When these reactions are unresponsive to diphenhydramine, benztropine mesylate I.V. 1-2 mg may be effective. These agents are generally effective within 2-5 minutes.

Drug Interactions Guanethidine's hypotensive effect may be decreased by thioxanthenes

Stability Protect all dosage forms from light, clear or slightly yellow solutions may be used; should be dispensed in amber or opaque vials/bottles. Solutions may be diluted or mixed with fruit juices or other liquids but must be administered immediately after mixing; do not prepare bulk dilutions or store bulk dilutions.

Mechanism of Action Blocks postsynaptic mesolimbic dopaminergic D_1 and D_2 receptors in the brain; exhibits a strong alpha-adrenergic blocking and anticholinergic effect; depresses the release of hypothalamic and hypophyseal hormones; believed to depress the reticular activating system thus affecting basal metabolism, body temperature, wakefulness, vasomotor tone, and emesis

Pharmacokinetics

Absorption: Oral absorption results in peak concentrations between 2-4 hours. Absorption may be affected by the inherent anticholinergic action on

(Continued)

Chlorprothixene *(Continued)*

the gastrointestinal tissue causing variable absorption. Absorption from tablets is erratic with less variation seen with solutions.

Distribution: Widely distributed in tissues with CNS concentrations exceeding that of plasma due to their lipophilic characteristics.

Protein binding: Antipsychotic agents are bound 90% to 99% to plasma proteins; highly bound to brain and lung tissue and other tissues with a high blood perfusion.

Elimination: Elimination occurs through hepatic metabolism (oxidation) where numerous active metabolites are produced; active metabolites excreted in urine; elimination half-lives of antipsychotics ranges from 20-40 hours which may be extended in elderly due to decline in oxidative hepatic reactions (phase I) with age. The biologic effect of a single dose persists for 24 hours. When the patient has accommodated to initial side effects (sedation), once daily dosing is possible due to the long half-life of antipsychotics.

Steady-state plasma concentrations are achieved in 4-7 days; therefore, if possible, do not make dose adjustments more than once in a 7-day period. Due to the long half-lives of antipsychotics, as needed (prn) use is ineffective since repeated doses are necessary to achieve therapeutic tissue concentrations in the CNS.

Usual Dosage

Geriatrics (nonpsychotic patient; dementia behavior): 10 mg 1-2 times/day; increase dose 10 mg/day at 4- to 7-day intervals; increase dosing intervals (bid, tid, etc) as necessary to control response or side effects; maximum daily dose: 300 mg; gradual increases (titration) may prevent some side effects or decrease their severity

Adults:
Oral: 25-50 mg 3-4 times/day, to be increased as needed; doses exceeding 600 mg/day are rarely required
I.M.: 25-50 mg up to 3-4 times/day
Not dialyzable (0% to 5%)

Monitoring Parameters Orthostatic blood pressures; tremors, gait changes, abnormal movement in trunk, neck, buccal area, or extremities; monitor target behaviors for which the agent is given

Test Interactions Increased cholesterol (S), glucose; decreased uric acid (S)

Patient Information Do not take antacid within 1 hour of taking drug; avoid alcohol; avoid excess sun exposure (use sun block); may cause drowsiness, rise slowly from recumbent position; use of supportive stockings may help prevent orthostatic hypotension

Nursing Implications Avoid skin contact with oral suspension or solution; may cause contact dermatitis; monitor orthostatic blood pressures 3-5 days after initiation of therapy or a dose increase; observe for tremor and abnormal movement or posturing (extrapyramidal symptoms)

Special Geriatric Considerations See Warnings.

Many elderly patients receive antipsychotic medications for inappropriate nonpsychotic behavior. Before initiating antipsychotic medication, the clinician should investigate any possible reversible cause; any stress or stress from any disease can cause acute "confusion" or worsening of baseline nonpsychotic behavior. Most commonly acute changes in behavior are due to increases in drug dose or addition of new drug to regimen; fluid electrolyte loss; infections; and changes in environment.

Any changes in disease status in any organ system can result in behavior changes.

In the treatment of agitated, demented, elderly patients, authors of meta-analysis of controlled trials of the response to the traditional antipsychotics (phenothiazines, butyrophenones) in controlling agitation have concluded that the use of neuroleptics results in a response rate of 18%. Clearly neuroleptic therapy for behavior control should be limited with frequent attempts to withdraw the agent given for behavior control.

Dosage Forms

Injection: 12.5 mg/mL (2 mL)
Tablet: 10 mg, 25 mg, 50 mg, 100 mg

References

Peabody CA, Warner MD, Whiteford HA, et al, "Neuroleptics and the Elderly," *J Am Geriatr Soc*, 1987, 35(3):233-8.

Risse SC and Barnes R, "Pharmacologic Treatment of Agitation Associated With Dementia," *J Am Geriatr Soc*, 1986, 34(5):368-76.

Saltz BL, Woerner MG, Kane JM, et al, "Prospective Study of Tardive Dyskinesia Incidence in the Elderly," *JAMA*, 1991, 266(17):2402-6.

Seifert RD, "Therapeutic Drug Monitoring: Psychotropic Drugs," *J Pharm Pract*, 1984, 6:403-16.

Chlorthalidone (klor THAL i done)

Brand Names Hygroton®; Thalitone®

Generic Available Yes

Therapeutic Category Diuretic, Miscellaneous

Use Management of mild to moderate hypertension, used alone or in combination with other agents; treatment of edema associated with congestive heart failure, or nephrotic syndrome

Contraindications Hypersensitivity to chlorthalidone or any component, cross-sensitivity with other thiazides or sulfonamides; do not use in anuric patients

Precautions Use with caution in hypokalemia, renal disease, hepatic disease, gout, lupus, erythematosus, diabetes mellitus

Adverse Reactions
Cardiovascular: Hypotension
Dermatologic: Photosensitivity, rash
Endocrine & metabolic: Fluid and electrolyte imbalances (hypokalemia, hypocalcemia, hypomagnesemia, hyponatremia), hyperglycemia
Genitourinary: Prerenal azotemia, polyuria
Hematologic: Rarely blood dyscrasias

Overdosage Symptoms of overdose include electrolyte depletion, volume depletion

Toxicology Treatment is primarily symptomatic and supportive; hypotension responds to fluids and Trendelenburg position; replace electrolytes as necessary

Drug Interactions
Decreased effect of oral hypoglycemics; decreased absorption with cholestyramine and colestipol
Decreased effect: NSAIDs
Increased effect with furosemide and other loop diuretics
Increased toxicity/levels of lithium; when given with digoxin, diuretic-induced hypokalemia increases the risk of digoxin toxicity

Mechanism of Action Inhibits sodium reabsorption in the distal tubules causing increased excretion of sodium and water as well as potassium and hydrogen ions

Pharmacodynamics
Peak clinical effect: Within 2-6 hours
Duration: 24-72 hours

Pharmacokinetics
Absorption: 65%
Metabolism: In the liver
Half-life: 35-55 hours and may be prolonged with renal impairment; (anuria): 81 hours
Elimination: ~50% to 65% of dose excreted unchanged in urine

Usual Dosage Oral:
Geriatrics: Initial: 12.5-25 mg/day or every other day; there is little advantage to using doses >25 mg/day
Adults: 25-100 mg/day or 100 mg 3 times/week

Monitoring Parameters Blood pressure (standing and sitting/supine), serum electrolytes, renal function, I & O, weight

Test Interactions Increased creatine phosphokinase [CPK] (S), ammonia (B), amylase (S), calcium (S), chloride (S), cholesterol (S), glucose, increased acid (S), decreased chloride (S), magnesium, potassium (S), sodium (S)

Patient Information Take in the morning; may cause increased sensitivity to sunlight; rise slowly from lying down or sitting

Nursing Implications Administer in the morning (see Monitoring Parameters); check patient for orthostasis

Special Geriatric Considerations Studies have found chlorthalidone effective in the treatment of isolated systolic hypertension in the elderly. The use of chlorthalidone as a step 1 medication reduced the incidence of stroke in the SHEP trial.

Dosage Forms
Tablet: 25 mg, 50 mg, 100 mg
Hygroton®: 25 mg, 50 mg, 100 mg
Thalitone®: 15 mg, 25 mg

References
Hulley SB, Furberg CD, Gurland B, et al, "Systolic Hypertension in the Elderly Program (SHEP): Antihypertensive Efficacy of Chlorthalidone," *Am J Cardiol*, 1985, 56(15):913-20.
SHEP Cooperative Research Group, "Prevention of Stroke by Antihypertensive Drug Treatment in Older Persons With Isolated Systolic Hypertension," *JAMA*, 1991, 265(24):3255-64.

Chlor-Trimeton® [OTC] *see* Chlorpheniramine *on page 208*

Chlorzoxazone (klor ZOKS a zone)

Brand Names Flexaphen®; Mus-Lax®; Paraflex®; Parafon Forte™ DSC
Synonyms Chlorzoxazone With Acetaminophen
Generic Available Yes
Therapeutic Category Centrally Acting Skeletal Muscle Relaxant; Skeletal Muscle Relaxant
Use Symptomatic treatment of muscle spasm and pain associated with acute musculoskeletal conditions
Contraindications Known hypersensitivity to chlorzoxazone; impaired liver function
Precautions If signs or symptoms of impaired liver dysfunction occur, discontinue drug
Adverse Reactions
Central nervous system: Drowsiness, dizziness, lightheadedness, headache
Dermatologic: Rash, urticaria
Gastrointestinal: Nausea, vomiting, diarrhea, GI bleeding
Hematologic: Anemia, granulocytopenia
Hepatic: Hepatitis, hepatic necrosis, hepatic failure
Neuromuscular & skeletal: Paresthesia
Overdosage Symptoms of overdose include nausea, vomiting, diarrhea, drowsiness, dizziness, headache, absent tendon reflexes, hypotension
Toxicology Treatment is supportive following attempts to enhance drug elimination. Hypotension should be treated with I.V. fluids and/or Trendelenburg positioning. Dialysis and hemoperfusion and osmotic diuresis have all been useful in reducing serum drug concentrations. The patient should be observed for possible relapses due to incomplete gastric emptying.
Drug Interactions Increased effect/CNS toxicity: Alcohol, CNS depressants
Mechanism of Action Acts on the spinal cord and subcortical levels by depressing polysynaptic reflexes; this results in reduced skeletal muscle spasm, relief of pain, and increased mobility of involved muscles
Pharmacodynamics
Onset of action: 60 minutes
Duration: 3-4 hours
Pharmacokinetics
Absorption: Oral: Readily absorbed
Metabolism: Extensive in the liver by glucuronidation; substrate CYP2E1
Elimination: In urine as conjugates
Usual Dosage Oral:
Geriatrics: Initial: 250 mg 2-4 times/day; increase as necessary to 750 mg 3-4 times/day
Adults: 250-500 mg 3-4 times/day up to 750 mg 3-4 times/day
Monitoring Parameters Liver function tests, relief of symptoms, mental status
Patient Information Avoid alcohol and CNS depressants; may cause drowsiness, dizziness, or lightheadedness; urine may turn orange or purple-red; take with food or milk
Nursing Implications Administer with food or milk if GI complaints occur; may discolor urine
Additional Information Not useful in the chronic spasticity associated with stroke or Parkinson's disease
Special Geriatric Considerations No data available on the use of skeletal muscle relaxants in the elderly. Start dosing low and increase as necessary. The FDA recently approved a stronger warning about hepatotoxicity in the labeling of chlorzoxazone. Because it can cause unpredictable, fatal hepatic toxicity, the use of chlorzoxazone should be avoided.
Dosage Forms
Caplet (Parafon Forte™ DSC): 500 mg
Capsule (Flexaphen®, Mus-Lax®): 250 mg with acetaminophen 300 mg
Tablet: Paraflex®: 250 mg

Chlorzoxazone With Acetaminophen *see* Chlorzoxazone *on this page*
Cholac® *see* Lactulose *on page 523*

Cholecalciferol (kole e kal SI fer ole)

Brand Names Delta-D®
Synonyms D_3
Generic Available No
Therapeutic Category Vitamin D Analog

Use Dietary supplement, treatment of vitamin D deficiency or prophylaxis of deficiency

Unlabeled use: Hypocalcemic tetany, hypoparathyroidism

Contraindications Hypercalcemia, hypersensitivity to cholecalciferol or any component; malabsorption syndrome; evidence of vitamin D toxicity, decreased renal function

Warnings Administer with extreme caution in patients with impaired renal function, heart disease, renal stones, or arteriosclerosis; maintain adequate fluid intake, calcium-phosphate product must not exceed 70%; avoid hypercalcemia; must administer with supplemental calcium; use caution in patients with renal impairment and hyperparathyroidism

Precautions Use with caution in coronary artery disease and elderly

Adverse Reactions
Cardiovascular: Hypertension, arrhythmias
Central nervous system: Drowsiness, irritability, headache, somnolence, seizures
Endocrine & metabolic: Acidosis
Gastrointestinal: Nausea, vomiting, anorexia, xerostomia, constipation, weight loss, metallic taste
Hematologic: Anemia
Hepatic: Elevated AST/ALT
Neuromuscular & skeletal: Myalgia, bone pain, weakness, metastatic calcifications
Ocular: Photophobia
Renal: Polyuria, polydipsia, nephrocalcinosis, renal damage

Overdosage Symptoms of overdose include hypercalcemia, anorexia, nausea, weakness, constipation, diarrhea, mental confusion, tinnitus, ataxia, depression, hallucinations, syncope, coma; polyuria, polydypsia, nocturia, hypercalciuria, irreversible renal insufficiency or proteinuria, azotemia; will spread tissue calcifications, hypertension

Toxicology Following withdrawal of the drug, treatment consists of bed rest, liberal intake of fluids, reduced calcium intake, and cathartic administration. Severe hypercalcemia requires I.V. hydration and forced diuresis with I.V. furosemide (20-40 mg I.V. every 4-6 hours). Urine output should be monitored and maintained at >3 mL/kg/hour. I.V. saline can quickly and significantly increase excretion of calcium into the urine. Calcitonin, cholestyramine, prednisone, sodium EDTA, and mithramycin have all been used successfully to treat the more resistant cases of vitamin D-induced hypercalcemia.

Drug Interactions
Vitamin D may increase absorption of magnesium from magnesium compounds; hypercalcemia may be precipitated by vitamin D and, therefore, may increase cardiac arrhythmias in patients taking digitalis glycosides and verapamil; hypoparathyroid patients may develop hypercalcemia when using thiazide diuretics

Phenytoin and barbiturates decrease half-life of vitamin D; mineral oil with prolonged use decreases vitamin D absorption; cholestyramine reduces absorption of vitamin D

Usual Dosage Geriatrics and Adults: Oral: 400-1000 units/day; general supplementation: 400 units (see Additional Information)

Monitoring Parameters Monitor renal function, serum calcium, and phosphate concentrations; if hypercalcemia is encountered, discontinue agent until serum calcium returns to normal

Reference Range Calcium (serum) 9-10 mg/dL (4.5-5 mEq/L); phosphate 2.5-5 mg/dL

Test Interactions Increases calcium (S), cholesterol (S); false increased serum cholesterol concentrations with the Zlavkis-Zak reaction

Patient Information Do not take more than the recommended amount. While taking this medication, your physician may want you to follow a special diet or take a calcium supplement. Follow this diet closely. Avoid taking magnesium supplements or magnesium-containing antacids. Early symptoms of hypercalcemia include weakness, fatigue, somnolence, headache, anorexia, dry mouth, metallic taste, nausea, vomiting, cramps, diarrhea, muscle pain, bone pain, and irritability.

Nursing Implications See Overdosage and Monitoring Parameters

Additional Information 1 mg of cholecalciferol = 40,000 units of vitamin D activity

Special Geriatric Considerations Recommended daily allowances (RDA) have not been developed for persons >65 years of age; vitamin D, folate, and B_{12} (cyanocobalamin) have decreased absorption with age, but the clinical significance is yet unknown. Calorie requirements decrease with age and, (Continued)

Cholecalciferol *(Continued)*

therefore, nutrient density must be increased to ensure adequate nutrient intake, including vitamins and minerals. Therefore, the use of a daily supplement with a multiple vitamin with minerals is recommended. Elderly consume less vitamin D, absorption may be decreased and many elderly have decreased sun exposure; therefore, elderly should receive supplementation with 800 units (20 mcg)/day. This is a recommendation of particular need to those with high risk for osteoporosis.

Dosage Forms Tablet: 400 units, 1000 units

References

Letsou AP and Price LS, "Health Aging and Nutrition: An Overview," *Clin Geriatr Med*, 1987, 3(2):253-60.

Myrianthopoulos M, "Dietary Treatment of Hyperlipidemia in the Elderly," *Clin Geriatr Med*, 1987, 3(2):343-59.

Riggs BL and Melton LJ, "The Prevention and Treatment of Osteoporosis," *N Engl J Med*, 1992, 327(9):620-7.

Cholera Vaccine (KOL er a vak SEEN)

Related Information

Immunization Guidelines *on page 1058*

Therapeutic Category Vaccine, Inactivated Bacteria

Use Primary immunization for cholera prophylaxis for individuals traveling or living in endemic or epidemic countries

Contraindications Acute respiratory or other active infections, immune deficiency states, known hypersensitivity to cholera vaccine

Warnings Do not inject I.V.; do not administer I.M. to persons with thrombocytopenia, coagulation defects, or receiving anticoagulants; hypersensitivity to vaccine, have epinephrine 1:1000 available to treat anaphylactic reactions

Precautions Aspirate syringe before delivering I.M. or S.C. dose to avoid accidental I.V. administration

Adverse Reactions

Cardiovascular: Local edema

Central nervous system: Malaise, fever, headache

Local: Pain, tenderness, erythema, and induration at injection site; may persist for 1-2 days

Drug Interactions Yellow fever vaccine; do not administer within 3 weeks of yellow fever vaccination

Stability Refrigerate at 2°C to 8°C (36°F to 46°C), avoid freezing

Mechanism of Action A sterile suspension of equal parts of phenol inactivated Ogawa and Inaba serotypes of *Vibrio cholerae*; 50% effective; protection lasts 3-6 months

Usual Dosage Geriatrics and Adults: I.M., S.C.: 0.5 mL in 2 doses one week to 1 month or more apart; administer boosters (0.5 mL) 6 months apart

Patient Information Local reactions can occur up to 2 days; avoid food and water which may be contaminated

Nursing Implications Defer immunization in individuals with moderate or severe febrile illness; do not administer I.V.; administer I.M., S.C., or intradermally

Special Geriatric Considerations Review history of elderly to assure no drug or disease is contraindicated with use of vaccine

Dosage Forms Injection: 8 billion killed organisms/mL (1.5 mL, 20 mL)

Cholestyramine Resin (koe LES tir a meen REZ in)

Brand Names Prevalite®; Questran®; Questran® Light

Therapeutic Category Antilipemic Agent

Use Adjunct in the management of primary hypercholesterolemia; pruritus associated with elevated levels of bile acids; diarrhea associated with excess fecal bile acids; binding toxicologic agents; pseudomembraneous colitis

Contraindications Avoid using in complete biliary obstruction

Warnings Questran® Light contains aspartame; caution patients with phenylketonuria

Precautions Use with caution in patients with constipation

Adverse Reactions

Dermatologic: Rash

Endocrine & metabolic: Hyperchloremic acidosis

Gastrointestinal: Constipation, nausea, vomiting, abdominal distention and pain, malabsorption of fat-soluble vitamins, bowel obstruction

Local: Irritation of perianal area, skin, or tongue

Renal: Increased urinary calcium excretion

Overdosage Symptoms of overdose include GI obstruction

Drug Interactions May decrease oral absorption of digitalis glycosides, warfarin, thyroid hormones, thiazide diuretics, propranolol, phenobarbital, acetaminophen, corticosteroids, glipizide, amiodarone, methotrexate, naproxen, piroxicam, and other drugs by binding to the drug in the intestine; compounded effect with other drugs that cause constipation

Mechanism of Action Forms a nonabsorbable complex with bile acids in the intestine, releasing chloride ions in the process; inhibits enterohepatic reuptake of intestinal bile salts and thereby increases the fecal loss of bile salt-bound low density lipoprotein cholesterol

Pharmacodynamics Peak effects: Within 21 days

Pharmacokinetics
Absorption: Not absorbed from GI tract
Elimination: In feces as an insoluble complex with bile acids

Usual Dosage Geriatrics and Adults: Oral (dosages are expressed in terms of anhydrous resin): 4 g 1-6 times/day to a maximum of 16-32 g/day in 2-4 divided doses

Monitoring Parameters Bowel function, plasma cholesterol (LDL and VLDL fractions)

Test Interactions Increased prothrombin time; decreased cholesterol (S), iron (B)

Patient Information Take before meals; mix with liquids, pulpy fruits, or soups; chew bars thoroughly and follow with fluids (at least 4 fluid oz); do not take concurrently with other medications; take other medications 1 hour before or 4-6 hours after binding resin; adhere to prescribed diet

Nursing Implications Do not administer the powder in its dry form; just prior to administration, mix with fluid or with applesauce; administer warfarin at least 1-2 hours prior to, or 6 hours after cholestyramine because cholestyramine may bind warfarin and decrease its total absorption. **Note:** Cholestyramine itself may cause hypoprothrombinemia in patients with impaired enterohepatic circulation; can be very constipating, monitor for bowel function to prevent fecal impaction.

Additional Information Overdose may result in GI obstruction; Questran® Light contains aspartame

Special Geriatric Considerations The definition of and, therefore, when to treat hyperlipidemia in the elderly is a controversial issue. The National Cholesterol Education Program recommends that all adults 20 years of age and older maintain a plasma cholesterol concentration <200 mg/dL. By this definition, 60% of all elderly would be considered to have an elevated plasma cholesterol. However, plasma cholesterol has been shown to be a less reliable predictor of coronary heart disease in the elderly. Therefore, it is the authors' belief that pharmacologic treatment be reserved for those who are unable to obtain a desirable plasma cholesterol concentration by diet alone and for whom the benefits of treatment are believed to outweigh the potential adverse effects, drug interactions, and cost of treatment.

Dosage Forms
Powder: 4 g of resin/9 g of powder (9 g, 378 g)
Powder, for oral suspension, with aspartame: 4 g of resin/5 g of powder (5 g, 210 g)
Powder, for oral suspension, with phenylalanine: 4 g of resin/5.5 g of powder (60s)

References
Leaf DA, "Lipid Disorders: Applying New Guidelines to Your Older Patients," *Geriatrics*, 1994, 49(5):35-41.

Choline Magnesium Trisalicylate
(KOE leen mag NEE zhum trye sa LIS i late)

Brand Names Tricosal®; Trilisate®

Generic Available Yes

Therapeutic Category Analgesic, Non-narcotic; Anti-inflammatory Agent; Antipyretic; Nonsteroidal Anti-inflammatory Agent (NSAID), Oral; Salicylate

Use Treatment of mild to moderate pain, inflammation and fever; management of rheumatic fever, rheumatoid arthritis, osteoarthritis, and gout (see Mechanism of Action)

Contraindications Bleeding disorders (factor VII or IX deficiencies), hypersensitivity to salicylates or other nonsteroidal anti-inflammatory drugs (NSAIDs); tartrazine dye and asthma

Warnings Tinnitus or impaired hearing may indicate toxicity; discontinue use 1 week prior to surgical procedures
(Continued)

Choline Magnesium Trisalicylate *(Continued)*

Precautions Use with caution in patients with platelet and bleeding disorders, renal dysfunction, hepatic disease, history of salicylate-induced gastric irritation, peptic ulcer disease, erosive gastritis, bleeding disorders, hypoprothrombinemia, and vitamin K deficiency; use cautiously in asthmatics, especially those with aspirin intolerance and nasal polyps

Adverse Reactions

Central nervous system: Dizziness, mental confusion, CNS depression, headache, lassitude, fever

Dermatologic: Rash, urticaria, angioedema

Gastrointestinal: Nausea, vomiting, GI distress, ulcers, thirst

Hematologic: Bleeding, inhibition of platelet aggregation, leukopenia, thrombocytopenia

Hepatic: Hepatotoxicity

Otic: Tinnitus

Respiratory: Pulmonary edema, bronchospasm, hyperventilation

Miscellaneous: Diaphoresis

Overdosage 10-30 g; symptoms of overdose include tinnitus, headache, dizziness, confusion, metabolic acidosis, hyperpyrexia, hyperpnea, tachypnea, nausea, vomiting, irritability, disorientation, hallucinations, lethargy, stupor, dehydration, hyperventilation, hyperthermia, hyperactivity, depression leading to coma, respiratory failure, and collapse; laboratory abnormalities include hypokalemia, hypoglycemia or hyperglycemia with alterations in pH

Toxicology The "Done" nomogram is very helpful for estimating the severity of aspirin poisoning and directing treatment using serum salicylate concentrations. Treatment can also be based upon symptomatology; see table.

Aspirin or Other Salicylate Toxicity

Toxic Symptoms	Treatment
Overdose	Induce emesis with ipecac, and/or lavage with saline, followed with activated charcoal
Dehydration	I.V. fluids with KCl (no D_5W only)
Metabolic acidosis (must be treated)	Sodium bicarbonate
Hyperthermia	Cooling blankets or sponge baths
Coagulopathy/hemorrhage	Vitamin K I.V.
Hypoglycemia (with coma, seizures, or change in mental status)	Dextrose 25 g I.V.
Seizures	Diazepam 5-10 mg I.V.

Drug Interactions

Antacids + Trilisate® may cause decreased salicylate concentration

Warfarin + Trilisate® may cause possible increased hypoprothrombinemic effect; ammonium chloride, vitamin C (high dose), methionine, antacids, urinary alkalinizers, carbonic anhydrase inhibitors, corticosteroids, nizatidine, alcohol, ACE inhibitors, beta-blockers, loop diuretics, methotrexate, probenecid, sulfinpyrazone, spironolactone

Mechanism of Action Inhibits prostaglandin synthesis; acts on the hypothalamus heat-regulating center to reduce fever through vasodilation of peripheral vessels; decreases pain receptor sensitivity. Other proposed mechanisms of action for salicylate anti-inflammatory action are lysosomal stabilization, inhibition of kinin and leukotriene production, alteration of chemotactic factors, and inhibition of neutrophil activation. This latter mechanism may be the most significant pharmacologic action to reduce inflammation. Nonacetylated salicylates are **not** as potent in prostaglandin synthesis inhibition and, therefore, tend to have less adverse effects on gastrointestinal and renal tissues. They do not inhibit platelet function as aspirin does since they are not acetylated and, therefore, cannot acetylate platelet cyclooxygenase.

Pharmacokinetics

Absorption: From the stomach and small intestine

Distribution: Readily into most body fluids and tissues

Half-life: Dose-dependent ranging from 2-3 hours at low doses to 30 hours at high doses

Time to peak plasma concentrations: Within ~2 hours

Usual Dosage Geriatrics and Adults (based on **total salicylate content**):

Oral: 500 mg to 1.5 g 1-3 times/day

Monitoring Parameters Serum concentrations, renal function; hearing changes or tinnitus; monitor for response (ie, pain, inflammation, range of motion, grip strength); observe for abnormal bleeding, bruising, weight gain

Reference Range

Salicylate blood concentrations for anti-inflammatory effect: 150-300 μg/mL (15-30 mg/dL)

Analgesia and antipyretic effect: 30-50 μg/mL (3-5 mg/dL)

Test Interactions False-negative results for glucose oxidase urinary glucose tests (Clinistix®); false-positives using the cupric sulfate method (Clinitest®); also, interferes with Gerhardt test (urinary ketone analysis), VMA determination; 5-HIAA, xylose tolerance test, and T_3 and T_4; increased PBI; increased uric acid

Patient Information Do not take with antacids; watch for any signs of bleeding (stool); take with food to minimize GI distress; report ringing in ears, persistent GI pain to physician or pharmacist

Nursing Implications Liquid may be mixed with fruit juice just before drinking; do not administer with antacids (see Monitoring Parameters, Reference Range, and Special Geriatric Considerations)

Additional Information Salicylate salts do not inhibit platelet aggregation and, therefore, should not be substituted for aspirin in the prophylaxis of thrombosis; use caution in patients with renal failure or reduced renal function (ie, elderly - magnesium accumulation)

Special Geriatric Considerations Elderly are a high-risk population for adverse effects from nonsteroidal anti-inflammatory agents. As much as 60% of elderly can develop peptic ulceration and/or hemorrhage asymptomatically. The concomitant use of H_2 blockers, omeprazole, and sucralfate is not effective as prophylaxis with the exception of NSAID-induced duodenal ulcers which may be prevented by the use of ranitidine. Misoprostol and proton pump inhibitors are the only agents proven to help prevent the development of NSAID-induced ulcers. Also, concomitant disease and drug use contribute to the risk for GI adverse effects. Avoid use of multiple drugs (OTCs) which contain salicylates (eg, bismuth subsalicylate with other salicylates). Use lowest effective dose for shortest period possible. Consider renal function decline with age. Use of NSAIDs can compromise existing renal function especially when Cl_{cr} is ≤30 mL/minute. There is the consideration that the use of choline magnesium salicylate may cause less gastrointestinal and renal adverse effects than ASA or other NSAIDs in the elderly. Tinnitus may be a difficult and unreliable indication of toxicity due to age-related hearing loss or eighth cranial nerve damage. CNS adverse effects such as confusion, agitation, and hallucination are generally seen in overdose or high dose situations, but elderly may demonstrate these adverse effects at lower doses than younger adults.

Dosage Forms See table.

Choline Magnesium Trisalicylate

Brand Name	Dosage Form	Total Salicylate	Choline Salicylate	Magnesium Salicylate
Trilisate®	Liquid	500 mg/5 mL	293 mg/5 mL	362 mg/5 mL
Trilisate 500®	Tablet	500 mg	293 mg	362 mg
Trilisate 750®	Tablet	750 mg	440 mg	544 mg
Trilisate 1000®	Tablet	1000 mg	587 mg	725 mg

References

Hawkey CJ, Karrasch JA, Szczepaski L, et al, "Omeprazole Compared With Misoprostrol for Ulcers Associated With Nonsteroidal Anti-inflammatory Drugs," *N Engl J Med*, 1998, 338(11):727-34.

Weissmann G, "Aspirin," *Sci Am*, 1991, 264(1):84-90.

Yeomans ND, Tulassay Z, Juhasz L, et al, "A Comparison of Omeprazole With Ranitidine for Ulcers Associated With Nonsteroidal Anti-inflammatory Drugs," *N Engl J Med*, 1998, 338(11):719-26.

Choline Salicylate *see* Salicylates (Various Salts) *on page 842*

Chooz® [OTC] *see* Calcium Salts (Oral) *on page 152*

Chronulac® *see* Lactulose *on page 523*

Cibacalcin® Injection *see* Calcitonin *on page 142*

Ciloxan™ Ophthalmic *see* Ciprofloxacin *on page 226*

Cimetidine (sye MET i deen)

Related Information

Antacid Drug Interactions *on page 1096*

(Continued)

Cimetidine *(Continued)*

I.V. Medication Recommendations *on page 1080*

Brand Names Tagamet®; Tagamet® HB [OTC]

Generic Available Yes

Therapeutic Category Histamine H_2 Antagonist

Use Short-term treatment of active duodenal ulcers and benign gastric ulcers; long-term prophylaxis of duodenal ulcer; gastric hypersecretory states; gastroesophageal reflux; prevention of upper GI bleeding in critically ill patients

Tagamet® HB [OTC]: Relief of symptoms of heartburn, acid indigestion, and sour stomach

Unlabeled use: Prevent aspiration pneumonitis, hyperparathyroidism, tinea capitis, herpes virus infection, hirsutism, chronic idiopathic urticaria, dermatologic symptoms of anaphylaxis, acetaminophen overdose, and dyspepsia

Contraindications Hypersensitivity to cimetidine or any component or other H_2 antagonists

Warnings Adjust dosages in renal/hepatic impairment; decline in renal function with age

Precautions Gastric malignancy may be masked

Adverse Reactions

Cardiovascular: Bradycardia, hypotension, cardiac arrhythmias

Central nervous system: Dizziness, mental confusion, agitation, headache, phytobezoar formation, depression, psychosis, hallucinations, anxiety

Dermatologic: Rash, exfoliative dermatitis, alopecia, epidermal necrolysis

Endocrine & metabolic: Gynecomastia

Gastrointestinal: Mild diarrhea, pancreatitis

Genitourinary: Urinary retention

Hematologic: Neutropenia, agranulocytosis, thrombocytopenia

Hepatic: Elevated AST and ALT

Neuromuscular & skeletal: Peripheral neuropathy, myalgia, arthralgia, polymyositis

Renal: Rare reversible nephritis, elevated creatinine

Respiratory: Bronchospasm

Overdose No experience with intentional overdose; reported ingestions of 20 g have had transient side effects seen with recommended doses; animal data have shown respiratory failure, tachycardia, muscle tremors, vomiting, restlessness, hypotension, salivation, emesis, and diarrhea

Toxicology Treatment is primarily symptomatic and supportive

Drug Interactions

Decreased elimination of lidocaine, theophylline, caffeine, calcium channel blockers, labetalol, carbamazepine, metoprolol, moricizine, pentoxifylline, phenytoin, propafenone, chloroquine sulfonylureas, metronidazole, triamterene, procainamide, quinidine and propranolol; inhibition of warfarin metabolism, tricyclic antidepressant metabolism, diazepam elimination and cyclosporine elimination; antacids may reduce the absorption of cimetidine

Increased absorption with cisapride

Stability I.V. infusion solution with NS or D_5W solution is stable for 48 hours at room temperature; do not refrigerate the injection since precipitation may occur

Mechanism of Action Competitive inhibition of histamine at H_2 receptors of the gastric parietal cells resulting in reduced gastric acid secretion; gastric volume and hydrogen ion concentration reduced

Pharmacodynamics 400 mg twice daily and 300 mg 4 times/day suppress nocturnal acid secretion 47% to 83% over a 6- to 8-hour interval; 800 mg at bedtime decreases acid secretion 85% over 8 hours; 1600 mg at bedtime gives 100% reduction over 8 hours

Pharmacokinetics

Protein binding: 13% to 25%

Bioavailability: 60% to 70%

Metabolism: Inhibitor of CYP1A2, 2C18, 2D6, and 3A4

Half-life: Adults with normal renal function: 2 hours

Time to peak serum concentrations: Oral: Within 1-2 hours

Elimination: Principally as unchanged drug by the kidney; some excretion in bile and feces

Usual Dosage Geriatrics and Adults (see Additional Information and Special Geriatric Considerations):

Short-term treatment of active ulcers:

Oral: 300 mg 4 times/day or 800 mg at bedtime or 400 mg twice daily for up to 8 weeks

I.M., I.V.: 300 mg every 6 hours or 37.5 mg/hour by continuous infusion; I.V. dosage should be adjusted to maintain an intragastric pH ≥5

Duodenal ulcer prophylaxis: Oral: 400-800 mg at bedtime

Gastric hypersecretory conditions: Oral, I.M., I.V.: 300-600 mg every 6 hours; dosage not to exceed 2.4 g/day

Tagamet® HB [OTC]: 200 mg as needed up to twice daily; do not take maximum dose for more than 14 days continuously, unless directed by a physician

Dosing interval in renal impairment:

Cl_{cr} >40 mL/minute: Administer 300 mg every 6 hours

Cl_{cr} 20-40 mL/minute: Administer 300 mg every 8 hours

Cl_{cr} 0-20 mL/minute: Administer 300 mg every 12 hours

Monitoring Parameters Signs and symptoms of peptic ulcer disease, occult blood with GI bleeding, gastric pH where necessary; monitor renal function to correct dose; monitor for side effects

Reference Range Therapeutic: >1 µg/mL (SI: 4 µmol/L); mental confusion reported with concentrations >1.25 µg/mL

Test Interactions Increased creatinine, AST, ALT

Patient Information Take with or immediately after meals; inform pharmacist and physician (nurse, practitioner) of any concomitant drug therapy; stagger doses with antacids.

Tagamet® HB [OTC]: Do not take maximum dose for more than 14 days continuously, unless directed by a physician.

Nursing Implications Administer with meals so that the peak effect occurs at the proper time (peak inhibition of gastric acid secretion occurs at 1 and 3 hours after dosing in fasting subjects and ~2 hours in nonfasting subjects; this correlates well with the time food is no longer in the stomach offering a buffering effect); modify dosage in patients with renal impairment

Additional Information All presently available H_2 blockers have equivalent healing properties for both DU and GU when dose at equivalent doses; practitioners should realize that when H_2 blocker doses are adjusted for renal function, it is **not** a "dose reduction" that results in less than therapeutic tissue concentration. Therapeutic concentrations are maintained with doses adjusted for renal function. When prophylaxing for gastric ulcers, must use full therapeutic dose; prophylaxis for DU can be reduced as indicated.

Special Geriatric Considerations Patients diagnosed with PUD should be evaluated for *Helicobacter pylori*. When H_2-blockers are indicated, they are the preferred drugs for treating PUD in elderly due to cost and ease of administration. These agents are no less or more effective than any other therapy. The preferred agents, due to side effects, drug interaction profile, and pharmacokinetics are ranitidine, famotidine, and nizatidine. Treatment for PUD in elderly is recommended for 12 weeks since their lesions are larger and, therefore, take longer to heal. Always adjust dose based upon creatinine clearance.

Dosage Forms

Infusion, as hydrochloride: 300 mg in 50 mL NS

Injection, as hydrochloride: 150 mg/mL (2 mL)

Liquid, oral, as hydrochloride: 300 mg/5 mL (5 mL, 240 mL)

Tablet: 200 mg, 300 mg, 400 mg, 800 mg

Tablet [OTC]: 100 mg

References

Fennerty MD and Higbee M, "Drug Therapy of Gastrointestinal Disease," *Geriatric Pharmacology*, Bressler R and Katz MD, eds, New York, NY: McGraw-Hill, 1993, 585-608.

Somogyi A and Gugler R, "Clinical Pharmacokinetics of Cimetidine," *Clin Pharmacokinet*, 1983, 8(6):463-95.

Somogyi A and Muirhead M, "Pharmacokinetic Interactions of Cimetidine 1987," *Clin Pharmacokinet*, 1987, 12(5):321-66.

Cinobac® Pulvules® *see* Cinoxacin *on this page*

Cinoxacin (sin OKS a sin)

Related Information

Antacid Drug Interactions *on page 1096*

Brand Names Cinobac® Pulvules®

Generic Available No

Therapeutic Category Antibiotic, Quinolone

Use Urinary tract infections caused by susceptible pathogens: *E. coli*, *P. mirabilis*, *P. vulgaris*, *K. pneumoniae*, *Klebsiella* sp, and *Enterobacter* sp

Contraindications History of convulsive disorders, hypersensitivity to cinoxacin or any component or other quinolones and nalidixic acid

(Continued)

Cinoxacin *(Continued)*

Warnings Dose should be adjusted in patients with renal impairment; use with caution in patients with a history of hepatic disease

Adverse Reactions

Central nervous system: Dizziness, insomnia, confusion, headache

Gastrointestinal: Nausea, vomiting, abdominal pain, diarrhea, heartburn, dysgeusia, flatulence, anorexia

Hematologic: Thrombocytopenia

Ocular: Photophobia

Otic: Tinnitus

Drug Interactions Probenecid will decrease renal secretion and increase serum concentrations; cimetidine may decrease clearance of cinoxacin; anticoagulants may have effects enhanced; fluoroquinolones increase nephrotoxic effects of cyclosporine; decreased clearance of theophylline

Mechanism of Action Inhibits microbial synthesis of DNA with resultant problems in protein synthesis

Pharmacokinetics

Absorption: Oral: Rapid and complete; food decreases peak serum concentrations by 30% but not total amount absorbed

Distribution: Concentrates in prostate tissue

Protein binding: 60% to 80%

Half-life: 1.5 hours

Time to peak serum concentration: Within 2-3 hours

Elimination: Prolonged in renal impairment, ~60% excreted as unchanged drug in urine

Usual Dosage Oral:

Geriatrics: Usual adult dose adjusted for renal function when appropriate

Adults: 1 g/day in 2-4 doses

Dosing adjustment in renal impairment following an initial 500 mg dose:

Cl_{cr} >80 mL/minute/1.73 m^2: Administer 500 mg every 12 hours

Cl_{cr} 50-80 mL/minute/1.73 m^2: Administer 250 mg every 8 hours

Cl_{cr} 20-50 mL/minute/1.73 m^2: Administer 250 mg every 12 hours

Cl_{cr} <20 mL/minute/1.73 m^2: Administer 250 mg every 24 hours

Monitoring Parameters Signs and symptoms of infection; cultures and sensitivities

Test Interactions BUN, AST, ALT, serum creatinine, and alkaline phosphatase have been reported to be elevated; hematocrit/hemoglobin have been reported to be reduced

Patient Information Complete entire course of therapy; may be taken with food or milk; may cause dizziness, use caution when driving or performing other tasks that require alertness; eyes may be sensitive to light

Special Geriatric Considerations Adjust dose for renal function in elderly (see Usual Dosage)

Dosage Forms Capsule: 250 mg, 500 mg

Ciprofloxacin *(sip roe FLOKS a sin)*

Related Information

Antacid Drug Interactions *on page 1096*

Cephalosporins, Aminoglycosides, Macrolides, & Quinolones *on page 1014*

I.V. Medication Recommendations *on page 1080*

Brand Names Ciloxan™ Ophthalmic; Cipro™ Injection; Cipro™ Oral

Generic Available No

Therapeutic Category Antibiotic, Ophthalmic; Antibiotic, Quinolone

Use Treatment of documented or suspected pseudomonal infection in home care patients; documented multidrug resistant gram-negative organisms; documented infectious diarrhea due to *Campylobacter jejuni*, *Shigella*, or *Salmonella*; osteomyelitis caused by susceptible organisms in which parenteral therapy is not feasible; used ophthalmically for superficial ocular infections due to strains of microorganisms susceptible to ciprofloxacin

Contraindications Hypersensitivity to ciprofloxacin, any component or other quinolones, and nalidixic acid

Warnings Prolonged use may result in superinfection; use with caution in patients with seizure disorders or renal impairment; modify dosage in patients with renal impairment

Precautions CNS stimulation may occur which may lead to tremor, restlessness, confusion and very rarely to hallucinations or convulsive seizures; use with caution in patients with known or suspected CNS disorders; phototoxicity

Adverse Reactions

Central nervous system: Restlessness, dizziness, confusion, seizures, headache, hallucinations, psychosis

Dermatologic: Rash

Gastrointestinal: Nausea, diarrhea, pseudomembranous colitis, vomiting, GI bleeding

Genitourinary: Vaginitis

Hematologic: Anemia

Hepatic: Increased liver enzymes

Neuromuscular & skeletal: Arthralgia, tremors

Renal: Acute renal failure, increased serum creatinine and BUN

Toxicology For acute overdose, empty stomach contents by inducing vomiting or gastric lavage; observe and treat the patient symptomatically; maintain fluid status

Drug Interactions Antacids, iron salts, sucralfate, and zinc salts may reduce absorption by up to 98%, if given at the same time; increased toxicity/serum concentrations of theophylline, cyclosporine, nitrofurantoin, anticoagulants, caffeine; increased toxicity/levels of ciprofloxacin with azlocillin, cimetidine, probenecid; decreased effectiveness/serum concentrations of phenytoin

Drug/Food Interactions Calcium-containing foods (milk, yogurt) may decrease absorption, best to avoid concomitant ingestion

Stability Stable up to 14 days at refrigerated or room temperature when diluted with NS, USP or D_5W, USP; protect from freezing

Mechanism of Action Inhibits DNA-gyrase in susceptible organisms; inhibits relaxation of supercoiled DNA and promotes breakage of double-stranded DNA

Pharmacokinetics

Protein binding: 16% to 43%

Metabolism: Partially in the liver to active metabolites; inhibitor CYP1A2

Bioavailability: Oral: 50% to 85%; in elderly, the bioavailability has been reported to be increased (70% to 80%), serum half-life is prolonged (4.8-6.8 hours) secondary to reduced renal clearance

Half-life (patients with normal renal function): 3-5 hours

Time to peak serum concentration: Oral: Within 0.5-2 hours

Elimination: 30% to 50% of dose excreted as unchanged drug in urine; 20% to 40% of a dose is excreted in feces primarily from biliary excretion

Only small amounts of ciprofloxacin are removed by dialysis (<10%)

Usual Dosage

Geriatrics: Normal adult dose adjusted for renal function

Adults:

Oral: 250-750 mg every 12 hours, depending on severity of infection and susceptibility

I.V.: 200-400 mg every 12 hours depending on severity of infection

Ophthalmic: 1-2 drops every 2 hours while awake for 2 days, then 1-2 drops every 4 hours for 5 days

Dosing adjustment in renal impairment:

Cl_{cr} >50 mL/minute (oral); ≥30 mL/minute (I.V.): Unchanged

Cl_{cr} 30-50 mL/minute: Administer 250-500 mg (oral) every 12 hours

Cl_{cr} 5-29 mL/minute: Administer 250-500 mg (oral) every 18 hours; 200-400 mg every 18-24 hours (I.V.)

Hemodialysis or peritoneal dialysis: 250-500 mg every 24 hours (after dialysis)

Only small amounts of ciprofloxacin are removed by dialysis (<10%)

Monitoring Parameters Patients receiving concurrent ciprofloxacin and theophylline should have serum concentrations of theophylline monitored; patients receiving concurrent warfarin should have prothrombin time or INR monitored; patients receiving cyclosporine should be watched for nephrotoxicity and have their cyclosporine concentrations monitored

Reference Range Therapeutic: 2.6-3 µg/mL; Toxic: >5 µg/mL

Patient Information May be taken with food to minimize upset stomach but avoid calcium-containing foods; avoid antacid use; drink fluid liberally; instruct patient on use of ophthalmic product

Nursing Implications Hold antacids for 3-4 hours after giving; administer around-the-clock rather than 2 times/day (ie, 9 and 9, not 9 and 5) to promote less variation in peak and trough serum concentrations; encourage fluids

Special Geriatric Considerations Ciprofloxacin should not be used as first-line therapy unless the culture and sensitivity findings show resistance to usual therapy; the interactions with caffeine and theophylline can result in serious toxicity in the elderly; adjust dose for renal function (see Pharmacokinetics and Usual Dosage)

(Continued)

Ciprofloxacin (Continued)

Dosage Forms
Ciprofloxacin hydrochloride:
  Infusion, in D_5W: 400 mg (200 mL)
  Infusion, in NS or D_5W: 200 mg (100 mL)
  Injection: 200 mg (20 mL); 400 mg (40 mL)
  Solution, ophthalmic: 3.5 mg/mL (2.5 mL, 5 mL)
  Tablet: 100 mg, 250 mg, 500 mg, 750 mg

References
Bayer A, Gajewska A, Stephens M, et al, "Pharmacokinetics of Ciprofloxacin in the Elderly," *Respiration*, 1987, 51(4):292-5.

Campoli-Richards DM, Monk JP, Price A, et al, "Ciprofloxacin: A Review of Its Antibacterial Activity, Pharmacokinetic Properties and Therapeutic Use," *Drugs*, 1988, 35(4):373-447.

Guay DRP, Awni WM, Peterson PK, et al, "Single and Multiple Dose Pharmacokinetics of Oral Ciprofloxacin in Elderly Patients," *Int J Clin Pharmacol Ther Toxicol*, 1988, 26(6):279-84.

Nilsson-Ehle I and Ljungberg B, "Quinolone Disposition in the Elderly: Practical Implications," *Drugs Aging*, 1991, 1(4):279-88.

Cipro™ Injection *see* Ciprofloxacin *on page 226*

Cipro™ Oral *see* Ciprofloxacin *on page 226*

Cisapride (SIS a pride)

Brand Names Propulsid®

Therapeutic Category Antiemetic; Cholinergic Agent

Use Treatment of nocturnal symptoms of gastroesophageal reflux disease (GERD), also demonstrated effectiveness for gastroparesis, refractory constipation, and nonulcer dyspepsia

Contraindications Hypersensitivity to cisapride or any of its components; GI hemorrhage, mechanical obstruction, GI perforation, or other situations when GI motility stimulation is dangerous

Warnings Serious cardiac arrhythmias, including ventricular tachycardia, ventricular fibrillation, torsade de pointes, and Q-T prolongation have been reported in patients taking cisapride with other drugs that inhibit cytochrome P-450 III A4, such as ketoconazole, itraconazole, fluconazole, miconazole IV, troleandomycin, erythromycin, and clarithromycin. Some of these events have been fatal.

Precautions Steady-state serum concentrations are often higher in geriatric patients due to increased elimination half-life, however, adverse effect rate is no greater than in younger adults

Adverse Reactions
Central nervous system: Headache, insomnia, anxiety, nervousness, migraine headache

Dermatological: Rash, pruritus

Gastrointestinal: Diarrhea, abdominal pain, nausea, constipation, flatulence, dyspepsia

Hematologic: Thrombocytopenia, pancytopenia, leukopenia, granulocytopenia, increased LFTs, aplastic anemia

Neuromuscular & skeletal: Tremors

Respiratory: Rhinitis, sinusitis, coughing, upper respiratory tract infection

Miscellaneous: Pain, fever, increased incidence of viral infection

Overdosage Acute toxicity may present with tremors, seizures, dyspnea, ptosis, catalepsy, catatonia, hypotonia, loss of righting reflex, diarrhea, retching, borborygmi, stool and urinary frequency, and flatulence

Toxicology Treat with gastric lavage or activated charcoal; general supportive measures

Drug Interactions
Decreased effect with atropine or other anticholinergics; cisapride may decrease the absorption of digoxin

Increased effect/toxicity of Coumadin® (warfarin), absorption of cimetidine, and ranitidine increased; increased serum concentration of cisapride with concomitant use of H_2-blockers; azole antifungals (ketoconazole, fluconazole, itraconazole, miconazole IV) and monolide antibiotics (troleandomycin, erythromycin, clarithromycin) inhibit cytochrome P-450 III A4 metabolism of cisapride (see Warnings)

Increased serum concentrations observed with alcohol and benzodiazepines

Mechanism of Action Enhances the release of acetylcholine at the myenteric plexus. *In vitro* studies have shown cisapride to have serotonin-4 receptor agonistic properties which may increase gastrointestinal motility and cardiac rate; increases lower esophageal sphincter pressure and lower esophageal peristalsis; accelerates gastric emptying of both liquids and solids.

Pharmacokinetics
Bioavailability: 35% to 40%
Protein binding: 97.5% to 98%
Metabolism: Extensive to norcisapride, which is eliminated in urine and feces; substrate CYP3A4
Half-life: 6-12 hours
Elimination: <10% of dose excreted into feces and urine

Usual Dosage Geriatrics and Adults: Oral: Initial: 10 mg 4 times/day at least 15 minutes before meals and at bedtime; in some patients the dosage will need to be increased to 20 mg to obtain a satisfactory result

Monitoring Parameters Symptoms of relief or GERD, abdominal complaints, diarrhea (see Adverse Reactions)

Patient Information May enhance effects of alcohol and benzodiazepines; take 15-30 minutes before meals

Special Geriatric Considerations Steady-state serum concentrations are higher than those in younger adults; however, the therapeutic dose and pharmacologic effects are the same as those in younger adults and no adjustment in dose recommended for elderly

Dosage Forms
Suspension, oral (cherry cream flavor): 1 mg/mL (450 mL)
Tablet, scored: 10 mg, 20 mg

Citracal® [OTC] *see* Calcium Salts (Oral) *on page 152*

Citrate of Magnesia *see* Magnesium Citrate *on page 563*

Cl-719 *see* Gemfibrozil *on page 421*

Cla *see* Clarithromycin *on this page*

Claforan® *see* Cefotaxime *on page 182*

Clarithromycin (kla RITH roe mye sin)

Related Information
Cephalosporins, Aminoglycosides, Macrolides, & Quinolones *on page 1014*
Prevention of Bacterial Endocarditis *on page 1062*
Regimens Used to Treat *Helicobacter pylori* and Ulcers *on page 1033*

Brand Names Biaxin™

Synonyms Cla

Generic Available No

Therapeutic Category Antibiotic, Macrolide

Use Treatment against most respiratory pathogens (eg, *S. pyogenes, S. pneumoniae, S. agalactiae, S. viridans, M. catarrhalis, C. trachomatis, Legionella* spp, *Mycoplasma pneumoniae, S. aureus*). Clarithromycin is highly active (MICs ≤0.25 mcg/mL) against *H. influenzae*, the combination of clarithromycin and its metabolite demonstrate an additive effect. Additionally, clarithromycin has shown activity against *C. pneumoniae* (including strain TWAR); treatment of peptic ulcers secondary to *H. pylori*; treatment of disseminated *Mycobacterium avium* complex

Contraindications Hypersensitivity to clarithromycin, erythromycin, or any macrolide antibiotic; concurrent use with terfenadine or astemizole is not advised (see Drug Interactions); use with pimozide

Warnings In presence of severe renal impairment with or without coexisting hepatic impairment, decreased dosage or prolonged dosing interval may be appropriate; antibiotic associated colitis has been reported with use of clarithromycin; elderly patients experienced increased incidents of adverse effects due to known age-related decreases in renal function

Adverse Reactions The incidence of adverse GI effects (diarrhea, nausea, vomiting, dyspepsia, abdominal pain) is lower (13%) compared to erythromycin-treated patients (32%)

Cardiovascular: Ventricular tachycardia, torsade de pointes
Central nervous system: Headache
Gastrointestinal: Diarrhea, flatulence, nausea, abdominal pain, dysgeusia, dyspepsia
Hematologic: Decreased white blood cell count, elevated prothrombin time
Hepatic: Elevated AST, alkaline phosphatase, and bilirubin
Renal: Elevated BUN and serum creatinine

Overdosage Symptoms of overdose include nausea, vomiting, diarrhea, prostration, reversible pancreatitis, hearing loss with or without tinnitus or vertigo

Toxicology General and supportive care only

Drug Interactions
Clarithromycin decreased clearance/increase risk of toxicity of astemizole, loratadine, cisapride
(Continued)

229

Clarithromycin *(Continued)*

Clarithromycin has been shown to increase serum **theophylline** concentrations by as much as 20%; digoxin serum concentrations have been elevated (approximately 10% of patients) producing abnormal EKG readings. **Carbamazepine** levels have been shown to increase after a single dose of clarithromycin. While other drug interactions (digoxin, anticoagulants, ergotamine, triazolam) known to occur with erythromycin have not been reported in clinical trials with clarithromycin, concurrent use of these drugs should be monitored closely.

Mechanism of Action Exerts its antibacterial action by binding to 50S ribosomal subunit resulting in inhibition of protein synthesis. The 14-OH metabolite of clarithromycin is twice as active as the parent compound.

Pharmacokinetics

Absorption: Highly stable in the presence of gastric acid (unlike erythromycin)

Distribution: Widely into most body tissues with the exception of the CNS

Metabolism: Partially converted to the microbiologically active metabolite, 14-OH clarithromycin; substrate and inhibitor CYP3A4

Bioavailability: 50% (250 mg tablet)

Half-life, elimination: 3-4 hours with a 250 mg dose; 5-7 hours with a 500 mg dose; 7.7 hours in healthy elderly

Time to peak serum concentration: Oral: 2-4 hours

Elimination: Following 250 mg or 500 mg doses every 12 hours, ~20% to 30% of unchanged parent drug is excreted in urine

Usual Dosage Geriatrics and Adults: Oral: Usual dose: 250-500 mg every 12 hours for 7-14 days

Upper respiratory tract: 250-500 mg every 12 hours for 10-14 days
  Pharyngitis/tonsillitis: 250 mg every 12 hours for 10 days
  Acute maxillary sinusitis: 500 mg every 12 hours for 14 days
  Mycobacterium avium complex: 500 mg every 12 hours

Lower respiratory tract: 250-500 mg every 12 hours for 7-14 days
  Acute exacerbation of chronic bronchitis due to:
    M. catarrhalis and *S. pneumoniae*: 250 mg every 12 hours for 7-14 days
    H. influenzae: 500 mg every 12 hours for 7-14 days
  Pneumonia due to *M. pneumoniae* and *S. pneumoniae*: 250 mg every 12 hours for 7-14 days

Uncomplicated skin and skin structure: 250 mg every 12 hours for 7-14 days

Helicobacter pylori: 500 mg three times/day for 2 weeks with omeprazole, 40 mg once daily for 2 weeks, then 20 mg once daily for 2 weeks (see Appendix for Regimens Used to Treat *Helicobacter pylori* and Ulcers)

Dosing adjustment in severe renal impairment: Decreased doses or prolonged dosing intervals are recommended

Patient Information May be taken with meals; finish all medication; do not skip doses

Nursing Implications Clarithromycin may be given with or without meals; administer every 12 hours rather than twice daily to avoid peak and trough variation in serum concentrations

Special Geriatric Considerations Considered one of the drugs of choice in the outpatient treatment of community-acquired pneumonia in older adults. After doses of 500 mg every 12 hours for 5 days, 12 healthy elderly had significantly increased C_{max} and C_{min}, elimination half-lives of clarithromycin and 14-OH clarithromycin compared to 12 healthy young subjects. These changes were attributed to a significant decrease in renal clearance; at a dose of 1000 mg twice daily, 100% of 13 older adults experienced an adverse event compared to only 10% taking 500 mg twice daily (see Usual Dosage and Pharmacokinetics).

Dosage Forms

Granules for oral suspension: 125 mg/5 mL (100 mL, 200 mL); 250 mg/5 mL (100 mL, 200 mL)

Tablet, film coated: 250 mg, 500 mg

References

American Thoracic Society, "Guidelines for the Initial Management of Adults With Community-Acquired Pneumonia: Diagnosis, Assessment of Severity, and Initial Antimicrobial Therapy," *Am Rev Respir Dis*, 1993, 148(5):1418-26.

Chu SY, Wilson DS, Guay DR, et al, "Clarithromycin Pharmacokinetics in Healthy Young and Elderly Volunteers," *J Clin Pharmacol*, 1992, 32(11):1045-9.

Wallace RJ Jr, Brown BA, and Griffith DE, "Drug Intolerance to High-Dose Clarithromycin Among Elderly Patients," *Diagn Microbiol Infect Dis*, 1993, 16(3):215-21.

Claritin® *see* Loratadine *on page 550*

Clear Away® **Disc [OTC]** *see* Salicylic Acid *on page 845*

Clear Eyes® **[OTC]** *see* Naphazoline *on page 653*

Clear Tussin® 30 *see Guaifenesin and Dextromethorphan on page 439*

Clemastine (KLEM as teen)
Brand Names Antihist-1® [OTC]; Tavist®; Tavist®-1 [OTC]
Generic Available No
Therapeutic Category Antihistamine
Use Perennial and seasonal allergic rhinitis and other allergic symptoms including urticaria
Contraindications Narrow-angle glaucoma, bladder neck obstruction, symptomatic prostate hypertrophy, asthmatic attacks, and stenosing peptic ulcer, hypersensitivity to clemastine or any component
Warnings Antihistamines are more likely to cause dizziness, excessive sedation, syncope, toxic confusional states, and hypotension in the elderly
Precautions Use with caution in patients with heart disease, hypertension, thyroid disease, and asthma
Adverse Reactions
Central nervous system: Sedation, paradoxical excitation
Gastrointestinal: Nausea, xerostomia
Ocular: Diplopia
Renal: Polyuria
Respiratory: Thick bronchial secretions
Overdosage Symptoms of overdose include dry mouth, flushed skin, dilated pupils, CNS depression
Toxicology There is no specific treatment for an antihistamine overdose, however, most of its clinical toxicity is due to anticholinergic effects. Cholinesterase inhibitors may be useful by reducing acetylcholinesterase. Acetylcholinesterase inhibitors include physostigmine, neostigmine, pyridostigmine, and edrophonium. For anticholinergic overdose with severe life-threatening symptoms, physostigmine 1-2 mg I.V., slowly may be given to reverse these effects.
Drug Interactions Increased toxicity (CNS depression): CNS depressants, MAO inhibitors, alcohol, tricyclic antidepressants, phenothiazines
Mechanism of Action Competes with histamine for H_1-receptor sites on effector cells in the gastrointestinal tract, blood vessels, and respiratory tract
Pharmacodynamics
Peak therapeutic effect: Within 5-7 hours
Duration of action: 10-12 hours; some patients experience therapeutic effects for 24 hours
Pharmacokinetics
Absorption: Almost 100% from GI tract
Metabolism: In the liver
Elimination: In urine
Usual Dosage Oral:
Geriatrics: 1.34 mg once or twice daily
Adults: 1.34 mg twice daily to 2.68 mg 3 times/day; do not exceed 8.04 mg/day
Monitoring Parameters Relief of symptoms
Patient Information May cause drowsiness; avoid CNS depressants and alcohol
Nursing Implications Monitor for relief of symptoms, side effects
Additional Information 1.34 mg of clemastine fumarate = 1 mg clemastine base. Clemastine offers no significant benefit over other antihistamines except that it may be dosed twice daily (in adults) as compared to other antihistamines with more frequent dosing.
Special Geriatric Considerations See Contraindications and Warnings
Dosage Forms
Clemastine fumarate:
Syrup (citrus flavor): 0.67 mg/5 mL with alcohol 5.5% (120 mL)
Tablet: 1.34 mg, 2.68 mg

Cleocin HCl® *see Clindamycin on next page*
Cleocin Pediatric® *see Clindamycin on next page*
Cleocin Phosphate® *see Clindamycin on next page*
Cleocin T® *see Clindamycin on next page*

Clidinium and Chlordiazepoxide
(kli DI nee um & klor dye az e POKS ide)
Brand Names Clindex®; Librax®
Synonyms Chlordiazepoxide and Clidinium
Generic Available Yes
(Continued)

Clidinium and Chlordiazepoxide *(Continued)*

Therapeutic Category Anticholinergic Agent

Use Adjunct treatment of peptic ulcer, treatment of irritable bowel syndrome

Usual Dosage Geriatrics and Adults: Oral: 1-2 capsules 3-4 times/day, before meals or food and at bedtime

Administration Should be administered before meals

Nursing Implications After extended therapy, abrupt discontinuation should be avoided and a gradual dose tapering schedule followed

Special Geriatric Considerations The use of anticholinergic agents may cause problems with bladder emptying, constipation or cause confusion. The addition of chlordiazepoxide may enhance confusion potential. Monitor closely initially.

Dosage Forms Capsule: Clidinium bromide 2.5 mg and chlordiazepoxide hydrochloride 5 mg

Climara® Transdermal *see* Estradiol *on page 350*

Clinda-Derm® Topical Solution *see* Clindamycin *on this page*

Clindamycin (klin da MYE sin)

Related Information

I.V. Medication Recommendations *on page 1080*

Penicillins, Penicillin-Related Antibiotics, & Other Antibiotics *on page 1010*

Prevention of Bacterial Endocarditis *on page 1062*

Brand Names Cleocin HCl®; Cleocin Pediatric®; Cleocin Phosphate®; Cleocin T®; Clinda-Derm® Topical Solution; C/T/S® Topical Solution

Generic Available Yes: Injection

Therapeutic Category Acne Products; Antibiotic, Anaerobic; Antibiotic, Miscellaneous

Use Treatment of aerobic and anaerobic streptococci (except enterococci), most staphylococci, *Bacteroides* sp. and *Actinomyces*; used topically in treatment of severe acne

Contraindications Hypersensitivity to clindamycin or any component; previous pseudomembranous colitis, hepatic impairment; do not use for the treatment of minor bacterial and viral infections

Warnings Can cause severe and possibly fatal colitis; characterized by severe persistent diarrhea, severe abdominal cramps and possibly, the passage of blood and mucus; discontinue drug if significant diarrhea occurs

Precautions Dosage adjustment may be necessary in patients with severe hepatic dysfunction; no change necessary with renal insufficiency; diarrhea may not be well tolerated in the frail elderly because of fluid and electrolyte loss; superinfection with prolonged therapy

Adverse Reactions

Cardiovascular: Hypotension

Dermatologic: Urticaria, rash, Stevens-Johnson syndrome

Gastrointestinal: Diarrhea, nausea, vomiting, pseudomembranous colitis

Hematologic: Eosinophilia, granulocytopenia, thrombocytopenia, neutropenia

Hepatic: Elevation of liver enzymes

Local: Sterile abscess at I.M. injection site, thrombophlebitis

Neuromuscular & skeletal: Polyarthritis

Renal: Rare renal dysfunction

Drug Interactions Increased duration of neuromuscular blockade from tubocurarine, pancuronium; erythromycin (*in vitro* antagonism)

Stability Do **not** refrigerate the reconstituted oral solution because it will thicken; oral solution stable for 2 weeks at room temperature following reconstitution; I.V. infusion solution in NS or D_5W solution is stable for 16 days at room temperature

Mechanism of Action Reversibly binds to 50S ribosomal subunits preventing peptide bond formation thus inhibiting bacterial protein synthesis; bacteriostatic or bactericidal depending on drug concentration, infection site, and organism

Pharmacokinetics

Absorption: Topical: ~10% absorbed systemically

Distribution: No significant concentrations seen in CSF, even with inflamed meninges

Protein binding: 94%

Bioavailability: Oral: ~90%

Half-life: 1.6-5.3 hours, average: 2-3 hours

Time to peak serum concentration:

Oral: Within 60 minutes

I.M.: Within 1-3 hours

Elimination: Most of the drug is eliminated by hepatic metabolism; 10% of an oral dose is excreted in urine and 3.6% is excreted in feces as active drug and metabolites

Usual Dosage

Geriatrics and Adults:

Oral: 150-450 mg/dose every 6-8 hours; maximum dose: 1.8 g/day

I.M., I.V.: 1.2-1.8 g/day in 2-3 divided doses; maximum dose: 3.6 g/day

Adults:

Topical: Apply twice daily

Pneumonitis carinii pneumonia:

Oral: 300-450 mg 4 times/day with primaquine

I.M., I.V.: 1200-2400 mg/day with pyrimethamine

I.V.: 600 mg 4 times/day with primaquine

Vaginal: One full applicator (100 mg) inserted intravaginally once daily before bedtime for 7 consecutive days

Dosing interval in renal impairment: No change necessary

Administration Administer oral dosage form with a full glass of water to minimize esophageal ulceration. Administer around-the-clock rather than 4 times/day, 3 times/day, etc (ie, 12-6-12-6, not 9-1-5-9) to promote less variation in peak and trough serum concentrations.

Monitoring Parameters Observe for changes in bowel frequency; during prolonged therapy monitor CBC, liver and renal function tests periodically

Patient Information Report any severe diarrhea immediately and do not take antidiarrheal medication; take each oral dose with a full glass of water; finish all medication; do not skip doses; **should not engage in sexual intercourse during treatment with vaginal product**; avoid contact of topical gel/solution with eyes, abraded skin, or mucous membranes

Nursing Implications See Administration

Special Geriatric Considerations Clindamycin has not been studied in the elderly; however, since it is eliminated principally by nonrenal mechanisms, major alteration in its pharmacokinetics are not expected (see Precautions)

Dosage Forms

Capsule, as hydrochloride: 75 mg, 150 mg, 300 mg

Granules for oral solution, as palmitate: 75 mg/5 mL (100 mL)

Clindamycin phosphate:

Gel, topical: 1% [10 mg/g] (7.5 g, 30 g)

Infusion, in D$_5$W: 300 mg (50 mL); 600 mg (50 mL)

Injection: 150 mg/mL (2 mL, 4 mL, 6 mL, 50 mL, 60 mL)

Solution, topical: 1% [10 mg/mL] (30 mL, 60 mL, 480 mL)

Cream, vaginal: 2% (40 g with 7 applicators)

Lotion: 1% [10 mg/mL] (60 mL)

References

Yoshikawa TT, "Antimicrobial Therapy for the Elderly Patient," *J Am Geriatr Soc*, 1990, 38(12):1353-72.

Clindex® *see* Clidinium and Chlordiazepoxide *on page 231*

Clinoril® *see* Sulindac *on page 881*

Clobetasol (kloe BAY ta sol)

Related Information

Corticosteroids Comparison, Topical *on page 1030*

Brand Names Temovate®

Generic Available Yes

Therapeutic Category Corticosteroid, Topical (Low Potency); Corticosteroid, Topical (Super High Potency)

Use Short-term relief (<2 weeks) of inflammatory and pruritic manifestations of corticosteroid-responsive dermatoses (super high potency topical)

Contraindications Viral, fungal, or tubercular skin lesions; known hypersensitivity to clobetasol or any component

Precautions Systemic absorption of topical corticosteroids has produced reversible HPA axis suppression. This is more likely to occur when the preparation is used on large surfaces or denuded areas for prolonged periods of time or with an occlusive dressing. Should not be used for longer than 2 weeks; should not be used on the face, axillae, or groin.

Adverse Reactions

Dermatologic: Acne, hypopigmentation, allergic dermatitis, maceration of the skin, skin atrophy, striae, miliaria, telangiectasia

Endocrine & metabolic: HPA suppression, Cushing's syndrome, growth retardation

Local: Burning, itching, irritation, dryness, folliculitis, hypertrichosis

(Continued)

Clobetasol *(Continued)*

Miscellaneous: Secondary infection

Mechanism of Action Topical corticosteroids have anti-inflammatory, anti-pruritic, vasoconstrictive, and antiproliferative actions

Pharmacokinetics Absorption: Percutaneous absorption variable and dependent upon many factors including vehicle used, integrity of epidermis, dose, and use of occlusive dressings

Usual Dosage Geriatrics and Adults: Topical: Apply in thin layer twice daily for up to 2 weeks with no more than 50 g/week

Monitoring Parameters Relief of symptoms

Patient Information Use only as prescribed and for no longer than the period prescribed; apply sparingly in a thin film and rub in lightly; avoid contact with eyes; notify physician if condition persists or worsens; do not use longer than 2 weeks

Nursing Implications Do not use on open or weeping wounds; apply sparingly

Additional Information Considered a super high potency steroid; avoid use on face

Special Geriatric Considerations Due to age-related changes in skin, limit use of topical glucocorticosteroids (see Precautions)

Dosage Forms
Clobetasol propionate:
Cream: 0.05% (15 g, 30 g, 45 g)
Cream, in emollient base: 0.05% (15 g, 30 g, 60 g)
Gel: 0.05% (15 g, 30 g, 45 g)
Ointment, topical: 0.05% (15 g, 30 g, 45 g)
Scalp application: 0.05% (25 mL, 50 mL)

Clocort® Maximum Strength *see* Hydrocortisone *on page 462*

Clofazimine (kloe FA zi meen)

Brand Names Lamprene®

Generic Available No

Therapeutic Category Antibiotic, Miscellaneous

Use Treatment of dapsone-resistant leprosy; multibacillary dapsone-sensitive leprosy; erythema nodosum leprosum; *Mycobacterium avium* - intracellular (MAI) infections

Contraindications Hypersensitivity to clofazimine or any component

Warnings Use with caution in patients with GI problems; well tolerated when administered in dosages ≤100 mg/day; dosages >100 mg/day should be used for as short a duration as possible; skin discoloration may lead to depression; two suicides have been reported

Adverse Reactions
Central nervous system: Dizziness, drowsiness
Dermatologic: Pink to brownish black discoloration of the skin and conjunctiva, dry skin, rash, pruritus
Endocrine & metabolic: Hyperglycemia
Gastrointestinal: Constipation, abdominal pain, diarrhea, nausea, vomiting, bowel obstruction, GI bleeding
Ocular: Irritation of the eyes

Toxicology Following GI decontamination, treatment is supportive

Drug Interactions Decreased effect with dapsone (unconfirmed)

Mechanism of Action Binds preferentially to mycobacterial DNA to inhibit mycobacterial growth; also has some anti-inflammatory activity through an unknown mechanism

Pharmacokinetics
Absorption: Oral: 45% to 70% of dose absorbed slowly
Distribution: Remains in tissues for prolonged periods
Metabolism: Partially in the liver to two metabolites
Half-life:
Terminal: 8 days
Tissue: 70 days
Elimination: Mainly in feces; only negligible amounts excreted unchanged in urine; small amounts excreted in sputum, saliva, and sweat

Usual Dosage Geriatrics and Adults: Oral:
Dapsone-resistant leprosy: 100 mg/day in combination with one or more antileprosy drugs for 3 years; then alone 100 mg/day
Dapsone-sensitive multibacillary leprosy: 100 mg/day in combination with 2 or more antileprosy drugs for at least 2 years and continue until negative skin

smears are obtained, then institute single drug therapy with appropriate agent

Erythema nodosum leprosum: 100-200 mg/day for up to 3 months or longer then taper dose to 100 mg/day when possible

Pyoderma gangrenosum: 300-400 mg/day for up to 12 months

Dosing adjustment in hepatic impairment: Should be considered in severe hepatic dysfunction

Monitoring Parameters GI complaints, signs and symptoms of infection

Test Interactions Increased ESR, increased glucose (S), increased albumin, increased bilirubin, increased AST

Patient Information Drug may cause a pink to brownish-black discoloration of the skin, conjunctiva, tears, sweat, urine, feces, and nasal secretions; although reversible, may take months to years to disappear after therapy is complete; take with meals

Nursing Implications Requires long-term therapy; encourage compliance and monitor for side effects, particularly GI and dermatologic; see Warnings

Special Geriatric Considerations No specific studies in the elderly; use with caution in diabetics (see Adverse Reactions)

Dosage Forms Capsule, as palmatate: 50 mg, 100 mg

Clofibrate (kloe FYE brate)

Brand Names Atromid-S®

Generic Available Yes

Therapeutic Category Antilipemic Agent

Use Adjunct to dietary therapy in the management of hyperlipidemias associated with high triglyceride levels (type III hyperlipidemia); primarily lowers triglycerides and very low density lipoprotein

Contraindications Hypersensitivity to clofibrate or any component, severe hepatic or renal impairment, primary biliary cirrhosis

Warnings Clofibrate has been shown to be tumorigenic in toxicity studies using rats; discontinue if lipid response is not obtained; no evidence substantiates a beneficial effect on cardiovascular mortality

Adverse Reactions The most frequent is nausea which usually decreases with continued therapy or reduction in dosage

Central nervous system: Fatigue, drowsiness, dizziness

Dermatologic: Skin rash, alopecia, dry skin, dry and brittle hair, urticaria, pruritus

Gastrointestinal: Nausea, vomiting, diarrhea, gastritis, weight gain, flatulence, abdominal pain

Genitourinary: Impotence

Hematologic: Leukopenia, eosinophilia, anemia

Hepatic: Hepatomegaly, increased liver function test

Neuromuscular & skeletal: Myalgia, weakness

Renal: Rhabdomyolysis-induced renal failure

Miscellaneous: Flu-like symptoms

Drug Interactions

May potentiate the anticoagulant effects of warfarin; insulin and sulfonylureas effects may be increased

Probenecid may increase the effects of clofibrate

Mechanism of Action Mechanism is unclear but thought to reduce cholesterol synthesis and triglyceride hepatic-vascular transference

Pharmacokinetics

Absorption: Occurs completely

Distribution: V_d: 5.5 L/kg

Protein binding: 95%

Metabolism: In the liver to an inactive glucuronide ester

Intestinal transformation is required to activate the drug

Half-life: 6-24 hours, increases significantly with reduced renal function

Anuria: 110 hours

Time to peak serum concentration: Within 3-6 hours

Elimination: 40% to 70% excreted in urine

Usual Dosage Geriatrics and Adults: Oral: 500 mg 4 times/day

Dosing interval in renal impairment:

Cl_{cr} 15-50 mL/minute: Administer every 12-18 hours

Cl_{cr} <10 mL/minute: Avoid use

Monitoring Parameters Serum lipid profile; triglycerides and fractionated cholesterol

Test Interactions Increased creatine phosphokinase [CPK] (S); decreased alkaline phosphatase (S), cholesterol (S), glucose, uric acid (S)

(Continued)

Clofibrate *(Continued)*

Patient Information May be taken with food if stomach upset occurs; contact your physician if severe stomach pain with nausea and vomiting occurs, fever or chills, chest pain, irregular heart rhythm, shortness of breath, weight gain, decreased urination, blood in urine, leg swelling; adhere to prescribed diet

Nursing Implications See Patient Information and Special Geriatric Considerations

Special Geriatric Considerations The definition of and, therefore, when to treat hyperlipidemia in the elderly is a controversial issue. The National Cholesterol Education Program recommends that all adults 20 years of age and older maintain a plasma cholesterol concentration <200 mg/dL. By this definition, 60% of all elderly would be considered to have an elevated plasma cholesterol. However, plasma cholesterol has been shown to be a less reliable predictor of coronary heart disease in the elderly. Therefore, it is the authors' belief that pharmacologic treatment be reserved for those who are unable to obtain a desirable plasma cholesterol concentration by diet alone and for whom the benefits of treatment are believed to outweigh the potential adverse effects, drug interactions, and cost of treatment. Adjust dose for renal function.

Dosage Forms Capsule: 500 mg

Clomipramine (kloe MI pra meen)

Related Information
Antidepressant Agents Comparison *on page 1021*
Antidepressant Medication Guidelines *on page 1075*

Brand Names Anafranil®

Generic Available No

Therapeutic Category Antidepressant, Tricyclic

Use Treatment of obsessive-compulsive disorder (OCD)

Unlabeled use: May also relieve depression, panic attacks, panic disorder, chronic pain

Contraindications Patients in acute recovery stage of recent myocardial infarction; not to be used within 14 days of MAO inhibitors

Warnings Seizures are likely and are dose-related; can be additive when coadministered with other drugs that can lower the seizure threshold; use with caution in patients with asthma, bladder outlet destruction, angle-closure glaucoma

Adverse Reactions

Cardiovascular: Orthostatic hypotension, tachycardia

Central nervous system: Seizures, drowsiness, dizziness, confusion, headache, delirium, hyperthermia, aggressive reaction

Dermatologic: Rash, dry skin

Gastrointestinal: Xerostomia, constipation, nausea, vomiting, increased appetite, weight gain

Genitourinary: Urinary retention, ejaculation failure

Hematologic: Agranulocytosis, anemia

Hepatic: Hepatitis

Neuromuscular & skeletal: Weakness

Ocular: Increased intraocular pressure, blurred vision

Otic: Vestibular disorder

Overdosage Symptoms of overdose include agitation, confusion, hallucinations, hyperthermia, CNS depression, dry mucous membranes, arrhythmias

Toxicology Following initiation of essential overdose management, toxic symptoms should be treated

Ventricular arrhythmias often respond to systemic alkalinization (sodium bicarbonate 0.5-2 mEq/kg I.V.) and/or phenytoin 15-20 mg/kg. Arrhythmias unresponsive to this therapy may respond to lidocaine 1 mg/kg I.V. followed by a titrated infusion. Physostigmine (1-2 mg I.V. slowly for adults) may be indicated in reversing cardiac arrhythmias that are life-threatening.

Seizures usually respond to diazepam I.V. boluses (5-10 mg for adults up to 30 mg). If seizures are unresponsive or recur, phenytoin or phenobarbital may be required.

Drug Interactions Cimetidine, fluoxetine, methylphenidate, and haloperidol may decrease the metabolism and/or increase TCA levels

Decreased effect with barbiturates, carbamazepine, phenytoin

Increased effect of alcohol, CNS depressants, anticholinergics, sympathomimetics

Increased toxicity: MAO inhibitors (increased temperature, seizures, coma, and death); antipsychotics (increased risk of hyperthermia)

Mechanism of Action Clomipramine appears to affect serotonin uptake while its active metabolite, desmethylclomipramine, affects norepinephrine uptake

Pharmacodynamics Onset of action: 1-3 weeks; 5-HT >NE

Pharmacokinetics

Absorption: Oral: Rapid

Metabolism: Extensive first-pass; metabolized to desmethylclomipramine (active) in the liver; substrate CYP1A2, 2C19, 2D6

Half-life: 20-30 hours

Usual Dosage Geriatrics and Adults: Oral: Initial: 25 mg/day and gradually increase, as tolerated, to 100 mg/day the first 2 weeks, may then be increased to a total of 250 mg/day maximum

Monitoring Parameters Signs and symptoms of disorder, plasma concentrations, blood pressure

Reference Range Therapeutic plasma concentration: 80-100 ng/mL

Test Interactions Elevated glucose

Patient Information May cause seizures; caution should be used in activities that require alertness like driving, operating machinery, or swimming; effect of drug may take several weeks to appear; avoid alcohol; do not discontinue abruptly; may cause dry mouth, constipation, blurred vision

Nursing Implications Monitor blood pressure and pulse rate prior to and during initial therapy; evaluate mental status; monitor weight, may increase appetite and possibly a craving for sweets

Special Geriatric Considerations Not approved as an antidepressant, clomipramine's anticholinergic and hypotensive effects limit its use versus other preferred antidepressants; elderly patients were found to have higher dose-normalized plasma concentrations as a result of decreased demethylation (decreased 50%) and hydroxylation (25%)

Dosage Forms Capsule, as hydrochloride: 25 mg, 50 mg, 75 mg

References
Bocksberger JP, Gex-Fabry M, Gauthey L, et al, "Clomipramine Therapy in the Geriatric Hospital: Experience With Therapeutic Drug Monitoring," *Ther Drug Monit*, 1994, 16(2):113-9.

Clonazepam (kloe NA ze pam)

Related Information

Antacid Drug Interactions *on page 1096*
Anxiolytic/Hypnotic Use in Long-Term Care Facilities *on page 1099*
Benzodiazepines Comparison *on page 1024*

Brand Names Klonopin™

Generic Available No

Therapeutic Category Antianxiety Agent; Anticonvulsant, Benzodiazepine; Benzodiazepine

Use Prophylaxis of absence (petit mal), petit mal variant (Lennox-Gastaut), akinetic, and myoclonic seizures

Unlabeled use: Restless legs syndrome, neuralgia (chronic pain syndromes), multifocal tic disorder, parkinsonian dysarthria, acute manic episodes in bipolar disorder, and adjunct therapy for schizophrenia

Restrictions C-IV

Contraindications Hypersensitivity to clonazepam, any component, or other benzodiazepines; severe liver disease, acute narrow-angle glaucoma

Precautions Use with caution in patients with chronic respiratory disease or impaired renal function; abrupt discontinuance may precipitate withdrawal symptoms, status epilepticus or seizures; use cautiously in depressed patients

Adverse Reactions

Cardiovascular: Hypotension

Central nervous system: Drowsiness, changes in behavior or personality, ataxia, vertigo, confusion, hallucinations, depression, disorientation, memory impairment, decreased concentration, headache, hypotonia, choreiform movements, staggering, falling

Dermatologic: Rash

Gastrointestinal: Nausea, xerostomia, vomiting, diarrhea, constipation, anorexia, hypersalivation

Hematologic: Thrombocytopenia, anemia, leukopenia, eosinophilia

Neuromuscular & skeletal: Tremors

Ocular: Nystagmus, blurred vision

Respiratory: Bronchial hypersecretion, respiratory depression, apnea

Miscellaneous: Physical and psychological dependence

Overdosage Symptoms of overdose include somnolence, confusion, ataxia, diminished reflexes, or coma

(Continued)

Clonazepam *(Continued)*

Toxicology Treatment for benzodiazepine overdose is supportive. Rarely is mechanical ventilation required. Flumazenil (Romazicon™) has been shown to selectively block the binding of benzodiazepines to CNS receptors, resulting in a reversal of benzodiazepine-induced CNS depression.

Drug Interactions Benzodiazepines may increase digoxin concentrations and may decrease the effect of levodopa; probenecid may increase onset of action and prolong the effect of benzodiazepine

Decreased metabolism: Cimetidine, fluoxetine

Increased metabolism: Rifampin

Increased toxicity: CNS depressants, alcohol

Mechanism of Action Suppresses the spike-and-wave discharge in absence seizures by depressing nerve transmission in the motor cortex

Pharmacodynamics

Onset of action: 20-60 minutes

Duration: 12 hours

Pharmacokinetics

Absorption: Oral: Well absorbed

Distribution: V_d: 1.5-4.4 L/kg

Protein binding 85%

Metabolism: Extensive

Half-life: 19-50 hours

Elimination: Metabolites excreted as glucuronide or sulfate conjugates; less than 2% excreted unchanged in urine

Usual Dosage Geriatrics and Adults: Oral: Initial daily dose not to exceed 1.5 mg given in 3 divided doses; may increase by 0.5-1 mg every third day until seizures are controlled or adverse effects seen; usual maintenance dose: 0.05-0.2 mg/kg; do not exceed 20 mg/day

Monitoring Parameters Monitor blood pressure, respiratory rate, motor coordination, mental status

Reference Range

Sample size: 2 mL serum or plasma (green top tube)

Therapeutic concentrations: 20-80 ng/mL; Toxic concentration: >80 ng/mL

Timing of serum samples: Peak serum concentrations occur 1-3 hours after oral ingestion; half-life: 20-40 hours; therefore, steady-state occurs in 5-7 days

Patient Information May cause drowsiness, dizziness, confusion. Avoid alcohol; use with caution when driving or performing tasks requiring alertness

Nursing Implications Observe patient for excess sedation, respiratory depression, orthostasis

Additional Information Ethosuximide or valproic acid may be preferred for treatment of absence (petit mal) seizures; clonazepam-induced behavioral disturbances may be more frequent in mentally handicapped patients; up to 30% of patients have demonstrated a loss of anticonvulsant control within several months which requires a dosage adjustment

Special Geriatric Considerations Hepatic clearance may be decreased allowing accumulation of active drug. Observe for signs of CNS and pulmonary toxicity (see Adverse Reactions)

Dosage Forms Tablet: 0.5 mg, 1 mg, 2 mg

Clonidine *(KLOE ni deen)*

Brand Names Catapres® Oral; Catapres-TTS® Transdermal; Duraclon® Injection

Generic Available Yes: Tablet

Therapeutic Category Alpha-Adrenergic Agonist

Use Management of mild to moderate hypertension; either used alone or in combination with other antihypertensives; not recommended for first-line therapy for hypertension

Unlabeled use: heroin withdrawal, smoking cessation therapy, prophylaxis of migraines, glaucoma, diabetic diarrhea, vasomotor symptoms of menopause, postherpetic neuralgia, ulcerative colitis

Contraindications Hypersensitivity to clonidine hydrochloride or any component

Warnings Do not abruptly discontinue; rapid increase in blood pressure, and symptoms of sympathetic overactivity (such as increased heart rate, tremor, agitation, anxiety, insomnia, sweating, palpitations) may occur; if need to discontinue, taper dose gradually over more than 1 week

Precautions Dosage modification may be required in patients with renal impairment; use with caution in cerebrovascular disease, coronary insufficiency, renal impairment, sinus node dysfunction; use with caution in patients unable to comply with the therapeutic regimen because of the risk of rebound hypertension

Adverse Reactions

Cardiovascular: Raynaud's phenomenon, hypotension, bradycardia, palpitation, tachycardia, congestive heart failure

Central nervous system: Drowsiness, headache, dizziness, fatigue, insomnia, anxiety, nightmares, hallucinations, delirium, nervousness, depression

Dermatologic: Rash

Endocrine & metabolic: Sodium and water retention, parotid pain

Gastrointestinal: Constipation, anorexia, xerostomia

Local: Skin reactions with patch

Overdosage Symptoms of overdose include bradycardia, CNS depression, hypothermia, diarrhea, respiratory depression, apnea

Toxicology Treatment is primarily supportive and symptomatic. Hypotension usually responds to I.V. fluids or Trendelenburg positioning. If unresponsive to these measures the use of a parenteral vasoconstrictor may be required (eg, norepinephrine 0.1-0.2 mcg/kg/minute titrated to response). Naloxone may be utilized in treating the hypotension, CNS depression and/or apnea and should be given I.V. 0.4-2 mg, with repeats as needed. Atropine 15 mcg/kg I.V. may be needed for symptomatic bradycardia.

Drug Interactions

Beta-blockers may potentiate bradycardia in patients receiving clonidine and may increase the rebound hypertension seen with clonidine withdrawal; discontinue beta-blocker several days before clonidine is tapered off

Other hypotensive agents may potentiate hypotensive effects

Tricyclic antidepressants antagonize hypotensive effects of clonidine

Mechanism of Action Stimulates alpha$_2$-adrenoreceptors in the brain stem, thus activating an inhibitory neuron, resulting in reduced sympathetic outflow, producing a decrease in vasomotor tone and heart rate

Pharmacodynamics

Onset of action: Oral: 30-60 minutes

Peak effect: Within 2-4 hours

Duration: 6-10 hours

Pharmacokinetics

Distribution: V_d: 2.1 L/kg

Metabolism: Hepatic to inactive metabolites; enterohepatic recirculation

Bioavailability: Oral: 75% to 95%

Half-life:

Normal renal function: 6-20 hours

Renal impairment: 18-41 hours

Elimination: 65% excreted in urine (32% unchanged and 22% excreted in feces)

Usual Dosage

Geriatrics: Oral: Initial: 0.1 mg once daily at bedtime; increase gradually as needed

Adults: Oral: Initial: 0.1 mg twice daily, usual maintenance dose: 0.2-1.2 mg/day in 2-4 divided doses; maximum recommended dose: 2.4 mg/day

Unlabeled route of administration: Sublingual clonidine 0.1-0.2 mg twice daily may be effective in patients unable to take oral medication

Clonidine tolerance test (test of growth hormone release from the pituitary): 0.15 mg/m^2 or 4 mcg/kg as a single dose

Transdermal: Initial: Catapres-TTS® 1 every week; maximum: 2 Catapres-TTS® 3 every week

Conversion from oral to transdermal:

Day 1: Place Catapres-TTS® 1; administer 100% of oral dose

Day 2: Administer 50% of oral dose

Day 3: Administer 25% of oral dose

Always start with Catapres-TTS® 1 unless the patient was on a large oral dose

Not dialyzable (0% to 5%)

Administration Catapres-TTS® comes in 2 parts - the small patch containing the drug and an overlay to keep the patch in place for 1 week; both parts should be used for maximum efficacy; it may be useful to note on the patch which day it should be changed

Monitoring Parameters Blood pressure, standing and sitting/supine; mental status

Reference Range Therapeutic: 1-2 ng/mL (SI: 4.4-8.7 nmol/L)

(Continued)

Clonidine *(Continued)*

Test Interactions Increased sodium (S); decreased catecholamines (U)

Patient Information Do not stop drug except on instruction of physician; check daily to be sure patch present; may cause drowsiness

Nursing Implications Patches should be applied weekly at bedtime to a clean, hairless area of the upper outer arm or chest; rotate patch sites weekly (see Administration)

Special Geriatric Considerations Because of its potential CNS adverse effects, clonidine may not be considered a drug of choice in the elderly. If the decision is to use clonidine, adjust dose based on response and adverse reactions.

Dosage Forms

Patch, transdermal: 1, 2, and 3 (0.1mg, 0.2 mg, 0.3 mg/day for 7-day duration)

Tablet, as hydrochloride: 0.1 mg, 0.2 mg, 0.3 mg

Clonidine and Chlorthalidone

(KLOE ni deen & klor THAL i done)

Related Information

Chlorthalidone *on page 217*

Clonidine *on page 238*

Brand Names Combipres®

Generic Available Yes

Therapeutic Category Antihypertensive, Combination

Special Geriatric Considerations Combination products are not recommended for first-line treatment and divided doses of diuretics may increase the incidence of nocturia in the elderly

Dosage Forms

Tablet:

0.1: Clonidine 0.1 mg and chlorthalidone 15 mg

0.2: Clonidine 0.2 mg and chlorthalidone 15 mg

0.3: Clonidine 0.3 mg and chlorthalidone 15 mg

Clopidogrel (kloh PID oh grel)

Brand Names Plavix®

Therapeutic Category Antiplatelet Agent

Use The reduction of atherosclerotic events (myocardial infarction, stroke, vascular deaths) in patients with atherosclerosis documented by recent myocardial infarctions, recent stroke or established peripheral arterial disease

Contraindications In patients with active pathologic bleeding, coagulation disorders, or who have shown hypersensitivity to the drug or any component of the drug and should be used with caution in patients with severe liver disease

Precautions Use with caution in patients with hypertension, hepatic or renal impairment, history of bleeding or drug-induced hematologic disorders, or patients scheduled for surgery

Adverse Reactions

Central nervous system: Intracranial bleeding

Dermatologic: Rash, urticaria

Gastrointestinal: Diarrhea, nausea, vomiting, bleeding

Hematologic: Neutropenia, prolonged bleeding time

Hepatic: Increased LFTs

Drug Interactions

At high concentrations *in vitro*, clopidogrel inhibits P-450 2C9. Therefore, it may interfere with the metabolism of phenytoin, tamoxifen, tolbutamide, warfarin, torsemide, fluvastatin, and some NSAIDs.

Clopidogrel and naproxen caused increased occult GI blood loss; clopidogrel prolongs bleeding time; use with caution with warfarin

Mechanism of Action Blocks the ADP receptor and in so doing, prevents the binding of fibrinogen to that site. Clopidrogel, however, does not alter the receptor, which suggests that it prevents the binding of fibrinogen in an indirect manner. This drug reduces the number of functional ADP receptors. The effect of clopidrogel continues for several days after discontinuing the drug and it effects decrease proportionally to platelet renewal.

Pharmacokinetics

Absorption: Well absorbed

Metabolism: CYP1A to active metabolite

Half-life: 7-8 hours (active metabolite)

Usual Dosage Geriatrics and Adults: Oral: 75 mg once daily; dose adjustment may be necessary for patients with moderate to severe hepatic disease

Patient Information May be taken with food; notify physician if bleeding or bruising occurs

Nursing Implications Monitor patients for signs of bleeding; blood pressure, pulse; see Precautions

Special Geriatric Considerations Because of the risk of neutropenia and its relative expense as compared with aspirin, clopidogrel should only be used in patients with a documented intolerance to aspirin (see Pharmacokinetics and Usual Dosage). Plasma concentrations of main metabolite of clopidogrel were significantly higher in the elderly (≥75 years). This was not associated with changes in bleeding time or platelet aggregation. No dosage adjustment is recommended.

Dosage Forms Tablet, as bisulfate: 75 mg

Clopra® see Metoclopramide on page 616

Clorazepate (klor AZ e pate)

Related Information
Antacid Drug Interactions on page 1096
Anxiolytic/Hypnotic Use in Long-Term Care Facilities on page 1099
Benzodiazepines Comparison on page 1024

Brand Names Gen-XENE®; Tranxene®

Generic Available Yes

Therapeutic Category Antianxiety Agent; Anticonvulsant, Benzodiazepine; Benzodiazepine; Sedative

Use Treatment of generalized anxiety and panic disorders; management of alcohol withdrawal; adjunct anticonvulsant in management of partial seizures

Restrictions C-IV

Contraindications Hypersensitivity to clorazepate dipotassium or any component; cross-sensitivity with other benzodiazepines may exist; avoid using in patients with pre-existing CNS depression, severe uncontrolled pain, or narrow-angle glaucoma

Precautions Use with caution in patients with hepatic or renal disease, or a history of drug dependence; abrupt discontinuation may cause withdrawal symptoms or seizures

Adverse Reactions
Cardiovascular: Hypotension
Central nervous system: Drowsiness, dizziness, confusion, amnesia, headache, depression, ataxia
Dermatologic: Rash
Gastrointestinal: Nausea, xerostomia
Ocular: Blurred vision
Miscellaneous: Physical and psychological dependence with long-term use; long-term use may also be associated with renal or hepatic injury and reduced hematocrit

Overdosage Symptoms of overdose include somnolence, confusion, ataxia, diminished reflexes, coma

Toxicology Treatment for benzodiazepine overdose is supportive; rarely is mechanical ventilation required; flumazenil has been shown to selectively block the binding of benzodiazepines to CNS receptors, resulting in a reversal of benzodiazepine-induced CNS depression, but not respiratory depression

Drug Interactions
Benzodiazepines may decrease the effect of levodopa
Decreased metabolism: Cimetidine, fluoxetine
Increased metabolism: Rifampin
Increased toxicity: CNS depressants, alcohol

Stability Unstable in water

Mechanism of Action Benzodiazepines appear to potentiate the effects of GABA and other inhibitory neurotransmitters by binding to specific benzodiazepine-receptor sites in various areas of the CNS

Pharmacodynamics Studies have shown that the elderly are more sensitive to the effects of benzodiazepines as compared to younger adults

Pharmacokinetics
Absorption: Rapidly decarboxylated to desmethyldiazepam (active) in acidic stomach prior to absorption
Metabolism: In the liver to oxazepam (active)
Half-life: Adults:
Desmethyldiazepam: 48-96 hours
Oxazepam: 6-8 hours
(Continued)

241

Clorazepate *(Continued)*

Time to peak serum concentration: Oral: Within 1 hour
Elimination: Metabolites excreted primarily in urine

Usual Dosage Oral:
Geriatrics: Anxiety: 7.5 mg 1-2 times/day
Adults:
Anxiety: 7.5-15 mg 2-4 times/day, or given as single dose of 15-22.5 mg at bedtime
Alcohol withdrawal: Initial: 30 mg, then 15 mg 2-4 times/day on first day; maximum daily dose: 90 mg; gradually decrease dose over subsequent days

Monitoring Parameters Respiratory, cardiovascular, and mental status

Reference Range Therapeutic: 0.12-1 µg/mL (SI: 0.36-3.01 µmol/L)

Patient Information Avoid alcohol and other CNS depressants; may cause drowsiness; avoid activities needing good psychomotor coordination until CNS effects are known; may cause physical or psychological dependence; avoid abrupt discontinuation after prolonged use

Nursing Implications Assist patient with ambulation during initiation of therapy; monitor for alertness

Additional Information Clorazepate offers no advantage over the other benzodiazepines

Special Geriatric Considerations Due to its long-acting metabolite, clorazepate is not considered a drug of choice in the elderly; (see Pharmacodynamics); long-acting benzodiazepines have been associated with falls in the elderly; interpretive guidelines from the Health Care Financing Administration (HCFA) discourage the use of this agent in residents of long-term care facilities

Dosage Forms
Clorazepate dipotassium:
Capsule: 3.75 mg, 7.5 mg, 15 mg
Tablet: dipotassium: 3.75 mg, 7.5 mg, 15 mg
Tablet, single dose: 11.25 mg, 22.5 mg

Clotrimazole *(kloe TRIM a zole)*

Brand Names Femizole-7® [OTC]; Gyne-Lotrimin® [OTC]; Lotrimin®; Lotrimin® AF Cream [OTC]; Lotrimin® AF Lotion [OTC]; Lotrimin® AF Solution [OTC]; Mycelex®; Mycelex®-7; Mycelex®-G

Generic Available Yes

Therapeutic Category Antifungal Agent, Oral Nonabsorbed; Antifungal Agent, Topical; Antifungal Agent, Vaginal

Use Treatment of susceptible fungal infections, including oropharyngeal candidiasis, dermatophytoses, superficial mycoses, and cutaneous candidiasis, as well as vulvovaginal candidiasis; limited data suggest that the use of clotrimazole troches may be effective for prophylaxis against oropharyngeal candidiasis in neutropenic patients

Contraindications Hypersensitivity to clotrimazole or any component

Precautions Clotrimazole troches should not be used for treatment of systemic fungal infection

Adverse Reactions
Gastrointestinal: Nausea and vomiting may occur in patients on clotrimazole troches
Hepatic: Abnormal liver function tests
Local: Mild burning, irritation, stinging to skin or vaginal area

Mechanism of Action Binds to phospholipids in the fungal cell membrane altering cell wall permeability resulting in loss of essential intracellular elements

Pharmacokinetics
Absorption: Negligible: Through intact skin when administered topically; following oral topical administration, salivary concentrations occur within 3 hours following 30 minutes of dissolution time in the mouth; high vaginal concentrations occur following vaginal cream administration within 8-24 hours and within 1-2 days following vaginal tablet administration
Metabolism: Inhibitor CYP3A4, 3A5-7
Elimination: As metabolites via bile

Usual Dosage Geriatrics and Adults:
Oral: 10 mg troche dissolved slowly 5 times/day for 14 days
Topical: Apply twice daily
Vaginal: 100 mg/day for 7 days or 200 mg/day for 3 days or 500 mg single dose or 5 g (= 1 applicatorful) of 1% vaginal cream daily for 7-14 days

Monitoring Parameters Periodic liver function tests during oral therapy with clotrimazole lozenges

Patient Information May cause irritation to the skin; avoid contact with the eyes; lozenge (troche) must be dissolved slowly in the mouth

Nursing Implications Administer around-the-clock rather than 4 times/day, 3 times/day, etc (ie, 12-6-12-6, not 9-1-5-9) to promote less variation in peak and trough serum concentrations

Special Geriatric Considerations Localized fungal infections frequently follow broad spectrum antimicrobial therapy; specifically, oral and vaginal infections due to *Candida*

Dosage Forms
Combination pack (Mycelex-7®): Vaginal tablet 100 mg (7's) and vaginal cream 1% (7 g)

Cream:
Topical (Lotrimin®, Lotrimin® AF, Mycelex®, Mycelex® OTC) : 1% (15 g, 30 g, 45 g, 90 g)
Vaginal (FemCare®, Femizole-7®, Gyne-Lotrimin®, Mycelex®-G): 1% (45 g, 90 g)

Lotion (Lotrimin®): 1% (30 mL)

Solution, topical (Lotrimin®, Lotrimin® AF, Mycelex®, Mycelex® OTC): 1% (10 mL, 30 mL)

Tablet, vaginal (Gyne-Lotrimin®, Mycelex®-G): 100 mg (7s); 500 mg (1s)

Troche (Mycelex®): 10 mg

Twin pack (Mycelex®): Vaginal tablet 500 mg (1's) and vaginal cream 1% (7 g)

Cloxacillin (kloks a SIL in)

Related Information
Penicillins, Penicillin-Related Antibiotics, & Other Antibiotics *on page 1010*

Brand Names Cloxapen®; Tegopen®

Generic Available Yes

Therapeutic Category Antibiotic, Penicillin

Use Treatment of susceptible bacterial infections, notably penicillinase-producing staphylococci (not methicillin-resistant) causing respiratory tract, skin and skin structure, bone and joint, urinary tract infections, endocarditis, septicemia, and meningitis

Contraindications Hypersensitivity to cloxacillin or any component, or penicillins

Precautions Use with caution in patients allergic to cephalosporins

Adverse Reactions
Central nervous system: Fever
Dermatologic: Rash
Gastrointestinal: Nausea, vomiting, diarrhea
Hematologic: Eosinophilia, leukopenia, neutropenia, thrombocytopenia, agranulocytosis
Hepatic: Serum sickness-like reactions, hepatotoxicity
Renal: Hematuria

Overdosage Symptoms of overdose include neuromuscular hypersensitivity, convulsions

Toxicology Many beta-lactam-containing antibiotics have the potential to cause neuromuscular hyperirritability or convulsive seizures. Hemodialysis may be helpful to aid in the removal of the drug from the blood, otherwise most treatment is supportive or symptom directed.

Drug Interactions
Increased serum concentrations with probenecid
Cloxacillin has been reported to decrease effect of warfarin in a small number of patients

Stability Refrigerate oral solution after reconstitution; discard after 14 days; stable for 3 days at room temperature

Mechanism of Action Interferes with bacterial cell wall synthesis during active multiplication causing cell death and resultant bactericidal activity against susceptible bacteria

Pharmacokinetics
Absorption: Oral: ~50%
Protein binding: 90% to 98%
Metabolism: Significant in the liver to active and inactive metabolites
Half-life: 30-90 minutes (prolonged with renal impairment); reported to be longer in the elderly, but is not considered clinically significant
Time to peak serum concentration: Oral: Within 0.5-2 hours
Elimination: In urine and through bile
(Continued)

Cloxacillin *(Continued)*

Usual Dosage Geriatrics and Adults: Oral: 250-500 mg every 6 hours
Not dialyzable (0% to 5%)

Monitoring Parameters Signs and symptoms of infection; mental status, WBC; PT for patients on warfarin

Test Interactions False-positive urine and serum proteins

Patient Information Complete full course of therapy; contact your physician or pharmacist if not improving or diarrhea develops

Nursing Implications Administer 1 hour before or 2 hours after meals

Special Geriatric Considerations Dosage change for renal function is not necessary (see Pharmacokinetics and Usual Dosage)

Dosage Forms
Cloxacillin sodium:
Capsule: 250 mg, 500 mg
Powder for oral suspension: 125 mg/5 mL (100 mL, 200 mL)

References
Bluhm G, Jacobson B, Julander I, et al, "Antibiotic Prophylaxis in Pacemaker Surgery - A Prospective Study," *Scand J Thorac Cardiovasc Surg,* 1984, 18(3):227-34.

Cloxapen® *see* Cloxacillin *on previous page*

Clozapine *(KLOE za peen)*

Related Information
Antipsychotic Agents Comparison *on page 1023*
Antipsychotic Medication Guidelines *on page 1076*
Federal OBRA Regulations Recommended Maximum Doses - Antipsychotics *on page 1056*

Brand Names Clozaril®

Generic Available No

Therapeutic Category Antipsychotic Agent; Neuroleptic Agent

Use Management of severely ill schizophrenic patients who fail to respond to standard antipsychotic therapy; not recommended at this time for nonpsychotic symptoms associated with dementia or other diseases in elderly

Contraindications In patients with WBC ≤3500 cells/mm^3 before therapy; if WBC falls to <3000 cells/mm^3 during therapy, the drug should be withheld until signs and symptoms of infection disappear and WBC rises to >3000 cells/mm^3 or granulocytes decrease (ANC) falls to <500/mm^2

Warnings Significant risk of agranulocytosis, potentially life-threatening; therefore, reserve clozapine for use in severely ill schizophrenic patients who fail therapy with standard antipsychotic therapy either because of insufficient effectiveness or inability to achieve effective dose due to intolerable ADRs; before initiating clozapine therapy, it is strongly recommended to attempt at least two trials, each with different standard antipsychotic agents at an adequate dose for an adequate period of time. Patients treated with clozapine must have a baseline WBC with differential, repeated weekly throughout treatment and for 4 weeks after discontinuing clozapine. No established risk factors have been established, however, a higher number of patients with Jewish background developed agranulocytosis in U.S. studies. The numbers were disproportionate to other ethnic groups; also caution should be used with women and elderly since these two groups have a higher incidence of agranulocytosis occurring with the use of antipsychotic therapy.

Seizures: Occurs with high doses
Cardiovascular disease: Use with caution; see changes seen with other antipsychotic agents (see Adverse Reactions)
Orthostatic hypotension: May occur, especially during initiation and rapid dose increases
Neuroleptic malignant syndrome (NMS): A potentially serious and fatal symptom complex associated with antipsychotic therapy. However, no cases of NMS due to clozapine alone have been reported to date. There has been reports with patients treated concomitantly with lithium or other CNS active agents
Tardive dyskinesia: No cases of tardive dyskinesia have been reported. However, it cannot be concluded that clozapine does not cause this symptom complex until more clinical use of this agent has been evaluated

Precautions Fever, transient elevations (>100.4°F) occur in the first 3 weeks of therapy; if fever persists, may need to stop therapy; evaluate for infection and agranulocytosis; if fever is high consider NMS (see Warnings)

Anticholinergic: May cause increased confusion in elderly; consider effects on bladder, bowel, and in patients with cardiovascular disease

CNS: Severe sedation may impair mental and physical abilities; especially in first few days of therapy; use gradual dose increases

Use with caution in patients with renal, hepatic, or cardiac disease due to limited experience with clozapine

Adverse Reactions

Cardiovascular: Hypotension, tachycardia, EKG changes, syncope

Central nervous system: Seizures, headache, dizziness, agitation, fatigue, insomnia, drowsiness, visual disturbances, fever, akathisia

Dermatologic: Rash

Gastrointestinal: Hypersalivation, xerostomia, nausea, vomiting, constipation, heartburn, abdominal discomfort, diarrhea, weight gain

Genitourinary: Incontinence

Hematologic: Agranulocytosis

Neuromuscular & skeletal: Tremors

Miscellaneous: Diaphoresis

Overdosage Symptoms of overdose include altered states of consciousness, tachycardia, hypotension, hypersalivation, respiratory depression

Toxicology Following initiation of essential overdose management, toxic symptom treatment and supportive treatment should be initiated. Hypotension usually responds to I.V. fluids or Trendelenburg positioning. If unresponsive to these measures the use of a parenteral inotrope may be required (eg, norepinephrine 0.1-0.2 mcg/kg/minute titrated to response). Do not use epinephrine. Seizures commonly respond to diazepam (I.V. 5-10 mg bolus every 15 minutes if needed up to a total of 30 mg) or to phenytoin or pheno-barbital. Also critical cardiac arrhythmias often respond to I.V. phenytoin (15 mg/kg up to 1 g), while other antiarrhythmics can be used. Neuroleptics often cause extrapyramidal symptoms (eg, dystonic reactions) requiring manage-ment with diphenhydramine 1-2 mg/kg up to a maximum of 50 mg I.M. or I.V. slow push followed by a maintenance dose for 48-72 hours. When these reactions are unresponsive to diphenhydramine, benztropine mesylate I.V. 1-2 mg may be effective. These agents are generally effective within 2-5 minutes.

Drug Interactions

Anticholinergic: Enhanced anticholinergic effect by clozapine

Antihypertensives: Augment hypotensive effect

CNS active drugs: Enhances CNS pharmacologic effects or CNS active drugs

Bone marrow suppressants: Clozapine may act synergistically with other bone marrow suppressing drugs

Protein binding: Clozapine highly bound to serum protein; use cautiously with other highly protein bound drugs (eg, warfarin, phenytoin, phenobarbital, etc)

Stability Dispensed in "clozapine patient system" packaging

Mechanism of Action Clozapine is a weak dopamine$_1$ and dopamine$_2$ receptor blocker; in addition, it blocks the serotonin$_2$, alpha-adrenergic, and histamine H$_1$ central nervous system receptors; clozapine appears to be preferentially more active in the limbic system than in striatal areas. Its low affinity for D$_1$ and D$_2$ receptors in striatal area may explain its relatively low EPS side effects. Clozapine, as does other antipsychotics, increases delta and theta activity but slows dominant alpha frequencies on EEG. REM sleep is increased.

Pharmacokinetics

Absorption: Well absorbed

Protein binding: 95% bound to serum proteins

Metabolism: Undergoes extensive metabolism primarily to unconjugated forms; substrate CYP1A2, 2D6

Bioavailability: Food does not appear to affect bioavailability

Half-life, elimination: (mean): 12 hours (range: 4-66 hours)

Time to peak: Occurs on an average of 2.5 hours after administration (range 1-6 hours)

Elimination: In urine

Usual Dosage Oral:

Geriatrics: Experience in elderly is limited; initial dose should be 25 mg/day; increase as tolerated by 25 mg/day to desired response; maximum daily dose in elderly should probably be 450 mg; dose titration to 300-450 mg/day may be attained in 2 weeks if tolerated; however, elderly may require slower titration and daily increases may not be tolerated

Adults: 25 mg once or twice daily initially and increased, as tolerated to a target dose of 300-450 mg/day, but may require doses as high as 600-900 mg/day

(Continued)

Clozapine *(Continued)*

Monitoring Parameters CBC (WBC), WBC testing should occur weekly for the duration of therapy and for 4 weeks after discontinuation of clozapine; orthostatic blood pressures; tremors; gait changes, abnormal movement in trunk, neck, buccal area, or extremities; monitor target behaviors for which the agent is given

Patient Information Report any lethargy, fever, sore throat, flu-like symptoms or any other signs or symptoms of infection; may cause drowsiness, orthostatic hypotension; inform patient of importance of weekly blood tests

Nursing Implications Benign, self-limiting temperature elevations sometimes occur during the first 3 weeks of treatment; monitor orthostatic blood pressures; observe for signs of infection; observe for motor abnormalities

Additional Information Medication should not be stopped abruptly; taper off over 1-2 weeks

Special Geriatric Considerations Not recommended for use in nonpsychotic patients (see Warnings).

Many elderly patients receive antipsychotic medications for inappropriate nonpsychotic behavior. Before initiating antipsychotic medication, the clinician should investigate any possible reversible cause; any stress or stress from any disease can cause acute "confusion" or worsening of baseline nonpsychotic behavior. Most commonly acute changes in behavior are due to increases in drug dose or addition of new drug to regimen; fluid electrolyte loss; infections; and/or changes in environment.

Any changes in disease status in any organ system can result in behavior changes.

In the treatment of agitated, demented, elderly patients, authors of meta-analysis of controlled trials of the response to the traditional antipsychotics (phenothiazines, butyrophenones) in controlling agitation have concluded that the use of neuroleptics results in a response rate of 18%. Clearly neuroleptic therapy for behavior control should be limited with frequent attempts to withdraw the agent given for behavior control.

Dosage Forms Tablet: 25 mg, 100 mg

References
Drug Facts and Comparisons, New York, NY: JB Lippincott, 1990, 265E-F.

Peabody CA, Warner MD, Whiteford HA, et al, "Neuroleptics and the Elderly," *J Am Geriatr Soc*, 1987, 35(3):233-8.

Risse SC and Barnes R, "Pharmacologic Treatment of Agitation Associated With Dementia," *J Am Geriatr Soc*, 1986, 34(5):368-76.

Saltz BL, Woerner MG, Kane JM, et al, "Prospective Study of Tardive Dyskinesia Incidence in the Elderly," *JAMA*, 1991, 266(17):2402-6.

Seifert RD, "Therapeutic Drug Monitoring: Psychotropic Drugs," *J Pharm Pract*, 1984, 6:403-16.

Clozaril® *see Clozapine on page 244*

Clysodrast® *see Bisacodyl on page 121*

Cobex® *see Cyanocobalamin on page 257*

Codeine *(KOE deen)*

Related Information
I.V. Push Recommended Guidelines *on page 1083*
Narcotic Agonist Comparative Pharmacology *on page 1036*
Pharmacokinetics of Narcotic Agonist Analgesics *on page 1037*

Synonyms Methylmorphine

Generic Available Yes

Therapeutic Category Analgesic, Narcotic; Antitussive

Use Treatment of mild to moderate pain; antitussive in lower doses

Restrictions C-II

Contraindications Hypersensitivity to codeine or any component

Warnings Some preparations contain sulfites which may cause allergic reactions

Precautions Use with caution in patients with hypersensitivity reactions to other phenanthrene derivative opioid agonists (morphine, hydrocodone, hydromorphone, levorphanol, oxycodone, oxymorphone); respiratory diseases including asthma, emphysema, COPD; or severe liver or renal insufficiency

Adverse Reactions
Cardiovascular: Palpitations, hypotension, bradycardia, peripheral vasodilation
Central nervous system: CNS depression, increased intracranial pressure
Dermatologic: Pruritus
Endocrine & metabolic: Antidiuretic hormone release

Gastrointestinal: Nausea, vomiting, constipation

Ocular: Miosis

Respiratory: Respiratory depression

Miscellaneous: Physical and psychological dependence, biliary or urinary tract spasm, histamine release

Overdosage Symptoms of overdose include CNS and respiratory depression, gastrointestinal cramping, constipation

Toxicology Treatment of an overdose includes support of patient's airway, establishment of an I.V. line, and naloxone 2 mg I.V. with repeat administration as necessary up to a total of 10 mg

Drug Interactions Increased toxicity: CNS depressants, phenothiazines, tricyclic antidepressants, alcohol; SSRIs and other CYP2D6 inhibitors may prevent metabolism to morphine (active)

Stability Store injection between 15°C to 30°C, avoid freezing; do not use if injection is discolored or contains a precipitate

Mechanism of Action Binds to opiate receptors in the CNS, causing inhibition of ascending pain pathways, altering the perception of and response to pain; causes cough supression by direct central action in the medulla; produces generalized CNS depression

Pharmacodynamics

Onset of action:

Oral: 30-60 minutes

I.M.: 10-30 minutes

Peak action:

Oral: 60-90 minutes

I.M.: 30-60 minutes

Duration of action: 4-6 hours; may be increased in the elderly; enhanced analgesia has been seen in elderly patients on therapeutic doses of narcotics

Pharmacokinetics

Absorption: Oral: Adequate

Protein binding: 7%

Metabolism: Hepatic metabolism to morphine (active); substrate and inhibitor CYP2D6, substrate 3A4

Half-life: 2.5-3.5 hours

Elimination: 3% to 16% excreted in urine as unchanged drug, norcodeine and free and conjugated morphine

Usual Dosage Doses should be titrated to appropriate analgesic effect; when changing routes of administration, note that oral dose is 66% as effective as parenteral dose

Analgesic: Oral, I.M., S.C.: Geriatrics and Adults: Usual: 30 mg/dose; range: 15-60 mg every 4-6 hours as needed; maximum: 360 mg/24 hours

Antitussive: Oral (for nonproductive cough): Adults: 10-20 mg/dose every 4-6 hours as needed; maximum: 120 mg/day

Dosing adjustment in renal impairment:

Cl_{cr} 10-50 mL/minute: Administer 75% of dose

Cl_{cr} <10 mL/minute: Administer 50% of dose

Dosing adjustment in hepatic impairment: Probably necessary in hepatic insufficiency

Monitoring Parameters Pain relief, respiratory and mental status, blood pressure

Reference Range Therapeutic: Not established; Toxic: >1.1 µg/mL

Test Interactions Increased aminotransferase [ALT (SGPT)/AST (SGOT)] (S)

Patient Information Avoid alcohol, may cause drowsiness; may cause GI upset, can take with food

Nursing Implications Observe patient for excessive sedation or confusion, respiratory depression, constipation

Additional Information May be habit-forming; dextromethorphan has equivalent antitussive activity but has much lower toxicity in accidental overdose

Special Geriatric Considerations The elderly may be particularly susceptible to CNS depression and confusion as well as the constipating effects of narcotics (see Pharmacodynamics)

Dosage Forms

Codeine phosphate:

Injection: 30 mg/mL (1 mL, 2 mL); 60 mg/mL (1 mL, 2 mL)

Tablet, soluble: 15 mg, 30 mg, 60 mg

Codeine sulfate:

Tablet: 15 mg, 30 mg, 60 mg

Tablet, soluble: 15 mg, 30 mg, 60 mg

(Continued)

Codeine *(Continued)*

References

Ferrell BA, "Pain Management in Elderly People," *J Am Geriatr Soc*, 1991, 39(1):64-73.

Kaiko RF, Wallenstein SL, Rogers AG, et al, "Narcotics in the Elderly," *Med Clin North Am*, 1982, 66(5):1079-89.

Codeine and Acetaminophen *see* Acetaminophen and Codeine *on page 18*

Codeine and Aspirin *see* Aspirin and Codeine *on page 87*

Codeine and Guaifenesin *see* Guaifenesin and Codeine *on page 438*

Codoxy® *see* Oxycodone and Aspirin *on page 706*

Cogentin® *see* Benztropine *on page 111*

Co-Gesic® *see* Hydrocodone and Acetaminophen *on page 461*

Cognex® Oral *see* Tacrine *on page 885*

Colace® [OTC] *see* Docusate *on page 312*

ColBENEMID® *see* Colchicine and Probenecid *on next page*

Colchicine *(KOL chi seen)*

Generic Available Yes: Tablet

Therapeutic Category Anti-inflammatory Agent

Use Treatment of acute gouty arthritis attacks and to prevent recurrences of such attacks; management of familial Mediterranean fever

Contraindications Hypersensitivity to colchicine or any component; severe renal, GI disease, cardiac disorders, or blood dyscrasias

Warnings Use cautiously in patients with hepatic dysfunction; elderly and debilitated patients are at risk for adverse effects

Precautions Severe local irritation can occur following S.C. or I.M. administration; GI side effects may cause difficulty in patients with peptic ulcer disease or spastic colon; colchicine-induced myoneuropathy after misdiagnosed as polymyositis or uremic neuropathy; reversible vitamin B_{12} malabsorption

Adverse Reactions

Dermatologic: Rash, alopecia, purpura

Gastrointestinal: Nausea, vomiting, diarrhea, abdominal pain

Genitourinary: Azoospermia

Hematologic: Agranulocytosis, aplastic anemia, bone marrow suppression

Hepatic: Hepatotoxicity, elevate alkaline phosphatase and AST

Neuromuscular & skeletal: Myopathy, peripheral neuritis

Overdosage Symptoms of overdose include burning in throat, watery to bloody diarrhea, nausea, vomiting, abdominal pain, hypotension, anuria, cardiovascular collapse, delirium, convulsions, shock, S-T segment elevation, muscle weakness, paralysis, respiratory failure, hepatic damage; by 5th day, leukopenia, thrombocytopenia, coagulopathy, alopecia, stomatitis

Toxicology Gastric lavage, treat for shock; hemodialysis or peritoneal dialysis effective; atropine and morphine relieve abdominal pain; use respiratory assistance as needed; administer general supportive care; deaths occur with 65 mg orally or 7 mg I.V.

Drug Interactions May decrease platelet counts

Stability Protect tablets from light; I.V. colchicine is incompatible with dextrose or I.V. solutions with preservatives

Mechanism of Action Decreases leukocyte motility, decreases phagocytosis in joints, and lactic acid production, thereby reducing the deposition of urate crystals that perpetuates the inflammatory response; interferes with kinin formation and reduces phagocytosis thereby decreasing inflammatory response

Pharmacodynamics Articular pain and swelling decrease within 12 hours; attack resolved in 1-2 days

Pharmacokinetics

Distribution: Partially deacetylated in the liver

Protein binding: 10% to 31%

Half-life: 12-30 minutes

Time to peak serum concentrations: Oral: Within 30-120 minutes then decline for 2 hours before increasing again due to enterohepatic recycling

Elimination: Primarily in feces via bile; 10% to 20% eliminated unchanged in urine

Usual Dosage Geriatrics and Adults:

Prophylaxis of familial Mediterranean fever: Oral: 1-2 mg/day in 2-3 divided doses

Gout:
Oral: Acute attacks: Initial: 0.5-1.2 mg, then 0.5-0.6 mg every 1-2 hours or 1-1.2 mg every 1-2 hours until relief or GI side effects occur; maximum total dose: 8 mg/day; wait 3 days before initiating a second course

I.V.: Initial: 1-3 mg, then 0.5 mg every 6 hours until response, not to exceed 4 mg/day; if pain recurs, it may be necessary to administer a daily dose of 1 to 2 mg for several days, however, do not administer more colchicine by any route for at least 7 days after a full course of I.V. therapy (4 mg), transfer to oral colchicine in a dose similar to that being given I.V. **Note:** Deaths have been reported by this route of administration. Avoid I.V. use if possible. The risk of adverse effects is much greater.

Prophylaxis of recurrent attacks: Oral:
Less than 1 attack per year: 0.5-0.6 mg/day for 3-4 days/week
More than 1 attack per year: 0.5-0.6 mg/day
Severe cases: 1-1.8 mg/day

Dosing interval in renal impairment: Cl_{cr} <10 mL/minute: Decrease dose by 50%

Not dialyzable (0% to 5%)

Monitoring Parameters GI effects, symptoms

Test Interactions May cause false-positive results in urine tests for erythrocytes or hemoglobin; may cause false-positive results when testing urine for blood or hemoglobin

Patient Information Discontinue if nausea or vomiting occur; avoid alcohol; if taking for acute attack, discontinue as soon as pain resolves; do not exceed 8 mg/day orally; notify physician if sore throat, persistent abdominal pain, nausea, diarrhea, fever, bleeding, bruising, tiredness, weakness, numbness, or tingling occurs

Nursing Implications Injection should be made over 2-5 minutes into tubing of free-flowing I.V. with compatible fluid; **incompatible with dextrose** (see Adverse Reactions); monitor for response; CBC, LFTs, renal function

Special Geriatric Considerations Colchicine appears to be more toxic in elderly, particularly in the presence of renal, gastrointestinal, or cardiac disease. The most predictable oral side effects are (gastrointestinal) vomiting, abdominal pain, and nausea. If colchicine is stopped at this point, other more severe adverse effects may be avoided, such as bone marrow suppression, peripheral neuritis, etc.

Dosage Forms
Injection: 0.5 mg/mL (2 mL)
Tablet: 0.5 mg, 0.6 mg, 0.65 mg

References
Emmerson BT, "The Management of Gout," *N Engl J Med*, 1996, 334(7):445-51.
Levy M, Spino M, and Read SE, "Colchicine: A State-of-the-Art Review," *Pharmacotherapy*, 1991, 11(3):196-211.

Colchicine and Probenecid (KOL chi seen & proe BEN e sid)
Related Information
Colchicine *on previous page*
Probenecid *on page 779*
Brand Names ColBENEMID®; Proben-C®
Synonyms Probenecid and Colchicine
Generic Available Yes
Therapeutic Category Uricosuric Agent
Use Treatment of chronic gouty arthritis when complicated by frequent, recurrent acute attacks of gout
Usual Dosage Geriatrics and Adults: Oral: 1 tablet daily for 1 week; then 1 tablet twice daily thereafter
Special Geriatric Considerations See monographs for individual agents
Dosage Forms Tablet: Colchicine 0.5 mg and probenecid 0.5 g

Cold & Allergy® Elixir [OTC] *see* Brompheniramine and Phenylpropanolamine *on page 130*

Colestid® *see* Colestipol *on this page*

Colestipol (koe LES ti pole)
Brand Names Colestid®
Therapeutic Category Antilipemic Agent
Use Adjunct in the management of primary hypercholesterolemia; to relieve pruritus associated with elevated levels of bile acids, possibly used to decrease plasma half-life of digoxin as an adjunct in the treatment of toxicity
Contraindications Hypersensitivity to colestipol or any component; avoid using in complete biliary obstruction
(Continued)

Colestipol *(Continued)*

Precautions Patients with high triglycerides, GI dysfunction (constipation); may be associated with increased bleeding tendency as a result of hypothrombinemia secondary to vitamin K deficiency; may cause depletion of vitamins A, D, and E

Adverse Reactions

Central nervous system: Dizziness, headache, anxiety, vertigo, drowsiness, fatigue

Dermatologic: Urticaria, dermatitis

Endocrine & metabolic: Increased serum phosphorous and chloride with decrease of sodium and potassium

Gastrointestinal: Constipation, abdominal pain and distention, belching, flatulence, nausea, vomiting, diarrhea, anorexia, peptic ulceration

Hepatic: Transient increases in serum AST (SGOT) and alkaline phosphatase concentrations

Neuromuscular & skeletal: Myalgia, arthralgia, arthritis, weakness

Respiratory: Shortness of breath

Overdosage Symptoms of overdose include GI obstruction, nausea, GI distress

Toxicology Treatment is supportive

Drug Interactions Since colestipol is an anion-exchange resin, it is capable of binding to a number of drugs (especially tetracycline, penicillin G, chlorothiazide, digoxin, and propranolol) in the GI tract and may delay or reduce their absorption; may prevent absorption of vitamin A, D, E, and K; oral supplements of vitamin A and D may be necessary

Mechanism of Action Binds with bile acids to form an insoluble complex that is eliminated in the feces; it thereby increases the fecal loss of bile acid-bound low density lipoprotein cholesterol

Pharmacokinetics Absorption: Oral: Not absorbed

Usual Dosage Geriatrics and Adults: 5-30 g/day in divided doses 2-4 times/day

Administration Dry powder should be added to at least 90 mL of liquid and stirred until completely mixed; other drugs should be administered at least 1 hour before or 4 hours after colestipol

Monitoring Parameters Serum lipid profile; plasma cholesterol (LDL and VLDL fractions); observe for gastrointestinal side effects

Test Interactions Increased prothrombin time; decreased cholesterol (S)

Patient Information Mix in liquids, cereals, soda, soup, or pulpy fruits; add at least 90 mL of liquid; do not take dry; stir well, powder will not dissolve; rinse glass with small amount of liquid to ensure full dose is taken

Nursing Implications See Administration

Special Geriatric Considerations The definition of and, therefore, when to treat hyperlipidemia in the elderly is a controversial issue. The National Cholesterol Education Program recommends that all adults 20 years of age and older maintain a plasma cholesterol concentration <200 mg/dL. By this definition, 60% of all elderly would be considered to have an elevated plasma cholesterol. However, plasma cholesterol has been shown to be a less reliable predictor of coronary heart disease in the elderly. Therefore, it is the authors' belief that pharmacologic treatment should be reserved for those who are unable to obtain a desirable plasma cholesterol concentration by diet alone and for whom the benefits of treatment are believed to outweigh the potential adverse effects, drug interactions, and cost of treatment.

Dosage Forms

Colestipol hydrochloride:

Granules: 5 g packet, 300 g, 500 g

Tablet: 1 g

Colistin, Neomycin, and Hydrocortisone

(koe LIS tin, nee oh MYE sin & hye droe KOR ti sone)

Brand Names Coly-Mycin® S Otic Drops

Generic Available No

Therapeutic Category Antibiotic/Corticosteroid, Otic

Use Treatment of superficial and susceptible bacterial infections of the external auditory canal; for treatment of susceptible bacterial infections of mastoidectomy and fenestration cavities

Usual Dosage Geriatrics and Adults: Otic: 4 drops in affected ear 3-4 times/day

Nursing Implications Shake well for 10 seconds before administering

Special Geriatric Considerations Many elderly will overuse eye drops or use for nonindicated reasons. Limit their use.

Dosage Forms Suspension, otic: Colistin sulfate 0.3%, neomycin sulfate 0.47%, and hydrocortisone acetate 1% (5 mL, 10 mL)

Collagenase (KOL la je nase)

Brand Names Biozyme-C®; Santyl®

Generic Available No

Therapeutic Category Enzyme, Topical Debridement

Use Promotes debridement of necrotic tissue in dermal ulcers and severe burns

Contraindications Known hypersensitivity to collagenase

Warnings For external use only; avoid contact with eyes

Precautions Monitor patients for signs or symptoms of systemic bacterial infections; apply collagenase only to lesion, slight erythema has occurred in surrounding tissue

Adverse Reactions Local: Pain and burning may occur at site of application

Toxicology Action of enzyme may be stopped by applying Burow's solution

Drug Interactions Decreased effect: Enzymatic activity is inhibited by detergents, benzalkonium chloride, hexachlorophene, nitrofurazone, tincture of iodine, and heavy metal ions (silver and mercury)

Mechanism of Action Collagenase is an enzyme derived from the fermentation of *Clostridium histolyticum* and differs from other proteolytic enzymes in that its enzymatic action has a high specificity for native and denatured collagen. Collagenase will not attack collagen in healthy tissue or newly formed granulation tissue. In addition, it does not act on fat, fibrin, keratin, or muscle.

Usual Dosage Topical: Apply once daily (or more frequently if the dressing becomes soiled)

Administration Prior to application, cleanse lesion of debris and digested material; when infection is present, neomycin-bacitracin-polymyxin B may be used with collagenase; excess ointment should be removed each time the dressing is changed; treatment should be discontinued when debridement is complete and granulation tissue is well established

Monitoring Parameters Healing of ulcer

Patient Information For external use only; avoid contact with eyes

Nursing Implications Do not introduce into major body cavities; monitor debilitated patients for systemic bacterial infections (see Administration)

Special Geriatric Considerations Preventive skin care should be instituted in all older patients at high risk for pressure ulcers; collagenase is indicated in stage 3 and 4 pressure ulcers

Dosage Forms Ointment, topical: 250 units/g (15 g, 30 g)

References
Chamberlain TM, Cali TS, Cuzzell J, et al, "Assessment and Management of Pressure Sores in Long-Term Care Facilities," *Consult Pharm*, 1992, 7(12)1328-40.

Collyrium Fresh® Ophthalmic [OTC] *see* Tetrahydrozoline *on page 901*

Coly-Mycin® S Otic Drops *see* Colistin, Neomycin, and Hydrocortisone *on previous page*

Combipres® *see* Clonidine and Chlorthalidone *on page 240*

Comfort® Ophthalmic [OTC] *see* Naphazoline *on page 653*

Comfort® Tears Solution [OTC] *see* Artificial Tears *on page 82*

Compazine® *see* Prochlorperazine *on page 782*

Compound E *see* Cortisone Acetate *on next page*

Compound F *see* Hydrocortisone *on page 462*

Compound W® [OTC] *see* Salicylic Acid *on page 845*

Compoz® Gel Caps [OTC] *see* Diphenhydramine *on page 302*

Compoz® Nighttime Sleep Aid [OTC] *see* Diphenhydramine *on page 302*

Conjugated Estrogens and Medroxyprogesterone Acetate, Combined *see* Estrogens and Medroxyprogesterone *on page 352*

Constilac® *see* Lactulose *on page 523*

Constulose® *see* Lactulose *on page 523*

Contac® Cough Formula Liquid [OTC] *see* Guaifenesin and Dextromethorphan *on page 439*

Control® [OTC] *see* Phenylpropanolamine *on page 741*

Cophene-B® *see* Brompheniramine *on page 129*

Cordarone® *see* Amiodarone *on page 58*

Coreg® *see* Carvedilol *on page 168*

Corgard® see Nadolol on page 646

CortaGel® [OTC] see Hydrocortisone on page 462

Cortaid® Maximum Strength [OTC] see Hydrocortisone on page 462

Cortaid® with Aloe [OTC] see Hydrocortisone on page 462

Cort-Dome® see Hydrocortisone on page 462

Cortef® see Hydrocortisone on page 462

Cortef® Feminine Itch see Hydrocortisone on page 462

Cortenema® see Hydrocortisone on page 462

Corticosteroids Comparison, Systemic see page 1029

Corticosteroids Comparison, Topical see page 1030

Cortifoam® see Hydrocortisone on page 462

Cortisol see Hydrocortisone on page 462

Cortisone Acetate (KOR ti sone AS e tate)

Related Information
Antacid Drug Interactions on page 1096
Corticosteroids Comparison, Systemic on page 1029

Brand Names Cortone® Acetate

Synonyms Compound E

Generic Available Yes

Therapeutic Category Adrenal Corticosteroid; Anti-inflammatory Agent; Corticosteroid, Systemic

Use Management of adrenocortical insufficiency

Contraindications Serious infections, except septic shock or tuberculous meningitis, idiopathic thrombocytopenia purpura (I.M. use), administration of live virus vaccines

Precautions Use with caution in patients with hypothyroidism, cirrhosis, hypertension, congestive heart failure, ulcerative colitis, thromboembolic disorders, osteoporosis, convulsive disorders, peptic ulcer, diabetes mellitus, myasthenia gravis

Adverse Reactions
Cardiovascular: Edema, hypertension, accelerated atherogenesis

Central nervous system: Vertigo, seizures, headache, psychosis, pseudo-tumor cerebri

Dermatologic: Acne, skin atrophy, impaired wound healing, hirsutism

Endocrine & metabolic: Cushing's syndrome, pituitary-adrenal axis suppression, growth suppression, glucose intolerance, hypokalemia, alkalosis, hot flashes, postmenopausal bleeding

Gastrointestinal: Peptic ulcer, nausea, vomiting, pancreatitis

Neuromuscular & skeletal: Muscle weakness, osteoporosis, fractures, aseptic necrosis of femoral and humeral heads, steroid myopathy

Ocular: Cataracts, glaucoma

Miscellaneous: Increased susceptibility to infections

Toxicology When consumed in excessive quantities for prolonged periods, systemic hypercorticism and adrenal suppression may occur; in those cases, discontinuation and withdrawal of the corticosteroid should be done judiciously

Drug Interactions
Steroids decrease the effect of anticholinesterases, isoniazid, salicylates, insulin, oral hypoglycemics

Decreased effect: Barbiturates, phenytoin, rifampin

Increased effect (hypokalemia) of potassium-depleting diuretics

Increased risk of digoxin toxicity (due to hypokalemia)

Increased effect: Estrogens, ketoconazole

Mechanism of Action Decreases inflammation by suppression of migration of polymorphonuclear leukocytes and reversal of increased capillary permeability; suppresses immune response with pharmacologic doses

Pharmacodynamics
Peak effect:
Oral: Within 2 hours
I.M.: Within 20-48 hours
Duration of action: 30-36 hours

Pharmacokinetics
Absorption: Slow
Distribution: To muscles, liver, skin, intestines, and kidneys
Metabolism: In the liver to inactive metabolites
Half-life: 30 minutes; biologic half-life: 8-12 hours
Elimination: In bile and urine

Usual Dosage Oral, I.M. (depends upon the condition being treated and the response of the patient) (see Additional Information):

Geriatrics: Use lowest effective dose
Adults: 20-300 mg/day

Monitoring Parameters Blood pressure, blood glucose, electrolytes, symptoms of fluid retention

Test Interactions Increased amylase (S), chloride (S), cholesterol (S), glucose, protein, sodium (S); decreased calcium (S), chloride (S), potassium (S), thyroxine (S)

Patient Information Take with food or milk; take single daily doses in the morning; do not stop abruptly; carry an identification card or bracelet advising that you are on steroids

Nursing Implications I.M. use only; shake vial before measuring out dose; withdraw gradually following long-term therapy

Additional Information Approximately 80% the potency of cortisol; the maximum activity of the adrenal cortex is between 2 AM and 8 AM and it is minimal between 4 PM and midnight; if possible, administer glucocorticoids before 9 AM to minimize adrenocortical suppression; prolonged therapy (>5 days) of pharmacologic doses of corticosteroids may lead to hypothalamic-pituitary-adrenal suppression, the degree of adrenal suppression varies with the degree and duration of glucocorticoid therapy; this must be taken into consideration when taking patients off steroids; supplemental doses may be warranted during times of stress in the course of withdrawal therapy

Special Geriatric Considerations Because of the risk of adverse effects, systemic corticosteroids should be used cautiously in the elderly, in the smallest possible dose, and for the shortest possible time.

Dosage Forms
Injection: 50 mg/mL (10 mL)
Tablet: 5 mg, 10 mg, 25 mg

Cortizone®-5 [OTC] see Hydrocortisone on page 462
Cortizone®-10 [OTC] see Hydrocortisone on page 462
Cortone® Acetate see Cortisone Acetate on previous page
Cotazym® see Pancrelipase on page 712
Cotazym-S® see Pancrelipase on page 712
Cotrim® see Co-Trimoxazole on this page
Cotrim® DS see Co-Trimoxazole on this page

Co-Trimoxazole (koe trye MOKS a zole)

Related Information
Penicillins, Penicillin-Related Antibiotics, & Other Antibiotics on page 1010

Brand Names Bactrim™; Bactrim™ DS; Cotrim®; Cotrim® DS; Septra®; Septra® DS; Sulfatrim®

Synonyms SMZ-TMP; Sulfamethoxazole and Trimethoprim; TMP-SMZ; Trimethoprim and Sulfamethoxazole

Generic Available Yes

Therapeutic Category Antibiotic, Sulfonamide Derivative

Use Oral treatment of urinary tract infections; acute exacerbations of chronic bronchitis in adults; prophylaxis of Pneumocystis carinii pneumonitis (PCP); I.V. treatment of documented PCP, empiric treatment of highly suspected PCP in immune compromised patients; treatment of documented or suspected shigellosis, typhoid fever, or Nocardia asteroides infection in patients who are NPO

Contraindications Hypersensitivity to any sulfa drug or any component; porphyria; megaloblastic anemia due to folate deficiency

Warnings Fatalities associated with sulfonamides, although rare, have occurred due to severe reactions including Stevens-Johnson syndrome, toxic epidermal necrolysis, hepatic necrosis, agranulocytosis, aplastic anemia and other blood dyscrasias; discontinue use at first sign of rash or any sign of adverse reaction

Precautions Use with caution in patients with G-6-PD deficiency, impaired renal or hepatic function; adjust dosage in patients with renal impairment

Adverse Reactions
Central nervous system: Confusion, depression, hallucinations, seizures, fever, ataxia
Dermatologic: Rash, erythema multiforme, Stevens-Johnson syndrome, epidermal necrolysis, photosensitivity, urticaria
(Continued)

Co-Trimoxazole *(Continued)*

Gastrointestinal: Nausea, vomiting, glossitis, stomatitis, diarrhea, pseudo-membranous colitis

Hematologic: Thrombocytopenia, megaloblastic anemia, granulocytopenia, aplastic anemia, hemolysis (with G-6-PD deficiency)

Hepatic: Hepatitis

Renal: Interstitial nephritis, increased serum creatinine due to trimethoprim's interference with creatinine's tubular secretion

Miscellaneous: Serum sickness

Overdosage Symptoms of overdose include anorexia, nausea, vomiting, dizziness, headache, loss of consciousness, toxic fever, acidosis, acute hemolytic anemia, hepatic jaundice, toxic neuritis

Drug Interactions

Decreased effect of cyclosporine

Increased effect of sulfonylureas and oral anticoagulants

Increased toxicity/levels of phenytoin and zidovudine

Increased toxicity by displacing methotrexate from protein binding sites

Increased nephrotoxicity of cyclosporine

Increased serum concentrations of dapsone and SMX-TMP may occur

Stability Do not refrigerate injection; is less soluble in more alkaline pH; protect from light; stability of parenteral admixture at room temperature (25°C): 5 mL/125 mL D_5W = 6 hours; 5 mL/100 mL D_5W = 4 hours; 5 mL/75 mL D_5W = 2 hours

Mechanism of Action Sulfamethoxazole interferes with bacterial folic acid synthesis and growth via inhibition of dihydrofolic acid formation from para-aminobenzoic acid; trimethoprim inhibits dihydrofolic acid reduction to tetra-hydrofolate resulting in sequential inhibition of enzymes of the folic acid pathway

Pharmacokinetics

Absorption: Oral: Almost completely, 90% to 100%

Protein binding:

SMX: 68%

TMP: 45%

Metabolism:

SMX is N-acetylated and glucuronidated

TMP is metabolized to oxide and hydroxylated metabolites

Half-life:

SMX: 9 hours

TMP: 6-17 hours, both are prolonged in renal failure

Time to peak serum concentration: Within 1-4 hours

Elimination: Both are excreted in urine as metabolites and unchanged drug

Effects of aging on the pharmacokinetics of both agents has been variable; increase in half-life and decreases in clearance have been associated with reduced creatinine clearance

Usual Dosage Geriatrics and Adults (dosage recommendations are based on the trimethoprim component):

Urinary tract infection, chronic bronchitis: Oral: 1 double strength tablet every 12 hours for 10-14 days

Sepsis: I.V.: 20 TMP/kg/day divided every 6 hours

Pneumocystis carinii:

Prophylaxis: Oral, I.V.: 10 mg TMP/kg/day divided every 12 hours up to 160 mg TMP/day or every other day

Treatment: I.V.: 20 mg TMP/kg/day divided every 6 hours

Dosing interval/adjustment in renal impairment:

Cl_{cr} 30-50 mL/minute: Administer every 12-18 hours or reduce dose by 25%

Cl_{cr} 15-30 mL/minute: Administer every 18-24 hours or reduce dose by 50%

Cl_{cr} <15 mL/minute: Not recommended

Administration Infuse over 60-90 minutes, must dilute well before giving; not for I.M. injection

Monitoring Parameters Signs and symptoms of infection including mental status

Test Interactions False-positive urine glucose tests that use Benedict's method

Patient Information Take oral medication with 8 oz of water on an empty stomach (1 hour before or 2 hours after meals) for best absorption; report any skin rashes immediately; complete full course of therapy

Nursing Implications Maintain adequate fluid intake to prevent crystalluria (see Administration)

Additional Information Do not use NS as a diluent; injection vehicle contains benzyl alcohol and sodium metabisulfite; the 5:1 ratio (SMX to TMP) remains constant in all dosage forms

Special Geriatric Considerations Elderly patients appear at greater risk for more severe adverse reactions (see Pharmacokinetics and Usual Dosage); adjust dose based on renal function

Dosage Forms

Injection: Sulfamethoxazole 80 mg and trimethoprim 16 mg per mL (5 mL, 10 mL, 20 mL, 30 mL, 50 mL)

Suspension, oral: Sulfamethoxazole 200 mg and trimethoprim 40 mg per 5 mL (20 mL, 100 mL, 150 mL, 200 mL, 480 mL)

Tablet: Sulfamethoxazole 400 mg and trimethoprim 80 mg

Tablet, double strength: Sulfamethoxazole 800 mg and trimethoprim 160 mg

References

Naber K, Vergin H, and Weigand W, "Pharmacokinetics of Co-trimoxazole and Co-tetroxazine in Geriatric Patients," *Infection*, 1981, 9(5):239-43.

Varoquaux O, Lajoie D, Gobert C, et al, "Pharmacokinetics of the Trimethoprim-Sulfamethoxazole Combination in the Elderly," *Br J Clin Pharmacol*, 1985, 20:575-81.

Coumadin® see Warfarin on page 989

Covera-HS® see Verapamil on page 986

Cozaar® see Losartan on page 553

CPM see Cyclophosphamide on page 260

Creon® see Pancreatin on page 711

Creon® 10 see Pancrelipase on page 712

Creon® 20 see Pancrelipase on page 712

Creo-Terpin® [OTC] see Dextromethorphan on page 278

Crolom® Ophthalmic Solution see Cromolyn Sodium on this page

Cromoglycic Acid see Cromolyn Sodium on this page

Cromolyn Sodium (KROE moe lin SOW dee um)

Related Information

Asthma Guidelines on page 1040

Inhaled Medications Comparison on page 1034

Brand Names Crolom® Ophthalmic Solution; Gastrocrom® Oral; Intal® Inhalation Capsule; Intal® Nebulizer Solution; Intal® Oral Inhaler; Nasalcrom® Nasal Solution [OTC]

Synonyms Cromoglycic Acid; Disodium Cromoglycate; DSCG

Therapeutic Category Inhalation, Miscellaneous

Use Adjunct in the prophylaxis of allergic disorders, including rhinitis, giant papillary conjunctivitis, and asthma; inhalation product may be used for relief and prevention of exercise-induced bronchospasm; systemic mastocytosis, food allergy, and treatment of inflammatory bowel disease; **cromolyn is a prophylactic drug with no benefit for acute situations**

Contraindications Hypersensitivity to cromolyn or any component; acute asthma attacks

Warnings Aerosol inhalant should not be used in patients with cardiac arrhythmias

Precautions Caution should be used when withdrawing the drug or tapering the dose as symptoms may reoccur; use with caution in patients with a history of cardiac arrhythmia; use with caution in patients with renal and hepatic impairment

Adverse Reactions

Central nervous system: Dizziness, headache

Dermatologic: Rash, urticaria

Gastrointestinal: Nausea, vomiting, diarrhea

Neuromuscular & skeletal: Arthralgia

Ocular: Ocular stinging, lacrimation

Respiratory: Coughing, wheezing, throat irritation, eosinophilic pneumonia, pulmonary infiltrates, hoarseness, nasal burning

Overdosage Symptoms of overdose include bronchospasm, laryngeal edema, dysuria

Stability Compatible with metaproterenol sulfate, isoproterenol hydrochloride, 0.25% isoetharine hydrochloride, epinephrine hydrochloride, terbutaline sulfate, and 20% acetylcysteine solution for at least 1 hour after their admixture

Mechanism of Action Prevents the mast cell release of histamine, leukotrienes, and slow-reacting substance of anaphylaxis by inhibiting degranulation after contact with antigens

(Continued)

Cromolyn Sodium *(Continued)*

Pharmacokinetics
Absorption:
Inhalation: ~8% of dose reaches the lungs upon inhalation of the powder and is well absorbed
Oral: Only 0.5% to 2%
Half-life: 80-90 minutes
Time to peak serum concentration: Inhalation: Within 15 minutes
Elimination: Absorbed cromolyn is equally excreted unchanged in urine and feces (via bile); small amounts are exhaled

Usual Dosage Geriatrics and Adults:
Inhalation: 20 mg 4 times/day (Spinhaler®) or nebulization solution, 2 inhalations 4 times/day by metered spray
For prevention of exercise-induced bronchospasm: Single dose of 2 inhalations (aerosol) or 20 mg (powder inhalation) just prior to exercise (no more than 1 hour)
Nasal: 1 spray in each nostril 3-4 times/day
Ophthalmic: Instill 1-2 drops 4-6 times/day
Systemic mastocytosis: Oral: 200 mg 4 times/day 30 minutes before meals and at bedtime
Food allergy and inflammatory bowel disease: Oral: 200 mg 4 times/day 15-20 minutes before meal, up to 400 mg 4 times/day (investigational)

Monitoring Parameters Pulmonary function tests, spirometry

Patient Information Do not discontinue abruptly; not effective for acute relief of symptoms; must be taken on a regularly scheduled basis; unless instructed otherwise, capsules are for inhalation, not oral ingestion; store nebulizer solution away from light; follow instructions that come with the product

Nursing Implications Advise patient to clear as much mucus as possible before inhalation treatments

Additional Information Oral administration is strictly investigational; cromolyn is a prophylactic drug with no benefit for acute situations

Special Geriatric Considerations Assess the patient's ability to empty the capsules via the Spinhaler®. Older persons often have difficulty with inhaled and ophthalmic dosage forms.

Dosage Forms
Capsule:
Oral (Gastrocrom®): 100 mg
Inhalation, oral (Intal®): 800 mcg/spray (8.1 g)
Solution, for nebulization:
10 mg/mL (2 mL)
Intal®: 10 mg/mL (2 mL)
Solution, nasal (Nasalcrom®): 40 mg/mL (13 mL)
Solution, ophthalmic (Crolom®): 4% (2.5 mL, 10 mL)

Crotamiton (kroe TAM i tonn)

Brand Names Eurax®

Generic Available No

Therapeutic Category Antipruritic, Topical; Pediculocide; Scabicidal Agent

Use Treatment of scabies and symptomatic treatment of pruritus

Contraindications Hypersensitivity to crotamiton or other components; patients who manifest a primary irritation response to topical medications

Precautions Avoid contact with face, eyes, mucous membranes, and urethral meatus; do not apply to acutely inflamed or raw skin

Adverse Reactions
Dermatologic: Pruritus, contact dermatitis
Local: Irritation, warm sensation

Overdosage Burning or irritation in the oral cavity may signify oral ingestion, burning of the esophagus and gastric mucosa, nausea, vomiting; no specific treatment

Usual Dosage Topical: Scabicide: Geriatrics and Adults: Wash thoroughly and scrub away loose scales, then towel dry; apply a thin layer and massage drug onto skin of the entire body from the neck to the toes (with special attention to skin folds, creases, and interdigital spaces). Repeat application in 24 hours; take a cleansing bath 48 hours after the final application.

Administration Lotion: Shake well before using; avoid contact with face, eyes, mucous membranes, and urethral meatus

Patient Information For topical use only; keep away from eyes and mucosa membranes, all contaminated clothing and bed linen should be washed to avoid reinfestation; shake lotion well

Nursing Implications See Administration

Additional Information Treatment may be repeated after 7-10 days if live mites are still present

Special Geriatric Considerations If cure is not achieved after 2 doses, use alternative therapy

Dosage Forms
Cream: 10% (60 g)
Lotion: 10% (60 mL, 454 mL)

Crystalline Penicillin *see* Penicillin G, Parenteral, Aqueous *on page 722*

Crystamine® *see* Cyanocobalamin *on this page*

Crysticillin® A.S. *see* Penicillin G Procaine *on page 723*

Crystodigin® *see* Digitoxin *on page 291*

CSA *see* Cyclosporine *on page 263*

CTM *see* Chlorpheniramine *on page 208*

C/T/S® Topical Solution *see* Clindamycin *on page 232*

CTX *see* Cyclophosphamide *on page 260*

Cuprimine® *see* Penicillamine *on page 719*

Curretab® Oral *see* Medroxyprogesterone Acetate *on page 578*

Cutivate™ *see* Fluticasone *on page 403*

CyA *see* Cyclosporine *on page 263*

Cyanocobalamin (sye an oh koe BAL a min)

Brand Names Berubigen®; Cobex®; Crystamine®; Cyanoject®; Cyomin®; Ener-B® [OTC]; Kaybovite-1000®; Redisol®; Rubramin-PC®; Sytobex®

Synonyms Vitamin B_{12}

Generic Available Yes

Therapeutic Category Vitamin, Water Soluble

Use Pernicious anemia; vitamin B_{12} deficiency; thyrotoxicosis, hemorrhage, malignancy, liver or kidney disease; hydroxocobalamin has been used to treat cyanide toxicity associated with nitroprusside

Contraindications Hypersensitivity to cyanocobalamin or any component, cobalt; patients with hereditary optic nerve atrophy

Warnings I.M. route used to treat pernicious anemia; vitamin B_{12} deficiency for >3 months results in irreversible degenerative CNS lesions; treatment of vitamin B_{12} megaloblastic anemia may result in severe hypokalemia, sometimes, fatal, when anemia corrects due to cellular potassium requirements

Precautions Folate doses exceeding 10 mcg/day may produce hematologic response in patients with folate deficiency. Indiscriminate folate use may mask the true diagnosis of pernicious anemia. Single deficiency is rare (except multiple deficiencies). Doses of folate >0.1 mg/day may reverse vitamin B_{12} hematologic abnormalities; however, the neurologic manifestations will not be treated or prevented, and irreversible neurologic damage will ensue; B_{12} deficiency masks signs of polycythemia vera; vegetarian diets may result in B_{12} deficiency; pernicious anemia occurs more often in gastric carcinoma than in general population.

Adverse Reactions
Cardiovascular: Peripheral vascular thrombosis
Dermatologic: Itching, urticaria
Gastrointestinal: Diarrhea
Miscellaneous: Anaphylaxis

Toxicology Excess vitamin B_{12} is excreted in urine; toxic doses not known

Drug Interactions
Aminosalicylic acid may reduce therapeutic action of vitamin B_{12}
Chloramphenicol may decrease the hematologic effect of vitamin B_{12} in patients with pernicious anemia
Colchicine and prolonged alcohol (>2 weeks) use may decrease absorption of vitamin B_{12}

Stability Clear pink to red solutions are stable at room temperature; protect from light; incompatible with chlorpromazine, phytonadione, prochlorperazine, warfarin, ascorbic acid, dextrose, heavy metals, oxidizing or reducing agents; avoid freezing

Mechanism of Action Coenzyme for various metabolic functions, including fat and carbohydrate metabolism and protein synthesis, used in cell replication, hematopoiesis, and myelin synthesis

Pharmacokinetics
Absorption: From the terminal ileum in the presence of calcium; for absorption to occur, gastric "intrinsic factor" must be present to transfer the compound across the intestinal mucosa

(Continued)

257

Cyanocobalamin *(Continued)*

Protein binding: Following absorption, bound to transcobalamin II (the major transport protein) and converted in the tissues to active coenzymes methylcobalamin and deoxyadenosylcobalamin; principally stored in the liver, also stored in the kidneys and adrenals. Hydroxocobalamin (vitamin B_{12a}) is bound highly to protein and is retained in the body longer than cyanocobalamin, but offers no clinical advantage.

Usual Dosage Geriatrics and Adults:

Pernicious anemia: I.M.: 100 mcg/day for at least 2 weeks; maintenance: 100 mcg/month; administer folic acid 1 mg/day for 1 month concomitantly

Vitamin B_{12} deficiency: I.M., S.C.: 100 mcg/day for 6-7 days followed by 100 mcg/month for life; maximal oral absorption: 2-3 mcg/day

Oral: RDA: 2 mcg

Nutritional deficiency: 25-250 mcg/day (oral not recommended for pernicious anemia due to lack of absorption)

Reference Range Normal range of serum B_{12} is 150-750 pg/mL; this represents 0.1% of total body content. Metabolic requirements are 2-5 µg/day; years of deficiency required before hematologic and neurologic signs and symptoms are seen. Most commercial methods have in the past undergone modification. The lower limit of normal (critical to the diagnosis of B_{12} deficiency/pernicious anemia) has not been firmly established. Clinical correlation and multiple test documentation of the etiology of macrocytic anemia is advised. Occasional patients with significant neuropsychiatric abnormalities may have no hematologic abnormalities and normal serum cobalamin concentrations, 200 pg/mL (SI: >150 pmol/L), or more commonly between 100-200 pg/mL (SI: 75-150 pmol/L).

Test Interactions Methotrexate, pyrimethamine, and most antibiotics interfere with microbiologic assays

Patient Information Patients with pernicious anemia will require monthly injections for life

Nursing Implications I.M. or deep S.C. are preferred routes of administration; oral therapy is markedly inferior to parenteral therapy; monitor potassium concentrations during early therapy; folate therapy may be necessary in first month B_{12} replacement

Additional Information Water-soluble vitamin with a wide margin of safety; oral therapy with hog mucosa intrinsic factor will not effectively or adequately treat pernicious anemia

Special Geriatric Considerations There exists evidence that people, particularly elderly whose serum cobalamin concentrations <300 pg/mL, should receive replacement parenteral therapy; this recommendation is based upon neuropsychiatric disorders and cardiovascular disorders associated with lower sodium cobalamin concentrations

Dosage Forms

Injection: 30 mcg/mL (30 mL); 1000 mcg/mL (1 mL, 10 mL, 30 mL)

Tablet: 25 mcg, 50 mcg, 100 mcg, 250 mcg, 500 mcg, 1000 mcg

References

Lindenbaum J, Healton EB, Savage DG, et al, "Neuropsychiatric Disorders Caused by Cobalamin Deficiency in the Absence of Anemia or Macrocytosis," *N Engl J Med*, 1988, 318(26):1720-8.

Olszewski AJ, Szostak WB, Bialkowska M, et al, "Reduction of Plasma Lipid and Homocysteine Levels by Pyridoxine, Folate, Cobalamin, Choline, Riboflavin, and Troxerutin in Atherosclerosis," *Atherosclerosis*, 1989, 75(1):1-6.

Regland B, Gottfries CG, and Lindstedt G, "Dementia Patients With Low Serum Cobalamin Concentration: Relationship to Atrophic Gastritis," *Aging Milano*, 1992, 4(1):35-41.

Cyanoject® *see Cyanocobalamin on previous page*

Cyclizine *(SYE kli zeen)*

Brand Names Marezine® [OTC]

Generic Available No

Therapeutic Category Antiemetic; Antihistamine

Use Prevention and treatment of nausea, vomiting and vertigo associated with motion sickness; control of postoperative nausea and vomiting

Contraindications Hypersensitivity to meclizine, cyclizine, or any component

Precautions Use with caution in patients with angle-closure glaucoma or prostatic hypertrophy; elderly may be at risk for anticholinergic side effects such as glaucoma, prostate hypertrophy, constipation, gastrointestinal obstructive disease

Adverse Reactions

Cardiovascular: Palpitations, tachycardia, hypotension

Central nervous system: Drowsiness, fatigue, restlessness, excitation, insomnia, confusion, euphoria, vertigo

Dermatologic: Rash, urticaria

Gastrointestinal: Xerostomia, anorexia, nausea, vomiting, diarrhea, constipation

Genitourinary: Polyuria, urinary retention, dysuria

Hepatic: Cholestatic jaundice

Ocular: Blurred vision, diplopia, visual hallucinations

Otic: Tinnitus, auditory hallucinations

Miscellaneous: Dry nose

Overdosage Excitation alternating with drowsiness, respiratory depression, hallucinations

Toxicology There is no specific treatment for an antihistamine overdose, however, most of its clinical toxicity is due to anticholinergic effects. Cholinesterase inhibitors may be useful by reducing acetylcholinesterase. Acetylcholinesterase inhibitors include physostigmine, neostigmine, pyridostigmine and edrophonium. For anticholinergic overdose with severe life-threatening symptoms, physostigmine 1-2 mg I.V., slowly may be given to reverse these effects.

Drug Interactions May enhance actions of drugs with similar adverse reactions and pharmacologic actions (see Adverse Reactions)

Mechanism of Action Has antiemetic, anticholinergic, and antihistaminic activity; has central anticholinergic action by blocking chemoreceptor trigger zone; decreases excitability of the middle ear labyrinth and blocks conduction in the middle ear vestibular-cerebellar pathways

Pharmacodynamics

Onset of action: Oral: Within 30-60 minutes

Duration: 4-6 hours

Pharmacokinetics

Metabolism: Reportedly in the liver

Half-life: 6 hours

Elimination: As metabolites in urine and as unchanged drug in feces

Usual Dosage Geriatrics and Adults:

Oral: 25-50 mg taken 30 minutes before departure, may repeat in 4-6 hours if needed, up to 200 mg/day

I.M.: 25-50 mg every 4-6 hours as needed

Monitoring Parameters Monitor for CNS side effects in elderly

Patient Information May impair ability to perform hazardous tasks; may cause drowsiness; may cause dry mouth, constipation, difficulty urinating, confusion

Nursing Implications See Precautions and Special Geriatric Considerations

Special Geriatric Considerations Due to anticholinergic action, use lowest dose in divided doses to avoid side effects and their inconvenience; limit use if possible; may cause confusion or aggravate symptoms of confusion in those with dementia; constipation and difficulty voiding urine may occur

Dosage Forms

Injection, as lactate: 50 mg/mL (1 mL)

Tablet, as hydrochloride: 50 mg

Cyclobenzaprine (sye kloe BEN za preen)

Brand Names Flexeril®

Generic Available Yes

Therapeutic Category Skeletal Muscle Relaxant

Use Treatment of muscle spasm associated with acute painful musculoskeletal conditions

Contraindications Hypersensitivity to cyclobenzaprine or any component; do not use concomitantly or within 14 days of MAO inhibitors; acute recovery phase of myocardial infarction, arrhythmias, heart block, conduction disturbances, congestive heart failure, or hyperthyroidism

Warnings Use only for short periods of time (2-3 weeks); cyclobenzaprine shares the toxic potentials of the tricyclic antidepressants; the usual precautions of tricyclic antidepressant therapy should be observed

Precautions Because it has anticholinergic effects, use with caution in patients with urinary hesitancy or angle-closure glaucoma

Adverse Reactions

Cardiovascular: Tachycardia, hypotension, arrhythmias

Central nervous system: Drowsiness, headache, dizziness, fatigue, nervousness, convulsions, confusion

Dermatologic: Rash

Gastrointestinal: Dyspepsia, nausea, constipation, xerostomia, vomiting, diarrhea, dysgeusia

Genitourinary: Polyuria, urinary retention

(Continued)

Cyclobenzaprine *(Continued)*

Hepatic: Abnormal liver function
Neuromuscular & skeletal: Weakness
Ocular: Blurred vision

Overdosage Symptoms of overdose include drowsiness, hypothermia, tachycardia, arrhythmias, dilated pupils, convulsions, severe hypotension, stupor, and coma

Toxicology Following initiation of essential overdose management, toxic symptoms should be treated. Ventricular arrhythmias often respond to systemic alkalinization (sodium bicarbonate 0.5-2 mEq/kg I.V.) and/or phenytoin 15-20 mg/kg. Arrhythmias unresponsive to this therapy may respond to lidocaine 1 mg/kg I.V. followed by a titrated infusion. Physostigmine 1-2 mg I.V. slowly may be indicated in reversing cardiac arrhythmias that are life-threatening. Seizures usually respond to 5-10 mg diazepam I.V. boluses. If seizures are unresponsive or recur, phenytoin or phenobarbital may be required.

Drug Interactions Do not use concomitantly or within 14 days after MAO inhibitors
Increased effect/toxicity with alcohol, barbiturates, CNS depressants
Increased toxicity with MAO inhibitors, TCAs, anticholinergics

Mechanism of Action Reduces tonic somatic motor activity influencing both alpha and gamma motor neurons

Pharmacodynamics
Onset of action: Commonly occurs within 1 hour
Duration: 12-24 hours

Pharmacokinetics
Absorption: Oral: Completely
Protein binding: 93%
Metabolism: Hepatic; may undergo enterohepatic recycling; metabolized to glucuronide-like conjugate
Half-life: 1-3 days
Time to peak serum concentration: Within 3-8 hours
Elimination: Renally as inactive metabolites and in feces (via bile) as unchanged drug

Usual Dosage Oral: **Note:** Do not use longer than 2-3 weeks
Geriatrics: See Special Geriatric Considerations
Adults: Initial: 10 mg 3 times/day; range: 20-40 mg/day in divided doses; maximum dose: 60 mg/day

Monitoring Parameters Relief of pain and muscle spasm, liver function tests, mental status

Patient Information May cause drowsiness, dizziness, or blurred vision; use caution performing activities requiring alertness; avoid alcohol and CNS depressants; may cause dry mouth

Nursing Implications Raise bed rails and institute safety measures; assist with ambulation

Special Geriatric Considerations High doses in the elderly caused drowsiness and dizziness; therefore, use the lowest dose possible. Because cyclobenzaprine causes anticholinergic effects, it may not be the skeletal muscle relaxant of choice in the elderly.

Dosage Forms Tablet, as hydrochloride: 10 mg

Cyclocort® *see* Amcinonide *on page 50*

Cyclophosphamide *(sye kloe FOS fa mide)*

Brand Names Cytoxan® Injection; Cytoxan® Oral; Neosar® Injection
Synonyms CPM; CTX; CYT; NSC 26271
Generic Available No
Therapeutic Category Antineoplastic Agent, Alkylating Agent (Nitrogen Mustard)
Use Management of Hodgkin's disease, malignant lymphomas, multiple myeloma, leukemias, small cell carcinoma of the lungs, mycosis fungoides, neuroblastoma, ovarian carcinoma, breast carcinoma, a variety of other tumors; nephrotic syndrome
Unlabeled uses: Lupus erythematosus, severe rheumatoid arthritis, rheumatoid vasculitis, multiple sclerosis, polyarteritis nodosa, and polymyositis
Contraindications Hypersensitivity to cyclophosphamide or any component, severely depressed bone marrow function
Warnings The U.S. Food and Drug Administration (FDA) currently recommends that procedures for proper handling and disposal of antineoplastic agents be considered.

Cardiac toxicity with necrosis: Reported with high doses (120-170 mg/kg given over a few days); no residual cardiac effects seen with EKG or echocardiogram

Genitourinary: Hemorrhagic cystitis occurs in 7% to 12% of patients; higher percentages have been reported. This sterile hemorrhagic cystitis is related to the concentration of metabolites in bladder (acrolein); may result in bladder telangiectasis fibrosis and bladder cancer.

Pulmonary: Pulmonary fibrosis has been reported

Skin: May interfere with normal wound healing

Hypersensitivity: Type I reactions have occurred; anaphylaxis is rare

Renal: Use cautiously in renal impairment since alterations in renal function may result in altered pharmacokinetics. No evidence for a need to alter dose for renal function; long-term free water clearance may be impaired

Carcinogenesis: Long-term follow up indicates an increased incidence of leukemia (myeloproliferative and lymphoproliferative malignancies); these secondary malignancies have occurred most frequently in patients with primary myeloproliferative/lymphoproliferative diseases; most frequent malignancies occur in the bladder; some cases of secondary malignancies have occurred years after discontinuation of cyclophosphamide

Precautions Use with caution in patients with bone marrow suppression and impaired renal or hepatic function

Adverse Reactions

Cardiovascular: Cardiotoxicity with high dose therapy

Dermatologic: Alopecia

Endocrine & metabolic: Hypokalemia, amenorrhea, SIADH, hyperuricemia

Gastrointestinal: Nausea, vomiting, dysgeusia

Genitourinary: Oligospermia

Hematologic: Leukopenia nadir at 8-15 days, hemolytic anemia, myelosuppression, positive Coombs' test

Renal: Hemorrhagic cystitis

Respiratory: Interstitial pulmonary fibrosis, nasal congestion

Overdosage Symptoms of overdose include myelosuppression, alopecia, nausea, vomiting, cystitis

Toxicology Institute general supportive care; cyclophosphamide and its metabolites are dialyzable; no specific antidote is known

Drug Interactions

Cardiotoxic drugs (eg, doxorubicin); drugs that affect hepatic microsomal enzymes (eg, phenobarbital, phenytoin, chloramphenicol); barbiturates, allopurinol, imipramine, phenothiazines, succinylcholine

Digoxin serum concentrations may decrease

Thiazide diuretics enhance leukopenia

Stability Reconstituted solution is stable for 24 hours at room temperature and 6 days when refrigerated; if powder for injection is not reconstituted with bacteriostatic water for injection, USP, use within 6 hours; does not contain antimicrobial agent; assure sterile preparation

Mechanism of Action Cyclophosphamide is converted through hepatic metabolism to active metabolites: non-nitrogen mustard and phosphoramide mustard. Acrolein is a significant metabolite thought to cause bladder toxicity. The active metabolites interfere with the normal function of DNA by alkylation and cross-linking the strands of DNA, and by possible protein modification.

Pharmacokinetics

Absorption: Completely from GI tract

Metabolism: In the liver to active metabolite; substrate CYP2B6, 3A4

Half-life: 3-12 hours

Time to peak serum concentrations: Oral: Within 1 hour

Elimination: In urine as unchanged drug (<30%) and as metabolites (85% to 90%)

Alkylating activity is lost 10 hours after oral administration

Usual Dosage

Geriatrics (refer to individual protocols): Initial and maintenance: 1-2 mg/kg/day; adjust for renal clearance

Adults with no hematologic problems:

Induction:

Oral: 1-5 mg/kg/day

I.V.: 40-50 mg/kg (1.5-1.8 g/m^2) in divided doses over 2-5 days

Maintenance:

Oral: 1-5 mg/kg/day

I.V.: 10-15 mg/kg (350-550 mg/m^2) every 7-10 days or 3-5 mg/kg (110-185 mg/m^2) twice weekly

(Continued)

Cyclophosphamide *(Continued)*

Dosing adjustment in renal impairment:
Cl_{cr} 25-50 mL/minute: Decrease dose by 50%
Cl_{cr} <25 mL/minute: Avoid use
Moderately dialyzable (20% to 50%)
Adults:
SLE: I.V.: 500-750 mg/m² every month; maximum: 1 g/m²
BMT-conditioning regimen: I.V.: 50 mg/kg/day once daily for 3-4 days
Nephrotic syndrome: Oral: 2-3 mg/kg/day every day for up to 12 weeks when corticosteroids are unsuccessful

Monitoring Parameters Monitor WBC and platelets; observe for signs of infection, bleeding, and bladder irritation; monitor urinalysis for blood (see Additional Information)

Test Interactions Increased prothrombin time, potassium (S)

Patient Information Drink plenty of fluids before and after doses; report any blood in the urine. May cause nausea, vomiting, and diarrhea. If these side effects persist, call physician; report any bruising, bleeding, chills, cough, shortness of breath, unusual lumps, seizures, sores in mouth, flank or joint pain.

Nursing Implications Encourage adequate hydration and frequent voiding to help prevent hemorrhagic cystitis (see Monitoring Parameters and Patient Information)

Additional Information Myelosuppressive effects:
WBC: Moderate
Platelets: Moderate
Onset (days): 7
Nadir (days): 10-14
Recovery (days): 21

Special Geriatric Considerations Toxicity to immunosuppressives is increased in elderly. Start with lowest recommended adult doses. Signs of infection, such as fever and WBC rise, may not occur. Lethargy and confusion may be more prominent signs of infection; adjust dose for renal function in elderly.

Dosage Forms
Injection: 100 mg, 200 mg, 500 mg, 1 g, 2 g
Tablet: 25 mg, 50 mg

References

Bostrom BC, Weisdorf DJ, Kim TH, et al, "Bone Marrow Transplantation for Advanced Acute Leukemia: A Pilot Study of High-Energy Total Body Irradiation, Cyclophosphamide and Continuous Infusion Etoposide," *Bone Marrow Transplant*, 1990, 5(2):83-9.

Hutchins LF and Lipschitz DA, "Cancer, Clinical Pharmacology, and Aging," *Clin Geriatr Med*, 1987, 3(3):483-503.

Kaplan HG, "Use of Cancer Chemotherapy in the Elderly," *Drug Treatment in the Elderly*, Vestal RE, ed, Boston, MA: ADIS Health Science Press, 1984, 338-49.

McCune WJ, Golbus J, Zeldes W, et al, "Clinical and Immunologic Effects of Monthly Administration of Intravenous Cyclophosphamide in Severe Systemic Lupus Erythematosus," *N Engl J Med*, 1988, 318(22):1423-31.

Cycloserine *(sye kloe SER een)*

Brand Names Seromycin® Pulvules®

Therapeutic Category Antibiotic, Miscellaneous; Antitubercular Agent

Use Adjunctive treatment in pulmonary or extrapulmonary tuberculosis; treatment of acute urinary tract infections caused by *E. coli* or *Enterobacter* sp when less toxic conventional therapy has failed or is contraindicated

Contraindications Known hypersensitivity to cycloserine; epilepsy, depression, severe anxiety or psychosis, severe renal insufficiency, chronic alcoholism

Precautions Adjust dosage with renal impairment

Adverse Reactions
Cardiovascular: Cardiac arrhythmias
Central nervous system: Drowsiness, headache, dizziness, vertigo, seizures, confusion, psychosis, coma, paresis
Dermatologic: Rash
Hepatic: Elevated liver enzymes
Neuromuscular & skeletal: Tremors
Miscellaneous: Vitamin B_{12} deficiency, folate deficiency

Overdosage Symptoms of overdose include confusion, CNS depression, psychosis, coma

Toxicology Seizures; decontaminate with activated charcoal; can be hemodialyzed; management is supportive; administer 100-300 mg/day of pyridoxine to reduce neurotoxic effects; acute toxicity can occur with ingestions >1 g

Drug Interactions Alcohol increases risk of seizures, isoniazid may increase cycloserine CNS side effects

Mechanism of Action Inhibits bacterial cell wall synthesis by competing with amino acid (D-alanine) for incorporation into the bacterial cell wall

Pharmacokinetics

Absorption: Oral: ~70% to 90% from GI tract

Half-life: Normal renal function: 10 hours

Time to peak serum concentration: Oral: Within 3-4 hours

Elimination: 60% to 70% of oral dose excreted unchanged in urine by glomerular filtration within 72 hours, small amounts excreted in feces, remainder is metabolized

Usual Dosage Oral:

Tuberculosis: Geriatrics and Adults: Initial: 250 mg every 12 hours for 14 days, then administer 500 mg to 1 g/day in 2 divided doses for 18-24 months (maximum daily dose: 1 g)

Urinary tract infection: Adults: 250 mg every 12 hours for 14 days; patients with impaired renal function should have their dose adjusted based upon serum concentrations (see Monitoring Parameters and Reference Range)

Dosing interval in renal impairment:

Cl_{cr} 10-50 mL/minute: Administer every 12-24 hours

Cl_{cr} <10 mL/minute: Administer every 24 hours

Monitoring Parameters Check serum concentrations weekly for patients with decreased renal function, receiving >500 mg/day, or when toxicity is suspected

Reference Range Adequate CSF penetration; toxicity is greatly increased at concentrations >30 µg/mL

Patient Information May cause drowsiness; notify physician if skin rash, mental confusion, dizziness, headache, or tremors occur

Nursing Implications Some of the neurotoxic effects may be relieved or prevented by the concomitant administration of pyridoxine

Additional Information Administer 100-300 mg/day of pyridoxine to relieve neurotoxic effects

Special Geriatric Considerations Adjust dose for renal function (see Usual Dosage)

Dosage Forms Capsule: 250 mg

Cyclosporin A see Cyclosporine on this page

Cyclosporine (SYE kloe spor een)

Related Information

Serum Drug Concentrations Commonly Monitored: Guidelines on page 1114

Brand Names Neoral® Oral; Sandimmune® Injection; Sandimmune® Oral

Synonyms CSA; CyA; Cyclosporin A

Generic Available No

Therapeutic Category Immunosuppressant Agent

Use Immunosuppressant used with corticosteroids to prevent graft versus host disease in patients with kidney, liver, heart, and bone marrow transplants.

Unlabeled use: Rheumatoid arthritis

Contraindications Hypersensitivity to cyclosporine or polyoxyethylated castor oil

Warnings Administer with adrenal corticosteroids; infection and possible development of lymphoma may result; make dose adjustments (to avoid toxicity or possible organ rejection) via cyclosporine blood levels because absorption is erratic

Precautions Dosage needs to be adjusted in patients with hepatic and renal dysfunction

Adverse Reactions

Cardiovascular: Hypertension, hypotension, tachycardia, warmth, flushing

Central nervous system: Seizure, headache

Dermatologic: Hirsutism

Endocrine & metabolic: Hyperkalemia, hypomagnesemia, hyperuricemia

Gastrointestinal: Abdominal discomfort, gingival hyperplasia

Hepatic: Hepatotoxicity

Neuromuscular & skeletal: Myositis, tremors, paresthesia

Renal: Nephrotoxicity, renal dysfunction

Respiratory: Respiratory distress

Miscellaneous: Increased susceptibility to infection, and sensitivity to temperature extremes

(Continued)

Cyclosporine *(Continued)*

Toxicology Minimal experience with overdosage; may see transient hepatotoxicity and nephrotoxicity; not dialyzable, not cleared well by charcoal hemoperfusion

Drug Interactions

Decreased levels: Carbamazepine, barbiturates, phenytoin, rifampin

Increased levels: Diltiazem, erythromycin, fluconazole, ketoconazole, nicardipine, imipenem-cilastatin, metoclopramide

Increased toxicity: Aminoglycosides, amphotericin B, NSAIDs, co-trimoxazole, digoxin (increased digoxin levels)

Increased risk of gingival hyperplasia when given with nifedipine

Stability Stability of injection of parenteral admixture at room temperature (25°C): 6 hours in PVC, 12 hours in glass; do not refrigerate; protect I.V. ampuls from light; use contents of oral solution within 2 months after opening

Mechanism of Action Inhibition of production and release of interleukin II and inhibits interleukin II-induced activation of resting T lymphocytes

Pharmacokinetics

Absorption: Oral: Incomplete and erratic

Protein binding: 90% of dose binds to blood proteins

Metabolism: By mixed function oxidase enzymes in the liver; substrate CYP3A4

Bioavailability: Gut dysfunction, commonly seen in BMT recipients reduces oral bioavailability further

Half-life: Adults: 19-40 hours

Time to peak serum concentration: 3-4 hours

Elimination: Primarily in bile, clearance is decreased in patients with liver disease

Usual Dosage Geriatrics and Adults (**Note:** Sandimmune® and Neoral® are not bioequivalent and cannot be used interchangeably without physician supervision):

Oral: Initial: 14-18 mg/kg/dose daily, beginning 4-12 hours prior to organ transplantation; maintenance: 5-10 mg/kg/day

I.V.: Initial: 5-6 mg/kg/day in divided doses every 12-24 hours; patients should be switched to oral cyclosporine as soon as possible

Rheumatoid arthritis: Oral: 5-10 mg/kg/day

Administration For I.V. use, dilute to a concentration of 50 mg per 20-100 mL; infuse over 2-6 hours; do not administer liquid from plastic or styrofoam cup; mixing with milk, chocolate milk, or orange juice preferably at room temperature, improves palatability; stir well and drink at once; do not allow to stand before drinking; rinse with more diluent to ensure that the total dose is taken; after use, dry outside of pipette; do not rinse with water or other cleaning agents

Monitoring Parameters Cyclosporine serum concentrations, serum electrolytes, renal function, hepatic function, blood pressure, pulse

Reference Range Reference ranges are **method dependent and specimen dependent**. Trough concentrations should be obtained 12-18 hours after oral dose (chronic usage), 12 hours after I.V., dose, or immediately prior to next dose.

Therapeutic: Not well defined, dependent on organ transplanted, time after transplant, organ function and CSA toxicity

Toxic: Not well defined, nephrotoxicity usually occurs at a serum concentration >400 ng/mL, but may occur at any concentration

Test Interactions Specific whole blood, HPLC assay for cyclosporine may be falsely elevated if sample is drawn from the same line through which dose was administered (even if flush has been administered and/or dose was given hours before)

Patient Information Use glass droppers or glass to hold dose; may mix with milk or juice for flavor; rinse container to get full dose

Nursing Implications May cause inflamed gums (see Administration)

Additional Information Should be mixed in glass containers; Sandimmune® and Neoral® are not bioequivalent

Special Geriatric Considerations Cyclosporine has not been specifically studied in the elderly; cyclosporine is being used in combination therapy for the treatment of severe rheumatoid arthritis

Dosage Forms

Capsule (Sandimmune®): 25 mg, 100 mg

Capsule, soft gel (Sandimmune®): 50 mg

Capsule, soft gel for microemulsion (Neoral®): 25 mg, 100 mg

Injection (Sandimmune®): 50 mg/mL (5 mL)

Solution, oral (Sandimmune®): 100 mg/mL (50 mL)
Solution, oral for microemulsion (Neoral®): 100 mg/mL (50 mL)

References

Burckart GJ, Canafax DM, and Yee GC, "Cyclosporine Monitoring," *Drug Intell Clin Pharm*, 1986, 20(9):649-52.

Wells G and Tugwell P, "Cyclosporin A in Rheumatoid Arthritis: Overview of Efficacy," *Br J Rheumatol*, 1993, 32(Suppl 1):51-6.

Cycrin® Oral *see* Medroxyprogesterone Acetate *on page 578*

Cyomin® *see* Cyanocobalamin *on page 257*

Cyproheptadine (si proe HEP ta deen)

Brand Names Periactin®

Generic Available Yes

Therapeutic Category Antihistamine

Use Perennial and seasonal allergic rhinitis and other allergic symptoms including cold urticaria

Unlabeled use: Appetite stimulant, vascular cluster headaches, migraine headache prophylaxis, reversal of antidepressant-induced impotence or sexual dysfunction

Contraindications Hypersensitivity to cyproheptadine or any component; narrow-angle glaucoma, bladder neck obstruction, asthmatic attack, stenosing peptic ulcer, GI tract obstruction, those on MAO inhibitors

Warnings Antihistamines are more likely to cause dizziness, excessive sedation, syncope, toxic confusional states, and hypotension in the elderly

Precautions Use with caution in patients with heart disease, hypertension, thyroid disease, and asthma

Adverse Reactions

Cardiovascular: Tachycardia

Central nervous system: Sedation, CNS stimulation, seizures

Gastrointestinal: Appetite stimulation, weight gain

Hematologic: Hemolytic anemia, leukopenia, thrombocytopenia

Miscellaneous: Allergic reactions

Overdosage Symptoms of overdose include CNS depression or stimulation, dry mouth, flushed skin, fixed and dilated pupils, apnea

Toxicology There is no specific treatment for an antihistamine overdose, however, most of its clinical toxicity is due to anticholinergic effects. Cholinesterase inhibitors may be useful by reducing acetylcholinesterase. Acetylcholinesterase inhibitors include physostigmine, neostigmine, pyridostigmine, and edrophonium. For anticholinergic overdose with severe life-threatening symptoms, physostigmine 1-2 mg I.V., slowly may be given to reverse these effects.

Drug Interactions Increased toxicity: MAO inhibitors, CNS depressants, alcohol

Mechanism of Action Competes with histamine for H_1-receptor sites on effector cells in the gastrointestinal tract, blood vessels, and respiratory tract; also has antiserotonin effects

Pharmacokinetics

Metabolism: Almost completely

Elimination: >50% excreted in urine (primarily as metabolites) and ~25% excreted in feces

Usual Dosage Oral:

Geriatrics: Initial: 4 mg twice daily

Adults: Initial: 4 mg 3 times/day; maximum: do not to exceed 0.5 mg/kg/day

Appetite stimulant: 4 mg 3-4 times/day

Dosing adjustment in hepatic impairment: Dosage should be reduced in patients with significant hepatic dysfunction

Monitoring Parameters Relief of symptoms, weight

Test Interactions Diagnostic antigen skin tests

Patient Information May cause drowsiness; avoid CNS depressants and alcohol

Nursing Implications Monitor relief of symptoms, weight, eating habits

Additional Information May stimulate appetite

Special Geriatric Considerations In case reports, cyproheptadine has promoted weight gain in anorexic adults, though it has not been specifically studied in the elderly. All cases of weight loss or decreased appetite should be adequately assessed. Cyproheptadine may cause less sedation than diphenhydramine or hydroxyzine and, therefore, may be useful for pruritus in the elderly; elderly may not tolerate anticholinergic effects.

(Continued)

Cyproheptadine (Continued)

Dosage Forms
Cyproheptadine hydrochloride:
Syrup: 2 mg/5 mL with alcohol 5% (473 mL)
Tablet: 4 mg

Cystospaz® see Hyoscyamine on page 471

Cystospaz-M® see Hyoscyamine on page 471

CYT see Cyclophosphamide on page 260

Cytomel® Oral see Liothyronine on page 539

Cytotec® see Misoprostol on page 632

Cytovene® see Ganciclovir on page 419

Cytoxan® Injection see Cyclophosphamide on page 260

Cytoxan® Oral see Cyclophosphamide on page 260

D₃ see Cholecalciferol on page 218

D-3-Mercaptovaline see Penicillamine on page 719

Dacodyl® [OTC] see Bisacodyl on page 121

Dakrina® Ophthalmic Solution [OTC] see Artificial Tears on page 82

Dalalone® see Dexamethasone on page 274

Dalalone D.P.® see Dexamethasone on page 274

Dalalone L.A.® see Dexamethasone on page 274

Dalmane® see Flurazepam on page 399

Dalteparin (dal TE pa rin)
Brand Names Fragmin®
Therapeutic Category Anticoagulant
Use Prevention of deep vein thrombosis which may lead to pulmonary embolism, in patients requiring abdominal surgery who are at risk for thromboembolism complications (ie, patients >40 years of age, obese, patients with malignancy, history of deep vein thrombosis or pulmonary embolism, and surgical procedures requiring general anesthesia and lasting longer than 30 minutes)

Contraindications Hypersensitivity to dalteparin or other low-molecular weight heparins or pork products; cerebrovascular disease or other active hemorrhage; cerebral aneurysm; severe uncontrolled hypertension

Warnings Use with caution in patients with pre-existing thrombocytopenia, recent childbirth, subacute bacterial endocarditis, peptic ulcer disease, pericarditis or pericardial effusion, liver or renal function impairment, recent lumbar puncture, vasculitis, concurrent use of aspirin (increased bleeding risk), previous hypersensitivity to heparin, heparin-associated thrombocytopenia

Adverse Reactions
Dermatologic: Allergic reactions (eg, pruritus, rash, fever, injection site reaction, bullous eruption), anaphylactoid reactions and skin necrosis
Hematologic: Bleeding, wound hematoma, injection site hematoma, thrombocytopenia
Local: Pain at injection site

Overdosage Symptoms include hemorrhage

Drug Interactions Increased toxicity: Caution should be used when using aspirin, other platelet inhibitors, and oral anticoagulants in combination with dalteparin due to an increased risk of bleeding

Stability Store at temperatures ≤25°C

Mechanism of Action Low molecular weight heparin analog with a molecular weight of 4000-6000 daltons; the commercial product contains 3% to 15% heparin with a molecular weight <3000 daltons; 65% to 78% with a molecular weight of 3000-8000 daltons and 14% to 26% with a molecular weight >8000 daltons; while dalteparin has been shown to inhibit both factor Xa and factor IIa (thrombin), the antithrombotic effect of dalteparin is characterized by a higher ratio of antifactor Xa to antifactor IIa activity (ratio = 4)

Pharmacodynamics T_{max}: S.C.: 2.3-3 hours after single injection

Pharmacokinetics Pharmacokinetics have not been shown to be significantly altered by age
Distribution: V_d: 40-60 mg/kg
Bioavailability: S.C.: 87%
Half-life:
Normal renal function: 1.82 hours
Patients with chronic renal insufficiency requiring hemodialysis: 5.7 hours
Elimination: Renal; clearance: 15-25 mL/minute

Usual Dosage Geriatrics and Adults: S.C.: 2500 units 1-2 hours prior to surgery, then once daily for 5-10 days postoperatively

Administration S.C. only, do not administer I.M.; patient should be sitting or lying down; administer by deep S.C. injection to the area around the navel, the upper outer thigh, or the upper outer area of the buttock

Monitoring Parameters Periodic CBC including platelet count; stool occult blood tests; urinalysis

Nursing Implications See Administration

Special Geriatric Considerations No specific recommendations are necessary for elderly (see Usual Dosage)

Dosage Forms Injection: Prefilled syringe: 2500 units (16 mg) in 0.2 mL

References
Simoneau G, Bergmann JF, Kher A, et al, "Pharmacokinetics of a Low Molecular Weight Heparin (Fragmin®) in Young and Elderly Subjects," *Thromb Res*, 1992, 66(5):603-7.

Danaparoid (da NAP a roid)

Brand Names Orgaran®

Therapeutic Category Anticoagulant

Use Prevention of postoperative deep vein thrombosis following elective hip replacement surgery

Contraindications Patients with severe hemorrhagic diathesis including active major bleeding, hemorrhagic stroke in the acute phase, hemophilia and idiopathic thrombocytopenic purpura; type II thrombocytopenia associated with a positive *in vitro* test for antiplatelet antibody in the presence of danaparoid, hypersensitivity to danaparoid or known hypersensitivity to pork products

Warnings Do not administer intramuscularly; use with extreme caution in patients with a history of bacterial endocarditis, hemorrhagic stroke, recent CNS or ophthalmological surgery, bleeding diathesis, uncontrolled arterial hypertension, or a history of recent gastrointestinal ulceration and hemorrhage. Danaparoid shows a low cross-sensitivity with antiplatelet antibodies in individuals with type II heparin-induced thrombocytopenia. This product contains sodium sulfite which may cause allergic-type reactions, including anaphylactic symptoms and life-threatening asthmatic episodes in susceptible people; this is seen more frequently in asthmatics.

Adverse Reactions
Cardiovascular: Peripheral edema, generalized edema
Central nervous system: Fever, insomnia, headache, dizziness
Dermatologic: Rash, pruritus
Gastrointestinal: Nausea, constipation, vomiting
Genitourinary: Urinary tract infections, urinary retention
Hematologic: Anemia, hemorrhage, hematoma
Local: Injection site pain
Neuromuscular & skeletal: Joint disorder, weakness

Overdosage Symptoms of overdose include hemorrhage

Toxicology Protamine zinc has been used to reverse effects

Drug Interactions Increased toxicity with oral anticoagulants, platelet inhibitors

Pharmacokinetics
Half-life, plasma: Mean terminal half-life: ~24 hours
Elimination: Primarily by the kidneys

Usual Dosage Geriatrics and Adults: S.C.: 750 anti-Xa units twice daily; beginning 1-4 hours before surgery and then not sooner than 2 hours after surgery and every 12 hours until the risk of DVT has diminished, the average duration of therapy is 7-10 days

Dosing adjustment in renal impairment: Adjustment may be necessary in elderly and patients with severe renal impairment; patients with serum creatinine concentrations ≥2.0 mg/dL should be carefully monitored

Administration Administer S.C., not I.M.; have patient lie down and administer by deep S.C. injection using a fine needle (25-26 gauge); rotate sites of injection

Monitoring Parameters Platelets, occult blood, and anti-Xa activity, if available; the monitoring of PT and/or PTT is not necessary; stool for occult blood; urinalysis

Nursing Implications See Administration

Special Geriatric Considerations Evaluation of elderly's creatinine serum concentrations is important before initiating therapy; See Usual Dosage and Monitoring Parameters

Dosage Forms Injection, as sodium: 750 anti-Xa units/0.6 mL

Dantrium® *see* Dantrolene *on next page*

Dantrolene (DAN troe leen)
Brand Names Dantrium®
Generic Available No
Therapeutic Category Antidote, Malignant Hyperthermia; Hyperthermia, Treatment; Skeletal Muscle Relaxant
Use Treatment of spasticity associated with spinal cord injury, stroke, cerebral palsy, or multiple sclerosis; also used as treatment of malignant hyperthermia
Unlabeled use: Neuroleptic malignant syndrome, heat stroke
Contraindications Active hepatic disease; should not be used where spasticity is used to maintain posture or balance
Warnings Has potential for hepatotoxicity; overt hepatitis has been most frequently observed between the third and twelfth month of therapy; hepatic injury appears to be greater in females and in patients >35 years of age
Precautions Use with caution in patients with impaired cardiac function or impaired pulmonary function
Adverse Reactions
Cardiovascular: Pleural effusion with pericarditis
Central nervous system: Seizures, drowsiness, dizziness, lightheadedness, confusion, headache
Dermatologic: Rash
Gastrointestinal: Diarrhea, nausea, vomiting
Hepatic: Hepatitis
Neuromuscular & skeletal: Muscle weakness
Overdosage Symptoms of overdose include CNS depression, nausea, vomiting; employ supportive measures, gastric lavage
Drug Interactions
Decreased protein binding: Warfarin, clofibrate
Definite drug interaction with estrogen has not been established, but increased hepatotoxicity is seen in women >35 years of age using both drugs
Increased hyperkalemia and cardiac depression with verapamil
Stability Add 60 mL of sterile water for injection USP (not **bacteriostatic water for injection**); protect from light; use within 6 hours
Mechanism of Action Acts directly on skeletal muscle by interfering with release of calcium ion from the sarcoplasmic reticulum; prevents or reduces the increase in myoplasmic calcium ion concentration that activates the acute catabolic processes associated with malignant hyperthermia
Pharmacokinetics
Absorption: Slow and incomplete from GI tract
Metabolism: Slowly in the liver
Half-life: 8.7 hours
Elimination: 25% in urine as metabolites and unchanged drug, and 45% to 50% in feces via bile
Usual Dosage Geriatrics and Adults:
Spasticity: Oral: 25 mg/day to start, increase frequency to 3-4 times/day, then increase dose by 25 mg every 4-7 days to a maximum of 100 mg 2-4 times/day or 400 mg/day
Hyperthermia:
Oral: 4-8 mg/kg/day in 4 divided doses
I.V.: 1 mg/kg; may repeat dose up to cumulative dose of 10 mg/kg (mean effective dose is 2.5 mg/kg), then switch to oral dosage
Monitoring Parameters Blood pressure, pulse, temperature, liver function tests, motor performance
Test Interactions Increased serum AST (SGOT), ALT (SGPT), alkaline phosphatase, LDH, BUN, and total serum bilirubin
Patient Information Avoid unnecessary exposure to sunlight (or use sunscreen, protective clothing); avoid alcohol and other CNS depressants; patients should use caution while driving or performing other tasks requiring alertness
Nursing Implications 36 vials needed for adequate hyperthermia therapy; exercise caution at meals on the day of administration because difficulty swallowing and choking has been reported
Additional Information Avoid glass bottles for I.V. infusion
Special Geriatric Considerations There is little experience with this drug in the elderly (see Warnings and Monitoring Parameters)
Dosage Forms
Dantrolene sodium:
Capsule: 25 mg, 50 mg, 100 mg
Powder for injection: 20 mg

Extemporaneous Preparations A suspension can be prepared by mixing 500 mg (from capsules) with 150 mg citric acid, 10 mL distilled water, and sufficient simple syrup to bring the total volume to 100 mL (final concentration 5 mg/mL)

Dapa® [OTC] *see* Acetaminophen *on page 16*

Dapiprazole (DA pi pray zole)

Brand Names Rēv-Eyes™
Generic Available No
Therapeutic Category Alpha-Adrenergic Blocking Agent, Ophthalmic
Use Reverse dilation due to drugs (adrenergic or parasympathomimetic) after eye exams
Contraindications In the presence of conditions where miosis is unacceptable, such as acute iritis and in patients with a history of hypersensitivity to any component of the formulation
Warnings For ophthalmic use only
Adverse Reactions
 Central nervous system: Headache
 Local: Burning sensation in the eyes, lid edema, ptosis, lid erythema, chemosis, itching, punctate keratitis, corneal edema
 Ocular: Photophobia
Stability After reconstitution, drops are stable at room temperature for 21 days
Mechanism of Action Dapiprazole is a selective alpha-adrenergic blocking agent, exerting effects primarily on alpha$_1$-adrenoceptors. It induces miosis via relaxation of the smooth dilator (radial) muscle of the iris, which causes pupillary constriction. It is devoid of cholinergic effects. Dapiprazole also partially reverses the cycloplegia induced with parasympatholytic agents such as tropicamide. Although the drug has no significant effect on the ciliary muscle per se, it may increase accommodative amplitude, therefore relieving the symptoms of paralysis of accommodation. Does not significantly alter intraocular pressure in eyes that are normotensive or with increased intraocular pressure.
Usual Dosage Geriatrics and Adults: Administer 2 drops followed 5 minutes later by an additional 2 drops applied to the conjunctiva of each eye; should not be used more frequently than once a week in the same patient
Administration Finger pressure should be applied to lacrimal sac for 1-2 minutes after instillation to decrease risk of absorption and systemic reactions; do not touch eye with dropper
Patient Information May still be sensitive to sunlight and sensitivity may return in 2 or more hours; store at room temperature
Nursing Implications See Administration and Patient Information
Special Geriatric Considerations No specific data in the elderly (see Usual Dosage)
Dosage Forms Powder, as hydrochloride, lyophilized: 25 mg [0.5% solution when mixed with supplied diluent]

Darvocet-N® *see* Propoxyphene and Acetaminophen *on page 796*
Darvocet-N® 100 *see* Propoxyphene and Acetaminophen *on page 796*
Darvon® *see* Propoxyphene *on page 795*
Darvon-N® *see* Propoxyphene *on page 795*
Datril® [OTC] *see* Acetaminophen *on page 16*
Daypro™ *see* Oxaprozin *on page 699*
DC 240® Softgels® [OTC] *see* Docusate *on page 312*
DDAVP® *see* Desmopressin Acetate *on page 273*
ddI *see* Didanosine *on page 286*
1-Deamino-8-D-Arginine Vasopressin *see* Desmopressin Acetate *on page 273*
Debrisan® [OTC] *see* Dextranomer *on page 278*
Debrox® Otic [OTC] *see* Carbamide Peroxide *on page 162*
Decadron® *see* Dexamethasone *on page 274*
Decadron®-LA *see* Dexamethasone *on page 274*
Decadron® Phosphate *see* Dexamethasone *on page 274*
Decaject® *see* Dexamethasone *on page 274*
Decaject-LA® *see* Dexamethasone *on page 274*
Declomycin® *see* Demeclocycline *on next page*
Decofed® Syrup [OTC] *see* Pseudoephedrine *on page 802*
Deficol® [OTC] *see* Bisacodyl *on page 121*
Degas® [OTC] *see* Simethicone *on page 856*

Degest® 2 Ophthalmic [OTC] *see* Naphazoline *on page 653*

Delatest® Injection *see* Testosterone *on page 895*

Delatestryl® Injection *see* Testosterone *on page 895*

Delaxin® *see* Methocarbamol *on page 604*

Delcort® *see* Hydrocortisone *on page 462*

Delestrogen® Injection *see* Estradiol *on page 350*

Del-Mycin® Topical *see* Erythromycin, Topical *on page 347*

Delsym® [OTC] *see* Dextromethorphan *on page 278*

Delta-Cortef® Oral *see* Prednisolone *on page 774*

Deltacortisone *see* Prednisone *on page 776*

Delta-D® *see* Cholecalciferol *on page 218*

Deltadehydrocortisone *see* Prednisone *on page 776*

Deltahydrocortisone *see* Prednisolone *on page 774*

Deltasone® *see* Prednisone *on page 776*

Delta-Tritex® *see* Triamcinolone *on page 949*

Demadex® *see* Torsemide *on page 942*

Demeclocycline (dem e kloe SYE kleen)

Brand Names Declomycin®

Synonyms Demethylchlortetracycline

Therapeutic Category Antibiotic, Tetracycline Derivative

Use Treatment of susceptible bacterial infections (acne, gonorrhea, pertussis and urinary tract infections) caused by both gram-negative and gram-positive organisms; used when penicillin is contraindicated; treatment of chronic syndrome of inappropriate secretion of antidiuretic hormone (SIADH)

Contraindications Hypersensitivity to demeclocycline, tetracyclines, or any component

Warnings Photosensitivity reactions occur frequently with this drug, avoid prolonged exposure to sunlight, do not use tanning equipment

Adverse Reactions

Cardiovascular: Pericarditis

Central nervous system: Increased intracranial pressure

Dermatologic: Pruritus, pigmentation of nails, exfoliative dermatitis, photosensitivity

Endocrine & metabolic: Diabetes insipidus syndrome

Gastrointestinal: Nausea, vomiting, diarrhea, esophagitis, anorexia, abdominal cramps

Genitourinary: Azotemia

Neuromuscular & skeletal: Paresthesia

Renal: Acute renal failure

Miscellaneous: Superinfections, anaphylaxis

Overdosage Symptoms of overdose include photosensitivity, diabetes insipidus, nausea, anorexia, diarrhea

Drug Interactions

Do not administer with antacids, milk or dairy products, zinc, and iron preparations which may decrease absorption

Carbamazepine, barbiturates, hydantoins may decrease effect

Increased effect of warfarin

Stability Tetracyclines form toxic products when outdated or when exposed to light, heat, or humidity (Fanconi-like syndrome)

Mechanism of Action Inhibits protein synthesis by binding with the 30S and possibly the 50S ribosomal subunit(s) of susceptible bacteria; may also cause alterations in the cytoplasmic membrane

Pharmacodynamics Onset of action for diuresis in SIADH: Several days

Pharmacokinetics

Absorption: ~50% to 80% from GI tract (food and dairy products reduce absorption)

Protein binding: 41% to 50%

Metabolism: Small amounts metabolized in the liver to inactive metabolites; enterohepatically recycled

Half-life: 10-17 hours (prolonged with reduced renal function)

Time to peak serum concentration: Oral: Within 3-6 hours

Elimination: As unchanged drug (42% to 50%) in urine

Usual Dosage Geriatrics and Adults: 150 mg 4 times/day or 300 mg twice daily

Uncomplicated gonorrhea (penicillin-sensitive): 600 mg stat, 300 mg every 12 hours for 4 days (3 g total)

SIADH: 900-1200 mg/day or 13-15 mg/kg/day divided every 6-8 hours initially, then decrease to 0.6-0.9 g/day

Administration Administer 1 hour before or 2 hours after food or milk with plenty of fluid; avoid administration within 2-3 hours of antacids

Monitoring Parameters CBC, renal and hepatic function; PT or INR in patients taking anticoagulants

Test Interactions May interfere with tests for urinary glucose (false-negative urine glucose using Clinistix®, Tes-Tape®); may suppress bacterial growth in blood and urine for several days after discontinuance

Patient Information Avoid prolonged exposure to sunlight or sunlamps; avoid taking antacids before tetracyclines

Nursing Implications See Administration and Patient Information

Special Geriatric Considerations Has not been studied exclusively in the elderly (see Usual Dosage)

Dosage Forms
Demeclocycline hydrochloride:
Capsule: 150 mg
Tablet: 150 mg, 300 mg

References
Troyer AD, "Demeclocycline. Treatment for Syndrome of Inappropriate Antidiuretic Hormone Secretion," *JAMA*, 1977, 237(25):2723-6.

Demerol® *see* Meperidine *on page 584*

Demethylchlortetracycline *see* Demeclocycline *on previous page*

Depacon® *see* Valproic Acid and Derivatives *on page 977*

Depakene® *see* Valproic Acid and Derivatives *on page 977*

Depakote® *see* Valproic Acid and Derivatives *on page 977*

depAndro® Injection *see* Testosterone *on page 895*

Depen® *see* Penicillamine *on page 719*

depGynogen® Injection *see* Estradiol *on page 350*

Depitol® *see* Carbamazepine *on page 160*

depMedalone® Injection *see* Methylprednisolone *on page 611*

Depo®-Estradiol Injection *see* Estradiol *on page 350*

Depogen® Injection *see* Estradiol *on page 350*

Depoject® Injection *see* Methylprednisolone *on page 611*

Depo-Medrol® Injection *see* Methylprednisolone *on page 611*

Deponit® Patch *see* Nitroglycerin *on page 677*

Depopred® Injection *see* Methylprednisolone *on page 611*

Depo-Provera® Injection *see* Medroxyprogesterone Acetate *on page 578*

Depotest® Injection *see* Testosterone *on page 895*

Depo®-Testosterone Injection *see* Testosterone *on page 895*

Deprenyl *see* Selegiline *on page 851*

Dermacort® *see* Hydrocortisone *on page 462*

Dermaflex® Gel *see* Lidocaine *on page 537*

Dermarest Dricort® *see* Hydrocortisone *on page 462*

Derma-Smoothe/FS® *see* Fluocinolone *on page 391*

Dermatop® *see* Prednicarbate *on page 773*

DermiCort® *see* Hydrocortisone *on page 462*

Dermolate® [OTC] *see* Hydrocortisone *on page 462*

Dermtex® HC with Aloe *see* Hydrocortisone *on page 462*

DES *see* Diethylstilbestrol *on page 287*

Desiccated Thyroid *see* Thyroid *on page 917*

Desipramine (des IP ra meen)

Related Information
Antidepressant Agents Comparison *on page 1021*
Antidepressant Medication Guidelines *on page 1075*
Federal OBRA Regulations Recommended Maximum Doses - Antidepressants *on page 1056*
Serum Drug Concentrations Commonly Monitored: Guidelines *on page 1114*

Brand Names Norpramin®

Synonyms Desmethylimipramine Hydrochloride

Generic Available Yes: Tablet

Therapeutic Category Antidepressant, Tricyclic

Use Treatment of various forms of depression, often in conjunction with psychotherapy; as an analgesic in chronic pain, peripheral neuropathies
(Continued)

Desipramine *(Continued)*

Unlabeled use: Facilitate cocaine withdrawal

Contraindications Hypersensitivity to desipramine (cross-sensitivity with other tricyclic antidepressants may occur); patients receiving MAO inhibitors within past 14 days; narrow-angle glaucoma

Warnings Some formulations contain tartrazine which may cause allergic reaction; do not discontinue abruptly in patients receiving long-term high dose therapy

Precautions Use with caution in patients with cardiovascular disease, conduction disturbances, urinary retention; seizure disorders, bipolar illness, renal or hepatic impairment, hyperthyroidism or those receiving thyroid replacement; an EKG prior to the start of therapy is advised

Adverse Reactions Less sedation and anticholinergic adverse effects than amitriptyline or imipramine

Cardiovascular: Arrhythmias, hypotension
Central nervous system: Sedation, confusion, delirium, dizziness, excitation, headache, seizures
Dermatologic: Photosensitivity
Endocrine & metabolic: SIADH
Gastrointestinal: Xerostomia, constipation, nausea, vomiting, increased appetite, weight gain, craving sweets, GE reflux, dysgeusia
Genitourinary: Urinary retention
Hematologic: Blood dyscrasias
Hepatic: Hepatitis, cholestatic jaundice, increased liver enzymes
Ocular: Increased intraocular pressure, blurred vision
Otic: Tinnitus
Miscellaneous: Hypersensitivity reactions, associated with falls, excessive diaphoresis

Overdosage Symptoms of overdose include agitation, confusion, hallucinations, hyperthermia, urinary retention, CNS depression, cyanosis, dry mucous membranes

Toxicology Following initiation of essential overdose management, toxic symptoms should be treated. Ventricular arrhythmias often respond to phenytoin 15-20 mg/kg with concurrent systemic alkalinization (sodium bicarbonate 0.5-2 mEq/kg I.V.). Arrhythmias unresponsive to this therapy may respond to lidocaine 1 mg/kg I.V. followed by a titrated infusion. Physostigmine (1-2 mg I.V. slowly) may be indicated in reversing cardiac arrhythmias that are due to vagal blockade or for anticholinergic effects. Seizures usually respond to diazepam I.V. boluses (5-10 mg, up to 30 mg). If seizures are unresponsive or recur, phenytoin or phenobarbital may be required.

Drug Interactions

May decrease effects of guanethidine and clonidine resulting in hypertensive crisis
May increase effects of CNS depressants, adrenergic agents, dicumarol, anticholinergic agents
With MAO inhibitors, hyperpyrexia, tachycardia, hypertension, seizures, and death may occur; interactions similar to other tricyclics may occur
Cimetidine, fluoxetine, methylphenidate, and haloperidol may decrease the metabolism and/or increase TCA levels
Phenobarbital may increase TCA metabolism

Mechanism of Action Traditionally believed to increase the synaptic concentration of norepinephrine in the central nervous system by inhibition of its reuptake by the presynaptic neuronal membrane. However, additional receptor effects have been found including desensitization of adenyl cyclase, down regulation of beta-adrenergic receptors, and down regulation of serotonin receptors.

Pharmacodynamics Onset of action: 1-3 weeks; norepinephrine only

Pharmacokinetics

Absorption: Well absorbed from GI tract
Protein binding: 90%
Metabolism: In the liver; substrate CYP1A2, 2D6
Half-life: 12-57 hours
    Plasma concentration and half-life have been found to positively correlate with age; mean half-life: >75 hours, twice that of young patients
Elimination: 70% excreted in urine

Usual Dosage Oral:

Geriatrics: Initial dose: 10-25 mg/day; increase by 10-25 mg every 3 days for inpatients and every week for outpatients if tolerated; usual maintenance dose: 75-100 mg/day, but doses up to 300 mg may be necessary

Adults: Initial: 75 mg/day in divided doses; increase gradually to 150-200 mg/day in divided or single dose; maximum: 300 mg/day

Cocaine withdrawal: 50-200 mg/day in divided or single dose

Monitoring Parameters Improvement in depressive symptoms; blood pressure, pulse

Reference Range
Therapeutic: 125-160 ng/mL
Possible toxicity: >300 ng/mL (SI: 1070 nmol/L)
Toxic: >1000 ng/mL (SI: >3750 nmol/L)
In geriatric patients the response rate is greatest with steady-state plasma concentrations >115 ng/mL

Test Interactions Increased glucose

Patient Information Avoid alcohol ingestion; do not discontinue medication abruptly; may cause urine to turn blue-green; may cause drowsiness, dry mouth, blurred vision or dizziness; rise slowly to prevent dizziness

Nursing Implications Monitor blood pressure and pulse rate prior to and during initial therapy; evaluate mental status; monitor weight, may increase appetite

Additional Information Avoid unnecessary exposure to sunlight

Special Geriatric Considerations Preferred agent because of its milder side effect profile; patients may experience excitation or stimulation, in such cases, administer as a single morning dose or divided dose. Data from a clinical trial comparing fluoxetine to tricyclics suggest that fluoxetine is significantly less effective than nortriptyline in hospitalized elderly patients with unipolar major affective disorder, especially those with melancholia and concurrent cardiovascular disease.

Dosage Forms Tablet, as hydrochloride (Norpramin®): 10 mg, 25 mg, 50 mg, 75 mg, 100 mg, 150 mg

References
Nelson JC, Jatlow PI, and Mazure C, "Desipramine Plasma Levels and Response in Elderly Melancholic Patients," *J Clin Psychopharmacol*, 1985, 5(4):217-20.
Nies A, Robinson DS, Friedman MS, et al, "Relationship Between Age and Tricyclic Antidepressant Plasma Levels," *Am J Psychiatry*, 1977, 134:790-3.
Roose SP, Glassman AH, Attia E, et al, "Comparative Efficacy of Selective Serotonin Reuptake Inhibitors and Tricyclics in the Treatment of Melancholia," *Am J Psychiatry*, 1994, 151(12):1735-9.

Desmethylimipramine Hydrochloride *see Desipramine on page 271*

Desmopressin Acetate (des moe PRES in AS e tate)

Brand Names DDAVP®; Stimate® Nasal

Synonyms 1-Deamino-8-D-Arginine Vasopressin

Therapeutic Category Antihemophilic Agent; Hemostatic Agent; Vasopressin Analog, Synthetic

Use Treatment of diabetes insipidus; control bleeding in certain types of hemophilia; primary nocturnal enuresis (intranasal)

Contraindications Hypersensitivity to desmopressin or any component; avoid using in patients with type IIB or platelet-type von Willebrand disease; or patients with <5% factor VIII activity level

Precautions Avoid overhydration especially when drug is used for its hemostatic effect; use with caution in patients with serious cardiovascular disease

Adverse Reactions
Cardiovascular: Facial flushing, increase in blood pressure, arrhythmias, decreased cardiac output
Central nervous system: Headache, dizziness
Endocrine & metabolic: Hyponatremia, water intoxication
Gastrointestinal: Nausea, abdominal cramps
Genitourinary: Vulval pain
Local: Pain at the injection site
Respiratory: Nasal congestion

Overdosage Symptoms of overdose include drowsiness, headache, confusion, anuria, water intoxication

Drug Interactions
Decreased effect: Demeclocycline, lithium can decrease ADH effect
Increased effect: Chlorpropamide, carbamazepine, fludrocortisone can increase ADH response

Stability Keep in refrigerator, avoid freezing; discard discolored solutions

Mechanism of Action Enhances reabsorption of water in the kidneys by increasing cellular permeability of the collecting ducts; possibly causes smooth muscle constriction with resultant vasoconstriction
(Continued)

Desmopressin Acetate *(Continued)*

Pharmacodynamics
Intranasal administration:
Onset of ADH effects: Within 1 hour
Peak effect: Within 1-5 hours
Duration: 5-21 hours
I.V. infusion:
Onset of increased factor VIII activity: Within 15-30 minutes
Peak effect: 0.75-3 hours

Pharmacokinetics
Absorption: Nasal: Slow, 10% to 20%
Metabolism: Unknown
Half-life: Terminal elimination: 75 minutes

Usual Dosage Geriatrics and Adults:
Diabetes insipidus:
Oral: Initial: 0.05 mg twice daily; titrate each dose to optimal therapeutic effect and diurinal effect; range 0.1-1.2 mg divided 2-3 times/day
Intranasal: 0.1-0.4 mL/day as a single dose or divided in 2-3 doses
I.V., S.C.: 0.5-1 mL/day in 2 divided doses or $1/10$ of the maintenance intranasal dose
Hemophilia:
Intranasal: 1 spray per nostril (300 mcg)
I.V.: 0.3 mcg/kg by slow infusion

Administration Infuse over 15-30 minutes; dilute in 10-50 mL 0.9% sodium chloride

Monitoring Parameters Blood pressure and pulse should be monitored during I.V. infusion
Diabetes insipidus: Fluid intake, urine volume, specific gravity, plasma and urine osmolality, serum electrolytes
Hemophilia: Factor VIII antigen levels, APTT

Test Interactions Decreased sodium (S)

Patient Information Avoid overhydration; notify physician if headache, shortness of breath, heartburn, nausea, abdominal cramps or vulval pain occurs; follow administration guidelines for intranasal products

Nursing Implications See Administration

Additional Information Manufacturer supplies a flexible tubing for administering the nasal solution

Special Geriatric Considerations Elderly patients should be cautioned not to increase their fluid intake beyond that sufficient to satisfy their thirst in order to avoid water intoxication and hyponatremia. Under experimental conditions, the elderly have been shown to have a decreased responsiveness to vasopressin with respect to its effects on water homeostasis.

Dosage Forms
Injection: 4 mcg/mL (1 mL)
Solution, nasal: 0.1 mg/mL (2.5 mL, 5 mL), 1.5 mg/mL
Tablet: 0.1 mg, 0.2 mg

References
Asplund R and Aberg H, "Desmopressin in Elderly Subjects With Increased Nocturnal Diuresis: A Two-Month Treatment Study," *Scand J Urol Nephrol*, 1993, 27(1):77-82.
Lindeman RD, Lee TD Jr, Yiengst MJ, et al, "Influence of Age, Renal Disease, Hypertension, Diuretics, and Calcium on the Antidiuretic Responses to Suboptimal Infusions of Vasopressin," *J Lab Clin Med*, 1966, 68(2):206-23.
Miller JH and Shock NW, "Age Differences in the Renal Tubular Response to Antidiuretic Hormone," *J Gerontol*, 1953, 8:446-50.

Desoxyphenobarbital *see* Primidone *on page 778*

Desyrel® *see* Trazodone *on page 948*

Devrom® [OTC] *see* Bismuth *on page 122*

Dexacidin® *see* Neomycin, Polymyxin B, and Dexamethasone *on page 661*

Dexacort® Phosphate in Respihaler *see* Dexamethasone *on this page*

Dexacort® Phosphate Turbinaire® *see* Dexamethasone *on this page*

Dex-A-Diet® [OTC] *see* Phenylpropanolamine *on page 741*

Dexamethasone (deks a METH a sone)
Related Information
Antacid Drug Interactions *on page 1096*
Corticosteroids Comparison, Systemic *on page 1029*
Corticosteroids Comparison, Topical *on page 1030*
Inhaled Medications Comparison *on page 1034*
I.V. Push Recommended Guidelines *on page 1083*

Tobramycin and Dexamethasone *on page 931*

Brand Names Aeroseb-Dex®; AK-Dex® Ophthalmic; Baldex®; Dalalone®; Dalalone D.P.®; Dalalone L.A.®; Decadron®; Decadron®-LA; Decadron® Phosphate; Decaject®; Decaject-LA®; Dexacort® Phosphate in Respihaler; Dexacort® Phosphate Turbinaire®; Dexasone®; Dexasone® L.A.; Dexone®; Dexone® LA; Dexotic®; Hexadrol®; Hexadrol® Phosphate; I-Methasone®; Maxidex®; Solurex®; Solurex L.A.®

Synonyms Dexamethasone Acetate; Dexamethasone Sodium Phosphate

Generic Available Yes

Therapeutic Category Adrenal Corticosteroid; Antiemetic; Anti-inflammatory Agent; Anti-inflammatory Agent, Ophthalmic; Corticosteroid, Inhalant; Corticosteroid, Ophthalmic; Corticosteroid, Systemic; Corticosteroid, Topical (Low Potency)

Use Systemically and locally for chronic inflammation, allergic, hematologic, neoplastic, and autoimmune diseases; may be used in management of cerebral edema, septic shock, and as a diagnostic agent

Contraindications Active untreated infections; viral, fungal, or tuberculous diseases of the eye

Warnings Fatalities have occurred due to adrenal insufficiency in asthmatic patients during and after transfer from systemic corticosteroids to aerosol steroids; during this period, aerosol steroids do **not** provide the systemic steroid needed to treat patients having trauma, surgery or infections

Precautions Use with caution in patients with hypothyroidism, cirrhosis, hypertension, congestive heart failure, nonspecific ulcerative colitis, thromboembolic disorders, and in patients with increased risk for peptic ulcer disease; gradually taper dose to withdraw therapy

Adverse Reactions

Cardiovascular: Hypertension, edema, accelerated atherogenesis

Central nervous system: Euphoria, mental changes, headache, vertigo, seizures, psychoses, pseudotumor cerebri

Dermatologic: Folliculitis, hypertrichosis, acneiform eruption, dermatitis, maceration, skin atrophy, acne, impaired wound healing, hirsutism, striae, miliaria, telangiectasia

Endocrine & metabolic: Growth suppression, Cushing's syndrome, pituitary-adrenal axis suppression, alkalosis, glucose intolerance, hypokalemia, postmenopausal bleeding, hot flashes

Gastrointestinal: Peptic ulcer, nausea, vomiting, pancreatitis

Local: Burning, irritation

Neuromuscular & skeletal: Muscle weakness, osteoporosis, fractures, aseptic necrosis of femoral and humeral heads, steroid myopathy

Ocular: Cataracts, glaucoma

Miscellaneous: Increased susceptibility to infection

Toxicology When consumed in excessive quantities for prolonged periods, systemic hypercorticism and adrenal suppression may occur; in those cases, discontinuation and withdrawal of the corticosteroid should be done judiciously

Drug Interactions

Steroids decrease the effect of anticholinesterases, isoniazid, salicylates, insulin, oral hypoglycemics

Decreased effect: Barbiturates, phenytoin, rifampin

Increased effect (hypokalemia) of potassium-depleting diuretics

Increased risk of digoxin toxicity (due to hypokalemia)

Increased effect: Estrogens, ketoconazole

Stability

Stability of injection of parenteral admixture at room temperature (25°C): 24 hours

Stability of injection of parenteral admixture at refrigeration temperature (4°C): 2 days; protect from light and freezing

Mechanism of Action Decreases inflammation by suppression of migration of polymorphonuclear leukocytes and reversal of increased capillary permeability; suppresses normal immune response

Pharmacodynamics Duration of metabolic effects: Can last for 72 hours

Pharmacokinetics

Metabolism: In the liver; substrate and inducer CYP3A4

Half-life: 1.8-3.5 hours; biologic half-life: 36-54 hours

Time to peak serum concentration:

Oral: Within 1-2 hours

I.M.: Within 8 hours

Elimination: In urine and bile

(Continued)

Dexamethasone *(Continued)*

Usual Dosage
Geriatrics: Use lowest effective dose
Adults:
Anti-inflammatory: Oral, I.M., I.V.: 0.75-9 mg/day in divided doses every 6-12 hours
Cerebral edema: I.V.: 10 mg stat, 4 mg I.M./I.V. every 6 hours until response is maximized, then switch to oral regimen, then taper off if appropriate
Inoperable brain tumor: Oral: 2 mg 2-4 times/day
Diagnosis for Cushing's syndrome: Oral: 1 mg at 11 PM, draw blood at 8 AM
Ophthalmic:
Suspension: Instill 1 drop 3-4 times/day
Ointment: Apply a thin layer 3-4 times/day, gradually taper dose
Inhalation: 3 inhalations 3-4 times/day; maximum: 12 inhalations/day
Nasal: 2 sprays in each nostril 2-3 times/day; maximum: 12 sprays/day
Topical: Apply 2-4 times/day

Monitoring Parameters Blood pressure, blood glucose, electrolytes, symptoms of fluid retention

Reference Range Dexamethasone suppression test, overnight: 8 AM cortisol <6 µg/100 mL (dexamethasone 1 mg)

Test Interactions Increased amylase (S), cholesterol (S), glucose, protein, sodium (S); decreased calcium (S), chloride (S), potassium (S), thyroxine (S)

Patient Information Notify physician of any signs of infection or injuries during therapy; inform physician or dentist before surgery if you are taking a corticosteroid; may cause GI upset; take with food or milk; do not stop abruptly. If on oral product, carry an identification card or bracelet advising that you are on steroid. For topical products, use a thin layer; do not overuse; follow instructions with inhaled products.

Nursing Implications Administer with meals to decrease GI upset; do not use topical products on open wounds; acetate injection is not for I.V. use

Special Geriatric Considerations Because of the risk of adverse effects, systemic corticosteroids should be used cautiously in the elderly in the smallest possible dose, and for the shortest possible time.

Dosage Forms
Aerosol:
Nasal, as sodium phosphate: 0.1 mg/spray (15 mg/12.6 g, 12.6 g)
Oral, as sodium phosphate: 0.01% (58 g); 0.04% (25 g)
Topical: 0.075 mg/spray (25 g)
Cream, as sodium phosphate: 0.1% (15 g)
Elixir: 0.5 mg/5 mL (100 mL, 273 mL)
Gel: 0.01% (30 g)
Injection, as acetate: 8 mg/mL (1 mL, 5 mL); 16 mg/mL (1 mL, 5 mL)
Injection, as sodium phosphate: 4 mg/mL (1 mL, 5 mL, 10 mL, 25 mL, 30 mL); 10 mg/mL (1 mL, 10 mL); 20 mg/mL (5 mL)
Ointment, ophthalmic, as sodium phosphate: 0.05% (3.5 g)
Solution:
Concentrate: 0.5 mg/0.5 mL (30 mL)
Oral: 0.5 mg/5 mL (5 mL, 20 mL, 500 mL)
Suspension, ophthalmic, as sodium phosphate: 0.1% with methylcellulose 0.5% (15 mL)
Tablet: 0.25 mg, 0.5 mg, 0.75 mg, 1 mg, 1.5 mg, 2 mg, 4 mg, 6 mg

Dexamethasone Acetate *see* Dexamethasone *on page 274*

Dexamethasone and Tobramycin *see* Tobramycin and Dexamethasone *on page 931*

Dexamethasone Sodium Phosphate *see* Dexamethasone *on page 274*

Dexasone® *see* Dexamethasone *on page 274*

Dexasone® L.A. *see* Dexamethasone *on page 274*

Dexasporin® *see* Neomycin, Polymyxin B, and Dexamethasone *on page 661*

Dexatrim® [OTC] *see* Phenylpropanolamine *on page 741*

Dexchlor® *see* Dexchlorpheniramine *on this page*

Dexchlorpheniramine (deks klor fen EER a meen)
Brand Names Dexchlor®; Poladex®; Polaramine®
Generic Available Yes
Therapeutic Category Antihistamine, H₁ Blocker

Use Perennial and seasonal allergic rhinitis and other allergic symptoms including urticaria

Contraindications Narrow-angle glaucoma, stenosing peptic ulcer, bladder neck obstruction, use with MAO inhibitors; hypersensitivity to dexchlorpheniramine or any component; not recommended in the treatment of lower respiratory infections

Warnings Bladder neck obstruction, symptomatic prostatic hypertrophy, asthmatic attack, stenosing peptic ulcer, pyloroduodenal obstruction, and lower respiratory tract infections

Precautions Use with caution in patients with heart disease, hypertension, thyroid disease, and asthma

Adverse Reactions
Cardiovascular: Edema, palpitations (bradycardia, tachycardia)
Central nervous system: Slight to moderate drowsiness (often tolerance develops), headache, fatigue, nervousness, dizziness, coordination dysfunction, depression, paradoxical excitability, restlessness, insomnia
Dermatologic: Angioedema, photosensitivity, rash
Gastrointestinal: Anorexia, appetite increase, weight gain, nausea, diarrhea, abdominal pain, xerostomia, constipation
Genitourinary: Urinary retention, dysuria, inhibition of ejaculation
Hematologic: Hemolytic anemia, agranulocytosis, leukopenia, thrombocytopenia, pancytopenia
Hepatic: Hepatitis
Neuromuscular & skeletal: Arthralgia, myalgia, paresthesia
Ocular: Blurred vision
Respiratory: Pharyngitis, dry throat, bronchospasm, epistaxis, thickening of bronchial secretions
Miscellaneous: Anaphylactic shock

Overdosage Symptoms of overdose include dry mouth, flushed skin, dilated pupils, CNS depression

Toxicology There is no specific treatment for an antihistamine overdose, however, most of its clinical toxicity is due to anticholinergic effects. For anticholinergic overdose with severe life-threatening symptoms, physostigmine 1-2 mg (0.5 or 0.02 mg/kg for children) I.V., slowly may be given to reverse these effects.

Drug Interactions Increased effect/toxicity: CNS depressants (alcohol, etc), MAO inhibitors, TCAs, phenothiazines, guanabenz

Mechanism of Action Competes with histamine for H_1-receptor sites on effector cells in the gastrointestinal tract, blood vessels, and respiratory tract

Pharmacodynamics
Peak effect: Oral: Within 3 hours
Duration: 3-6 hours

Pharmacokinetics
Absorption: Well absorbed from GI tract
Distribution: Small amounts appear in breast milk
Metabolism: In the liver
Elimination: In urine within 24 hours as inactive metabolites

Usual Dosage Geriatrics and Adults: Oral: 2 mg every 4-6 hours or 4-6 mg timed release at bedtime or every 8-10 hours

Monitoring Parameters Monitor mental function, bowel function, and urinary retention

Test Interactions May interfere with a methacholine bronchial challenge

Patient Information May cause drowsiness, dry mouth, confusion; swallow whole, do not crush or chew sustained release product; avoid alcohol, may impair coordination and judgment

Nursing Implications Raise bed rails, institute safety measures, assist with ambulation; monitor for mental function changes, constipation, urinary retention

Special Geriatric Considerations Anticholinergic action may cause significant confusional symptoms, constipation, or problems voiding urine (see Contraindications, Warnings, and Usual Dosage)

Dosage Forms
Dexchlorpheniramine maleate:
Syrup (orange flavor): 2 mg/5 mL with alcohol 6% (480 mL)
Tablet: 2 mg
Tablet, sustained action: 4 mg, 6 mg

Dexferrum® Injection see Iron Dextran Complex on page 497

Dexone® see Dexamethasone on page 274

Dexone® LA see Dexamethasone on page 274

Dexotic® *see Dexamethasone on page 274*

Dextranomer (deks TRAN oh mer)
Brand Names Debrisan® [OTC]
Generic Available No
Therapeutic Category Topical Skin Product
Use Clean exudative ulcers and wounds such as venous stasis ulcers, decubitus ulcers, and infected traumatic and surgical wounds; no controlled studies have found dextranomer to be more effective than conventional therapy
Contraindications Deep fistulas, sinus tracts, hypersensitivity to any component
Precautions Do not use in deep fistulas or any area where complete removal is not assured; do not use on dry wounds (ineffective); avoid contact with eyes
Adverse Reactions
Dermatologic: Maceration may occur
Local: Transitory pain, bleeding, blistering, erythema
Mechanism of Action Dextranomer is a network of dextran-sucrose beads possessing a great many exposed hydroxy groups; when this network is applied to an exudative wound surface, the exudate is drawn by capillary forces generated by the swelling of the beads, with vacuum forces producing an upward flow of exudate into the network
Usual Dosage Geriatrics and Adults: Apply to affected area once or twice daily in a ¼" layer; apply a dressing and seal on all four sides
Administration Sprinkle beads into ulcer (or apply paste) to ¼" thickness; change dressings 1-4 times/day depending on drainage; change dressing before it is completely dry to facilitate removal. Remove beads or paste when they become saturated. Occasionally vigorous irrigation, soaking, or whirlpool may be needed to remove the product. Each container should only be used for one patient to avoid cross-contamination.
Patient Information Avoid contact with eyes; for external use only
Nursing Implications Discontinue treatment when the area is free of exudate and edema or when healthy granulation tissue is present
Special Geriatric Considerations Preventive skin care should be instituted in all older patients at high risk for decubitus ulcers. Debrisan® is indicated in stage 3 and 4 decubitus ulcers.
Dosage Forms
Beads: 4 g, 25 g, 60 g, 120 g
Paste, premixed and sterile: 10 g foil packets
References
Chamberlain TM, Cali TJ, Cuzzell J, et al, "Assessment and Management of Pressure Sores in Long-Term Care Facilities," *Consult Pharm*, 1992, 7(12):1328-40.

Dextromethorphan (deks troe meth OR fan)
Brand Names Benylin DM® [OTC]; Benylin® Pediatric [OTC]; Children's Hold® [OTC]; Creo-Terpin® [OTC]; Delsym® [OTC]; Drixoral® Cough Liquid Caps [OTC]; Hold® DM [OTC]; Pertussin® CS [OTC]; Pertussin® ES [OTC]; Robitussin® Cough Calmers [OTC]; Robitussin® Pediatric [OTC]; Scot-Tussin DM® Cough Chasers [OTC]; Silphen DM® [OTC]; St. Joseph® Cough Suppressant [OTC]; Sucrets® Cough Calmers [OTC]; Suppress® [OTC]; Trocal® [OTC]; Vicks Formula 44® [OTC]; Vicks Formula 44® Pediatric Formula [OTC]
Generic Available Yes
Therapeutic Category Antitussive
Use Symptomatic relief of coughs caused by minor viral upper respiratory tract infections or inhaled irritants; most effective for a chronic nonproductive cough
Contraindications Hypersensitivity to dextromethorphan or any component
Warnings Should not be used for chronic productive coughs
Adverse Reactions
Central nervous system: Drowsiness, dizziness, coma
Gastrointestinal: Nausea, constipation
Respiratory: Respiratory depression
Overdosage Symptoms of overdose include nausea, vomiting, drowsiness, blurred vision, nystagmus, urinary retention, stupor, hallucinations
Toxicology Naloxone 2 mg I.V. with repeat administration as necessary up to a total of 10 mg
Drug Interactions
Decreased metabolism: Quinidine, amiodarone
Increased toxicity: MAO inhibitors, selegiline, alcohol, CNS depressants

Mechanism of Action Chemical relative of morphine lacking narcotic properties; controls cough by depressing the medullary cough center

Pharmacodynamics
Onset of antitussive action: Within 15-30 minutes
Duration: Up to 6 hours; higher doses may have longer duration

Pharmacokinetics
Metabolism: In the liver; substrate CYP2D6, 3A4
Elimination: Principally in urine

Usual Dosage Geriatrics and Adults: Oral: 10-20 mg every 4 hours or 30 mg every 6-8 hours; extended release: 60 mg twice daily; maximum: 120 mg/day

Monitoring Parameters Cough, mental status

Patient Information May cause drowsiness; avoid CNS depressants and alcohol; do not use for persistent or chronic cough

Nursing Implications See Monitoring Parameters

Additional Information Dextromethorphan is considered approximately half as potent as codeine as an antitussive; dextromethorphan is a component in many cough and cold preparations

Special Geriatric Considerations See Warnings

Dosage Forms
Capsule (Drixoral® Cough Liquid Caps): 30 mg
Liquid:
Pertussin® CS: 3.5 mg/5 mL (120 mL)
Robitussin® Pediatric, St. Joseph® Cough Suppressant: 7.5 mg/5 mL (60 mL, 120 mL, 240 mL)
Pertussin® ES, Vicks Formula 44®: 15 mg/5 mL (120 mL, 240 mL)
Liquid, sustained release, as polistirex (Delsym®): 30 mg/5 mL (89 mL)
Lozenges:
Scot-Tussin DM® Cough Chasers: 2.5 mg
Children's Hold®, Hold® DM, Robitussin® Cough Calmers, Sucrets® Cough Calmers: 5 mg
Suppress®, Trocal®: 7.5 mg
Syrup:
Benylin DM®, Silphen DM®: 10 mg/5 mL (120 mL, 3780 mL)
Vicks Formula 44® Pediatric Formula: 15 mg/15 mL (120 mL)

Dextromethorphan and Guaifenesin see Guaifenesin and Dextromethorphan on page 439

Dextropropoxyphene see Propoxyphene on page 795

Dey-Dose® Isoproterenol see Isoproterenol on page 501

Dey-Dose® Metaproterenol see Metaproterenol on page 596

Dey-Lute® Isoetharine see Isoetharine on page 499

D.H.E. 45® Injection see Dihydroergotamine on page 295

DHPG Sodium see Ganciclovir on page 419

DHT™ see Dihydrotachysterol on page 296

Diaβeta® see Glyburide on page 428

Diabetic Tussin DM® [OTC] see Guaifenesin and Dextromethorphan on page 439

Diabetic Tussin EX® [OTC] see Guaifenesin on page 437

Diabinese® see Chlorpropamide on page 212

Dialose® [OTC] see Docusate on page 312

Dialose® Plus Capsule [OTC] see Docusate and Casanthranol on page 313

Dialume® [OTC] see Aluminum Hydroxide on page 41

Diamine T.D.® [OTC] see Brompheniramine on page 129

Diamox® see Acetazolamide on page 19

Diamox Sequels® see Acetazolamide on page 19

Diapid® see Lypressin on page 559

Diar-aid® [OTC] see Loperamide on page 548

Diasorb® [OTC] see Attapulgite on page 94

Diastat® Rectal Delivery System see Diazepam on this page

Diazemuls® Injection see Diazepam on this page

Diazepam (dye AZ e pam)

Related Information
Antacid Drug Interactions on page 1096
Anxiolytic/Hypnotic Use in Long-Term Care Facilities on page 1099
Benzodiazepines Comparison on page 1024
Federal OBRA Regulations Recommended Maximum Doses - Anxiolytics on page 1057
(Continued)

Diazepam (Continued)

I.V. Push Recommended Guidelines *on page 1083*

Brand Names Diastat® Rectal Delivery System; Diazemuls® Injection; Diazepam Intensol®; Dizac® Injectable Emulsion; Valium® Injection; Valium® Oral

Generic Available Yes

Therapeutic Category Antianxiety Agent; Anticonvulsant, Benzodiazepine; Benzodiazepine; Sedative

Use Management of general anxiety disorders, panic disorders, and to provide preoperative sedation, light anesthesia, and amnesia; treatment of status epilepticus, alcohol withdrawal symptoms; used as a skeletal muscle relaxant

Restrictions C-IV

Contraindications Hypersensitivity to diazepam or any component; there may be a cross-sensitivity with other benzodiazepines; do not use in a comatose patient, in those with pre-existing CNS depression, respiratory depression, narrow-angle glaucoma, or severe uncontrolled pain

Precautions Use with caution in patients receiving other CNS depressants, patients with low albumin, hepatic dysfunction, in patients with a history of drug dependence, and in the elderly

Adverse Reactions

Cardiovascular: Cardiac arrest, hypotension, bradycardia, cardiovascular collapse

Central nervous system: Drowsiness, confusion, dizziness, ataxia, amnesia, slurred speech, paradoxical excitement or rage

Local: Phlebitis, pain with injection

Neuromuscular & skeletal: Impaired coordination

Ocular: Blurred vision, diplopia

Respiratory: Decrease in respiratory rate, apnea, laryngospasm

Miscellaneous: Physical and psychological dependence with prolonged use

Overdosage Symptoms of overdose include somnolence, confusion, coma, hypoactive reflexes, dyspnea, hypotension, slurred speech, impaired coordination

Toxicology Treatment for benzodiazepine overdose is supportive. Rarely is mechanical ventilation required. Flumazenil has been shown to selectively block the binding of benzodiazepines to CNS receptors, resulting in a reversal of benzodiazepine-induced CNS depression, but not respiratory depression.

Drug Interactions Diazepam may increase digoxin concentrations and may decrease the effect of levodopa

Decreased metabolism: Cimetidine, fluoxetine

Increased metabolism: Rifampin

Increased toxicity: CNS depressants, alcohol

Stability Protect parenteral dosage form from light; potency is retained for up to 3 months when kept at room temperature; most stable at pH 4-8, hydrolysis occurs at pH <3; do not mix I.V. product with other medications

Mechanism of Action Benzodiazepines appear to potentiate the effects of GABA and other inhibitory neurotransmitters by binding to specific benzodiazepine-receptor sites in various areas of the CNS

Pharmacodynamics

Onset of action: Almost immediate with short duration of action (20-30 minutes) when given I.V. for status epilepticus

Studies have shown that the elderly are more sensitive to the effects of benzodiazepines as compared to younger adults

Pharmacokinetics

Absorption: Oral: 85% to 100%

Distribution: V_d: Increased in elderly

Protein binding: 98%

Metabolism: In liver; active major metabolite is desmethyldiazepam; substrate CYP2C8, 2C19, 3A4

Half-life: 20-50 hours, increased half-life in elderly (~90 hours) and those with severe hepatic disorders; desmethyldiazepam has a half-life of 50-100 hours and can be prolonged in the elderly; accumulation of diazepam is extensive

Usual Dosage

Geriatrics:

Anxiety: Oral: Initial: 1-2 mg 1-2 times/day; increase gradually as needed, rarely need to use >10 mg/day

Skeletal muscle relaxation: 2-5 mg 2-4 times/day

Adults:

Anxiety:

Oral: 2-10 mg 2-4 times/day

I.M., I.V.: 2-10 mg, may repeat in 3-4 hours if needed

Skeletal muscle relaxation:

Oral: 2-10 mg 2-4 times/day

I.M., I.V.: 5-10 mg, may repeat in 2-4 hours

Status epilepticus: I.V.: 5-10 mg every 10-20 minutes up to 30 mg in an 8-hour period; may repeat in 2-4 hours

Reference Range Therapeutic: Diazepam: 0.2-1.5 µg/mL (SI: 0.7-5.3 µmol/L); N-desmethyldiazepam (nordiazepam): 0.1-0.5 µg/mL (SI: 0.35-1.8 µmol/L)

Test Interactions False-negative urinary glucose determinations when using Clinistix® or Diastix®

Patient Information Avoid alcohol and other CNS depressants; may cause drowsiness; avoid activities needing good psychomotor coordination until CNS effects are known; may cause physical or psychological dependence; avoid abrupt discontinuation after prolonged use

Nursing Implications Do not exceed 5 mg/minute IVP; provide safety measures (ie, side rails, night light, and call button); remove smoking materials from area; supervise ambulation

Additional Information Oral absorption more reliable than I.M.

Special Geriatric Considerations Due to its long-acting metabolite, diazepam is not considered a drug of choice in the elderly (see Pharmacodynamics and Pharmacokinetics); long-acting benzodiazepines have been associated with falls in the elderly; interpretive guidelines from the Health Care Financing Administration (HCFA) discourage the use of this agent in residents of long-term care facilities

Dosage Forms

Gel, rectal delivery system (Diastat®):

Adult rectal tip (6 cm): 5 mg/mL (10 mg, 15 mg, 20 mg) [twin packs]

Injection: 5 mg/mL (1 mL, 2 mL, 5 mL, 10 mL)

Injection, emulsified:

Dizac®: 5 mg/mL (3 mL)

Diazemuls®: 5 mg/mL (2 mL)

Solution, oral (wintergreen-spice flavor): 5 mg/5 mL (5 mL, 10 mL, 500 mL)

Solution, oral concentrate (Diazepam Intensol®): 5 mg/mL (30 mL)

Tablet: 2 mg, 5 mg, 10 mg

References

Klotz U, Avant GR, Hoyumpa A, et al, "The Effects of Age and Liver Disease on the Disposition and Elimination of Diazepam in Adult Man," *J Clin Invest*, 1975, 55(2):347-59.

Pomara N, Stanley B, Block R, et al, "Increased Sensitivity of the Elderly to the Central Depressant Effects of Diazepam," *J Clin Psychiatry*, 1985, 46(5):185-7.

Reidenberg MM, Levy M, Warner H, et al, "Relationship Between Diazepam Dose, Plasma Level, Age, and Central Nervous System Depression," *Clin Pharmacol Ther*, 1978, 23(4):371-4.

Diazepam Intensol® *see* Diazepam *on page 279*

Dibent® Injection *see* Dicyclomine *on page 285*

Dibenzyline® *see* Phenoxybenzamine *on page 739*

Dicarbosil® [OTC] *see* Calcium Salts (Oral) *on page 152*

Dichysterol *see* Dihydrotachysterol *on page 296*

Diclofenac (dye KLOE fen ak)

Brand Names Cataflam® Oral; Voltaren® Ophthalmic; Voltaren® Oral; Voltaren-XR® Oral

Generic Available No

Therapeutic Category Analgesic, Non-narcotic; Anti-inflammatory Agent; Anti-inflammatory Agent, Ophthalmic; Antipyretic; Nonsteroidal Anti-inflammatory Agent (NSAID), Ophthalmic; Nonsteroidal Anti-inflammatory Agent (NSAID), Oral

Use Acute and chronic treatment of rheumatoid arthritis, ankylosing spondylitis, and osteoarthritis; also used for gout, mild to moderate pain relief, acute painful shoulder, sunburn; ophthalmic used for treatment of postoperative inflammation following cataract removal

Contraindications Known hypersensitivity to diclofenac, any component, aspirin or other nonsteroidal anti-inflammatory drugs (NSAIDs); porphyria

Warnings Hypersensitivity to diclofenac or any component of product used; GI toxicity (bleeding, ulceration, perforation); systemic effects from ocular absorption may occur (ie, bleeding); CNS effects may occur (headaches, confusion, depression); hypersensitivity, anaphylactoid reactions (intermittent tolmetin use more often); cross-sensitivity with aspirin and other NSAIDs exists; renal function decline, acute renal insufficiency, interstitial nephritis, dysuria, cystitis, hematuria, nephrotic syndrome, hyperkalemia in acute renal insufficiency, hyponatremia, papillary necrosis, hepatic function impairment; elderly have increased risk for adverse reactions to NSAIDs. **Note:** Use

(Continued)

Diclofenac *(Continued)*

caution with ophthalmic solutions if patient wears soft contact lenses; eye irritation, burning, and redness reported (see Special Geriatric Considerations).

Precautions Use with caution in patients with congestive heart failure, hypertension, decreased renal or hepatic function, history of GI disease (bleeding or ulcers), or those receiving anticoagulants; perform ophthalmologic evaluation for those who develop eye complaints during therapy (blurred vision, diminished vision, changes in color vision, retinal changes); NSAIDs may mask signs/symptoms of infections; photosensitivity reported

Adverse Reactions

Cardiovascular: Congestive heart failure, angina, hypertension, hypotension, arrhythmias, edema

Central nervous system: Headache, drowsiness, vertigo, dizziness, fatigue, hallucinations, confusion, depression, emotional lability, psychotic behavior, pyrexia

Dermatologic: Rash, urticaria, angioedema, Stevens-Johnson syndrome, exfoliative dermatitis, bruising, petechiae, purpura

Endocrine & metabolic: Hyperglycemia, hypoglycemia, hyperkalemia, gynecomastia, hyponatremia, fluid retention

Gastrointestinal: Dyspepsia, heartburn, nausea, diarrhea, constipation, flatulence, stomatitis, vomiting, abdominal pain, peptic ulcer, GI bleeding, GI perforation, gingival ulcers, pancreatitis, proctitis, paralytic ulcers, colitis, anorexia, weight loss, dry mucous membranes

Genitourinary: Azotemia, impotence, dysuria

Hematologic: Neutropenia, anemia, agranulocytosis, bone marrow suppression, hemolytic anemia, hemorrhage, inhibition of platelet aggregation

Hepatic: Hepatitis, elevated LFTs, cholestatic jaundice

Neuromuscular & skeletal: Involuntary muscle movements, muscle weakness, tremors, weakness

Ocular: Vision changes, burning, redness, irritation, keratitis, elevated IOP, anterior chamber reaction, ocular allergy

Otic: Tinnitus

Renal: Polyuria, pyuria, oliguria, anuria, acute renal failure

Respiratory: Exacerbation of asthma, dyspnea

Miscellaneous: Thirst, diaphoresis

Overdosage Acute renal failure (2.5 g); symptoms include drowsiness, lethargy, disorientation, confusion, dizziness, numbness, paresthesia, nausea, vomiting, gastric irritation, abdominal pain, headache, tinnitus, sweating, blurred vision, muscle twitching, seizures, coma, acute renal failure, increased BUN and serum creatinine, hypotension, tachycardia, and metabolic acidosis

Toxicology Management of a nonsteroidal anti-inflammatory agent (NSAID) intoxication is primarily supportive and symptomatic. Fluid therapy is commonly effective in managing the hypotension that may occur following an acute NSAID overdose, except when this is due to an acute blood loss. Seizures tend to be very short-lived and often do not require drug treatment although recurrent seizures should be treated with I.V. diazepam. Since many of the NSAIDs undergo enterohepatic cycling, multiple doses of charcoal may be needed to reduce the potential for delayed toxicities. NSAIDs are highly bound to plasma proteins, therefore hemodialysis and peritoneal dialysis are not useful.

Drug Interactions

May increase nephrotoxicity of cyclosporin

Diclofenac + potassium-sparing diuretics may increase serum K^+

Concomitant insulin or oral hypoglycemic agents may increase or decrease serum glucose

May increase digoxin, methotrexate, and lithium serum concentrations

Aspirin or other salicylates may decrease NSAID serum concentrations

Other NSAIDs may increase adverse GI effects; increased prothrombin time with anticoagulants

Decreased antihypertensive effects of ACE inhibitors, beta-blockers, and thiazide diuretics

Increased response to sympathomimetics

Probenecid may increase toxicity of NSAIDs by increase in serum concentrations

Effects of loop diuretics may decrease

Concomitant use with loop diuretics may enhance azotemia in elderly

Mechanism of Action Inhibits prostaglandin synthesis, acts on the hypothalamus heat-regulating center to reduce fever, blocks prostaglandin synthetase action which prevents formation of the platelet-aggregating substance thromboxane A_2; decreases pain receptor sensitivity. Other proposed mechanisms of action are lysosomal stabilization, inhibition of kinin and leukotriene production, alteration of chemotactic factors, and inhibition of neutrophil activation. This latter mechanism may be the most significant pharmacologic action to reduce inflammation. In animals, prostaglandins are mediators of intraocular inflammation; prostaglandins produce disruption of the blood-aqueous humor barrier, increased vascular permeability, vasodilation, leukocytosis, and increased intraocular pressure (IOP).

Pharmacokinetics
  Absorption: Completely
  Protein binding: 99%
  Metabolism: In the liver to inactive metabolites; substrate CYP2C8, 2C9
  Half-life: 1-2 hours
  Time to peak serum concentrations: Within 2-3 hours
  Elimination: Primarily in urine

Usual Dosage Geriatrics and Adults:
  Oral (maximum daily dose: 200 mg):
    Rheumatoid arthritis: 150-200 mg/day in 2-4 divided doses (do not exceed 200 mg/day)
    Osteoarthritis: 100-150 mg/day in 2-3 divided doses
    Ankylosing spondylitis: 100-125 mg/day in 4-5 divided doses
    Mild to moderate pain: 25 mg 3-4 times/day
  Ophthalmic: Instill 1 drop to affected eye 4 times/day starting 24 hours after cataract surgery and continue for 2 weeks of postoperative care

Monitoring Parameters Monitor response (pain, range of motion, grip strength, mobility, ADL function), inflammation; observe for weight gain, edema; monitor renal function; observe for bleeding, bruising; evaluate gastrointestinal effects (abdominal pain, bleeding, dyspepsia); mental confusion, disorientation, CBC, serum, creatinine, BUN, liver function tests

Patient Information Do not crush delayed release (enteric coated) tablets. Serious gastrointestinal bleeding can occur as well as ulceration and perforation. Pain may or may not be present. Avoid aspirin and aspirin-containing products while taking this medication. If gastric upset occurs, take with food, milk, or antacid. If gastric adverse effects persist, contact physician. May cause drowsiness, dizziness, blurred vision, and confusion. Use caution when performing tasks which require alertness (eg, driving). Do not take for more than 3 days for fever or 10 days for pain without physician advice.

Nursing Implications Do not crush enteric coated tablets (see Monitoring Parameters, Overdosage, Patient Information, and Special Geriatric Considerations)

Additional Information There are no clinical guidelines to predict which NSAID will give response in a particular patient. Trials with each must be initiated until response determined. Consider dose, patient convenience, and cost.

Special Geriatric Considerations Elderly are a high-risk population for adverse effects from nonsteroidal anti-inflammatory agents. As much as 60% of elderly can develop peptic ulceration and/or hemorrhage asymptomatically. The concomitant use of H_2 blockers, omeprazole, and sucralfate is not effective as prophylaxis with the exception of NSAID-induced duodenal ulcers which may be prevented by the use of ranitidine. Misoprostol and proton pump inhibitors are the only agents proven to help prevent the development of NSAID-induced ulcers. Also, concomitant disease and drug use contribute to the risk for GI adverse effects. Use lowest effective dose for shortest period possible. Consider renal function decline with age. Use of NSAIDs can compromise existing renal function especially when Cl_{cr} is ≤30 mL/minute. Tinnitus may be a difficult and unreliable indication of toxicity due to age-related hearing loss or eighth cranial nerve damage. CNS adverse effects such as confusion, agitation, and hallucination are generally seen in overdose or high dose situations, but elderly may demonstrate these adverse effects at lower doses than younger adults.

Dosage Forms
  Diclofenac sodium:
    Solution, ophthalmic (Voltaren®): 0.1% (2.5 mL, 5 mL)
    Tablet, enteric coated (Voltaren®): 25 mg, 50 mg, 75 mg
    Tablet, extended release (Voltaren-XR®): 100 mg
  Tablet, as potassium (Cataflam®): 50 mg

References
Brooks PM, Day RO, "Nonsteroidal Anti-inflammatory Drugs - Differences and Similarities," *N Engl J Med*, 1991, 324(24):1716-25.
  (Continued)

Diclofenac (Continued)

Clinch D, Banerjee AK, Ostick G, "Absence of Abdominal Pain in Elderly Patients With Peptic Ulcer," Age Ageing, 1984, 13:120-3.

Clive DM, Stoff JS, "Renal Syndromes Associated With Nonsteroidal Anti-inflammatory Drugs," N Engl J Med, 1984, 310(9):563-72.

Graham DY, "Prevention of Gastroduodenal Injury Induced by Chronic Nonsteroidal Anti-inflammatory Drug Therapy," Gastroenterology, 1989, 96(2 Pt 2 Suppl):675-81.

Gurwitz JH, Avorn J, Ross-Degnan D, et al, "Nonsteroidal Anti-Inflammatory Drug-Associated Azotemia in the Very Old," JAMA, 1990, 264(4):471-5.

Hawkey CJ, Karrasch JA, Szczepaski L, et al, "Omeprazole Compared With Misoprostrol for Ulcers Associated With Nonsteroidal Anti-inflammatory Drugs," N Engl J Med, 1998, 338(11):727-34.

Knodel LC, "Preventing NSAID-Induced Ulcers: The Role of Misoprostol," Consult Pharm, 1989, 4:37-41.

Pounder R, "Silent Peptic Ulceration: Deadly Silence or Golden Silence?" Gastroenterology, 1989, 96(2 Pt 2 Suppl):626-31.

Yeomans ND, Tulassay Z, Juhasz L, et al, "A Comparison of Omeprazole With Ranitidine for Ulcers Associated With Nonsteroidal Anti-inflammatory Drugs," N Engl J Med, 1998, 338(11):719-26.

Dicloxacillin (dye kloks a SIL in)

Related Information

Penicillins, Penicillin-Related Antibiotics, & Other Antibiotics on page 1010

Brand Names Dycill®; Dynapen®; Pathocil®

Generic Available Yes

Therapeutic Category Antibiotic, Penicillin

Use Treatment of systemic infections such as pneumonia, skin and soft tissue infections and osteomyelitis caused by penicillinase-producing staphylococci

Contraindications Known hypersensitivity to dicloxacillin, penicillin, or any components

Precautions Use with caution in patients with cephalosporin allergy

Adverse Reactions

Central nervous system: Fever

Dermatologic: Rash

Gastrointestinal: Nausea, vomiting, diarrhea

Hematologic: Eosinophilia, neutropenia, leukopenia, thrombocytopenia

Hepatic: Elevation in liver enzymes

Miscellaneous: Serum sickness-like reaction

Overdosage Symptoms of overdose include neuromuscular hypersensitivity, convulsions

Toxicology Many beta-lactam-containing antibiotics have the potential to cause neuromuscular hyperirritability or convulsive seizures. Hemodialysis may be helpful to aid in the removal of the drug from the blood, otherwise most treatment is supportive or symptom directed.

Drug Interactions

Decreased effect of warfarin

Increased effect with probenecid

Drug/Food Interactions Food decreases rate and extent of absorption

Stability Refrigerate suspension after reconstitution; discard after 14 days if refrigerated or 7 days if kept at room temperature

Mechanism of Action Interferes with bacterial cell synthesis during active multiplication causing cell death and resultant bactericidal activity against susceptible bacteria

Pharmacokinetics

Absorption: 35% to 76% from GI tract

Half-life: 0.6-0.8 hours, half-life is slightly prolonged in patients with renal impairment Protein binding: 96%

Time to peak serum concentration: Within 0.5-2 hours

Elimination: Partially by the liver and excreted in bile, 56% to 70% is eliminated in urine as unchanged drug

The percent unbound has been reported to be increased in the elderly compared to young healthy volunteers (8.8% vs 7.3%), but this is not felt to be clinically significant

Usual Dosage Geriatrics and Adults: Oral: 125-500 mg every 6 hours

Not dialyzable (0% to 5%)

Administration Administer 1 hour before or 2 hours after meals; administer around-the-clock rather than 4 times/day, 3 times/day, etc (ie, 12-6-12-6, not 9-1-5-9) to promote less variation in peak and trough serum concentrations

Monitoring Parameters Signs and symptoms of infection; mental status; monitor PT or INR if patient concurrently on warfarin

Reference Range

Level guidelines: 10-25 µg/mL

Panic value: >100 µg/mL
Time to obtain blood for serum concentrations: 2 hours after dose
Test Interactions Increased protein
Patient Information Complete full course of therapy; report diarrhea or if symptoms not improving to physician or pharmacist
Nursing Implications See Administration and Monitoring Parameters
Additional Information
Sodium content of 250 mg capsule: 13 mg (0.6 mEq)
Sodium content of suspension 65 mg/5 mL: 27 mg (1.2 mEq)
Special Geriatric Considerations No dosage adjustment for renal function is necessary (see Pharmacokinetics)
Dosage Forms
Dicloxacillin sodium:
Capsule: 125 mg, 250 mg, 500 mg
Powder for oral suspension: 62.5 mg/5 mL (80 mL, 100 mL, 200 mL)
References
Pacifici GM, Viani A, Taddeucci-Brunelli G, et al, "Plasma Protein Binding of Dicloxacillin: Effects of Age and Diseases," *Int J Clin Pharmacol Ther Toxicol*, 1987, 25(11):622-6.

Dicyclomine (dye SYE kloe meen)

Brand Names Antispas® Injection; Bentyl® Hydrochloride Injection; Bentyl® Hydrochloride Oral; Byclomine® Injection; Dibent® Injection; Dilomine® Injection; Di-Spaz® Injection; Di-Spaz® Oral; Or-Tyl® Injection; Spasmoject® Injection
Synonyms Dicycloverine Hydrochloride
Generic Available Yes
Therapeutic Category Antispasmodic Agent, Gastrointestinal
Use Treatment of functional disturbances of GI motility such as irritable bowel syndrome
Unlabeled use: Urinary incontinence
Contraindications Hypersensitivity to any anticholinergic drug; narrow-angle glaucoma, tachycardia, GI obstruction, obstruction of the urinary tract, myasthenia gravis
Precautions Use with caution in patients with hepatic or renal disease, ulcerative colitis, hyperthyroidism, cardiovascular disease, hypertension
Adverse Reactions
Cardiovascular: Tachycardia, palpitations
Central nervous system: Seizures, coma, nervousness, excitement, confusion, insomnia, headache (**the elderly may be at increased risk for confusion and hallucinations**)
Gastrointestinal: Nausea, vomiting, constipation, xerostomia
Genitourinary: Urinary retention
Neuromuscular & skeletal: Muscular hypotonia
Ocular: Blurred vision
Respiratory: Respiratory distress, asphyxia
Overdosage Symptoms of overdose include CNS stimulation followed by depression, confusion, delusions, nonreactive pupils, tachycardia, hypertension
Toxicology Anticholinergic toxicity is caused by strong binding of the drug to cholinergic receptors. Cholinesterase inhibitors reduce acetylcholinesterase, the enzyme that breaks down acetylcholine and thereby allows acetylcholine to accumulate and compete for receptor binding with the offending anticholinergic. For anticholinergic overdose with severe life-threatening symptoms, physostigmine 1-2 mg S.C. or I.V., slowly may be given to reverse these effects.
Drug Interactions
Decreased effect of phenothiazines, anti-Parkinson's drugs, haloperidol, sustained release dosage forms, metoclopramide, cisapride; decreased effect with antacids
Increased effect/toxicity with anticholinergics, amantadine, narcotic analgesics, type I antiarrhythmics, antihistamines, phenothiazines, tricyclic antidepressants
Antagonistic effect: Tacrine, donepezil
Mechanism of Action Blocks the action of acetylcholine at parasympathetic sites in smooth muscle, secretory glands, and the CNS
Pharmacodynamics
Onset of action: 1-2 hours
Duration: Up to 4 hours
Pharmacokinetics
Absorption: Oral: Well absorbed
(Continued)

Dicyclomine *(Continued)*

Metabolism: Extensive

Elimination: In urine with only a small amount excreted as unchanged drug

Usual Dosage

Geriatrics: 10-20 mg 4 times/day; increasing as necessary to 160 mg/day

Adults:

Oral: Begin with 80 mg/day in 4 equally divided doses, then increase up to 160 mg/day; if no effects after 2 weeks, discontinue the medication

I.M. **(should not be used I.V.):** 80 mg/day in 4 divided doses (20 mg/dose); do not use for longer than 1-2 days

Monitoring Parameters Pulse, anticholinergic effects, urinary output, GI symptoms

Patient Information Take 30-60 minutes before a meal; may cause drowsiness, dizziness, or blurred vision; may cause dry mouth, difficult urination, or constipation

Nursing Implications Do not administer I.V.

Special Geriatric Considerations Long-term use of antispasmodics should be avoided in the elderly. The potential for a toxic reaction is greater than the potential benefit. In addition, the anticholinergic effects of dicyclomine are not well tolerated in the elderly (see Adverse Reactions).

Dosage Forms

Dicyclomine hydrochloride:

Capsule: 10 mg, 20 mg

Injection: 10 mg/mL (2 mL, 10 mL)

Syrup: 10 mg/5 mL (118 mL, 473 mL, 946 mL)

Tablet: 20 mg

References

Beers MH, Ouslander JG, Rollingher I, et al, "Explicit Criteria for Determining Inappropriate Medication Use in Nursing Home Residents," *Arch Intern Med,* 1991, 151(9):1825-32.

Dicycloverine Hydrochloride *see* Dicyclomine *on previous page*

Didanosine *(dye DAN oh seen)*

Brand Names Videx® Oral

Synonyms ddI

Generic Available No

Therapeutic Category Antiviral Agent, Oral

Use Treatment of advanced HIV infection in patients who are intolerant of zidovudine therapy or who have demonstrated significant clinical or immunologic deterioration during zidovudine therapy

Contraindications Hypersensitivity to any component

Warnings Didanosine is indicated for treatment of HIV infection only in patients intolerant of zidovudine or who have failed zidovudine. Patients receiving didanosine may still develop opportunistic infections. Peripheral neuropathy occurs in ~35% of patients receiving the drug; pancreatitis, which in some cases can be fatal, occurs in ~17% of patients receiving didanosine; patients should undergo retinal examination every 6 months to 1 year. Use with caution in patients with decreased renal or hepatic function; in high concentrations, didanosine is mutagenic; use with caution in patients with edema or congestive heart failure; use with caution in patients with hyperuricemia.

Adverse Reactions

Central nervous system: Anxiety, headache (32% to 36%), irritability, insomnia, restlessness, seizures

Gastrointestinal: Abdominal pain, nausea, diarrhea (18%), pancreatitis (9%)

Hematologic: Anemia, granulocytopenia, leukopenia, thrombocytopenia

Hepatic: Elevated liver enzymes, hepatic failure

Neuromuscular & skeletal: Peripheral neuropathy

Ocular: Retinal depigmentation

Miscellaneous: Hypersensitivity

Overdosage Chronic overdose may cause pancreatitis, peripheral neuropathy, diarrhea, hyperuricemia, and hepatic impairment

Toxicology There is no known antidote for didanosine overdose

Drug Interactions

Decreased absorption of tetracyclines and quinolones if given together; administer drugs whose absorption is pH dependent at least 2 hours prior to dosing

H_2 antagonists and antacids may increase absorption

Drug/Food Interactions Food decreases extent of absorption and peak concentration by 50%

Mechanism of Action Didanosine, a purine nucleoside analogue and the deamination product of dideoxyadenosine (ddA), inhibits HIV replication *in vitro* in both T cells and monocytes. Didanosine is converted within the cell to the monophosphates, diphosphates, and triphosphates of ddA. These ddA-triphosphates act as substrate and inhibitor of HIV reverse transcriptase substrate and inhibitor of HIV reverse transcriptase thereby blocking viral DNA synthesis and suppressing HIV replication.

Pharmacokinetics

Absorption: 20% to 25% more bioavailable from the tablet than the powder form; absolute: 30% to 33%

Distribution: V_d: 22-103 L; CSF concentrations equal 21% of serum concentrations

Half-life:

Serum: 0.8 hours

Intracellular: Much longer

Usual Dosage Geriatrics and Adults: Oral (administer on an empty stomach), dosing is based on patient weight:

<60 kg: 125 mg tablets twice daily or 167 mg buffered powder twice daily

>60 kg: 200 mg tablets twice daily or 250 mg buffered powder twice daily

Note: Adults should receive 2 tablets per dose for adequate buffering and absorption; tablets should be chewed

Dosing adjustment in renal impairment: Should be considered in patients with Cl_{cr} <60 mL/minute

Dosing adjustment in hepatic impairment: Should be considered

Administration Administer on an empty stomach; administer liquified powder immediately after dissolving

Monitoring Parameters Serum potassium, uric acid, creatinine, hemoglobin, CBC with neutrophil and platelet count, CD4 cells, liver function tests, amylase, weight gain; perform dilated retinal exam every 6 months

Patient Information Thoroughly chew tablets or manually crush or disperse 2 tablets in 1 oz of water prior to taking; for powder, open packet and pour contents into 4 oz of liquid; do not mix with fruit juice or other acid-containing liquid; stir until dissolved, drink immediately; do not take with meals

Nursing Implications Avoid creating dust if powder spilled, use wet mop or damp sponge (see Administration)

Additional Information Sodium content of buffered tablets: 264.5 mg (11.5 mEq)

Special Geriatric Considerations Since the elderly often have a creatinine clearance <60 mL/minute, monitor closely for adverse reactions (see Adverse Reactions and Monitoring Parameters); adjust dose accordingly to maintain efficacy (CD4 counts)

Dosage Forms

Powder for oral solution: Buffered (single dose packet): 100 mg, 167 mg, 250 mg, 375 mg

Tablet, buffered, chewable (mint flavor): 25 mg, 50 mg, 100 mg, 150 mg

Didronel® *see Etidronate Disodium* on page 362

Diethylstilbestrol (dye eth il stil BES trole)

Brand Names Stilphostrol®

Synonyms DES; Stilbestrol

Generic Available Yes

Therapeutic Category Estrogen Derivative

Use Management of severe vasomotor symptoms of menopause, for estrogen replacement, and for palliative treatment of inoperable metastatic prostatic carcinoma

Contraindications Undiagnosed vaginal bleeding, during pregnancy; breast cancer except in select patients with metastatic disease

Warnings Estrogens have been reported to increase the risk of endometrial carcinoma; this risk can be reduced by cycling with a progestin (ie, medroxy-progesterone) for the last 10-13 days of each month

Precautions Use with caution in patients with a history of breast cancer, thromboembolism, stroke, myocardial infarction (especially >40 years of age who smoke), liver tumor, hypertension, cardiac, renal or hepatic insufficiency

Adverse Reactions

Cardiovascular: Hypertension, thromboembolism, stroke, myocardial infarction, edema

Central nervous system: Migraine, dizziness, anxiety, depression, headache

Dermatologic: Chloasma, melasma, rash

(Continued)

287

Diethylstilbestrol *(Continued)*

Endocrine & metabolic: Decreased glucose tolerance, alterations in frequency and flow of menses, breast tenderness or enlargement, breast tumors

Gastrointestinal: Nausea, GI distress, anorexia, vomiting, diarrhea

Genitourinary: Increased libido (female), decreased libido (male)

Hepatic: Increased triglycerides and LDL, cholestatic jaundice

Miscellaneous: Increased susceptibility to *Candida* infection, intolerance to contact lenses

Overdosage Symptoms of overdose include nausea

Drug Interactions

Estrogens may reduce the effects of anticoagulants, alter the effects of antidepressants; estrogen effects may be reduced by barbiturates, rifampin, and other agents that induce hepatic microsomal enzymes

Corticosteroids may decrease the clearance and increase the half-life of estrogens

Mechanism of Action Competes with estrogenic and androgenic compounds for binding onto tumor cells and thereby inhibits their effects on tumor growth

Pharmacokinetics

Metabolism: In the liver

Elimination: In urine and feces

Usual Dosage Geriatrics and Adults:

Menopausal symptoms: Oral: 0.1-2 mg/day for 3 weeks and then off 1 week

Postmenopausal breast carcinoma: Oral: 15 mg/day

Prostate carcinoma: Oral: 1-3 mg/day

Prostatic cancer: I.V.: 0.5 g to start, then 1 g every 2-5 days followed by 0.25-0.5 g 1-2 times/week as maintenance

Diphosphate:

Oral: 50 mg 3 times/day; increase up to 200 mg or more 3 times/day

I.V.: Administer 0.5 g, dissolved in 250 mL of saline or D_5W, administer slowly the first 10-15 minutes then adjust rate so that the entire amount is given in 1 hour

Monitoring Parameters Mammography should be performed in all women prior to starting estrogen therapy and then annually; blood pressure, Pap smear annually

Test Interactions

Increased prothrombin and factors VII, VIII, IX, X

Decreased antithrombin III

Increased platelet aggregability

Increased thyroid binding globulin

Increased total thyroid hormone (T_4)

Decreased serum folate concentration

Increased serum triglycerides/phospholipids

Patient Information Patients should inform their physicians if signs or symptoms of any of the following occur: thromboembolic or thrombotic disorders including sudden severe headache or vomiting, disturbance of vision or speech, loss of vision, numbness or weakness in an extremity, sharp or crushing chest pain, calf pain, shortness of breath, severe abdominal pain or mass, mental depression or unusual bleeding. Women should perform regular self-exams on breasts.

Nursing Implications Administer 0.5 g I.V., dissolved in 250 mL of saline or D_5W, administer slowly the first 10-15 minutes then adjust rate so that the entire amount is given in 1 hour

Special Geriatric Considerations The benefits of postmenopausal estrogen therapy may be substantial for some women. Diethylstilbestrol is not the drug of choice for vasomotor symptoms, to prevent bone loss, or to treat vaginal atrophy or urinary incontinence secondary to estrogen deficiency. Diethylstilbestrol does have a role in the treatment of inoperable, progressive prostatic carcinoma and inoperable, progressive breast cancer in select men and women.

Dosage Forms

Injection: 50 mg/mL (5 mL)

Injection, as diphosphate sodium (Stilphostrol®): 0.25 g (5 mL)

Tablet: 0.25 mg, 0.5 mg, 1 mg, 5 mg

Tablet, enteric coated: 0.1 mg, 0.25 mg, 0.5 mg, 1 mg, 5 mg

Tablet (Stilphostrol®): 50 mg

Diflucan® *see* Fluconazole *on page 387*

Diflunisal (dye FLOO ni sal)
Brand Names Dolobid®
Generic Available No
Therapeutic Category Analgesic, Non-narcotic; Anti-inflammatory Agent; Antipyretic; Nonsteroidal Anti-inflammatory Agent (NSAID), Oral
Use Management of inflammatory disorders usually including rheumatoid arthritis and osteoarthritis; can be used as an analgesic for treatment of mild to moderate pain
Contraindications Hypersensitivity to diflunisal or any component, may be a cross-sensitivity with other nonsteroidal anti-inflammatory agents including aspirin; should not be used in patients with active GI bleeding; factor VII or IX deficiencies; may cause reaction in patients with tartrazine dye sensitivity
Warnings Tinnitus or impaired hearing may indicate toxicity; discontinue use 1 week prior to surgical procedures
Precautions Ophthalmologic effects; impaired renal function, use lower dosage; peripheral edema; elevation in liver tests; use with caution in patients with platelet and bleeding disorders, renal dysfunction, hepatic disease, history of salicylate-induced gastric irritation, peptic ulcer disease, erosive gastritis, bleeding disorders, hypoprothrombinemia, and vitamin K deficiency; use cautiously in asthmatics, especially those with aspirin intolerance and nasal polyps

Adverse Reactions
Cardiovascular: Palpitations, chest pain, syncope
Central nervous system: Headache, dizziness, somnolence, nervousness, hallucinations, confusion, depression, insomnia, vertigo, fatigue
Dermatologic: Rash, pruritus, TEN, Stevens-Johnson syndrome, photosensitivity, urticaria
Gastrointestinal: Nausea, dyspepsia, GI pain, diarrhea, vomiting, constipation, flatulence, GI bleeding/perforation, dry mucous membranes
Genitourinary: Dysuria
Hematologic: Agranulocytosis (rare)
Neuromuscular & skeletal: Muscle cramps, weakness
Ocular: Blurred vision
Otic: Tinnitus
Renal: Interstitial nephritis, proteinuria, hematuria
Respiratory: Dyspnea
Miscellaneous: Diaphoresis

Overdosage 10-30 g; symptoms of overdose include tinnitus, headache, dizziness, confusion, metabolic acidosis, hyperpyrexia, hyperpnea, tachypnea, nausea, vomiting, irritability, disorientation, hallucinations, lethargy, stupor, dehydration, hyperventilation, hyperthermia, hyperactivity, depression leading to coma, respiratory failure, and collapse; laboratory abnormalities include hypokalemia, hypoglycemia or hyperglycemia with alterations in pH
Toxicology Lowest fatal dose: 15 g
The "Done" nomogram is very helpful for estimating the severity of aspirin poisoning and directing treatment using serum salicylate concentrations. Treatment can also be based upon symptomatology. See table.

Aspirin or Other Salicylate Toxicity

Toxic Symptoms	Treatment
Overdose	Induce emesis with ipecac, and/or lavage with saline, followed with activated charcoal
Dehydration	I.V. fluids with KCl (no D_5W only)
Metabolic acidosis (must be treated)	Sodium bicarbonate
Hyperthermia	Cooling blankets or sponge baths
Coagulopathy/hemorrhage	Vitamin K I.V.
Hypoglycemia (with coma, seizures, or change in mental status)	Dextrose 25 g I.V.
Seizures	Diazepam 5-10 mg I.V.

Drug Interactions
Diflunisal - digoxin may cause increased digoxin plasma concentration
Diflunisal - methotrexate may cause increased methotrexate plasma concentrations
Diflunisal - anticoagulants may cause increased prothrombin time
Hydantoins, sulfonamides, and sulfonylureas may be displayed may cause increased activity
(Continued)

Diflunisal *(Continued)*

Lithium - diflunisal may cause increased lithium level

Diflunisal - anticoagulants and thrombolytics increased bleeding without increased PT or PTT but with increased bleeding time

Increased acetaminophen levels, hydrochlorothiazide levels, indomethacin levels

Decreased hyperuricemic effects of hydrochlorothiazide

Decreased levels of sulindac

Aspirin or other salicylates may decrease serum concentrations of NSAIDs

Effects of loop diuretics may be decreased; may increase azotemia when used with loop diuretics

Mechanism of Action Unknown; proposed that is inhibits prostaglandin synthesis by decreasing the activity of the enzyme, cyclo-oxygenase, which results in decreased formation of prostaglandin precursors (see Additional Information)

Pharmacodynamics

Onset of analgesia: Within 60 minutes

Duration of action: 8-12 hours

Pharmacokinetics

Absorption: Well absorbed from GI tract

Plasma protein binding: >90% bound

Metabolism: Extensive in the liver

Half-life: 8-12 hours, prolonged with renal impairment

Time to peak serum concentrations: Oral: Within 2-3 hours

Elimination: In urine within 72-96 hours, ~3% as unchanged drug and 90% as glucuronide conjugates

Usual Dosage Geriatrics and Adults: Oral (see Additional Information):

Pain: Initial: 500-1000 mg followed by 250-500 mg every 8-12 hours

Osteoarthritis: 500-750 mg/day in divided doses

Inflammatory condition: 500-1000 mg/day in 2 divided doses; do not exceed doses of 1.5 g/day

Monitoring Parameters Fecal blood loss, renal function; hearing changes or tinnitus; monitor for response (ie, pain, inflammation, range of motion, grip strength); observe for abnormal bleeding, bruising, weight gain

Test Interactions Increased chloride (S), glucose, ketone (U), uric acid (S), sodium (S); decreased uric acid (S), catecholamines (U), glucose, potassium (S), prothrombin time, uric acid (S)

Patient Information May cause GI upset, take with water, milk, or meals; do not take aspirin with diflunisal, swallow tablets whole, do not crush or chew

Nursing Implications See Monitoring Parameters, Patient Information, Additional Information, and Special Geriatric Considerations

Additional Information Diflunisal is a salicylic acid derivative which is chemically different than aspirin and is not metabolized to salicylic acid. Diflunisal 500 mg is equal in analgesic efficacy to aspirin 650 mg, acetaminophen 650 mg, and acetaminophen 650 mg/propoxyphene napsylate 100 mg, but has a longer duration of effect (8-12 hours). Not recommended as an antipyretic. Not found to be clinically useful to treat fever; at doses of ≥2 g/day, platelets are reversibly inhibited in function. Diflunisal is uricosuric at 500-750 mg/day; causes less GI and renal toxicity than aspirin and other NSAIDs; fecal blood loss is ½ that of aspirin at 2.6 g/day.

Special Geriatric Considerations Elderly are a high-risk population for adverse effects from nonsteroidal anti-inflammatory agents. As much as 60% of elderly can develop peptic ulceration and/or hemorrhage asymptomatically. The concomitant use of H_2 blockers, omeprazole, and sucralfate is not effective as prophylaxis with the exception of NSAID-induced duodenal ulcers which may be prevented by the use of ranitidine. Misoprostol and proton pump inhibitors are the only agents proven to help prevent the development of NSAID-induced ulcers. Also, concomitant disease and drug use contribute to the risk for GI adverse effects. Use lowest effective dose for shortest period possible. Consider renal function decline with age. Use of NSAIDs can compromise existing renal function especially when Cl_{cr} is ≤30 mL/minute. Tinnitus may be a difficult and unreliable indication of toxicity due to age-related hearing loss or eighth cranial nerve damage. CNS adverse effects such as confusion, agitation, and hallucination are generally seen in overdose or high dose situations, but elderly may demonstrate these adverse effects at lower doses than younger adults.

Dosage Forms Tablet: 250 mg, 500 mg

References

Gurwitz JH, Avorn J, Ross-Degnan D, et al, "Nonsteroidal Anti-Inflammatory Drug-Associated Azotemia in the Very Old," *JAMA*, 1990, 264(4):471-5.

Hawkey CJ, Karrasch JA, Szczepaski L, et al, "Omeprazcle Compared With Misoprostrol for Ulcers Associated With Nonsteroidal Anti-inflammatory Drugs," *N Engl J Med*, 1998, 338(11):727-34.

Yeomans ND, Tulassay Z, Juhasz L, et al, "A Comparison of Omeprazole With Ranitidine for Ulcers Associated With Nonsteroidal Anti-inflammatory Drugs," *N Engl J Med*, 1998, 338(11):719-26.

Di-Gel® [OTC] *see* Aluminum Hydroxide, Magnesium Hydroxide, and Simethicone *on page 44*

Digepepsin® *see* Pancreatin *on page 711*

Digitoxin (di ji TOKS in)

Brand Names Crystodigin®

Generic Available Yes

Therapeutic Category Antiarrhythmic Agent, Miscellaneous; Cardiac Glycoside

Use Treatment of congestive heart failure; slows the ventricular rate in tachyarrhythmias; atrial fibrillation; atrial flutter; paroxysmal atrial tachycardia; and cardiogenic shock

Contraindications Hypersensitivity to digitoxin or any component (rare); digitalis toxicity, beriberi heart disease, A-V block, idiopathic hypertrophic subaortic stenosis, constrictive pericarditis, ventricular fibrillation, or tachycardia

Warnings Use with caution in patients with hypoxia, hypothyroidism, acute myocarditis, suspected digitalis toxicity must be ruled out; do not use to treat obesity; patients with incomplete A-V block (Stokes-Adams attack) may progress to complete block with digitalis drug administration; use with caution in patients with acute myocardial infarction, severe pulmonary disease, advanced heart failure, idiopathic hypertrophic subaortic stenosis, Wolff-Parkinson-White syndrome, sick sinus syndrome (bradyarrhythmias), amyloid heart disease, and constrictive cardiomyopathies; adjust dose with renal impairment and aged patients; elderly may develop exaggerated serum/tissue concentrations due to decreased lean body mass, total body water, and age-related reduction in renal function; hepatic disease or failure requires dose reduction

Precautions When changing from oral (tablets or liquid) or I.M. to I.V. therapy, dosage should be reduced by 20% to 25%; use with caution in patients with hypoxia, myxedema, hypokalemia, hypomagnesemia, hypercalcemia, hypothyroidism, acute myocarditis

Adverse Reactions

Cardiovascular: Sinus bradycardia, A-V block, S-A block, atrial or nodal ectopic beats, ventricular arrhythmias, bigeminy, trigeminy, atrial tachycardia with A-V block

Central nervous system: Drowsiness, fatigue, headache, lethargy, vertigo, disorientation, restlessness, delirium, hallucinations, psychosis, apathy, depression, confusion, seizures, neuralgia

Endocrine & metabolic: Hyperkalemia with acute toxicity

Gastrointestinal: Vomiting, nausea, anorexia, abdominal pain, diarrhea

Neuromuscular & skeletal: Weakness

Ocular: Blurred vision, halos, yellow or green vision, diplopia, photophobia, flashing lights

Overdosage Symptoms of overdose include anorexia, nausea, vomiting, diarrhea, abdominal discomfort, headache, weakness, drowsiness, visual disturbances, mental depression, confusion, restlessness, disorientation, seizures, hallucinations; cardiac abnormalities include ventricular tachycardia, unifocal or multifocal PVCs (bigeminal, trigeminal); paroxysmal nodal rhythms, A-V dissociation; excessive slowing of the pulse, A-V block of varying degree; P-R prolongation, S-T depression; occasional atrial fibrillation; ventricular fibrillation is common cause of death (alterations in cardiac rate an rhythm can result in any type or known arrhythmia)

Toxicology Antidote: Life-threatening digitoxin toxicity is treated with Digibind®; discontinue digitalis preparation; administer potassium 40-80 mEq in divided doses in D_5W at 20 mEq/hour I.V.; do not administer potassium with complete heart block secondary to digitalis product or in cases of renal failure; digitalis-induced arrhythmias not responsive to potassium may be treated with phenytoin (0.5 mg/kg I.V. at 50 mg/minute), lidocaine (1 mg/kg over 5 minutes); cholestyramine, colestipol, activated charcoal may decrease absorption; other agents to consider, based on EKG and clinical assessment are atropine, quinidine, procainamide, and propranolol. **Note:** Other antiarrhythmics appear more dangerous to use in toxicity.

(Continued)

Digitoxin *(Continued)*

Drug Interactions
Aminosalicylic acid, antacids, cholestyramine; colestipol, kaolin and pectin, metoclopramide, sulfasalazine, and some combinations of antineoplastic agents decrease gastrointestinal absorption

Aminoglutethimide, rifampin, phenylbutazone, barbiturates, and hydantoins increase metabolism of digitoxin

Nondepolarizing muscle relaxants, succinylcholine have increased toxic effect

Potassium-sparing diuretics increase toxic effects

Diuretics enhance toxicity due to potassium decrease

Thyroid replacement may decrease effect of digitoxin

Mechanism of Action
Digitalis binds to and inhibits magnesium and adenosine triphosphate dependent sodium and potassium ATPase thereby increasing the influx of calcium ions, from extracellular to intracellular cytoplasm due to the inhibition of sodium and potassium ion movement across the myocardial membranes; this increase in calcium ions results in a potentiation of the activity of the contractile heart muscle fibers and an increase in the force of myocardial contraction (positive inotropic effect); digitalis may also increase intracellular entry or calcium via slow calcium channel influx; stimulates release and blocks reuptake of norepinephrine; decreases conduction through the S-A and A-V nodes

Pharmacodynamics
Onset: 1-4 hours

Pharmacokinetics
Absorption: 90% to 100%

Protein binding: 90% to 97%

Half-life: 7-8 days

Time to peak serum concentration: 8-12 hours

Elimination:
Hepatic: 50% to 70%
Renal: Metabolites (digoxin)

Usual Dosage
Geriatrics and Adults: Oral:
Rapid loading dose: Initial: 0.6 mg followed by 0.4 mg and then 0.2 mg at intervals of 4-6 hours

Slow loading dose: 0.2 mg twice daily for a period of 4 days followed by a maintenance dose

Maintenance: 0.05-0.3 mg/day

Most common dose: 0.15 mg/day

Not dialyzable (0% to 5%)

Monitoring Parameters
Monitor apical pulse, peripheral pulse, serum concentrations, EKG in critical cases of toxicity or arrhythmias

Reference Range
Therapeutic: 20-35 ng/mL; Toxic: >45 ng/mL

Test Interactions
Will give confusing and misleading results if a digoxin concentration is measured; **must** measure digitoxin concentration

Patient Information
Do not discontinue medication without physician's advice; instruct patients to notify physician if they suffer loss of appetite, visual changes, nausea, vomiting, weakness, drowsiness, headache, confusion, or depression

Nursing Implications
Check apical pulse before administering; can monitor with EKG if patient is critical

Special Geriatric Considerations
Digitalis preparations (primarily digoxin) are frequently used to treat common cardiac diseases in elderly (congestive heart failure, atrial fibrillation). Elderly are at risk for toxicity due to age-related changes; volume of distribution is diminished significantly; half-life is increased as a result of decreased total body clearance. Additionally, elderly frequently have concomitant diseases which affect the pharmacokinetics in digitalis glycosides; hypo- and hyperthyroidism and renal function decline will affect clearance of digoxin. Must be observant for noncardiac signs of toxicity in elderly such as anorexia, vision changes (blurred), confusion, and depression.

Dosage Forms
Injection: 0.2 mg/mL

Tablet: 0.05 mg, 0.1 mg, 0.15 mg, 0.2 mg

References
Nolan PE and Mooradian AD, "Digoxin," Bressler R and Katz MD eds, *Geriatric Pharmacology*, New York, NY: McGraw-Hill, 1993, 7:151-63.

Digoxin *(di JOKS in)*

Related Information
Antacid Drug Interactions *on page 1096*

I.V. Push Recommended Guidelines *on page 1083*
Serum Drug Concentrations Commonly Monitored: Guidelines *on page 1114*

Brand Names Lanoxicaps®; Lanoxin®

Generic Available Yes: Tablet

Therapeutic Category Antiarrhythmic Agent, Miscellaneous; Cardiac Glycoside

Use Treatment of congestive heart failure; slows the ventricular rate in tachyarrhythmias such as atrial fibrillation, atrial flutter, supraventricular tachycardia (paroxysmal atrial tachycardia), cardiogenic shock

Contraindications Hypersensitivity to digoxin or any component (rare); digitalis toxicity, beriberi, heart disease, A-V block, idiopathic hypertrophic subaortic stenosis, constrictive pericarditis, ventricular fibrillation, or tachycardia

Warnings Use with caution in patients with hypoxia, hypothyroidism, acute myocarditis, suspected digitalis toxicity must be ruled out; do not use to treat obesity; patients with incomplete A-V block (Stokes-Adams attack) may progress to complete block with digitalis drug administration; use with caution in patients with acute myocardial infarction, severe pulmonary disease, advanced heart failure, idiopathic hypertrophic subaortic stenosis, Wolff-Parkinson-White syndrome, sick sinus syndrome (bradyarrhythmias), amyloid heart disease, and constrictive cardiomyopathies; adjust dose with renal impairment and aged patients; elderly may develop exaggerated serum/tissue concentrations due to decreased lean body mass, total body water, and age-related reduction in renal function

Precautions When changing from oral (tablets or liquid) or I.M. to I.V. therapy, dosage should be reduced by 20% to 25%

Adverse Reactions

Cardiovascular: Sinus bradycardia, A-V block, S-A block, atrial or nodal ectopic beats, ventricular arrhythmias, bigeminy, trigeminy, atrial tachycardia with A-V block

Central nervous system: Drowsiness, fatigue, headache, lethargy, vertigo, disorientation, restlessness, delirium, hallucinations, psychosis, apathy, depression, confusion, seizures, neuralgia

Endocrine & metabolic: Hyperkalemia with acute toxicity

Gastrointestinal: Vomiting, nausea, anorexia, abdominal pain, diarrhea

Neuromuscular & skeletal: Weakness

Ocular: Blurred vision, halos, yellow or green vision, diplopia, photophobia, flashing lights

Overdosage Symptoms of overdose include anorexia, nausea, vomiting, diarrhea, abdominal discomfort, headache, weakness, drowsiness, visual disturbances, mental depression, confusion, restlessness, disorientation, seizures, hallucinations; cardiac abnormalities include ventricular tachycardia, unifocal or multifocal PVCs (bigeminal, trigeminal); paroxysmal nodal rhythms, A-V dissociation; excessive slowing of the pulse, A-V block of varying degree; P-R prolongation, S-T depression; occasional arterial fibrillation; ventricular fibrillation is common cause of death (alterations in cardiac rate an rhythm can result in any type or known arrhythmia)

Toxicology Antidote: Life-threatening digoxin toxicity is treated with Digibind®; discontinue digitalis preparation; administer potassium 40-80 mEq in divided doses in D_5W at 20 mEq/hour I.V.; do not administer potassium with complete heart block secondary to digitalis product or in cases of renal failure; digitalis-induced arrhythmias not responsive to potassium may be treated with phenytoin (0.5 mg/kg I.V. at 50 mg/minute), lidocaine (1 mg/kg over 5 minutes); cholestyramine, colestipol, activated charcoal may decrease absorption; other agents to consider, based on EKG and clinical assessment are atropine, quinidine, procainamide, and propranolol. **Note:** Other antiarrhythmics appear more dangerous to use in toxicity.

Drug Interactions

Antacids, psyllium, kaolin-pectin, aminosalicylic acid, colestipol, sulfasalazine, antineoplastics, cholestyramine, and metoclopramide may decrease absorption of digoxin

Quinidine, indomethacin, verapamil (20% to 30% decrease in clearance of digoxin), nifedipine, diltiazem, esmolol, flecainide, hydroxychloroquine, ibuprofen, quinine, tolbutamide, amiodarone, erythromycin, tetracycline, and spironolactone (25% decrease in digoxin clearance) may increase digoxin serum concentration; penicillamine may decrease digoxin's pharmacologic effects

Captopril, diltiazem decreased renal clearance

Anticholinergics increased absorption

(Continued)

Digoxin (Continued)

Disopyramide, nondepolarizing muscle relaxants, succinylcholine, potassium-sparing diuretics

Amiloride may decrease inotropic effects

Triamterene may increase pharmacologic effects

Diuretics decrease potassium

Thyroid replacement and penicillamine may decrease therapeutic effects

Stability Protect elixir and injection from light; solution compatibility: D_5W, $D_{10}W$, NS, sterile water for injection (when diluted fourfold or greater)

Mechanism of Action Digitalis binds to and inhibits magnesium and adenosine triphosphate dependent sodium and potassium ATPase thereby increasing the influx of calcium ions, from extracellular to intracellular cytoplasm due to the inhibition of sodium and potassium ion movement across the myocardial membranes; this increase in calcium ions results in a potentiation of the activity of the contractile heart muscle fibers and an increase in the force of myocardial contraction (positive inotropic effect); digitalis may also increase intracellular entry or calcium via slow calcium channel influx; stimulates release and blocks reuptake of norepinephrine; decreases conduction through the S-A and A-V nodes

Pharmacodynamics

Onset of effects:
Oral: 1-2 hours
I.V.: 5-30 minutes
Peak effect:
Oral: 2-8 hours
I.V.: 1-4 hours
Duration: 3-4 days

Pharmacokinetics

Distribution: V_d: Geriatrics: 194 L (range: 129-314 L)
Protein binding: 25%
Bioavailability: Dependent upon formulation:
Elixir: 70% to 85%
Tablets: 60% to 80% (76% in elderly)
Capsules: 90% to 100%
Half-life:
Geriatrics: 69 hours (average)
Adults: 38-48 hours
Anephric Adults: >4.5 days
Time to peak serum concentration:
Oral: 2-6 hours
I.V.: 1-5 hours
Elimination: Renal

Usual Dosage Geriatrics and Adults (based on lean body weight and normal renal function for age. Decrease dose in patients with decreased renal function)

Total digitalizing dose: Administer ½ as initial dose, then administer ¼ of the total digitalizing dose (TDD) in each of 2 subsequent doses at 8- to 12-hour intervals. Obtain EKG 6 hours after each dose to assess potential toxicity.
Oral: 0.75-1.5 mg
I.M., I.V.: 0.5-1 mg
Daily maintenance dose:
Oral: 0.125-0.5 mg
I.M., I.V.: 0.1-0.4 mg

Monitoring Parameters Monitor apical pulse, peripheral pulse, serum concentrations, EKG in critical cases of toxicity or arrhythmias

Reference Range Therapeutic: 1-2 ng/mL (SI: 1.3-2.6 nmol/L); <0.5 ng/mL (SI: <0.6 nmol/L) probably indicates underdigitalization unless there are special circumstances; Toxic: >2 ng/mL (SI: >2.6 nmol/L)

Test Interactions Endogenous digoxin-like immunoreactive substances (DLISs) and metabolites of digoxin may accumulate to cross-react with the antibodies used in immunoassays. This occurs in renal impairment, uremic states, and hepatic disease; need to communicate with laboratory to use another more specific assay (ie, monoclonal antibody assay as a radioimmunoassay with a double antibody system to eliminate cross-reactivity problems).

Patient Information Do not discontinue medication without physician's advice; instruct patients to notify physician if they suffer loss of appetite, visual changes, nausea, vomiting, weakness, drowsiness, headache, confusion, or depression

Nursing Implications Check apical pulse before giving; monitor blood pressure and EKG closely

Additional Information The AHCPR Clinical Practice Guideline for Heart Failure recommends that digoxin should be saved for patients who do not respond to ACE inhibitors and diuretics or who present with severe dyspnea on exertion. Digoxin is useful in systolic dysfunction, but not diastolic dysfunction.

Special Geriatric Considerations Digitalis preparations (primarily digoxin) are frequently used to treat common cardiac diseases in elderly (congestive heart failure, atrial fibrillation). Elderly are at risk for toxicity due to age-related changes; volume of distribution is diminished significantly; half-life is increased as a result of decreased total body clearance. Additionally, elderly frequently have concomitant diseases which affect the pharmacokinetics in digitalis glycosides; hypo- and hyperthyroidism and renal function decline will affect clearance of digoxin. Exercise in elderly will reduce serum concentrations of digoxin due to increased skeletal muscle uptake. Therefore, a knowledge of the physical activity of the elderly helps interpret serum assays. Must be observant for noncardiac signs of toxicity in elderly such as anorexia, vision changes (blurred), confusion, and depression. Changes in dose may be necessary with declining renal function with age; monitor closely.

Dosage Forms
Capsule: 0.05 mg, 0.1 mg, 0.2 mg
Injection: 0.25 mg/mL (1 mL, 2 mL)
Tablet: 0.125 mg, 0.25 mg, 0.5 mg

References
Agency for Health Care Policy and Research, Clinical Practice Guidelines, "Heart Failure: Evaluation and Care of Patients With Left-Ventricular Systolic Dysfunction," *U.S. Department of Health and Human Services*, Pub No 94-0612, June 1994.
Nolan PE and Mooradian AD, "Digoxin," Bressler R and Katz MD eds, *Geriatric Pharmacology*, New York, NY: McGraw-Hill, 1993, 7:151-63.

Dihydrex® Injection *see* Diphenhydramine *on page 302*

Dihydroergotamine (dye hye droe er GOT a meen)

Brand Names D.H.E. 45® Injection; Migranal®
Generic Available Yes
Therapeutic Category Ergot Alkaloid
Use Aborts or prevents vascular headaches
Contraindications Hypersensitivity to dihydroergotamine or any component; peripheral vascular disease, hepatic or renal dysfunction, hypertension, CAD, or severe pruritus
Precautions Use with caution in hypertension, angina, peripheral vascular disease, impaired renal or hepatic function; avoid prolonged use; dependence is a potential for patients taking for extended periods
Adverse Reactions
Cardiovascular: Localized edema, peripheral vascular effects (numbness and tingling of fingers and toes), precordial distress and pain, transient tachycardia or bradycardia
Central nervous system: Drowsiness, dizziness
Gastrointestinal: Xerostomia, diarrhea, nausea, vomiting
Neuromuscular & skeletal: Muscle pain in the extremities, weakness in the legs

Overdosage Symptoms of overdose include nausea, vomiting, leg weakness, pain in lumbar, numbness/tingling of toes and fingers, precordial pain, tachycardia or bradycardia, hypotension, hypertension, itching, localized edema, muscle pain in movement, and cold, pale, numbness in feet or hands; ergotamine toxicity can be manifested by confusion, drowsiness, depression, and seizures; impaired renal or hepatic function predisposes a patient to overdosage

Toxicology Treatment consisting of drug withdrawal and general care is initially instituted; anticoagulants, low molecular weight dextran, and vasodilators may be helpful; I.V. nitroprusside administration has been shown to reverse vasoconstriction

Drug Interactions Increased toxicity with erythromycin, clarithromycin, nitroglycerin, propranolol, troleandomycin

Stability Store in refrigerator

Mechanism of Action Ergot alkaloid alpha-adrenergic blocker directly stimulates vascular smooth muscle to vasoconstrict peripheral and cerebral vessels; also has effects on serotonin receptors

Pharmacodynamics
Onset of action: Within 15-30 minutes
(Continued)

Dihydroergotamine (Continued)

Duration: 3-4 hours

Pharmacokinetics
Distribution: V_d: 14.5 L/kg
Protein binding: 90%
Metabolism: Extensively in the liver
Half-life: 1.3-3.9 hours
Time to peak serum concentration: I.M.: Within 15-30 minutes
Elimination: Predominately into bile and feces and 10% excreted in urine, mostly as metabolites

Usual Dosage Geriatrics and Adults:
I.M.: 1 mg at first sign of headache; repeat hourly to a maximum dose of 3 mg total
I.V.: Up to 2 mg maximum dose for faster effects; maximum dose: 6 mg/week
Intranasal: 1 spray (0.5 mg) of nasal spray should be administered into each nostril; if the condition has not sufficiently improved ~15 minutes later, an additional spray should be administered to each nostril. The usual dosage required to obtain optimal efficacy is a total dosage of 4 sprays (2 mg); nasal spray is exclusively indicated for the symptomatic treatment of migraine attacks; no more than 4 sprays (2 mg) should be administered for any single migraine attack; an interval of at least 6-8 hours should be observed before treating another migraine attack with the nasal spray or any drug containing dihydroergotamine or ergotamine; no more than 8 sprays (4 mg) (corresponding to the use of 2 ampuls) should be administered during any 24-hour period; maximum weekly dosage: 24 sprays (12 mg)

Monitoring Parameters Monitor blood pressure, heart rate, signs of tingling or numbness

Reference Range Minimum concentration for vasoconstriction is reportedly 0.06 ng/mL

Patient Information Rare feelings of numbness or tingling of fingers, toes, or face may occur; avoid using this medication if you are pregnant, have heart disease, hypertension, liver disease, infection, itching

Nursing Implications Do not exceed doses above (see Monitoring Parameters)

Special Geriatric Considerations Monitor cardiac and peripheral effects closely in elderly since they often have cardiovascular disease and peripheral vascular impairment (ie, diabetes mellitus, PVD) that will complicate therapy and monitoring for adverse effects

Dosage Forms
Injection, as mesylate: 1 mg/mL (1 mL)
Spray, nasal: 4 mg/mL [0.5 mg/spray] (1 mL)

Dihydroergotoxine see Ergoloid Mesylates on page 342
Dihydrogenated Ergot Alkaloids see Ergoloid Mesylates on page 342
Dihydrohydroxycodeinone see Oxycodone on page 703
Dihydromorphinone see Hydromorphone on page 464

Dihydrotachysterol (dye hye droe tak IS ter ole)

Brand Names DHT™; Hytakerol®

Synonyms Dichysterol

Generic Available Yes

Therapeutic Category Vitamin D Analog

Use Treatment of hypocalcemia associated with hypoparathyroidism; prophylaxis of hypocalcemic tetany following thyroid surgery

Contraindications Hypercalcemia, known hypersensitivity to dihydrotachysterol, vitamin D toxicity, malabsorption syndrome, decreased renal function

Warnings Must administer concomitant calcium supplementation; maintain adequate fluid intake; calcium-phosphate product (serum calcium and phosphorus) must not exceed 70; avoid hypercalcemia; renal function impairment with secondary hyperparathyroidism

Precautions Use with caution in coronary artery disease, decreased renal function, renal stones, and elderly

Adverse Reactions
Cardiovascular: Cardiac arrhythmias
Central nervous system: Somnolence
Endocrine & metabolic: Hypercalcemia
Gastrointestinal: Nausea, vomiting, anorexia, weight loss, convulsions, constipation, metallic taste, xerostomia

Hematologic: Anemia

Hepatic: Elevated AST/ALT

Neuromuscular & skeletal: Metastatic calcification, myalgia, bone pain, weakness

Ocular: Photophobia

Renal: Renal damage, polyuria, polydipsia

Overdosage Symptoms of overdose include hypercalcemia, anorexia, nausea, weakness, constipation, diarrhea, vague aches, mental confusion, tinnitus, ataxia, depression, hallucinations, syncope, coma; polyuria, polydypsia, nocturia, hypercalciuria, irreversible renal insufficiency or proteinuria, azotemia; will spread tissue calcifications, hypertension

Toxicology Following withdrawal of the drug, treatment consists of bed rest, liberal intake of fluids, reduced calcium intake, and cathartic administration. Severe hypercalcemia requires I.V. hydration and forced diuresis with I.V. furosemide (20-40 mg I.V. every 4-6 hours). Urine output should be monitored and maintained at >3 mL/kg/hour. I.V. saline can quickly and significantly increase excretion of calcium into the urine. Calcitonin, cholestyramine, prednisone, sodium EDTA, and mithramycin have all been used successfully to treat the more resistant cases of vitamin D-induced hypercalcemia.

Drug Interactions

Vitamin D may increase absorption of magnesium from magnesium compounds; hypercalcemia may be precipitated by vitamin D and, therefore, may increase cardiac arrhythmias in patients taking digitalis glycosides and verapamil; hypoparathyroid patients may develop hypercalcemia when using thiazide diuretics

Phenytoin and barbiturates decrease half-life of vitamin D; mineral oil with prolonged use decreases vitamin D absorption; cholestyramine reduces absorption of vitamin D

Stability Protect from light

Mechanism of Action Stimulates calcium and phosphate absorption from the small intestine, promotes secretion of calcium from bone to blood (calcium hemostasis); promotes renal tubule resorption or phosphate

Pharmacodynamics

Onset of action: Maximum hypercalcemic effects occur within 2-4 weeks

Duration: Can be as long as 9 weeks

Pharmacokinetics

Absorption: Well from GI tract

Elimination: In bile and feces; stored in liver, fat, skin, muscle, and bone

Usual Dosage Geriatrics and Adults: Oral:

Hypoparathyroidism: 0.5-1 mg/day

Nutritional rickets: 0.5 mg as a single dose or 13-50 mcg/day until healing occurs

Renal osteodystrophy: 0.6-6 mg/24 hours; maintenance: 0.25-0.6 mg/24 hours adjusted as necessary to achieve normal serum calcium concentrations and promote bone healing. 1 mg is equal to 3 mg vitamin D_2 (120,000 IU) not recommended for daily supplementation due to dosage form strengths; not easily divided to deliver 800 IU

Monitoring Parameters Monitor renal function, serum calcium and phosphate concentrations; if hypercalcemia is encountered, discontinue agent until serum calcium returns to normal

Reference Range Calcium (serum) 9-10 mg/dL (4.5-5 mEq/L); phosphate 2.5-5 mg/dL

Test Interactions Increased calcium (S), cholesterol (S)

Patient Information Do not take more than the recommended amount. While taking this medication, your physician may want you to follow a special diet or take a calcium supplement. Follow this diet closely. Avoid taking magnesium supplements or magnesium containing antacids. Early symptoms of hypercalcemia include weakness, fatigue, somnolence, headache, anorexia, dry mouth, metallic taste, nausea, vomiting, cramps, diarrhea, muscle pain, bone pain, and irritability.

Nursing Implications Monitor calcium and phosphate levels closely; monitor symptoms of hypercalcemia (see Adverse Reactions)

Additional Information Synthetic analog of vitamin D with a faster onset of action; dose adjustment should be based on serum calcium level

Special Geriatric Considerations Recommended daily allowances (RDA) have not been developed for persons >65 years of age; vitamin D, folate, and B_{12} (cyanocobalamin) have decreased absorption with age, but the clinical significance is yet unknown. Calorie requirements decrease with age and therefore, nutrient density must be increased to ensure adequate nutrient

(Continued)

Dihydrotachysterol *(Continued)*

intake, including vitamins and minerals. Therefore, the use of a daily supplement with a multiple vitamin with minerals is recommended. Elderly consume less vitamin D, absorption may be decreased, and many elderly have decreased sun exposure; therefore, elderly should receive supplementation with 800 units of vitamin D (20 mcg)/day. This is a recommendation of particular need to those with high risk for osteoporosis.

Dosage Forms
Capsule: 0.125 mg
Solution: 0.25 mg/mL in oil (15 mL); 0.2 mg/5 mL (500 mL)
Solution, concentrate: 0.2 mg/mL (30 mL)
Tablet: 0.125 mg, 0.2 mg, 0.4 mg

References
Letsou AP and Price LS, "Health Aging and Nutrition: An Overview," *Clin Geriatr Med*, 1987, 3(2):253-60.
Myrianthopoulos M, "Dietary Treatment of Hyperlipidemia in the Elderly," *Clin Geriatr Med*, 1987, 3(2):343-59.
Riggs BL and Melton LJ, "The Prevention and Treatment of Osteoporosis," *N Engl J Med*, 1992, 327(9):620-7.

1,25 Dihydroxycholecalciferol *see* Calcitriol *on page 143*

Diiodohydroxyquin *see* Iodoquinol *on page 494*

Dilacor™ XR *see* Diltiazem *on this page*

Dilantin® *see* Phenytoin *on page 742*

Dilatrate®-SR *see* Isosorbide Dinitrate *on page 503*

Dilaudid® *see* Hydromorphone *on page 464*

Dilaudid-5® *see* Hydromorphone *on page 464*

Dilaudid-HP® *see* Hydromorphone *on page 464*

Dilocaine® *see* Lidocaine *on page 537*

Dilomine® Injection *see* Dicyclomine *on page 285*

Diltiazem *(dil TYE a zem)*

Related Information
Calcium Channel Blocking Agents Comparison *on page 1027*
I.V. Push Recommended Guidelines *on page 1083*

Brand Names Cardizem® CD; Cardizem® Injectable; Cardizem® SR; Cardizem® Tablet; Dilacor™ XR; Tiamate®; Tiazac®

Generic Available Yes

Therapeutic Category Antianginal Agent; Calcium Channel Blocker

Use Management of angina pectoris due to coronary insufficiency (chronic, stable) Raynaud's syndrome; SR preparation: angina pectoris (chronic, stable, and vasospastic); hypertension; diltiazem I.V.: arrhythmias

Unlabeled use: Prevent non-Q-wave myocardial infarction, tardive dyskinesia; diastolic dysfunction

Contraindications Severe hypotension or second and third degree heart block; hypersensitivity to other calcium channel blockers, adenosine; atrial and ventricular arrhythmias; acute myocardial infarction, and pulmonary congestion

Warnings Monitor EKG and blood pressure closely in patients receiving I.V. therapy; hypotension, congestive heart failure; cardiac conduction defects, PVCs, idiopathic hypertrophic subaortic stenosis; may cause platelet intubation; do not abruptly withdraw (chest pain); hepatic dysfunction, renal function impairment, increased angina, increased intracranial pressure with cranial tumors; elderly may have greater hypotensive effect

The FDA's Cardiovascular and Renal Drug Advisory Committee reviewed current data regarding the risk of heart attacks in patients treated with calcium channel blockers and determined that as a class, the calcium channel antagonists are safe; however, they warned that short-acting nifedipine could increase the risk of myocardial infarction in some patients. The committee was in agreement with a statement issued September, 1995 by the National Heart Lung, and Blood Institute of the National Institute of Health, that warned that short-acting nifedipine should be used with great caution especially at higher doses.

Precautions Sick sinus syndrome, severe left ventricular dysfunction, congestive heart failure, hepatic or renal impairment, hypertrophic cardiomyopathy (especially obstructive), concomitant therapy with beta-blockers or digoxin, edema

Adverse Reactions
Cardiovascular: Tachycardia, hypotension, bradycardia, first, second, or third degree A-V block, worsening heart failure, palpitations, congestive heart

failure, myocardial infarction, angina, bundle-branch block, peripheral edema

Central nervous system: Amnesia, dizziness, headache, fatigue, seizures (occasionally with I.V. use), lightheadedness, psychotic symptoms, insomnia

Dermatologic: Bruising

Gastrointestinal: Thirst, constipation (more of a problem in elderly), nausea, abdominal discomfort, diarrhea, gingival hyperplasia, xerostomia

Genitourinary: Urinary incontinence

Hematologic: Petechiae, bruising, purpura

Hepatic: Increase in hepatic enzymes

Neuromuscular & skeletal: Gait abnormality, paresthesia, weakness

Ocular: Amblyopia, eye irritation, blurred vision

Respiratory: May precipitate insufficiency of respiratory muscle function in Duchenne muscular dystrophy

Miscellaneous: Gingival swelling and inflammation

Overdosage Symptoms of overdose include heartblock, hypotension, asystole

Toxicology Ipecac-induced emesis can hypothetically worsen calcium antagonist toxicity, since it can produce vagal stimulation. The potential for seizures precipitously following acute ingestion of large doses of a calcium antagonist may also contraindicate the use of ipecac. Supportive and symptomatic treatment, including I.V. fluids and Trendelenburg positioning, should be initiated as intoxication may cause hypotension. Although calcium (calcium chloride I.V. 1-2 g) has been used as an "antidote" for acute intoxications, there is limited experience to support its routine use, and should be reserved for those cases where definite signs of myocardial depression are evident. Heart block may respond to isoproterenol, glucagon, atropine and/or calcium, although a temporary pacemaker may be required.

Drug Interactions

Calcium channel blockers (CCB) and H_2 blockers may increase bioavailability CCB

CCB and beta-blockers may increase cardiac depressant effects on A-V conduction

CCB and carbamazepine may increase carbamazepine levels (nifedipine does not appear to interact with carbamazepine)

CCB and cyclosporine may increase cyclosporine levels

CCB and digitalis may increase digitalis levels

CCB and theophylline may increase pharmacologic actions of theophylline

Stability Store injections in refrigerator at 2°C to 8°C (36°F to 46°F); stable for 24 hours

Mechanism of Action Inhibits calcium ion from entering the "slow channels" or select voltage-sensitive areas of vascular smooth muscle and myocardium during depolarization, producing a relaxation of coronary vascular smooth muscle and coronary vasodilation; increases myocardial oxygen delivery in patients with vasospastic angina

Pharmacodynamics

Onset of action: 30-60 minutes after oral administration (including sustained release)

Peak effects: 2-3 hours for plain tablets, 6-11 hours for sustained release

Pharmacokinetics

Absorption: 80% to 90%

Distribution: V_d: 1.7 L/kg

Protein binding: 77% to 85%

Metabolism: Extensive in the liver; inhibitor CYP1A2, 3A4; substrate CYP3A4

Bioavailability: Around 40% to 65% due to a significant first-pass effect following oral administration

Half-life: 4-6 hours (may increase with renal impairment), 5-7 hours for sustained release

Time to peak serum concentrations: Within 2-3 hours

Elimination: In urine and in bile mostly as metabolites

Usual Dosage Geriatrics and Adults:

Oral: Initial dose: 30 mg 3-4 times/day, then 30-120 mg 3-4 times/day; dosage should be increased gradually, at 1- to 2-day intervals until optimum response is obtained; not to exceed 360 mg/day

Sustained-release capsules: Initial dose: 60-120 mg twice daily; increase dose at 14-day intervals

Cardizem® CD and Dilacor™ XR: 180-240 mg once daily; increase dose at 14-day intervals

(Continued)

Diltiazem *(Continued)*

    Parenteral: Initial dose: 0.25 mg/kg as a bolus over 2 minutes (20 mg is an average dose); second bolus: 0.35 mg/kg over 2 minutes (25 mg is an average dose)

    Continuous I.V.: After bolus, 5-10 mg/hour (see Additional Information)

Dosing adjustment in renal impairment: None

Monitoring Parameters Heart rate, blood pressure, signs and symptoms of congestive heart failure

Reference Range Therapeutic: 50-200 ng/mL

Patient Information Sustained release products should be taken with food and not crushed; limit caffeine intake; avoid alcohol; notify physician if angina pain is not reduced when taking this drug, irregular heartbeat, shortness of breath, swelling, dizziness, constipation, nausea, or hypotension occur; do not stop therapy without advice of physician

Nursing Implications Do not crush sustained release capsules (see Warnings, Precautions, Monitoring Parameters, and Special Geriatric Considerations)

Additional Information Mix injection for continuous infusion in D_5W, NS, $D_5\frac{1}{2}NS$

Special Geriatric Considerations Elderly may experience a greater hypotensive response; constipation may be more of a problem in elderly; calcium channel blockers are no more effective in elderly than other therapies; however, they do not cause significant CNS effects which is an advantage over some antihypertensive agents.

Dosage Forms

Capsule, sustained release:

    Cardizem® CD: 120 mg, 180 mg, 240 mg, 300 mg

    Cardizem® SR: 60 mg, 90 mg, 120 mg

    Dilacor™ XR: 180 mg, 240 mg

    Tiazac®: 120 mg, 180 mg, 240 mg, 300 mg, 360 mg

Injection: 5 mg/mL (5 mL, 10 mL)

    Cardizem®: 5 mg/mL (5 mL, 10 mL)

Tablet (Cardizem®): 30 mg, 60 mg, 90 mg, 120 mg

Tablet, extended release (Tiamate®): 120 mg, 180 mg, 240 mg

Dimaphen® Elixir [OTC] *see* Brompheniramine and Phenylpropanolamine *on page 130*

Dimaphen® Tablets [OTC] *see* Brompheniramine and Phenylpropanolamine *on page 130*

Dimenhydrinate *(dye men HYE dri nate)*

Brand Names Calm-X® Oral [OTC]; Dimetabs® Oral; Dinate® Injection; Dramamine® Oral [OTC]; Dramilin® Injection; Dramoject® Injection; Dymenate® Injection; Hydrate® Injection; Marmine® Injection; Marmine® Oral [OTC]; Tega-Vert® Oral; TripTone® Caplets® [OTC]

Generic Available Yes

Therapeutic Category Antiemetic; Antihistamine

Use Treatment and prevention of nausea, vertigo, and vomiting associated with motion sickness

Contraindications Hypersensitivity to dimenhydrinate or any component; chlorotheophylline and theophylline

Warnings Use with caution when giving with antibiotics which may cause ototoxicity since dimenhydrinate may mask signs of ototoxicity (vestibular toxicity)

Precautions Use with caution with prostatic hypertrophy, peptic ulcer, pyloroduodenal obstruction, bladder neck obstruction, narrow-angle glaucoma, bronchial asthma, and cardiac arrhythmias

Adverse Reactions

Cardiovascular: Hypotension

Central nervous system: Drowsiness, headache, paradoxical CNS stimulation, dizziness, confusion, nervousness, restlessness, insomnia, vertigo, lassitude

Gastrointestinal: Anorexia, dry mucous membranes

Genitourinary: Polyuria

Local: Pain at the injection site

Neuromuscular & skeletal: Heaviness and weakness of hands

Ocular: Blurred vision, diplopia

Otic: Tinnitus

Respiratory: Chest tightness, wheezing, thickening of bronchial secretions

Overdosage Toxicity may resemble atropine overdosage; CNS depression or stimulation; convulsions, coma, respiratory depression with massive overdosage

Toxicology There is no specific treatment for an antihistamine overdose, however, most of its clinical toxicity is due to anticholinergic effects. Cholinesterase inhibitors may be useful by reducing acetylcholinesterase. Acetylcholinesterase inhibitors include physostigmine, neostigmine, pyridostigmine, and edrophonium. For anticholinergic overdose with severe life-threatening symptoms, physostigmine 1-2 mg I.V. slowly may be given to reverse these effects; treat convulsions with diazepam.

Drug Interactions CNS depressants, drugs with anticholinergic effects, ototoxic drugs, alcohol

Mechanism of Action Competes with histamine for H_1-receptor sites on effector cells in the gastrointestinal tract, blood vessels, and respiratory tract; blocks chemoreceptor trigger zone, diminishes vestibular stimulation and depresses labyrinthine function through its central anticholinergic activity

Pharmacodynamics
Onset of action: Oral: Within 15-30 minutes following administration
Duration: ~4-6 hours

Pharmacokinetics
Absorption: Well absorbed from GI tract
Metabolism: Extensive in the liver

Usual Dosage Geriatrics and Adults: Oral, I.M., I.V.: 50-100 mg every 4-6 hours, not to exceed 400 mg/day; start elderly at lowest dose recommended; do not inject intra-arterially (see Nursing Implications)

Monitoring Parameters Monitor for anticholinergic side effects; emetic episodes and nausea

Patient Information May cause drowsiness

Nursing Implications I.V. injection must be diluted to 10 mL with NS and given at 25 mg/minute over at least 2 minutes

Special Geriatric Considerations Monitor for anticholinergic side effects (confusion, constipation, etc); limit use if possible to short-term therapy

Dosage Forms
Capsule: 50 mg
Injection: 50 mg/mL (1 mL, 5 mL, 10 mL)
Liquid: 12.5 mg/4 mL; 15.62 mg/5 mL
Tablet: 50 mg
Tablet, chewable: 50 mg

Dimetabs® Oral see Dimenhydrinate on previous page

Dimetane® Extentabs® [OTC] see Brompheniramine on page 129

Dimetapp® 4-Hour Liqui-Gel Capsule [OTC] see Brompheniramine and Phenylpropanolamine on page 130

Dimetapp® Elixir [OTC] see Brompheniramine and Phenylpropanolamine on page 130

Dimetapp® Extentabs® [OTC] see Brompheniramine and Phenylpropanolamine on page 130

Dimetapp® Tablet [OTC] see Brompheniramine and Phenylpropanolamine on page 130

Dimethoxyphenyl Penicillin Sodium see Methicillin on page 602

β,β-Dimethylcysteine see Penicillamine on page 719

Dinate® Injection see Dimenhydrinate on previous page

Diocto® [OTC] see Docusate on page 312

Diocto C® [OTC] see Docusate and Casanthranol on page 313

Diocto-K® [OTC] see Docusate on page 312

Diocto-K Plus® [OTC] see Docusate and Casanthranol on page 313

Dioctolose Plus® [OTC] see Docusate and Casanthranol on page 313

Dioctyl Calcium Sulfosuccinate see Docusate on page 312

Dioctyl Potassium Sulfosuccinate see Docusate on page 312

Dioctyl Sodium Sulfosuccinate see Docusate on page 312

Dioeze® [OTC] see Docusate on page 312

Dioval® Injection see Estradiol on page 350

Diovan® see Valsartan on page 979

Dipentum® see Olsalazine on page 692

Diphenacen-50® Injection see Diphenhydramine on next page

Diphen® Cough [OTC] see Diphenhydramine on next page

Diphenhist [OTC] see Diphenhydramine on next page

Diphenhydramine (dye fen HYE dra meen)

Related Information
Anxiolytic/Hypnotic Use in Long-Term Care Facilities *on page 1099*
Federal OBRA Regulations Recommended Maximum Doses - Hypnotics *on page 1057*
I.V. Push Recommended Guidelines *on page 1083*

Brand Names AllerMax® Oral [OTC]; Banophen® Oral [OTC]; Belix® Oral [OTC]; Benadryl® Injection; Benadryl® Oral [OTC]; Benadryl® Topical; Ben-Allergin-50® Injection; Benylin® Cough Syrup [OTC]; Bydramine® Cough Syrup [OTC]; Compoz® Gel Caps [OTC]; Compoz® Nighttime Sleep Aid [OTC]; Dihydrex® Injection; Diphenacen-50® Injection; Diphen® Cough [OTC]; Diphenhist [OTC]; Dormarex® 2 Oral [OTC]; Dormin® Oral [OTC]; Genahist® Oral; Hydramyn® Syrup [OTC]; Hyrexin-50® Injection; Maximum Strength Nytol® [OTC]; Miles Nervine® Caplets [OTC]; Nidryl® Oral [OTC]; Nordryl® Injection; Nordryl® Oral; Nytol® Oral [OTC]; Phendry® Oral [OTC]; Siladryl® Oral [OTC]; Silphen® Cough [OTC]; Sleep-eze 3® Oral [OTC]; Sleepinal® [OTC]; Sleepwell 2-nite® [OTC]; Sominex® Oral [OTC]; Tusstat® Syrup; Twilite® Oral [OTC]; Uni-Bent® Cough Syrup; 40 Winks® [OTC]

Generic Available Yes

Therapeutic Category Antidote, Hypersensitivity Reactions; Antihistamine; Anti-Parkinson's Agent; Sedative

Use Symptomatic relief of allergic symptoms caused by histamine release which include nasal allergies and allergic dermatosis; mild nighttime sedation, prevention of motion sickness, antitussive
Unlabeled use: Parkinson's disease (anticholinergic effects)

Contraindications Hypersensitivity to diphenhydramine or any component; should not be used in acute attacks of asthma

Warnings Antihistamines are more likely to cause dizziness, excessive sedation, syncope, toxic confusional states, and hypotension in the elderly

Precautions Use with caution in patients with angle-closure glaucoma, peptic ulcer, urinary tract obstruction, hyperthyroidism; some preparations contain sodium bisulfite; syrup contains alcohol

Adverse Reactions
Cardiovascular: Hypotension, palpitations
Central nervous system: Sedation, dizziness, paradoxical excitement, fatigue, insomnia
Gastrointestinal: Nausea, vomiting, dry mucous membranes
Genitourinary: Urinary retention
Neuromuscular & skeletal: Tremors
Ocular: Blurred vision

Overdosage Symptoms of overdose include CNS depression or stimulation, dry mouth, flushed skin, fixed and dilated pupils, apnea

Toxicology There is no specific treatment for an antihistamine overdose, however, most of its clinical toxicity is due to anticholinergic effects. Cholinesterase inhibitors may be useful by reducing acetylcholinesterase. Acetylcholinesterase inhibitors include physostigmine, neostigmine, pyridostigmine, and edrophonium. For anticholinergic overdose with severe life-threatening symptoms, physostigmine 1-2 mg I.V., slowly may be given to reverse these effects.

Drug Interactions Increased effect/toxicity: CNS depressants, alcohol, tricyclic antidepressants, monoamine oxidase inhibitors; elixir should not be given to patients taking drugs that can cause disulfiram reactions (ie, metronidazole, chlorpropamide) due to alcohol content

Stability Protect from light

Mechanism of Action Competes with histamine for H_1-receptor sites on effector cells in the gastrointestinal tract, blood vessels, and respiratory tract

Pharmacodynamics Duration of action: 4-7 hours

Pharmacokinetics
Absorption: Oral: ~65%
Metabolism: Extensive in the liver, and to smaller degrees in the lung and kidneys
Half-life:
  Elderly: 13.5 hours
  Adults: 2-8 hours
Time to peak serum concentration: 2-4 hours; one study showed significant increase in peak concentration in elderly
Elimination: Total body clearance is decreased in elderly

Usual Dosage
Geriatrics: Initial: 25 mg 2-3 times/day increasing as needed

Dosing interval in renal impairment:
   Cl_{cr} 10-50 mL/minute: Increase dosing interval to 6-12 hours
   Cl_{cr} <10 mL/minute: Increase dosing interval to 12-18 hours
Adults:
   Oral:
      Antihistamine: 25-50 mg every 4-6 hours
      Antitussive: 25 mg every 4 hours
      Antiemetic: 25-50 mg 3-4 times/day
      Parkinson's disease: 25-50 mg 3-4 times/day
      Sleep aid: 50 mg at bedtime (maximum)
   I.M., I.V.: 10-50 mg in a single dose every 2-4 hours, not to exceed 400 mg/day
   Topical: Apply to affected area for not longer than 7 days

Monitoring Parameters Relief of symptoms, mental alertness

Reference Range Therapeutic: Not established; Toxic: >0.1 µg/mL

Test Interactions May suppress the wheal and flare reactions to skin test antigens

Patient Information May cause drowsiness; avoid CNS depressants and alcohol

Nursing Implications I.V. must be given slowly; monitor patient for sedation

Additional Information Has antinauseant and topical anesthetic properties

Special Geriatric Considerations Diphenhydramine has high sedative and anticholinergic properties, so it may not be considered the antihistamine of choice for prolonged use in the elderly. Its use as a sleep aid is discouraged due to its anticholinergic effects; interpretive guidelines issued by the Health Care Financing Administration (HCFA) discourage the use of diphenhydramine as a sedative or anxiolytic in long-term care facilities (see Pharmacokinetics).

Dosage Forms
Diphenhydramine hydrochloride:
   Capsule: 25 mg, 50 mg
   Cream: 1%, 2%
   Elixir: 12.5 mg/5 mL (5 mL, 10 mL, 20 mL, 120 mL, 480 mL, 3780 mL)
   Injection: 10 mg/mL (10 mL, 30 mL); 50 mg/mL (1 mL, 10 mL)
   Lotion: 1% (75 mL)
   Solution, topical spray: 1% (60 mL)
   Syrup: 12.5 mg/5 mL (5 mL, 120 mL, 240 mL, 480 mL, 3780 mL)
   Tablet: 25 mg, 50 mg

References
Simons KJ, Watson WT, Martin TJ, et al, "Diphenhydramine: Pharmacokinetics and Pharmacodynamics in Elderly Adults, Young Adults, and Children," *J Clin Pharmacol*, 1990, 30(7):665-71.

Diphenoxylate and Atropine (dye fen OKS i late & A troe peen)

Brand Names Lofene®; Logen®; Lomanate®; Lomodix®; Lomotil®; Lonox®; Low-Quel®

Synonyms Atropine and Diphenoxylate

Generic Available Yes

Therapeutic Category Antidiarrheal

Use Adjunctive treatment of diarrhea

Restrictions C-V

Contraindications Hypersensitivity to diphenoxylate, atropine or any component; severe liver disease, jaundice, dehydrated patient, and narrow-angle glaucoma, diarrhea due to pseudomembranous enterocolitis or enterotoxin-producing bacteria

Warnings Reduction of intestinal motility may be deleterious in diarrhea resulting from *Shigella*, *Salmonella*, toxigenic strains of *E. coli* and from pseudomembranous enterocolitis associated with broad spectrum antibiotics; diphenoxylate may induce toxic megacolon in patients with ulcerative colitis; discontinue use if abdominal distention occurs; hepatic coma may be precipitated when used in patients with significant or severe hepatic disease

Precautions High doses may cause addiction; use with caution in patients with ulcerative colitis, dehydration, and hepatic dysfunction; use with caution in patients performing hazardous tasks (driving, etc)

Adverse Reactions
Cardiovascular: Tachycardia
Central nervous system: Sedation, dizziness, euphoria, headache, anaphylaxis, headache, confusion, delirium, sedation, malaise, lethargy, restlessness, hyperthermia
Dermatologic: Pruritus, urticaria, dry skin, angioneurotic edema
(Continued)

Diphenoxylate and Atropine *(Continued)*

Gastrointestinal: Nausea, vomiting, abdominal discomfort, paralytic ileus, pancreatitis, xerostomia, toxic megacolon

Genitourinary: Urinary retention

Neuromuscular & skeletal: Weakness

Ocular: Blurred vision

Respiratory: Respiratory depression

Miscellaneous: Edema

Overdosage Symptoms of overdose include drowsiness, hypotension, blurred vision (mydriasis), flushing, dry mouth, miosis, dry mucous membranes, restlessness, hyperthermia, tachycardia, lethargy; and then coma, hypotonic reflexes, nystagmus, respiratory depression; respiratory depression may occur 12-30 hours after ingestion

Toxicology Naloxone 2 mg I.V. with repeat administration as necessary to maintain respiration, up to a total of 10 mg. Duration of diphenoxylate is longer than naloxone. Repeated doses necessary. Monitor closely for 48 hours. For the anticholinergic overdose with severe life-threatening symptoms, physostigmine 1-2 mg S.C. or I.V., slowly may be given to reverse these effects. Administration of activated charcoal will reduce bioavailability of diphenoxylate. Gastric lavage can be used in place of activated charcoal therapy.

Drug Interactions Diphenoxylate may precipitate hypertensive crises with monoamine oxidase inhibitors; diphenoxylate may increase CNS depressant effects of barbiturates, alcohol, major and minor tranquilizers

Stability Protect liquid from light

Mechanism of Action Diphenoxylate inhibits excessive GI motility and GI propulsion; this is both a peripheral and central mechanism of action; commercial preparations contain a subtherapeutic amount of atropine to discourage abuse; diphenoxylate is a congener of meperidine but lacks analgesic activity; high doses (40-60 mg) exhibit opioid activity

Pharmacodynamics

Onset of action: Within 45-60 minutes

Duration: 3-4 hours

Pharmacokinetics

Absorption: Oral: Well absorbed

Metabolism: Diphenoxylate is extensively metabolized in the liver to diphenoxylic acid (active)

Half-life:

Diphenoxylate: 2.5 hours

Diphenoxylic acid (difenoxin): 12-14 hours

Time to peak plasma concentrations: 2 hours

Elimination: Primarily in feces (via bile) and ~14% excreted in urine; <1% excreted unchanged in urine

Usual Dosage Geriatrics and Adults: Oral (as diphenoxylate): 15-20 mg/day in 3-4 divided doses initially; reduce dosage as soon as symptoms are controlled; maintenance dose is 1/4 of initial dose (see Additional Information)

Monitoring Parameters Monitor number and consistency of stools; observe for signs of toxicity, fluid and electrolyte loss, hypotension, and respiratory depression

Patient Information Drowsiness, dizziness, dry mouth; use caution while driving or performing hazardous tasks; avoid alcohol or other CNS depressants; do not exceed prescribed dose; report persistent diarrhea, fever, or palpitations to physician

Nursing Implications Watch for signs of atropinism (dryness of skin and mucous membranes, tachycardia, thirst, flushing), hypotension, respiratory depression, confusion (see Monitoring Parameters)

Additional Information If there is no response within 48 hours, the drug is unlikely to be effective and should be discontinued. If chronic diarrhea is not improved symptomatically within 10 days at maximum dosage of 20 mg/day, control is unlikely with further use. Diarrhea should also be treated with dietary measures (ie, clear liquids), and avoid milk products and high sodium foods such as bouillon and soups.

Special Geriatric Considerations Elderly are particularly sensitive to fluid and electrolyte loss. This generally results in lethargy, weakness, and confusion. Repletion and maintenance of electrolytes and water are essential in the treatment of diarrhea. Drug therapy must be limited in order to avoid toxicity with this agent.

Dosage Forms
Solution, oral: Diphenoxylate hydrochloride 2.5 mg and atropine sulfate 0.025 mg per 5 mL (60 mL)

Tablet: Diphenoxylate hydrochloride 2.5 mg and atropine sulfate 0.025 mg

Diphenylan Sodium® *see* Phenytoin *on page 742*

Diphenylhydantoin *see* Phenytoin *on page 742*

Diphtheria and Tetanus Toxoid
(dif THEER ee a & TET a nus TOKS oyd)

Related Information
Immunization Guidelines *on page 1058*

Synonyms DT; Td; Tetanus and Diphtheria Toxoid

Therapeutic Category Toxoid

Use Active immunity against diphtheria and tetanus

Contraindications Patients receiving immunosuppressive agents, prior anaphylactic, allergic, or systemic reactions, hypersensitivity to diphtheria and tetanus toxoid or any component

Warnings Do not use to treat active tetanus or diphtheria infections

Precautions Hypersensitivity may occur; primary immunization should be postponed until the second year of life due to possibility of CNS damage or convulsion

Adverse Reactions
Cardiovascular: Flushing, tachycardia, hypotension, especially those who have received many booster injections

Central nervous system: Drowsiness, malaise, neurologic symptoms are uncommon (ie, radial nerve paralysis, dysphagia, etc), severe fever, convulsions rarely

Dermatologic: Urticaria, rash, pruritus, redness

Gastrointestinal: Anorexia, vomiting

Local: Pain, tenderness, palpable nodules and sterile abscesses may occur at injection site

Neuromuscular & skeletal: Generalized aches and pains

Miscellaneous: Arthus-type hypersensitivity reactions, edema

Drug Interactions Immunosuppressive agents

Stability Refrigerate

Usual Dosage Geriatrics and Adults: I.M.: Two primary doses of 0.5 mL each, given at an interval of 4-6 weeks; third (reinforcing) dose of 0.5 mL 6-12 months later; boosters every 10 years

Patient Information A nodule may be palpable at the injection site for a few weeks

Nursing Implications Shake well before giving, advise patient of adverse reactions; must be given I.M.; do not inject the same site more than once; federal law requires that the date of administration, the vaccine manufacturer, lot number of vaccine, and the administering person's name, title, and address be entered into the patient's permanent medical record

Dosage Forms See table.

Diphtheria and Tetanus Toxoid

Manufacturer	Diphtheria in Lf units per 0.5 mL	Tetanus in Lf units per 0.5 mL
Connaught Td	2	5
Lederle Td	2	5
Sclavo Td	2	10
Wyeth Td	1.5	5

Td — adult use.

Special Geriatric Considerations Tetanus is a rare disease in U.S. with <100 cases annually; 66% of cases occur in persons >50 years of age; protective tetanus and diphtheria antibodies decline with age; it is estimated that <50% of elderly are protected.

Elderly are at risk because:
Many lack proper immunization maintenance
Higher case fatality ratio

(Continued)

Diphtheria and Tetanus Toxoid *(Continued)*

Immunizations are not available from childhood

Indications for vaccination:

Primary series with combined tetanus-diphtheria (Td) should be given to all elderly lacking a clear history of vaccination

Boosters should be given at 10-year intervals; earlier for wounds

Elderly are more likely to require tetanus immune globulin with infection of tetanus due to lower antibody titer

References
Bentley DW, "Vaccinations," *Clin Geriatr Med*, 1992, 8(4):745-60.
Gardner P and Schaffner W, "Immunization of Adults," *N Engl J Med*, 1993, 328(17):1242-8.

Dipivalyl Epinephrine *see* Dipivefrin *on this page*

Dipivefrin *(dye PI ve frin)*
Related Information
Glaucoma Drug Therapy Comparison *on page 1032*
Brand Names AKPro® Ophthalmic; Propine® Ophthalmic
Synonyms Dipivalyl Epinephrine; DPE
Generic Available No
Therapeutic Category Adrenergic Agonist Agent, Ophthalmic; Ophthalmic Agent, Vasoconstrictor
Use Reduce elevated intraocular pressure in chronic open-angle glaucoma; also used to treat ocular hypertension, low tension, and secondary glaucomas
Contraindications Hypersensitivity to dipivefrin, ingredients in the formulation, or epinephrine; contraindicated in patients with angle-closure glaucoma
Warnings Contains sulfites which cause allergic-type reactions in susceptible persons
Precautions Use with caution in patients with vascular hypertension or cardiac disorders and in aphakic patients
Adverse Reactions
Cardiovascular: Tachycardia, arrhythmia, hypertension
Central nervous system: Headache
Local: Burning, stinging
Ocular: Ocular congestion, photophobia, mydriasis, blurred vision, ocular pain, bulbar conjunctival follicles, blepharoconjunctivitis, cystoid macular edema
Drug Interactions Effects when used with other agents to lower intraocular pressure may be additive or synergistic; cyclopropane and halothane (general anesthetics) sensitize the heart to sympathomimetics; chymotrypsin is inactivated by epinephrine, exaggerated adrenergic pressor effects with monoamine oxidase inhibitors and tricyclic antidepressants
Stability Avoid exposure to light and air, discolored or darkened solutions indicate loss of potency
Mechanism of Action Dipivefrin is a prodrug of epinephrine which is the active agent that stimulates alpha- and/or beta-adrenergic receptors increasing aqueous humor outflow
Pharmacodynamics
Ocular pressure effects: Within 30 minutes
Duration: 12 hours or longer; mydriasis may occur within 30 minutes and last for several hours
Pharmacokinetics Absorption: Rapid into the aqueous humor; converted to epinephrine
Usual Dosage Geriatrics and Adults: Ophthalmic: Initial: Instill 1 drop every 12 hours
Monitoring Parameters Intraocular pressure; heart rate and blood pressure
Patient Information Discolored solutions should be discarded; do not touch dropper to eye; slight amount of discomfort may follow instillation; headache or browache may occur at start of therapy; report any change in vision to physician immediately
Nursing Implications Instruct on how to administer eye drops
Additional Information Contains sodium metabisulfite
Special Geriatric Considerations Use with caution in patients with heart disease. Assess patient's ability to self-administer drops.
Dosage Forms Solution, ophthalmic, as hydrochloride: 0.1% (5 mL, 10 mL, 15 mL)

Diprolene® *see* Betamethasone *on page 114*

Diprolene® AF *see* Betamethasone *on page 114*
Dipropylacetic Acid *see* Valproic Acid and Derivatives *on page 977*
Diprosone® *see* Betamethasone *on page 114*

Dipyridamole (dye peer ID a mole)
Brand Names Persantine®
Generic Available Yes
Therapeutic Category Antiplatelet Agent; Vasodilator, Coronary
Use Maintain patency after surgical grafting procedures including coronary artery bypass; with warfarin to decrease thrombosis in patients after artificial heart valve replacement; for chronic management of angina pectoris; with aspirin to prevent coronary artery thrombosis; in combination with aspirin or warfarin to prevent other thromboembolic disorders
Contraindications Hypersensitivity to dipyridamole or any component
Warnings Use with caution in patients with hypotension
Precautions May further decrease blood pressure in patients with hypotension due to peripheral vasodilation
Adverse Reactions
  Cardiovascular: Vasodilatation, flushing, syncope
  Central nervous system: Dizziness, headache
  Dermatologic: Rash, pruritus, bruising
  Gastrointestinal: Abdominal distress
  Hematologic: Bleeding
  Neuromuscular & skeletal: Weakness
Overdosage Symptoms of overdose include hypotension, peripheral vasodilation
Drug Interactions Decreased vasodilation from I.V. dipyridamole when given to patients taking theophylline; enhances bleeding of anticoagulated patients (aspirin, heparin, Coumadin®)
Mechanism of Action Inhibits the activity of adenosine deaminase and phosphodiesterase, which causes an accumulation of adenosine, adenine nucleotides, and cyclic AMP; these mediators then inhibit platelet aggregation and may cause vasodilation; may also stimulate release of prostacyclin or PGD_2
Pharmacokinetics
  Absorption: Readily from GI tract
  Distribution: V_d: Adults: 2-3 L/kg
  Protein binding: 91% to 99%
  Metabolism: Concentrated and metabolized in the liver
  Bioavailability: Ranges from 37% to 66%
  Half-life (terminal): 10-12 hours
  Time to peak serum concentrations: Within 2-2.5 hours
  Elimination: In feces via bile as glucuronide conjugates and unchanged drug
Usual Dosage Geriatrics and Adults: Oral: 75-400 mg/day in 3-4 divided doses before meals (see Additional Information)
Additional Information Dipyridamole may also be given 2 days prior to open heart surgery to prevent platelet activation by extracorporeal bypass pump; differences in bioavailability between products observed; evidence exists that doses of 400-600 mg/day have been shown to have **no effect** on platelet aggregation; this casts doubt on clinical usefulness as an antiplatelet agent
Special Geriatric Considerations Since evidence suggests that clinically used doses are ineffective for prevention of platelet aggregation, consideration for low dose aspirin (81-325 mg/day) alone may be necessary; this will decrease cost as well as inconvenience
Dosage Forms Tablet: 25 mg, 50 mg, 75 mg
References
  Fitzgerald GA, "Dipyridamole," *N Engl J Med*, 1987, 316(20):1247-57.

Dirithromycin (dye RITH roe mye sin)
Related Information
  Cephalosporins, Aminoglycosides, Macrolides, & Quinolones *on page 1014*
Brand Names Dynabac®
Generic Available No
Therapeutic Category Antibiotic, Macrolide
Use Treatment of mild to moderate upper and lower respiratory tract infections due to *Moraxella catarrhalis*, *Streptococcus pneumoniae*, *Legionella pneumophila*, or *S. pyogenes* (ie, acute exacerbation of chronic bronchitis, secondary bacterial infection of acute bronchitis, community-acquired pneumonia, pharyngitis/tonsillitis, not proven to be effective in prevention of potentially
(Continued)

Dirithromycin *(Continued)*

subsequent rheumatic fever), and uncomplicated infections of the skin and skin structure due to *Staphylococcus aureus*

Note: Serum concentrations of dirithromycin are not adequate to treat bacteremias due to other sensitive strains; **empiric** treatment of acute bacterial exacerbations of chronic or secondary bronchitis is not recommended since resistance of the frequently causative agent, *H. influenzae*, occurs

Contraindications Hypersensitivity to dirithromycin or other macrolides; use with pimozide

Precautions Contrary to potential serious consequences with other macrolides (eg, cardiac arrhythmias), the combination of terfenadine and dirithromycin has not shown alteration of terfenadine metabolism; however, caution should be taken during coadministration of dirithromycin and terfenadine; pseudomembranous colitis has been reported and should be considered in patients presenting with diarrhea subsequent to therapy with dirithromycin

Adverse Reactions

Central nervous system: Headache, dizziness

Dermatologic: Skin rash, urticaria

Gastrointestinal: Abdominal pain, nausea, diarrhea, vomiting, dyspepsia, flatulence

Hepatic: Increased LFTs, alkaline phosphatase

Neuromuscular & skeletal: Weakness

Renal: Nephrotoxicity

Overdosage Symptoms of overdose include nausea, vomiting, abdominal pain, diarrhea

Toxicology Treatment is supportive; dialysis has not been found effective

Drug Interactions

Increased effect: Absorption of dirithromycin is slightly enhanced with concomitant antacids and H₂-antagonists; dirithromycin may, like erythromycin, increase the effect of alfentanil, anticoagulants, bromocriptine, carbamazepine, cyclosporine, digoxin, disopyramide, ergots, methylprednisolone, and triazolam

Note: Interactions with nonsedating antihistamines (eg, terfenadine) and theophylline are not known to occur, however, caution is advised with coadministration

Drug/Food Interactions Take with food; food may increase bioavailability

Mechanism of Action Converted to erythromycylamine which exhibits RNA-dependent protein synthesis at the chain elongation step; binds to the 50S ribosomal subunit blocking transpeptidation

Pharmacokinetics

Distribution: V_d: ~800 L

Protein binding 15% to 30% (primarily as erythromycylamine)

Metabolism: Converted via hydrolysis to erythromycylamine during absorption and distribution

Bioavailability 6% to 14%

Half-life: 20-50 hours (erythromycylamine)

Elimination: 1% to 4% excreted unchanged in urine

Usual Dosage Geriatrics and Adults: Oral: 500 mg once daily, with food or within 1 hour of eating, for 7-14 days

Dosing adjustment in renal impairment: None necessary

Dosing adjustment in severe hepatic impairment: Potential need for dose adjustment

Monitoring Parameters Signs and symptoms of infection; temperature, CBC

Patient Information Take with food or within an hour following a meal; do not cut, chew, or crush tablets; entire course of medication should be taken to ensure eradication of organism

Nursing Implications Monitor tolerance to medication; do not administer concurrently with aluminum or magnesium antacids (see Drug Interactions); monitor respiratory, cardiac, and fluid status of nursing home patients being treated for pneumonia; do not alter enteric coated dosage form

Special Geriatric Considerations Dosage adjustment does not appear to be necessary in the elderly (see Usual Dosage and Pharmacokinetics); considered an appropriate choice in the outpatient treatment of community-acquired pneumonia in older adults (see Warnings)

Dosage Forms Tablet, enteric coated: 250 mg

References

Niederman MS, Bass JB Jr, Campbell GD, et al, "Guidelines for the Initial Management of Adults With Community-Acquired Pneumonia: Diagnosis, Assessment of Severity, and Initial Antimicrobial Therapy," *Am Rev Respir Dis*, 1993, 148(5):1418-26.

Disalcid® *see* Salsalate *on page 847*

Disalicylic Acid *see* Salsalate *on page 847*

Disanthrol® [OTC] *see* Docusate and Casanthranol *on page 313*

Disodium Cromoglycate *see* Cromolyn Sodium *on page 255*

d-Isoephedrine Hydrochloride *see* Pseudoephedrine *on page 802*

Disonate® [OTC] *see* Docusate *on page 312*

Disopyramide (dye soe PEER a mide)

Brand Names Norpace®

Generic Available Yes

Therapeutic Category Antiarrhythmic Agent, Class I-A

Use Suppression and prevention of unifocal and multifocal premature ventricular complexes, coupled ventricular tachycardia considered to be life-threatening; also effective in the conversion of atrial fibrillation, atrial flutter, and paroxysmal atrial tachycardia to normal sinus rhythm and prevention of the recurrence of these arrhythmias after conversion by other methods

Contraindications Pre-existing second or third degree A-V block; cardiogenic shock or known hypersensitivity to the drug

Warnings Demonstrates proarrhythmic effect to the extent it is not recommended for arrhythmias capable of being treated with less toxic, more traditional therapy, has not been shown to increase survival; negative inotropic action may result in congestive heart failure or hypotension; QRS widening, Q-T$_c$ prolongation; atrial arrhythmias; use with caution in sick sinus syndrome, Wolff-Parkinson-White syndrome, and patients with heart block; hypoglycemia reported; disopyramide has strong anticholinergic activity; use with caution and reduce dosage in renal (Cl$_{cr}$ ≤40 mL/minute) and hepatic impairment

Precautions Pre-existing urinary retention, family history or existing angle-closure glaucoma, myasthenia gravis, hypotension during initiation of therapy, congestive heart failure unless caused by an arrhythmias, widening of QRS complex during therapy or Q-T interval (>25% to 50% of baseline QRS complex or Q-T interval), sick sinus syndrome or WPW, renal or hepatic impairment require decrease in dosage; disopyramide ineffective in hypokalemia and potentially toxic with hyperkalemia

Adverse Reactions

Cardiovascular: Hypotension, congestive heart failure, edema, chest pain, syncope, conduction disturbances including A-V block, widening QRS complex and lengthening of Q-T interval

Central nervous system: Nervousness, acute psychosis, depression, dizziness, fatigue, headache, malaise, pain

Dermatologic: Generalized rashes

Endocrine & metabolic: Hypoglycemia, increased cholesterol and triglycerides; hyperkalemia may enhance toxicities

Gastrointestinal: Constipation, xerostomia, weight gain, nausea, vomiting, diarrhea, gas, anorexia

Genitourinary: Urinary retention, urinary hesitancy

Neuromuscular & skeletal: Weakness

Ocular: Blurred vision

Respiratory: Dyspnea

Miscellaneous: Dry nose, eyes, and throat

Overdosage Symptoms of overdose include anticholinergic effects, hypotension, loss of consciousness, respiratory arrest, cardiac conduction disturbances, arrhythmias, widening of the QRS complex and Q-T interval, bradycardia, congestive heart failure, asystole, and seizures

Toxicology General supportive care: Induce emesis or perform gastric lavage followed by cathartic or activated charcoal; use of pressor agents (isoproterenol, dopamine), diuretics, cardiac glycosides, intra-aortic balloon counterpulsation, mechanical ventilation may be necessary as indicated; hemodialysis and charcoal hemoperfusion are effective to help eliminate disopyramide

Drug Interactions

Hepatic microsomal enzyme inducing agents (ie, phenytoin, phenobarbital, rifampin) may increase metabolism of disopyramide

Erythromycin may increase disopyramide serum concentrations

Anticoagulants may have decreased PTs after discontinuation of disopyramide

Digoxin and quinidine serum concentrations may be increased, and drugs with anticholinergic effects will be augmented

(Continued)

Disopyramide *(Continued)*

Mechanism of Action Class IA antiarrhythmic: Decreases myocardial excitability and conduction velocity; reduces disparity in refractory between normal and infarcted myocardium; possesses anticholinergic, peripheral vasoconstrictive, and negative inotropic effects

Pharmacodynamics
Onset of action: 0.5-3.5 hours
Duration of effect: 1.5-8.5 hours

Pharmacokinetics
Protein binding: Concentration-dependent ranging from 20% to 60%
Metabolism: In the liver to inactive metabolites
Bioavailability: 60% to 83%
Half-life: 4-10 hours with Cl_{cr} <40 mL/minute; half-life: 8-18 hours; increased half-life with hepatic or renal disease
Time to peak concentrations: 1-2 hours
Elimination: 40% to 60% unchanged in urine and 10% to 15% in feces
Total body clearance of unbound disopyramide averages 3.2-5.4 mL/minute/kg; total disopyramide clearance range: 0.7-1.2 mL/minute/kg; the total body clearance (bound and unbound) is decreased in elderly

Usual Dosage Oral (initiate therapy in hospital):
Geriatrics and Adults:
Initial loading: 300 mg (<50 kg: 200 mg); follow with 200 mg every 6 hours (if no toxicity or response after 6 hours); if no response in 48 hours, increase carefully to 250 mg every 6 hours or stop drug
<50 kg: 100 mg every 6 hours or 200 mg every 12 hours (controlled release)
>50 kg: 150 mg every 6 hours or 300 mg every 12 hours (controlled release); if no response, may increase to 200 mg every 6 hours; most adults respond to 600 mg/day; maximum dose required for patients with severe refractory ventricular tachycardia may be 400 mg every 6 hours. When switching from immediate release to controlled release dosage form, initiate controlled release dose 6 hours following last dose of immediate release preparation.

Dosing adjustment in renal impairment: Adults: 100 mg (nonsustained release) given at the following intervals; see table.

Creatinine Clearance (mL/min)	Dosage Interval
30-40	q8h
15-30	q12h
<15	q24h

Monitoring Parameters Congestive heart failure, hypotension and urinary retention; monitor EKG, blood pressure, pulse, and serum concentrations

Reference Range
Therapeutic:
Atrial arrhythmias: 2.8-3.2 µg/mL (SI: 8.3-9.4 µmol/L)
Ventricular arrhythmias: 3.3-7.5 µg/mL (SI: 9.7-22 µmol/L)
Toxic: >7 µg/mL (SI: >20.7 µmol/L)

Test Interactions Decreased glucose

Patient Information May cause dry mouth, difficulty with urination, dizziness, dyspnea, blurred vision, and constipation; do not break or chew sustained release capsules

Nursing Implications Administer around-the-clock rather than 4 times/day, 3 times/day, etc (ie, 12-6-12-6, not 9-1-5-9) to promote less variation in peak and trough serum concentrations; do not crush controlled release capsules

Special Geriatric Considerations Due to changes in total clearance (decreased) in elderly, monitor closely; the anticholinergic action may be intolerable and require discontinuation; monitor for CNS anticholinergic effects (confusion, agitation, hallucinations, etc). **Note:** Dose needs to be altered with Cl_{cr} <40 mL/minute which may be found frequently in elderly.

Dosage Forms
Disopyramide phosphate:
Capsule: 100 mg, 150 mg
Capsule, sustained action: 100 mg, 150 mg

References
Fenster PE and Nolan PE, "Antiarrhythmic Drugs," *Geriatric Pharmacology*, Bressler R and Katz MD, eds, New York, NY: McGraw-Hill, 1993, 6:105-49.

Di-Spaz® Injection *see* Dicyclomine *on page 285*

Di-Spaz® Oral *see* Dicyclomine *on page 285*

Dispos-a-Med® Isoproterenol *see* Isoproterenol *on page 501*

Ditropan® *see* Oxybutynin *on page 702*

Diurigen® *see* Chlorothiazide *on page 207*

Diuril® *see* Chlorothiazide *on page 207*

Divalproex Sodium *see* Valproic Acid and Derivatives *on page 977*

Dizac® Injectable Emulsion *see* Diazepam *on page 279*

Dizmiss® [OTC] *see* Meclizine *on page 574*

***dl*-Norephedrine Hydrochloride** *see* Phenylpropanolamine *on page 741*

D-Med® Injection *see* Methylprednisolone *on page 611*

Dobutamine (doe BYOO ta meen)

Related Information
I.V. Medication Recommendations *on page 1080*

Brand Names Dobutrex® Injection

Generic Available Yes

Therapeutic Category Adrenergic Agonist Agent

Use Short-term management of patients with cardiac decompensation due to depressed contractility

Contraindications Hypersensitivity to sulfites (commercial preparation contains sodium bisulfite); patients with idiopathic hypertrophic subaortic stenosis (IHSS)

Warnings Potent drug, must be diluted prior to use; patient's hemodynamic status should be monitored

Precautions Continuously monitor EKG and blood pressure; hypovolemia should be corrected prior to use; infiltration causes local inflammatory changes, extravasation may cause dermal necrosis; use with extreme caution following myocardial infarction

Adverse Reactions
Cardiovascular: Ectopic heartbeats, increased heart rate, chest pain, angina, palpitations, elevation in blood pressure; in higher doses ventricular tachycardia or arrhythmias may be seen. **Patients with atrial fibrillation or flutter are at risk of developing a rapid ventricular response.**

Central nervous system: Headache

Gastrointestinal: Nausea, vomiting

Neuromuscular & skeletal: Mild leg cramps, paresthesia

Respiratory: Dyspnea

Overdosage Symptoms of overdose include fatigue, nervousness, tachycardia, hypertension, arrhythmias

Toxicology Reduce rate of administration or discontinue infusion until condition stabilizes

Drug Interactions
General anesthetics (ie, halothane or cyclopropane) and usual doses of dobutamine have resulted in ventricular arrhythmias in animals. In animals, the cardiac effects of dobutamine are antagonized by beta-adrenergic blockers, resulting in predominance of alpha-adrenergic effects and increased peripheral resistance.

Bretylium and tricyclic antidepressants may potentiate dobutamine's effects

Stability Incompatible with alkaline solutions (sodium bicarbonate); store reconstituted solution under refrigeration for 48 hours or 6 hours at room temperature; after dilution, the solution is stable for 24 hours at room temperature; pink discoloration of solution indicates slight oxidation but **no** significant loss of potency.

Mechanism of Action Stimulates beta$_1$-adrenergic receptors, causing increased cardiac output, with little effect on beta$_2$- or alpha-receptors; heart rate is not usually increased; dobutamine does not cause the release of norepinephrine

Pharmacodynamics
Onset of action: I.V.: 1-10 minutes following administration
Peak effect: Within 10-20 minutes

Pharmacokinetics
Metabolism: In tissues and liver to inactive metabolites
Half-life: 2 minutes
Elimination: In urine

Usual Dosage Geriatrics and Adults: I.V. infusion: 2.5-15 mcg/kg minute; maximum: 40 mcg/kg/minute, titrate to desired response; administer with an infusion device to control the flow rate

(Continued)

Dobutamine *(Continued)*

Administration Do not administer through same I.V. line as heparin, hydrocortisone sodium succinate, cefazolin, or penicillin; administer into large vein; use infusion device to control rate of flow

Monitoring Parameters EKG, blood pressure, pulse, hemodynamic status

Nursing Implications See Administration

Additional Information Most clinical experience with dobutamine is short-term (several hours)
Standard diluent: 250 mg/500 mL D_5W
Minimum volume: 500 mg/250 mL D_5W

Special Geriatric Considerations A recent study demonstrated beneficial hemodynamic effects in elderly patients; monitor closely (see Adverse Reactions - Cardiovascular)

Dosage Forms Injection, as hydrochloride: 12.5 mg/mL (20 mL)

References
Rich MN, Woods WL, Davila-Roman VG, et al, "A Randomized Comparison of Intravenous Amrinone Versus Dobutamine in Older Patients With Decompensated Congestive Heart Failure," *J Am Geriatr Soc*, 1995, 43(3):271-4.

Dobutrex® Injection *see Dobutamine on previous page*

Docusate *(DOK yoo sate)*

Brand Names Colace® [OTC]; DC 240® Softgels® [OTC]; Dialose® [OTC]; Diocto® [OTC]; Diocto-K® [OTC]; Dioeze® [OTC]; Disonate® [OTC]; DOK® [OTC]; DOS® Softgel® [OTC]; D-S-S® [OTC]; Kasof® [OTC]; Modane® Soft [OTC]; Pro-Cal-Sof® [OTC]; Regulax SS® [OTC]; Sulfalax® [OTC]; Surfak® [OTC]

Synonyms Dioctyl Calcium Sulfosuccinate; Dioctyl Potassium Sulfosuccinate; Dioctyl Sodium Sulfosuccinate; DOSS; DSS

Generic Available Yes

Therapeutic Category Laxative, Surfactant; Stool Softener

Use Stool softener in patients who should avoid straining during defecation and constipation associated with hard, dry stools; prophylaxis for straining (Valsalva) following myocardial infarction

Contraindications Concomitant use of mineral oil; intestinal obstruction, acute abdominal pain, nausea, vomiting; hypersensitivity to docusate or any component

Warnings Excessive use may lead to fluid and electrolyte imbalance

Adverse Reactions
Dermatologic: Rash
Gastrointestinal: Diarrhea, abdominal cramping
Miscellaneous: Throat irritation

Drug Interactions Mineral oil

Mechanism of Action Reduces surface tension of the oil-water interface of the stool resulting in enhanced incorporation of water and fat allowing for stool softening in small and large intestine; may also cause increased intestinal secretion

Pharmacodynamics Onset of action: 12-72 hours

Usual Dosage Geriatrics and Adults:
Oral: 100-400 mg/day in 1-4 divided doses
Rectal: Add 50-100 mg of docusate liquid to enema fluid (saline or water); administer as retention or flushing enema

Patient Information Patients should assure proper dietary fiber and fluid intake with adequate exercise if medically appropriate; do not use if abdominal pain, nausea, or vomiting are present; laxative use should be used for a short period of time (<1 week); prolonged use may result in abuse, dependence, as well as fluid and electrolyte loss; notify physician if bleeding occurs or if constipation is not relieved

Nursing Implications Docusate liquid can be given with milk or fruit juice to mask the bitter taste

Additional Information Docusate salts are interchangeable; the amount of sodium, calcium, or potassium per dosage unit is clinically insignificant; should institute nonpharmacologic therapy (ie, fluid, fiber, exercise)

Special Geriatric Considerations A safe agent to be used in elderly; some evidence that doses <200 mg are ineffective; stool softeners are unnecessary if stool is well hydrated or "mushy" and soft; shown to be ineffective used long-term

Dosage Forms
Capsule, as calcium:
DC 240® Softgels®, Pro-Cal-Sof®, Sulfalax®: 240 mg

Surfak®: 50 mg, 240 mg
Capsule, as potassium:
  Diocto-K®: 100 mg
  Kasof®: 240 mg
Capsule, as sodium:
  Colace®: 50 mg, 100 mg
  Dioeze®: 250 mg
  Disonate®: 100 mg, 240 mg
  DOK®: 100 mg, 250 mg
  DOS® Softgel®: 100 mg, 250 mg
  D-S-S®: 100 mg
  Modane® Soft: 100 mg
  Regulax SS®: 100 mg, 250 mg
Liquid, as sodium (Diocto®, Colace®, Disonate®, DOK®): 150 mg/15 mL (30 mL, 60 mL, 480 mL)
Solution, oral, as sodium (Doxinate®): 50 mg/mL with alcohol 5% (60 mL, 3780 mL)
Syrup, as sodium:
  50 mg/15 mL (15 mL, 30 mL)
  Colace®, Diocto®, Disonate®, DOK®: 60 mg/15 mL (240 mL, 480 mL, 3780 mL)
Tablet, as sodium (Dialose®): 100 mg

Docusate and Casanthranol (DOK yoo sate & ka SAN thra nole)

Related Information
Docusate *on previous page*

Brand Names Dialose® Plus Capsule [OTC]; Diocto C® [OTC]; Diocto-K Plus® [OTC]; Dioctolose Plus® [OTC]; Disanthrol® [OTC]; DSMC Plus® [OTC]; Genasoft® Plus [OTC]; Peri-Colace® [OTC]; Pro-Sof® Plus [OTC]; Regulace® [OTC]; Silace-C® [OTC]

Synonyms Casanthranol and Docusate; DSS With Casanthranol

Generic Available Yes

Therapeutic Category Laxative, Surfactant; Stool Softener

Use Treatment of constipation generally associated with dry, hard stools and decreased intestinal motility

Contraindications Concomitant use of mineral oil; intestinal obstruction; acute abdominal pain; nausea, vomiting, appendicitis, acute surgical abdomen; hypersensitivity to docusate or casanthranol

Warnings Do not use when abdominal pain, nausea, or vomiting are present; excessive use may lead to fluid and electrolyte imbalance

Precautions Drug is habit-forming and may result in laxative dependence and loss of normal bowel function with prolonged use; rectal bleeding and failure to respond to therapy may require further evaluation; discoloration of urine may occur

Adverse Reactions
Gastrointestinal: Diarrhea, abdominal cramping, griping, nausea, vomiting, bloating, flatulence
Miscellaneous: Throat irritation, diaphoresis

Overdosage Symptoms of overdose include fluid/electrolyte loss, hypotension, fatigue, lethargy, diarrhea, abdominal pain, nausea, vomiting

Drug Interactions Mineral oil

Stability Store in tight, light-resistant containers

Mechanism of Action Casanthranol has direct action on intestinal mucosa (colon) which stimulates the myenteric plexus, increases water and electrolyte secretion into intestine

Pharmacodynamics Onset of action: 6-12 hours after administration but may require up to 24 hours

Usual Dosage Adults: Oral: 1-2 capsules or 15-30 mL syrup at bedtime, may be increased to 2 capsules or 30 mL twice daily or 3 capsules at bedtime

Monitoring Parameters Monitor stools daily or weekly; fluid/electrolyte status

Patient Information Patients should assure proper dietary fiber and fluid intake with adequate exercise if medically appropriate; do not use if abdominal pain, nausea, or vomiting are present; laxative use should be used for a short period of time (<1 week); prolonged use may result in abuse, dependence, as well as fluid and electrolyte loss; notify physician if bleeding occurs or if constipation is not relieved

Nursing Implications See Contraindications and Special Geriatric Considerations

Special Geriatric Considerations The chronic use of stimulant cathartics is inappropriate and should be avoided; although constipation is a common
(Continued)

313

Docusate and Casanthranol (Continued)

complaint from elderly, such complaints require evaluation; short-term use of stimulants is best; if prophylaxis is desired, this can be accomplished with bulk agents (psyllium), stool softeners, and hyperosmotic agents (sorbitol 70%); stool softeners are unnecessary if stools are well hydrated, soft, or "mushy"

Dosage Forms

Capsule (Dialose® Plus, Diocto-K Plus®, Dioctolose Plus®, DSMC Plus®): Docusate potassium 100 mg and casanthranol 30 mg

Capsule (Disanthrol®, Genasoft® Plus, Peri-Colace®, Pro-Sof® Plus, Regulace®): Docusate sodium 100 mg and casanthranol 30 mg

Syrup (Diocto C®, Peri-Colace®, Silace-C®): Docusate sodium 60 mg and casanthranol 30 mg per 15 mL with alcohol 10% (240 mL, 480 mL, 4000 mL)

DOK® [OTC] see Docusate on page 312

Doktors® Nasal Solution [OTC] see Phenylephrine on page 740

Dolacet® see Hydrocodone and Acetaminophen on page 461

Dolasetron (dol A se tron)

Brand Names Anzemet®

Therapeutic Category Antiemetic; Serotonin Antagonist, Antiemetic

Use

Oral: The prevention of nausea and vomiting associated with moderately-emetogenic cancer chemotherapy, including initial and repeat courses; the prevention of postoperative nausea and vomiting.

Parenteral: The prevention of nausea and vomiting associated with initial and repeat courses of emetogenic cancer chemotherapy, including high dose cisplatin; the prevention of postoperative nausea and vomiting; as with other antiemetics, routine prophylaxis is not recommended for patients in whom there is little expectation that nausea and/or vomiting will occur postoperatively; in patients where nausea and/or vomiting must be avoided postoperatively, injection is recommended even where the incidence of postoperative nausea and/or vomiting is low; the treatment of postoperative nausea and/or vomiting

Contraindications In patients known to have hypersensitivity to the drug

Warnings Can cause EKG interval changes (P-R, Q-T$_c$, JT prolongation and QRS widening). These changes are related in magnitude and frequency to blood concentrations of the active metabolite. These changes are self-limiting with declining blood concentrations. Some patients have interval prolongation for 24 hours or longer. Interval prolongation could lead to cardiovascular consequences, including heart block or cardiac arrhythmias. These have rarely been reported. Dolasetron should be administered with caution in patients who have or may develop prolongation of cardiac conduction intervals, particularly Q-T$_c$. These include patients with hypokalemia or hypomagnesemia, patients taking diuretics with potential for inducing electrolyte abnormalities, patients with congenital Q-T syndrome, patients taking antiarrhythmic drugs or other drugs which lead to Q-T prolongation, and cumulative high dose anthracycline therapy. Use with caution in patients with hypertension, CAD, arrhythmias or CHF, seizures or other neurological conditions.

Adverse Reactions

Cardiovascular: Hypotension, hypertension, EKG changes

Central nervous system: Nervousness, paresthesias, dizziness, lightheadedness, somnolence, fatigue, headache, sleep disturbance, fever/chills with I.V. administration

Gastrointestinal: Hunger, increased appetite, diarrhea, taste alterations, nausea, constipation

Hepatic: Mild LFT increases

Local: Pain at injection site, erythema

Ophthalmic: Blurred vision

Mechanism of Action Dolasetron mesylate and its active metabolite, hydrodolasetron (MDL 74,156), are selective serotonin 5-HT3 receptor antagonists not shown to have activity at other known serotonin receptors and with low affinity for dopamine receptors.

Usual Dosage Geriatrics and Adults:

Oral:

Prevention of cancer chemotherapy-induced nausea and vomiting: 100 mg given within 1 hour before chemotherapy

Use in renal failure patients or hepatically impaired patients: No dosage adjustment is recommended

Prevention of postoperative nausea and vomiting: 100 mg within 2 hours before surgery

    Use in renal failure patients or hepatically impaired patients: No dosage adjustment is recommended

Parenteral (injection):

Prevention of cancer chemotherapy-induced nausea and vomiting: From clinical trials, the dose is 1.8 mg/kg given as a single dose approximately 30 minutes before chemotherapy; alternatively, for most patients, a fixed dose of 100 mg can be administered over 30 seconds

    Use in renal failure patients or in hepatically impaired patients: No dosage adjustment is recommended

Prevention of postoperative nausea and/or vomiting 12.5 mg given as a single dose approximately 15 minutes before the cessation of anesthesia (prevention) or as soon as nausea or vomiting presents (treatment)

Additional Information A single I.V. dose of dolasetron mesylate (1.8 or 2.4 mg/kg) has comparable safety and efficacy to a single 32-mg IV dose of ondansetron in patients receiving cisplatin chemotherapy.

Special Geriatric Considerations No dosage adjustment necessary (see Warnings)

Dosage Forms

Dolasetron mesylate:

Injection: 20 mg/mL (0.625 mL, 5 mL)

Tablet: 50 mg, 100 mg

References

Dempsey E, Bourque S, Spenard J, et al, "Pharmacokinetics of Single Intravenous and Oral Doses of Dolasetron Mesylate in Healthy Elderly Volunteers," *J Clin Pharmacol*, 1996, 36(10):903-10.

Dolene® *see* Propoxyphene *on page 795*

Dolobid® *see* Diflunisal *on page 289*

Dolophine® *see* Methadone *on page 599*

Domeboro® Topical [OTC] *see* Aluminum Acetate and Calcium Acetate *on page 41*

Donepezil (don EH pa zil)

Brand Names Aricept®

Synonyms E2020

Generic Available No

Therapeutic Category Cholinergic Agent; Cholinesterase Inhibitor

Use Treatment of mild to moderate dementia of the Alzheimer's type

Contraindications Known hypersensitivity to donepezil or to piperidine derivatives

Precautions Use with caution in patients with sick sinus syndrome or supraventricular cardiac conduction conditions; use with caution in patients with history of peptic ulcer disease or those receiving concurrent NSAID therapy (due to increased gastric acid secretion); due to its cholinergic activity, use with caution in patients with bladder outflow obstruction, seizures, or obstructive pulmonary disease; donepezil may exaggerate succinylcholine-type muscle relaxation during anesthesia

Adverse Reactions

Cardiovascular: Syncope

Central nervous system: Insomnia, fatigue, headache, dizziness, depression, abnormal dreams

Dermatologic: Bruising

Gastrointestinal: Nausea, diarrhea, vomiting, anorexia

Genitourinary: Polyuria

Neuromuscular & skeletal: Muscle cramps, arthritis

Overdosage Symptoms of overdose (seen in animals) include reduced spontaneous movement, prone position, staggering gait, lacrimation, clonic convulsions, depressed respiration, salivation, miosis, tremors, fasciculations, and lower body surface temperature

Toxicology Treat overdose with atropine at an initial dose of 1-2 mg I.V. with subsequent doses based upon clinical response

Drug Interactions Ketoconazole and quinidine inhibit donepezil metabolism *in vitro*, it is unknown whether this results in any clinical effect; donepezil decreases the activity of anticholinergic medications; synergistic effect is expected when donepezil is administered with succinylcholine, similar neuromuscular blocking agents, or bethanechol

(Continued)

Donepezil *(Continued)*

Mechanism of Action Donepezil enhances cholinergic function by increasing the concentration of acetylcholine through reversible inhibition of its hydrolysis by acetylcholinesterase; there is no evidence that donepezil alters the course of the underlying dementing process

Pharmacokinetics Note: No formal pharmacokinetic studies have been done in geriatric patients though mean donepezil plasma concentrations were no different in elderly Alzheimer patients as compared to younger adults

Absorption: Well absorbed

Protein binding: 96% mainly to albumin (75%) and alpha$_1$ acid glycoprotein (21%)

Metabolism: By CYP450 isoenzymes 2D6 and 3A4 and undergoes glucuronidation

Bioavailability: 100%

Half-life: 70 hours

Steady-state: 15 days

Time to peak plasma concentration: 3-4 hours

Elimination: Unchanged in urine and extensively metabolized to four major metabolites, two of which are active

Usual Dosage Geriatrics and Adults: Initial: 5 mg at bedtime; may be increased to 10 mg at bedtime after 4-6 weeks; a 10 mg dose may provide additional benefit for some patients

Monitoring Parameters Behavior, mood, bowel function

Patient Information May be taken with or without food; donepezil is not a cure for Alzheimer's disease, but may slow the progression of symptoms

Nursing Implications See Monitoring Parameters

Additional Information At the current time, the company is offering a Patient Assistance Program, which is supplying donepezil to eligible patients in need, call 1-800-226-2072

Special Geriatric Considerations Donepezil is a new anticholinesterase for the treatment of Alzheimer's disease. It has been shown to cause an improvement in the ADAS-cog scores. As compared to tacrine, donepezil does **not** cause elevations in liver function tests and does not require routine laboratory monitoring. In addition, it is dosed once a day versus tacrine's four doses per day. Because of these reasons, donepezil may be preferred over tacrine in the treatment of mild to moderate dementia of the Alzheimer's type.

Dosage Forms Tablet: 5 mg, 10 mg

References

Rogers SL and Friedhoff LT, "The Efficacy and Safety of Donepezil in Patients With Alzheimer's Disease: Results of a U.S. Multicentre, Randomized, Double-Blind, Placebo-Controlled Trial," *Dementia,* 1996, 7(6):293-303.

Dopamine *(DOE pa meen)*

Brand Names Intropin® Injection

Generic Available Yes

Therapeutic Category Adrenergic Agonist Agent

Use Adjunct in the treatment of shock which persists after adequate fluid volume replacement; dose related inotropic and vasopressor effects; stimulates dopaminergic, beta- and alpha-receptors

Contraindications Hypersensitivity to sulfites (commercial preparation contains sodium bisulfite); pheochromocytoma, ventricular fibrillation, or uncorrected tachyarrhythmias

Warnings Potent drug; must be diluted prior to use. Patient's hemodynamic status should be monitored.

Precautions Hypovolemia should be corrected by appropriate plasma volume expanders before administration; closely monitor patients with a history of occlusive vascular disease; extravasation may cause tissue necrosis

Adverse Reactions

Cardiovascular: Ectopic heartbeats, tachycardia, vasoconstriction, hypotension, cardiac conduction abnormalities, widened QRS complex, bradycardia, hypertension, ventricular arrhythmias, gangrene of the extremities

Central nervous system: Anxiety, headache

Gastrointestinal: Nausea, vomiting

Genitourinary: Decreased urine output, azotemia

Neuromuscular & skeletal: Piloerection

Respiratory: Dyspnea

Overdosage Symptoms of overdose include severe hypertension, cardiac arrhythmias, acute renal failure

Toxicology Reduce rate of administration or discontinue infusion until condition stabilizes

Drug Interactions

Decreased effect: Tricyclic antidepressants

Increased effect/toxicity: MAO inhibitors, alpha- and beta-adrenergic blockers, general anesthetics, phenytoin

Stability Do not mix with alkaline solutions (bicarbonate); protect from light; do **not** use if solution is discolored

Stability of parenteral admixture at room temperature (25°C): 2 days (prepared); manufacturer's expiration date (premixed)

Stability of parenteral admixture at refrigeration temperature (4°C): 7 days (prepared)

Mechanism of Action Stimulates both adrenergic and dopaminergic receptors, lower doses are mainly dopaminergic stimulating and produces renal and mesenteric vasodilation, higher doses stimulate both dopaminergic and beta$_1$-adrenergic and produces cardiac stimulation and renal vasodilation, large doses stimulate alpha-adrenergic receptors

Pharmacodynamics

Onset of action: 5 minutes upon administration

Duration of action: <10 minutes

Pharmacokinetics

Metabolism: In plasma, kidneys, and liver 75% to inactive metabolites by monoamine oxidase and 25% to norepinephrine (active)

Half-life: 2 minutes

Elimination: In urine; clearance is more prolonged with combined hepatic and renal dysfunction

Usual Dosage I.V. infusion:

Geriatrics and Adults: 1 mcg/kg/minute up to 50 mcg/kg/minute, titrate to desired response; administer with an infusion device to control flow rate

If dosages >20-30 mcg/kg/minute are needed, a more direct-acting pressor may be more beneficial (ie, epinephrine, norepinephrine)

The hemodynamic effects of dopamine are dose-dependent:

Low dose: 1-5 mcg/kg/minute, increased renal blood flow and urine output

Intermediate dose: 5-15 mcg/kg/minute, increased renal blood flow, heart rate, cardiac contractility, and cardiac output

High dose: >15 mcg/kg/minute, alpha-adrenergic effects begin to predominate, vasoconstriction, increased blood pressure

Administration Administer into large vein to prevent the possibility of extravasation; monitor continuously for free flow; use infusion device to control rate of flow; add 200-400 mg to 250-500 mL of D$_5$W, NS, D$_5$NS, D$_5$½NS, D$_5$LR, LR, or Normosol® to dilute

Monitoring Parameters Urine output, cardiac hemodynamic status, blood pressure, EKG, pulse

Nursing Implications When discontinuing the infusion, gradually decrease the dose of dopamine

Additional Information Important: Antidote for peripheral ischemia: To prevent sloughing and necrosis in ischemic areas, the area should be infiltrated as soon as possible with 10-15 mL of saline solution containing from 5-10 mg of Regitine® (brand of phentolamine), an adrenergic blocking agent. A syringe with a fine hypodermic needle should be used, and the solution liberally infiltrated throughout the ischemic area. Sympathetic blockade with phentolamine causes immediate and conspicuous local hyperemic changes if the area is infiltrated within 12 hours. Therefore, phentolamine should be given as soon as possible after the extravasation is noted.

Special Geriatric Considerations Has not been specifically studied in the elderly; monitor closely, especially due to increase in cardiovascular disease with age

(Continued)

Dopamine *(Continued)*

Dosage Forms

Dopamine hydrochloride:

Infusion: 0.8 mg/mL in D_5W (250 mL, 500 mL); 1.6 mg/mL in D_5W (250 mL, 500 mL); 3.2 mg/mL in D_5W (250 mL, 500 mL)

Injection: 40 mg/mL (5 mL, 10 mL, 20 mL); 80 mg/mL (5 mL, 20 mL); 160 mg/mL (5 mL)

Dopar® *see* Levodopa *on page 530*

Dopram® Injection *see* Doxapram *on next page*

Doral® *see* Quazepam *on page 808*

Dorcol® [OTC] *see* Acetaminophen *on page 16*

Dormarex® 2 Oral [OTC] *see* Diphenhydramine *on page 302*

Dormin® Oral [OTC] *see* Diphenhydramine *on page 302*

Doryx® Oral *see* Doxycycline *on page 322*

Dorzolamide *(dor ZOLE a mide)*

Related Information

Glaucoma Drug Therapy Comparison *on page 1032*

Brand Names Trusopt®

Therapeutic Category Carbonic Anhydrase Inhibitor

Use Treatment of elevated intraocular pressure in patients with ocular hypertension or open-angle glaucoma

Contraindications Hypersensitivity to any component of the product; contains benzalkonium chloride as a preservative

Warnings Dorzolamide is a sulfonamide and may provoke the same allergic response as other sulfonamides; no information on use in patients with severe renal impairment, hence, its use is not advised in these patients; use with caution in patients with hepatic impairment

Precautions Effects are unknown or have not been studied on corneal endothelium or acute angle glaucoma; concomitant use with oral carbonic anhydrase inhibitors is not recommended; not for use with soft contact lenses

Adverse Reactions

Endocrine & metabolic: Acidosis, electrolyte imbalance

Gastrointestinal: Bitter taste, nausea

Neuromuscular & skeletal: Weakness/fatigue (infrequent)

Ocular: Local burning or stinging, conjunctivitis, blurred vision, tearing, dry eyes, photophobia, superficial punctate keratitis

Toxicology Electrolyte imbalance, acidosis, and CNS effects

Drug Interactions None have been reported; theoretically, agents which are affected by a change in systemic pH (salicylates) or cause electrolyte imbalance are potential interacting agents

Mechanism of Action Topical application inhibits carbonic anhydrase isoenzyme II resulting in the inhibition of bicarbonate in the ciliary body of the eye; the net effect is a decreased production of aqueous humor and a lowering of intraocular pressure (IOP)

Pharmacodynamics

Mean peak decrease in IOP: 2 hours

Mean peak lowering IOP: 18%

Mean trough lowering IOP: 13%

Pharmacokinetics

Absorption: Topical: Reaches the systemic circulation where it accumulates in RBCs during chronic dosing as a result of binding to CA-11

Protein binding: Moderately to plasma proteins (~33%)

Metabolism: Forms a single metabolite which is less potent but also accumulates in RBCs where it binds primarily to CA-1

Half-life: 120 days

Elimination: Dorzolamide and its metabolite (N-desethyl) are excreted in the urine. After dosing is stopped, dorzolamide washes out of RBCs nonlinearly, resulting in a rapid decline of drug concentration initially, followed by a slower elimination phase with a half-life of about 4 months.

Usual Dosage Geriatrics and Adults: Ophthalmic: One drop in eye(s) three times daily

Administration See Patient Information

Monitoring Parameters Ophthalmic exams and IOP periodically

Patient Information May sting on instillation; do not touch dropper to eye; visual acuity may be decreased after administration; distance vision may be altered; assess patient's or caregiver's ability to administer; apply gentle pressure to lacrimal sac during and immediately following instillation (1 minute) to avoid systemic absorption

Nursing Implications Teach patient proper instillation of eye drops

Special Geriatric Considerations The oral carbonic anhydrase inhibitors are useful for patients who have difficulty administering ophthalmic drops, who do not achieve sufficient lowering of IOP, or who cannot tolerate other agents; dorzolamide is an important addition that may be useful in the latter two groups, but with better tolerance than its oral counterpart

Dosage Forms Solution, ophthalmic, as hydrochloride: 2%

References

Biollaz J, Munafo A, Buclin T, et al, "Whole Blood Pharmacokinetics and Metabolic Affects of the Topical Carbonic Anhydrase Inhibitor Dorzolamide," *Eur J Clin Pharmacol*, 1995, 47(5):455-60.

Wilkerson M, Cyrlin M, Lippa EA, et al, "Four-Week Safety and Efficacy Study of Dorzolamide, a Novel, Active, Topical Carbonic Anhydrase Inhibitor," *Arch Ophthalmol*, 1993, 111(10):1343-50.

DOSS *see* Docusate *on page 312*

DOS® Softgel® [OTC] *see* Docusate *on page 312*

Dovonex® *see* Calcipotriene *on page 141*

Doxapram (DOKS a pram)

Brand Names Dopram® Injection

Therapeutic Category Central Nervous System Stimulant, Nonamphetamine; Respiratory Stimulant

Use Respiratory and CNS stimulant; stimulate respiration in patients with drug-induced CNS depression or postanesthesia respiratory depression; in hospitalized patients with COPD associated with acute hypercapnia

Contraindications Hypersensitivity to doxapram or any component; epilepsy, cerebral edema, head injury, severe pulmonary disease, pheochromocytoma, cardiovascular disease, hypertension, hyperthyroidism

Warnings Assure an adequate airway and oxygenation; may only serve as an adjunct therapy in persons with severe respiratory depression

Precautions May cause severe CNS toxicity, seizures

Adverse Reactions

Cardiovascular: Hypertension (dose related), tachycardia, ectopic beats, arrhythmias, hypotension, flushing, feeling of warmth, vasoconstriction

Central nervous system: CNS stimulation, restlessness, lightheadedness, jitters, hallucinations, irritability, seizures, headache, hyperpyrexia

Gastrointestinal: Abdominal distension, nausea, vomiting, retching

Genitourinary: Urinary retention

Hematologic: Hemolysis

Local: Phlebitis

Neuromuscular & skeletal: Hyper-reflexia, bilateral Babinski, tremors

Ocular: Lacrimation, mydriasis

Respiratory: Coughing, laryngospasm, dyspnea

Miscellaneous: Diaphoresis

Overdosage Symptoms of overdose include tachycardia, dyspnea, hypertension

Toxicology Supportive care is the preferred treatment; seizures are unlikely and can be treated with benzodiazepines

Drug Interactions Sympathomimetic drugs and MAO inhibitors may cause significant elevation in blood pressure; doxapram may mask effects of muscle relaxants; halothane, cyclopropane, and enflurane may sensitize the myocardium to catecholamine and epinephrine which is released at the initiation of doxapram, hence, separate discontinuation of anesthetics and start of doxapram by at least 10 minutes

Stability Incompatible with aminophylline, thiopental, or sodium bicarbonate (alkali drugs)

Mechanism of Action Stimulates respiration through action on peripheral carotid chemoreceptors and at higher doses on respiratory center in medulla

Pharmacodynamics

Onset of respiratory stimulation: I.V.: 20-40 seconds

Peak effect: Within 1-2 minutes

Duration: 5-12 minutes

Pharmacokinetics

Metabolism: In the liver

Half-life: Mean: 3.4 hours

Elimination: In urine as metabolites within 24-48 hours

Usual Dosage Geriatrics and Adults: I.V.:

Respiratory depression following anesthesia:

Initial: 0.5-1 mg/kg; may repeat at 5-minute intervals; maximum total dose: 2 mg/kg

(Continued)

Doxapram *(Continued)*

I.V. infusion: Initial: 5 mg/minute until adequate response or adverse effects seen; decrease to 1-3 mg/minute; usual total dose: 0.5-4 mg/kg; maximum: 300 mg

Drug-induced CNS depression: Priming dose of 2 mg/kg and repeat in 5 minutes; repeat every 1-2 hours until patient wakes up; if patient relapses, then resume injections every 1-2 hours until patient awakens or maximum daily dose of 3 g is given

COPD with acute hypercapnia: Start an infusion of 1-2 mg/minute and increase to a maximum of 3 mg/minute

Administration Dilute to 1 mg/mL in D₅W or NS for continuous infusion; rotate infusion site on a regular basis to prevent phlebitis

Monitoring Parameters Blood pressure and deep tendon reflexes; arterial blood gas, respiratory rate

Nursing Implications See Administration

Special Geriatric Considerations Has not been studied in the elderly (see Adverse Reactions and Warnings)

Dosage Forms Injection, as hydrochloride: 20 mg/mL (20 mL)

Doxazosin (doks AYE zoe sin)

Brand Names Cardura®

Generic Available No

Therapeutic Category Alpha-Adrenergic Blocking Agent, Oral

Use Alpha-blocking agent for treatment of hypertension; symptoms of benign prostatic hypertrophy (BPH)

Contraindications Hypersensitivity to doxazosin or any component

Warnings Can cause marked hypotension and syncope with sudden loss of consciousness with the first few doses. Anticipate a similar effect if therapy is interrupted for a few days, if dosage is increased rapidly, or if another antihypertensive drug is introduced.

Precautions Use with caution in patients with renal impairment, patients receiving first dose, or dosage increase of doxazosin

Adverse Reactions

Cardiovascular: Syncope, palpitations, edema, tachycardia

Central nervous system: Dizziness, lightheadedness, drowsiness, headache

Dermatologic: Rash

Gastrointestinal: Nausea, xerostomia

Genitourinary: Polyuria, incontinence

Neuromuscular & skeletal: Weakness

Overdosage Symptoms of overdose include severe hypotension, drowsiness, tachycardia

Toxicology Hypotension usually responds to I.V. fluids or Trendelenburg positioning. If unresponsive to these measures, the use of a parenteral vasoconstrictor may be required (eg, norepinephrine 0.1-0.2 mcg/kg/minute titrated to response). Treatment is primarily supportive and symptomatic.

Drug Interactions Increased effect with other antihypertensive agents

Mechanism of Action Competitively inhibits postsynaptic alpha-adrenergic receptors which results in vasodilation of veins and arterioles and a decrease in total peripheral resistance and blood pressure; in BPH, doxazosin relaxes the smooth muscle of the bladder neck, thus reducing bladder outlet obstruction

Pharmacodynamics

Peak effect: Occurs 2-6 hours after a dose

Duration of effect: 24 hours

Pharmacokinetics Increased age does not significantly affect pharmacokinetics of doxazosin

Protein binding: 98%

Metabolism: Extensive in the liver

Half-life: 22 hours

Time to peak serum concentration: 2-3 hours

Usual Dosage Oral:

Hypertension:

Geriatrics: Initial: 0.5 mg once daily

Adults: 1 mg once daily, may be increased to 2 mg once daily thereafter up to 16 mg if needed

Benign prostatic hypertrophy: Geriatrics and Adults: Initial: 1 mg once daily increasing every 1-2 weeks as necessary to a maximum of 8 mg/day

Monitoring Parameters Blood pressure, standing and sitting/supine, urinary symptoms

Patient Information Rise from sitting/lying carefully; may cause dizziness; take the first dose at bedtime

Nursing Implications Syncope may occur, usually within 90 minutes of the initial dose

Additional Information First-dose hypotension occurs less frequently with doxazosin as compared to prazosin; this may be due to its slower onset of action

Special Geriatric Considerations Adverse reactions such as dry mouth and urinary problems can be particularly bothersome in the elderly (see Warnings)

Dosage Forms Tablet: 1 mg, 2 mg, 4 mg, 8 mg

Doxepin (DOKS e pin)

Related Information

Antidepressant Agents Comparison *on page 1021*
Antidepressant Medication Guidelines *on page 1075*
Federal OBRA Regulations Recommended Maximum Doses - Antidepressants *on page 1056*

Brand Names Adapin® Oral; Sinequan® Oral; Zonalon® Topical Cream

Generic Available Yes

Therapeutic Category Antianxiety Agent; Antidepressant, Tricyclic

Use Treatment of various forms of depression, usually in conjunction with psychotherapy; treatment of anxiety disorders; analgesic for certain chronic and neuropathic pain

Unlabeled use: Peptic ulcer disease, chronic urticaria, angioedema, and nocturnal pruritus

Topical: Short-term (<8 days) management of moderate pruritus in adults with atopic dermatitis or lichen simplex chronicus

Contraindications Hypersensitivity to doxepin or any component (cross-sensitivity with other tricyclic antidepressants may occur); narrow-angle glaucoma

Warnings Do not discontinue abruptly in patients receiving chronic high dose therapy

Precautions Use with caution in patients with cardiovascular disease, conduction disturbances, seizure disorders, urinary retention, hyperthyroidism or those receiving thyroid replacement; an EKG prior to the start of therapy is advised

Adverse Reactions Pronounced sedation and anticholinergic adverse effects may occur

Cardiovascular: Hypotension, arrhythmias
Central nervous system: Sedation, confusion, dizziness, delirium
Dermatologic: Photosensitivity
Endocrine & metabolic: SIADH
Gastrointestinal: Constipation, nausea, vomiting, xerostomia, weight gain
Genitourinary: Urinary retention
Hematologic: Blood dyscrasias
Hepatic: Hepatitis
Neuromuscular & skeletal: Associated with falls
Ocular: Blurred vision, increased intraocular pressure
Otic: Tinnitus
Miscellaneous: Hypersensitivity

Overdosage Symptoms of overdose include confusion, hallucinations, seizure, urinary retention, hypothermia, hypotension, tachycardia, cyanosis

Toxicology Following initiation of essential overdose management, toxic symptoms should be treated. Ventricular arrhythmias often respond to phenytoin 15-20 mg/kg with concurrent systemic alkalinization (sodium bicarbonate 0.5-2 mEq/kg I.V.). Arrhythmias unresponsive to this therapy may respond to lidocaine 1 mg/kg I.V. followed by a titrated infusion. Physostigmine (1-2 mg I.V. slowly) may be indicated in reversing cardiac arrhythmias that are due to vagal blockade or for anticholinergic effects. Seizures usually respond to diazepam I.V. boluses (5-10 mg, up to 30 mg). If seizures are unresponsive or recur, phenytoin or phenobarbital may be required.

Drug Interactions

Decreased effect of bretylium, guanethidine, clonidine, levodopa; decreased effect with ascorbic acid, cholestyramine

Increased effect/toxicity of carbamazepine, amphetamines, thyroid preparations, sympathomimetics

Increased toxicity with fluoxetine (seizures), thyroid preparations, MAO inhibitors, albuterol, CNS depressants (ie, benzodiazepines, opiate analgesics, phenothiazines, alcohol), anticholinergics, cimetidine

Stability Protect from light

(Continued)

Doxepin *(Continued)*

Mechanism of Action Traditionally believed to increase the synaptic concentration of serotonin and/or norepinephrine in the central nervous system by inhibition of their reuptake by the presynaptic neuronal membrane. However, additional receptor effects have been found including desensitization of adenyl cyclase, down regulation of beta-adrenergic receptors, and down regulation of serotonin receptors.

Pharmacodynamics Maximum antidepressant effects usually occur after more than 2 weeks; anxiolytic effects may occur sooner; 5-HT >NE

Pharmacokinetics

Protein binding: 80% to 85%

Metabolism: Hepatically to metabolites, including desmethyldoxepin (active)

Half-life: 6-8 hours

Elimination: Renal

Usual Dosage Oral:

Geriatrics: Initial: 10-25 mg at bedtime; increase by 10-25 mg every 3 days for inpatients and weekly for outpatients if tolerated; rarely does the maximum dose required exceed 75 mg/day; a single bedtime dose is recommended

Adults: Initial: 30-150 mg/day at bedtime or in 2-3 divided doses; may increase up to 300 mg/day; single dose should not exceed 150 mg; select patients may respond to 25-50 mg/day

Chronic urticaria, angioedema, nocturnal pruritus: 10-30 mg/day

Topical: Apply in a thin film 4 times/day

Dosing adjustment in hepatic impairment: Use a lower dose and adjust gradually

Monitoring Parameters Improvement of depressive symptoms; blood pressure, pulse; may need to use serum concentrations to help monitor response

Reference Range Therapeutic: >110 ng/mL for sum of doxepin and desmethyl-doxepin; Toxic: >500 ng/mL

Test Interactions Elevated glucose

Patient Information Avoid unnecessary exposure to sunlight; avoid alcohol ingestion; do not discontinue medication abruptly; may cause urine to turn blue-green; may cause drowsiness, dry mouth, sedation, urinary retention, blurred vision; rise slowly to prevent dizziness

Nursing Implications Monitor sitting and standing blood pressure and pulse rate prior to and during initial therapy; evaluate mental status; monitor weight, may increase appetite

Additional Information Entire daily dose may be given at bedtime; avoid unnecessary exposure to sunlight

Special Geriatric Considerations Preferred agent when sedation is a desired property; less anticholinergic than amitriptyline and less orthostatic hypotension than imipramine. The pharmacokinetics of doxepin have not been studied in older patients. Data from a clinical trial comparing fluoxetine to tricyclics suggest that fluoxetine is significantly less effective than nortriptyline in hospitalized elderly patients with unipolar major affective disorder, especially those with melancholia and concurrent cardiovascular disease.

Dosage Forms

Capsule, as hydrochloride: 10 mg, 25 mg, 50 mg, 75 mg, 100 mg, 150 mg

Concentrate, oral, as hydrochloride: 10 mg/mL (120 mL)

Cream: 5% (30 g)

References

Lakshmanan M, Mion LC, and Frengley JD, "Effective Low Dose Tricyclic Antidepressant Treatment for Depressed Geriatric Rehabilitation Patients. A Double-Blind Study," *J Am Geriatr Soc*, 1986, 34(6):421-6.

Roose SP, Glassman AH, Attia E, et al, "Comparative Efficacy of Selective Serotonin Reuptake Inhibitors and Tricyclics in the Treatment of Melancholia," *Am J Psychiatry*, 1994, 151(12):1735-9.

Doxychel® Injection *see* Doxycycline *on this page*

Doxychel® Oral *see* Doxycycline *on this page*

Doxycycline *(doks i SYE kleen)*

Related Information

I.V. Medication Recommendations *on page 1080*

Brand Names Bio-Tab® Oral; Doryx® Oral; Doxychel® Injection; Doxychel® Oral; Doxy® Oral; Monodox® Oral; Vibramycin® Injection; Vibramycin® Oral; Vibra-Tabs®

Generic Available Yes

Therapeutic Category Antibiotic, Tetracycline Derivative

Use Principally in the treatment of infections caused by susceptible *Rickettsia*, *Chlamydia*, and *Mycoplasma* along with uncommon susceptible gram-negative and gram-positive organisms

Unlabeled use: Treatment for syphilis in penicillin allergic patients or traveler's diarrhea

Contraindications Hypersensitivity to doxycycline, tetracycline, or any component; severe hepatic dysfunction

Warnings Photosensitivity reaction may occur with this drug; avoid prolonged exposure to sunlight or tanning equipment

Precautions Prolonged use may result in superinfection

Adverse Reactions

Central nervous system: Increased intracranial pressure

Dermatologic: Rash, photosensitivity

Gastrointestinal: Nausea, diarrhea, esophagitis

Hematologic: Neutropenia, eosinophilia

Hepatic: Hepatotoxicity

Local: Phlebitis

Overdosage Symptoms of overdose include photosensitivity, nausea, anorexia, diarrhea

Toxicology Following GI decontamination, supportive care only; fluid support may be required for hypotension

Drug Interactions

Antacids containing aluminum, calcium or magnesium, iron and bismuth subsalicylate may decrease doxycycline bioavailability

Barbiturates, phenytoin, and carbamazepine decrease doxycycline's half-life

Effects of warfarin may be increased

Digoxin concentrations may be increased in selected individuals

May increase effects of insulin

Stability Tetracyclines form toxic products when outdated or when exposed to light, heat, or humidity; reconstituted solution is stable for 72 hours (refrigerated); for I.V. infusion in NS or D_5W solution, complete infusion should be completed within 12 hours; discard remaining solution

Mechanism of Action Inhibits protein synthesis by binding with the 30S and possibly the 50S ribosomal subunits of susceptible bacteria; may also cause alterations in the cytoplasmic membrane

Pharmacokinetics

Absorption: Almost completely from GI tract; can be reduced by food or milk by 20%

Protein binding: 90%

Metabolism: Not metabolized in the liver, instead partially inactivated in GI tract by chelate formation

Half-life: 12-15 hours (usually increases to 22-24 hours with multiple dosing); may be slightly increased and serum and tissue concentrations have been reported to be higher in the elderly

Time to peak serum concentration: Within 1.5-4 hours

Elimination: Urine (23%), feces (30%)

Usual Dosage Geriatrics and Adults: Oral, I.V.: 100-200 mg/day in 1-2 divided doses

Sclerosing agent for pleural effusion injection: 500 mg as a single dose in 30-50 mL of NS or SWI

Not dialyzable (0% to 5%)

Administration Infuse I.V. doxycycline over 1 hour; do not administer with antacids, iron products, or dairy products when administering orally

Monitoring Parameters Signs and symptoms of infection including mental status; blood glucose in diabetics

Test Interactions False-negative urine glucose using Clinistix®, Tes-Tape®

Patient Information Avoid unnecessary exposure to sunlight; do not take with antacids, iron products, or dairy products; complete full course of therapy

Nursing Implications See Administration

Additional Information

Doxycycline hyclate: Oral suspension

Doxycycline monohydrate: Capsule, tablet, and injection

Special Geriatric Considerations Dose adjustment for renal function is not necessary (see Pharmacokinetics)

Dosage Forms

Doxycycline hycalate:

Capsule: 50 mg, 100 mg

Capsule, coated pellets: 100 mg

Injection: 100 mg, 200 mg

Tablet: hyclate: 50 mg, 100 mg

(Continued)

Doxycycline (Continued)

Suspension, as monohydrate: 25 mg/5 mL (60 mL)
Syrup, as calcium: 50 mg/5 mL (30 mL, 473 mL)

References

Böcker R, Mühlberg W, Platt D, et al, "Serum Level, Half-Life and Apparent Volume of Distribution of Doxycycline in Geriatric Patients," *Eur J Clin Pharmacol*, 1986, 30(1):105-8.

Ljungberg B and Nilsson-Ehle I, "Pharmacokinetics of Antimicrobial Agents in the Elderly," *Rev Infect Dis*, 1987, 9(2):250-64.

Doxy®️ Oral *see* Doxycycline *on page 322*

DPA *see* Valproic Acid and Derivatives *on page 977*

DPE *see* Dipivefrin *on page 306*

D-Penicillamine *see* Penicillamine *on page 719*

DPH *see* Phenytoin *on page 742*

Dramamine®️ II [OTC] *see* Meclizine *on page 574*

Dramamine®️ Oral [OTC] *see* Dimenhydrinate *on page 300*

Dramilin®️ Injection *see* Dimenhydrinate *on page 300*

Dramoject®️ Injection *see* Dimenhydrinate *on page 300*

Drisdol®️ Oral *see* Ergocalciferol *on page 340*

Dristan®️ Long Lasting Nasal Solution [OTC] *see* Oxymetazoline *on page 706*

Dristan®️ Saline Spray [OTC] *see* Sodium Chloride *on page 860*

Drixoral®️ Cough Liquid Caps [OTC] *see* Dextromethorphan *on page 278*

Drixoral®️ Non-Drowsy [OTC] *see* Pseudoephedrine *on page 802*

Droperidol (droe PER i dole)

Related Information

I.V. Push Recommended Guidelines *on page 1083*

Brand Names Inapsine®️

Generic Available Yes

Therapeutic Category Antiemetic; Antipsychotic Agent; Neuroleptic Agent

Use Tranquilizer and antiemetic in surgical and diagnostic procedures; antiemetic for cancer chemotherapy; preoperative medication

Contraindications Hypersensitivity to droperidol or any component of droperidol; since this is a butyrophenone derivative, caution should be used in patients with a hypersensitivity to haloperidol

Warnings

Tardive dyskinesia: Prevalence rate may be 40% in elderly; elderly women especially at risk; embarrassment from dyskinesias may lead to greater social isolation; development of the syndrome and the irreversible nature are proportional to duration and total cumulative dose over time. May be reversible if diagnosed early in therapy; intermittent use of antipsychotics (not proven use) helps decrease total cumulative dose.

EPS: Extrapyramidal reactions are more common in elderly with up to 50% developing these reactions after age 60. These reactions may be more common in dementia patients. Drug-induced **Parkinson's syndrome** occurs often. Discontinuation usually resolves symptoms but may take weeks to months (12+) to clear. **Akathisia** is the most common EPS reaction in elderly. The symptoms of motor restlessness are difficult to diagnose in demented elderly; increased nervousness, assertiveness, restlessness with constant movement may indicate this adverse event. Consider decreasing dose if antipsychotic to treat as well as diagnose problem; usually see this reaction within 2-3 months of initiating antipsychotic drug.

Anticholinergic effects: These side effects most common with low potency antipsychotics (eg, thioridazine, chlorpromazine). CNS toxicity occurs more frequently and severely in elderly; increased confusion, memory loss, psychotic behavior, and agitation frequently occur as a consequence of anticholinergic effects to antipsychotic agents. Peripheral anticholinergic action troublesome to elderly; most peripheral anticholinergic effects last only 2-3 weeks (see Adverse Reactions).

Orthostatic hypotension: More common with low potency agents (eg, thioridazine, chlorpromazine, and clozapine) but of concern with all antipsychotic agents; orthostasis due to alpha-receptor blockade by antipsychotic agents. Elderly present many risk factors for orthostatic hypotension: blunted baroreceptor reflexes, decreased vascular tone, decreased vascular volume, and possible presence of cardiac diseases which result in decreased cardiac output.

Sedation: Common side effect with antipsychotic therapy; should not be used as a hypnotic unless insomnia is associated with target behavior symptoms treated with antipsychotic medications (see Special Geriatric Considerations). Anecdotal reports suggesting antipsychotic sedation in nonpsychotic patients is extremely unpleasant due to feelings of depersonalization, derealization, and dysphoria. Due to the long duration of action with antipsychotic drugs, these reactions may last up to 24 hours and result in decreased daytime function.

Cardiac toxicity: Life-threatening arrhythmias have occurred at therapeutic doses of antipsychotics. Thioridazine more commonly demonstrates EKG changes than other antipsychotics; suggested to use high potency antipsychotic agents (ie, haloperidol) in patients with cardiac conduction defects.

Precautions May cause severe hypotension; use with caution in patients with hepatic or renal insufficiency; watch for hypotension when administering I.M. or I.V.; use with caution in patients with cardiovascular disease, seizures, and Parkinson's disease; benefits of therapy must be weighed against risks of therapy

Adverse Reactions

Cardiovascular: Hypotension, tachycardia

Central nervous system: Dystonic reactions, akathisia, anxiety, hyperactivity, drowsiness, dizziness, hallucinations, chills

Ocular: Oculogyric crisis

Respiratory: Laryngospasm, bronchospasm, respiratory depression

Overdosage Symptoms of overdose include hypotension, tachycardia, hallucinations, extrapyramidal symptoms; administer O_2 if hypoventilation or apnea present; assist respiratory function as needed; maintain fluid intake; maintain body warmth; observe for 24 hours (see Toxicology)

Toxicology Following initiation of essential overdose management, toxic symptom treatment and supportive treatment should be initiated. Hypotension usually responds to I.V. fluids or Trendelenburg positioning. If unresponsive to these measures the use of a parenteral inotrope may be required (eg, norepinephrine 0.1-0.2 mcg/kg/minute titrated to response). Do not use epinephrine. Seizures commonly respond to diazepam (I.V. 5-10 mg bolus every 15 minutes if needed up to a total of 30 mg) or to phenytoin or phenobarbital. Also critical cardiac arrhythmias often respond to I.V. phenytoin (15 mg/kg up to 1 g), while other antiarrhythmics can be used. Neuroleptics often cause extrapyramidal symptoms (eg, dystonic reactions) requiring management with diphenhydramine 1-2 mg/kg up to a maximum of 50 mg I.M. or I.V. slow push followed by a maintenance dose for 48-72 hours. When these reactions are unresponsive to diphenhydramine, benztropine mesylate I.V. 1-2 mg may be effective. These agents are generally effective within 2-5 minutes.

Drug Interactions

Other CNS depressants may cause additive effects (CNS, respiratory depression, etc)

Droperidol plus fentanyl or other other analgesics may increase blood pressure

Induction anesthesia may increase hypotension; droperidol plus epinephrine may decrease blood pressure due to alpha-adrenergic blockade effects of droperidol

Stability Stable in D_5W for injection; 0.9% sodium chloride for injection and lactated Ringer's for injection for 7-10 days in glass bottles and 7 days for plastic bags

Mechanism of Action Alters the action of dopamine in the CNS, at subcortical levels, to produce sedation; produces mild alpha-adrenergic blockade resulting in decreased peripheral blood pressure and possibly pulmonary artery pressure; may reduce epinephrine-induced arrhythmias

Pharmacodynamics

Onset of action: I.M., I.V.: 3-10 minutes

Peak effect: Parenteral: Within 30 minutes

Duration: 2-4 hours (may extend to 12 hours)

Pharmacokinetics

Metabolism: In the liver

Half-life: 2.3 hours

Elimination: In urine (75%) and feces (22%); ~1% excreted in urine unchanged

Usual Dosage

Geriatrics: Elderly patients should be started on lowest dose recommendations for adults; titrate carefully to desired effect

Adults:

Premedication: I.M.: 2.5-10 mg 30 minutes to 1 hour preoperatively

Adjunct to general anesthesia: I.V. induction: 0.22-0.275 mg/kg; maintenance: 1.25-2.5 mg/dose

Alone in diagnostic procedures: I.M.: Initial: 2.5-10 mg 30 minutes to 1 hour before; then 1.25-2.5 mg if needed

Nausea and vomiting: I.M., I.V.: 2.5-5 mg/dose every 3-4 hours as needed

Monitoring Parameters Monitor blood pressure, respiratory rate; observe for dystonias, extrapyramidal side effects, and temperature changes

Nursing Implications Administration recommendations for all doses: I.V.: Over 2-5 minutes (see Monitoring Parameters)

Additional Information Has good antiemetic effect as well as sedative and anti-anxiety effects

Special Geriatric Considerations See Warnings.

Many elderly patients receive antipsychotic medications for inappropriate nonpsychotic behavior although the use of droperidol is seldom used for this indication. Before initiating antipsychotic medication, the clinician should investigate any possible reversible cause; any stress or stress from any disease can cause

(Continued)

Droperidol *(Continued)*

acute "confusion" or worsening of baseline nonpsychotic behavior. Most commonly acute changes in behavior are due to increases in drug dose or addition of new drug to regimen; fluid electrolyte loss; infections; and changes in environment.

Any changes in disease status in any organ system can result in behavior changes. Care should be exercised with droperidol in that the elderly are more likely to experience adverse effects from the anticholinergic action and are more likely to develop EPS side effects.

Dosage Forms Injection: 2.5 mg/mL (1 mL, 2 mL, 5 mL, 10 mL)

References

Peabody CA, Warner MD, Whiteford HA, et al, "Neuroleptics and the Elderly," *J Am Geriatr Soc,* 1987, 35(3):233-8.

Risse SC and Barnes R, "Pharmacologic Treatment of Agitation Associated With Dementia," *J Am Geriatr Soc,* 1986, 34(5):368-76.

Saltz BL, Woerner MG, Kane JM, et al, "Prospective Study of Tardive Dyskinesia Incidence in the Elderly," *JAMA,* 1991, 266(17):2402-6.

Seifert RD, "Therapeutic Drug Monitoring: Psychotropic Drugs," *J Pharm Pract,* 1984, 6:403-16.

Dr Scholl's Athlete's Foot [OTC] *see* Tolnaftate *on page 939*

Dr Scholl's® Cracked Heel Relief Cream [OTC] *see* Lidocaine *on page 537*

Dr Scholl's® Disk [OTC] *see* Salicylic Acid *on page 845*

Dr Scholl's Maximum Strength Tritin [OTC] *see* Tolnaftate *on page 939*

Dr Scholl's® Wart Remover [OTC] *see* Salicylic Acid *on page 845*

Dry Eyes® Ophthalmic Ointment [OTC] *see* Ocular Lubricant *on page 688*

Dry Eyes® Solution [OTC] *see* Artificial Tears *on page 82*

Dry Eye® Therapy Solution [OTC] *see* Artificial Tears *on page 82*

DSCG *see* Cromolyn Sodium *on page 255*

DSMC Plus® [OTC] *see* Docusate and Casanthranol *on page 313*

DSS *see* Docusate *on page 312*

D-S-S® [OTC] *see* Docusate *on page 312*

DSS With Casanthranol *see* Docusate and Casanthranol *on page 313*

DT *see* Diphtheria and Tetanus Toxoid *on page 305*

Dulcolax® [OTC] *see* Bisacodyl *on page 121*

Dull-C® [OTC] *see* Ascorbic Acid *on page 82*

DuoCet™ *see* Hydrocodone and Acetaminophen *on page 461*

DuoFilm® [OTC] *see* Salicylic Acid *on page 845*

DuoPlant® Gel [OTC] *see* Salicylic Acid *on page 845*

Duo-Trach® *see* Lidocaine *on page 537*

DuP 753 *see* Losartan *on page 553*

Duphalac® *see* Lactulose *on page 523*

Duraclon® Injection *see* Clonidine *on page 238*

Duradyne DHC® *see* Hydrocodone and Acetaminophen *on page 461*

Dura-Estrin® Injection *see* Estradiol *on page 350*

Duragen® Injection *see* Estradiol *on page 350*

Duragesic® Transdermal *see* Fentanyl *on page 374*

Duralone® Injection *see* Methylprednisolone *on page 611*

Duramist Plus® [OTC] *see* Oxymetazoline *on page 706*

Duramorph® Injection *see* Morphine Sulfate *on page 640*

Duratears® Naturale® Ophthalmic Ointment [OTC] *see* Ocular Lubricant *on page 688*

Duratest® Injection *see* Testosterone *on page 895*

Durathate® Injection *see* Testosterone *on page 895*

Duration® Nasal Solution [OTC] *see* Oxymetazoline *on page 706*

Duratuss-G® *see* Guaifenesin *on page 437*

Duricef® *see* Cefadroxil *on page 173*

Durrax® *see* Hydroxyzine *on page 470*

Duvoid® *see* Bethanechol *on page 117*

Dwelle® Ophthalmic Solution [OTC] *see* Artificial Tears *on page 82*

Dyazide® *see* Hydrochlorothiazide and Triamterene *on page 460*

Dycill® *see* Dicloxacillin *on page 284*

Dymelor® *see* Acetohexamide *on page 21*

Dymenate® Injection *see* Dimenhydrinate *on page 300*

Dynabac® *see* Dirithromycin *on page 307*

Dynacin® Oral *see* Minocycline *on page 629*

DynaCirc® *see* Isradipine *on page 508*

Dyna-Hex® Topical [OTC] *see* Chlorhexidine Gluconate *on page 206*
Dynapen® *see* Dicloxacillin *on page 284*
Dyrenium® *see* Triamterene *on page 951*
E2020 *see* Donepezil *on page 315*
Easprin® *see* Aspirin *on page 84*

Echothiophate Iodide (ek oh THYE oh fate EYE oh dide)
Related Information
Glaucoma Drug Therapy Comparison *on page 1032*
Brand Names Phospholine Iodide® Ophthalmic
Synonyms Ecostigmine Iodide
Therapeutic Category Ophthalmic Agent, Miotic
Use Reverse toxic CNS effects caused by anticholinergic drugs; used as miotic in treatment of open-angle glaucoma; may be useful in specific case of narrow-angle glaucoma; accommodative esotropia
Contraindications Hypersensitivity to echothiophate or any component; most cases of angle-closure glaucoma; active uveal inflammation or any inflammatory disease of the iris or ciliary body, glaucoma associated with iridocyclitis; GI or GU obstruction, asthma, diabetes, gangrene
Warnings Tolerance may develop after prolonged use; a rest period restores response to the drug
Adverse Reactions
Dermatologic: Eczematoid dermatitis
Local: Stinging, burning
Ocular: Lacrimation, activation of latent iritis or uveitis may occur, lens opacities, paradoxical increase in intraocular pressure, retinal detachment, vitreous hemorrhage, conjunctival thickening, iris cysts may form, myopia, follicular conjunctivitis
Overdosage Symptoms of overdose include excessive salivation, urinary incontinence, dyspnea, diarrhea, profuse sweating
Toxicology If systemic effects occur, administer parenteral atropine; for severe muscle weakness, pralidoxime may be used in addition to atropine
Drug Interactions Increased toxicity: Carbamate or organophosphate insecticides and pesticides; succinylcholine; systemic acetylcholinesterases may increase neuromuscular effects
Stability Reconstituted solutions remain stable for 30 days at room temperature or 6 months when refrigerated
Mechanism of Action Produces miosis and changes in accommodation by inhibiting cholinesterase, thereby preventing the breakdown of acetylcholine; acetylcholine is therefore allowed to continuously stimulate the iris and ciliary muscles of the eye
Pharmacodynamics
Onset of action: Following ophthalmic instillation, miosis occurs within 10-30 minutes and a decrease in intraocular pressure (IOP) occurs within 4-8 hours
Duration: Miosis and IOP reduction can persist for 1-4 weeks
Usual Dosage Geriatrics and Adults: Ophthalmic:
Glaucoma: Instill 1 drop in affected eye(s) 1-2 times/day (twice daily preferred); some patients may have an adequate response with every other day dosing
Accommodative esotropia:
Diagnosis: Instill 1 drop of 0.125% once daily into both eyes at bedtime for 2-3 weeks
Treatment: Use lowest concentration and frequency which gives satisfactory response, with a maximum dose of 0.125% once daily, although more intensive therapy may be used for short periods of time
Monitoring Parameters Intraocular pressure
Patient Information Be sure of solution expiration date; local irritation and headache may occur; notify physician if abdominal cramps, diarrhea, or salivation occurs; use caution if driving at night or performing hazardous tasks; do not touch dropper to eye; report any change in vision to physician
Nursing Implications Instruct patient on how to administer drops
Special Geriatric Considerations Assess patient's ability to self-administer eye drops
Dosage Forms Solution, ophthalmic: 0.03% = 1.5 mg/5 mL (5 mL) ; 0.06% = 3 mg/5 mL (5 mL); 0.125% = 6.25 mg/5 mL (5 mL); 0.25% = 12.5 mg/5 mL (5 mL)

Econopred® Ophthalmic *see* Prednisolone *on page 774*
Econopred® Plus Ophthalmic *see* Prednisolone *on page 774*
Ecostigmine Iodide *see* Echothiophate Iodide *on this page*
Ecotrin® [OTC] *see* Aspirin *on page 84*
Ecotrin® Low Adult Strength [OTC] *see* Aspirin *on page 84*
Edecrin® *see* Ethacrynic Acid *on page 354*
Edex® Injection *see* Alprostadil *on page 38*

Edrophonium (ed roe FOE nee um)

Brand Names Enlon®; Reversol®; Tensilon®

Generic Available No

Therapeutic Category Antidote, Neuromuscular Blocking Agent; Cholinergic Agent; Diagnostic Agent, Myasthenia Gravis

Use Diagnosis of myasthenia gravis; differentiation of cholinergic crises from myasthenia crises; reversal of nondepolarizing neuromuscular blockers; treatment of paroxysmal atrial tachycardia; adjunct in treating respiratory depression by curare overdosage; **not** indicated for maintenance therapy due to its short duration of action

Contraindications Hypersensitivity to edrophonium or any component, GI or GU obstruction, hypersensitivity to sulfite agents, peritonitis

Warnings Does **not** antagonize and may prolong the phase I block of depolarizing muscle relaxants (eg, succinylcholine); use with caution in patients with epilepsy, asthma, bradycardia, hyperthyroidism, cardiac arrhythmias, or peptic ulcer; adequate facilities should be available for cardiopulmonary resuscitation when testing and adjusting dose for myasthenia gravis; have atropine and epinephrine ready to treat hypersensitivity reactions; overdosage may result in cholinergic crisis, this must be distinguished from myasthenic crisis; anticholinesterase insensitivity can develop for brief or prolonged periods

Precautions Patients may become insensitive to pharmacologic action; this may be brief or prolonged; reduce dose or withhold dose until patient regains sensitivity; monitor respiratory route

Adverse Reactions

Cardiovascular: Bradycardia, A-V block

Central nervous system: Seizures, headache, drowsiness, dysphoria

Gastrointestinal: Nausea, vomiting, diarrhea, excessive salivation, stomach cramps

Genitourinary: Polyuria

Local: Thrombophlebitis

Neuromuscular & skeletal: Weakness, muscle cramps, muscle spasms

Ocular: Small pupils, lacrimation, diplopia, miosis

Respiratory: Increased bronchial secretions, laryngospasm, bronchospasm, respiratory paralysis

Miscellaneous: Diaphoresis (increased), hypersensitivity, hyper-reactive cholinergic responses

Overdosage Symptoms of overdose include muscle weakness, nausea, vomiting, miosis, bronchospasm, respiratory paralysis, blurred vision, excessive sweating, salivation, hypertension

Toxicology Maintain adequate airway; antidote is atropine for muscarinic symptoms; pralidoxime (2-PAM) may also be needed to reverse severe muscle weakness or paralysis; skeletal muscle effects of edrophonium not alleviated by atropine.

Drug Interactions

Decreased effect: Atropine, nondepolarizing muscle relaxants, procainamide, quinidine, magnesium

Increased effect: Succinylcholine, digoxin, I.V. acetazolamide, neostigmine, physostigmine, aminoglycoside, antibiotics

Mechanism of Action Inhibits destruction of acetylcholine by acetylcholinesterase. This facilitates transmission of impulses across myoneural junction and results in increased cholinergic responses such as miosis, increased tonus of intestinal and skeletal muscles, bronchial and ureteral constriction, bradycardia, and increased salivary and sweat gland secretions.

Pharmacodynamics

I.M.:

Onset of effect: Within 2-10 minutes

Duration: 5-30 minutes

I.V.:

Onset of effect: Within 30-60 seconds

Duration: 10 minutes

Pharmacokinetics

Distribution: V_d: 1.1 L/kg

Half-life: 1.8 hours

Usual Dosage Usually administered I.V., however, if not possible, I.M. or S.C. may be used:

Geriatrics and Adults:

Diagnosis:

I.V.: 2 mg test dose administered over 15-30 seconds; 8 mg given 45 seconds later if no response is seen; test dose may be repeated after 30 minutes

I.M.: Initial: 10 mg; if no cholinergic reaction occurs, administer 2 mg 30 minutes later to rule out false-negative reaction

Titration of oral anticholinesterase therapy: 1-2 mg given 1 hour after oral dose of anticholinesterase; if strength improves, an increase in neostigmine or pyridostigmine dose is indicated

Reversal of nondepolarizing neuromuscular blocking agents (neostigmine with atropine usually preferred): I.V.: 10 mg over 30-45 seconds; may repeat every 5-10 minutes up to 40 mg

Termination of paroxysmal atrial tachycardia: I.V. rapid injection: 5-10 mg

Differentiation of cholinergic from myasthenic crisis: I.V.: 1 mg; may repeat after 1 minute. **Note:** Intubation and controlled ventilation may be required if patient has cholinergic crisis

Dosing adjustment in renal impairment: Dose may need to be reduced in patients with chronic renal failure

Administration When giving for reversal of neuromuscular blockade, keep patient well ventilated until recovered

Monitoring Parameters Monitor blood pressure, pulse, respiratory rate; monitor for muscle strength, fasiculations, and side effects (see Adverse Reactions)

Test Interactions ↑ aminotransferase [ALT (SGPT)/AST (SGOT)] (S), amylase (S)

Nursing Implications In the diagnosis of myasthenia gravis, all anticholinesterase medications should be discontinued for at least 8 hours before administering neostigmine; monitor for signs of cholinergic crisis

Special Geriatric Considerations Many elderly will have diseases which may influence the use of edrophonium (see Warnings). Also, many elderly will need doses reduced 50% due to creatinine clearances in the 10-50 mL/minute range (common in the aged); side effects or concomitant disease may warrant use of pyridostigmine.

Dosage Forms Injection, as chloride: 10 mg/mL (1 mL, 10 mL, 15 mL)

References
Rossen RN, Krikorian J, and Hancock EW, "Ventricular Asystole After Edrophonium Chloride Administration," *JAMA*, 1976, 235(10):1041-2.
Youngberg JA, "Cardiac Arrest Following Treatment of Paroxysmal Atrial Tachycardia With Edrophonium," *Anesthesiology*, 1979, 50(3):234-5.

ED-SPAZ® *see* Hyoscyamine *on page 471*

E.E.S.® Oral *see* Erythromycin *on page 344*

Effer-Syllium® [OTC] *see* Psyllium *on page 804*

Effexor® *see* Venlafaxine *on page 984*

Efidac/24® [OTC] *see* Pseudoephedrine *on page 802*

EHDP *see* Etidronate Disodium *on page 362*

Elavil® *see* Amitriptyline *on page 60*

Eldecort® *see* Hydrocortisone *on page 462*

Eldepryl® *see* Selegiline *on page 851*

Eldocort® *see* Hydrocortisone *on page 462*

Elimite™ Cream *see* Permethrin *on page 730*

Elixomin® *see* Theophylline *on page 902*

Elixophyllin® *see* Theophylline *on page 902*

Elocon® *see* Mometasone Furoate *on page 638*

Eltroxin® *see* Levothyroxine *on page 534*

Emete-Con® *see* Benzquinamide Hydrochloride *on page 110*

Emgel™ Topical *see* Erythromycin, Topical *on page 347*

Empirin® [OTC] *see* Aspirin *on page 84*

Empirin® With Codeine *see* Aspirin and Codeine *on page 87*

Emulsoil® [OTC] *see* Castor Oil *on page 171*

E-Mycin® Oral *see* Erythromycin *on page 344*

Enalapril (e NAL a pril)

Related Information

ACE Inhibitors Comparison *on page 1019*

Brand Names Vasotec® I.V.; Vasotec® Oral

Synonyms Enalaprilat

Generic Available No

Therapeutic Category Angiotensin-Converting Enzyme (ACE) Inhibitors

Use Management of hypertension; treatment of systolic congestive heart failure and asymptomatic left ventricular dysfunction; diabetic nephropathy; postmyocardial infarction for prevention of ventricular failure

Unlabeled use: Hypertensive crisis, hypertension secondary to scleroderma renal crisis

Contraindications Hypersensitivity to enalapril, enalaprilat or any component or any ACE inhibitor

Warnings Neutropenia, agranulocytosis, angioedema, decreased renal function (hypertension, renal artery stenosis, congestive heart failure), hepatic dysfunction (activation; elimination; enalapril is a prodrug which requires liver activation; may be inactive in severe liver failure), proteinuria, first-dose hypotension (hypovolemia, congestive heart failure, dehydrated patients at risk, eg, diuretic use, elderly), elderly (due to renal function changes)

Precautions Use with caution and modify dosage in patients with renal impairment (especially renal artery stenosis), hyponatremia, hypovolemia, severe congestive heart failure or with coadministered diuretic therapy; valvular stenosis, hyperkalemia (>5.7 mEq/L), anesthesia

(Continued)

Adverse Reactions

Cardiovascular: Hypotension, syncope, orthostatic hypotension, arrhythmias, tachycardia, atrial fibrillation, bradycardia, cardiac arrest, CVA, myocardial infarction, chest pain, palpitations, angina, vasculitis

Central nervous system: Fatigue, vertigo, insomnia, dizziness, headache, somnolence, ataxia, confusion, depression, nervousness, fever

Dermatologic: Rash, alopecia, urticaria, pemphigus, erythema multiforme, exfoliative dermatitis, flushing, Stevens-Johnson syndrome, photosensitivity, angioedema

Endocrine & metabolic: Hypoglycemia, hyperkalemia

Gastrointestinal: Nausea, ileus, diarrhea, xerostomia, dyspepsia, glossitis, abdominal pain, vomiting, dysgeusia, anorexia, constipation, pancreatitis, ageusia

Genitourinary: Impotence

Hematologic: Agranulocytosis, neutropenia, anemia, eosinophilia, thrombocytopenia

Hepatic: Hepatitis, cholestatic jaundice

Neuromuscular & skeletal: Muscle cramps, myalgia, arthralgia, arthritis, paresthesia, weakness

Ocular: Blurred vision

Otic: Tinnitus

Renal: Deterioration in renal function (20%), especially with renal artery stenosis, oliguria

Respiratory: Chronic cough (nonproductive, persistent; more often in women and seen in 15% to 30% of patients), asthma, bronchitis, bronchospasm, dyspnea, pulmonary embolism

Miscellaneous: Diaphoresis

Overdosage Symptoms of overdose include severe hypotension

Toxicology Following initiation of essential overdose management, toxic symptom treatment and supportive treatment should be initiated. Hypotension usually responds to I.V. fluids or Trendelenburg positioning. If unresponsive to these measures, the use of a parenteral inotrope may be required (eg, norepinephrine 0.1-0.2 mcg/kg/minute titrated to response). Seizures commonly respond to diazepam (I.V. 5-10 mg bolus in adults every 15 minutes if needed up to a total of 30 mg) or to phenytoin or phenobarbital.

Drug Interactions

Hypotensive agent or diuretics may increase hypotensive effect

Enalapril and potassium-sparing diuretics may cause additive hyperkalemic effect

Enalapril and indomethacin or nonsteroidal anti-inflammatory agents may cause reduced antihypertensive response to enalapril

Allopurinol and enalapril may cause neutropenia

Antacids and ACE inhibitors may decrease absorption of ACE inhibitors

Phenothiazines and ACE inhibitors may increase ACE inhibitor effect

Probenecid and ACE inhibitors (enalapril) may increase ACE inhibitors (enalapril) levels

Rifampin and ACE inhibitors (enalapril) may decrease ACE inhibitor effect

Digoxin and ACE inhibitors may increase serum digoxin concentrations

Lithium and ACE inhibitors may increase lithium serum concentration

Tetracycline and ACE inhibitors (enalapril) may decrease tetracycline absorption (up to 37%)

Food decreases enalapril absorption (see Additional Information)

Stability Solutions for I.V. infusion mixed in NS, D_5NS, D_5LR, or D_5W and Isolyte® E are stable for 24 hours at room temperature

Mechanism of Action Competitive inhibitor of angiotensin-converting enzyme (ACE); prevents conversion of angiotensin I to angiotensin II, a potent vasoconstrictor; results in lower levels of angiotensin II which causes an increase in plasma renin activity and a reduction in aldosterone secretion; a CNS mechanism may also be involved in hypotensive effect as angiotensin II increases adrenergic outflow from CNS; vasoactive kallikreins may be decreased in conversion to active hormones by ACE inhibitors, thus reducing blood pressure

Pharmacodynamics

Onset of action: Oral: ~1 hour following administration

Peak effect: 4-8 hours

Duration: 12-24 hours

Pharmacokinetics

Absorption: Oral: 55% to 75% (enalapril)

Protein binding: 50% to 60%

Enalapril is a prodrug and undergoes biotransformation to enalaprilat in the liver

Half-life:

Enalapril: 1-2 hours

Enalapril half-life (CHF): 3.4-5.8 hours

Enalaprilat half-life: 11 hours

Time to peak serum concentrations:

Enalapril: Within 0.5-1.5 hours

Enalaprilat (active): Within 3-4.5 hours

Elimination: Principally in urine (60% to 80%) with some fecal excretion

Usual Dosage Use lower listed initial dose in patients with hyponatremia, hypovolemia, severe congestive heart failure, decreased renal function, or in those receiving diuretics

Geriatrics and Adults:

Oral: **Enalapril:** 2.5-5 mg/day then increase as required in 2.5-5 mg increments at 1- to 2-week intervals; daily dose range is usually 10-40 mg/day in 1-2 divided doses

I.V.: **Enalaprilat:** 0.625-1.25 mg/dose, given over 5 minutes every 6 hours; for conversion from I.V. to oral, administer 2.5 mg orally once daily for those who responded to 0.625 mg I.V. every 6 hours

Asymptomatic left ventricular dysfunction: 2.5 mg twice daily; titrate carefully as tolerated to a recommended 20 mg/day in divided doses

Congestive heart failure: Initial: 2.5 mg once or twice daily; titrate slowly (several weeks) to a "target dose" of 10 mg twice daily; maximum dose: 20 mg twice daily; twice daily dosing is recommended

Dosing interval in renal impairment:
Cl$_{cr}$ 10-50 mL/minute: Administer 75% to 100% of the usual dose
Cl$_{cr}$ <10 mL/minute: Administer 50% of the usual dose
Enalaprilat is dialyzable (62 mL/minute)

Monitoring Parameters Blood pressure, serum potassium concentrations, BUN, serum creatinine, renal function, and WBC

Test Interactions Increased potassium (S); increased serum creatinine/BUN

Patient Information Do not stop therapy except under prescriber advice; notify physician if you develop sore throat, fever, swelling of hands, feet, face, eyes, lips, and tongue; difficult breathing, irregular heartbeats, chest pains, or cough. May cause dizziness, fainting, and lightheadedness, especially in first week of therapy, sit and stand up slowly; may cause changes in taste or rash; do not add a salt substitute (potassium) without advice of physician.

Nursing Implications May cause depression in some patients; discontinue if angioedema of the face, extremities, lips, tongue, or glottis occurs; watch for hypotensive effect within 1-3 hours of first dose or new higher dose (see Precautions, Warnings, Monitoring Parameters, and Special Geriatric Considerations)

Additional Information Severe hypotension may occur in patients who are sodium and/or volume depleted; initiate lower doses and monitor closely when starting therapy in these patients

Special Geriatric Considerations Due to frequent decreases in glomerular filtration (also creatinine clearance) with aging, elderly patients may have exaggerated responses to ACE inhibitors; differences in clinical response due to hepatic changes are not observed. ACE inhibitors may be preferred agents in elderly patients with congestive heart failure and diabetes mellitus. Diabetic proteinuria is reduced and insulin sensitivity is enhanced. In general, the side effect profile is favorable in elderly and causes little or no CNS confusion; use lowest dose recommendations initially; adjust dose for renal function in elderly.

Dosage Forms
Injection, as enalaprilat: 1.25 mg/mL (1 mL, 2 mL)
Tablet, as maleate: 2.5 mg, 5 mg, 10 mg, 20 mg

References

Konstam MA, Drakup K, Baker DW, et al, "Heart Failure: Evaluation and Care of Patients With Left Ventricular Systolic Dysfunction," *Clinical Practice Guideline No 11*, Rockville, MD: Agency for Health Care Policy and Research, Public Health Service, U.S. Department of Health and Human Services, 1994.

McAreavey D and Robertson JIS, "Angiotensin Converting Enzyme Inhibitors and Moderate Hypertension," *Drugs*, 1990, 40(3):326-45.

Williams JF, Bristow MR, Fowler MB, et al, "Guidelines for the Evaluation and Management of Heart Failure: Report of the American College of Cardiology/American Heart Association Task Force on Practice Guidelines (Committee on Evaluation and Management of Heart Failure)," *J Am Coll Cardiol*, 1995, 26:1376-8.

Enalaprilat *see* Enalapril *on page 329*

Endep® *see* Amitriptyline *on page 60*

Ener-B® [OTC] *see* Cyanocobalamin *on page 257*

Engerix-B® *see* Hepatitis B Vaccine *on page 453*

Enhanced-potency Inactivated Poliovirus Vaccine *see* Poliovirus Vaccine, Inactivated *on page 761*

Enlon® *see* Edrophonium *on page 328*

Enovil® *see* Amitriptyline *on page 60*

Encainide (en KAY nide)

Brand Names Enkaid®

Generic Available No

Therapeutic Category Antiarrhythmic Agent, Class I-C

Use Life-threatening sustained ventricular arrhythmias. **Note:** Manufacturer has withdrawn from market due to implications of CAST study; however, the drug is available for those who responded to it and physician does not believe a substitution should occur (contact Bristol-Myers-Squibb 1-800-332-2056). See Additional Information.

Contraindications Hypersensitivity to encainide or any component; second or third degree A-V block; premature ventricular complexes; symptomatic nonsustained ventricular arrhythmias; cardiogenic shock

(Continued)

Encainide *(Continued)*

Warnings Can worsen existing arrhythmias; such proarrhythmic effects range from an increase in frequency of PVCs to the development of more severe ventricular tachycardia (ie, tachycardia that is more sustained or more resistant to conversion to sinus rhythm), with potentially fatal consequences; may aggravate or cause congestive heart failure; electrolyte abnormalities alter drug response, therefore, correct any electrolyte abnormalities prior to therapy; use with caution in patients with sick sinus syndrome, and renal and hepatic dysfunction (caution when Cl_{cr} <20 mL/minute); see note under Use

Precautions Use with caution in patients with a history of congestive heart failure or myocardial dysfunction; use is recommended only on patients with life-threatening arrhythmias

Adverse Reactions
Cardiovascular: Arrhythmogenic effects range from an increased frequency of ventricular premature complexes (VPCs) to the development of new and/or more severe and potentially fatal ventricular tachyarrhythmias (~10% of patients); bradycardia, first degree A-V block; negative inotropic effect, chest pain, congestive heart failure, palpitations, peripheral edema
Central nervous system: Dizziness, headache, insomnia, nervousness, somnolence
Dermatologic: Rash
Gastrointestinal: Abdominal pain, constipation, nausea, vomiting, diarrhea, xerostomia, dyspepsia, anorexia
Neuromuscular & skeletal: Generalized pain, tremors
Ocular: Visual disturbances (blurred vision)
Respiratory: Cough, dyspnea

Overdosage Symptoms of overdose include second or third degree A-V block, sinus arrest, hypotension, convulsions, widening of QRS complex

Toxicology Cardiac dysrhythmias and hypotension often respond to bolus I.V. injections of hypertonic sodium bicarbonate 1-2 mEq/kg, while conventional type IA antiarrhythmics tend to worsen conduction defects, especially ventricular arrhythmias. In those patients displaying seizures along with conduction defects, phenytoin may be most effective in reducing these symptoms.

Mechanism of Action Encainide is a class IC agent that blocks the sodium channel of the Purkinje fibers

Pharmacokinetics
Metabolism: Extensively metabolized in the liver to two active metabolites, o-dimethyl encainide (ODE) and 3-methoxy-o-dimethyl encainide (MODE)
Half-life: 1-2.7 hours; ODE: 3-4 hours; MODE: 6-12 hours
Elimination: In urine and bile

Usual Dosage Geriatrics and Adults: Oral (hospitalization is necessary to initiate therapy): 25 mg every 8 hours; may increase to 35 mg every 8 hours after 3-5 days if needed; increase to 50 mg every 8 hours in another 3-5 days if response is not achieved

Monitoring Parameters EKG, heart rate, blood pressure

Additional Information Based on adverse outcomes noted with encainide in the CAST trial, the FDA recommends that use of encainide be limited to patients with life-threatening ventricular arrhythmias

Special Geriatric Considerations Prolonged half-life of the two active metabolites ODE and MODE; consider age changes in renal and hepatic function since this may alter clearance (see Warnings)

Dosage Forms Capsule, as hydrochloride: 25 mg, 35 mg, 50 mg

Enoxacin *(en OKS a sin)*

Related Information
Antacid Drug Interactions *on page 1096*

Brand Names Penetrex™ Oral

Generic Available No

Therapeutic Category Antibiotic, Quinolone

Use Complicated and uncomplicated urinary tract infections caused by susceptible gram-negative and gram-positive bacteria; uncomplicated urethral or cervical gonorrhea

Contraindications Hypersensitivity to enoxacin, the fluoroquinolones, or the quinolone group

Warnings Prolonged use may result in superinfection, including pseudomembranous colitis; use with caution in patients with seizure disorders or renal impairment; not effective for syphilis, may mask signs or symptoms and patients treated for gonorrhea should have serologic testing in 3 months

Precautions Modify dosage in patients with renal insufficiency; CNS stimulation may occur and manifest as tremor, restlessness, confusion, and very rarely seizures. Use with caution in patients with known or suspected CNS disorders; phototoxicity (patients may need sunglasses)

Adverse Reactions

Central nervous system: Restlessness, dizziness, confusion, seizures, headache, confusion, depersonalization, hypertonia, seizures

Dermatologic: Rash, photosensitivity

Gastrointestinal: Nausea, diarrhea, vomiting, GI bleeding, anorexia, pseudomembranous colitis

Genitourinary: Vaginitis

Hematologic: Anemia

Hepatic: Increased liver enzymes

Neuromuscular & skeletal: Arthralgia, myalgia, tremors

Renal: Acute renal failure

Overdosage Symptoms of overdose include acute renal failure, seizures

Toxicology GI decontamination and supportive care; for acute overdose, empty stomach contents by inducing vomiting or gastric lavage; observe and treat the patient symptomatically; maintain fluid status; diazepam for seizures; not removed by peritoneal or hemodialysis

Drug Interactions

Antacids, iron salts, sucralfate, and zinc salts may reduce absorption if given at the same time

Antineoplastic agents may decrease fluoroquinolone serum concentrations

Bismuth subsalicylate decreased enoxacin's bioavailability

Cimetidine decreased elimination

Probenecid decreased clearance

Caffeine's clearance is reduced

Digoxin serum concentrations may be increased

Anticoagulant effects may be increased

Cyclosporine may increase nephrotoxic effects when used with a quinolone

Decreased theophylline clearance and increased serum concentrations

Mechanism of Action Exerts a broad spectrum antimicrobial effect. The primary target of the fluoroquinolones is DNA gyrase (topoisomerase II) an essential bacterial enzyme that maintains the superhelical structure of DNA. DNA gyrase is required for DNA replication and transcription, DNA repair, recombination, and transposition.

Pharmacodynamics Bactericidal

Pharmacokinetics

Absorption: Peak plasma concentration in 1-3 hours; 98%

Distribution: Concentrations in the cervix, fallopian tube, and myometrium 1-2 times greater than plasma concentrations; renal and prostate concentrations 2-4 times greater than plasma concentrations

Metabolism: 15% to 20% of dose metabolized to 1 of 5 metabolites; inhibits selected cytochrome P-450 isoenzymes resulting in the decreased metabolism of certain drugs (see Drug Interactions)

Elimination: Renal, clearance: 2.28 mL/minute/kg in young adults

Half-life: 7.34 hours

In the elderly, mean peak serum concentrations were 50% greater than younger adults, statistically, a nonsignificant finding. One study found a significantly reduced renal clearance in the elderly, compared to younger adults (1.39 vs 2.28 mL/minute/kg); the mean half-life in older subjects has been reported to be 6.11-7.3 hours which is similar to younger adults. A dosage adjustment is recommended if the patient's estimated Cl_{cr} ≤30 mL/minute/1.73 m^2 (see Usual Dosage).

Usual Dosage Oral:

Geriatrics: Normal adult dose adjusted for renal function

Adults:

Uncomplicated urinary tract infection: 200 mg every 12 hours for 7 days

Complicated urinary tract infection: 400 mg every 12 hours for 14 days

Uncomplicated gonorrhea: 400 mg as a single dose

Dosing adjustment in renal impairment: Cl_{cr} ≤30 mL/minute/1.73 m^2: For all indications, administer normal initial dose, then 1/2 the recommended dose every 12 hours for the prescribed duration

Monitoring Parameters Signs and symptoms of infection (temperature, WBC, mental status, appetite); urinalysis; appropriate cultures and sensitivity; patients receiving concurrent theophylline should have their serum concentrations monitored; patients receiving concurrent warfarin therapy should have their prothrombin time or INR monitored; patients receiving cyclosporine should be monitored for nephrotoxicity

Patient Information Complete full course of therapy; take on empty stomach (1 hour before or 2 hours after meals); drink fluids liberally; warn of potential phototoxicity and sensitivity

(Continued)

Enoxacin *(Continued)*

Nursing Implications Hold antacids for 3-4 hours before or after giving; administer on an empty stomach; encourage fluids

Special Geriatric Considerations Adjust dose for renal function (see Pharmacokinetics and Usual Dosage)

Dosage Forms Tablet: 200 mg, 400 mg

References

Dobbs BR, Gazeley LR, Campbell AJ, et al, "The Effect of Age on the Pharmacokinetics of Enoxacin," *Eur J Clin Pharmacol*, 1987, 33(1):101-4.

Wise R, Baker SL, Misra M, et al, "The Pharmacokinetics of Enoxacin in Elderly Patients," *J Antimicrob Chemother*, 1987, 19(3):343-50.

Enoxaparin *(e noks ah PAIR in)*

Brand Names Lovenox® Injection

Therapeutic Category Anticoagulant

Use Prevention of deep vein thrombosis following hip or knee replacement surgery during and following hospitalization or abdominal surgery in patients at risk for thromboembolic complications; prevention of thromboembolism following knee replacement surgery

Unlabeled use: Treatment of acute proximal deep vein thrombosis

Contraindications Active major bleeding or hemophilia; hypersensitivity to heparin or pork products; drug-induced thrombocytopenia

Warnings Heparin-induced thrombocytopenia, bacterial endocarditis, congenital or acquired bleeding disorders, active ulceration and angiodysplastic gastrointestinal disease, hemorrhagic stroke, status post brain, spinal, or ophthalmological surgery, uncontrolled arterial hypertension, recent CNS surgery, elderly, and lactation. Never administer by intramuscular injection. Conventional heparin has possibly been associated with an increased risk of bleeding in females >60 years of age; it is unknown whether low molecular weight heparins pose the same risk; these agents should be used with caution in this population.

Adverse Reactions

Cardiovascular: Edema

Central nervous system: Confusion

Dermatologic: Bruising, erythema

Hematologic: Hemorrhage, thrombocytopenia, hematoma, hypochromic anemia

Gastrointestinal: Nausea

Hepatic: Asymptomatic increases in liver transaminases (AST, ALT)

Miscellaneous: Local irritation, pain, fever

Overdosage Symptoms of overdose include hemorrhage

Toxicology Protamine zinc has been used to reverse effects

Drug Interactions Increased toxicity with oral anticoagulants, platelet inhibitors

Pharmacodynamics

Peak effect: 3 hours

Duration: 275 minutes

Pharmacokinetics

Half-life: 275 minutes

Elimination: In the kidney

Usual Dosage S.C.:

Geriatrics and Adults: 30 mg within 24 hours of surgery, then twice daily for 7-10 days; 14 days maximum; a single daily dose of 40 mg has also been shown to be safe and effective in prevention of thromboembolism in patients undergoing orthopedic or gynecologic surgical procedures

Treatment of DVT: 1 mg/kg twice daily

Administration S.C. only; do not administer I.M. injection

Monitoring Parameters Periodic CBC including platelets, occult blood, and anti-Xa activity, if available

Nursing Implications See Administration

Special Geriatric Considerations No specific recommendations (see Usual Dosage). Treatment of DVT is not an approved indication, but clinical trials show comparable efficacy to unfractionated heparin.

Dosage Forms Injection, as sodium, preservative free: 30 mg/0.3 mL

References

Levine JM, Gent M, Hirsh J, et al, "A Comparison of Low-Molecular-Weight Heparin Administered Primarily at Home With Unfractionated Heparin Administered in the Hospital for Proximal Deep Vein Thrombosis," *N Engl J Med*, 1996, 334(11):677-81.

Simonneau G, Charbonnier B, Decousus H, et al, "Subcutaneous Low-Molecular-Weight Heparin Compared With Continuous Intravenous Unfractionated Heparin in the Treatment of Proximal Deep Vein Thrombosis," *Arch Intern Med*, 1993, 153(13):1541-6.

Enulose® *see Lactulose on page 523*

Ephedrine (e FED rin)

Brand Names Kondon's Nasal® [OTC]; Pretz-D® [OTC]

Generic Available Yes

Therapeutic Category Adrenergic Agonist Agent; Bronchodilator; Decongestant, Nasal

Use Bronchial asthma; nasal congestion (topical only); acute bronchospasm
  Unlabeled use: Carotid sinus syncope; malignant vasovagal syndrome

Contraindications Hypersensitivity to ephedrine or any component, cardiac arrhythmias, angle-closure glaucoma, patients on other sympathomimetic agents

Warnings Use caution in patients with unstable vasomotor symptoms, diabetes, hyperthyroidism, prostatic hypertrophy, or a history of seizures; also use caution in the elderly and those patients with cardiovascular disorders such as coronary artery disease, arrhythmias, and hypertension. Ephedrine may cause hypertension resulting in intracranial hemorrhage. Long-term use may cause anxiety and symptoms of paranoid schizophrenia.

Adverse Reactions
  Cardiovascular: Tachycardia, palpitations, elevation or depression of blood pressure
  Central nervous system: CNS-stimulating effects, nervousness, anxiety, apprehension, fear, tension, agitation, excitation, restlessness, irritability, insomnia, hyperactivity
  Gastrointestinal: Nausea, anorexia, GI upset
  Genitourinary: Dysuria; urinary retention may occur in men with enlarged prostates
  Neuromuscular & skeletal: Tremors (more common in the elderly), weakness

Overdosage Symptoms of overdose include dysrhythmias, CNS excitation, respiratory depression, vomiting, convulsions

Toxicology There is no specific antidote for ephedrine intoxication and the bulk of the treatment is supportive. Hyperactivity and agitation usually respond to reduced sensory input, however with extreme agitation, haloperidol may be required. Hyperthermia is best treated with external cooling measures, or when severe or unresponsive, muscle paralysis with pancuronium may be needed. Hypertension is usually transient and generally does not require treatment unless severe. For diastolic blood pressures >110 mm Hg, a nitroprusside infusion should be initiated. Seizures usually respond to diazepam I.V. and/or phenytoin maintenance regimens.

Drug Interactions
  Decreased effect of guanethidine; decreased effect with alpha-blockers, beta-blockers, methyldopa, reserpine
  Increased effect/toxicity with acetazolamide, sympathomimetics, theophylline, MAO inhibitors (increased blood pressure), atropine (increased blood pressure), digoxin, general anesthetics, albuterol, sodium bicarbonate

Stability Protect all dosage forms from light

Mechanism of Action Releases tissue stores of epinephrine and thereby produces an alpha- and beta-adrenergic stimulation. It is longer-acting but less potent than epinephrine.

Pharmacodynamics
  Onset of bronchodilation: Oral: 15-60 minutes
  Duration: 3-6 hours

Pharmacokinetics
  Metabolism: Little hepatic metabolism
  Half-life: 3-6 hours
  Elimination: 60% to 77% of dose excreted as unchanged drug in urine within 24 hours; renal excretion is dependent on urine pH; decreased excretion with alkaline urine

Usual Dosage
  Adults:
    I.M., S.C.: 25-50 mg
    I.V.: 10-25 mg slow I.V. push; repeat every 5-10 minutes, not to exceed 150 mg/24 hours
    Topical: Nasal congestion: Dosage is product specific

Monitoring Parameters Blood pressure, pulse, mental status

Patient Information May cause wakefulness or nervousness; available over-the-counter, but elderly patients should consult physician before using

Nursing Implications Protect from light; do not administer unless solution is clear; monitor mental status, vital signs
(Continued)

Ephedrine *(Continued)*

Additional Information Ephedrine is generally not used as a bronchodilator since newer beta₂-specific agents are less toxic

Special Geriatric Considerations Oral formulation was recently removed from the market; avoid as a bronchodilator. Use caution since it crosses the blood-brain barrier and may cause confusion (see Warnings, Adverse Reactions)

Dosage Forms

Ephedrine sulfate:
Capsule: 25 mg, 50 mg
Injection: 25 mg/mL (1 mL); 50 mg/mL (1 mL, 10 mL)
Spray (Pretz-D®): 0.25% (15 mL)
Jelly, as alkaloid (Kondon's Nasal®): 1% (20 g)

Epifrin® *see Epinephrine on this page*

E-Pilo-x® Ophthalmic *see Pilocarpine and Epinephrine on page 749*

Epinephrine (ep i NEF rin)

Related Information

Asthma Guidelines *on page 1040*
Glaucoma Drug Therapy Comparison *on page 1032*
Inhaled Medications Comparison *on page 1034*
I.V. Push Recommended Guidelines *on page 1083*

Brand Names Adrenalin®; AsthmaHaler®; AsthmaNefrin® [OTC]; Bronitin®; Bronkaid® Mist [OTC]; Epifrin®; EpiPen® Auto-Injector; EpiPen® Jr Auto-Injector; Glaucon®; microNefrin®; Primatene® Mist [OTC]; Sus-Phrine®; Vaponefrin®

Synonyms Adrenaline

Generic Available Yes

Therapeutic Category Adrenergic Agonist Agent; Adrenergic Agonist Agent, Ophthalmic; Antidote, Hypersensitivity Reactions; Bronchodilator; Decongestant, Nasal

Use Bronchospasm; anaphylactic reactions; cardiac arrest; management of open-angle (chronic simple) glaucoma

Contraindications Hypersensitivity to epinephrine or any component; cardiac arrhythmias, angle-closure glaucoma

Precautions Use with caution in geriatric patients, patients with diabetes mellitus or cardiovascular diseases, thyroid disease, or cerebral arteriosclerosis

Adverse Reactions

Cardiovascular: Pallor, tachycardia, hypertension, increased myocardial oxygen consumption, cardiac arrhythmias, sudden death
Central nervous system: Anxiety, headache, insomnia, dizziness
Gastrointestinal: Nausea, vomiting
Neuromuscular & skeletal: Weakness, tremors
Ocular: Precipitation of or exacerbation of narrow-angle glaucoma
Renal: Decreased renal and splanchnic blood flow, acute urinary retention in patients with bladder outflow obstruction
Miscellaneous: Increased diaphoresis

Rapid I.V. infusion may cause death from cerebrovascular hemorrhage or cardiac arrhythmias

Overdosage Symptoms of overdose include hypertension which may result in subarachnoid hemorrhage and hemiplegia; arrhythmias, unusually large pupils, pulmonary edema, renal failure, metabolic acidosis

Toxicology There is no specific antidote for epinephrine intoxication and the bulk of the treatment is supportive. Hyperactivity and agitation usually respond to reduced sensory input, however, with extreme agitation haloperidol may be required. Hyperthermia is best treated with external cooling measures, or when severe or unresponsive, muscle paralysis with pancuronium may be needed. Hypertension is usually transient and generally does not require treatment unless severe. For diastolic blood pressures >110 mm Hg, a nitroprusside infusion should be initiated. Seizures usually respond to diazepam I.V. and/or phenytoin maintenance regimens.

Drug Interactions

Hypertension may occur if administered with beta-blockers, guanethidine, tricyclic antidepressants
Arrhythmias may occur if administered with bretylium, halogenated hydrocarbon anesthetics
Epinephrine decreases the effect of hypoglycemic agents

Stability Protect from light, oxidation turns drug pink, then a brown color; solutions should not be used if they are discolored or contain a precipitate; stability of injection of parenteral admixture at room temperature and refrigeration: 24 hours; do not use D_5W as a diluent; D_5W is incompatible with epinephrine

Mechanism of Action Stimulates alpha-, beta$_1$- and beta$_2$-adrenergic receptors; small doses can cause vasodilation via beta$_2$ vascular receptors; decreases production of aqueous humor and increases aqueous outflow; dilates the pupil by contracting the dilator muscle

Pharmacodynamics

Onset of action:

S.C.: Bronchodilation occurs within 3-5 minutes following administration

Inhalation: Within 1 minute

Following conjunctival instillation, intraocular pressures fall within 1 hour with a maximal response occurring within 4-8 hours

Duration: Ocular effects persist for 12-24 hours; decreased beta-receptor responsiveness has been seen in the elderly

Pharmacokinetics

Absorption: Oral: Degraded in the GI tract and, therefore, is not useful

Metabolism: Following administration, drug is taken up into the adrenergic neuron and metabolized by monoamine oxidase and catechol-o-methyl-transferase, circulating drug is metabolized in the liver

Elimination: Inactive metabolites (metanephrine and the sulfate and hydroxy derivatives of mandelic acid) and a small amount of unchanged drug is excreted in urine

Usual Dosage Geriatrics and Adults:

Bronchodilator: I.M., S.C.: 0.1-0.5 mg every 10-15 minutes; I.V.: 0.1-0.25 mg (single dose maximum: 1 mg)

Nebulizer: Instill 8-15 drops into nebulizer reservoir; administer 1-3 inhalations 4-6 times/day

Cardiac arrest: I.V., intracardiac: 0.1-1 mg every 5 minutes as needed; intratracheal: 1 mg

Hypersensitivity reaction: I.M., S.C.: 0.2-0.5 mg every 20 minutes to 4 hours (single dose maximum: 1 mg)

Ophthalmic: Instill 1-2 drops in eye(s) once or twice daily

Monitoring Parameters Pulmonary function, blood pressure, pulse, intraocular pressure

Reference Range Therapeutic: 31-95 pg/mL (SI: 170-520 pmol/L)

Test Interactions Increased bilirubin (S), catecholamines (U), glucose, uric acid (S)

Patient Information Instruct patient on proper instillation of ophthalmic preparation; after instilling, apply pressure on the side of the nose near the eye to minimize systemic absorption; stinging may occur upon instillation; headache or aching in the brow area may occur

Nursing Implications Protect from light; oxidation turns dark pink, then brown - solutions should not be used if they are discolored or contain a precipitate; epinephrine is unstable in alkaline solution

Additional Information Oral inhalation of epinephrine is **not** the preferred route of administration. Patients should be cautioned to avoid the use of over-the-counter epinephrine inhalation products. Beta$_2$-adrenergic agents for inhalation are preferred.

Epinephrine: Primatene® Mist, Bronkaid® Mist, Sus-Phrine®

Epinephrine bitartrate: AsthmaHaler®, Bronitin®, Epitrate®, Medihaler-Epi®; Primatene® Mist

Epinephrine hydrochloride: Adrenalin®, Epifrin®, EpiPen®, EpiPen® Jr.

Racemic epinephrine: AsthmaHaler®, Breatheasy®, microNefrin®, Vaponefrin®

Epinephryl borate: Epinal®

Special Geriatric Considerations The use of epinephrine in the treatment of acute exacerbations of asthma was studied in older adults. A dose of 0.3 mg S.C. every 20 minutes for three doses was well tolerated in older patients with no history of angina or recent myocardial infarction. There was no significant difference in the incidence of ventricular arrhythmias in older adults versus younger adults (see Pharmacodynamics and Additional Information).

Dosage Forms

Aerosol, oral:

Bitartrate (AsthmaHaler®, Bronitin®, Medihaler-Epi®, Primatene® Suspension): 0.3 mg/spray [epinephrine base 0.16 mg/spray] (10 mL, 15 mL, 22.5 mL)

Bronkaid®: 0.5% (10 mL, 15 mL, 22.5 mL)

(Continued)

Epinephrine *(Continued)*

Primatene®: 0.2 mg/spray (15 mL, 22.5 mL)

Auto-injector:
EpiPen®: Delivers 0.3 mg I.M. of epinephrine 1:1000 (2 mL)
EpiPen® Jr.: Delivers 0.15 mg I.M. of epinephrine 1:2000 (2 mL)

Solution:
Inhalation:
Adrenalin®: 1% [10 mg/mL, 1:100] (7.5 mL)
AsthmaNefrin®, microNefrin®, Nephron®, S-2®: Racepinephrine 2% [epinephrine base 1.125%] (7.5 mL, 15 mL, 30 mL)
Vaponefrin®: Racepinephrine 2% [epinephrine base 1%] (15 mL, 30 mL)

Injection:
Adrenalin®: 0.01 mg/mL [1:100,000] (5 mL); 0.1 mg/mL [1:10,000] (3 mL, 10 mL); 1 mg/mL [1:1000] (1 mL, 2 mL, 30 mL)
Suspension (Sus-Phrine®): 5 mg/mL [1:200] (0.3 mL, 5 mL)

Nasal (Adrenalin®): 0.1% [1 mg/mL, 1:1000] (30 mL)
Ophthalmic, as borate (Epinal®): 0.5% (7.5 mL); 1% (7.5 mL)
Ophthalmic, as hydrochloride (Epifrin®, Glaucon®): 0.1% (1 mL, 30 mL); 0.5% (15 mL); 1% (1 mL, 10 mL, 15 mL); 2% (10 mL, 15 mL)
Topical (Adrenalin®): 0.1% [1 mg/mL, 1:1000] (10 mg, 30 mL)

References
Cydulka R, Davison R, Grammer L, et al, "The Use of Epinephrine in the Treatment of Older Adult Asthmatics," *Ann Emerg Med*, 1988, 17(4):322-6.

EpiPen® Auto-Injector *see* Epinephrine *on page 336*

EpiPen® Jr Auto-Injector *see* Epinephrine *on page 336*

Epitol® *see* Carbamazepine *on page 160*

EPO *see* Epoetin Alfa *on this page*

Epoetin Alfa (e POE e tin AL fa)

Brand Names Epogen®; Procrit®
Synonyms EPO; Erythropoietin; rHuEPO-α
Therapeutic Category Recombinant Human Erythropoietin
Use
Anemia associated with end stage renal disease (FDA-approved indication)
Anemia related to therapy with AZT-treated HIV-infected patients (FDA-approved indication)
Endogenous serum erythropoietin (EPO) concentration which are inappropriately low for hemoglobin level (anemia of neoplasia) (FDA approved indication)
Patients undergoing autologous blood donation prior to surgery - EPO may accelerate recovery of hemoglobin level and, in some cases, permit more units of blood to be donated
rHuEPO-α is not beneficial in the acute treatment of anemia (onset of reticulocyte response does not appear until 7-10 days and hemoglobin rise appears over 2-6 weeks after starting therapy). Therefore, emergency/stat orders for the drug are not appropriate.

Contraindications Known hypersensitivity to human albumin; uncontrolled hypertension

Warnings Use with caution in patients with porphyria, hypertension, or a history of seizures; prior to and during therapy, iron stores must be evaluated

Adverse Reactions
Cardiovascular: Hypertension, edema, chest pain, myocardial infarction
Central nervous system: Fatigue, dizziness, headache, seizure, CVA/TIA
Dermatologic: Rash
Gastrointestinal: Nausea
Hematologic: Clotted access
Neuromuscular & skeletal: Arthralgias
Miscellaneous: Hypersensitivity reactions

Overdosage Symptoms of overdose include polycythemia

Toxicology Adequate airway and other supportive measures and agents for treating anaphylaxis should be present when I.V. drug is given

Stability Do not shake; refrigerate; vials are stable 2 weeks at room temperature

Mechanism of Action Induces erythropoiesis by stimulating the division and differentiation of committed erythroid progenitor cells; induces the release of reticulocytes from the bone marrow into the bloodstream, where they mature to erythrocytes

Pharmacodynamics

Onset on action: Increase in reticulocyte count in 10 days, with an increase in RBC count, hemoglobin, and hematocrit within 2-6 weeks

Peak effect: 2-3 weeks

Pharmacokinetics

Distribution: V_d: 9 L; rapid in the plasma compartment; majority of drug is taken up by the liver, kidneys, and bone marrow

Metabolism: Some metabolic degradation does occur

Bioavailability: S.C.: ~21% to 31%; intraperitoneal epoetin in a few patients demonstrated a bioavailability of only 3%

Half-life: Circulating: 4-13 hours in patients with chronic renal failure; 20% shorter in patients with normal renal function

Time to peak serum concentration: S.C.: 2-8 hours after administration

Elimination: Small amounts recovered in the urine; majority hepatically eliminated; 10% excreted unchanged in the urine of normal volunteers

Usual Dosage Geriatrics and Adults:

In patients on dialysis epoetin alfa usually has been administered as an I.V. bolus 3 times/week. While the administration is independent of the dialysis procedure, it may be administered into the venous line at the end of the dialysis procedure to obviate the need for additional venous access; in patients with CRF not on dialysis, epoetin alfa may be given either as an I.V. or S.C. injection. See table.

Epoetin Alfa: General Therapeutic Guidelines

Starting dose	50-100 units/kg 3 times/week I.V.: Dialysis patients I.V. or S.C.: Nondialysis CRF patients
Reduce dose when	1. Target range is reached, or 2. Hematocrit increases >4 points in any 2-week period
Increase dose if	Hematocrit does not increase by 5-6 points after 8 weeks of therapy, and hematocrit is below target range
Maintenance dose	Individualize. General dosage range: 25 units/kg (3 times/week)
Target hematocrit range	30%-33% (maximum: 36%)

AZT-treated HIV-infected patients: I.V., S.C.: Initial: 100 units/kg/dose 3 times/week for 8 weeks; after 8 weeks of therapy the dose can be adjusted by 50-100 units/kg increments 3 times/week to a maximum dose of 300 units/kg 3 times/week; if the hematocrit exceeds 40%, the dose should be discontinued until the hematocrit drops to 36%

Cancer patients on chemotherapy: S.C.: Initial: 150 units/kg 3 times/week; if after 8 weeks results are unsatisfactory, the dose can be increased up to 200 units/kg 3 times/week

Monitoring Parameters

Careful monitoring of blood pressure is indicated; problems with hypertension have been noted in renal failure patients treated with rHuEPO-α. Other patients are less likely to develop this complication.

Follow serum ferritin and serum transferrin saturation monthly

Hematocrit should be determined twice weekly until stabilization within the target range (30% to 33%), and twice weekly at least 2-6 weeks after a dose increase

Baseline and follow-up of blood urea nitrogen (BUN), uric acid, serum creatinine, phosphorous, and potassium

Reference Range Hematocrit: 30% to 33%

Patient Information Frequent blood tests are needed to determine the correct dose; notify physician if any severe headache develops

Nursing Implications Monitor for access clotting, blood pressure (see Stability)

Additional Information Epogen® reimbursement hotline number for information regarding coverage of epoetin alfa is 1-800-2-PAY-EPO. ProCrit™ reimbursement hotline is 1-800-441-1366. Assure there are adequate iron stores or iron intake while using epoetin alfa. Supplementation may be necessary.

Special Geriatric Considerations There is limited information about the use of epoetin alfa in the elderly. Endogenous erythropoietin secretion has been reported to be decreased in older adults with normocytic or iron deficiency anemias or those with a serum hemoglobin concentration <12 g/dL; one study did not find such a relationship in elderly with chronic anemia. A blunted (Continued)

Epoetin Alfa (Continued)

erythropoietin response to anemia has been reported in patients with cancer, rheumatoid arthritis, and AIDS.

Dosage Forms Injection, preservative free: 2000 units (1 mL); 3000 units (1 mL); 4000 units (1 mL); 10,000 units (1 mL)

References

Carpenter MA, Kendall RG, O'Brien AE, et al, "Reduced Erythropoietin Response to Anaemia in Elderly Patients With Normocytic Anaemia," *Eur J Haematol*, 1992, 49(3):119-21.

Erslev AJ, "Erythropoietin," *N Engl J Med*, 1991, 324(19):1339-44.

Goodnough LT, Price TH, Parvin CA, "The Indigenous Erythropoietin Response and the Erythropoietic Response to Blood Loss Anemia: The Effects of Age and Gender," *J Lab Clin Med*, 1995, 126(1):57-64.

Joosten E, Van Hove L, Lesaffre E, et al, "Serum Erythropoietin Levels in Elderly Inpatients With Anemia of Chronic Disorders and Iron Deficiency Anemia," *J Am Geriatr Soc*, 1993, 41(12):1301-4.

Kario K, Matsuo T, and Nakao K, "Serum Erythropoietin Levels in the Elderly," *Gerontology*, 1991, 37(6):345-8.

Nafziger J, Pailla K, Luciani L, et al, "Decreased Erythropoietin Responsiveness to Iron Deficiency Anemia in the Elderly," *Am J Hematol*, 1993, 43(3):172-6.

Powers JS, Krantz SB, Collins JC, et al, "Erythropoietin Response to Anemia as a Function of Age," *J Am Geriatr Soc*, 1991, 39(1):30-2.

Epogen® see Epoetin Alfa on page 338

Epsom Salt [OTC] see Magnesium Salts (Various Salts) on page 568

Equalactin® Chewable Tablet [OTC] see Calcium Polycarbophil on page 151

Equanil® see Meprobamate on page 588

Equilet® [OTC] see Calcium Salts (Oral) on page 152

Ercaf® see Ergotamine on page 343

Ergocalciferol (er goe kal SIF e role)

Brand Names Calciferol™ Injection; Calciferol™ Oral; Drisdol® Oral

Synonyms Activated Ergosterol; Viosterol; Vitamin D_2

Generic Available Yes

Therapeutic Category Vitamin D Analog

Use Refractory rickets; hypophosphatemia; hypoparathyroidism

Contraindications Hypercalcemia, hypersensitivity to ergocalciferol or any component; malabsorption syndrome; evidence of vitamin D toxicity, decreased renal function

Warnings Administer with extreme caution in patients with impaired renal function, heart disease, renal stones, or arteriosclerosis; must administer concomitant calcium supplementation for adequate response to vitamin D; maintain adequate fluid intake; calcium-phosphate product (serum calcium and phosphorus) must not exceed 70; avoid hypercalcemia; renal function impairment with secondary hyperparathyroidism

Adverse Reactions

Cardiovascular: Hypertension, arrhythmias

Central nervous system: Drowsiness, irritability, headache, convulsions, somnolence

Endocrine & metabolic: Acidosis, polydipsia

Gastrointestinal: Nausea, vomiting, anorexia, xerostomia, constipation, weight loss, metallic taste

Genitourinary: Reversible azotemia

Hematologic: Anemia

Hepatic: Elevated AST/ALT

Neuromuscular & skeletal: Weakness, myalgia, bone pain, metastatic calcification

Ocular: Photophobia

Renal: Polyuria, nephrocalcinosis, renal damage

Miscellaneous: Ectopic calcifications

Overdosage Symptoms of overdose include hypercalcemia, hypercalciuria, hyperphosphatemia

Toxicology Following withdrawal of the drug, treatment consists of bed rest, liberal intake of fluids, reduced calcium intake, and cathartic administration. Severe hypercalcemia requires I.V. hydration and forced diuresis with I.V. furosemide (20-40 mg I.V. every 4-6 hours). Urine output should be monitored and maintained at >3 mL/kg/hour. I.V. saline can quickly and significantly increase excretion of calcium into the urine. Calcitonin, cholestyramine, prednisone, sodium EDTA, and mithramycin have all been used successfully to treat the more resistant cases of vitamin D-induced hypercalcemia.

Drug Interactions
Vitamin D may increase absorption of magnesium from magnesium compounds; hypercalcemia may be precipitated by vitamin D and, therefore, may increase cardiac arrhythmias in patients taking digitalis glycosides and verapamil; hypoparathyroid patients may develop hypercalcemia when using thiazide diuretics

Phenytoin and barbiturates decrease half-life of vitamin D; mineral oil with prolonged use decreases vitamin D absorption; cholestyramine reduces absorption of vitamin D

Stability Protect from light

Mechanism of Action Stimulates calcium and phosphate absorption from the small intestine, promotes secretion of calcium from bone to blood (calcium homeostasis); promotes renal tubule phosphate resorption

Pharmacodynamics Peak effect: Within a month following daily doses

Pharmacokinetics
Absorption: Readily from GI tract; absorption requires intestinal levels of bile
Inactive until hydroxylated in the liver and the kidney to calcifediol and then to calcitriol (most active form)

Usual Dosage Geriatrics and Adults (see Special Geriatric Considerations and Additional Information):
RDA: 400 IU/day; many elderly require 800 IU/day (see Special Geriatric Considerations)
Renal failure: Oral: 0.5 mg/day (20,000 units)
Hypoparathyroidism: Oral: 625 mcg to 5 mg/day (25,000-200,000 units) and calcium supplements (500 mg elemental calcium 6 times/day)
Vitamin D-dependent rickets: Oral: 250 mcg to 1.5 mg/day (10,000-60,000 units)
Nutritional rickets and osteomalacia: Oral: Adults (with normal absorption): 25 mcg/day (1000 units)
Familial phosphatemia: 10,000-80,000 IU/day and phosphorus 1-2 g/day
I.M. therapy may be required with liver, gastrointestinal, or biliary disease

Monitoring Parameters Measure serum calcium, BUN, and phosphorus every 1-2 weeks; obtain bone x-rays monthly; monitor until medical condition is corrected/stabilized and serum calcium remains between 9-10 mg/dL

Reference Range Serum calcium times phosphorus should not exceed 70 mg/dL to avoid ectopic calcification; serum calcium should be maintained between 9-10 mg/dL; phosphorus 2.5-5 mg/dL

Test Interactions Increased calcium (S), cholesterol (S); false increased serum cholesterol concentrations with the Zlavkis-Zak reaction

Patient Information Early symptoms of hypercalcemia include weakness, fatigue, somnolence, headache, anorexia, dry mouth, metallic taste, nausea, vomiting, cramps, diarrhea, muscle pain, bone pain, and irritability; do not take more than the recommended amount. While taking this medication, your physician may want you to follow a special diet or take a calcium supplement. Follow this diet closely. Avoid taking magnesium supplements or magnesium containing antacids.

Nursing Implications Parenteral injection for I.M. use only; monitor serum calcium, phosphorus, and BUN every 2 weeks; administer with extreme caution in patients with impaired renal function, heart disease, renal stones, or arteriosclerosis (see Warnings and Reference Range)

Additional Information 1.25 mg ergocalciferol provides 50,000 units of vitamin D activity

Special Geriatric Considerations Recommended daily allowances (RDA) have not been developed for persons >65 years of age; vitamin D, folate, and B_{12} (cyanocobalamin) have decreased absorption with age, but the clinical significance is yet unknown, although studies in ill elderly have demonstrated that low serum concentrations of vitamin D result in greater bone loss. Calorie requirements decrease with age and therefore, nutrient density must be increased to ensure adequate nutrient intake, including vitamins and minerals. Therefore, the use of a daily supplement with a multiple vitamin with minerals is recommended. Elderly consume less vitamin D, absorption may be decreased and many elderly have decreased sun exposure; therefore, elderly should receive supplementation with 800 units (20 mcg)/day. This is a recommendation of particular need to those with high risk for osteoporosis. A recent study gives evidence which supports the recommendation to give sick adults and older adults 800-1000 IU daily as supplemental vitamin D to the diet to prevent bone loss.

Dosage Forms
Capsule: 50,000 units = 1.25 mg
Injection: 500,000 units/mL = 12.5 mg/mL
(Continued)

Ergocalciferol *(Continued)*

Solution: 8000 units/mL = 200 mcg/mL
Tablet: 50,000 units = 1.25 mg

References

Letsou AP and Price LS, "Health Aging and Nutrition: An Overview," *Clin Geriatr Med*, 1987, 3(2):253-60.

Myrianthopoulos M, "Dietary Treatment of Hyperlipidemia in the Elderly," *Clin Geriatr Med*, 1987, 3(2):343-59.

Riggs BL and Melton LJ, "The Prevention and Treatment of Osteoporosis," *N Engl J Med*, 1992, 327(9):620-7.

Thomas MK, Lloyd-Jones, DM, Thadhani RI, et al, "Hypovitaminosis D in Medical Inpatients," *N Engl J Med*, 1998, 338(12):777-83.

Ergoloid Mesylates (ER goe loid MES i lates)

Brand Names Germinal®; Hydergine®; Hydergine® LC

Synonyms Dihydroergotoxine; Dihydrogenated Ergot Alkaloids

Generic Available Yes

Therapeutic Category Ergot Alkaloid

Use Age-related mental capacity declines related to primary progressive dementia, Alzheimer's dementia, senile onset, and multi-infarct dementia

Contraindications Acute or chronic psychosis, hypersensitivity to ergot or any component

Warnings Exclude possibility that signs and symptoms of illness are from a potentially reversible and treatable condition

Precautions Periodically reassess the diagnosis and benefit of current therapy to the patient

Adverse Reactions Adverse effects are minimal; most common include transient nausea, gastrointestinal disturbances and sublingual irritation with SL tablets; other common side effects include:

Cardiovascular: Orthostatic hypotension, bradycardia
Dermatologic: Skin rash, flushing
Ocular: Blurred vision
Respiratory: Nasal congestion

Overdosage Signs and symptoms of overdose include sinus bradycardia, blurred vision, headache, stomach cramps; chronic overdose usually manifests as signs and symptoms of extremity or organ ischemia

Toxicology Nitroprusside has been shown to reverse the vasoconstriction associated with ergot toxicity

Drug Interactions Increased toxicity with dopamine (peripheral ischemia)

Mechanism of Action Exact mechanism in dementia is unknown; originally classed as peripheral and cerebral vasodilator, now considered a "metabolic enhancer"

Pharmacokinetics

Absorption: Rapid yet incomplete
Metabolism: Significant first-pass metabolism
Half-life: 3.5 hours
Time to peak serum concentration: Within 1 hour

Usual Dosage Geriatrics and Adults: Oral: 1 mg 3 times/day up to 4.5-12 mg/day; up to 6 months of therapy may be necessary, using doses of at least 6 mg/day

Monitoring Parameters Blood pressure, heart rate, mental status

Patient Information Do not chew or crush sublingual tablets, allow to dissolve under tongue

Nursing Implications See Monitoring Parameters

Special Geriatric Considerations The efficacy of ergoloid mesylates in the treatment of dementia is controversial. Many clinicians regard it as no better than placebo and most patients do not experience significant benefits. Improvement in social function has been shown in some studies, but no consistent improvement in memory or cognitive function has been reported. If ergoloid mesylates are to be used, an oral dose of 6 mg/day for at least 6 months should be utilized. If no improvement after this time, the drug should be discontinued.

Dosage Forms

Capsule, liquid (Hydergine® LC): 1 mg
Liquid (Hydergine®): 1 mg/mL (100 mL)
Tablet:
  Oral:
    0.5 mg
    Gerimal®, Hydergine®: 1 mg
  Sublingual: Gerimal®, Hydergine®: 0.5 mg, 1 mg

Ergomar® *see* Ergotamine *on this page*

Ergotamine (er GOT a meen)

Brand Names Bellergal-S®; Cafatine®; Cafatine-PB®; Cafergot®; Cafetrate®; Ercaf®; Ergomar®; Phenerbel-S®; Wigraine®

Synonyms Ergotamine Tartrate and Caffeine; Ergotamine Tartrate With Belladonna Alkaloids, and Phenobarbital

Generic Available Yes

Therapeutic Category Adrenergic Blocking Agent; Ergot Alkaloid

Use Vascular headache, such as migraine or cluster

Contraindications Hypersensitivity to ergotamine, caffeine or any component; peripheral vascular disease, hepatic or renal disease, hypertension, peptic ulcer disease, sepsis, coronary artery disease

Precautions Avoid prolonged administration or excessive dosage because of the danger of ergotism and gangrene; patients who take ergotamine for extended periods of time may become dependent on it

Adverse Reactions
Cardiovascular: Tachycardia, bradycardia, arterial spasm, claudication and vasoconstriction
Dermatologic: Pruritus
Gastrointestinal: Nausea, vomiting, diarrhea
Neuromuscular & skeletal: Weakness in the legs, abdominal pain, myalgia, paresthesia
Miscellaneous: Rebound headache may occur with sudden withdrawal of the drug in patients on prolonged therapy, vasospasm, local edema

Overdosage Symptoms include vasospastic effects, nausea, vomiting, lassitude, impaired mental function, hypotension, hypertension, unconsciousness, seizures, shock and death.

Toxicology Treatment includes general supportive therapy, gastric lavage, or induction of emesis, activated charcoal, saline cathartic; keep extremities warm. Activated charcoal is effective at binding certain chemicals, and this is especially true for ergot alkaloids; treatment is symptomatic with heparin, vasodilators (nitroprusside); vasodilators should be used with caution to avoid exaggerating any pre-existing hypotension.

Drug Interactions
Decreased antianginal effect with nitrates
Increased toxicity: Beta-blockers, macrolide antibiotics
Increased pressor effects with vasodilators

Mechanism of Action Ergot alkaloid alpha-adrenergic blockade directly stimulates vascular smooth muscle to vasoconstrict peripheral and cerebral vessels; may also have antagonist effects on serotonin; may inhibit receptor reuptake of norepinephrine

Pharmacokinetics
Absorption:
Oral, rectal: Erratic; enhanced by caffeine coadministration
Inhalation: Rapid and complete
Metabolism: Extensive in the liver
Bioavailability: Poor overall (<5%)
Time to peak serum concentration: Within 0.5-3 hours following administration
Elimination: In bile as metabolites (90%)

Usual Dosage Geriatrics and Adults:
Oral:
Cafergot®: 2 tablets at onset of attack; then 1 tablet every 30 minutes as needed; maximum: 6 tablets per attack; do not exceed 10 tablets/week
Ergomar®: 1 tablet under tongue at first sign, then 1 tablet every 30 minutes if necessary; maximum: 3 tablets/24 hours; do not exceed 5 tablets/week
Rectal (Cafergot® suppositories, Wigraine® suppositories, Cafatine® P-B suppositories): 1 at first sign of an attack; follow with second dose after 1 hour, if needed; maximum: 2 per attack; do not exceed 5/week

Monitoring Parameters Relief of symptoms, blood pressure, pulse, peripheral circulation

Patient Information Any symptoms such as nausea, vomiting, numbness or tingling, and chest, muscle, or abdominal pain should be reported to the physician. Initiate therapy at first sign of attack. Do **not** exceed recommended dosage.

Nursing Implications Do not crush sublingual drug product

Additional Information
Ergotamine tartrate and caffeine: Cafergot®
Ergotamine, caffeine, belladonna alkaloids and pentobarbital: Cafertine® P-B
(Continued)

Ergotamine *(Continued)*

Special Geriatric Considerations May be harmful due to reduction in cerebral blood flow; may precipitate angina, myocardial infarction, or aggravate intermittent claudication; therefore, not considered a drug of choice in the elderly (see Contraindications and Precautions)

Dosage Forms

Suppository, rectal (Cafatine®, Cafergot®, Cafetrate®, Wigraine®): Ergotamine tartrate 2 mg and caffeine 100 mg (12s)

Tablet (Ercaf®, Wigraine®): Ergotamine tartrate 1 mg and caffeine 100 mg

Tablet:

Extended release:

Bellergal-S®: Ergotamine tartrate 0.6 mg with belladonna alkaloids 0.2 mg, and phenobarbital 40 mg

Cafatine-PB®: Ergotamine tartrate 1 mg with belladonna alkaloids 0.125 mg, caffeine 100 mg, and pentobarbital 30 mg

Sublingual (Ergomar®): Ergotamine tartrate 2 mg

Ergotamine Tartrate and Caffeine *see* Ergotamine *on previous page*

Ergotamine Tartrate With Belladonna Alkaloids, and Phenobarbital *see* Ergotamine *on previous page*

E•R•O Ear [OTC] *see* Carbamide Peroxide *on page 162*

Erycette® Topical *see* Erythromycin, Topical *on page 347*

Eryc® Oral *see* Erythromycin *on this page*

EryDerm® Topical *see* Erythromycin, Topical *on page 347*

Erygel® Topical *see* Erythromycin, Topical *on page 347*

Erymax® Topical *see* Erythromycin, Topical *on page 347*

EryPed® Oral *see* Erythromycin *on this page*

Ery-sol® Topical *see* Erythromycin, Topical *on page 347*

Ery-Tab® Oral *see* Erythromycin *on this page*

Erythrocin® Oral *see* Erythromycin *on this page*

Erythromycin *(er ith roe MYE sin)*

Related Information

Cephalosporins, Aminoglycosides, Macrolides, & Quinolones *on page 1014*

I.V. Medication Recommendations *on page 1080*

Brand Names E.E.S.® Oral; E-Mycin® Oral; Eryc® Oral; EryPed® Oral; Ery-Tab® Oral; Erythrocin® Oral; Ilosone® Oral; PCE® Oral

Generic Available Yes

Therapeutic Category Antibacterial, Topical; Antibiotic, Macrolide; Antibiotic, Ophthalmic

Use Treatment of susceptible bacterial infections including *M. pneumoniae*, *Legionella* pneumonia, diphtheria, pertussis, chancroid, *Chlamydia*, and *Campylobacter* gastroenteritis; used in conjunction with neomycin for decontaminating the bowel

Unlabeled use: Gastroparesis

Contraindications Hepatic impairment, known hypersensitivity to erythromycin or its any components, concurrent use with terfenadine or astemizole (see Drug Interactions); use with pimozide

Warnings Hepatic impairment with or without jaundice has occurred, it may be accompanied by malaise, nausea, vomiting, abdominal colic, and fever; discontinue use if these occur

Precautions Use with caution in patients with hepatic dysfunction

Adverse Reactions

Cardiovascular: Ventricular arrhythmias

Central nervous system: Fever

Dermatologic: Skin rash

Gastrointestinal: Abdominal pain, cramping, nausea, vomiting, diarrhea, hypertrophic pyloric stenosis

Hematologic: Eosinophilia

Hepatic: Cholestatic hepatitis

Local: Thrombophlebitis

Otic: Ototoxicity

Miscellaneous: Allergic reactions

Overdosage Symptoms of overdose include nausea, vomiting, diarrhea, prostration, reversible pancreatitis, hearing loss with or without tinnitus or vertigo

Toxicology General and supportive care only

Drug Interactions

Erythromycin decreased clearance of carbamazepine, cyclosporine, terfenadine, astemizole, loratadine, triazolam, and cisapride

Increased effects of anticoagulants, increased bromocriptine, cyclosporine, disopyramide, digoxin, methylprednisolone, and ergot alkaloid serum concentrations have been reported; erythromycin may decrease theophylline clearance and increased theophylline's half-life by up to 60% (patients on high dose theophylline and erythromycin or who have received erythromycin for >5 days may be at higher risk)

Stability
Erythromycin lactobionate should be reconstituted with sterile water for injection without preservatives to avoid gel formation; the reconstituted solution is stable for 2 weeks when refrigerated or 24 hours at room temperature. Erythromycin I.V. infusion solution is stable at pH 6-8. Do not use D_5W as a diluent unless sodium bicarbonate is added to solution.

Mechanism of Action
Inhibits RNA-dependent protein synthesis at the chain elongation step; binds to the 50S ribosomal subunit resulting in blockage of transpeptidation

Pharmacokinetics

Absorption: Variable but better with salt forms than with base form; 18% to 45% absorbed orally

Protein binding: 75% to 90%

Metabolism: In the liver by demethylation; inhibitor of CYP1A2, 3A4; substrate CYP3A4

Half-life: 1.5-2 hours, prolonged with reduced renal function

Time to peak concentration: 4 hours for the base, 3 hours for the stearate, 0.5-2.5 hours for the ethylsuccinate, 2-4 hours for the estolate; after oral administration peak serum concentrations occur within 4 hours (delayed in the presence of food except when using the estolate)

Elimination: 2% to 15% excreted as unchanged drug in urine and major excretion in feces (via bile)

Usual Dosage
Geriatrics and Adults:

Ophthalmic: Instill 1 or more times/day depending on the severity of the infection

Oral:

Base: 333 mg every 8 hours

Estolate, stearate or base: 250-500 mg every 6-12 hours

Ethylsuccinate: 400-800 mg every 6-12 hours

Preop bowel preparation: 1 g erythromycin base at 1, 2, and 11 PM on the day before surgery combined with mechanical cleansing of the large intestine and oral neomycin

I.V.: 2-4 g/day divided every 6 hours

Bacterial endocarditis prophylaxis: Oral: 1 g 2 hours before procedure, then 500 mg 6 hours after initial dose

Administration
Can administer with food to decrease GI upset; tablets should be swallowed whole, do not crush or chew; burning at I.V. site and phlebitis, change I.V. site frequently (see Stability)

Monitoring Parameters
Signs and symptoms of infection

Test Interactions
False-positive urinary catecholamines

Patient Information
Complete full course of therapy, do not skip doses; refrigerate after reconstitution; chewable tablets should not be swallowed whole; notify physician or pharmacist if GI side effects are intolerable, diarrhea develops, or symptoms are not improving

Nursing Implications
GI upset, including diarrhea, is common

Additional Information

Erythromycin base: E-Mycin®, Eryc®, Ery-Tab®, PCE®, Ilotycin®, Robimycin® Erythromycin estolate: Ilosone®

Erythromycin ethylsuccinate: E.E.S.®, E-Mycin® E, EryPed®, Wyamycin® E

Erythromycin glucceptate: Ilotycin® Gluceptate

Erythromycin lactobionate: Erythrocin® Lactobionate-IV

Erythromycin stearate: Eramycin®, Erypar®, Erythrocin®, Ethril®, Wintrocin®, Wyamycin® S

Due to differences in absorption, 200 mg erythromycin ethylsuccinate produces the same serum concentrations as erythromycin base or estolate; do not use D_5W as a diluent unless sodium bicarbonate is added to solution; infuse over 30 minutes

Sodium content of oral suspension (ethyl succinate) 200 mg/5 mL: 29 mg (1.3 mEq)

Sodium content of base Filmtab® 250 mg: 70 mg (3 mEq)

(Continued)

Erythromycin *(Continued)*

Special Geriatric Considerations Dose of erythromycin does not need to be adjusted in the elderly unless there is severe renal impairment or hepatic dysfunction; has not been studied in the elderly

Dosage Forms

Erythromycin base:
Capsule, delayed release: 250 mg
Capsule, delayed release, enteric coated pellets (Eryc®): 250 mg
Tablet, delayed release: 333 mg
Tablet, enteric coated (E-Mycin®, Ery-Tab®, E-Base®): 250 mg, 333 mg, 500 mg
Tablet, film coated: 250 mg, 500 mg
Tablet, polymer coated particles (PCE®): 333 mg, 500 mg

Erythromycin estolate:
Capsule (Ilosone® Pulvules®): 250 mg
Suspension, oral (Ilosone®): 125 mg/5 mL (480 mL); 250 mg/5 mL (480 mL)
Tablet (Ilosone®): 500 mg

Erythromycin ethylsuccinate:
Granules for oral suspension (EryPed®): 400 mg/5 mL (60 mL, 100 mL, 200 mL)
Powder for oral suspension (E.E.S.®): 200 mg/5 mL (100 mL, 200 mL)
Suspension, oral (E.E.S.®, EryPed®): 200 mg/5 mL (5 mL, 100 mL, 200 mL, 480 mL); 400 mg/5 mL (5 mL, 60 mL, 100 mL, 200 mL, 480 mL)
Suspension, oral [drops] (EryPed®): 100 mg/2.5 mL (50 mL)
Tablet (E.E.S.®): 400 mg
Tablet, chewable (EryPed®): 200 mg

Erythromycin gluceptate:
Injection: 1000 mg (30 mL)

Erythromycin lactobionate:
Powder for injection: 500 mg, 1000 mg

Erythromycin stearate:
Tablet, film coated (Eramycin®, Erythrocin®): 250 mg, 500 mg

References
Yoshikawa TT, "Antimicrobial Therapy for the Elderly Patient," *J Am Geriatr Soc*, 1990, 38(12):1353-72.

Erythromycin and Sulfisoxazole
(er ith roe MYE sin & sul fi SOKS a zole)

Related Information
Erythromycin *on page 344*
Sulfisoxazole *on page 880*

Brand Names Eryzole®; Pediazole®

Synonyms Sulfisoxazole and Erythromycin

Generic Available Yes

Therapeutic Category Antibiotic, Macrolide; Antibiotic, Sulfonamide Derivative

Use Treatment of susceptible bacterial infections of the upper and lower respiratory tract; and other infections in patients allergic to penicillin

Contraindications Hepatic dysfunction, known hypersensitivity to erythromycin or sulfonamides; patients with porphyria

Precautions Use with caution in patients with impaired renal or hepatic function, G-6-PD deficiency (hemolysis may occur)

Adverse Reactions
Central nervous system: Headache
Dermatologic: Rash, Stevens-Johnson syndrome, toxic epidermal necrolysis
Gastrointestinal: Abdominal cramping, nausea, vomiting, diarrhea
Hematologic: Agranulocytosis, aplastic anemia
Hepatic: Hepatic necrosis
Renal: Toxic nephrosis, crystalluria

Overdosage Symptoms of overdose include nausea, vomiting, diarrhea, prostration, reversible pancreatitis, hearing loss with or without tinnitus or vertigo

Toxicology General and supportive care only; keep patient well hydrated

Drug Interactions
Erythromycin may decrease theophylline clearance and increase theophylline's half-life by up to 60% (patients on high doses of theophylline and erythromycin or on >5 days of erythromycin may be at higher risk)
Increased effect/toxicity/levels of alfentanil, anticoagulants, cisapride, astemizole, terfenadine, loratadine, bromocriptine, carbamazepine, cyclosporine, digoxin, disopyramide, triazolam, and warfarin

Stability Reconstituted suspension is stable for 14 days when refrigerated

Mechanism of Action Erythromycin inhibits bacterial protein synthesis; sulfisoxazole competitively inhibits bacterial synthesis of folic acid from para-aminobenzoic acid

Pharmacokinetics
Erythromycin ethylsuccinate:
    Absorption: Well from the GI tract
    Protein binding: 75% to 90%
    Metabolism: In the liver
    Half-life: 1-1.5 hours
    Elimination: Unchanged drug excreted and concentrated in bile
Sulfisoxazole acetyl:
    Hydrolyzed in GI tract to sulfisoxazole which is readily absorbed
    Protein binding: 85%
    Half-life: 6 hours, prolonged in renal impairment
    Elimination: 50% excreted in urine as unchanged drug

Usual Dosage Geriatrics and Adults: Oral (dosage recommendation is based on the product's erythromycin content): 400 mg erythromycin and 1200 mg sulfisoxazole every 6 hours

Dosing adjustment in renal impairment (sulfisoxazole must be adjusted in renal impairment):
    Cl_{cr} 10-50 mL/minute: Administer every 8-12 hours
    Cl_{cr} <10 mL/minute: Administer every 12-24 hours

Monitoring Parameters CBC and periodic liver function test

Test Interactions False-positive urinary protein

Patient Information Maintain adequate fluid intake; avoid prolonged exposure to sunlight; discontinue if rash appears

Special Geriatric Considerations See individual agents; not recommended for use in the elderly (see Usual Dosage); adjust dose for renal function

Dosage Forms Suspension, oral: Erythromycin ethylsuccinate 200 mg and sulfisoxazole acetyl 600 mg per 5 mL (100 mL, 150 mL, 200 mL)

Erythromycin, Topical (er ith roe MYE sin TOP i kal)

Brand Names Akne-Mycin® Topical; A/T/S® Topical; Del-Mycin® Topical; Emgel™ Topical; Erycette® Topical; EryDerm® Topical; Erygel® Topical; Erymax® Topical; Ery-sol® Topical; E-Solve-2® Topical; ETS-2%® Topical; Ilotycin® Ophthalmic; Staticin® Topical; T-Stat® Topical

Therapeutic Category Acne Products; Antibiotic, Topical

Use Topical treatment of acne vulgaris

Contraindications Known hypersensitivity to erythromycin

Precautions External use only

Adverse Reactions Dermatologic: Erythema, desquamation, dryness, pruritus

Drug Interactions Antagonism with clindamycin, inactivated by acids; sodium alginate, pectin, bentonite, calamine, silicate, and polysorbate 80 all decrease activity

Mechanism of Action Erythromycin works by binding to the bacterial 50S ribosomal subunit, apparently interfering with the translocation reaction in which the growing peptide chain is moved from the receptor to the donor site; this causes disruption of protein synthesis

Usual Dosage Geriatrics and Adults: Apply twice daily

Patient Information Contains benzoyl peroxide which may stain or bleach clothing

Special Geriatric Considerations Not for infected wounds or pressure sores

Dosage Forms
Gel: 2% (30 g, 60 g)
Gel (A/T/S®, Emgel™, Erygel®): 2% (27 g, 30 g, 60 g)
Ointment:
    Ophthalmic (Ilotycin®, AK-Mycin®): 0.5% (1 g, 3.5 g, 3.75 g)
    Topical (Akne-Mycin®): 2% (25 g)
Pad (T-Stat®): 2% (60s)
Solution, topical:
    Staticin®: 1.5% (60 mL)
    Akne-Mycin®, A/T/S®, Del-Mycin®, EryDerm®, Ery-sol®, ETS-2%®, Romycin®, Theramycin Z®, T-Stat®: 2% (60 mL, 66 mL, 120 mL)
Swab (Erycette®): 2% (60s)

Erythropoietin see Epoetin Alfa on page 338

Eryzole® see Erythromycin and Sulfisoxazole on previous page

Eserine Salicylate see Physostigmine on page 745

Esidrix® *see* Hydrochlorothiazide *on page 458*
Eskalith® *see* Lithium *on page 545*

Esmolol (ES moe lol)

Related Information
Beta-Blockers Comparison *on page 1026*

Brand Names Brevibloc®

Therapeutic Category Antianginal Agent; Antiarrhythmic Agent, Class II; Beta-Adrenergic Blocker

Use Supraventricular tachycardia (primarily to control ventricular rate) and sinus tachycardia

Contraindications Sinus bradycardia or heart block, uncompensated congestive heart failure, cardiogenic shock, hypersensitivity to esmolol, any component, or other beta-blockers

Warnings Caution should be exercised when discontinuing esmolol infusions to avoid withdrawal effects; although esmolol primarily blocks $beta_1$-receptors, high doses can result in $beta_2$-receptor blockade. Abrupt withdrawal of beta-blockers may result in an exaggerated cardiac beta-adrenergic responsiveness in coronary artery disease, however, this has not been reported with esmolol. Symptomatology has included reports of tachycardia, hypertension, ischemia, angina, myocardial infarction, and sudden death.

Precautions Use with extreme caution in patients with hyper-reactive airway disease; use lowest dose possible and discontinue infusion if bronchospasm occurs; use with caution in diabetes mellitus, hypoglycemia, renal failure; avoid extravasation, if extravasation occurs, use another I.V. site. Avoid use of butterfly needles.

Adverse Reactions
Cardiovascular: Hypotension (especially with higher doses), bradycardia, Raynaud's phenomena

Central nervous system: Dizziness, somnolence, confusion, lethargy, depression, headache

Gastrointestinal: Nausea, vomiting

Local: Skin necrosis after extravasation, phlebitis

Respiratory: Bronchoconstriction (less than propranolol, but more likely with higher doses)

Miscellaneous: Diaphoresis, cold extremities

Overdosage Symptoms of overdose include hypotension

Toxicology Sympathomimetics (eg, epinephrine or dopamine), glucagon or a pacemaker can be used to treat the toxic bradycardia, asystole, and/or hypotension. Initially, fluids may be the best treatment for toxic hypotension. Patients should remain supine; serum glucose and potassium should be measured. Use supportive measures: lavage, syrup of ipecac; atenolol may be removed by hemodialysis. I.V. glucose should be administered for hypoglycemia; seizures may be treated with phenytoin or diazepam intravenously; continuous monitoring of blood pressure and EKG is necessary. If PVCs occur, treat with lidocaine or phenytoin; avoid quinidine, procainamide, and disopyramide since these agents further depress myocardial function. Bronchospasm can be treated with theophylline or $beta_2$ agonists (epinephrine).

Drug Interactions
Pharmacologic action of beta antagonists may be decreased by aluminum compounds, calcium salts, barbiturates, cholestyramine, colestipol, NSAIDs, penicillins (ampicillin), rifampin, salicylates, sulfinpyrazone, thyroid hormones; hypoglycemic effect of sulfonylureas may be blunted

Pharmacologic effect of beta antagonists may be enhanced with concomitant use of calcium channel blockers, oral contraceptives, flecainide (bioavailability and effect of flecainide also enhanced), haloperidol (hypotensive effects of both drugs), H_2 antagonists (decreased metabolism), hydralazine (both drugs hypotensive effects increased), loop diuretics (increased serum concentrations of beta-blockers except atenolol), MAO inhibitors, phenothiazines, propafenone, quinidine, quinolones, thioamines

Beta-blockers may decrease clearance of acetaminophen; beta-blockers may increase anticoagulant effects of warfarin (propranolol)

Benzodiazepine effects enhanced by the lipophilic beta-blockers (atenolol does not interact)

Significant and fatal increases in blood pressure have occurred after decrease in dose or discontinuation of clonidine in patients receiving both clonidine and beta-blockers together (reduce doses of each cautiously with small decreases)

Peripheral ischemia of ergot alkaloids enhanced by beta-blockers

Beta-blockers increase serum concentration of lidocaine; beta-blockers increase hypotensive effect of prazosin

Stability Diluted I.V. infusion solution is stable for 24 hours at room temperature; compatible with the following I.V. solutions: 5% dextrose injection, 5% dextrose in lactated Ringer's injection, 5% dextrose in Ringer's injection, 5% dextrose and 0.9% **or** 0.45% sodium chloride injection, lactated Ringer's injection, potassium chloride (40 mEq/L) in 5% dextrose injection, and 0.9% or 0.45% sodium chloride injection. Esmolol is **not** compatible with 5% sodium bicarbonate injection.

Mechanism of Action Class II antiarrhythmic: Competitively blocks response to beta$_1$-adrenergic receptors, with little or no effect on beta$_2$-receptors except at high doses

Pharmacodynamics
Onset of action: Beta blockade occurs within 2-10 minutes following initiation of I.V. administration (onset of effects is quickest when loading doses are administered)
Duration: Short (10-30 minutes)

Pharmacokinetics
Protein binding: 55%
Metabolism: By esterase in cytosol or red blood cells
Half-life: 9 minutes
Elimination: ~69% of dose excreted in urine as metabolites and 2% as unchanged drug

Usual Dosage Must be adjusted to individual response and tolerance
Geriatrics and Adults: I.V.: Loading dose: 500 mcg/kg over 1 minute; follow with a 50 mcg/kg/minute infusion for 4 minutes; if response is inadequate, rebolus with another 500 mcg/kg loading dose over 1 minute, and increase the maintenance infusion to 100 mcg/kg/minute. Repeat this process until a therapeutic effect has been achieved or to a maximum recommended maintenance dose of 200 mcg/kg/minute. Usual dosage range: 50-200 mcg/kg/minute with average dose = 100 mcg/kg/minute.

Monitoring Parameters Blood pressure, apical and peripheral pulse, EKG

Test Interactions Increased cholesterol (S), glucose

Nursing Implications The 250 mg/mL ampul is **not** for direct I.V. injection, but rather must first be diluted to a final concentration of 10 mg/mL (ie, 2.5 g in 250 mL or 5 g in 500 mL)

Special Geriatric Considerations Due to alterations in the beta-adrenergic autonomic nervous system, beta-adrenergic blockade may result in less hemodynamic response than seen in younger adults. Studies indicate that despite decreased sensitivity to the chronotropic effects of beta blockade with age, there appears to be an increased myocardial sensitivity to the negative inotropic effect during stress (ie, exercise). Controlled trials have shown the overall response rate for propranolol to be only 20% to 50% in elderly populations. Therefore, all beta-adrenergic blocking drugs may result in a decreased response as compared to younger adults.

Dosage Forms Injection, as hydrochloride: 10 mg/mL (10 mL); 250 mg/mL (10 mL)

References
Vincent RN, Click LA, Williams HM, et al, "Esmolol As an Adjunct in the Treatment of Systemic Hypertension After Operative Repair of Coarctation of the Aorta," *Am J Cardiol*, 1990, 65(13):941-3.

E-Solve-2® Topical *see Erythromycin, Topical on page 347*

Estazolam (es TA zoe lam)

Related Information
Antacid Drug Interactions *on page 1096*
Anxiolytic/Hypnotic Use in Long-Term Care Facilities *on page 1099*
Benzodiazepines Comparison *on page 1024*

Brand Names ProSom™

Generic Available No

Therapeutic Category Benzodiazepine; Hypnotic; Sedative

Use Short-term management of insomnia

Restrictions C-IV

Contraindications Hypersensitivity to estazolam, cross-sensitivity with other benzodiazepines may occur, severe uncontrolled pain, pre-existing CNS depression, narrow-angle glaucoma, sleep apnea

Warnings Abrupt discontinuance may precipitate withdrawal or rebound insomnia

Precautions Potential for drug dependence and abuse; use with caution in patients with the potential for drug dependence
(Continued)

Estazolam (Continued)

Adverse Reactions
Central nervous system: Drowsiness, amnesia, confusion, dizziness, headache, ataxia, impaired coordination

Gastrointestinal: Nausea, vomiting, xerostomia

Hepatic: Cholestatic jaundice

Miscellaneous: Physical and psychological dependence may occur with prolonged use

Overdosage Symptoms of overdose include somnolence, confusion, coma, and diminished reflexes

Toxicology Treatment for benzodiazepine overdose is supportive; rarely is mechanical ventilation required; flumazenil has been shown to selectively block the binding of benzodiazepines to CNS receptors, resulting in a reversal of benzodiazepine-induced sedation; however, its use may not alter the course of overdose

Drug Interactions
Decreased effect: Benzodiazepines may decrease the effect of levodopa

Increased toxicity: CNS depressants, alcohol

Mechanism of Action Benzodiazepines appear to potentiate the effects of GABA and other inhibitory neurotransmitters by binding to specific benzodiazepine-receptor sites in various areas of the CNS

Pharmacodynamics Studies have shown that the elderly are more sensitive to the effects of benzodiazepines as compared to younger adults

Pharmacokinetics
Metabolism: Rapid and extensive in the liver to inactive metabolites

Half-life: 10-24 hours (no significant changes in the elderly)

Time to peak serum concentration: 0.5-1.6 hours

Elimination: <5% excreted unchanged in urine

Usual Dosage Oral:
Geriatrics: Initial: 0.5-1 mg at bedtime

Adults: 1-2 mg at bedtime

Monitoring Parameters Respiratory, cardiovascular, and mental status

Patient Information Avoid alcohol and other CNS depressants; may cause drowsiness; avoid activities needing good psychomotor coordination until CNS effects are known; may cause physical or psychological dependence; avoid abrupt discontinuation after prolonged use

Nursing Implications Provide safety measures (ie, side rails, night light, and call button); remove smoking materials from area; supervise ambulation

Special Geriatric Considerations Because of its lack of active metabolites, estazolam would be a reasonable choice for elderly patients when a benzodiazepine hypnotic is indicated (see Pharmacodynamics)

Dosage Forms Tablet: 1 mg, 2 mg

Estimated Comparative Daily Dosages for Inhaled Corticosteroids see page 1045

Estinyl® see Ethinyl Estradiol on page 357

Estivin® II Ophthalmic [OTC] see Naphazoline on page 653

Estrace® Oral see Estradiol on this page

Estraderm® Transdermal see Estradiol on this page

Estra-D® Injection see Estradiol on this page

Estradiol (es tra DYE ole)

Brand Names Climara® Transdermal; Delestrogen® Injection; depGynogen® Injection; Depo®-Estradiol Injection; Depogen® Injection; Dioval® Injection; Dura-Estrin® Injection; Duragen® Injection; Estrace® Oral; Estraderm® Transdermal; Estra-D® Injection; Estra-L® Injection; Estring®; Estro-Cyp® Injection; Estroject-L.A.® Injection; Gynogen L.A.® Injection; Valergen® Injection; Vivelle® Transdermal

Synonyms Estradiol Transdermal

Generic Available Yes

Therapeutic Category Estrogen Derivative

Use Treatment of atrophic vaginitis, urinary incontinence secondary to estrogen deficiency, atrophic dystrophy of vulva, menopausal symptoms, female hypogonadism, oophorectomy, ovariectomy, primary ovarian failure, inoperable breast cancer, inoperable prostatic cancer, mild to severe vasomotor symptoms associated with menopause, prevention of osteoporosis

Contraindications Undiagnosed genital bleeding, diplopia, active liver disease; carcinoma of the breast (with certain exceptions), estrogen-dependent tumor, present or past thromboembolic disease, cerebrovascular disease

Warnings Estrogens have been reported to increase the risk of endometrial carcinoma; this risk can be reduced by cycling with a progestin (ie, medroxy-progesterone) for the last 10-13 days of estrogen therapy each month or administering daily throughout the month

Precautions Use with caution in patients with renal or hepatic insufficiency; in patients with a history of thromboembolism, stroke, liver tumor, hypertension

Adverse Reactions

Cardiovascular: Increase in blood pressure, edema, thromboembolic disorders

Central nervous system: Depression, headache

Dermatologic: Chloasma, melasma, scalp alopecia

Endocrine & metabolic: Hypercalcemia, folate deficiency, breakthrough bleeding, spotting, endometrial carcinoma

Gastrointestinal: Nausea, vomiting, bloating

Genitourinary: Increased libido (female), decreased libido (male)

Hepatic: Cholestatic jaundice, increased LDL and triglycerides

Local: Pain at injection site, enlargement of breasts (female and male), breast tenderness

Overdosage Symptoms of overdose include fluid retention, jaundice, thrombophlebitis

Toxicology Toxicity is unlikely following single exposures of excessive doses, any treatment following emesis and charcoal administration should be supportive and symptomatic

Drug Interactions

Rifampin, barbiturates, cigarette smoking, and other agents that induce hepatic metabolism can increase estrogen clearance and decrease serum concentrations

Increased toxicity (potential) with anticoagulants, tricyclic antidepressants, corticosteroids

Mechanism of Action Increases the synthesis of DNA, RNA, and various proteins in target tissues; reduces the release of gonadotropin-releasing hormone from the hypothalamus; reduces FSH and LH release from the pituitary

Pharmacokinetics

Absorption: Readily through skin and GI tract

Protein binding: 80%

Half-life: 50-60 minutes

Elimination: Principally degraded in the liver and excreted in urine as conjugates; small amounts excreted in feces via bile, reabsorbed from the GI tract and enterohepatically recycled

Usual Dosage Geriatrics and Adults (all doses need to be adjusted based upon the patient's response):

Male:

Prostate cancer: Valerate: I.M.: ≥30 mg or more every 1-2 weeks

Prostate cancer (androgen-dependent, inoperable, progressing): Oral: 10 mg 3 times/day for at least 3 months

Female:

Hypogonadism:

Oral: 1-2 mg/day

I.M.: Valerate: 10-20 mg/month

Transdermal: 0.05 mg patch initially (titrate dosage to response) applied twice weekly

Osteoporosis prevention:

Oral: 0.5 mg/day

Transdermal: 0.05 mg patch initially (titrate dosage to response) applied twice weekly

Breast cancer (inoperable, progressing): Oral: 10 mg 3 times/day for at least 3 months

Atrophic vaginitis, kraurosis vulvae: Vaginal: Insert 2-4 g/day for 2 weeks then gradually reduce to 1/2 the initial dose for 2 weeks followed by a maintenance dose of 1 g 1-3 times/week

Moderate to severe vasomotor symptoms: I.M.:

Cypionate: 1-5 mg every 3-4 weeks

Valerate: 10-20 mg every 4 weeks

Monitoring Parameters Mammography should be performed in all women prior to starting estrogen therapy and then every 18-24 months; blood pressure; Pap smear at baseline and then every 2 years; clinical breast exam annually

(Continued)

Estradiol *(Continued)*

Reference Range Male: 10-50 pg/mL (SI: 37-184 pmol/L); postmenopausal female: 0-30 pg/mL (SI: 0-110 pmol/L)

Test Interactions Increased chloride (S), glucose, iron (B), sodium (S), thyroxine (S); decreased protein, prothrombin time

Patient Information Women should inform their physicians if signs or symptoms of any of the following occur: thromboembolic or thrombotic disorders including sudden severe headache or vomiting, disturbance of vision or speech, loss of vision, numbness or weakness in an extremity, sharp or crushing chest pain, calf pain, shortness of breath, severe abdominal pain or mass, mental depression or unusual bleeding. Women should perform regular self exams on breasts. Notify physician if area under dermal patch becomes irritated or a rash develops.

Nursing Implications May also be administered intramuscularly; administer at bedtime to minimize occurrence of adverse effects; when given I.V., drug should be administered slowly to avoid the occurrence of a flushing reaction (see Patient Information)

Special Geriatric Considerations Before prescribing estrogen therapy to postmenopausal women, the risks and benefits must be weighed for each patient. Long-term estrogen use has been associated with reduced all-cause mortality, principally due to cardiovascular benefits in postmenopausal women. Data in women 80 years and older are minimal and it is unclear if the reduced risk is applicable to women in this age group. Women should be informed of these risks and benefits, as well as possible side effects and the return of menstrual bleeding (when cycled with a progestin), and be involved in the decision to prescribe. Oral therapy may be more convenient for vaginal atrophy and urinary incontinence.

Dosage Forms

Cream, vaginal (Estrace®): 0.1 mg/g (42.5 g)

Injection, as cypionate (depGynogen®, Depo®-Estradiol, Depogen®, Dura-Estrin®, Estro-Cyp®, Estroject-L.A.®): 5 mg/mL (5 mL, 10 mL)

Injection, as valerate:

Delestrogen®, Valergen®: 10 mg/mL (5 mL, 10 mL); 20 mg/mL (1 mL, 5 mL, 10 mL); 40 mg/mL (5 mL, 10 mL)

Dioval®, Duragen®, Estra-L®, Gynogen L.A.®: 20 mg/mL (10 mL); 40 mg/mL (10 mL)

Tablet, micronized (Estrace®): 1 mg, 2 mg

Transdermal system (Estraderm®):

0.05 mg/24 hours [10 cm^2], total estradiol 4 mg

0.1 mg/24 hours [20 cm^2], total estradiol 8 mg

References

American College of Physicians, "Guidelines for Counseling Postmenopausal Women About Preventive Hormone Therapy," *Ann Intern Med*, 1992, 117(12):1038-41.

Belchetz PE, "Hormone Treatment for Postmenopausal Women," *N Engl J Med*, 1994, 330(15):1062-71.

Ettinger B, Friedman GD, Bush T, et al, "Reduced Mortality Associated with Long-Term Postmenopausal Estrogen Therapy," *Obstet Gynecol*, 1996, 87(1):6-12.

Estradiol Transdermal *see* Estradiol *on page 350*

Estra-L® Injection *see* Estradiol *on page 350*

Estring® *see* Estradiol *on page 350*

Estro-Cyp® Injection *see* Estradiol *on page 350*

Estrogenic Substances, Conjugated *see* Estrogens, Conjugated *on next page*

Estrogens and Medroxyprogesterone

(ES troe jenz & me DROKS ee proe JES te rone)

Brand Names Premphase™; Prempro™

Synonyms Conjugated Estrogens and Medroxyprogesterone Acetate, Combined

Therapeutic Category Estrogen and Androgen Combination

Use Women with an intact uterus for the treatment of moderate to severe vasomotor symptoms associated with the menopause; treatment of atrophic vaginitis; primary ovarian failure; osteoporosis prophylactic

Additional Information See individual agents

Dosage Forms

Premphase™: Two separate tablets in therapy pack: Conjugated estrogens 0.625 mg [Premarin®] (28s) taken orally for 28 days and medroxyprogesterone acetate [Cycrin®] 5 mg (14s) which are taken orally with a Premarin® tablet on days 15 through 28

Prempro™: Conjugated estrogens 0.625 mg and medroxyprogesterone acetate 2.5 mg (14s)

Estrogens, Conjugated (ES troe jenz KON joo gate ed)
Brand Names Premarin®
Synonyms C.E.S.; Estrogenic Substances, Conjugated
Generic Available No
Therapeutic Category Estrogen Derivative
Use Atrophic vaginitis; atrophic dystrophy of vulva, urinary incontinence secondary to estrogen deficiency; hypogonadism; primary ovarian failure; vasomotor symptoms of menopause; prostatic carcinoma; prevention of osteoporosis, inoperable breast cancer
Contraindications Undiagnosed vaginal bleeding; hypersensitivity to estrogens or any component; thrombophlebitis, liver disease, breast cancer (with certain exceptions)
Warnings Estrogens have been reported to increase the risk of endometrial carcinoma; this risk can be reduced by cycling with a progestin (ie, medroxyprogesterone) for the last 10-13 days of estrogen therapy each month or administer progestin continuously
Precautions Use with caution in patients with asthma, epilepsy, migraine, diabetes, cardiac or renal dysfunction
Adverse Reactions
Cardiovascular: Increase in blood pressure, edema, thromboembolic disorder
Central nervous system: Depression, headache
Dermatologic: Chloasma, melasma, scalp alopecia
Endocrine & metabolic: Breast tenderness, hypercalcemia, breakthrough bleeding, spotting, endometrial carcinoma
Gastrointestinal: Nausea, vomiting
Hepatic: Cholestatic jaundice
Local: Pain at injection site
Overdosage Symptoms of overdose include fluid retention, jaundice, thrombophlebitis
Toxicology Toxicity is unlikely following single exposures of excessive doses, any treatment following emesis and charcoal administration should be supportive and symptomatic
Drug Interactions
Rifampin, barbiturates, cigarette smoking, and other agents that induce hepatic metabolism can increase estrogen clearance and decrease serum concentrations
Increased toxicity (potential) with anticoagulants, tricyclic antidepressants, corticosteroids
Stability Refrigerate injection
Mechanism of Action Increases the synthesis of DNA, RNA, and various proteins in target tissues; reduces the release of gonadotropin-releasing hormone from the hypothalamus; reduces FSH and LH release from the pituitary
Pharmacokinetics
Absorption: Readily from GI tract
Metabolism: To inactive compounds occurs in the liver
Elimination: In bile and urine
Usual Dosage Geriatrics and Adults:
Abnormal uterine bleeding:
Oral: 2.5-5 mg/day for 7-10 days; then decrease to 1.25 mg/day for 2 weeks
I.V.: 25 mg every 6-12 hours until bleeding stops
Osteoporosis: Oral: 0.625 mg/day chronically
Vasomotor symptoms: 0.3-1.25 mg/day; recommended duration: 5 years
Vaginal atrophy/urinary continence:
Oral: 0.3-0.625 mg/day; treat for 3 months and repeat as necessary
Cream: 2-4 g/day (1/2 to 1 applicatorful)
Monitoring Parameters Mammography should be performed in all women prior to starting estrogen therapy and then annually; blood pressure; Pap smear annually
Reference Range Male: 15-40 µg/24 hours (SI: 52-139 µmol/day); Female, postmenopausal: <20 µg/24 hours (SI: 69 µmol/day) (values at Mayo Medical Laboratories)
Test Interactions Increased chloride (S), glucose, iron (B), sodium (S), thyroxine (S); decreased protein, prothrombin time; endocrine function test may be altered
Patient Information Women should inform their physicians if signs or symptoms of any of the following occur: thromboembolic or thrombotic disorders
(Continued)

Estrogens, Conjugated *(Continued)*

including sudden severe headache or vomiting, disturbance of vision or speech, loss of vision, numbness or weakness in an extremity, sharp or crushing chest pain, calf pain, shortness of breath, severe abdominal pain or mass, mental depression or unusual bleeding; women should perform regular self-exams on breasts

Nursing Implications May also be administered intramuscularly; administer at bedtime to minimize occurrence of adverse effects; when given I.V., drug should be administered slowly to avoid the occurrence of a flushing reaction (see Patient Information and Additional Information)

Additional Information If using for osteoporosis or prevention of osteoporosis, assure adequate calcium supplement intake is administered. Studies have shown that postmenopausal estrogen use reduces the risk of severe coronary heart disease. This may be related to an estrogen-induced increase in HDL cholesterol levels.

Special Geriatric Considerations Before prescribing estrogen therapy to postmenopausal women, the risks and benefits must be weighed for each patient. Long-term estrogen use has been associated with reduced all-cause mortality, principally due to cardiovascular benefits in postmenopausal women. Data in women 80 years and older are minimal and it is unclear if the reduced risk is applicable to women in this age group. Women should be informed of these risks and benefits, as well as possible side effects and the return of menstrual bleeding (when cycled with a progestin), and be involved in the decision to prescribe. Oral therapy may be more convenient for vaginal atrophy and urinary incontinence.

Dosage Forms

Cream, vaginal: 0.625 mg/g (42.5 g)

Injection: 25 mg (5 mL)

Tablet: 0.3 mg, 0.625 mg, 0.9 mg, 1.25 mg, 2.5 mg

References

American College of Physicians, "Guidelines for Counseling Postmenopausal Women About Preventive Hormone Therapy," *Ann Intern Med*, 1992, 117(12):1038-41.

Belchetz PE, "Hormonal Treatment of Postmenopausal Women," *N Engl J Med*, 1994, 330 (15): 1062-71.

Ettinger B, Friedman GD, Bush T, et al, "Reduced Mortality Associated with Long-Term Postmenopausal Estrogen Therapy," *Obstet Gynecol*, 1996, 87(1):6-12.

The Writing Group for the PEPI Trial, "Effects of Estrogen or Estrogen/Progestin Regimens on Heart Disease Risk Factors in Postmenopausal Women," *JAMA*, 1995, 273(3):199-208.

Estroject-L.A.® Injection *see* Estradiol *on page 350*

Ethacrynic Acid *(eth a KRIN ik AS id)*

Brand Names Edecrin®

Generic Available No

Therapeutic Category Diuretic, Loop

Use Management of edema associated with congestive heart failure; hepatic cirrhosis or renal disease; short-term management of ascites due to malignancy, idiopathic edema, and lymphedema

Contraindications Hypersensitivity to ethacrynic acid or any component; anuria, hypotension, dehydration with low serum sodium concentrations; metabolic alkalosis with hypokalemia, or history of severe, watery diarrhea from ethacrynic acid

Warnings Loop diuretics are potent diuretics; excess amount can lead to profound diuresis with fluid and electrolyte loss; close medical supervision and dose evaluation is required, particularly in the elderly

Precautions Use with caution in patients with advanced hepatic cirrhosis or diabetes mellitus

Adverse Reactions

Cardiovascular: Hypotension

Central nervous system: Headache

Dermatologic: Rash

Endocrine & metabolic: Fluid and electrolyte imbalances (fluid depletion, hypokalemia, hyponatremia), hyperuricemia

Gastrointestinal: GI irritation, diarrhea

Hematologic: Thrombocytopenia, neutropenia, agranulocytosis

Hepatic: Abnormal liver function tests

Ocular: Blurred vision

Otic: Ototoxicity

Renal: Renal injury

Overdosage Symptoms of overdose include electrolyte depletion, volume depletion, dehydration, circulatory collapse

Toxicology Following GI decontamination, treatment is supportive; hypotension responds to fluids and Trendelenburg position

Drug Interactions
Decreased effect: Indomethacin, other NSAIDs
Increased hypotensive effect: Other antihypertensives
Increased level of lithium
Increased risk of ototoxicity: Aminoglycosides, other loop diuretics, vancomycin
Increased effect/toxicity of warfarin, lithium
When given with digoxin, diuretic-induced hypokalemia increases the risk of digoxin toxicity

Mechanism of Action Inhibits reabsorption of sodium and chloride in the ascending loop of Henle and distal renal tubule, interfering with the chloride-binding cotransport system, thus causing increased excretion of water, sodium, chloride, magnesium, and calcium

Pharmacodynamics
Onset of action:
Oral: Following administration diuretic effects occur within 30 minutes and peak in 2 hours
I.V.: Diuresis occurs in 5 minutes and peaks in 30 minutes
Duration of action:
Oral: 12 hours
I.V.: 2 hours

Pharmacokinetics
Absorption: Oral: Rapid
Metabolism: In the liver to active cysteine conjugate
Elimination: In bile and urine

Usual Dosage
Geriatrics: Oral: Initial: 25-50 mg/day
Adults:
Oral: Initial: 50-200 mg/day in 1-2 divided doses; increase by 25-50 mg/day to desired response
I.V.: 0.5-1 mg/kg/dose (maximum: 50 mg/dose); repeat doses not recommended

Administration Injection should **not** be given S.C. or I.M. due to local pain and irritation; single I.V. doses should not exceed 100 mg; use a new injection site if a second dose is needed, to avoid possible thrombophlebitis

Monitoring Parameters Blood pressure (both standing and sitting/supine), serum electrolytes, renal function, auditory function, weight, I & O

Test Interactions Increased ammonia (B), amylase (S), glucose, uric acid (S); decreased calcium (S); chloride (S), magnesium, sodium (S)

Patient Information May be taken with food or milk; get up slowly from a lying or sitting position to minimize dizziness, lightheadedness, or fainting; also use extra care when exercising, standing for long periods of time and during hot weather; take in the morning; take the last dose of multiple doses before 6 PM unless instructed otherwise

Nursing Implications See Monitoring Parameters and Administration

Additional Information Injection form may be given orally while hospitalized; ethacrynic acid should be saved for patients who are either allergic or resistant to furosemide, bumetanide, or torsemide

Special Geriatric Considerations Ethacrynic acid is rarely used because of its increased incidence of ototoxicity as compared to the other loop diuretics (see Additional Information)

Dosage Forms
Injection, as ethacrynate sodium: 1 mg/mL (50 mL)
Tablet: 25 mg, 50 mg

Ethambutol (e THAM byoo tole)
Brand Names Myambutol®
Generic Available No
Therapeutic Category Antitubercular Agent
Use Treatment of tuberculosis and other mycobacterial diseases in conjunction with other antituberculosis agents
Contraindications Hypersensitivity to ethambutol or any component; optic neuritis
Precautions Dosage modification required in patients with renal insufficiency
Adverse Reactions
Central nervous system: Malaise, mental confusion, fever, headache
Dermatologic: Rash, pruritus
Endocrine & metabolic: Elevated uric acid levels
(Continued)

Ethambutol *(Continued)*

Gastrointestinal: Nausea, vomiting, abdominal pain, anorexia
Hepatic: Abnormal liver function tests
Neuromuscular & skeletal: Peripheral neuritis
Ocular: Optic neuritis
Miscellaneous: Anaphylaxis, acute gout

Overdosage Symptoms of overdose include decrease in visual acuity, anorexia, joint pain, numbness of the extremities, toxic epidermal necrolysis

Toxicology Following GI decontamination, treatment is supportive

Drug Interactions Aluminum salts may delay absorption; take separately

Mechanism of Action Suppresses mycobacteria multiplication by interfering with RNA synthesis

Pharmacokinetics
Absorption: Oral: ~80%
Distribution: Well throughout the body with high concentrations in kidneys, lungs, saliva and red blood cells
Protein binding: 20% to 30%
Metabolism: 20% by the liver to inactive metabolite
Half-life: 2.5-3.6 hours (up to 7 hours or longer with renal impairment)
Time to peak serum concentration: 2-4 hours
Elimination: ~50% in urine and 20% excreted in feces as unchanged drug

Usual Dosage Geriatrics and Adults: Oral: 15-25 mg/kg/day once daily, not to exceed 2.5 g/day

Dosing interval in renal impairment:
Cl_{cr} 10-50 mL/minute: Administer every 24-36 hours
Cl_{cr} <10 mL/minute: Administer every 48 hours and/or reduce daily dose

Monitoring Parameters Perform eye testing (color testing also) before therapy and periodically while treated with ethambutol; both eyes and individual eyes need testing; periodic (monthly) visual testing in patients receiving more than 15 mg/kg/day; periodic renal, hepatic, and hematopoietic tests

Test Interactions Increased uric acid (S)

Patient Information Report any vision, visual, or color changes to physician; may cause stomach upset, take with food

Nursing Implications Reinforce compliance (see Patient Information)

Special Geriatric Considerations Since most elderly patients acquired their tuberculosis before current antituberculin regimens were available, ethambutol is only indicated when patients are from areas where drug resistant *M. tuberculosis* is endemic, in HIV-infected elderly patients, and when drug resistant *M. tuberculosis* is suspected (see dose adjustments for renal impairment)

Dosage Forms Tablet, as hydrochloride: 100 mg, 400 mg

References
Yoshikawa TT, "Tuberculosis in Aging Adults," *J Am Geriatr Soc*, 1992, 40(2):178-87.

Ethchlorvynol *(eth klor VI nole)*

Related Information
Anxiolytic/Hypnotic Use in Long-Term Care Facilities *on page 1099*
Federal OBRA Regulations Recommended Maximum Doses - Hypnotics *on page 1057*

Brand Names Placidyl®

Generic Available No

Therapeutic Category Hypnotic; Sedative

Use Short-term management of insomnia (should not exceed 7 days use)
Unlabeled use: Sedative

Contraindications Porphyria, hypersensitivity to ethchlorvynol or any component

Warnings Administer with caution to depressed or suicidal patients or to patients with a history of drug abuse; intoxication symptoms may appear with prolonged daily doses of as little as 1 g; withdrawal symptoms may be seen upon abrupt discontinuation and may be seen as late as 9 days after discontinuation; symptoms of withdrawal include slurred speech, delirium, memory loss, insomnia, ataxia, anxiety, tremors, agitation, nausea, vomiting, muscle twitching, sweating, and seizures; therefore, reductions should be gradual; some products may contain tartrazine

Precautions May impair motor coordination and cause instability to perform hazardous tasks (ie, driving); do not use in patients who have a diagnosis or a condition which results in unpredictable behavior since this drug may result in similar behaviors being exhibited; use with caution in the elderly and in patients with hepatic or renal dysfunction; use with caution in patients who have a history of paradoxical restlessness to barbiturates or alcohol

Adverse Reactions

Cardiovascular: Bradycardia, hypotension, syncope without hypotension

Central nervous system: Dizziness, mild hangover, nervousness, excitement, ataxia, confusion, drowsiness (daytime), hyperthermia, slurred speech

Dermatologic: Rash, urticaria

Gastrointestinal: Indigestion, nausea, vomiting, stomach pain, unpleasant aftertaste

Hematologic: Thrombocytopenia

Hepatic: Cholestatic jaundice

Neuromuscular & skeletal: Weakness, trembling, weakness (severe)

Ocular: Blurred vision

Respiratory: Shortness of breath

Overdosage
Symptoms of overdose include prolonged deep coma, respiratory depression, hypothermia, bradycardia, hypotension, nystagmus

Toxicology
Treatment is supportive in nature; immediate gastric evacuation for unconscious patients; hemoperfusion is most effective in enhancing elimination while hemodialysis and peritoneal dialysis are not as effective

Drug Interactions

Decreased effect of oral anticoagulants

Increased toxicity (CNS depression) with alcohol, CNS depressants, MAO inhibitors, TCAs (delirium)

Stability
Capsules should not be crushed and should not be refrigerated

Mechanism of Action
Causes nonspecific depression of the reticular activating system

Pharmacodynamics

Onset of action: 15-60 minutes

Duration: 5 hours

Pharmacokinetics

Absorption: Rapid from GI tract

Metabolism: In the liver; metabolites and the secondary alcohol of ethchlorvynol are excreted in urine (40% of dose); extensive enterohepatic recirculation of parent compound and metabolites

Half-life: 10-20 hours

Time to peak serum concentration: 2 hours

Usual Dosage
Oral:

Geriatrics: Use smallest effective dose; initial: 200 mg (see Special Geriatric Considerations)

Adults: 500-1000 mg at bedtime

Dosing adjustment in renal impairment: Cl_{cr} <50 mL/minute: Avoid use

Monitoring Parameters
Cardiac and respiratory function and abuse potential

Reference Range
Therapeutic: 2-9 µg/mL; Toxic: >20 µg/mL

Patient Information
May cause drowsiness, can impair judgment and coordination; avoid alcohol and other CNS depressants; ataxia can be reduced if taken with food, do not crush or refrigerate capsules

Nursing Implications
Raise bed rails, institute safety measures, assist with ambulation

Special Geriatric Considerations
This medication should be avoided in the elderly. The addiction potential, withdrawal problems, and side effect profile are undesirable for use in elderly. Also, many elderly have creatinine clearances <50 mL/minute. Less problematic agents are available for sleep induction. If used, use lowest effective dose for not more than 7 days.

Dosage Forms
Capsule: 200 mg, 500 mg, 750 mg

References
Kathpalia SC, Haslitt JH, and Lim VS, "Charcoal Hemoperfusion for Treatment of Ethchlorvynol Overdose," *Artif Organs*, 1983, 7(2):246-8.

Kelner MJ and Bailey DN, "Ethchlorvynol Ingestion: Interpretation of Blood Concentrations and Clinical Findings," *J Toxicol Clin Toxicol*, 1983-84, 21(3):399-408.

Yell RP, "Ethchlorvynol Overdose," *Am J Emerg Med*, 1990, 8(3):246-50.

Ethinyl Estradiol (ETH in il es tra DYE ole)

Brand Names
Estinyl®

Generic Available
No

Therapeutic Category
Estrogen Derivative

Use
Hypogonadism, primary ovarian failure, vasomotor symptoms of menopause, prostatic carcinoma, breast cancer

Contraindications
Thrombophlebitis, undiagnosed vaginal bleeding, hypersensitivity to ethinyl estradiol or any component, known or suspected pregnancy, carcinoma of the breast, estrogen-dependent tumor

Warnings
Use with caution in patients with asthma, seizure disorders, migraine, cardiac, renal or hepatic impairment, cerebrovascular disorders or
(Continued)

Ethinyl Estradiol *(Continued)*

history of breast cancer, past or present thromboembolic disease, smokers >35 years of age

Adverse Reactions

Cardiovascular: Peripheral edema, hypertension, thromboembolism, myocardial infarction, edema

Central nervous system: Headache, stroke, depression, dizziness, anxiety

Dermatologic: Chloasma, melasma, rash

Endocrine & metabolic: Enlargement of breasts, breast tenderness, bloating, increased libido, breast tumors, amenorrhea, alterations in frequency and flow of menses, decreased glucose tolerance, increased triglycerides and LDL

Gastrointestinal: Nausea, anorexia, vomiting, diarrhea, GI distress

Hepatic: Cholestatic jaundice

Ocular: Intolerance to contact lenses

Miscellaneous: Increased susceptibility to *Candida* infection

Overdosage Signs and symptoms include fluid retention, jaundice, thrombophlebitis, nausea toxicity is unlikely following single exposures of excessive doses

Toxicology Any treatment following emesis and charcoal administration should be supportive and symptomatic

Drug Interactions

Decreased effect: Rifampin decreases estrogen serum concentrations

Increased toxicity:

Hydrocortisone increases corticosteroid toxic potential

Anticoagulants: Increases potential for thromboembolic events with anticoagulants

Carbamazepine, tricyclic antidepressants, and corticosteroids; increased thromboembolic potential with oral anticoagulants

Mechanism of Action Increases the synthesis of DNA, RNA, and various proteins in target tissues; reduces the release of gonadotropin-releasing hormone from the hypothalamus; reduces FSH and LH release from the pituitary

Pharmacokinetics

Absorption: Absorbed well from GI tract

Protein binding: 50% to 80%

Metabolism: Inactivated by liver; substrate CYP3A4, 3A5-7

Elimination: By the kidneys

Usual Dosage Geriatrics and Adults: Oral:

Male: Prostatic cancer (inoperable, progressing): 0.15-2 mg/day for palliation

Female:

Hypogonadism: 0.05 mg 1-3 times/day for 2 weeks of a theoretical menstrual cycle followed by progesterone for 3-6 months

Vasomotor symptoms: 0.02-0.05 mg for 21 days, off 7 days and repeat

Breast cancer (inoperable, progressing): 1 mg 3 times/day for palliation

Osteoporosis: 0.02 mg/day, cycle with medroxyprogesterone for the last 12-14 days or as continuous therapy; 0.02 mg is equivalent to 0.625 mg conjugated estrogen

Monitoring Parameters Weight, blood pressure, glucose

Reference Range Peak plasma concentration of ethinyl estradiol after a 0.05 mg dose: 100-200 pg/mL

Test Interactions

Decreased antithrombin III

Decreased serum folate concentration

Increased prothrombin and factors VII, VIII, IX, X

Increased platelet aggregability

Increased thyroid binding globulin

Increased total thyroid hormone (T_4)

Increased serum triglycerides/phospholipids

Patient Information Inform your physician if signs or symptoms of any of the following occur: Thromboembolic or thrombotic disorders including sudden severe headache or vomiting, disturbance of vision or speech, loss of vision, numbness or weakness in an extremity, sharp or crushing chest pain, calf pain, shortness of breath, severe abdominal pain or mass, mental depression or unusual bleeding. Women should perform regular self-breast exams.

Nursing Implications Administer at bedtime to minimize occurrence of adverse effects (see Adverse Reactions)

Additional Information Estrinyl® contains tartrazine which can cause allergic reactions; 17-beta-estradiol modulates acetylcholine-induced coronary artery responses in postmenopausal women; if using for osteoporosis or prevention of osteoporosis, assure adequate calcium supplement intake is administered; studies have shown that postmenopausal estrogen use reduces the risk of severe coronary heart disease; this may be related to an estrogen-induced increase in HDL cholesterol levels

Special Geriatric Considerations Before prescribing estrogen therapy to postmenopausal women, the risks and benefits must be weighed for each patient. Long-term estrogen use has been associated with reduced all-cause mortality, principally due to cardiovascular benefits in postmenopausal women. Data in women 80 years and older are minimal and it is unclear if the reduced risk is applicable to women in this age group. Women should be informed of these risks and benefits, as well as possible side effects and the return of menstrual bleeding (when cycled with a progestin), and be involved in the decision to prescribe. Oral therapy may be more convenient for vaginal atrophy and urinary incontinence.

Dosage Forms Tablet: 0.02 mg, 0.05 mg, 0.5 mg

References

American College of Physicians, "Guidelines for Counseling Postmenopausal Women About Preventive Hormone Therapy," *Ann Intern Med*, 1992, 117(12):1038-41.

Belchetz PE, "Hormonal Treatment of Postmenopausal Women," *N Engl J Med*, 1994, 330 (15): 1062-71.

Ettinger B, Friedman GD, Bush T, et al, "Reduced Mortality Associated with Long-Term Postmenopausal Estrogen Therapy," *Obstet Gynecol*, 1996, 87(1):6-12.

The Writing Group for the PEPI Trial, "Effects of Estrogen or Estrogen/Progestin Regimens on Heart Disease Risk Factors in Postmenopausal Women," *JAMA*, 1995, 273(3):199-208.

Ethionamide (e thye on AM ide)

Brand Names Trecator®-SC

Therapeutic Category Antitubercular Agent

Use In conjunction with other antituberculosis agents in the treatment of tuberculosis and other mycobacterial diseases

Contraindications Contraindicated in patients with severe hepatic impairment or in patients who are hypersensitive to the drug

Precautions Use with caution in diabetic patients and patients receiving cycloserine or isoniazid

Adverse Reactions

Cardiovascular: Postural hypotension

Central nervous system: Drowsiness, dizziness, optic neuritis, seizures, headache

Dermatologic: Rash, stomatitis

Endocrine & metabolic: Hypoglycemia, goiter, gynecomastia

Gastrointestinal: Nausea, vomiting, abdominal pain, diarrhea, anorexia, metallic taste

Hematologic: Thrombocytopenia

Hepatic: Hepatitis

Neuromuscular & skeletal: Peripheral neuritis

Overdosage Symptoms of overdose include peripheral neuropathy, anorexia, joint pain

Toxicology Following GI decontamination, treatment is supportive; pyridoxine may be given to prevent peripheral neuropathy

Mechanism of Action Inhibits peptide synthesis

Pharmacokinetics

Protein binding: 10%

Bioavailability: 80%

Half-life: 2-3 hours

Time to peak serum concentration: Oral: Within 3 hours

Elimination: Metabolized and excreted as metabolites (active and inactive) and parent drug in urine

Usual Dosage Geriatrics and Adults: Oral: 500-1000 mg/day in 1-3 divided doses

Dosing adjustment in renal impairment: Cl_{cr} <50 mL/minute: Administer 50% of dose

Monitoring Parameters Initial and periodic serum AST and ALT

Test Interactions Decreased thyroxine (S)

Patient Information Take with meals, may cause upset stomach and loss of appetite, metallic taste or salivation

Nursing Implications Neurotoxic effects may be relieved by the administration of pyridoxine

Special Geriatric Considerations Since many elderly have Cl_{cr} <50 mL/minute, adjust dose for renal function (see Usual Dosage and Overdosage)

Dosage Forms Tablet: 250 mg

Ethmozine® *see Moricizine on page 638*

Ethopropazine (eth oh PROE pa zeen)

Brand Names Parsidol®

Generic Available No

Therapeutic Category Anticholinergic Agent; Anti-Parkinson's Agent

Use Treatment of parkinsonism, drug-induced extrapyramidal reactions

Contraindications Patients with narrow-angle glaucoma; hypersensitivity to any component; pyloric or duodenal obstruction, stenosing peptic ulcers; bladder neck obstructions; achalasia; myasthenia gravis

Precautions Use with caution in hot weather or during exercise. Elderly patients frequently develop increased sensitivity and require strict dosage regulation - side effects may be more severe in elderly patients with athero-sclerotic changes. Use with caution in patients with tachycardia, cardiac arrhythmias, hypertension, hypotension, prostatic hypertrophy (especially in the elderly) or any tendency toward urinary retention, liver or kidney disorders and obstructive disease of the GI or GU tract. May exacerbate mental symptoms and precipitate a toxic psychosis when used to treat extrapyramidal reactions resulting from phenothiazines. When given in large doses or to susceptible patients, may cause weakness and inability to move particular muscle groups. Anticholinergic agents can aggravate tardive dyskinesia caused by neuroleptic agents.

Adverse Reactions
Cardiovascular: Tachycardia
Central nervous system: Coma, nervousness, drowsiness, seizures, memory loss (**the elderly may be at increased risk for confusion and hallucinations**)
Dermatologic: Pigmentation of the skin
Gastrointestinal: Nausea, vomiting, constipation, xerostomia
Genitourinary: Urinary retention
Hepatic: Jaundice
Ocular: Blurred vision, mydriasis, pigmentation of the cornea, lens, retina
Miscellaneous: Heat intolerance

Overdosage Symptoms of overdose include CNS depression, confusion, nervousness, hallucinations, dizziness, blurred vision, nausea, vomiting, hyperthermia

Toxicology Anticholinergic toxicity is caused by strong binding of the drug to cholinergic receptors. Cholinesterase inhibitors reduce acetylcholinesterase, the enzyme that breaks down acetylcholine and thereby allows acetylcholine to accumulate and compete for receptor binding with the offending anticholinergic. For anticholinergic overdose with severe life-threatening symptoms, physostigmine 1-2 mg S.C. or I.V., slowly may be given to reverse these effects.

Drug Interactions
Decreased effect of levodopa (decreased absorption)
Increased toxicity (central anticholinergic syndrome): Narcotic analgesics, phenothiazines, and other antipsychotics, tricyclic antidepressants, some antihistamines, quinidine, disopyramide
Antagonistic effect: Tacrine, donepezil

Mechanism of Action Phenothiazine-derivative with strong atropine-like blocking effects on parasympathetic-innervated peripheral structures; also exhibits antihistamine activity

Pharmacokinetics No data available

Usual Dosage Geriatrics and Adults: Oral: Initial: 50 mg once or twice daily, increasing gradually; severe cases may need up to 600 mg/day

Monitoring Parameters Symptoms of EPS or Parkinson's, pulse, anticholinergic effects (ie, CNS, bowel and bladder function)

Patient Information Take after meals or with food if GI upset occurs; do not discontinue drug abruptly; notify physician if adverse GI effects, rapid or pounding heartbeat, confusion, eye pain, rash, fever or heat intolerance occurs. Observe caution when performing hazardous tasks or those that require alertness such as driving, as may cause drowsiness. Avoid alcohol and other CNS depressants. May cause dry mouth - adequate fluid intake or hard sugar-free candy may relieve. Difficult urination or constipation may occur - notify physician if effects persist; may increase susceptibility to heat stroke.

Nursing Implications Do not discontinue drug abruptly

Additional Information Ethopropazine is a phenothiazine with prominent anticholinergic effects. It is less effective than the synthetic anticholinergic agents. High doses of ethopropazine are relatively well tolerated in adults.

Special Geriatric Considerations Anticholinergic agents are generally not well tolerated in the elderly and their use should be avoided when possible (see Precautions and Adverse Reactions). In the elderly, anticholinergic agents should not be used as prophylaxis against extrapyramidal symptoms.

Dosage Forms Tablet, as hydrochloride: 10 mg, 50 mg

References
Feinberg M, "The Problems of Anticholinergic Adverse Effects in Older Patients," *Drugs Aging*, 1993, 3(4):335-48.

Ethosuximide (eth oh SUKS i mide)

Related Information
Serum Drug Concentrations Commonly Monitored: Guidelines on page 1114

Brand Names Zarontin®

Generic Available No

Therapeutic Category Anticonvulsant, Succinimide

Use Management of absence (petit mal) seizures, myoclonic seizures, and akinetic epilepsy; considered to be drug of choice for simple absence seizures

Contraindications Known hypersensitivity to ethosuximide or any succinimide

Warnings Use with caution in patients with hepatic or renal disease; abrupt withdrawal of the drug may precipitate absence status; ethosuximide may increase tonic-clonic seizures in patients with mixed seizure disorders; ethosuximide must be used in combination with other anticonvulsants in patients with both absence and tonic-clonic seizures

Precautions Proceed slowly when increasing or decreasing dose of ethosuximide; use caution and monitor closely when adding or eliminating other medications

Adverse Reactions
Central nervous system: Sedation, fatigue, dizziness, lethargy, euphoria, ataxia, irritability, nervousness, hallucinations, insomnia, agitation, behavioral changes, headache, sleep disturbances, loss of concentration, confusion, depression, aggressiveness

Dermatologic: Rashes, urticaria, Stevens-Johnson syndrome, erythema multiforme, alopecia

Gastrointestinal: Nausea, vomiting, anorexia, abdominal pain, cramps, diarrhea, constipation

Genitourinary: Vaginal bleeding, polyuria, hematuria (also microscopic hematuria)

Hematologic: Rarely: Leukopenia, aplastic anemia, thrombocytopenia, eosinophilia, granulocytopenia, monocytosis, pancytopenia

Ocular: Blurred vision, periorbital edema

Miscellaneous: Rarely SLE, edema of tongue, gingival hypertrophy, hiccups

Overdosage Acute overdosage can cause CNS depression, ataxia, stupor, coma, hypotension; chronic overdose can cause skin rash, confusion, ataxia, proteinuria, hepatic dysfunction, hematuria

Toxicology Treatment is supportive; hemoperfusion and hemodialysis may be useful

Drug Interactions
May increase serum concentrations of hydantoins (phenytoin)
Decreases serum concentrations of phenobarbital and primidone
Serum concentrations of valproic acid may increase or decrease

Mechanism of Action Increases the seizure threshold and suppresses paroxysmal spike-and-wave pattern in absence seizures; depresses nerve transmission in the motor cortex

Pharmacokinetics
Absorption: Well absorbed from GI tract
Distribution: Adults: V_d: 0.62-0.72 L/kg
Metabolism: ~80% in the liver to three inactive metabolites
Half-life: 50-60 hours
Time to peak serum concentration:
 Capsule: Within 3-7 hours
 Syrup: <2-4 hours
Elimination: Slowly excreted in urine as metabolites (50%) and as unchanged drug (10% to 20%); small amounts excreted in feces

Usual Dosage Geriatrics and Adults: Oral: Initial: 250 mg twice daily; increase by 250 mg as needed every 4-7 days up to 1.5 g/day in 2 divided doses

Monitoring Parameters CBC, platelets, liver enzymes, trough ethosuximide serum concentration
(Continued)

Ethosuximide *(Continued)*

Reference Range Therapeutic: 40-100 µg/mL (SI: 280-710 µmol/L); Toxic: >150 µg/mL (SI: >1062 µmol/L)

Test Interactions Increased alkaline phosphatase (S); positive Coombs' [direct]; decreased calcium (S)

Patient Information Take with food; do not discontinue abruptly; may cause drowsiness and impair judgment; patient should have a "Medic Alert" identification; call physician if experiencing rash, fever, sore throat, bleeding, dizziness, blurred vision

Nursing Implications Observe patient for excess sedation; maintain serum concentrations; monitor for bruising and bleeding

Additional Information Considered to be drug of choice for simple absence seizures

Special Geriatric Considerations No specific studies with the use of this medication in elderly; consider renal function and proceed slowly with dosing increases; monitor closely (see elimination under Pharmacokinetics)

Dosage Forms
Capsule: 250 mg
Syrup (raspberry flavor): 250 mg/5 mL (473 mL)

Ethoxynaphthamido Penicillin Sodium *see* Nafcillin *on page 648*

Etidronate Disodium (e ti DROE nate dye SOW dee um)

Brand Names Didronel®

Synonyms EHDP; Sodium Etidronate

Therapeutic Category Antidote, Hypercalcemia; Bisphosphonate Derivative

Use Symptomatic treatment of Paget's disease and heterotopic ossification due to spinal cord injury or after total hip replacement, hypercalcemia associated with malignancy
Unlabeled use: Postmenopausal osteoporosis

Contraindications Hypersensitivity to biphosphonates; patients with serum creatinine >5 mg/dL

Warnings Response may be slow; therefore, do not increase therapy prematurely or resume therapy before there is evidence of reactivation of disease process; renal dysfunction in hypercalcemic treatment (reversible)

Precautions Use with caution in patients with restricted calcium and vitamin D intake; dosage modification required in renal impairment; must maintain adequate calcium and vitamin D intake; do not administer during bouts of enterocolitis since it may aggravate or induce diarrhea; osteoid formation may delay mineralization, therefore, withhold therapy in patients with fractured bone until callus is evident; Paget's disease may fracture if doses are >20 mg/kg/day or are continuous for >6 months; hypocalcemia may occur during therapy; proximal renal tubular damage

Adverse Reactions
Central nervous system: Fever, seizures
Dermatologic: Angioedema, urticaria, rash, pruritus
Endocrine & metabolic: Hypocalcemia, hypophosphatemia, hypomagnesemia
Gastrointestinal: Diarrhea, nausea, vomiting constipation, ulcerative stomatitis, dysgeusia
Hepatic: Elevated hepatic enzymes
Neuromuscular & skeletal: Pain, increased risk of fractures
Renal: Nephrotoxicity, fluid overload, elevated serum creatinine and BUN
Respiratory: Dyspnea
Miscellaneous: Occult blood in stools, hypersensitivity reactions

Overdosage Symptoms of overdose include diarrhea, nausea, hypocalcemia; parenteral: EKG changes, bleeding, paresthesia, carpopedal spasm; renal insufficiency

Toxicology Gastric lavage, treat hypocalcemia (I.V. calcium); general supportive care, hypotension, and fever may be treated with corticosteroids

Drug Interactions Oral: Calcium, food decrease absorption

Stability Avoid heat >104°F (40°C)

Mechanism of Action Decreases bone resorption by inhibiting osteocystic osteolysis; decreases mineral release and matrix or collagen breakdown in bone

Pharmacodynamics
Onset of action: Within 1-3 months of therapy
Duration: 12 months without continuous therapy

Pharmacokinetics
Absorption: Oral: Dependent upon dose (1% at 5 mg/kg/day to 6% at 20 mg/kg/day) administered
Half-life:
Serum: 5-7 hours
Bone: >90 days
Metabolism: Not metabolized
Elimination: Excreted as unchanged drug primarily in urine with unabsorbed oral drug being eliminated in feces

Usual Dosage Geriatrics and Adults: Oral:
Paget's disease: Initial: 5 mg/kg/day given every day for no more than 6 months; may administer 10-20 mg/kg/day for up to 3 months. Daily dose may be divided if adverse GI effects occur; do not exceed 20 mg/kg/day.
Heterotropic ossification complications following total hip replacement: 20 mg/kg/day for 1 month preoperatively, followed by 20mg/kg/day for 3 months postoperatively
Heterotropic ossification with spinal cord injury: 20 mg/kg/day for 2 weeks, then 10 mg/kg/day for 10 weeks
Hypercalcemia associated with malignancy: I.V.: 7.5 mg/kg/day for 3 days; repeat treatment must be given at 7 days between treatments; oral therapy may be started following parenteral treatment, 20 mg/kg/day for 1 month; use for >90 days is recommended
Postmenopausal osteoporosis (unlabeled use): 400 mg/day for 2 weeks followed by a 13-week period with no etidronate, then repeat cycle; maintain adequate calcium and vitamin D intake during entire 15-week treatment cycle

Monitoring Parameters Serum calcium, phosphorous, potassium
Reference Range Calcium (total): Adults: 9.0-11.0 mg/dL (2.05-2.54 mmol/L), may slightly decrease with aging; phosphorus: 2.5-4.5 mg/dL (0.81-1.45 mmol/L)
Patient Information Maintain adequate intake of calcium and vitamin D; take medicine on an empty stomach; do not take with calcium, separate by 2 hours
Nursing Implications Dilute I.V. dose in at least 250 mL NS, ensure adequate hydration; dosage modification required in renal insufficiency
Special Geriatric Considerations Monitor serum electrolytes periodically since elderly are often receiving diuretics which can result in decreases in serum calcium, potassium, and magnesium
Dosage Forms
Injection: 50 mg/mL (6 mL)
Tablet: 200 mg, 400 mg

References
Storm T, Thamsborg G, Steiniche T, et al, "Effect of Intermittent Cyclical Etidronate Therapy on Bone Mass and Fracture Rate in Women With Postmenopausal Osteoporosis," *N Engl J Med*, 1990, 322(18):1265-71.
Watts NB, Harris ST, Genant HK, et al, "Intermittent Cyclical Etidronate Treatment of Postmenopausal Osteoporosis," *N Engl J Med*, 1990, 323(2):73-9.

Etodolac (ee toe DOE lak)
Brand Names Lodine®; Lodine® XL
Generic Available No
Therapeutic Category Analgesic, Non-narcotic; Anti-inflammatory Agent; Antipyretic; Nonsteroidal Anti-inflammatory Agent (NSAID), Oral
Use Acute and long-term use in the management of signs and symptoms of osteoarthritis and management of pain; rheumatoid arthritis
Unlabeled use: Ankylosing spondylitis, tendonitis, bursitis, acute painful shoulder, acute gout
Contraindications Hypersensitivity to etodolac, aspirin or other NSAIDs
Warnings GI toxicity (bleeding, ulceration, perforation); CNS effects may occur (headaches, confusion, depression); hypersensitivity, anaphylactoid reactions (intermittent tolmetin use more often); renal function decline, acute renal insufficiency, interstitial nephritis, dysuria, cystitis, hematuria, nephrotic syndrome, hyperkalemia in acute renal insufficiency, hyponatremia, papillary necrosis, hepatic function impairment; elderly have increased risk for adverse reactions to NSAIDs (see Special Geriatric Considerations)
Precautions Use with caution in patients with congestive heart failure, hypertension, decreased renal or hepatic function, history of GI disease (bleeding or ulcers), or those receiving anticoagulants; perform ophthalmologic evaluation for those who develop eye complaints during therapy (blurred vision, diminished vision, changes in color vision, retinal changes); NSAIDs may mask signs/symptoms of infections; photosensitivity reported
(Continued)

Etodolac *(Continued)*

Adverse Reactions

Cardiovascular: Congestive heart failure, angina, hypertension, hypotension, arrhythmias, edema

Central nervous system: Headache, drowsiness, vertigo, dizziness, fatigue, hallucinations, confusion, depression, emotional lability, psychotic behavior, pyrexia

Dermatologic: Rash, urticaria, angioedema, Stevens-Johnson syndrome, exfoliative dermatitis, bruising, petechiae, purpura

Endocrine & metabolic: Hyperglycemia, hypoglycemia, hyperkalemia, gynecomastia, hyponatremia, fluid retention

Gastrointestinal: Dyspepsia, heartburn, nausea, diarrhea, constipation, flatulence, stomatitis, vomiting, abdominal pain, peptic ulcer, GI bleeding, GI perforation, gingival ulcers, pancreatitis, proctitis, paralytic ulcers, colitis, anorexia, weight loss, dry mucous membranes

Genitourinary: Impotence, azotemia, dysuria

Hematologic: Neutropenia, anemia, agranulocytosis, bone marrow suppression, hemolytic anemia, hemorrhage, inhibition of platelet aggregation

Hepatic: Hepatitis, elevated LFTs, cholestatic jaundice

Neuromuscular & skeletal: Involuntary muscle movements, muscle weakness, tremors, weakness

Ocular: Vision changes

Otic: Tinnitus

Renal: Polyuria, pyuria, oliguria, anuria, acute renal failure

Respiratory: Exacerbation of asthma, dyspnea

Miscellaneous: Thirst, diaphoresis

Overdosage

Symptoms include drowsiness, lethargy, disorientation, confusion, dizziness, numbness, paresthesia, nausea, vomiting, gastric irritation, abdominal pain, headache, tinnitus, sweating, blurred vision, muscle twitching, seizures, coma, acute renal failure, increased BUN and serum creatinine, hypotension, tachycardia, and metabolic acidosis

Toxicology

Management of a nonsteroidal anti-inflammatory drug (NSAID) intoxication is primarily supportive and symptomatic. Fluid therapy is commonly effective in managing the hypotension that may occur following an acute NSAID overdose, except when this is due to an acute blood loss. Seizures tend to be very short-lived and often do not require drug treatment although recurrent seizures should be treated with I.V. diazepam. Since many of the NSAIDs undergo enterohepatic cycling, multiple doses of charcoal may be needed to reduce the potential for delayed toxicities. NSAIDs are highly bound to plasma proteins, therefore hemodialysis and peritoneal dialysis are not useful.

Drug Interactions

NSAIDs may decrease effect of loop diuretics

Cyclosporine may increase nephrotoxicity of both agents; may increase digoxin, methotrexate, and lithium serum concentrations

Aspirin or other salicylates may decrease NSAID serum concentrations

Other NSAIDs may increase adverse GI effects

Increased prothrombin time with anticoagulants

Decreased antihypertensive effects of ACE inhibitors, beta-blockers, and thiazide diuretics

Increased response to sympathomimetics

Probenecid may increase toxicity of NSAIDs by increase in serum concentrations

Concomitant use with loop diuretics may enhance azotemia in elderly

Stability

Protect from moisture

Mechanism of Action

Inhibits prostaglandin synthesis, acts on the hypothalamus heat-regulating center to reduce fever, blocks prostaglandin synthetase action which prevents formation of the platelet-aggregating substance thromboxane A_2; decreases pain receptor sensitivity. Other proposed mechanisms of action for salicylate anti-inflammatory action are lysosomal stabilization, inhibition of kinin and leukotrienes production, alteration of chemotactic factors, and inhibition of neutrophil activation. This latter mechanism may be the most significant pharmacologic action to reduce inflammation.

Pharmacodynamics

Onset of analgesic action: Within 30 minutes to 1 hour

Duration: 4-12 hours

Pharmacokinetics

Absorption: Oral: Well absorbed

Distribution: V_d: 0.4 L/kg

Protein binding: Highly protein-bound

Half-life: 7 hours

Time to peak serum concentration: Within 1-2 hours

Usual Dosage Geriatrics and Adults: Oral:

Acute pain: 200-400 mg every 6-8 hours, as needed, not to exceed total daily doses of 1200 mg; extended release dose: one tablet daily

Osteoarthritis: Initial: 800-1200 mg/day given in divided doses: 400 mg 2 or 3 times/day; 300 mg 2, 3 or 4 times/day; 200 mg 3 or 4 times/day; total daily dose should not exceed 1200 mg; for patients weighing <60 kg, total daily dose should not exceed 20 mg/kg

Rheumatoid arthritis: 500 mg twice daily

Monitoring Parameters Monitor CBC, liver enzymes; monitor BUN/serum creatinine in patients receiving diuretics; monitor response (pain, range of motion, grip strength, mobility, ADL function), inflammation; observe for weight gain, edema; monitor renal function; observe for bleeding, bruising; evaluate gastrointestinal effects (abdominal pain, bleeding, dyspepsia); mental confusion, disorientation

Test Interactions False-positive for urinary bilirubin and ketone

Patient Information Take with food, milk, or water; report any signs of blood in stool; serious gastrointestinal bleeding can occur as well as ulceration and perforation. Pain may or may not be present. Avoid aspirin and aspirin-containing products while taking this medication. If gastric upset occurs, take with food, milk, or antacid. If gastric adverse effects persist, contact physician. May cause drowsiness, dizziness, blurred vision, and confusion. Use caution when performing tasks which require alertness (eg, driving). Do not take for more than 3 days for fever or 10 days for pain without physician's advice.

Nursing Implications See Overdosage, Monitoring Parameters, Patient Information, and Special Geriatric Considerations

Additional Information Single dose of 76-100 mg is comparable to the analgesic effect of aspirin 650 mg; there are no clinical guidelines to predict which NSAID will give response in a particular patient. Trials with each must be initiated until response determined. Consider dose, patient convenience, and cost.

Special Geriatric Considerations Elderly are a high-risk population for adverse effects from nonsteroidal anti-inflammatory agents. As much as 60% of elderly who experience GI side effects can develop peptic ulceration and/or hemorrhage asymptomatically. The concomitant use of H_2 blockers, omeprazole, and sucralfate is not effective as prophylaxis with the exception of NSAID-induced duodenal ulcers which may be prevented by the use of ranitidine. Misoprostol and proton pump inhibitors are the only agents proven to help prevent the development of NSAID-induced ulcers. Also, concomitant disease and drug use contribute to the risk for GI adverse effects. Use lowest effective dose for shortest period possible. Consider renal function decline with age. Use of NSAIDs can compromise existing renal function especially when Cl_{cr} is ≤30 mL/minute. Tinnitus may be a difficult and unreliable indication of toxicity due to age-related hearing loss or eighth cranial nerve damage. CNS adverse effects such as confusion, agitation, and hallucination are generally seen in overdose or high dose situations, but elderly may demonstrate these adverse effects at lower doses than younger adults. In patients ≥65 years, no substantial differences in the pharmacokinetics or side-effects profile were seen compared with the general population.

Dosage Forms

Capsule (Lodine®): 200 mg, 300 mg

Tablet: 400 mg

Lodine®: 400 mg

Tablet, extended release (Lodine® XL): 400 mg, 600 mg

References

Brooks PM, Day RO, "Nonsteroidal Anti-inflammatory Drugs - Differences and Similarities," *N Engl J Med*, 1991, 324(24):1716-25.

Clinch D, Banerjee AK, Ostick G, "Absence of Abdominal Pain in Elderly Patients With Peptic Ulcer," *Age Ageing*, 1984, 13:120-3.

Clive DM, Stoff JS, "Renal Syndromes Associated With Nonsteroidal Anti-inflammatory Drugs," *N Engl J Med*, 1984, 310(9):563-72.

Graham DY, "Prevention of Gastroduodenal Injury Induced by Chronic Nonsteroidal Anti-inflammatory Drug Therapy," *Gastroenterology*, 1989, 96(2 Pt 2 Suppl):675-81.

Gurwitz JH, Avorn J, Ross-Degnan D, et al, "Nonsteroidal Anti-Inflammatory Drug-Associated Azotemia in the Very Old," *JAMA*, 1990, 264(4):471-5.

Hawkey CJ, Karrasch JA, Szczepaski L, et al, "Omeprazole Compared With Misoprostol for Ulcers Associated With Nonsteroidal Anti-inflammatory Drugs," *N Engl J Med*, 1998, 338(11):727-34.

Knodel LC, "Preventing NSAID-Induced Ulcers: The Role of Misoprostol," *Consult Pharm*, 1989, 4:37-41.

Pounder R, "Silent Peptic Ulceration: Deadly Silence or Golden Silence?" *Gastroenterology*, 1989, 96(2 Pt 2 Suppl):626-31.

(Continued)

Etodolac *(Continued)*

Yeomans ND, Tulassay Z, Juhasz L, et al, "A Comparison of Omeprazole With Ranitidine for Ulcers Associated With Nonsteroidal Anti-inflammatory Drugs," *N Engl J Med*, 1998, 338(11):719-26.

Etrafon® *see* Amitriptyline and Perphenazine *on page 62*

ETS-2%® Topical *see* Erythromycin, Topical *on page 347*

Eulexin® *see* Flutamide *on page 403*

Eurax® *see* Crotamiton *on page 256*

Evac-Q-Mag® [OTC] *see* Magnesium Citrate *on page 563*

Evalose® *see* Lactulose *on page 523*

Everone® Injection *see* Testosterone *on page 895*

E-Vista® *see* Hydroxyzine *on page 470*

Evista® *see* Raloxifene *on page 820*

Excedrin® IB [OTC] *see* Ibuprofen *on page 475*

Exidine® Scrub [OTC] *see* Chlorhexidine Gluconate *on page 206*

Extra Action Cough Syrup [OTC] *see* Guaifenesin and Dextromethorphan *on page 439*

Extra Strength Adprin-B® [OTC] *see* Aspirin *on page 84*

Extra Strength Bayer® Enteric 500 Aspirin [OTC] *see* Aspirin *on page 84*

Extra Strength Bayer® Plus [OTC] *see* Aspirin *on page 84*

Extra Strength Doan's® [OTC] *see* Salicylates (Various Salts) *on page 842*

Eye-Lube-A® Solution [OTC] *see* Artificial Tears *on page 82*

Eye-Sed® Ophthalmic [OTC] *see* Zinc Sulfate *on page 995*

Eyesine® Ophthalmic [OTC] *see* Tetrahydrozoline *on page 901*

Ezide® *see* Hydrochlorothiazide *on page 458*

F_3T *see* Trifluridine *on page 958*

Famciclovir *(fam SYE kloe veer)*

Brand Names Famvir™

Therapeutic Category Antiviral Agent, Oral

Use Management of acute herpes zoster (shingles); treatment of recurrent episodes of genital herpes

Contraindications Hypersensitivity to famciclovir

Warnings Has not been studied in immunocompromised patients or patients with ophthalmic or disseminated zoster

Precautions Adjust dose based on patient's renal function and in patients with noncompensated hepatic disease; should be started within 72 hours of initial lesion

Adverse Reactions

Central nervous system: Headache, fatigue, fever, dizziness, somnolence

Gastrointestinal: Nausea, diarrhea, vomiting, constipation, anorexia, abdominal pain

Neuromuscular & skeletal: Rigors, paresthesia

Toxicology Supportive and symptomatic care is recommended; hemodialysis may enhance elimination

Drug Interactions Increased effect/toxicity:

Cimetidine: Penciclovir (active metabolite) AUC may increase due to impaired metabolism

Digoxin: C_{max} of digoxin may increase by ~19%

Probenecid: Penciclovir serum concentrations significantly increase

Theophylline: Penciclovir AUC/C_{max} may increase and renal clearance decrease, although not clinically significant

Mechanism of Action Famciclovir is a prodrug which is rapidly biotransformed to the active metabolite, penciclovir, which is phosphorylated by viral thymidine kinase in HSV-1, HSV-2, and VZV-infected cells to a monophosphate form; this is then converted to penciclovir triphosphate and competes with deoxyguanosine triphosphate to inhibit HSV-2 polymerase (ie, herpes viral DNA synthesis/replication is selectively inhibited)

Pharmacokinetics

Absorption: Food decreases the maximum peak concentration and delays the time to peak; AUC remains the same

Distribution: V_{dss}: 0.98-1.08 L/kg

Protein binding: 20%

Metabolism: Rapidly deacetylated and oxidized to penciclovir (not by cytochrome P-450)

Bioavailability: 77%; T_{max}: 0.9 hours

Half-life: Penciclovir: 2-3 hours (10, 20, and 7 hours in HSV-1, HSV-2, and VZV-infected cells); linearly decreased with reductions in renal function

Elimination: >90% of penciclovir is eliminated unchanged in urine; C_{max} and T_{max} are decreased and prolonged, respectively in patients with noncompensated hepatic impairment

Usual Dosage Geriatrics and Adults: Oral:

Herpes zoster: 500 mg every 8 hours for 7 days

Herpes zoster dosing interval in renal impairment:
Cl_{cr} ≥60 mL/minute: Administer 500 mg every 8 hours
Cl_{cr} 40-59 mL/minute: Administer 500 mg every 12 hours
Cl_{cr} 20-39 mL/minute: Administer 500 mg every 24 hours
Cl_{cr} <20 mL/minute: Administer 250 mg every 48 hours

Genital herpes (recurrent episodes): 125 mg twice daily for 5 days

Genital herpes (recurrent) dosing interval in renal impairment:
Cl_{cr} ≥40 mL/minute: Administer 125 mg every 12 hours
Cl_{cr} 20-39 mL/minute: Administer 125 mg every 24 hours
Cl_{cr} <20 mL/minute: Administer 125 mg every 48 hours

Patient Information Patient may take medication without regard to meals; contagious only when viral shedding is occurring; avoid sexual intercourse when lesions are visible; begin medication at first sign or symptom of genital herpes or at diagnosis of herpes zoster

Special Geriatric Considerations For herpes zoster (shingles) infections, famciclovir should be started within 72 hours of the appearance of the rash to be effective. Famciclovir has been shown to accelerate healing, reduce the duration of viral shedding, and resolve posthepatic neuralgia faster than placebo. Comparison trials to acyclovir or valacyclovir are not available. Adjust dose for estimated renal function.

Dosage Forms Tablet: 125 mg, 250 mg, 500 mg

References
Pue MA and Benet LZ, "Pharmacokinetics of Famciclovir in Man," *Antiviral Chem Chemother*, 1993, 4(Suppl 1):47-55.
Tyring S, Barbarash RA, Nahlik JE, et al, "Famciclovir for the Treatment of Acute Herpes Zoster: Effects on Acute Disease and Postherpetic Neuralgia," *Ann Intern Med*, 1995, 123(2):89-96.

Famotidine (fa MOE ti deen)

Related Information
I.V. Medication Recommendations *on page 1080*
I.V. Push Recommended Guidelines *on page 1083*

Brand Names Pepcid®; Pepcid® AC Acid Controller [OTC]

Generic Available No

Therapeutic Category Histamine H_2 Antagonist

Use Therapy and treatment of duodenal ulcer, gastric ulcer, gastroesophageal reflux, pathological hypersecretory conditions, control gastric pH in critically ill patients

Pepcid® AC Acid Controller [OTC]: Relief and prevention of symptoms of heartburn, acid indigestion, or sour stomach

Unlabeled use: Prevent upper GI bleeding, prevent aspiration pneumonitis, symptomatic relief in gastritis, and active benign ulcer

Contraindications Hypersensitivity to famotidine or other H_2 antagonist

Warnings Adjust dosages in renal/hepatic impairment; elderly due to renal decline with age

Precautions Gastric malignancy may be masked, gynecomastia; cardiac arrhythmias and hypotension (I.V.); CNS side effects (confusion, depression, psychosis, hallucinations, anxiety)

Adverse Reactions
Cardiovascular: Flushing, palpitation, hypertension
Central nervous system: Headache, dizziness, fever, fatigue, hallucinations, anxiety, seizure, insomnia, drowsiness, depression
Dermatologic: Rash, acne, pruritus, urticaria, dry skin
Gastrointestinal: Constipation, anorexia, xerostomia, diarrhea, nausea, pancreatitis, abdominal discomfort, flatulence, belching
Genitourinary: Impotence, loss of libido
Hematologic: Thrombocytopenia
Neuromuscular & skeletal: Pain, weakness, paresthesia
Ocular: Orbital edema, conjunctival injection
Renal: Proteinuria, increases in BUN and creatinine
Respiratory: Bronchospasm

Overdosage No experience with intentional overdose; reported ingestions of 20 g have had transient side effects seen with recommended doses; animal data have shown respiratory failure, tachycardia, muscle tremors, vomiting, restlessness, hypotension, salivation, emesis, and diarrhea
(Continued)

Famotidine *(Continued)*

Toxicology Treatment is primarily symptomatic and supportive; food may increase absorption

Drug Interactions

Binds weakly to cytochrome P-450 and, therefore, does not cause significant inhibition of drug metabolism

Antacids may decrease absorption; decreased absorption of diazepam may occur (ranitidine)

Increased serum concentrations of procainamide (ranitidine)

Increased hypoglycemic effects observed with sulfonylureas; serum concentrations may be increased (case reports with ranitidine)

May decrease warfarin clearance and increase anticoagulant effect (ranitidine) but conflicting data are available

Stability Reconstituted I.V. solution is stable for 48 hours at room temperature; I.V. infusion in NS or D_5W solution is stable for 48 hours at room temperature; reconstituted oral solution is stable for 30 days at room temperature. Do not store powder in temperatures >40°C (104°F); after reconstitution, store in refrigerator <30°C (86°F); do not freeze; discard unused suspension in 30 days; store I.V. at 2°C to 8°C (36°F to 46°F).

Mechanism of Action Competitive inhibition of histamine at H_2 receptors of the gastric parietal cells, which inhibits gastric acid secretion; gastric volume and hydrogen ion concentration reduced

Pharmacodynamics

Onset of action: Oral: Gastrointestinal effects can be observed within 60 minutes following administration

Peak effects: Oral: Within 1-3 hours after doses

Duration: 10-12 hours

Duodenal ulcer healing rates at 40 mg/day: 4 weeks: 67% to 77%: 8 weeks: 82% to 95% in young adults

Pharmacokinetics

Protein binding: 15% to 20%

Metabolism: 30% to 35%

Bioavailability: Oral: 40% to 50%

Half-life: 2.5-3.5 hours (increases with renal impairment; oliguric half-life: 20 hours)

Elimination: Excreted as unchanged drug in urine 25% to 30% oral and 65% to 70% I.V.; excreted in bile and feces

Usual Dosage Geriatrics and Adults: Oral:

Duodenal ulcer and gastric ulcer: 40 mg/day at bedtime for 4-8 weeks for adults, 12 weeks for elderly; prophylaxis: 20 mg at bedtime

Pathological hypersecretory conditions: 20 mg every 6 hours, higher doses may be needed; 160 mg every 6 hours have been used for Zollinger-Ellison syndrome

GERD: 20 mg every 6 hours for 6 weeks

Erosive esophagitis: 20-40 mg twice daily for 12 weeks

Pepcid® AC Acid Controller [OTC] (do not take maximum dose for more than 14 days continuously unless directed by physician):

Relief of symptoms: 10 mg as needed up to twice daily

Prevention of symptoms: 10 mg 1 hour before eating a meal that is expected to cause symptoms; may take up to twice daily

Dosing interval in renal impairment: Cl_{cr} <10 mL/minute: Dose may have to be reduced to 20 mg at bedtime

Monitoring Parameters Signs and symptoms of peptic ulcer disease, occult blood with GI bleeding, gastric pH where necessary; monitor renal function to correct dose; monitor for side effects

Patient Information Take with or immediately after meals; inform pharmacist and physician (nurse, practitioner) of any concomitant drug therapy; stagger doses with antacids; for OTC use, do not take maximum dose for more than 14 days continuously unless directed by physician

Nursing Implications Injection must be diluted prior to administration to a concentration of 20 mg/mL; reduce dosage in decreased renal function

Additional Information The expensive parenteral route should only be used when a patient is unable to take oral medication

Special Geriatric Considerations H_2 blockers are the preferred drugs for treating PUD in elderly due to cost and ease of administration. These agents are no less or more effective than any other therapy. The preferred agents (due to side effects, drug interaction profile, and pharmacokinetics) are raniti-dine, famotidine, and nizatidine. Treatment for PUD in elderly is recom-mended for 12 weeks since their lesions are larger; therefore, take longer to heal. Always adjust dose based upon creatinine clearance.

Dosage Forms
Injection: 10 mg/mL (2 mL); 20 mg/50 mL (0.9% NaCl)
Powder, for oral suspension: 40 mg/5 mL
Tablet, film coated: 20 mg, 40 mg
Tablet [OTC]: 10 mg

References
Fennerty MD and Higbee M, "Drug Therapy of Gastrointestinal Disease," *Geriatric Pharmacology*, Bressler R and Katz MD, eds, New York, NY: McGraw-Hill, 1993, 585-608.

Famvir™ *see* Famciclovir *on page 366*

5-FC *see* Flucytosine *on page 388*

Federal OBRA Regulations Recommended Maximum Doses - Antidepres-sants *see page 1056*

Federal OBRA Regulations Recommended Maximum Doses - Antipsy-chotics *see page 1056*

Federal OBRA Regulations Recommended Maximum Doses - Anxiolytics *see page 1057*

Federal OBRA Regulations Recommended Maximum Doses - Hypnotics *see page 1057*

Felbamate (FEL ba mate)
Related Information
Antiepileptic Drug Interactions Comparison *on page 1022*
Brand Names Felbatol™
Generic Available No
Therapeutic Category Anticonvulsant, Miscellaneous
Use Monotherapy and adjunctive therapy in patients 14 years of age and older with partial and secondarily generalized seizures
Contraindications Patients with known hypersensitivity to felbamate or its ingredients; it should be used with caution in those patients who have demon-strated hypersensitivity reactions to other carbamates
Warnings Use with caution in patients allergic to other carbamates (eg, meprobamate); antiepileptic drugs should not be suddenly discontinued because of the possibility of increasing seizure frequency; **reported 10 cases of aplastic anemia in the U.S. after 2¹/₂ to 6 months of therapy**; Carter Wallace and the FDA recommended the use of this agent be suspended unless withdrawal of the product would place a patient at greater risk as compared to the frequently fatal form of anemia
Adverse Reactions
Central nervous system: Anxiety, headache, fatigue, dizziness, drowsiness, insomnia, clumsiness, depression or behavior changes, slurred speech, clouded sensorium, lethargy
Dermatologic: Acne, skin rash, alopecia
Gastrointestinal: Nausea, diarrhea, anorexia, vomiting, constipation, weight gain, gum bleeding, hyperplasia
Neuromuscular & skeletal: Muscle twitches
Ocular: Blurred vision, diplopia, uncontrollable eye movements
Respiratory: Cough
Overdosage No serious adverse reactions have been reported
Toxicology Treatment is symptomatic
Drug Interactions
Increased effect/toxicity of phenytoin, valproate
Decreased effect with phenytoin and carbamazepine; valproate does not significantly effect felbamate levels
Felbamate may decrease carbamazepine levels and increase levels of active metabolite of carbamazepine (these changes may offset each other)
Stability Store medication in tightly closed container at room temperature away from excessive heat
Mechanism of Action Mechanism of action is unknown but has properties in common with other marketed anticonvulsants; has weak inhibitory effects on GABA-receptor binding, benzodiazepine receptor binding, and is devoid of activity at the MK-801 receptor binding site of the NMDA receptor-ionophore complex.
Pharmacokinetics
Absorption: Oral: Rapidly and almost completely absorbed after oral adminis-tration, food has no effect upon the tablet's absorption
(Continued)

Felbamate *(Continued)*

Peak serum concentrations: Within 3 hours

V_d: 0.7-1 L/kg

Protein binding: 22% to 25%

Metabolism: Inhibitor CYP2C19

Half-life: 20-23 hours average

Elimination: Cleared renally 40% to 50% as unchanged drug and 40% as inactive metabolites in the urine

Note: Reduced clearance and prolonged half-life have been reported in persons 66-78 years of age compared to persons 18-45 years of age

Usual Dosage Geriatrics and Adults: Oral:

Monotherapy: Initial: 1200 mg/day in divided doses 3 or 4 times/day; titrate previously untreated patients under close clinical supervision, increasing the dosage in 600 mg increments every 2 weeks to 2400 mg/day based on clinical response and thereafter to 3600 mg/day in clinically indicated

Conversion to monotherapy: Initiate at 1200 mg/day in divided doses 3 or 4 times/day, reduce the dosage of the concomitant anticonvulsant(s) by 20% to 33% at the initiation of felbamate therapy; at week 2, increase the felbamate dosage to 2400 mg/day while reducing the dosage of the other anticonvulsant(s) up to an additional 33% of their original dosage; at week 3, increase the felbamate dosage up to 3600 mg/day and continue to reduce the dosage of the other anticonvulsant(s) as clinically indicated

Monitoring Parameters Monitor serum concentrations of concomitant anticonvulsant therapy

Reference Range Not necessary to routinely monitor serum drug concentrations, since dose should be titrated to clinical response

Test Interactions Blood urea nitrogen is slightly lower (1.25 mg/dL); may cause slightly elevated serum cholesterol concentration (about 7 mg/dL) in patients receiving about 2.6 g/day

Patient Information Shake oral suspension well before using

Nursing Implications Monitor patient for signs of anemia; monitor seizures; see Warnings

Additional Information Monotherapy has not been associated with gingival hyperplasia, impaired concentration, weight gain, or abnormal thinking

Special Geriatric Considerations Clinical studies have not included large numbers of patients >65 years of age; due to decreased hepatic and renal function, dosing should start at the lower end of the dosage range (see Usual Dosage and Pharmacokinetics)

Dosage Forms

Suspension, oral: 600 mg/5 mL (240 mL, 960 mL)

Tablet: 400 mg, 600 mg

References

Richens A, Banfield CR, Salfi M, et al, "Single and Multiple Dose Pharmacokinetics of Felbamate in the Elderly," *Br J Clin Pharmacol,* 1997, 44(2):129-34.

Felbatol™ *see Felbamate on previous page*

Feldene® *see Piroxicam on page 757*

Felodipine *(fe LOE di peen)*

Related Information

Calcium Channel Blocking Agents Comparison *on page 1027*

Brand Names Plendil®

Generic Available No

Therapeutic Category Calcium Channel Blocker

Use Hypertension

Unlabeled uses: Congestive heart failure, Raynaud's syndrome

Contraindications Hypersensitivity to the drug

Warnings Use with caution in titrating dosages for impaired hepatic function patients; use with caution in patients with congestive heart failure; may increase frequency, severity, duration of angina during initiation of therapy; do not abruptly withdraw therapy; use with caution in elderly due to greater propensity to hypotension

The FDA's Cardiovascular and Renal Drug Advisory Committee reviewed current data regarding the risk of heart attacks in patients treated with calcium channel blockers and determined that as a class, the calcium channel antagonists are safe; however, they warned that short-acting nifedipine could increase the risk of myocardial infarction in some patients. The committee was in agreement with a statement issued September, 1995 by the National Heart Lung, and Blood Institute of the National Institute of

Health, that warned that short-acting nifedipine should be used with great caution especially at higher doses.

Precautions Severe left ventricular dysfunction, congestive heart failure, hepatic or renal impairment, hypertrophic cardiomyopathy (especially obstructive), concomitant therapy with beta-blockers or digoxin, edema

Adverse Reactions

Cardiovascular: Arrhythmia, bradycardia, hypotension, palpitations, tachycardia, congestive heart failure, myocardial infarction, peripheral edema

Central nervous system: Dizziness, headache, fatigue, insomnia

Dermatologic: Rash

Gastrointestinal: Nausea, diarrhea, constipation, xerostomia

Genitourinary: Urinary incontinence

Hepatic: Mild to marked elevations in liver function tests

Ocular: Blurred vision

Respiratory: Shortness of breath

Miscellaneous: Gingival swelling and inflammation

Overdosage Symptoms of overdose include hypotension

Toxicology Ipecac-induced emesis can hypothetically worsen calcium antagonist toxicity since it can produce vagal stimulation. The potential for seizures precipitously following acute ingestion of large doses of a calcium antagonist may also contraindicate the use of ipecac. Supportive and symptomatic treatment, including I.V. fluids and Trendelenburg positioning, should be initiated as intoxication may cause hypotension. Although calcium (calcium chloride I.V. 1-2 g with repeats as needed) has been used as an "antidote" for acute intoxications, there is limited experience to support its routine use and should be reserved for those cases where definite signs of myocardial depression are evident. Heart block may respond to isoproterenol, glucagon, atropine, and/or calcium although a temporary pacemaker may be required.

Drug Interactions

Beta-blockers (increased cardiac and A-V conduction depression); fentanyl (increased volume requirements and hypotension); although this drug is new, other drug interactions not reported to the same degree as older agents; however, should be suspect of any drug interaction reported with other calcium channel blockers

Cimetidine, ranitidine may increase bioavailability

Digoxin levels may increase

Felodipine metabolism may be inhibited by erythromycin, ketoconazole, itraconazole, protease inhibitors; induced by rifampin, rifabutin

Mechanism of Action Inhibits calcium ion from entering the "slow channels" or select voltage-sensitive areas of vascular smooth muscle and myocardium during depolarization, producing a relaxation of coronary vascular smooth muscle and coronary vasodilation; increases myocardial oxygen delivery in patients with vasospastic angina

Pharmacodynamics Onset of action: 2-5 hours

Pharmacokinetics

Absorption: 98% to 100%

Protein bound: 99%

Metabolism: Substrate CYP3A4

Bioavailability: Due to first-pass elimination, absolute bioavailability is ~20%

Time to peak serum concentrations: Oral: 2-5 hours

Usual Dosage Oral:

Geriatrics: Initial dose: 2.5 mg/day

Adults: Initial: 5 mg once daily; dosage range: 2.5-10 mg once daily; may increase dose up to a maximum of 10 mg

Dosing adjustment in hepatic impairment: Use initial dose of 2.5 mg/day; do not use doses >10 mg/day

Monitoring Parameters Heart rate, blood pressure

Reference Range None described

Patient Information Do not crush or chew tablets; do not discontinue abruptly; report any dizziness, shortness of breath, palpitations, or edema occurs

Nursing Implications Do not crush sustained release capsules (see Warnings, Precautions, Monitoring Parameters, and Special Geriatric Considerations)

Special Geriatric Considerations Elderly may experience a greater hypotensive response; constipation may be more of a problem in elderly; calcium channel blockers are no more effective in elderly than other therapies; however, they do not cause significant CNS effects which is an advantage over some antihypertensive agents.

Dosage Forms Tablet, extended release: 2.5 mg, 5 mg, 10 mg

Femiron® [OTC] *see Ferrous Fumarate on page 376*
Femizole-7® [OTC] *see Clotrimazole on page 242*
Fenesin™ *see Guaifenesin on page 437*
Fenesin DM® *see Guaifenesin and Dextromethorphan on page 439*

Fenoprofen (fen oh PROE fen)

Brand Names Nalfon®

Generic Available Yes

Therapeutic Category Analgesic, Non-narcotic; Anti-inflammatory Agent; Antipyretic; Nonsteroidal Anti-inflammatory Agent (NSAID), Oral

Use Symptomatic treatment of acute and chronic rheumatoid arthritis and osteoarthritis; relief of mild to moderate pain, sunburn, migraine headache prophylaxis

Contraindications Renal impairment, known hypersensitivity to fenoprofen or other NSAIDs including aspirin and other salicylates

Warnings GI toxicity (bleeding, ulceration, perforation); CNS effects may occur (headaches, confusion, depression); hypersensitivity, anaphylactoid reactions (intermittent tolmetin use more often); renal function decline, acute renal insufficiency, interstitial nephritis, dysuria, cystitis, hematuria, nephrotic syndrome, hyperkalemia in acute renal insufficiency, hyponatremia, papillary necrosis, hepatic function impairment; elderly have increased risk for adverse reactions to NSAIDs (see Special Geriatric Considerations)

Precautions Use with caution in patients with congestive heart failure, hypertension, decreased renal or hepatic function, history of GI disease (bleeding or ulcers), or those receiving anticoagulants; perform ophthalmologic evaluation for those who develop eye complaints during therapy (blurred vision, diminished vision, changes in color vision, retinal changes); NSAIDs may mask signs/symptoms of infections; photosensitivity reported

Adverse Reactions

Cardiovascular: Congestive heart failure, angina, hypertension, hypotension, arrhythmias, edema

Central nervous system: Headache, drowsiness, vertigo, dizziness, fatigue, hallucinations, confusion, depression, emotional lability, psychotic behavior, pyrexia

Dermatologic: Rash, urticaria, angioedema, Stevens-Johnson syndrome, exfoliative dermatitis, bruising, petechiae, purpura

Endocrine & metabolic: Hyperglycemia, hypoglycemia, hyperkalemia, gynecomastia, hyponatremia, fluid retention

Gastrointestinal: Dyspepsia, heartburn, nausea, diarrhea, constipation, flatulence, anorexia, stomatitis, vomiting, abdominal pain, peptic ulcer, GI bleeding, GI perforation, gingival ulcers, pancreatitis, proctitis, paralytic ulcers, colitis, weight loss, dry mucous membranes

Genitourinary: Impotence, azotemia

Hematologic: Neutropenia, anemia, agranulocytosis, bone marrow suppression, hemolytic anemia, hemorrhage, inhibition of platelet aggregation

Hepatic: Hepatitis, elevated LFTs, cholestatic jaundice

Neuromuscular & skeletal: Involuntary muscle movements, muscle weakness, tremors, weakness

Ocular: Vision changes

Otic: Tinnitus

Renal: Dysuria, polyuria, pyuria, oliguria, anuria, acute renal failure

Respiratory: Exacerbation of asthma, dyspnea

Miscellaneous: Thirst, diaphoresis

Overdosage Symptoms include drowsiness, lethargy, disorientation, confusion, dizziness, numbness, paresthesia, nausea, vomiting, gastric irritation, abdominal pain, headache, tinnitus, sweating, blurred vision, muscle twitching, seizures, coma, acute renal failure, increased BUN and serum creatinine, hypotension, tachycardia, and metabolic acidosis

Toxicology Management of a nonsteroidal anti-inflammatory agent (NSAID) intoxication is primarily supportive and symptomatic. Fluid therapy is commonly effective in managing the hypotension that may occur following an acute NSAID overdose, except when this is due to an acute blood loss. Seizures tend to be very short-lived and often do not require drug treatment although recurrent seizures should be treated with I.V. diazepam. Since many of the NSAIDs undergo enterohepatic cycling, multiple doses of charcoal may be needed to reduce the potential for delayed toxicities.

Drug Interactions

Cyclosporine may increase nephrotoxicity of both agents; may increase digoxin, methotrexate, and lithium serum concentrations

Aspirin and other salicylates may decrease NSAID serum concentrations

Other NSAIDs may increase adverse GI effects

Increased prothrombin time with anticoagulants

Decreased antihypertensive effects of ACE inhibitors, beta-blockers, and thiazide diuretics

Increased response to sympathomimetics

Probenecid may increase toxicity of NSAIDs by increase in serum concentrations

NSAIDs may decrease effects of loop diuretics

May enhance azotemia in elderly receiving loop diuretics

Mechanism of Action Inhibits prostaglandin synthesis, acts on the hypothalamus heat-regulating center to reduce fever, blocks prostaglandin synthetase action which prevents formation of the platelet-aggregating substance thromboxane A_2; decreases pain receptor sensitivity. Other proposed mechanisms of action for salicylate anti-inflammatory action are lysosomal stabilization, inhibition of kinin and leukotriene production, alteration of chemotactic factors, and inhibition of neutrophil activation. This latter mechanism may be the most significant pharmacologic action to reduce inflammation.

Pharmacodynamics

Onset of anti-inflammatory action: 2 days

Maximum response: 2-3 weeks

Pharmacokinetics

Absorption: Rapid (to 80%) from upper GI tract

Protein binding: 99%

Metabolism: Extensive in the liver

Half-life: 2.5-3 hours

Time to peak serum concentration: Within 1-2 hours

Elimination: In urine 2% to 5% as unchanged drug; small amounts appear in feces

Usual Dosage Geriatrics and Adults: Oral:

Arthritis: 300-600 mg 3-4 times/day up to 3.2 g/day; maximum response may take 2-3 weeks

Pain: 200 mg every 4-6 hours as needed; do not exceed 3.2 g/day

Monitoring Parameters Monitor response (pain, range of motion, grip strength, mobility, ADL function), inflammation; observe for weight gain, edema; monitor renal function; observe for bleeding, bruising; evaluate gastrointestinal effects (abdominal pain, bleeding, dyspepsia); mental confusion, disorientation, CBC, serum, creatinine, BUN, liver function tests

Reference Range Therapeutic: 20-65 µg/mL (SI: 82-268 µmol/L)

Test Interactions Increased chloride (S), increased sodium (S)

Patient Information Serious gastrointestinal bleeding can occur as well as ulceration and perforation. Pain may or may not be present. Avoid aspirin and aspirin-containing products while taking this medication. If gastric upset occurs, take with food, milk, or antacid. If gastric adverse effects persist, contact physician. May cause drowsiness, dizziness, blurred vision, and confusion. Use caution when performing tasks which require alertness (eg, driving). Do not take for more than 3 days for fever or 10 days for pain without physician advice.

Nursing Implications See Monitoring Parameters, Overdosage, Patient Information, and Special Geriatric Considerations

Additional Information There are no clinical guidelines to predict which NSAID will give response in a particular patient. Trials with each must be initiated until response determined. Consider dose, patient convenience, and cost.

Special Geriatric Considerations Elderly are a high-risk population for adverse effects from nonsteroidal anti-inflammatory agents. As much as 60% of elderly can develop peptic ulceration and/or hemorrhage asymptomatically. The concomitant use of H_2 blockers, omeprazole, and sucralfate is not effective as prophylaxis with the exception of NSAID-induced duodenal ulcers which may be prevented by the use of ranitidine. Misoprostol and proton pump inhibitors are the only agents proven to help prevent the development of NSAID-induced ulcers. Also, concomitant disease and drug use contribute to the risk for GI adverse effects. Use lowest effective dose for shortest period possible. Consider renal function decline with age. Use of NSAIDs can compromise existing renal function especially when Cl_{cr} is ≤30 mL/minute. Tinnitus may be a difficult and unreliable indication of toxicity due to age-related hearing loss or eighth cranial nerve damage. CNS adverse effects such as confusion, agitation, and hallucination are generally seen in overdose or high-dose situations, but elderly may demonstrate these adverse effects at lower doses than younger adults.

(Continued)

Fenoprofen *(Continued)*

Dosage Forms
Fenoprofen calcium:
Capsule: 200 mg, 300 mg
Tablet: 600 mg

References
Brooks PM, Day RO, "Nonsteroidal Anti-inflammatory Drugs - Differences and Similarities," *N Engl J Med*, 1991, 324(24):1716-25.

Clinch D, Banerjee AK, Ostick G, "Absence of Abdominal Pain in Elderly Patients With Peptic Ulcer," *Age Ageing*, 1984, 13:120-3.

Clive DM, Stoff JS, "Renal Syndromes Associated With Nonsteroidal Anti-inflammatory Drugs," *N Engl J Med*, 1984, 310(9):563-72.

Graham DY, "Prevention of Gastroduodenal Injury Induced by Chronic Nonsteroidal Anti-inflammatory Drug Therapy," *Gastroenterology*, 1989, 96(2 Pt 2 Suppl):675-81.

Gurwitz JH, Avorn J, Ross-Degnan D, et al, "Nonsteroidal Anti-Inflammatory Drug-Associated Azotemia in the Very Old," *JAMA*, 1990, 264(4):471-5.

Hawkey CJ, Karrasch JA, Szczepaski L, et al, "Omeprazole Compared With Misoprostrol for Ulcers Associated With Nonsteroidal Anti-inflammatory Drugs," *N Engl J Med*, 1998, 338(11):727-34.

Knodel LC, "Preventing NSAID-Induced Ulcers: The Role of Misoprostol," *Consult Pharm*, 1989, 4:37-41.

Pounder R, "Silent Peptic Ulceration: Deadly Silence or Golden Silence?" *Gastroenterology*, 1989, 96(2 Pt 2 Suppl):626-31.

Yeomans ND, Tulassay Z, Juhasz L, et al, "A Comparison of Omeprazole With Ranitidine for Ulcers Associated With Nonsteroidal Anti-inflammatory Drugs," *N Engl J Med*, 1998, 338(11):719-26.

Fentanyl (FEN ta nil)

Related Information
Narcotic Agonist Comparative Pharmacology *on page 1036*
Pharmacokinetics of Narcotic Agonist Analgesics *on page 1037*

Brand Names Duragesic® Transdermal; Fentanyl Oralet®; Sublimaze® Injection

Generic Available Yes: Injection

Therapeutic Category Analgesic, Narcotic; General Anesthetic

Use Sedation; relief of pain; preoperative medication; adjunct to general or regional anesthesia; management of chronic pain (transdermal product)

Restrictions C-II

Contraindications Hypersensitivity to fentanyl or any component; increased intracranial pressure; severe respiratory depression; severe liver or renal insufficiency;

Transmucosal is contraindicated in unmonitored settings where a risk of unrecognized hypoventilation exists or in treating acute or chronic pain

Warnings Rapid I.V. infusion may result in skeletal muscle and chest wall rigidity which leads to impaired ventilation causing respiratory distress including apnea, bronchoconstriction, laryngospasm; inject slowly over 3-5 minutes; nondepolarizing skeletal muscle relaxant may be required. Transdermal product: Patients who experience adverse reactions should be monitored for at least 12 hours after the removal of the product. Transmucosal product is not recommended for use in those who have received MAO inhibitors within 14 days.

Precautions Fentanyl shares the toxic potentials of opiate agonists, and precautions of opiate agonist therapy should be observed; use with caution in patients with bradycardia

Adverse Reactions
Cardiovascular: Hypotension, bradycardia
Central nervous system: CNS depression, drowsiness, dizziness, sedation
Dermatologic: Erythema, pruritus
Endocrine & metabolic: ADH release
Gastrointestinal: Nausea, vomiting, constipation
Local: Edema (transdermal system)
Neuromuscular & skeletal: Skeletal and thoracic muscle rigidity especially following rapid I.V. administration
Ocular: Miosis
Respiratory: Respiratory depression
Miscellaneous: Physical and psychological dependence with prolonged use, biliary or urinary tract spasm

Overdosage Symptoms of overdose include CNS depression, respiratory depression, miosis

Toxicology Treatment of an overdose includes support of the patient's airway, establishment of an I.V. line and administration of naloxone 2 mg I.V. with repeat administration as necessary up to a total of 10 mg.

Drug Interactions Increased toxicity: CNS depressants, phenothiazines, tricyclic antidepressants

Stability Protect from light

Mechanism of Action Binds with stereospecific receptors at many sites within the CNS, increases pain threshold, alters pain reception, inhibits ascending pain pathways

Pharmacodynamics

Onset of analgesia:
I.M.: 7-15 minutes
I.V.: Almost immediate

Duration:
I.M.: 1-2 hours
I.V.: 30-60 minutes; respiratory depressant effect may last longer than analgesic effect; duration of action may be increased in the elderly; enhanced analgesia has been seen in elderly patients on therapeutic doses of narcotics

Transmucosal:
Onset of effect: 5-15 minutes with a maximum reduction in activity/apprehension
Peak analgesia: Within 20-30 minutes
Duration: Related to serum concentration of the drug

Pharmacokinetics

Absorption: Transmucosal: Rapid, ~25% from the buccal mucosa; 75% swallowed with saliva and slowly absorbed from gastrointestinal tract

Metabolism: In the liver

Half-life: 2-4 hours; transmucosal: 6.6 hours (range: 5-15 hours)

Elimination: In urine primarily as metabolites and 10% as unchanged drug

In the elderly, the clearance of fentanyl is decreased and the half-life increased; it is unknown how this affects the kinetics of the transdermal system

Transdermal: Serum concentrations increase gradually, leveling off between 12-24 hours with peak levels occurring 24-72 hours after application; after 72-hour application, steady-state fentanyl concentration is reached

Usual Dosage A wide range of doses may be used; when choosing a dose, take into consideration the following patient factors; age, weight, physical status, underlying disease states, other drugs used, type of anesthesia used, and the surgical procedure to be performed.

Geriatrics and Adults:
Preoperative sedation, adjunct to regional anesthesia, postoperative pain:
I.M., I.V.: 50-100 mcg/dose
Adjunct to general anesthesia: I.M., I.V.: 2-50 mcg/kg depending on the procedure to be performed
General anesthesia without additional anesthetic agents: I.V. 50-100 mcg/kg with O_2 and skeletal muscle relaxant
Transdermal: Initial: 25 mcg/hour system applied every 72 hours (3 days); maximum dose: 300 mcg/hour, increase if necessary after 3 days; may take 6 days to reach equilibrium on new dose; if currently receiving

Corresponding Doses of Oral/Intramuscular Morphine and Duragesic™

Oral 24-Hour Morphine (mg/d)	I.M. 24-Hour Morphine (mg/d)	Duragesic™ Dose (mcg/h)
45-134	8-22	25
135-224	28-37	50
225-314	38-52	75
315-404	53-67	100
405-494	68-82	125
495-584	83-97	150
585-674	98-112	175
675-764	113-127	200
765-854	128-142	225
855-944	143-157	250
945-1034	158-172	275
1035-1124	173-187	300

Product information, Duragesic™ — Janssen Pharmaceutica, January, 1991.

(Continued)

Fentanyl *(Continued)*

opiates, calculate the 24-hour analgesia requirements and convert it to the equianalgesic oral morphine dose; use the table to choose the appropriate Duragesic™ dose.

Transmucosal:

Geriatrics: 2.5-5 mcg/kg; suck on lozenge vigorously approximately 20-40 minutes before the start of procedure

Adults: 5 mcg/kg; suck on lozenge as above

Administration Transmucosal product should begin 20-40 minutes prior to the anticipated start of surgery, diagnostic, or therapeutic procedure; foil overwrap should be removed just prior to administration; once removed, patient should place the unit in mouth and suck (not chew) it; unit should be removed after it is consumed or if patient has achieved an adequate sedation and anxiolytic level, and/or shows signs of respiratory depression

Monitoring Parameters Respiratory, cardiovascular status, mental status

Patient Information Transdermal system: Apply to intact skin on the upper torso; clip hair at application site (do not shave) before applying system. If cleansing skin before application, use clear water and allow skin to dry completely before applying system; leave system in place for 72 hours; dispose of system by folding it (medication side in) and flushing down the toilet; may cause dizziness or drowsiness, avoid alcohol, and CNS depressants.

Nursing Implications May cause rebound respiratory depression postoperatively

Transdermal system: See Patient Information for instructions on applying the transdermal system. If gel from the patch contacts the health worker's skin, wash the area with water; do not use soap or solvents as this will enhance the drug's ability to penetrate the skin; during initiation of therapy, short-acting analgesics may be needed until the full effects of the system are obtained; monitor patients for at least 12 hours after the removal of the patch

Transmucosal: See Administration

Special Geriatric Considerations The elderly may be particularly susceptible to the CNS depressant and constipating effects of narcotics (see Pharmacodynamics, Pharmacokinetics, and Usual Dosage).

Dosage Forms

Injection, as citrate: 0.05 mg/mL (2 mL, 5 mL, 10 mL, 20 mL, 50 mL)

Lozenge, oral transmucosal (raspberry flavored): 200 mcg, 300 mcg, 400 mcg

Transdermal system: 25 mcg/hour [10 cm^2]; 50 mcg/hour [20 cm^2]; 75 mcg/hour [30 cm^2]; 100 mcg/hour [40 cm^2] (all available in 5s)

Fentanyl Oralet® *see Fentanyl on page 374*

Feosol® [OTC] *see Ferrous Sulfate on page 379*

Feostat® [OTC] *see Ferrous Fumarate on this page*

Feratab® [OTC] *see Ferrous Sulfate on page 379*

Fergon® [OTC] *see Ferrous Gluconate on page 378*

Fer-In-Sol® [OTC] *see Ferrous Sulfate on page 379*

Fer-Iron® [OTC] *see Ferrous Sulfate on page 379*

Fero-Gradumet® [OTC] *see Ferrous Sulfate on page 379*

Ferospace® [OTC] *see Ferrous Sulfate on page 379*

Ferralet® [OTC] *see Ferrous Gluconate on page 378*

Ferralyn® Lanacaps® [OTC] *see Ferrous Sulfate on page 379*

Ferra-TD® [OTC] *see Ferrous Sulfate on page 379*

Ferro-Sequels® [OTC] *see Ferrous Fumarate on this page*

Ferrous Fumarate *(FER us FYOO ma rate)*

Brand Names Femiron® [OTC]; Feostat® [OTC]; Ferro-Sequels® [OTC]; Fumasorb® [OTC]; Fumerin® [OTC]; Hemocyte® [OTC]; Ircon® [OTC]; Nephro-Fer™ [OTC]; Span-FF® [OTC]

Therapeutic Category Iron Salt

Use Prevention and treatment of iron deficiency anemias

Contraindications Hemochromatosis, hemolytic anemia, known hypersensitivity to iron salts

Precautions Avoid using for longer than 6 months except in patients with conditions that require prolonged therapy; avoid in patients with peptic ulcer, enteritis, or ulcerative colitis

Adverse Reactions

Gastrointestinal: GI irritation, epigastric pain, nausea, diarrhea, dark stool, vomiting

Genitourinary: Urine discoloration

Miscellaneous: Liquid preparations may temporarily stain the teeth

Overdosage Symptoms of overdose include lethargy, tarry stools, hypotension, acidosis, pulmonary edema, hyperthermia, convulsions

Toxicology Following treatment for fluid losses, metabolic acidosis, and shock, a severe iron overdose (when the serum iron concentration exceeds the total iron-binding capacity) may be treated with deferoxamine. Deferoxamine may be administered I.V. (80 mg/kg over 24 hours) or I.M. (40-90 mg/kg every 8 hours).

Drug Interactions

Absorption of oral preparation of iron and tetracyclines are decreased when both of these drugs are given together; concurrent administration of antacids or H_2 antagonists may decrease iron absorption; iron may decrease absorption of levodopa, methyldopa, quinolones, and penicillamine when given at the same time

Iron absorption may be increased in patients receiving chloramphenicol; concurrent administration ≥200 mg vitamin C per 30 mg elemental iron increases absorption of oral iron

Drug/Food Interactions Milk and eggs may decrease absorption of iron

Mechanism of Action Replaces iron found in hemoglobin, myoglobin, and other enzymes; allows the transportation of oxygen via hemoglobin

Pharmacodynamics

Onset of action: Hematologic response to oral iron in red blood cells form and color changes occur within 3-10 days

Peak action: Within 5-10 days, and hemoglobin values increase within 2-4 weeks

Pharmacokinetics

Absorption: Iron is absorbed in the duodenum and upper jejunum; in persons with normal iron stores 10% of an oral dose is absorbed, this is increased to 20% to 30% in persons with inadequate iron stores. Food and achlorhydria will decrease absorption; aging has not been shown to affect absorption, but the percent uptake by red cells decreases from 91.2% in healthy young adults to 60% in healthy older adults.

Elimination: Iron is largely bound to serum transferrin and excreted in the urine, sweat, sloughing of intestinal mucosa, and by menstrual bleeding.

Usual Dosage Oral (to avoid GI upset, start with a single daily dose and increase by 1 tablet/day each week or as tolerated until desired daily dose is achieved):

Geriatrics and Adults: 200 mg 3-4 times/day

Administration Administer 2 hours prior to or 4 hours after antacids

Monitoring Parameters Hemoglobin, hematocrit, ferritin, reticulocyte count

Reference Range Therapeutic: Male: 75-175 µg/dL (SI: 13.4-31.3 µmol/L); Female: 65-165 µg/dL (SI: 11.6-29.5 µmol/L); ranges may vary by laboratory

Test Interactions Increased serum iron

Patient Information May color stool black, take between meals for maximum absorption; may take with food if GI upset occurs, do not take with milk or antacids

Nursing Implications See Administration

Additional Information The elemental iron content in ferrous fumarate is 33% (ie, 200 mg ferrous fumarate is equivalent to 66 mg ferrous iron). Administration of iron for longer than 6 months should be avoided except in patients with continuous bleeding or menorrhagia.

Special Geriatric Considerations Anemia in the elderly is often caused by "anemia of chronic disease", a result of aging changes in the bone marrow, or associated with inflammation rather than blood loss. Iron stores are usually normal or increased, with a serum ferritin >50 ng/mL and a decreased total iron binding capacity. Hence, the anemia is not secondary to iron deficiency but the inability of the reticuloendothelial system to use available iron stores. Timed release iron preparations should be avoided due to their erratic absorption. Products combined with a laxative or stool softener should not be used unless the need for the combination is demonstrated.

Dosage Forms

Drops: 45 mg/0.6 mL

Tablet: 200 mg, 325 mg

Tablet, timed release (Ferro-Sequels®): Ferrous fumarate 150 mg and docusate sodium 100 mg

(Continued)

Ferrous Fumarate *(Continued)*

See table.

Elemental Iron Content of Iron Salts

Iron Salt	% Iron
Ferrous sulfate	20
Ferrous sulfate, exsiccated	~30
Ferrous gluconate	11.6
Ferrous fumarate	33

References

Lipschitz DA, "The Anemia of Chronic Disease," *J Am Geriatr Soc*, 1990, 38(11):1258-64.
Marx JJM, "Normal Iron Absorption and Decreased Red Cell Iron Uptake in the Aged," *Blood*, 1979, 53:204-11.

Ferrous Gluconate (FER us GLOO koe nate)

Brand Names Fergon® [OTC]; Ferralet® [OTC]; Simron® [OTC]

Therapeutic Category Iron Salt

Use Prevention and treatment of iron deficiency anemias

Contraindications Hemochromatosis, hemolytic anemia; known hypersensitivity to iron salts

Precautions Avoid using for longer than 6 months, except in patients with conditions that require prolonged therapy

Adverse Reactions

Gastrointestinal: GI irritation, epigastric pain, nausea, diarrhea, dark stool
Miscellaneous: Liquid preparations may temporarily stain the teeth

Overdosage Symptoms of overdose include lethargy, tarry stools, hypotension, acidosis, pulmonary edema, hyperthermia, convulsions

Toxicology Following treatment for fluid losses, metabolic acidosis, and shock, a severe iron overdose (when the serum iron concentration exceeds the total iron-binding capacity) may be treated with deferoxamine. Deferoxamine may be administered I.V. (80 mg/kg over 24 hours) or I.M. (40-90 mg/kg every 8 hours)

Drug Interactions

Absorption of oral preparation of iron and tetracyclines are decreased when both of these drugs are given together; concurrent administration of antacids or H_2 antagonists may decrease iron absorption; iron may decrease absorption of levodopa, methyldopa, quinolones, and penicillamine when given at the same time

Iron absorption may be increased in patients receiving chloramphenicol; concurrent administration ≥200 mg vitamin C per 30 mg elemental iron increases absorption of oral iron

Drug/Food Interactions Milk and eggs may decrease absorption of iron

Mechanism of Action Replaces iron, found in hemoglobin, myoglobin, and enzymes; allows the transportation of oxygen via hemoglobin

Pharmacodynamics

Onset of action: Hematologic response to either oral or parenteral iron salts is essentially the same; red blood cell form and color changes within 3-10 days

Peak effect: Within 5-10 days, and hemoglobin values increase within 2-4 weeks

Pharmacokinetics

Absorption: Iron is absorbed in the duodenum and upper jejunum; in persons with normal iron stores 10% of an oral dose is absorbed, this is increased to 20% to 30% in persons with inadequate iron stores. Food and achlorhydria will decrease absorption; aging has not been shown to affect absorption, but the percent uptake by red cells decreases from 91.2% in healthy young adults to 60% in healthy older adults.

Elimination: Iron is largely bound to serum transferrin and excreted in the urine, sweat, sloughing of intestinal mucosa, and by menstrual bleeding

Usual Dosage Oral (to avoid GI upset, start with a single daily dose and increase by 1 tablet/day each week or as tolerated until desired daily dose is achieved):

Dose expressed in terms of elemental iron (see Additional Information):
Geriatrics and Adults:
Iron deficiency: 60 mg iron twice daily up to 60 mg iron 4 times/day
Prophylaxis: 60 mg iron/day

Administration Administer 2 hours before or 4 hours after antacids

Monitoring Parameters Hemoglobin, hematocrit, ferritin, reticulocyte count

Reference Range Therapeutic: Male: 75-175 µg/dL (SI: 13.4-31.3 µmol/L); Female: 65-165 µg/dL (SI: 11.6-29.5 µmol/L); ranges may vary by laboratory

Test Interactions Increased serum iron

Patient Information May color the stool black; take between meals for maximum absorption; may take with food if GI upset occurs; do **not** take with milk or antacid

Nursing Implications See Administration

Additional Information Gluconate contains 12% elemental iron (ie, 300 mg ferrous gluconate is equivalent to 34 mg ferrous iron); administration of iron for longer than 6 months should be avoided except in patients with continued bleeding or menorrhagia

Special Geriatric Considerations Anemia in the elderly is often caused by "anemia of chronic disease", a result of aging changes in the bone marrow, or associated with inflammation rather than blood loss. Iron stores are usually normal or increased, with a serum ferritin >50 ng/mL and a decreased total iron binding capacity. Hence, the anemia is not secondary to iron deficiency but the inability of the reticuloendothelial system to use available iron stores. Timed release iron preparations should be avoided due to their erratic absorption. Products combined with a laxative or stool softener should not be used unless the need for the combination is demonstrated.

Dosage Forms
Capsule: 86 mg, 325 mg, 435 mg
Elixir: 300 mg/5 mL (473 mL)
Tablet: 300 mg, 320 mg, 325 mg

References
Lipschitz DA, "The Anemia of Chronic Disease," *J Am Geriatr Soc*, 1990, 38(11):1258-64.
Marx JJM, "Normal Iron Absorption and Decreased Red Cell Iron Uptake in the Aged," *Blood*, 1979, 53:204-11.

Ferrous Sulfate (FER us SUL fate)

Brand Names Feosol® [OTC]; Feratab® [OTC]; Fer-In-Sol® [OTC]; Fer-Iron® [OTC]; Fero-Gradumet® [OTC]; Ferospace® [OTC]; Ferralyn® Lanacaps® [OTC]; Ferra-TD® [OTC]; Mol-Iron® [OTC]; Slow FE® [OTC]

Synonyms FeSO$_4$

Generic Available Yes

Therapeutic Category Iron Salt

Use Prevention and treatment of iron deficiency anemias

Contraindications Hemochromatosis, hemolytic anemia; known hypersensitivity to iron salts

Precautions Avoid using for longer than 6 months, except in patients with conditions that require prolonged therapy

Adverse Reactions
Gastrointestinal: GI irritation, epigastric pain, nausea, diarrhea, dark stool
Miscellaneous: Liquid preparations may temporarily stain the teeth

Overdosage Symptoms of overdose include acute GI irritation; erosion of GI mucosa, hepatic and renal impairment, coma, hematemesis, lethargy, acidosis

Toxicology Following treatment for fluid losses, metabolic acidosis, and shock, a severe iron overdose (when the serum iron concentration exceeds the total iron-binding capacity) may be treated with deferoxamine. Deferoxamine may be administered I.V. (80 mg/kg over 24 hours) or I.M. (40-90 mg/kg every 8 hours). Lethal dose of elemental iron is 180-300 mg/kg.

Drug Interactions
Absorption of oral preparation of iron and tetracyclines are decreased when both of these drugs are given together; concurrent administration of antacids or H$_2$ antagonists may decrease iron absorption; iron may decrease absorption of levodopa, methyldopa, quinolones, and penicillamine when given at the same time
Iron absorption may be increased in patients receiving chloramphenicol; concurrent administration ≥200 mg vitamin C per 30 mg elemental iron increases absorption of oral iron

Drug/Food Interactions Milk and eggs may decrease absorption of iron

Mechanism of Action Replaces iron, found in hemoglobin, myoglobin, and other enzymes; allows the transportation of oxygen via hemoglobin

Pharmacodynamics
Onset of action: Hematologic response to either oral or parenteral iron salts is essentially the same; red blood cell form and color changes within 3-10 days

(Continued)

Ferrous Sulfate *(Continued)*

Peak effect: Reticulocytosis occurs in 5-10 days, and hemoglobin values increase within 2-4 weeks

Pharmacokinetics

Absorption: Iron is absorbed in the duodenum and upper jejunum; in persons with normal serum iron stores, 10% of an oral dose is absorbed; this is increased to 20% to 30% in persons with inadequate iron stores. Food and achlorhydria will decrease absorption; aging has not been shown to affect absorption, but the percent uptake by red cells decreases from 91.2% in healthy young adults to 60% in healthy older adults.

Elimination: Iron is largely bound to serum transferrin and excreted in the urine, sweat, sloughing of the intestinal mucosa, and by menstrual bleeding

Usual Dosage Oral (to avoid GI upset, start with a single daily dose and increase by 1 tablet/day each week or as tolerated until desired daily dose is achieved):

Dose expressed in terms of elemental iron (see Additional Information):
Geriatrics and Adults:
Iron deficiency: 60 mg iron twice daily up to 60 mg iron 4 times/day or 50 mg iron (extended release) 1-2 times/day
Prophylaxis: 60 mg iron/day

Administration Administer 2 hours prior to or 4 hours after antacids

Monitoring Parameters Hemoglobin, hematocrit, ferritin, reticulocyte count

Reference Range Therapeutic: Male: 75-175 µg/dL (SI: 13.4-31.3 µmol/L); Female: 65-165 µg/dL (SI: 11.6-29.5 µmol/L); values may vary by laboratory

Test Interactions Increased serum iron

Patient Information May color stool black, take between meals for maximum absorption; may take with food if GI upset occurs, do not take with milk or antacids

Nursing Implications See Administration

Additional Information The elemental iron content of ferrous sulfate is 20% (ie, 300 mg ferrous sulfate is equivalent to 60 mg ferrous iron). Administration of iron for longer than 6 months should be avoided except in patients with continued bleeding, or menorrhagia

Special Geriatric Considerations Anemia in the elderly is often caused by "anemia of chronic disease", a result of aging changes in the bone marrow, or associated with inflammation rather than blood loss. Iron stores are usually normal or increased, with a serum ferritin >50 ng/mL and a decreased total iron binding capacity. Hence, the anemia is not secondary to iron deficiency but the inability of the reticuloendothelial system to use available iron stores. Timed release iron preparations should be avoided due to their erratic absorption. Products combined with a laxative or stool softener should not be used unless the need for the combination is demonstrated.

Dosage Forms

Capsule, timed release: 150 mg, 250 mg, 390 mg
Drops: 75 mg/0.6 mL (50 mL); 125 mg/mL (50 mL)
Elixir: 220 mg/5 mL (473 mL, 4000 mL)
Liquid: 300 mg/5 mL unit dose
Syrup: 90 mg/5 mL; 300 mg/5 mL (480 mL)
Tablet: 325 mg
Tablet, timed release: 525 mg

References

Lipschitz DA, "The Anemia of Chronic Disease," *J Am Geriatr Soc*, 1990, 38(11):1258-64.
Marx JJM, "Normal Iron Absorption and Decreased Red Cell Iron Uptake in the Aged," *Blood*, 1979, 53:204-11.

FeSO₄ *see Ferrous Sulfate on previous page*

Feverall™ [OTC] *see Acetaminophen on page 16*

Fexofenadine *(feks oh FEN a deen)*

Brand Names Allegra®

Generic Available No

Therapeutic Category Antihistamine

Use A nonsedating antihistamine indicated for the relief of seasonal allergic rhinitis

Contraindications Known hypersensitivity to fexofenadine or any of its components

Warnings See Drug Interactions

Adverse Reactions

Central nervous system: Drowsiness, fatigue
Gastrointestinal: Nausea, dyspepsia

Genitourinary: Dysmenorrhea

Miscellaneous: Viral infection (cold, flu)

Toxicology Not effectively removed by hemodialysis; doses up to 690 mg twice daily were administered for 1 month without significant adverse effects; GI tract decontamination and supportive measures are recommended

Drug Interactions Erythromycin and ketoconazole increased C_{max} and AUC_{ss} of fexofenadine when administered concomitantly; however, neither drug significantly affected adverse effects or Q-T_c intervals; mechanism of action is unknown and the effect of other macrolide agents or -azoles has not been investigated

Mechanism of Action Fexofenadine is an active metabolite of terfenadine and like terfenadine it competes with histamine for H_1-receptor sites on effector cells in the gastrointestinal tract, blood vessels and respiratory tract; it appears that fexofenadine does not cross the blood brain barrier to any appreciable degree, resulting in a greatly reduced potential for sedation

Pharmacokinetics

Absorption: Rapid

Protein binding: 60% to 70% bound to albumin and alpha$_1$-acid glycoprotein

Metabolism: ~5%

Half-life, mean: 14.4 hours

Pharmacokinetics in renal impairment:

Cl_{cr} 41-80 mL/minute:

Peak concentration: 87% higher

Half-life: 59% longer

Cl_{cr} 11-40 mL/minute:

Peak concentration: 111% higher

Half-life: 72% longer

Time to peak plasma concentration: 2.6 hours; peak plasma fexofenadine concentrations were 99% higher in elderly patients as compared to younger volunteers; no unusual adverse effects were seen with these elevated concentrations

Elimination: 80% in feces; 11% in urine

Usual Dosage Geriatrics and Adults: Oral: 60 mg twice daily

Dosing adjustment in renal impairment: Cl_{cr} <80 mL/minute: 60 mg once daily

Monitoring Parameters Symptoms of allergic rhinitis

Patient Information Do not exceed recommended dose

Special Geriatric Considerations See Pharmacokinetics and Usual Dosage

Dosage Forms Capsule, as hydrochloride: 60 mg

Fiberall® Chewable Tablet [OTC] see Calcium Polycarbophil on page 151

Fiberall® Powder [OTC] see Psyllium on page 804

Fiberall® Wafer [OTC] see Psyllium on page 804

FiberCon® Tablet [OTC] see Calcium Polycarbophil on page 151

Fiber-Lax® Tablet [OTC] see Calcium Polycarbophil on page 151

Filgrastim (fil GRA stim)

Brand Names Neupogen®

Synonyms G-CSF; Granulocyte Colony Stimulating Factor

Generic Available No

Therapeutic Category Colony Stimulating Factor

Use Decreases the period of neutropenia and the associated risk of infection in patients with nonmyeloid malignancies receiving myelosuppressive chemotherapeutic regimens associated with a significant incidence of severe neutropenia with fever; it has also been used in AIDS patients on zidovudine and in patients with noncancer chemotherapy-induced neutropenia

Contraindications Hypersensitivity to E. coli derived proteins or G-CSF

Warnings Complete blood count and platelet count should be obtained prior to chemotherapy. Do not use G-CSF in the period 24 hours before to 24 hours after administration of cytotoxic chemotherapy because of the potential sensitivity of rapidly dividing myeloid cells to cytotoxic chemotherapy. Precaution should be exercised in the usage of G-CSF in any malignancy with myeloid characteristics. G-CSF can potentially act as a growth factor for any tumor type, particularly myeloid malignancies. Tumors of nonhematopoietic origin may have surface receptors for G-CSF.

Adverse Reactions

Cardiovascular: Transient decrease in blood pressure, vasculitis

Central nervous system: Fever

(Continued)

Filgrastim (Continued)

Dermatologic: Exacerbation of pre-existing skin disorders

Endocrine & metabolic: Reversible increase in uric acid, lactate dehydrogenase, alkaline phosphatase

Gastrointestinal: Splenomegaly, nausea

Hematologic: Thrombocytopenia

Neuromuscular & skeletal: Medullary bone pain (24% incidence) is generally dose related, localized to the lower back, posterior iliac crests, and sternum, osteoporosis

Renal: Hematuria, proteinuria

Toxicology Leukocytosis which was not associated with any clinical adverse effects; after discontinuing the drug there is a 50% decrease in circulating levels of neutrophils within 1-2 days, return to pretreatment levels within 1-7 days. No clinical adverse effects seen with high-dose producing ANC >10,000/mm³.

Stability Store at 2°C to 8°C (36°F to 46°F); do not expose to freezing or dry ice. Prior to administration, filgrastim may be allowed to be at room temperature for a maximum of 24 hours. It may be diluted in dextrose 5% in water to a concentration of ≥15 mcg/mL for I.V. infusion administration. Minimum concentration is 15 mcg/mL; concentrations <15 mcg/mL require addition of albumin (1 mL of 5%) to the bag to prevent absorption. This diluted solution is stable for 7 days under refrigeration or at room temperature. **Filgrastim is incompatible with 0.9% sodium chloride (normal saline).**

Standard diluent: ≥375 mcg/25 mL D₅W

Mechanism of Action Stimulates the production, maturation, and activation of neutrophils, G-CSF activates neutrophils to increase both their migration and cytotoxicity. Natural proteins which stimulate hematopoietic stem cells to proliferate, prolong cell survival, stimulate cell differentiation, and stimulate functional activity of mature cells. CSFs are produced by a wide variety of cell types. Specific mechanisms of action are not yet fully understood, but possibly work by a second-messenger pathway with resultant protein production. See table.

Proliferation/Differentiation	G-CSF (Filgrastim)	GM-CSF (Sargramostim)
Neutrophils	Yes	Yes
Eosinophils	No	Yes
Macrophages	No	Yes
Neutrophil migration	Enhanced	Inhibited

Pharmacodynamics

Onset of action: Rapid elevation in neutrophil counts within the first 24 hours, reaching a plateau in 3-5 days

Duration: ANC decreases by 50% within 2 days after discontinuing G-CSF white counts return to the normal range in 4-7 days

Pharmacokinetics

Absorption: S.C.: 100%; peak plasma concentrations can be maintained for up to 12 hours

Distribution: V_d: 150 mL/kg; no evidence of drug accumulation over a 11- to 20-day period

Metabolism: Systemic

Bioavailability: Oral: Not bioavailable

Half-life: 1.8-3.5 hours

Time to peak serum concentration: S.C.: Within 2-6 hours

Usual Dosage Geriatrics and Adults:

Initial dosing recommendations: 5 mcg/kg/day administered S.C. or I.V. as a single daily infusion over 20-30 minutes

Doses may be increased in increments of 5 mcg/kg for each chemotherapy cycle, according to the duration and severity of the absolute neutrophil count (ANC) nadir. In phase III trials, efficacy was observed at doses of 4-6 mcg/kg/day. Discontinue therapy if the ANC count is >10,000/mm³ after the ANC nadir has occurred.

Length of therapy:

Bone marrow transplant patients: G-CSF should be administered daily for up to 30 days, until the ANC has reached 1000/mm³ for 3 consecutive days following the expected chemotherapy-induced neutrophil nadir.

Chemotherapy-treated patients: G-CSF may be administered daily for up to 2 weeks until the ANC has reached 10,000/mm³ following the expected chemotherapy-induced neutrophil nadir. Duration of therapy needed to attenuate chemotherapy-induced neutropenia may be dependent on the myelosuppressive potential of the chemotherapy regimen employed. Duration of therapy in clinical studies has ranged from 2 weeks to 3 years. Safety and efficacy of chronic administration have not been established. Premature discontinuation of G-CSF therapy prior to the time of recovery from the expected neutrophil is generally not recommended; a transient increase in neutrophil counts is typically seen 1-2 days after initiation of therapy

Administration Infuse I.V. dose over 20-30 minutes

Monitoring Parameters Complete blood cell count and platelet count should be obtained twice weekly. Leukocytosis (white blood cell counts ≥100,000/mm^3) have been observed in ~2% of patients receiving G-CSF at doses >5 mcg/kg/day. Monitor platelets and hematocrit regularly. Monitor patients with pre-existing cardiac conditions closely as cardiac events (myocardial infarctions, arrhythmias) have been reported in premarketing clinical studies.

Reference Range No clinical benefit seen with ANC >10,000/mm^3

Patient Information Possible bone pain

Nursing Implications Do not mix with sodium chloride solutions (see Administration)

Additional Information Reimbursement hotline: 1-800-28-AMGEN

Special Geriatric Considerations No specific data available for the elderly (see Usual Dosage and Monitoring Parameters)

Dosage Forms Injection, preservative free: 300 mcg/mL (1 mL, 1.6 mL)

Finasteride (fi NAS teer ide)

Brand Names Propecia®; Proscar®

Generic Available No

Therapeutic Category Antiandrogen; Urinary Tract Product

Use

Proscar®: Early data indicate that finasteride is useful in the treatment of symptomatic benign prostatic hyperplasia (BPH)

Propecia®: Treatment of male pattern hair loss in **men only**; safety and efficacy were demonstrated in men between 18-41 years of age

Unlabeled use: Adjuvant monotherapy after radical prostatectomy in the treatment of prostatic cancer

Contraindications History of hypersensitivity to drug

Warnings Women who are pregnant or who may become pregnant should not handle crushed finasteride tablets because of potential effects on a male fetus; pregnant women should also avoid exposure to the semen of a patient on finasteride

Precautions Use with caution in patients with impaired hepatic function; patients should be evaluated for prostate cancer before initiating therapy with finasteride

Adverse Reactions Genitourinary: <4% incidence of impotence, decreased libido, decreased volume of ejaculate

Drug Interactions Finasteride decreased theophylline half-life by 10%, but this was not clinically significant

Mechanism of Action

Finasteride is a 4-azo analog of testosterone and is a competitive inhibitor of both tissue and hepatic 5-alpha reductase. This results in inhibition of the conversion of testosterone to dihydrotestosterone and markedly suppresses serum dihydrotestosterone concentration; depending on dose and duration, serum testosterone concentrations may or may not increase. Testosterone-dependent processes such as fertility, muscle strength, potency, and libido are not affected by finasteride.

Pharmacodynamics

Onset of clinical effect: Within 12 weeks to 6 months of ongoing therapy

Duration of action:

After a single oral dose as small as 0.5 mg: 65% depression of plasma dihydrotestosterone levels persists 5-7 days

After 6 months of treatment with 5 mg/day: Circulating dihydrotestosterone levels are reduced to castration levels without significant effects on circulating testosterone; levels return to normal within 14 days of discontinuation of treatment

Pharmacokinetics

Absorption: Oral: Extent of absorption may be reduced if administered with food

Bioavailability: Mean: 63%

Half-life:

Elderly: 8 hours

Adults: 6 hours (3-16)

(Continued)

Finasteride *(Continued)*

Protein binding: 90%

Elimination: Excreted as metabolites in urine and feces; elimination rate is decreased in the elderly, but no dosage adjustment is needed

Usual Dosage Geriatrics and Adults: Oral:

Proscar®: 5 mg/day as a single dose; clinical response occurs within 12 weeks to 6 months of initiation of therapy; long-term administration is recommended for maximal response

Propecia®: 1 mg once daily

Monitoring Parameters Objective and subjective signs of relief of benign prostatic hyperplasia, including improvement in urinary flow, reduction in symptoms of urgency, and relief of difficulty in micturition

Test Interactions Finasteride does not influence plasma FSH, LH, cortisol, or estradiol concentration; plasma dihydrotestosterone and prostate specific antigen concentration is suppressed; plasma testosterone concentration is usually increased; no clinically significant effects on serum concentration

Patient Information Explain that it may take 6-12 months to see a response; in patients who respond, treatment is for life (see Warnings)

Nursing Implications See Warnings

Additional Information Finasteride may be useful in men with moderately symptomatic BPH who either refuse prostatectomy or are poor surgical candidates. Risk:benefit ratio and cost must be explained to the patient. Currently, there is no way to predict which men will respond to finasteride. A recent study found finasteride to be no more effective than placebo in men with BPH. When added to terazosin (an alpha antagonist), the combination was no more effective than terazosin alone.

Propecia®: Daily use for 3 or more months is necessary before benefit is observed. Withdrawal of treatment leads to reversal of effect within 12 months.

Special Geriatric Considerations Clearance of finasteride is decreased in the elderly, but no dosage reductions are necessary (see Precautions)

Dosage Forms

Tablet:

Propecia®: 1 mg

Proscar®: 5 mg

References

Lepor H, Williford WO, Barry MJ, et al, "The Efficacy of Terazosin, Finasteride, or Both in Benign Prostatic Hyperplasia," *N Engl J Med*, 1996, 335(8):533-9.

Fisalamine *see* Mesalamine *on page 591*

Flagyl® Oral *see* Metronidazole *on page 620*

Flatulex [OTC] *see* Simethicone *on page 856*

Flavorcee® [OTC] *see* Ascorbic Acid *on page 82*

Flavoxate *(fla VOKS ate)*

Brand Names Urispas®

Generic Available No

Therapeutic Category Antispasmodic Agent, Urinary

Use Antispasmodic to provide symptomatic relief of dysuria, nocturia, suprapubic pain, urgency, and incontinence due to detrusor instability and hyperreflexia in elderly with cystitis, urethritis, urethrocystitis, urethrotrigonitis, and prostatitis

Contraindications Pyloric or duodenal obstruction, GI hemorrhage, GI obstruction; ileus; achalasia; obstructive uropathies of lower urinary tract (BPH)

Warnings Glaucoma

Precautions May cause drowsiness, vertigo, and ocular disturbances; administer cautiously in patients with suspected glaucoma

Adverse Reactions

Cardiovascular: Tachycardia, palpitation

Central nervous system: Nervousness, fatigue, mental confusion (especially in geriatrics), vertigo, headache, drowsiness (>10%), hyperpyrexia

Dermatologic: Urticaria, other dermatoses

Gastrointestinal: Constipation, nausea, vomiting, xerostomia (>10%)

Hematologic: Eosinophilia; one case of reversible leukopenia has been reported

Ocular: Blurred vision, increased ocular tension (<1%)

Renal: Dysuria

Miscellaneous: Dry throat (>10%)

Overdosage Symptoms of overdose include clumsiness, dizziness, drowsiness, flushing, hallucinations, irritability

Toxicology Treatment is general supportive care

Drug Interactions May enhance the anticholinergic effects of drugs exhibiting anticholinergic pharmacologic action (see Adverse Reactions)

Mechanism of Action Synthetic antispasmotic with similar actions to that of propantheline; it exerts a direct relaxant effect on smooth muscles via phosphodiesterase inhibition, providing relief to a variety of smooth muscle spasms; it is especially useful for the treatment of bladder spasticity, whereby it produces an increase in urinary capacity

Pharmacodynamics Onset of action: 55-60 minutes

Pharmacokinetics
  Metabolism: To methyl- flavone carboxylic acid active
  Elimination: 10% to 30% in urine within 6 hours

Usual Dosage Geriatrics and Adults: Oral: 100-200 mg 3-4 times/day; reduction of dose may be possible with symptomatic improvement

Monitoring Parameters Monitor incontinence episodes; postvoid residual (PVR); monitor for anticholinergic side effects

Patient Information May cause drowsiness, dizziness, or visual disturbances; use with caution if performing tasks requiring coordination or mental alertness; avoid other substances that may cause similar effects (eg, alcohol)

Nursing Implications Monitor incontinence and PVR (see Adverse Reactions, Overdosage)

Special Geriatric Considerations Caution should be used in elderly due to anticholinergic activity (eg, confusion, constipation, blurred vision, and tachycardia)

Dosage Forms Tablet, film coated, as hydrochloride: 100 mg

Flecainide (fle KAY nide)
Related Information
  Antacid Drug Interactions *on page 1096*
Brand Names Tambocor™
Generic Available No
Therapeutic Category Antiarrhythmic Agent, Class I-C
Use Prevention and suppression of documented life-threatening ventricular arrhythmias (ie, sustained ventricular tachycardia); controlling symptomatic, disabling supraventricular tachycardias in patients without structural heart disease
Contraindications Pre-existing second or third degree A-V block; right bundle-branch block associated with left hemiblock (bifascicular block) or trifascicular block; cardiogenic shock, myocardial depression; known hypersensitivity to the drug
Warnings Due to the results of the CAST study, the manufacturer and FDA recommend that this drug be reserved for life-threatening ventricular arrhythmias unresponsive to conventional therapy. Its use for symptomatic nonsustained ventricular tachycardia, frequent premature ventricular complexes (PVCs), uniform and multiform PVCs and/or coupled PVCs is no longer recommended. Flecainide can worsen or cause arrhythmias with an associated risk of death. Proarrhythmic effects range from an increased number of PVCs to more severe ventricular tachycardias (eg, tachycardias that are more sustained or more resistant to conversion to sinus rhythm). Electrolyte abnormalities alter effects of drug; correct abnormalities prior to treatment (see Adverse Reactions).
Precautions Pre-existing sinus node dysfunction, sick sinus syndrome, history of congestive heart failure or myocardial dysfunction; increases in P-R interval ≥300 MS, QRS ≥180 MS, Q-T$_c$ interval increases and/or new bundle-branch block; patients with pacemakers, renal impairment and/or hepatic impairment
Adverse Reactions
  Cardiovascular: Bradycardia, heart block, increased P-R, QRS duration, worsening ventricular arrhythmias, congestive heart failure, palpitations, chest pain, edema, syncope
  Central nervous system: Dizziness, fatigue, nervousness, headache, lightheadedness, hypoesthesia
  Dermatologic: Rashes
  Gastrointestinal: Nausea, constipation, abdominal pain, diarrhea, anorexia, dyspepsia, flatulence, dysgeusia, xerostomia
  Hematologic: Blood dyscrasias
  Hepatic: Possible hepatic dysfunction
  Neuromuscular & skeletal: Tremors, paresthesia
(Continued)

Flecainide *(Continued)*

Ocular: Blurred vision

Respiratory: Dyspnea

Overdosage Increases in P-R, QRS, Q-T intervals and amplitude of the T wave, reduced heart rate and myocardial contractility, conduction disturbances, hypotension and death

Toxicology Supportive monitoring, charcoal hemoperfusion; may be useful as well as acidification of the urine; flecainide-induced ventricular tachycardia should be treated with ventricular pacing, antiarrhythmic drugs and/or cardioversion, however it is commonly refractory to these measures

Drug Interactions

Digoxin (increased plasma digoxin concentrations), beta-blockers (possible additive negative inotropic effects)

Alkalinizing agents (high-dose antacids, carbonic anhydrase inhibitors or sodium bicarbonate) may decrease flecainide's clearance

Mechanism of Action Class IC antiarrhythmic; slows conduction in cardiac tissue by altering transport of ions across cell membranes; causes slight prolongation of refractory periods; decreases the rate of rise of the action potential without affecting its duration; increases electrical stimulation threshold of ventricle, HIS-Purkinje system; possesses local anesthetic and moderate negative inotropic effects

Pharmacokinetics

Absorption: Oral: Rapid

Distribution: V_d: Adults: 5-13.4 L/kg

Protein binding: 40% to 50% (alpha$_1$ glycoprotein)

Metabolism: In the liver; substrate CYP2D6

Bioavailability: 85% to 90%

Half-life: Adults: 7-22 hours (average: 14 hours); increased half-life with congestive heart failure or renal dysfunction

Time to peak serum concentrations: Within 1.5-3 hours

Elimination: 80% to 90% in urine as unchanged drug and metabolites (10% to 50%)

Usual Dosage Geriatrics and Adults: Oral:

Ventricular arrhythmias: Initial: 100 mg every 12 hours, increase by 50 mg/day (given in 2 doses/day) every 4 days to maximum of 400 mg/day; for patients receiving 400 mg/day who are not controlled and have trough concentrations <0.6 µg/mL, dosage may be increased to 600 mg/day

Supraventricular arrhythmias: 50 mg every 12 hours; increase by 50 mg twice daily at 4-day intervals; maximum daily dose: 300 mg

Dosing interval in severe renal impairment: Cl$_{cr}$ <35 mL/minute/1.73 m²: Decrease the usual dose by 25% to 50%

When transferring from another antiarrhythmic agent, allow for 2-4 half-lives of the agent to pass before initiating flecainide therapy

Monitoring Parameters EKG, blood pressure, pulse, periodic serum concentrations, especially in patients with renal or hepatic impairment

Reference Range Therapeutic: 0.2-1 µg/mL (SI: 0.4-2 µmol/L)

Patient Information Take as directed; do not change dose except from advice of your physician; report any chest pain or irregular heartbeats

Nursing Implications Administer around-the-clock rather than 4 times/day, 3 times/day, etc (ie, 12-6-12-6, not 9-1-5-9) to promote less variation in peak and trough serum concentrations

Special Geriatric Considerations Decreased clearance and, therefore, prolonged half-life is possible; however, studies have shown no difference in response to usual doses in elderly despite slight decrease in clearance; calculate or measure Cl$_{cr}$ since many elderly have Cl$_{cr}$ <35 mL/minute (see Usual Dosage)

Dosage Forms Tablet, as acetate: 50 mg, 100 mg, 150 mg

References

Fenster PE and Nolan PE, "Antiarrhythmic Drugs," *Geriatric Pharmacology*, Bressler R and Katz MD, eds, New York, NY: McGraw-Hill, 1993, 6:105-49.

Fleet® Babylax® Rectal [OTC] *see* Glycerin *on page 429*

Fleet® Enema [OTC] *see* Sodium Phosphates *on page 862*

Fleet® Flavored Castor Oil [OTC] *see* Castor Oil *on page 171*

Fleet® Laxative [OTC] *see* Bisacodyl *on page 121*

Fleet® Mineral Oil Enema [OTC] *see* Mineral Oil *on page 628*

Fleet® Phospho®-Soda [OTC] *see* Sodium Phosphates *on page 862*

Flexaphen® *see* Chlorzoxazone *on page 218*

Flexeril® *see* Cyclobenzaprine *on page 259*

Flomax™ *see* Tamsulosin *on page 888*

Flonase™ *see* Fluticasone *on page 403*

Florical® **[OTC]** *see* Calcium Salts (Oral) *on page 152*

Florinef® Acetate *see* Fludrocortisone Acetate *on page 389*

Flovent® *see* Fluticasone *on page 403*

Floxin® *see* Ofloxacin *on page 688*

Flubenisolone *see* Betamethasone *on page 114*

Fluconazole (floo KOE na zole)

Related Information
I.V. Medication Recommendations *on page 1080*

Brand Names Diflucan®

Generic Available No

Therapeutic Category Antifungal Agent, Systemic

Use Treatment of susceptible fungal infections including oropharyngeal and esophageal candidiasis; treatment of systemic candidal infections including urinary tract infection, peritonitis, and pneumonia; treatment of cryptococcal meningitis

Contraindications Known hypersensitivity to fluconazole or other azoles

Warnings Patients who develop abnormal liver function tests during fluconazole therapy should be monitored closely for the development of more severe hepatic injury; if clinical signs and symptoms consistent with liver disease develop that may be attributable to fluconazole, fluconazole should be discontinued

Precautions Should be used with caution in patients with renal and hepatic dysfunction or previous hepatotoxicity from other azole derivatives

Adverse Reactions
Cardiovascular: Pallor
Central nervous system: Dizziness, headache
Dermatologic: Skin rash, exfoliative skin disorders
Endocrine & metabolic: Hypokalemia
Gastrointestinal: Nausea, abdominal pain, vomiting, diarrhea
Hepatic: Elevated AST, ALT, or alkaline phosphatase

Overdosage Symptoms of overdose include decreased lacrimation, salivation, respiration, and GI motility; urinary incontinence, cyanosis

Toxicology Hemodialysis for 3 hours reduces plasma concentration by ~50%

Drug Interactions
May increase cyclosporine levels when high doses used, may increase phenytoin serum concentration; fluconazole may also inhibit warfarin's metabolism
Rifampin decreased concentrations of fluconazole
Cimetidine has been reported to decrease fluconazole's absorption
Hydrochlorothiazide has been reported to increase fluconazole's absorption
Fluconazole may increase ethinyl estradiol absorption; fluconazole given concurrently with tolbutamide, glyburide, and glipizide has resulted in increased maximum concentrations and AUC of the oral hypoglycemics with hypoglycemia
Increased levels of cisapride

Stability Do not add other medications to I.V. unit

Mechanism of Action Interferes with cytochrome P-450 activity, decreasing ergosterol synthesis (principal sterol in fungal cell membrane) and inhibiting cell membrane formation

Pharmacokinetics
Protein binding, plasma: 11% to 12%
Metabolism: Inhibitor CYP2C9 and 3A4
Bioavailability: Oral: >90%
Half-life: Normal renal function: 25-30 hours
Time to peak: Oral: Within 2-4 hours
Elimination: 80% of dose excreted unchanged in urine

Indication	Day 1	Daily Therapy	Minimum Duration of Therapy
Oropharyngeal candidiasis	200 mg	100 mg	14 d
Esophageal candidiasis	200 mg	100 mg	21 d
Systemic candidiasis	400 mg	200 mg	28 d
Cryptococcal meningitis acute	400 mg	200 mg	10-12 wk after CSF culture becomes negative
relapse	200 mg	200 mg	10-12 wk after CSF culture becomes negative

(Continued)

Fluconazole *(Continued)*

Usual Dosage Oral and I.V. daily dose of fluconazole is the same
  Geriatrics and Adults: Oral, I.V.: For once daily dosing, see table.
    Vaginal candidiasis: 150 mg as a single dose
  Dosing adjustment in renal impairment: Cl$_{cr}$ 11-50 mL/minute: Administer 50% of recommended dose

Administration Parenteral fluconazole must be administered by I.V. infusion over ~1-2 hours; do not exceed 200 mg/hour when giving I.V. infusion

Monitoring Parameters AST, ALT, and alkaline phosphatase, potassium

Patient Information Complete full course of therapy; contact physician or pharmacist if side effects develop

Nursing Implications Monitor renal function as dosage adjustments are required with significant changes in renal function; do not unwrap unit until ready for use; do not use if cloudy or precipitated (see Administration and Stability)

Additional Information An expensive oral alternative to I.V. amphotericin B infusions; in some clinical studies it has been as effective as amphotericin B, but is less likely to cause serious adverse reactions

Special Geriatric Considerations Has not been specifically studied in the elderly (see Usual Dosage and dosing in renal impairment)

Dosage Forms
  Injection: 2 mg/mL (100 mL, 200 mL)
  Powder, for oral suspension: 10 mg/mL, 40 mg/mL when reconstituted
  Tablet: 50 mg, 100 mg, 150 mg, 200 mg

References
Grant SM and Clissold SP, "Fluconazole: A Review of Its Pharmacodynamic and Pharmacokinetic Properties and Therapeutic Potential in Superficial and Systemic Mycoses," *Drugs*, 1990, 39(6):877-916.

Flucytosine *(floo SYE toe seen)*

Brand Names Ancobon®
Synonyms 5-FC; 5-Flurocytosine
Therapeutic Category Antifungal Agent, Systemic
Use Treatment of susceptible fungal infections, usually strains of *Candida* or *Cryptococcus*
  Unlabeled use: Treatment of chromomycosis
Contraindications Hypersensitivity to flucytosine or any component
Warnings Use with extreme caution in patients with renal impairment, bone marrow suppression; patients with AIDS
Precautions Dosage modification required in patients with impaired renal function
Adverse Reactions
  Cardiovascular: Cardiac arrest
  Central nervous system: Confusion, sedation, parkinsonism, hallucinations, psychosis, headache, ataxia
  Dermatologic: Rash, photosensitivity
  Endocrine & metabolic: Hypoglycemia, hypokalemia
  Gastrointestinal: Nausea, vomiting, diarrhea, abdominal pain, loss of appetite
  Hematologic: Bone marrow suppression, anemia, leukopenia, thrombocytopenia
  Hepatic: Elevated liver enzymes, jaundice
  Neuromuscular & skeletal: Paresthesia
  Otic: Hearing loss
  Respiratory: Respiratory arrest
Overdosage Symptoms of overdose include nausea, vomiting, diarrhea
Toxicology Treatment is supportive
Drug Interactions Amphotericin dose must be reduced when used at the same time; cytosine may inactivate flucytosine
Stability Protect from light
Mechanism of Action Penetrates fungal cells and is converted to fluorouracil which competes with uracil interfering with fungal RNA and protein synthesis
Pharmacokinetics
  Absorption: Oral: 75% to 90%
  Protein binding: 2% to 4%
  Metabolism: Minimal
  Half-life: 3-8 hours (may be as long as 200 hours in anuria)

Time to peak serum concentration: Within 2-6 hours
Elimination: 75% to 90% excreted unchanged in urine by glomerular filtration

Usual Dosage Geriatrics and Adults: Oral: 50-150 mg/kg/day in divided doses every 6 hours

Dosing interval in renal impairment:
Cl_{cr} >50 mL/minute: Administer every 12 hours
Cl_{cr} 10-50 mL/minute: Administer every 16 hours
Cl_{cr} <10 mL/minute: Administer every 24 hours
Dialyzable (50% to 100%)

Monitoring Parameters Serum creatinine, BUN, alkaline phosphatase, AST, ALT, CBC; serum flucytosine concentrations

Reference Range Therapeutic: 25-100 µg/mL (SI: 195-775 µmol/L)

Test Interactions Flucytosine causes markedly false elevations in serum creatinine values when the Ektachem® analyzer is used

Patient Information Take capsules a few at a time with food over a 15-minute period

Nursing Implications Administer around-the-clock rather than 4 times/day, 3 times/day, etc (ie, 12-6-12-6, not 9-1-5-9) to promote less variation in peak and trough serum concentration; perform hematologic, renal and hepatic function tests

Special Geriatric Considerations Adjust for renal function (see Usual Dosage)

Dosage Forms Capsule: 250 mg, 500 mg

Fludrocortisone Acetate (floo droe KOR ti sone AS e tate)

Related Information
Corticosteroids Comparison, Systemic *on page 1029*

Brand Names Florinef® Acetate

Synonyms Fluohydrisone Acetate; Fluohydrocortisone Acetate; 9α-Fluorohydrocortisone Acetate

Generic Available No

Therapeutic Category Adrenal Corticosteroid; Mineralocorticoid

Use Addison's disease; partial replacement therapy for adrenal insufficiency and for treatment of salt-losing forms of congenital adrenogenital syndrome
Unlabeled use: Severe orthostatic hypotension; Shy-Drager syndrome

Contraindications Known hypersensitivity to fludrocortisone; congestive heart failure, systemic fungal infections

Precautions Addison's disease, sodium retention and potassium loss, infection

Adverse Reactions
Cardiovascular: Hypertension, edema, congestive heart failure
Central nervous system: Convulsions, headache
Dermatologic: Acne, rash, bruising
Endocrine & metabolic: Hypokalemic alkalosis, suppression of growth, hyperglycemia, HPA suppression
Gastrointestinal: Peptic ulcer
Neuromuscular & skeletal: Muscle weakness, steroid myopathy
Ocular: Cataracts, glaucoma

Overdosage Symptoms of overdose include hypertension, edema, hypokalemia, and weight gain; muscle weakness may develop due to hypokalemia

Toxicology Treat by discontinuing medication; administer potassium supplement, if necessary

Drug Interactions
Steroids decrease the effect of anticholinesterases, isoniazid, salicylates, insulin, oral hypoglycemics
Decreased effect: Barbiturates, phenytoin, rifampin
Increased effect (hypokalemia) of potassium-depleting diuretics
Increased effect: Estrogens, ketoconazole
Increased risk of digoxin toxicity (due to hypokalemia)

Mechanism of Action Promotes increased reabsorption of sodium and loss of potassium from distal tubules

Pharmacodynamics Duration of action: 1-2 days

Pharmacokinetics
Absorption: Rapid and completely from GI tract
Protein binding: 42%
Metabolism: In the liver
Half-life: 30-35 minutes; biological: 18-36 hours
Time to peak serum concentration: 1-7 hours

Usual Dosage Geriatrics and Adults: Oral: 0.05-0.2 mg/day
Orthostatic hypotension: 0.1 mg 2-3 times/day
(Continued)

Fludrocortisone Acetate *(Continued)*

Monitoring Parameters Blood pressure, standing and sitting/lying down, signs of edema, electrolytes

Test Interactions Increased amylase (S), chloride (S), increased cholesterol (S), increased glucose, increased protein, increased sodium (S); decreased calcium (S), decreased chloride (S), decreased potassium (S), decreased thyroxine (S)

Patient Information Notify physician if dizziness, severe or continuing headaches, swelling of feet or lower legs or unusual weight gain occur

Nursing Implications See Monitoring Parameters

Additional Information Very potent mineralocorticoid with high glucocorticoid activity

Special Geriatric Considerations The most common use of fludrocortisone in the elderly is orthostatic hypotension that is unresponsive to more conservative measures; attempt nonpharmacologic measures (hydration, support stockings etc) before starting drug therapy

Dosage Forms Tablet: 0.1 mg

Flu-Imune® *see* Influenza Virus Vaccine *on page 487*

Flumadine® *see* Rimantadine *on page 833*

Flunisolide (floo NIS oh lide)

Related Information

Asthma Guidelines *on page 1040*

Estimated Comparative Daily Dosages for Inhaled Corticosteroids *on page 1045*

Inhaled Medications Comparison *on page 1034*

Brand Names AeroBid®-M Oral Aerosol Inhaler; AeroBid® Oral Aerosol Inhaler; Nasalide® Nasal Aerosol; Nasarel® Nasal Spray

Generic Available No

Therapeutic Category Anti-inflammatory Agent; Corticosteroid, Inhalant

Use Steroid-dependent asthma; intranasal product is used for seasonal or perennial rhinitis

Contraindications Known hypersensitivity to flunisolide, acute status asthmaticus; viral, tuberculosis, fungal or bacterial respiratory infections

Warnings Fatalities have occurred due to adrenal insufficiency in asthmatic patients during and after transfer from systemic corticosteroids to aerosol steroids; several months may be required for recovery of this syndrome; during this period, aerosol steroids do **not** provide the systemic steroid needed to treat patients having trauma, surgery or infections

Precautions Use with caution in patients with hypothyroidism, cirrhosis, hypertension, congestive heart failure, ulcerative colitis, thromboembolic disorders; do not stop medication abruptly if on prolonged therapy

Adverse Reactions

Central nervous system: Dizziness, headache

Endocrine & metabolic: Adrenal suppression

Gastrointestinal: Sore throat, bitter taste

Respiratory: Nasal burning, nasal congestion, nasal dryness, sneezing, atrophic rhinitis, *Candida* infections of the nose or pharynx

Toxicology When consumed in excessive quantities for prolonged periods, systemic hypercorticism and adrenal suppression may occur; in those cases, discontinuation and withdrawal of the corticosteroid should be done judiciously

Drug Interactions Although there have been no reported drug interactions to date, one would expect flunisolide could potentially interact with drugs known to interact with other corticosteroids

Mechanism of Action Decreases inflammation by suppression of migration of polymorphonuclear leukocytes and reversal of increased capillary permeability; does not depress hypothalamus; in asthma, flunisolide may enhance effectiveness of beta-adrenergic drugs, inhibit bronchoconstrictor mechanisms, or produce direct smooth muscle relaxation

Pharmacokinetics

Absorption: Nasal inhalation: ~50%

Metabolism: Rapid in the liver to active metabolites

Half-life: 1.8 hours

Elimination: Equally excreted in urine and feces

Usual Dosage Geriatrics and Adults:

Oral inhalation: 2 inhalations twice daily up to 8 inhalations/day

Nasal: 2 sprays in each nostril twice daily; maximum: 8 sprays/day in each nostril; after desired effect is obtained, decrease dose to the smallest one possible; some patients may be maintained on 1 spray per nostril per day

Monitoring Parameters Relief of symptoms

Patient Information Follow instructions that accompany the product; do not exceed recommended dosage; do not confuse or interchange oral and nasal inhalers

Nursing Implications Shake well before giving; do not use Nasalide® orally; dispose of product after it has been opened for 3 months; allow at least 1 minute between inhalations

Additional Information Does not contain fluorocarbons; contains polyethylene glycol vehicle

Special Geriatric Considerations Many elderly patients have difficulty using metered dose inhalers, which can limit their effectiveness. Assess technique in all older patients. A spacer device may be useful for the oral inhaler.

Dosage Forms
Inhalant:
Nasal (Nasalide®): 25 mcg/actuation [200 sprays] (25 mL)
Oral:
AeroBid®: 250 mcg/actuation [100 metered doses] (7 g)
AeroBid-M® (menthol flavor): 250 mcg/actuation [100 metered doses] (7 g)

Fluocinolone (floo oh SIN oh lone)
Related Information
Corticosteroids Comparison, Topical *on page 1030*

Brand Names Derma-Smoothe/FS®; Fluonid®; Flurosyn®; FS Shampoo®; Synalar®; Synalar-HP®; Synemol®

Generic Available Yes

Therapeutic Category Corticosteroid, Topical (Medium Potency); Corticosteroid, Topical (High Potency)

Use Relief of the inflammatory and pruritic manifestations of corticosteroid-responsive dermatoses

Contraindications Fungal infection, hypersensitivity to fluocinolone or any component, TB of skin, herpes (including varicella)

Precautions Systemic absorption of topical corticosteroids has produced reversible HPA axis suppression. This is more likely to occur when the preparation is used on large surfaces or denuded areas for prolonged periods of time or with an occlusive dressing.

Adverse Reactions
Dermatologic: Acne, hypopigmentation, allergic dermatitis, maceration of the skin, skin atrophy, striae, miliaria, telangiectasia
Endocrine & metabolic: HPA suppression, Cushing's syndrome, growth retardation
Local: Burning, itching, irritation, dryness, folliculitis, hypertrichosis
Miscellaneous: Secondary infection

Mechanism of Action Topical corticosteroids have anti-inflammatory, antipruritic, vasoconstrictive, and antiproliferative actions

Usual Dosage Topical: Apply thin layer to affected areas 2-4 times/day

Monitoring Parameters Relief of symptoms

Patient Information Use only as prescribed and for no longer than the period prescribed; apply sparingly in a thin film and rub in lightly; avoid contact with eyes; notify physician if condition persists or worsens

Nursing Implications Use sparingly

Additional Information Considered a moderate-potency steroid; avoid prolonged use on the face, may cause atrophic changes

Special Geriatric Considerations Due to age-related changes in skin, limit use of topical glucocorticosteroids (see Precautions)

Dosage Forms
Fluocinolone acetonide:
Cream: 0.01% (15 g, 60 g); 0.025% (15 g, 60 g)
Flurosyn®, Synalar®: 0.01% (15 g, 30 g, 60 g, 425 g)
Flurosyn®, Synalar®, Synemol®: 0.025% (15 g, 60 g, 425 g)
Synalar-HP®: 0.2% (12 g)
Ointment, topical: 0.025% (15 g, 60 g)
Flurosyn®, Synalar®: 0.025% (15 g, 30 g, 60 g, 425 g)
Oil (Derma-Smoothe/FS®): 0.01% (120 mL)
Shampoo (FS Shampoo®): 0.01% (180 mL)
(Continued)

Fluocinolone *(Continued)*

Solution, topical: 0.01% (20 mL, 60 mL)
Fluonid®, Synalar®: 0.01% (20 mL, 60 mL)

Fluocinonide (floo oh SIN oh nide)

Related Information

Corticosteroids Comparison, Topical *on page 1030*

Brand Names Lidex®; Lidex-E®

Generic Available Yes

Therapeutic Category Corticosteroid, Topical (High Potency)

Use Relief of the inflammatory and pruritic manifestations of corticosteroid-responsive dermatoses

Contraindications Viral, fungal, or tubercular skin lesions, herpes simplex, known hypersensitivity to fluocinonide

Precautions Systemic absorption of topical corticosteroids has produced reversible HPA axis suppression. This is more likely to occur when the preparation is used on large surfaces or denuded areas for prolonged periods of time or with an occlusive dressing.

Adverse Reactions

Dermatologic: Acne, hypopigmentation, allergic dermatitis, maceration of the skin, skin atrophy, striae, miliaria, telangiectasia

Endocrine & metabolic: HPA suppression, Cushing's syndrome, growth retardation

Local: Burning, itching, irritation, dryness, folliculitis, hypertrichosis

Miscellaneous: Secondary infection

Mechanism of Action Topical corticosteroids have anti-inflammatory, antipruritic, vasoconstrictive, and antiproliferative actions

Usual Dosage Topical: Apply thin layer to affected area 2-4 times/day depending on the severity of the condition

Monitoring Parameters Relief of symptoms

Patient Information Use only as prescribed and for no longer than the period prescribed; apply sparingly in a thin film and rub in lightly; avoid contact with eyes; notify physician if condition persists or worsens

Nursing Implications Use sparingly

Additional Information Considered a high potency steroid; avoid prolonged use on the face; may cause atrophic changes

Special Geriatric Considerations Due to age-related changes in skin, limit use of topical glucocorticosteroids (see Precautions)

Dosage Forms

Cream: 0.05% (15 g, 30 g, 60 g, 120 g)
Anhydrous, emollient (Lidex®): 0.05% (15 g, 30 g, 60 g, 120 g)
Aqueous, emollient (Lidex-E®): 0.05% (15 g, 30 g, 60 g, 120 g)
Gel, topical: 0.05% (15 g, 60 g)
Lidex®: 0.05% (15 g, 30 g, 60 g, 120 g)
Ointment, topical: 0.05% (15 g, 30 g, 60 g)
Lidex®: 0.05% (15 g, 30 g, 60 g, 120 g)
Solution, topical: 0.05% (20 mL, 60 mL)
Lidex®: 0.05% (20 mL, 60 mL)

Fluogen® *see* Influenza Virus Vaccine *on page 487*

Fluohydrisone Acetate *see* Fludrocortisone Acetate *on page 389*

Fluohydrocortisone Acetate *see* Fludrocortisone Acetate *on page 389*

Fluonid® *see* Fluocinolone *on previous page*

Fluoride (FLOR ide)

Brand Names ACT® [OTC]; Fluorigard® [OTC]; Fluorinse®; Fluoritab®; Flura®; Flura-Drops®; Flura-Loz®; Gel Kam®; Gel-Tin® [OTC]; Karidium®; Karigel®; Karigel®-N; Listermint® with Fluoride [OTC]; Luride®; Luride® Lozi-Tab®; Luride®-SF Lozi-Tab®; Minute-Gel®; Pediaflor®; Pharmaflur®; Phos-Flur®; Point-Two®; PreviDent®; Stop® [OTC]; Thera-Flur®; Thera-Flur-N®

Synonyms Acidulated Phosphate Fluoride; Sodium Fluoride; Stannous Fluoride

Generic Available Yes

Therapeutic Category Mineral, Oral; Mineral, Oral Topical

Use Prevention of dental caries

Unlabeled use: Treatment of osteoporosis

Contraindications Hypersensitivity to fluoride or any component; when fluoride content of drinking water exceeds 0.7 ppm

Precautions Prolonged ingestion with excessive doses may result in dental fluorosis and osseous changes; do **not** exceed recommended dosage

Adverse Reactions

Dermatologic: Rash

Gastrointestinal: GI upset, nausea, vomiting, especially with large doses for treatment of bone diseases

Neuromuscular & skeletal: Pain in lower extremities

Respiratory: Ulceration of mucous membranes

Miscellaneous: Stannous fluoride may stain the teeth

Overdosage

Hypersalivation, salty or soapy taste, epigastric pain, nausea, vomiting, diarrhea, rash muscle weakness, tremor, seizure, cardiac failure, respiratory arrest, shock, death

Treatment of overdose: Gastric lavage with calcium chloride or $Ca(OH)_2$ solution; administer large quantity of milk at frequent intervals; $Al(OH)_3$ may also bind the fluoride ion

Toxicology Fatal dose not known; adults: 7-140 mg/kg

Drug Interactions Magnesium-, aluminum-, and calcium-containing products (including foods) may decrease absorption of fluoride

Stability Store in tight plastic containers (not glass)

Mechanism of Action Reduces acid production by dental bacteria; increases tooth resistance to acid dissolution by formation of fluorohydroxyapatite; direct stimulation of osteoblasts

Pharmacokinetics

Absorption: In the GI tract, lungs and skin; 50% of fluoride is deposited in teeth and bone after ingestion; topical application works superficially on enamel and plaque

Elimination: In urine and feces

Usual Dosage Recommended daily fluoride supplement: Not recommended for persons >14 years of age

Geriatrics and Adults: Oral:

Dental rinse or gel: 10 mL rinse or apply to teeth and spit daily after brushing

Treatment of osteoporosis: 50-75 mg/day in divided doses

Patient Information Take with food (but not milk) to eliminate GI upset; with dental rinse or dental gel do **not** swallow, do **not** eat or drink for 30 minutes after use; notify physician of GI or lower extremity complaints

Nursing Implications Avoid giving with milk or dairy products, antacids

Additional Information 2.2 mg of sodium fluoride is equivalent to 1 mg of fluoride ion

Special Geriatric Considerations Postmenopausal women taking high doses of sodium fluoride have increased their bone density in the lumbar spine by 35% with a smaller increase in the femoral neck. In spite of these increases, the overall rate of vertebral fracture did not decline significantly while the rate of hip fracture increased. The results of a randomized, placebo-controlled trial using an investigational slow-release fluoride formulation at a lower dose (50 mg/day) are encouraging. Patients who received fluoride for 1 year or more had a lower vertebral fracture rate and substantial increase in L2-L4 bone mass and femoral neck bone density compared to placebo. Both groups took calcium. At the present time, restricted to investigational protocols.

Dosage Forms

Gel, as sodium: 1.1% (24 g, 125 g)

Gel, oral topical, as stannous: 0.4%

Gel, oral topical, acidulated phosphate: 1.1% (480 mL)

Paste, as sodium: 33.3%

Solution:

Oral, as acidulated phosphate: 0.044% (250 mL, 500 mL)

Oral, as sodium: 1.1 mg/mL (50 mL); 4.4 mg/mL (30 mL); 4.97 mg/mL (50 mL); 12.3 mg/mL (24 mL); 13 mg/mL (19 mL)

Rinsing: 0.02%, 0.05%, 0.2%

Tablet, as sodium: 2.2 mg

Tablet, chewable, as sodium: 0.55 mg, 1.1 mg, 2.2 mg

References

Pak CYS, Sakhaee K, Adams-Huet B, et al, "Treatment of Postmenopausal Osteoporosis With Slow-Release Sodium Fluoride: Final Report of a Randomized Controlled Trial," *Ann Intern Med*, 1995, 123(6):401-8.

Riggs BL, Hodgson SF, O'Fallon WM, et al, "Effect of Fluoride Treatment on the Fracture Rate in Postmenopausal Women With Osteoporosis," *N Engl J Med*, 1990, 322(12):802-9.

Fluorigard® [OTC] *see* Fluoride *on previous page*

Fluorinse® *see* Fluoride *on page 392*

Fluoritab® *see* Fluoride *on page 392*

9α-Fluorohydrocortisone Acetate *see* Fludrocortisone Acetate *on page 389*

Fluoxetine (floo OKS e teen)

Related Information
Antidepressant Agents Comparison *on page 1021*
Antidepressant Medication Guidelines *on page 1075*

Brand Names Prozac®

Generic Available No

Therapeutic Category Antidepressant; Selective Serotonin Reuptake Inhibitor (SSRI)

Use Treatment of major depression

Contraindications Hypersensitivity to fluoxetine; patients receiving MAO inhibitors currently or in past 2 weeks; concurrent use with terfenadine or astemizole is not advised (see Drug Interactions)

Precautions Due to limited experience, use with caution in patients with renal or hepatic impairment, seizure disorders, diabetes mellitus; use with caution in patients at high risk for suicide

Adverse Reactions
Cardiovascular: Chest pain
Central nervous system: Headache, nervousness, insomnia, abnormal dreams, drowsiness, anxiety, dizziness, fatigue, sedation, seizures, extrapyramidal reactions (rare)
Dermatologic: Rash, pruritus
Endocrine & metabolic: Hypoglycemia, hyponatremia (elderly or volume-depleted patients), SIADH
Gastrointestinal: Nausea, diarrhea, xerostomia, anorexia, dyspepsia, constipation, vomiting, weight loss
Genitourinary: Frequent urination, ejaculation problems
Neuromuscular & skeletal: Tremors, myalgia, weakness
Ocular: Visual disturbances
Respiratory: Nasal congestion
Miscellaneous: Swollen glands, excessive diaphoresis

Overdosage Symptoms of overdose include nausea, vomiting, agitation, hypomania, seizures

Toxicology Following initiation of essential overdose management (emesis, lavage, activated charcoal), toxic symptoms should be treated. Seizures usually respond to diazepam I.V. boluses (5-10 mg, up to 30 mg). If seizures are unresponsive or recur, phenytoin or phenobarbital may be required.

Drug Interactions
Fluoxetine decreased clearance of terfenadine and potentially astemizole, loratadine, and cisapride
Increased effect with tricyclics (2 times increased plasma concentration)
Increased/decreased effect of lithium (both increased and decreased level has been reported)
Increased toxicity of diazepam, alprazolam, clonazepam, trazodone via decreased clearance; increased toxicity with MAO inhibitors including selegiline (hyperpyrexia, tremors, seizures, delirium, coma); increased toxicity with dexfenfluramine (possible)
Displace protein bound drugs
Cyproheptadine may decrease or reverse effect of fluoxetine
Carbamazepine, hydantoin, and haloperidol levels may be increased, increasing pharmacologic effects and risk of toxicity
May inhibit metabolism of codeine and tramadol to active metabolites

Mechanism of Action Inhibits CNS neuron serotonin uptake; minimal or no effect on reuptake of norepinephrine or dopamine; does not significantly bind to alpha-adrenergic, histamine or cholinergic receptors; may therefore be useful in patients at risk from sedation, hypotension and anticholinergic effects of tricyclic antidepressants

Pharmacodynamics Peak antidepressant effects: Usually occur after more than 4 weeks; due to long half-life, resolution of adverse reactions after discontinuation may be slow

Pharmacokinetics
Absorption: Oral: Well absorbed
Metabolism: To norfluoxetine (active); inhibitor CYP2C19, 2D6, 3A4; substrate CYP2D6
Half-life (adults): 2-3 days
Time to peak serum concentration: Within 4-8 hours
Elimination: In urine as fluoxetine (2.5% to 5%) and norfluoxetine (10%)

Geriatrics: Similar to younger patients after a single dose; has not been evaluated under steady-state conditions

Usual Dosage Oral:

Geriatrics: Some patients may require an initial dose of 10 mg/day with dosage increases of 10 and 20 mg every several weeks as tolerated; should not be taken at night unless patient experiences sedation

Adults: 20 mg/day in the morning; may increase after several weeks by 20 mg/day increments; maximum: 80 mg/day; doses >20 mg should be divided into morning and noon doses. **Note:** Lower doses of 5 mg/day have been used for initial treatment.

Dosing adjustment in hepatic impairment:

Cirrhosis patients: Administer a lower dose or less frequent dosing interval

Compensated cirrhosis without ascites: Administer 50% of normal dose

Monitoring Parameters Signs and symptoms of depression, anxiety, sleep, appetite, and weight; signs of EPS in patients taking haloperidol

Reference Range Therapeutic: Fluoxetine 100-800 ng/mL (SI: 289-2314 nmol/L); norfluoxetine 100-600 ng/mL (SI: 289-1735 nmol/L); not well correlated

Test Interactions Increased albumin in urine

Patient Information Use sugarless hard candy for dry mouth; avoid alcoholic beverages, may cause drowsiness or insomnia, improvement may take several weeks; rise slowly to prevent dizziness

Nursing Implications Offer patient sugarless hard candy for dry mouth

Special Geriatric Considerations Fluoxetine's favorable side effect profile makes it a useful alternative to the traditional tricyclic antidepressants; its potential stimulating and anorexic effects may be bothersome to some patients; has not been shown to be superior in efficacy to the traditional tricyclic antidepressants or other SSRIs; the long half-life in the elderly makes it less attractive compared to other SSRIs. Data from a clinical trial comparing fluoxetine to tricyclics suggest that fluoxetine is significantly less effective than nortriptyline in hospitalized elderly patients with unipolar major affective disorder, especially those with melancholia and concurrent cardiovascular diseases.

Dosage Forms

Fluoxetine hydrochloride:

Capsule: 10 mg, 20 mg

Liquid (mint flavor): 20 mg/5 mL (120 mL)

Extemporaneous Preparations A 20 mg capsule may be mixed with 4 oz of water, apple juice, or Gatorade to provide a solution that is stable for 14 days under refrigeration

References

Beasley CM, Bosomworth JC, and Wernicke JF, "Fluoxetine: Relationships Among Dose, Response, Adverse Events, and Plasma Concentrations in the Treatment of Depression," *Psychopharmacol Bull*, 1990, 26(1):18-24.

Feighner JP and Cohn JB, "Double-blind Comparative Trials of Fluoxetine and Doxepin in Geriatric Patients With Major Depressive Disorder," *J Clin Psychiatry*, 1985, 46(3 Pt 2):20-5.

Lemberger L, Bergstrom RF, Wolen RL, et al, "Fluoxetine: Clinical Pharmacology and Physiologic Disposition," *J Clin Psychiatry*, 1985, 46(3 Pt 2):14-9.

Roose SP, Glassman AH, Attia E, et al, "Comparative Efficacy of Selective Serotonin Reuptake Inhibitors and Tricyclics in the Treatment of Melancholia," *Am J Psychiatry*, 1994, 151(12):1735-9.

Schone W and Ludwig M, "A Double-Blind Study of Paroxetine Compared With Fluoxetine in Geriatric Patients With Major Depression," *J Clin Psychopharmacol*, 1993, 13(6 Suppl 2):34S-9S.

Fluphenazine (floo FEN a zeen)

Related Information

Antacid Drug Interactions *on page 1096*
Antipsychotic Agents Comparison *on page 1023*
Antipsychotic Medication Guidelines *on page 1076*
Federal OBRA Regulations Recommended Maximum Doses - Antipsychotics *on page 1056*

Brand Names Permitil® Oral; Prolixin Decanoate® Injection; Prolixin Enanthate® Injection; Prolixin® Injection; Prolixin® Oral

Generic Available Yes

Therapeutic Category Antipsychotic Agent; Neuroleptic Agent; Phenothiazine Derivative

Use Management of manifestations of psychotic disorders; depressive neurosis; alcohol withdrawal; nausea and vomiting; nonpsychotic symptoms associated with dementia in elderly, Tourette's syndrome; Huntington's chorea; spiromatic torticollis and Reye's syndrome (see Special Geriatric Considerations)

(Continued)

Fluphenazine *(Continued)*

Contraindications Hypersensitivity to fluphenazine or any component, cross-sensitivity with other phenothiazines may exist; avoid use in patients with narrow-angle glaucoma, bone marrow suppression, severe liver or cardiac disease; subcortical brain damage; circulatory collapse, severe hypotension or hypertension

Warnings

Tardive dyskinesia: Prevalence rate may be 40% in elderly; elderly women especially at risk; embarrassment from dyskinesias may lead to greater social isolation; development of the syndrome and the irreversible nature are proportional to duration and total cumulative dose over time. May be reversible if diagnosed early in therapy; intermittent use of antipsychotics (not proven use) helps decrease total cumulative dose.

EPS: Extrapyramidal reactions are more common in elderly with up to 50% developing these reactions after age 60. These reactions may be more common in dementia patients. Drug-induced **Parkinson's syndrome** occurs often. Discontinuation usually resolves symptoms but may take weeks to months (12+) to clear. **Akathisia** is the most common EPS reaction in elderly. The symptoms of motor restlessness are difficult to diagnose in demented elderly; increased nervousness, assertiveness, restlessness with constant movement may indicate this adverse event. Consider decreasing dose if antipsychotic to treat as well as diagnose problem; usually see this reaction within 2-3 months of initiating antipsychotic drug.

Anticholinergic effects: These side effects most common with low potency antipsychotics (eg, thioridazine, chlorpromazine). CNS toxicity occurs more frequently and severely in elderly; increased confusion, memory loss, psychotic behavior, and agitation frequently occur as a consequence of anticholinergic effects to antipsychotic agents. Peripheral anticholinergic action troublesome to elderly; most peripheral anticholinergic effects last only 2-3 weeks (see Adverse Reactions).

Orthostatic hypotension: More common with low potency agents (eg, thioridazine, chlorpromazine, and clozapine) but of concern with all antipsychotic agents; orthostasis due to alpha-receptor blockade by antipsychotic agents. Elderly present many risk factors for orthostatic hypotension: blunted baroreceptor reflexes, decreased vascular tone, decreased vascular volume, and possible presence of cardiac diseases which result in decreased cardiac output.

Sedation: Common side effect with antipsychotic therapy; should not be used as a hypnotic unless insomnia is associated with target behavior symptoms treated with antipsychotic medications (see Special Geriatric Considerations). Anecdotal reports suggesting antipsychotic sedation in nonpsychotic patients is extremely unpleasant due to feelings of depersonalization, derealization, and dysphoria. Due to the long duration of action with antipsychotic drugs, these reactions may last up to 24 hours and result in decreased daytime function.

Cardiac toxicity: Life-threatening arrhythmias have occurred at therapeutic doses of antipsychotics. Thioridazine more commonly demonstrates EKG changes than other antipsychotics; suggested to use high potency antipsychotic agents (ie, haloperidol) in patients with cardiac conduction defects.

Precautions Use with caution in patients with cardiovascular disease, seizures, and Parkinson's disease; benefits of therapy must be weighed against risks of therapy; adverse effects may be of longer duration with Depot® form

Adverse Reactions

Cardiovascular: EKG changes, orthostatic hypotension, tachycardia, arrhythmias, abnormal T waves with prolonged ventricular repolarization

Central nervous system: Sedation, drowsiness, restlessness, anxiety, extrapyramidal reactions, pseudoparkinsonian signs and symptoms, tardive dyskinesia, neuroleptic malignant syndrome, seizures, altered central temperature regulation

Dermatologic: Hyperpigmentation, pruritus, rash, photosensitivity (rare)

Endocrine & metabolic: Amenorrhea, galactorrhea, gynecomastia

Gastrointestinal: GI upset, xerostomia (problem for denture users), constipation, adynamic ileus, weight gain

Genitourinary: Urinary retention, overflow incontinence, priapism, impotence, sexual dysfunction (up to 60%)

Hematologic: Agranulocytosis, leukopenia (usually in patients with large doses for prolonged periods), thrombocytopenia, hemolytic anemia, eosinophilia

Hepatic: Cholestatic jaundice (rare)

Ocular: Retinal pigmentation (more common than with chlorpromazine), blurred vision, decreased visual acuity (may be irreversible)

Miscellaneous: Anaphylactoid reactions

Overdosage Symptoms of overdose include deep sleep, coma, extrapyramidal symptoms, abnormal involuntary muscle movements, hypotension or hypertension; agitation, restlessness, fever, hypothermia or hyperthermia, seizures, cardiac arrhythmias, EKG changes

Toxicology Following initiation of essential overdose management, toxic symptom treatment and supportive treatment should be initiated. Hypotension usually responds to I.V. fluids or Trendelenburg positioning. If unresponsive to these measures the use of a parenteral inotrope may be required (eg, norepinephrine 0.1-0.2 mcg/kg/minute titrated to response). Do not use epinephrine. Seizures commonly respond to diazepam (I.V. 5-10 mg bolus in adults every 15 minutes if needed up to a total of 30 mg) or to phenytoin or phenobarbital. Also critical cardiac arrhythmias often respond to I.V. phenytoin (15 mg/kg up to 1 g), while other antiarrhythmics can be used. Neuroleptics often cause extrapyramidal symptoms (eg, dystonic reactions) requiring management with diphenhydramine 1-2 mg/kg up to a maximum of 50 mg I.M. or I.V. slow push followed by a maintenance dose for 48-72 hours. When these reactions are unresponsive to diphenhydramine, benztropine mesylate I.V. 1-2 mg may be effective. These agents are generally effective within 2-5 minutes.

Drug Interactions

Alcohol may increase CNS sedation

Anticholinergic agents may decrease pharmacologic effects; increase anticholinergic side effects; may enhance tardive dyskinesia

Aluminum salts may decrease absorption of phenothiazines

Barbiturates may decrease phenothiazine serum concentrations

Bromocriptine may have decreased efficacy when administered with phenothiazines

Guanethidine's hypotensive effect is decreased by phenothiazines

Lithium administration with phenothiazines may increase disorientation

Meperidine and phenothiazine coadministration increases sedation and hypotension

Methyldopa administration with phenothiazine (trifluoperazine) may significantly increase blood pressure

Norepinephrine, epinephrine have decreased pressor effect when administered with chlorpromazine; therefore, be aware of possible decreased effectiveness or when any phenothiazine is used

Phenytoin serum concentrations may increase or decrease with phenothiazines; tricyclic antidepressants may have increased serum concentrations with concomitant administration with phenothiazines

Propranolol administered with phenothiazines may increase serum concentrations of both drugs

Valproic acid may have increased half-life when administered with phenothiazines (chlorpromazine)

Stability Avoid freezing; protect all dosage forms from light, clear or slightly yellow solutions may be used; should be dispensed in amber or opaque vials/bottles. Solutions may be diluted or mixed with fruit juices or other liquids but must be administered immediately after mixing; do not prepare bulk dilutions or store bulk dilutions.

Mechanism of Action Blocks postsynaptic mesolimbic dopaminergic D_1 and D_2 receptors in the brain; exhibits a strong alpha-adrenergic blocking and anticholinergic effect, depresses the release of hypothalamic and hypophyseal hormones; believed to depress the reticular activating system thus affecting basal metabolism, body temperature, wakefulness, vasomotor tone, and emesis

Pharmacodynamics

Onset of action: I.M., S.C.: 24-72 hours

Peak effects: 48-96 hours; derivative dependent; the hydrochloride salt acts quickly and persists briefly, while the decanoate lasts the longest and requires more time for onset

Following hydrochloride derivative administration, the onset of activity occurs within 1 hour yet persists for only 6-8 hours

(Continued)

Fluphenazine *(Continued)*

Pharmacokinetics

Absorption: Oral: May be affected by the inherent anticholinergic action on the gastrointestinal tissue causing variable absorption. Absorption from tablets is erratic with less variation seen with solutions. These agents are widely distributed in tissues with CNS concentrations exceeding that of plasma due to their lipophilic characteristics.

Protein binding: Antipsychotic agents are bound 90% to 99% to plasma or proteins; highly bound to brain and lung tissue and other tissues with a high blood perfusion

Metabolism: Substrate and inhibitor CYP2D6

Half-life (derivative dependent):
  Enanthate: 84-96 hours
  Hydrochloride: 33 hours
  Decanoate: 163-232 hours

Time to peak serum concentrations: 2-4 hours

Elimination: Excretion occurs through hepatic metabolism (oxidation) where numerous active metabolites are produced; active metabolites excreted in urine; elimination half-lives of antipsychotics ranges from 20-40 hours which may be extended in elderly due to decline in oxidative hepatic reactions (phase I) with age.

The biologic effect of a single dose persists for 24 hours. When the patient has accommodated to initial side effects (sedation), once daily dosing is possible due to the long half-life of antipsychotics.

Steady-state plasma concentrations are achieved in 4-7 days; therefore, if possible, do not make dose adjustments more than once in a 7-day period.

Due to the long half-lives of antipsychotics, as needed (prn) use is ineffective since repeated doses are necessary to achieve therapeutic tissue concentrations in the CNS

Usual Dosage

Geriatrics: Initial (nonpsychotic patient; dementia behavior): 1-2.5 mg/day; increase dose at 4- to 7-day intervals by 1-2.5 mg/day; increase dosing intervals (bid, tid) as necessary to control response or side effects. Maximum daily dose: 20 mg; gradual increases (titration) may prevent some side effects or decrease their severity.

Adults:
  Oral: 0.5-10 mg/day; dose is 2-3 times the parenteral dose
  I.M.: 2.5-10 mg/day
  I.M., S.C. (Decanoate®): 12.5 mg every 3 weeks
  I.M., S.C. (Enanthate®): 12.5-25 mg every 3 weeks

Conversion ratio from hydrochloride salt to decanoate salt is ~0.5 mL (12.5 mg) decanoate every 3 weeks for every 10 mg of hydrochloride salt daily.

Not dialyzable (0% to 5%)

Monitoring Parameters Orthostatic blood pressures; tremors, gait changes, abnormal movement in trunk, neck, buccal area, or extremities; monitor target behaviors for which the agent is given

Reference Range Therapeutic: 0.13-2.8 ng/mL; correlation of serum concentrations and efficacy is controversial; most often dosed to best response

Test Interactions Increased cholesterol (S), increased glucose; decreased uric acid (S)

Patient Information Oral concentrate must be diluted in 2-4 oz of liquid (water, fruit juice, carbonated drinks, milk, or pudding); do not take antacid within 1 hour of taking drug; avoid alcohol; avoid excess sun exposure (use sun block); may cause drowsiness, rise slowly from recumbent position; use of supportive stockings may help prevent orthostatic hypotension

Nursing Implications Watch for hypotension when administering I.M. or I.V.; Dilute the oral concentrate with water or juice before administration; avoid skin contact with oral suspension or solution; may cause contact dermatitis; monitor orthostatic blood pressures 3-5 days after initiation of therapy or a dose increase; observe for tremor and abnormal movement or posturing (extrapyramidal symptoms)

Additional Information Oral liquid to be diluted in the following **only**: water, saline, 7-UP, homogenized milk, carbonated orange beverages, pineapple, apricot, prune, orange, V-8 juice, tomato, and grapefruit juices; do not mix with beverages containing caffeine, tannins, or pectin (ie, coffee, tea, apple juice)

Special Geriatric Considerations See Warnings.

Many elderly patients receive antipsychotic medications for inappropriate nonpsychotic behavior. Before initiating antipsychotic medication, the clinician should investigate any possible reversible cause; any stress or stress from any disease can cause acute "confusion" or worsening of baseline nonpsychotic behavior. Most commonly acute changes in behavior are due to increases in drug dose or addition of new drug to regimen; fluid electrolyte loss; infections; and changes in environment.

Any changes in disease status in any organ system can result in behavior changes.

In the treatment of agitated, demented, elderly patients, authors of meta-analysis of controlled trials of the response to the traditional antipsychotics (phenothiazines, butyrophenones) in controlling agitation have concluded that the use of neuroleptics results in a response rate of 18%. Clearly neuroleptic therapy for behavior control should be limited with frequent attempts to withdraw the agent given for behavior control.

Dosage Forms
Fluphenazine hydrochloride:
    Concentrate: 5 mg/mL with alcohol 14% (120 mL)
    Elixir: 2.5 mg/5 mL with alcohol 14% (60 mL)
    Injection: 2.5 mg/mL (10 mL)
    Tablet: 1 mg, 2.5 mg, 5 mg, 10 mg
Injection, as decanoate ester: 25 mg/mL (1 mL, 5 mL)
Injection, as enanthate: 25 mg/mL (5 mL)

References
Peabody CA, Warner MD, Whiteford HA, et al, "Neuroleptics and the Elderly," *J Am Geriatr Soc*, 1987, 35(3):233-8.

Risse SC and Barnes R, "Pharmacologic Treatment of Agitation Associated With Dementia," *J Am Geriatr Soc*, 1986, 34(5):368-76.

Saltz BL, Woerner MG, Kane JM, et al, "Prospective Study of Tardive Dyskinesia Incidence in the Elderly," *JAMA*, 1991, 266(17):2402-6.

Seifert RD, "Therapeutic Drug Monitoring: Psychotropic Drugs," *J Pharm Pract*, 1984, 6:403-16.

Flura® *see* Fluoride *on page 392*

Flura-Drops® *see* Fluoride *on page 392*

Flura-Loz® *see* Fluoride *on page 392*

Flurazepam (flure AZ e pam)

Related Information
Antacid Drug Interactions *on page 1096*
Anxiolytic/Hypnotic Use in Long-Term Care Facilities *on page 1099*
Benzodiazepines Comparison *on page 1024*
Federal OBRA Regulations Recommended Maximum Doses - Hypnotics *on page 1057*

Brand Names Dalmane®

Generic Available Yes

Therapeutic Category Benzodiazepine; Hypnotic; Sedative

Use Short-term treatment of insomnia

Restrictions C-IV

Contraindications Hypersensitivity to flurazepam or any component; there may be cross-sensitivity with other benzodiazepines; pre-existing CNS depression, respiratory depression, narrow-angle glaucoma

Precautions Use with caution in patients receiving other CNS depressants, patients with low albumin, and hepatic dysfunction, or a history of drug dependence

Adverse Reactions
Cardiovascular: Hypotension
Central nervous system: Drowsiness, dizziness, confusion, residual daytime sedation, paradoxical reactions, hyperactivity and excitement (rare), ataxia, hallucinations
Respiratory: Decrease in respiratory rate, apnea, laryngospasm
Miscellaneous: Physical and psychological dependence with prolonged use, falls in the elderly

Toxicology Treatment for benzodiazepine overdose is supportive. Rarely is mechanical ventilation required. Flumazenil has been shown to selectively block the binding of benzodiazepines to CNS receptors, resulting in a reversal of benzodiazepine-induced CNS depression, but not respiratory depression.

Drug Interactions
Decreased effect: Benzodiazepines may decrease the effect of levodopa
Decreased metabolism: Cimetidine, fluoxetine
Increased metabolism: Rifampin
Increased toxicity: CNS depressants, alcohol

Stability Store in light-resistant containers
(Continued)

Flurazepam *(Continued)*

Mechanism of Action Benzodiazepines appear to potentiate the effects of GABA and other inhibitory neurotransmitters by binding to specific benzodiazepine-receptor sites in various areas of the CNS

Pharmacodynamics Because of a long-acting metabolite, residual, daytime sedation or "hangover effect" may occur, particularly in the elderly. Studies have shown that the elderly are more sensitive to the effects of benzodiazepines as compared to younger adults.

Hypnotic effects:
Onset of action: 15-20 minutes
Peak effect: 3-6 hours
Duration of action: 7-8 hours

Pharmacokinetics
Metabolism: In liver to N-desalkylflurazepam (active)
Half-life (active metabolite): Adults: 40-114 hours
Elimination: Prolonged in elderly; accumulation of the parent drug and its metabolite occurs

Usual Dosage Oral:
Geriatrics: 15 mg at bedtime
Adults: 15-30 mg at bedtime

Monitoring Parameters Respiratory, cardiovascular, and mental status

Reference Range Therapeutic: 0-4 ng/mL (SI: 0-9 nmol/L); metabolite N-desalkylflurazepam: 20-110 ng/mL (SI: 43-240 nmol/L); Toxic: >0.12 µg/mL

Patient Information Avoid alcohol and other CNS depressants, may cause drowsiness or "hangover" effect; avoid activities needing good psychomotor coordination until CNS effects are known; may cause physical or psychological dependence; avoid abrupt discontinuation after prolonged use

Nursing Implications Provide safety measures (ie, side rails, night light, and call button); remove smoking materials from area; supervise ambulation; avoid abrupt discontinuance in patients with prolonged therapy or seizure disorders; observe for orthostasis

Special Geriatric Considerations Due to its long-acting metabolite, flurazepam is not considered a drug of choice in the elderly (see Pharmacodynamics and Pharmacokinetics); long-acting benzodiazepines have been associated with falls in the elderly; interpretive guidelines from the Health Care Financing Administration (HCFA) discourage the use of this agent in residents of long-term care facilities

Dosage Forms Capsule, as hydrochloride: 15 mg, 30 mg

References
Maletta G, Mattox KM, and Dysken M, "Guidelines for Prescribing Psychoactive Drugs in the Elderly: Part 1," *Geriatrics*, 1991, 46(9):40-7.
Reidenberg MM, Levy M, Warner H, et al, "Relationship Between Diazepam Dose, Plasma Level, Age, and Central Nervous System Depression," *Clin Pharmacol Ther*, 1978, 23(4):371-4.

Flurbiprofen *(flure BI proe fen)*

Brand Names Ansaid® Oral; Ocufen® Ophthalmic

Generic Available Tablet: No

Therapeutic Category Analgesic, Non-narcotic; Anti-inflammatory Agent; Anti-inflammatory Agent, Ophthalmic; Nonsteroidal Anti-inflammatory Agent (NSAID), Ophthalmic

Use Acute or long-term treatment of signs and symptoms of rheumatoid arthritis and osteoarthritis; inhibition of intraoperative miosis; topical treatment of cystoid macular edema; postcataract surgery inflammation and uveitis syndromes

Unlabeled use: Ankylosing spondylitis, mild to moderate pain, tendonitis, bursitis, acute painful shoulder, acute gout, sunburn, for aborting acute migraine headache attacks; ophthalmic: prevention and management of postoperative ocular inflammation and postoperative cystoid macular edema

Contraindications Hypersensitivity to flurbiprofen or any component; hypersensitivity to aspirin or other NSAIDs; dendritic keratitis

Warnings Potential cross-sensitivity to aspirin and other NSAIDs exists; systemic effects from ocular absorption may occur (ie, bleeding): GI toxicity (bleeding, ulceration, perforation); CNS effects may occur (headaches, confusion, depression); hypersensitivity, anaphylactoid reactions (intermittent tolmetin use more often); renal function decline, acute renal insufficiency, interstitial nephritis, dysuria, cystitis, hematuria, nephrotic syndrome, hyperkalemia in acute renal insufficiency, hyponatremia, papillary necrosis, hepatic function impairment; should be used with caution in patients with a history of herpes simplex, keratitis, and patients who might be affected by inhibition of platelet aggregation; patients in whom asthma, rhinitis, or urticaria is precipitated by aspirin or other NSAIDs; systemic absorption occurs with ocular application; elderly have increased risk for adverse reactions to NSAIDs (see Special Geriatric Considerations)

Precautions Use with caution in patients with congestive heart failure, hypertension, decreased renal or hepatic function, history of GI disease (bleeding or ulcers), or those receiving anticoagulants; perform ophthalmologic evaluation for those who develop eye complaints during therapy (blurred vision, diminished vision, changes in color vision, retinal changes); should be used with caution in patients with a history of herpes simplex, keratitis, and patients who might be affected by inhibition of platelet aggregation; slowing of corneal wound healing; NSAIDs may mask signs/symptoms of infections; photosensitivity reported

Adverse Reactions

Cardiovascular: Congestive heart failure, angina, hypertension, hypotension, arrhythmias, edema

Central nervous system: Headache, drowsiness, vertigo, dizziness, fatigue, hallucinations, confusion, depression, emotional lability, psychotic behavior, pyrexia

Dermatologic: Rash, urticaria, angioedema, Stevens-Johnson syndrome, exfoliative dermatitis, bruising, petechiae, purpura, slowing of corneal wound healing

Endocrine & metabolic: Hyperglycemia, hypoglycemia, hyperkalemia, gynecomastia, hyponatremia, fluid retention

Gastrointestinal: Dyspepsia, heartburn, nausea, diarrhea, constipation, flatulence, anorexia, stomatitis, vomiting, abdominal pain, peptic ulcer, GI bleeding, GI perforation, gingival ulcers, pancreatitis, proctitis, paralytic ulcers, colitis, weight loss, dry mucous membranes

Genitourinary: Impotence, azotemia

Hematologic: Neutropenia, anemia, agranulocytosis, bone marrow suppression, hemolytic anemia, hemorrhage, inhibition of platelet aggregation

Hepatic: Hepatitis, elevated LFTs, cholestatic jaundice

Neuromuscular & skeletal: Tremors, weakness

Ocular: Vision changes, transient stinging, burning, ocular irritation

Otic: Tinnitus

Renal: Dysuria, polyuria, pyuria, oliguria, anuria, acute renal failure

Respiratory: Exacerbation of asthma, dyspnea

Miscellaneous: Thirst, diaphoresis

Overdosage Symptoms include drowsiness, lethargy, disorientation, confusion, dizziness, numbness, paresthesia, nausea, vomiting, gastric irritation, abdominal pain, headache, tinnitus, sweating, blurred vision, muscle twitching, seizures, coma, acute renal failure, increased BUN and serum creatinine, hypotension, tachycardia, and metabolic acidosis

Toxicology Management of a nonsteroidal anti-inflammatory drug (NSAID) intoxication is primarily supportive and symptomatic. Fluid therapy is commonly effective in managing the hypotension that may occur following an acute NSAID overdose, except when this is due to an acute blood loss. Seizures tend to be very short-lived and often do not require drug treatment although recurrent seizures should be treated with I.V. diazepam. Since many of the NSAIDs undergo enterohepatic cycling, multiple doses of charcoal may be needed to reduce the potential for delayed toxicities. NSAIDs are highly bound to plasma proteins; therefore, hemodialysis and peritoneal dialysis are not useful.

Drug Interactions

May increase digoxin, methotrexate, and lithium serum concentrations

Aspirin or other salicylates may decrease NSAID serum concentrations

Other NSAIDs may increase adverse GI effect

Increased prothrombin time with anticoagulants; decreased antihypertensive effects of ACE inhibitors, beta-blockers, and thiazide diuretics; increased response to sympathomimetics

Probenecid may increase toxicity of NSAIDs by increase in serum concentrations

Effects of loop diuretics may be decreased

When used concurrently with flurbiprofen, acetylcholine chloride and carbachol may be ineffective

Mechanism of Action Inhibits prostaglandin synthesis by decreasing the activity of the enzyme, cyclo-oxygenase, which results in decreased formation of prostaglandin precursors; acts on the hypothalamus heat-regulating center to reduce fever, blocks prostaglandin synthetase action which prevents (Continued)

Flurbiprofen *(Continued)*

formation of the platelet-aggregating substance, thromboxane A_2; decreases pain receptor sensitivity. Other proposed mechanisms of action for salicylate anti-inflammatory action are lysosomal stabilization, inhibition of kinin and leukotriene production, alteration of chemotactic factors, and inhibition of neutrophil activation. This latter mechanism may be the most significant pharmacologic action to reduce inflammation; prostaglandins are believed to play a role in constricting the iris sphincter during ocular surgery. In animals, prostaglandins are mediators of intraocular inflammation. Prostaglandins produce disruption of the blood-aqueous humor barrier, increased vascular permeability, vasodilation, leukocytosis, and increased intraocular pressure (IOP).

Pharmacodynamics Onset of action: Within 1-2 hours

Pharmacokinetics
Absorption: Oral: Rapid
Protein binding: 99%
Metabolism: Metabolized in the liver
Half-life: 5-6 hours
Time to peak serum concentration: Within 1-2 hours
Elimination: Excreted by kidneys primarily as glucuronides and sulfates

Usual Dosage Geriatrics and Adults:
Oral: Rheumatoid arthritis and osteoarthritis: Initial: 50 mg 4 times/day to 100 mg 3 times/day; do not administer more than 100 mg for any single dose; maximum dose: 300 mg/day
Ophthalmic: Instill 1 drop every 30 minutes, 2 hours prior to surgery (total of 4 drops to each affected eye)

Monitoring Parameters Monitor response (pain, range of motion, grip strength, mobility, ADL function), inflammation; observe for weight gain, edema; monitor renal function; observe for bleeding, bruising; evaluate gastrointestinal effects (abdominal pain, bleeding, dyspepsia); mental confusion, disorientation, CBC, serum creatinine, BUN, liver function tests

Test Interactions Increased chloride (S), increased sodium (S)

Patient Information Serious gastrointestinal bleeding can occur as well as ulceration and perforation. Pain may or may not be present. Avoid aspirin and aspirin-containing products while taking this medication. If gastric upset occurs, take with food, milk, or antacid. If gastric adverse effects persist, contact physician. May cause drowsiness, dizziness, blurred vision, and confusion. Use caution when performing tasks which require alertness (eg, driving). Do not take for more than 3 days for fever and 10 days for pain without physician's advice.

Ophthalmic: May sting on instillation; do not touch dropper to eye; visual acuity may be decreased after administration; assess patient's or caregiver's ability to administer

Nursing Implications See Monitoring Parameters, Overdosage, Patient Information, and Special Geriatric Considerations

Additional Information There are no clinical guidelines to predict which NSAID will give response in a particular patient. Trials with each must be initiated until response is determined. Consider dose, patient convenience, and cost.

Special Geriatric Considerations Elderly are a high-risk population for adverse effects from nonsteroidal anti-inflammatory agents. As much as 60% of elderly can develop peptic ulceration and/or hemorrhage asymptomatically. The concomitant use of H_2 blockers, omeprazole, and sucralfate is not effective as prophylaxis with the exception of NSAID-induced duodenal ulcers which may be prevented by the use of ranitidine. Misoprostol and proton pump inhibitors are the only agents proven to help prevent the development of NSAID-induced ulcers. Also, concomitant disease and drug use contribute to the risk for GI adverse effects. Use lowest effective dose for shortest period possible. Consider renal function decline with age. Use of NSAIDs can compromise existing renal function especially when Cl_{cr} is ≤30 mL/minute. Tinnitus may be a difficult and unreliable indication of toxicity due to age-related hearing loss or eighth cranial nerve damage. CNS adverse effects such as confusion, agitation, and hallucination are generally seen in overdose or high-dose situations, but elderly may demonstrate these adverse effects at lower doses than younger adults.

Dosage Forms
Flurbiprofen sodium:
Solution, ophthalmic (Ocufen®): 0.03% (2.5 mL, 5 mL, 10 mL)
Tablet (Ansaid®): 50 mg, 100 mg

References

Brooks PM, Day RO, "Nonsteroidal Anti-inflammatory Drugs - Differences and Similarities," *N Engl J Med*, 1991, 324(24):1716-25.

Clinch D, Banerjee AK, Ostick G, "Absence of Abdominal Pain in Elderly Patients With Peptic Ulcer," *Age Ageing*, 1984, 13:120-3.

Clive DM, Stoff JS, "Renal Syndromes Associated With Nonsteroidal Anti-inflammatory Drugs," *N Engl J Med*, 1984, 310(9):563-72.

Graham DY, "Prevention of Gastroduodenal Injury Induced by Chronic Nonsteroidal Anti-inflammatory Drug Therapy," *Gastroenterology*, 1989, 96(2 Pt 2 Suppl):675-81.

Hawkey CJ, Karrasch JA, Szczepaski L, et al, "Omeprazole Compared With Misoprostrol for Ulcers Associated With Nonsteroidal Anti-inflammatory Drugs," *N Engl J Med*, 1998, 338(11):727-34.

Knodel LC, "Preventing NSAID-Induced Ulcers: The Role of Misoprostol," *Consult Pharm*, 1989, 4:37-41.

Pounder R, "Silent Peptic Ulceration: Deadly Silence or Golden Silence?" *Gastroenterology*, 1989, 96(2 Pt 2 Suppl):626-31.

Yeomans ND, Tulassay Z, Juhasz L, et al, "A Comparison of Omeprazole With Ranitidine for Ulcers Associated With Nonsteroidal Anti-inflammatory Drugs," *N Engl J Med*, 1998, 338(11):719-26.

5-Flurocytosine *see* Flucytosine *on page 388*

Flurosyn® *see* Fluocinolone *on page 391*

Flutamide (FLOO ta mide)
Brand Names Eulexin®
Generic Available No
Therapeutic Category Antiandrogen
Use In combination therapy with LHRH agonistic (leuprolide) in treatment of metastatic prostatic carcinoma (see Additional Information)
Contraindications Known hypersensitivity to flutamide or any component
Warnings Animal data (based on using doses higher than recommended for humans) produced testicular interstitial cell adenoma
Precautions Do not discontinue therapy without physician's advice
Adverse Reactions
  Cardiovascular: Edema, hypertension
  Central nervous system: Drowsiness, nervousness, depression, anxiety, confusion
  Endocrine & metabolic: Gynecomastia, hot flashes
  Gastrointestinal: Diarrhea, nausea, anorexia
  Genitourinary: Impotence, loss of libido
  Hepatic: Elevated LFTs (usually transient)
Overdosage Symptoms of overdose include hypoactivity, ataxia, anorexia, vomiting, piloerection, decreased respiration, tranquilization, lacrimation
Toxicology Induce vomiting; general supportive care; dialysis not effective
Mechanism of Action Inhibiting androgen uptake or inhibits binding of androgen in target tissues
Pharmacokinetics
  Absorption: Oral: Rapid and complete
  Metabolism: Extensive to more than 10 metabolites
  Half-life: 5-6 hours
  Elimination: All excreted primarily in urine
Usual Dosage Geriatrics and Adults: Oral: 2 capsules (250 mg) every 8 hours
Monitoring Parameters LFTs, tumor reduction, testosterone/estrogen, and phosphatase serum concentration
Patient Information Do not discontinue therapy without physician's advice
Nursing Implications See Monitoring Parameters
Additional Information To achieve benefit to combination therapy, both drugs need to be started simultaneously; most common side effect with this dual therapy is diarrhea
Special Geriatric Considerations A study has shown that the addition of flutamide to leuprolide therapy in patients with advanced prostatic cancer increased median actuarial survival time to 34.9 months versus 27.9 months with leuprolide alone. No specific dose alterations are necessary in elderly.
Dosage Forms Capsule: 125 mg
References
Crawford ED, Eisenberger MA, McLeod DG, et al, "A Controlled Trial of Leuprolide With and Without Flutamide in Prostatic Carcinoma," *N Engl J Med* , 1989, 321(7):419-24.

Flutex® *see* Triamcinolone *on page 949*

Fluticasone (floo TIK a sone)
Related Information
  Asthma Guidelines *on page 1040*
  Corticosteroids Comparison, Topical *on page 1030*
(Continued)

Fluticasone *(Continued)*

Estimated Comparative Daily Dosages for Inhaled Corticosteroids *on page 1045*

Brand Names Cutivate™; Flonase™; Flovent®

Generic Available No

Therapeutic Category Corticosteroid, Inhalant; Corticosteroid, Nasal; Corticosteroid, Topical (Medium Potency)

Use

Inhalation: Maintenance treatment of asthma as prophylactic therapy. It is also indicated for patients requiring oral corticosteroid therapy for asthma to assist in total discontinuation or reduction of total oral dose. NOT indicated for the relief of acute bronchospasm.

Intranasal: Management of seasonal and perennial allergic rhinitis in patients ≥12 years of age

Topical: Relief of inflammation and pruritus associated with corticosteroid-responsive dermatoses [medium potency topical corticosteroid]

Contraindications Hypersensitivity to any component, bacterial infections, ophthalmic use

Warnings Adverse systemic effects may occur when used on large areas of the body, denuded areas, for prolonged periods of time, and/or with an occlusive dressing

Adverse Reactions

Dermatologic: Acne, hypopigmentation, allergic dermatitis, maceration of the skin, skin atrophy, striae, miliaria, telangiectasia

Endocrine & metabolic: HPA suppression, Cushing's syndrome, growth retardation

Local: Burning, itching, irritation, dryness, folliculitis, hypertrichosis

Miscellaneous: Secondary infection

Overdosage When consumed in excessive quantities, systemic hypercorticism and adrenal suppression may occur

Toxicology Discontinuation and withdrawal of the corticosteroid should be done judiciously

Mechanism of Action Fluticasone belongs to a new group of corticosteroids which utilizes a fluorocarbothioate ester linkage at the 17 carbon position; extremely potent vasoconstrictive and anti-inflammatory activity; has a weak hypothalamic-pituitary-adrenocortical axis (HPA) inhibitory potency when applied topically, which gives the drug a high therapeutic index. Although HPA suppression does occur after I.V. administration, fluticasone is inactive when administered orally due to first-pass hydrolysis of the carbothioate ester to the corresponding carboxylic acid, which is inactive.

Usual Dosage Geriatrics and Adults:

Topical: Apply sparingly in a thin film twice daily

Inhalation, Oral:

Recommended Oral Inhalation Doses

Previous Therapy	Recommended Starting Dose	Highest Recommended Dose
Bronchodilator Alone	88 mcg twice daily	440 mcg twice daily
Inhaled Corticosteroids	88–220 mcg twice daily	440 mcg twice daily
Oral Corticosteroids	880 mcg twice daily	880 mcg twice daily

Intranasal: Initially 2 sprays (50 mcg/spray) per nostril once daily. After the first few days, dosage may be reduced to 1 spray per nostril once daily for maintenance therapy. Maximum total daily dose should not exceed 4 sprays (200 mcg)/day.

Monitoring Parameters Relief of symptoms

Patient Information Use only as prescribed, and for no longer than the period prescribed; apply topical product sparingly in light film, rub in lightly, avoid contact with eyes; notify physician if condition being treated persists or worsens; for intranasal and oral inhalers, follow the instructions accompanying the medication; do not confuse or interchange intranasal and oral inhalers

Nursing Implications Use sparingly; spray is for intranasal use only

Special Geriatric Considerations No specific geriatric information is available

Dosage Forms
Fluticasone propionate:
Spray, aerosol, oral inhalation (Flovent®): 44 mcg/actuation (7.9 g = 60 actuations or 13 g = 120 actuations), 110 mcg/actuation (13 g = 120 actuations); 220 mcg/actuation (13 g = 120 actuations)
Spray, intranasal (Flonase™): 50 mcg/actuation (16 g = 120 actuations)
Topical (Cutivate™):
Cream: 0.05% (15 g, 30 g, 60 g)
Ointment: 0.005% (15 g, 60 g)

Fluvastatin (FLOO va sta tin)
Brand Names Lescol®
Therapeutic Category Antilipemic Agent; HMG-CoA Reductase Inhibitor
Use Adjunct to dietary therapy to decrease elevated serum total and LDL cholesterol concentrations in primary hypercholesterolemia
Contraindications Active liver disease or unexplained persistent elevations of LFTs, hypersensitivity to fluvastatin or other HMG-CoA reductase inhibitors
Warnings Musculoskeletal effects include myopathy (myalgia and/or muscle weakness accompanied by markedly elevated CR concentrations), rash and/or pruritus
Precautions May elevate aminotransferases; LFTs should be performed before and every 4- 6 weeks during the first 12-15 months of therapy and periodically thereafter; serum cholesterol and triglyceride concentrations should be determined prior to and regularly during therapy; use with caution in patients who consume large quantities of alcohol
Adverse Reactions
Central nervous system: Headache, dizziness, insomnia, fatigue
Dermatologic: Rash, pruritus
Gastrointestinal: Nausea, vomiting, diarrhea, abdominal cramps, constipation, flatulence, dyspepsia
Neuromuscular & skeletal: Muscle cramps, back pain, arthropathy
Respiratory: Upper respiratory infection, rhinitis, cough, pharyngitis, sinusitis, bronchitis
Miscellaneous: Influenza, allergy
Overdosage Few cases have been reported; no patients were symptomatic and all recovered without adverse effects
Drug Interactions Increased anticoagulant effect of warfarin; concurrent use of niacin, gemfibrozil, erythromycin, and cyclosporine increases the risk of rhabdomyolysis or myopathy
Mechanism of Action Acts by competitively inhibiting 3-hydroxyl-3-methyl-glutaryl-coenzyme A (HMG-CoA) reductase, the enzyme that catalyzes the rate-limiting step in cholesterol biosynthesis
Pharmacokinetics
Protein binding: >98%
Metabolism: Extensive first-pass metabolism; metabolized to active and inactive metabolites although the active forms do not circulate systemically; inhibitor CYP2C9
Bioavailability: Absolute (24%)
T_{max}: ≤1 hour
Half-life: 1.2 hours
Elimination: Urine (5%), feces (90%)
Usual Dosage Geriatrics and Adults: Oral: 20 mg at bedtime; maximum: 40 mg/day
No dose adjustment needed in mild to moderate renal impairment
Administration May be taken without regard to meals; if concomitant therapy with a bile acid resin, take at least 2 hours later
Monitoring Parameters Serum cholesterol (total and fractionated), CPK serum concentrations; LFTs before and every 4-6 weeks during the first 12-15 months of therapy and periodically thereafter or LFTs before and every 4-6 weeks during the first 3 months of therapy and then every 6-12 weeks during the next 12 months and periodically thereafter
Patient Information Promptly report any unexplained muscle pain, tenderness or weakness, especially if accompanied by malaise or fever; follow prescribed diet; take with meals
Nursing Implications The best effect is seen when administered at night; monitor for symptoms of adverse effects (see Adverse Reactions and Special Geriatric Considerations)
Special Geriatric Considerations The definition of and, therefore, when to treat hyperlipidemia in the elderly is a controversial issue. The National Cholesterol Education Program recommends that all adults 20 years of age
(Continued)

Fluvastatin *(Continued)*

and older maintain a plasma cholesterol <200 mg/dL. By this definition, 60% of all elderly would be considered to have a borderline high (200-239 mg/dL) or high (≥240 mg/dL) plasma cholesterol. However, plasma cholesterol has been shown to be a less reliable predictor of coronary heart disease in the elderly. Therefore, it is the authors' belief that pharmacologic treatment be reserved for those who are unable to obtain a desirable plasma cholesterol concentration by diet alone and for whom the benefits of treatment are believed to outweigh the potential adverse effects, drug interactions, and cost of treatment.

Dosage Forms Capsule: 20 mg, 40 mg

References

"Summary of the Second Report of the National Cholesterol Education Program (NCEP) Expert Panel on Detection, Evaluation, and Treatment of High Blood Cholesterol in Adults (Adult Treatment Panel II)," *JAMA*, 1993, 269(23):3015-23.

Fluvoxamine (floo VOKS ah meen)

Related Information

Antidepressant Agents Comparison *on page 1021*
Antidepressant Medication Guidelines *on page 1075*

Brand Names Luvox®

Therapeutic Category Antidepressant; Selective Serotonin Reuptake Inhibitor (SSRI)

Use Treatment of obsessive-compulsive disorder (OCD); effective in the treatment of major depression; may be useful for the treatment of panic disorder

Contraindications Concomitant terfenadine or astemizole; during or within 14 days of MAO inhibitors; hypersensitivity to fluvoxamine or any congeners (eg, fluoxetine)

Warnings Use with caution in patients with liver dysfunction, suicidal tendencies, history of seizures, mania, or drug abuse, ECT, cardiovascular disease, and the elderly

Adverse Reactions

Cardiovascular: Palpitations

Central nervous system: Somnolence, headache, insomnia, dizziness, nervousness, mania, hypomania, vertigo, abnormal thinking, agitation, anxiety, malaise, amnesia, seizures, extrapyramidal reactions (rare)

Dermatologic: Toxic epidermal necrolysis

Endocrine & metabolic: Decreased libido

Gastrointestinal: Xerostomia, abdominal pain, vomiting, dyspepsia, constipation, diarrhea, dysgeusia, anorexia

Hematologic: Thrombocytopenia

Hepatic: Hepatic dysfunction

Neuromuscular & skeletal: Tremors, weakness

Renal: Increases in serum creatinine

Miscellaneous: Diaphoresis, extrapyramidal reactions

Overdosage Symptoms of overdose include drowsiness, nausea, vomiting, abdominal pain, tremors, sinus bradycardia, and seizures

Toxicology Specific antidote does not exist; treatment is supportive. Although vomiting has not been extensive in overdose to date, patients should be monitored for fluid and electrolyte loss, and appropriate replacement therapy instituted when necessary.

Drug Interactions Because fluvoxamine inhibits cytochrome P-450 isozymes 1A2, 2C9, 2CA, 3A4, 2D6, it is associated with numerous significant drug interactions

Increased toxicity: Dexfenfluramine (possible); terfenadine, astemizole, and cisapride are metabolized by the cytochrome P-450 IIIA4 isozyme; increased levels of these drugs have been associated with prolongation of the Q-T interval and potentially fatal, torsade de pointes ventricular arrhythmias. Since fluvoxamine inhibits the enzyme responsible for their clearance, the concomitant use of these agents is contraindicated.

Potentiates triazolam and alprazolam (dose should be reduced by at least 50%), hypertensive crisis with MAO inhibitors, theophylline (doses should be reduced by 1/3 and plasma concentrations monitored), warfarin (reduce its dose and monitor PT/INR), carbamazepine (monitor levels), tricyclic antidepressants (monitor effects and reduce doses accordingly), haloperidol, methadone, beta-blockers (reduce dose of propranolol or metoprolol), diltiazem. Caution with other benzodiazepines, phenytoin, lithium, clozapine, alcohol, other CNS drugs, quinidine, ketoconazole.

Mechanism of Action Inhibits CNS neuron serotonin uptake, thereby enhancing serotonergic activity and inhibiting adrenergic activity in the locus ceruleus; minimal or no effect on reuptake of norepinephrine or dopamine; does not significantly bind to alpha-adrenergic, histamine or cholinergic receptors

Pharmacodynamics

Maximum effect: Requires at least 4-6 weeks of treatment

Pharmacokinetics The pharmacokinetics of fluvoxamine do not appear to be affected by age

Absorption: Oral: Readily complete in the fasting and nonfasting state

Distribution: V_d: >5-20 L/kg

Protein binding: 77%

Metabolism: Via oxidative pathways to 14 inactive compounds which are renally (see Drug Interactions)

Bioavailability, systemic: 53%

Half-life: 16 hours after multiple dosing

Peak plasma concentration: Within 2-8 hours after a single dose

Time to steady-state: ~10 days

Elimination: ~3% recovered unchanged in the urine

Usual Dosage

Geriatrics: See Special Geriatric Considerations

Adults: Initial: 50 mg at bedtime; adjust in 50 mg increments at 4- to 7-day intervals; usual dose range: 100-300 mg/day; divide total daily dose into 2 doses; administer larger portion at bedtime

Dosing adjustment in hepatic impairment: Reduce dose, titrate slowly

Monitoring Parameters Signs and symptoms of depression, anxiety, weight gain or loss, nutritional intake, sleep

Reference Range A therapeutic range has not been established

Patient Information Avoid alcoholic beverages; its favorable side effect profile makes it a useful alternative to the traditional agents; use sugarless hard candy for dry mouth; avoid alcoholic beverages, may cause drowsiness; improvement may take several weeks; rise slowly to prevent dizziness. As with all psychoactive drugs, fluvoxamine may impair judgment, thinking, or motor skills, so use caution when operating hazardous machinery, including automobiles, especially early on into therapy. Inform your physician of any concurrent medications you may be taking or antidepressants you have been taking.

Nursing Implications Best tolerated as a single bedtime dose; can be taken with or without food

Special Geriatric Considerations Given fluvoxamine's approved indication (OCD), the number of drug interactions, and the limited information available on its use in the elderly, it may be best to select a different agent when treating depression (see Pharmacokinetics). Data from a clinical trial comparing fluoxetine to tricyclics suggest that fluoxetine is significantly less effective than nortriptyline in hospitalized elderly patients with unipolar major affective disorder, especially those with melancholia and concurrent cardiovascular diseases.

Dosage Forms Tablet: 50 mg, 100 mg

References

de Vries MH, Raghoebar M, Mathlener IS, et al, "Single and Multiple Oral Dose Fluvoxamine Kinetics in Young and Elderly Subjects," *Ther Drug Monit*, 1992, 14(6):493-8.

Grimsley SR and Jann MW, "Paroxetine, Sertraline, and Fluvoxamine: New Selective Serotonin Reuptake Inhibitors," *Clin Pharm*, 1992, 11(11):930-57.

Roose SP, Glassman AH, Attia E, et al, "Comparative Efficacy of Selective Serotonin Reuptake Inhibitors and Tricyclics in the Treatment of Melancholia," *Am J Psychiatry*, 1994, 151(12):1735-9.

Fluzone® *see* Influenza Virus Vaccine *on page 487*

Folacin *see* Folic Acid *on this page*

Folate *see* Folic Acid *on this page*

Folex® PFS *see* Methotrexate *on page 605*

Folic Acid (FOE lik AS id)

Brand Names Folvite®

Synonyms Folacin; Folate; Pteroylglutamic Acid

Generic Available Yes

Therapeutic Category Vitamin, Water Soluble

Use Treatment of megaloblastic and macrocytic anemias due to folate deficiency

Contraindications Pernicious, aplastic, or normocytic anemias

(Continued)

Folic Acid *(Continued)*

Warnings Large doses may mask the hematologic effects of B_{12} deficiency, thus obscuring the diagnosis of pernicious anemia while allowing the neurologic complications due to B_{12} deficiency to progress; injection contains benzyl alcohol (1.5%) as preservative

Precautions Doses >0.1 mg/day may obscure pernicious anemia; patients with pernicious anemia may show hematologic improvement with doses as low as 0.25 mg/day with continuing irreversible nerve damage progression. Resistance to treatment may occur with depressed hematopoiesis, alcoholism, deficiencies of other vitamins; should rule out pernicious anemia with Schilling Test and serum vitamin concentration.

Adverse Reactions
  Dermatologic: Pruritus
  Miscellaneous: Allergic reaction

Overdosage Not described (see Additional Information)

Toxicology Not described (see Additional Information)

Drug Interactions In folate-deficient patients, folic acid therapy may increase phenytoin metabolism resulting in decreased phenytoin serum concentrations. Phenytoin, primidone, para-aminosalicylic acid, and sulfasalazine have been reported to decrease serum folate concentrations and may cause deficiency. Concurrent administration of chloramphenicol and folic acid in these patients may result in antagonism of the hematopoietic response to folic acid.

Stability Incompatible with oxidizing and reducing agents and heavy metal ions

Mechanism of Action Folic acid is necessary for formation of a number of coenzymes in many metabolic systems, particularly for purine and pyrimidine synthesis; required for nucleoprotein synthesis and maintenance in erythropoiesis; stimulates WBC and platelet production in folate deficiency anemia

Pharmacodynamics Peak effects: Oral: Within 30-60 minutes

Pharmacokinetics Absorption: In the proximal part of the small intestine

Usual Dosage Geriatrics and Adults: RDA: 0.4 mg
  Folic acid deficiency: Oral, I.M., I.V., S.C.: Initial: 1 mg/day; replacement requires only 2-3 weeks; maintenance dose: 0.5 mg/day; 1 mg/day may be needed for patients taking anticonvulsant therapy (see Special Geriatric Considerations)

Monitoring Parameters Reticulocyte count within 5-10 days of initiation of therapy; hematocrit, hemoglobin, RBC count at monthly intervals; diarrheal episodes should stop in 2-3 days of therapy; monitor seizure activity, serum phenytoin concentration should be monitored more often

Reference Range Therapeutic: 0.005-0.015 µg/mL

Test Interactions Falsely low serum concentrations may occur with the *Lactobacillus casei* assay method in patients on anti-infectives (eg, tetracycline)

Patient Information Take folic acid replacement only under recommendation of physician

Nursing Implications Oral, but may also be administered by deep I.M., S.C., or I.V. injection; a diluted solution for oral or for parenteral administration may be prepared by diluting 1 mL of folic acid injection (5 mg/mL), with 49 mL sterile water for injection; resulting solution is 0.1 mg folic acid per 1 mL (see Monitoring Parameters)

Additional Information Water-soluble vitamin with a wide margin of safety

Special Geriatric Considerations Elderly frequently have combined nutritional deficiencies; must rule out vitamin B_{12} deficiency before initiating folate therapy; elderly RDA requirements from 1989 RDA are 200 mcg minimum (0.2 mg). Elderly, due to decreased nutrient intake, may benefit from daily intake of a multiple vitamin with minerals.

Dosage Forms
  Injection, as sodium folate: 5 mg/mL (10 mL); 10 mg/mL (10 mL)
  Tablet: 0.1 mg, 0.4 mg, 0.8 mg, 1 mg

References
Olszewski AJ, Szostak WB, Bialkowska M, et al, "Reduction of Plasma Lipid and Homocysteine Levels by Pyridoxine, Folate, Cobalamin, Choline, Riboflavin, and Troxerutin in Atherosclerosis," *Atherosclerosis*, 1989, 75(1):1-6.

Folvite® *see Folic Acid on previous page*

Formula Q® *see Quinine on page 817*

Fortaz® *see Ceftazidime on page 188*

Fosamax® *see Alendronate on page 31*

Foscarnet (fos KAR net)

Related Information
I.V. Medication Recommendations *on page 1080*

Brand Names Foscavir®

Synonyms PFA; Phosphonoformate; Phosphonoformic Acid

Generic Available No

Therapeutic Category Antiviral Agent, Parenteral

Use Alternative to ganciclovir for treatment of CMV retinitis and other CMV infections; alternative to acyclovir for treatment of acyclovir-resistant HSV infections

Contraindications Hypersensitivity to foscarnet; a Cl_{cr} <0.4 mL/minute/kg during therapy

Warnings Impairment of renal function is the major toxicity and is experienced to some extent in most patients, thus renal function should be closely monitored (see Monitoring Parameters). Imbalance of serum electrolytes or minerals occurs in 6% to 18% of patients (hypocalcemia, low ionized calcium, hypo- or hyperphosphatemia, hypomagnesemia or hypokalemia). Patients with a low ionized calcium may experience perioral tingling, numbness, paresthesias, tetany, and seizures. Seizures have been experienced by up to 10% of AIDS patients. Risk factors for seizures include a low baseline absolute neutrophil count (ANC), impaired baseline renal function and low total serum calcium. Some patients who have experienced seizures have died, while others have been able to continue or resume foscarnet treatment after their mineral or electrolyte abnormality has been corrected, their underlying disease state treated or their dose decreased. Foscarnet has been shown to be mutagenic *in vitro* and in mice at very high doses.

Precautions Diagnosis of CMV retinitis should be made by an ophthalmologist familiar with the presentation and differentiation of CMV from other ophthalmic conditions with similar presentations (ie, candidiasis, toxoplasmosis, etc); local irritation at the infusion site and penile and vulvovaginal ulcerations have been reported. The risk of these irritations may be minimized by infusion into a large enough vein for quick dilution and maintaining adequate hydration, respectively.

Adverse Reactions
Central nervous system: Headache, seizures, fever, dizziness, anxiety, hypothermia, confusion, fatigue
Endocrine & metabolic: Electrolyte imbalance
Gastrointestinal: Diarrhea, nausea, vomiting
Neuromuscular & skeletal: Rigors
Renal: Renal impairment

Overdosage Symptoms of overdose include seizures, coma, renal impairment, paresthesias, hypocalcemia and hypo- or hyperphosphatemia

Toxicology No specific antidote is available; in overdose situations, maintain hydration and monitor renal function and electrolytes; hydration and hemodialysis may be useful but have not been well studied.

Drug Interactions
Concurrent treatment with aminoglycosides, amphotericin B, or I.V. pentamidine or other potential nephrotoxic drugs; foscarnet's elimination may be decreased by drugs that block renal tubular secretion (ie, probenecid)
I.V. pentamidine (hypocalcemia); zidovudine (anemia); any drug that may influence serum calcium concentration (ie, furosemide) may increase risk for hypocalcemia or lower serum ionized calcium levels

Stability Administer in normal saline or 5% dextrose solution; administer no other drug or supplement concurrently via the same catheter. Incompatible with 30% dextrose, amphotericin B, and calcium-containing solutions such as Ringer's lactate and TPN. See package insert for a complete list of incompatibilities.

Mechanism of Action Pyrophosphate analogue which acts as a noncompetitive inhibitor of many viral RNA and DNA polymerases as well as HIV reverse transcriptase. Inhibitory effects occur at concentrations which do not affect host cellular DNA polymerases; however, some human cell growth suppression has been observed with high *in vitro* concentrations. Similar to ganciclovir, foscarnet is a virostatic agent; foscarnet does not require activation by thymidine kinase.

Pharmacokinetics
Absorption: Oral: Poor; I.V. therapy is needed for the treatment of viral infections in AIDS patients
Distribution: Up to 28% of cumulative I.V. dose may be deposited in bone
Metabolism: Biotransformation does not occur
(Continued)

Foscarnet *(Continued)*

Half-life: ~3 hours
Elimination: Up to 28% excreted unchanged in urine

Usual Dosage I.V.:

Geriatrics: Adjust dose based upon estimated renal function

Adults:

Induction treatment: 60 mg/kg at a constant rate of infusion over at least 1 hour every 8 hours for 2-3 weeks

Maintenance treatment: 90-120 mg/kg/day at a constant rate of infusion over 2 hours

Dosing adjustment in renal impairment: See tables.

Dose Adjustment for Renal Impairment

The induction dose of foscarnet should be adjusted according to creatinine clearance as follows:

Creatinine Clearance (mL/min/kg)	Foscarnet Induction Dose (mg/kg q8h)
1.6	60
1.5	57
1.4	53
1.3	49
1.2	46
1.1	42
1	39
0.9	35
0.8	32
0.7	28
0.6	25
0.5	21
0.4	18

The maintenance dose of foscarnet should be adjusted according to creatinine clearance as follows:

Creatinine Clearance (mL/min/kg)	Foscarnet Maintenance Dose (mg/kg/day)
1.4	90-120
1.2-1.4	78-104
1-1.2	75-100
0.8-1	71-94
0.6-0.8	63-84
0.4-0.6	57-75

Administration Do not administer by rapid or bolus I.V. injection; an infusion pump must be used to avoid overdose. Administer diluted to 12 mg/mL through a peripheral line; may be administered undiluted through a central line (see Stability and Usual Dosage)

Monitoring Parameters Measure serum electrolytes, minerals, creatinine and estimated creatinine clearance at baseline, 2-3 times/week during induction therapy, and at least once every 1-2 weeks during maintenance therapy. More frequent monitoring and dosage adjustments may be necessary in patients with fluctuating renal function. A 24-hour creatinine clearance in selected patients; serum electrolytes and minerals should be monitored at the time (or as close as possible) that a patient experiences symptoms of electrolyte abnormalities.

Patient Information Close monitoring is important and any symptom of electrolyte abnormalities should be reported immediately; maintain adequate fluid intake and hydration; regular ophthalmic examinations are necessary. Foscarnet is not a cure for CMV retinitis; progression may occur during or following treatment.

Nursing Implications See Administration, Monitoring Parameters, and Stability

Special Geriatric Considerations Information on the use of foscarnet is lacking in the elderly; dose adjustments and proper monitoring must be performed because of the decreased renal function common in older patients (see Warnings and Usual Dosage)

Dosage Forms Injection: 24 mg/mL (250 mL, 500 mL)

Foscavir® *see* Foscarnet *on page 409*

Fosinopril (foe SIN oh pril)

Related Information
ACE Inhibitors Comparison *on page 1019*

Brand Names Monopril®

Generic Available No

Therapeutic Category Angiotensin-Converting Enzyme (ACE) Inhibitors

Use Treatment of hypertension, either alone or in combination with other antihypertensive agents; management of systolic congestive heart failure

Contraindications Renal impairment, collagen vascular disease, hypersensitivity to fosinopril, any component, or other angiotensin-converting enzyme inhibitors

Warnings Use with caution and modify dosage in patients with renal impairment (decrease dosage) (especially renal artery stenosis); severe congestive heart failure or with coadministered diuretic therapy. Severe hypotension may occur in patients who are sodium and/or volume depleted, initiate lower doses and monitor closely when starting therapy in these patients; observe for hyperkalemia (>5.7 mEq/L) first-dose hypotension, proteinuria, neutropenia, agranulocytosis, and angioedema.

Adverse Reactions
Cardiovascular: Hypotension, tachycardia, arrhythmias, orthostatic blood pressure changes, angina, palpitations, chest pain, CVA, myocardial infarction, syncope, flushing, hypertensive crisis, claudication

Central nervous system: Nervousness, depression, confusion, somnolence, fatigue, dizziness, headache, insomnia, vertigo

Dermatologic: Rash, urticaria, photosensitivity, pruritus, angioedema

Endocrine & metabolic: Hyperkalemia, hypoglycemia

Gastrointestinal: Pancreatitis, constipation, anorexia, nausea, heartburn, flatulence, vomiting, diarrhea, abdominal pain, xerostomia, dysphagia, abdominal distention, ageusia

Genitourinary: Azotemia, impotence, decreased libido

Hematologic: Anemia, neutropenia, leukopenia, eosinophilia, agranulocytosis

Hepatic: Hepatitis

Neuromuscular & skeletal: Myalgia, arthralgia, muscle cramps, paresthesia

Ocular: Blurred vision

Otic: Tinnitus

Renal: Proteinuria, oliguria, deterioration in renal function, increased BUN and serum creatinine

Respiratory: Cough, dyspnea, asthma, bronchospasm, sinusitis

Miscellaneous: Diaphoresis

Overdosage Symptoms of overdose include severe hypotension

Toxicology Following initiation of essential overdose management, toxic symptom treatment and supportive treatment should be initiated. Hypotension usually responds to I.V. fluids or Trendelenburg positioning. If unresponsive to these measures, the use of a parenteral inotrope may be required (eg, norepinephrine 0.1-0.2 mcg/kg/minute titrated to response). Seizures commonly respond to diazepam (I.V. 5-10 mg bolus in adults every 15 minutes if needed up to a total of 30 mg) or to phenytoin or phenobarbital.

Drug Interactions
Fosinopril and potassium-sparing diuretics may cause additive hyperkalemic effect

Fosinopril and indomethacin or nonsteroidal anti-inflammatory agents may cause reduced antihypertensive response to fosinopril

Allopurinol and fosinopril may cause neutropenia

Antacids and ACE inhibitors may decrease absorption of ACE inhibitors

Phenothiazines and ACE inhibitors may increase ACE inhibitor effect

Probenecid and ACE inhibitors (fosinopril) may increase ACE inhibitors (fosinopril) levels

Rifampin and ACE inhibitors (enalapril) may decrease ACE inhibitor effect

Digoxin and ACE inhibitors may increase serum digoxin concentrations

Lithium and ACE inhibitors may increase lithium serum concentration

Tetracycline and ACE inhibitors (quinapril) may decrease tetracycline absorption (up to 37%)

Food decreases fosinopril absorption (see Additional Information)

Mechanism of Action Competitive inhibitor of angiotensin-converting enzyme (ACE); prevents conversion of angiotensin I to angiotensin II, a potent vasoconstrictor; results in lower levels of angiotensin II which causes an increase in plasma renin activity and a reduction in aldosterone secretion; a CNS mechanism may also be involved in hypotensive effect as angiotensin
(Continued)

Fosinopril *(Continued)*

II increases adrenergic outflow from CNS; vasoactive kallikreins may be decreased in conversion to active hormones by ACE inhibitors, thus reducing blood pressure

Pharmacodynamics Duration of effect: ~12-24 hours

Pharmacokinetics

Absorbed: 36%

Metabolism: Fosinopril is a prodrug and is hydrolyzed to its active metabolite fosinoprilat by intestinal wall and hepatic esterases

Half-life, serum (fosinoprilat): 12 hours

Time to peak serum concentration: ~3 hours

Elimination: In the urine and bile as fosinoprilat and it conjugates in roughly equal proportions (45% to 50%)

Usual Dosage Geriatrics and Adults: Oral: Initial: 10 mg/day and increase to a maximum dose of 40 mg/day; most patients are maintained on 20-40 mg/day (see Additional Information)

Congestive heart failure: Initial: 10 mg/day; titrate slowly (over several weeks), as tolerated, to a "target dose" of 20-40 mg/day; do not exceed 40 mg/day (see Additional Information)

Moderately dialyzable (20% to 50%)

Monitoring Parameters Serum potassium concentration, BUN, serum creatinine, renal function, WBC

Test Interactions Increases BUN, creatinine, potassium, positive Coombs' [direct]; decreases cholesterol (S); may cause false-positive results in urine acetone determinations using sodium nitroprusside reagent

Patient Information Notify physician if vomiting, diarrhea, excessive perspiration, or dehydration should occur; also if swelling of face, lips, tongue, or difficulty in breathing occurs or if persistent cough develops; may be taken with meals; do not stop therapy or add a potassium salt replacement without physician's advice

Nursing Implications May cause depression in some patients; discontinue if angioedema of the face, extremities, lips, tongue, or glottis occurs; watch for hypotensive effects within 1-3 hours of first dose or new higher dose (see Precautions and Special Geriatric Considerations)

Additional Information Some patients may have a decreased hypotensive effect between 12-16 hours; consider dividing total daily dose into 2 doses 12 hours apart; if patient is receiving a diuretic, a potential for first-dose hypotension is increased; to decrease this potential, stop diuretic for 2-3 days prior to initiating fosinopril if possible; continue diuretic if needed to control blood pressure

Special Geriatric Considerations Due to frequent decreases in glomerular filtration (also creatinine clearance) with aging, elderly patients may have exaggerated responses to ACE inhibitors; differences in clinical response due to hepatic changes are not observed. ACE inhibitors may be preferred agents in elderly patients with congestive heart failure and diabetes mellitus. Diabetic proteinuria is reduced and insulin sensitivity is enhanced. In general, the side effect profile is favorable in elderly and causes little or no CNS confusion; use lowest dose recommendations initially.

Dosage Forms Tablet: 10 mg, 20 mg

References

Konstam MA, Drakup K, Baker DW, et al, "Heart Failure: Evaluation and Care of Patients With Left Ventricular Systolic Dysfunction," *Clinical Practice Guideline No 11*, Rockville, MD: Agency for Health Care Policy and Research, Public Health Service, U.S. Department of Health and Human Services, 1994.

McAreavey D and Robertson JIS, "Angiotensin Converting Enzyme Inhibitors and Moderate Hypertension," *Drugs*, 1990, 40(3):326-45.

Williams JF, Bristow MR, Fowler MB, et al, "Guidelines for the Evaluation and Management of Heart Failure: Report of the American College of Cardiology/American Heart Association Task Force on Practice Guidelines (Committee on Evaluation and Management of Heart Failure)," *J Am Coll Cardiol*, 1995, 26:1376-8.

Fosphenytoin *(FOS fen i toyn)*

Related Information

I.V. Push Recommended Guidelines *on page 1083*

Brand Names Cerebyx®

Synonyms 3-Phosphoryloxymethyl Phenytoin Disodium

Generic Available No

Therapeutic Category Anticonvulsant, Hydantoin

Use Indicated for short-term parenteral administration when other means of phenytoin administration are unavailable, inappropriate or deemed less advantageous; the safety and effectiveness of fosphenytoin in this use has not been systematically evaluated for more than 5 days; may be used for the control of generalized convulsive status epilepticus and prevention and treatment of seizures occurring during neurosurgery

Contraindications Hypersensitivity to phenytoin or fosphenytoin; occurrence of any rash while on treatment; the drug should not be resumed if rash is exfoliative, purpuric, or bullous; do not use in patients with A-V block (second and third degree), sinoatrial block, sinus bradycardia, or patients with Adams-Stokes syndrome; use with caution in patients with hypotension and myocardial insufficiency

Warnings Avoid abrupt discontinuation; dosing should be slowly reduced to avoid precipitation of seizures; increased toxicity with nephrotic syndrome patient; may increase frequency of petit mal seizures

Precautions Use with caution in patients with severe cardiovascular, hepatic, renal disease or diabetes mellitus; I.V. form may cause hypotension, skin necrosis at I.V. site; avoid I.V. administration in small veins; use with caution in patients with porphyria, fever, or hypothyroidism; discontinue if rash or lymphadenopathy occurs; consider phosphate load in patients with severe renal impairment

Adverse Reactions

Cardiovascular: Facial edema, hypotension, bradycardia, arrhythmia

Central nervous system: Slurred speech, dizziness, drowsiness, choreoathetosis, fever, visual hallucinations, ataxia, confusion, mood changes, lethargy

Dermatologic: Rash, exfoliative dermatitis, erythema multiforme, acne, hirsutism, coarsening of facial features

Endocrine & metabolic: Folic acid depletion, osteomalacia, hyperglycemia, reduced plasma testosterone, gynecomastia

Gastrointestinal: Nausea, vomiting, gingival hyperplasia

Genitourinary: Peyronie's disease, urinary retention, oliguria, polyuria, urinary incontinence, vaginitis, dysuria

Hematologic: Lymphadenopathy, neutropenia, thrombocytopenia, anemia (megaloblastic), leukopenia, pancytopenia, agranulocytosis

Local: Pain on injection; due to the fact that fosphenytoin is water soluble and has a lower pH (8.8) than phenytoin (12), necrosis or irritation at injection site is reduced

Neuromuscular & skeletal: Sensory paresthesia (long-term treatment), dyskinesias

Ocular: Nystagmus, blurred vision, diplopia

Renal: Nephrotic syndrome

Overdosage Signs and symptoms of toxicity include unsteady gait, tremors, hyperglycemia, chorea (extrapyramidal), gingival hyperplasia, gynecomastia, myoglobinuria, nephrotic syndrome, slurred speech, mydriasis, myoclonus, confusion, encephalopathy, hyperthermia, drowsiness, nausea, hypothermia, fever, hypotension, respiratory depression, leukopenia; neutropenia; agranulocytosis; granulocytopenia; hyper-reflexia, coma, systemic lupus erythematosus (SLE), ophthalmoplegia

Toxicology Treatment is supportive for hypotension; treat with I.V. fluids and place patient in Trendelenburg position; seizures may be controlled with lorazepam or diazepam 5-10 mg (0.25-0.4 mg/kg in children); intravenous albumin (25 g every 6 hours has been used to increase bound fraction of drug). Multiple dosing of activated charcoal may be effective; peritoneal dialysis, diuresis, hemodialysis, hemoperfusion, and plasmapheresis is of little value

Drug Interactions

No drug interaction noted with diazepam

Phenytoin may decrease the serum concentration or effectiveness of lamotrigine, valproic acid, ethosuximide, primidone, warfarin, corticosteroids, cyclosporin, theophylline, chloramphenicol, rifampin, doxycycline, quinidine, mexiletine, disopyramide, dopamine, or nondepolarizing skeletal muscle relaxants

Protein binding of phenytoin can be affected by valproic acid or salicylates

Serum phenytoin concentrations may be increased by cimetidine, chloramphenicol, INH, trimethoprim, or sulfonamides and decreased by rifampin, cisplatin, vinblastine, bleomycin, folic acid, or continuous NG feeds; do not use extended release capsules for enteral feeding (NG)

Stability Refrigerated vials are stable for 2 years; I.V. solutions are stable for one day when refrigerated; do not store at room temperature for more than 48 hours

(Continued)

Fosphenytoin *(Continued)*

Compatible with all diluents and does not require propylene glycol or ethanol for solubility

Mechanism of Action Diphosphate ester salt of phenytoin which acts as a water soluble prodrug of phenytoin; after administration, plasma esterases convert fosphenytoin to phosphate, formaldehyde and phenytoin as the active moiety; phenytoin works by stabilizing neuronal membranes and decreasing seizure activity by increasing efflux or decreasing influx of sodium ions across cell membranes in the motor cortex during generation of nerve impulses

Pharmacokinetics

Fosphenytoin is a prodrug of phenytoin and its anticonvulsant effects are attributable to phenytoin

Absorption/bioavailability: I.M.: Completely bioavailable

Distribution: V_d: Increases with fosphenytoin dose and rate, ranges 4.3-10.8 L

Protein binding: 95% to 99% (albumin), can displace phenytoin and increase free fraction (up to 30% unbound) during the period required for conversion of fosphenytoin to phenytoin

Conversion to phenytoin: Following I.V. administration conversion half-life is 15 minutes; following I.M. administration peak phenytoin levels are reached in 3 hours

Phenytoin:

Distribution: V_d: Adults: 0.6-0.7 L/kg

Protein binding: 90% to 95%; increased free fraction can occur in patients with hyperbilirubinemia, hypoalbuminemia, uremia

Metabolism: Metabolism follows dose-dependent (Michaelis-Menten) pharmacokinetics with increased Vmax in infants >6 months and children vs adults; inducer CYP2B6, 3A4, 3A5-7; substrate 2C9

Elimination: Highly variable clearance dependent upon intrinsic hepatic function and dose administered; increased clearance and decreased serum concentrations with febrile illness; <5% excreted unchanged in urine; major metabolite (via oxidation) HPPA undergoes enterohepatic recycling and elimination in urine as glucuronides

Usual Dosage The dose, concentration in solutions, and infusion rates for fosphenytoin are expressed as phenytoin sodium equivalents; fosphenytoin should always be prescribed and dispensed in phenytoin sodium equivalents

Dilute in D_5W or 0.9% NS for injection. Concentrations can range from 1.5-25 mg/mL.

Status epilepticus: Geriatrics and Adults: I.V.: Loading dose: Phenytoin equivalent: 15-20 mg/kg I.V. administered at 100-150 mg/minute

Nonemergent loading and maintenance dosing: Geriatrics and Adults: I.V. or I.M.:

Loading dose: Phenytoin equivalent: 10-20 mg/kg I.V. or I.M. (maximum I.V. rate: 150 mg/minute)

Initial daily maintenance dose: Phenytoin equivalent: 4-6 mg/kg/day I.V. or I.M.

Since hypertension is a risk, administer at a rate <150 mg/minute.

I.M. or I.V. substitution for oral phenytoin therapy: May be substituted for oral phenytoin sodium at the same total daily dose, however, Dilantin® capsules are ~90% bioavailable by the oral route; phenytoin, supplied as fosphenytoin, is 100% bioavailable by both the I.M. and I.V. routes; for this reason, plasma phenytoin concentrations may increase when I.M. or I.V. fosphenytoin is substituted for oral phenytoin sodium therapy; in clinical trials I.M. fosphenytoin was administered as a single daily dose utilizing either 1 or 2 injection sites; some patients may require more frequent dosing

Dosing adjustments in renal/hepatic impairment: Phenytoin clearance may be substantially reduced in cirrhosis and plasma concentration monitoring with dose adjustment advisable; free phenytoin levels should be monitored closely in patients with renal or hepatic disease or in those with hypoalbuminemia; furthermore, fosphenytoin clearance to phenytoin may be increased without a similar increase in phenytoin in these patients leading to increase frequency and severity of adverse events

Administration Since there is no precipitation problem with fosphenytoin, no I.V. filter is required

Monitoring Parameters Blood pressure, EKG, respiratory rate for 10-20 minutes after completion of administration; plasma concentration monitoring, CBC, liver function tests; monitor gait, CNS effects, speech

Reference Range

Therapeutic: 10-20 µg/mL (SI: 40-79 µmol/L); toxicity is measured clinically, and some patients require serum concentrations outside the suggested therapeutic range

Toxic: 30-50 µg/mL (SI: 120-200 µmol/L)

Lethal: >100 µg/mL (SI: >400 µmol/L)

Manifestations of toxicity:

Nystagmus: 20 µg/mL (SI: 79 µmol/L)

Ataxia: 30 µg/mL (SI: 118.9 µmol/L)

Decreased mental status: 40 µg/mL (SI: 159 µmol/L)

Coma: 50 µg/mL (SI: 200 µmol/L)

Peak serum phenytoin concentration after a 375 mg I.M. fosphenytoin dose in healthy males: 5.7 µg/mL

Peak serum fosphenytoin concentrations and phenytoin concentrations after a 1.2 g infusion (I.V.) in healthy subjects over 30 minutes were 129 µg/mL and 17.2 µg/mL respectively

Do not obtain serum for analysis 8-12 hours after administration; spurious elevations will be seen due to slow distribution of phenytoin

Test Interactions Increases glucose, alkaline phosphatase (S); decreases thyroxine (S), calcium (S); serum sodium increases in overdose setting

Nursing Implications I.V. injections should be followed by normal saline flushes through the same needle or I.V. catheter to avoid local irritation of the vein; must be diluted to concentrations <6 mg/mL, in normal saline, for I.V. infusion; monitor vital signs for 10-20 minutes after completion of I.V. administration; do not obtain serum for concentration analysis for 8-12 hours after completion of administration

Additional Information 1.5 mg fosphenytoin is approximately equivalent to 1 mg phenytoin; equimolar fosphenytoin dose is 375 mg (75 mg/mL solution) to phenytoin 250 mg (50 mg/mL); 0.0037 mmol phosphate/mg PE fosphenytoin Water solubility: 142 mg/mL at pH of 9

Antiarrhythmic effects may be similar to phenytoin; parenteral product contains no propylene sterol; this should allow for rapid intravenous bolus dosing without cardiovascular complications; formaldehyde production is not expected to be clinically consequential (about 200 mg) if used for one week

Special Geriatric Considerations No significant changes in fosphenytoin pharmacokinetics with age have been noted. Phenytoin clearance is decreased in elderly and lower doses may be needed. Elderly may have reduced hepatic clearance due to age decline in phase I metabolism. Elderly may have low albumin which will increase free fraction and, therefore, pharmacologic response. Monitor closely in those who are hypoalbuminemic. Free fraction measurements advised, also elderly may display a higher incidence of adverse effects (cardiovascular) when using the I.V. loading regimen; therefore, recommended to decrease loading I.V. dose to 25 mg/minute (see Warnings).

Dosage Forms Injection, as sodium: 150 mg [equivalent to phenytoin sodium 100 mg] in 2 mL vials; 750 mg [equivalent to phenytoin sodium 500 mg] in 10 mL vials

References

Bebin M and Bleck TP, "New Anticonvulsant Drugs. Focus on Flunarizine, Fosphenytoin, Midazolam, and Stiripentol," *Drugs*, 1994, 48(2):153-71.

Jamerson BD, Dukes GE, Brouwer KL, et al, "Venous Irritation Related to Intravenous Administration of Phenytoin Versus Fosphenytoin," *Pharmacotherapy*, 1994, 14(1):47-52.

Leppik IE, Boucher R, Wilder BJ, et al, "Phenytoin Prodrug: Preclinical and Clinical Studies," *Epilepsia*, 1989, 30(Suppl 2):S22-6.

Fragmin® see Dalteparin *on page 266*

Freezone® Solution [OTC] see Salicylic Acid *on page 845*

Frusemide see Furosemide *on next page*

FS Shampoo® see Fluocinolone *on page 391*

Fulvicin® P/G see Griseofulvin *on page 436*

Fulvicin-U/F® see Griseofulvin *on page 436*

Fumasorb® [OTC] see Ferrous Fumarate *on page 376*

Fumerin® [OTC] see Ferrous Fumarate *on page 376*

Fungizone® see Amphotericin B *on page 69*

Fungoid® Creme see Miconazole *on page 625*

Fungoid® Tincture see Miconazole *on page 625*

Furadantin® see Nitrofurantoin *on page 676*

Furalan® see Nitrofurantoin *on page 676*

Furan® see Nitrofurantoin *on page 676*

Furanite® *see* Nitrofurantoin *on page 676*

Furazolidone (fyoor a ZOE li done)
Brand Names Furoxone®
Therapeutic Category Antibiotic, Miscellaneous; Antidiarrheal; Antiprotozoal
Use Treatment of bacterial or protozoal diarrhea and enteritis caused by susceptible organisms: *Giardia lamblia* and *Vibrio cholerae*
Contraindications Known hypersensitivity to furazolidone; concurrent use of alcohol; MAO inhibitors, tyramine-containing foods
Precautions Use caution in patients with G-6-PD deficiency
Adverse Reactions
  Cardiovascular: Orthostatic hypotension, hypotension
  Central nervous system: Dizziness, drowsiness, malaise, fever, headache
  Dermatologic: Rash, dermatologic, residular morbilliform rash
  Endocrine & metabolic: Hypoglycemia, disulfiram-like reaction after alcohol ingestion
  Gastrointestinal: Nausea, vomiting
  Hematologic: Agranulocytosis, hemolysis in patients with G-6-PD deficiency
Overdosage Hypertensive crisis after doses greater than recommended or if taken for more than 5 days
Drug Interactions MAO inhibitors, indirect-acting sympathomimetic amines, levodopa, guanethidine, tricyclic antidepressant, meperidine, sedatives, antihistamines, narcotics, insulin, and sulfonylureas
Drug/Food Interactions Alcohol, tyramine-containing food (MAO inhibitor)
Mechanism of Action Inhibits several vital enzymatic reactions causing antibacterial and antiprotozoal action; also exhibits a disulfiram reaction with alcohol; has MAO inhibition (see Drug Interactions)
Pharmacokinetics
  Absorption: Oral: Poor
  Elimination: 33% of oral dose excreted in urine as active drug and metabolites
Usual Dosage Geriatrics and Adults: Oral: 100 mg 4 times/day; not more than 8.8 mg/kg/day; treatment duration: 7 days
Test Interactions False-positive results for urine glucose with Clinitest®
Patient Information May discolor urine to a brown tint; avoid drinking alcohol with or within 4 days of taking furazolidone or eating tyramine-containing foods; avoid medications containing sympathomimetics (cold and allergy medications, etc); if result not achieved at the end of treatment contact physician
Nursing Implications See Patient Information
Special Geriatric Considerations See Adverse Reactions and Usual Dosage
Dosage Forms
  Liquid: 50 mg/15 mL (60 mL, 473 mL)
  Tablet: 100 mg

Furazosin *see* Prazosin *on page 772*

Furosemide (fyoor OH se mide)
Related Information
  I.V. Push Recommended Guidelines *on page 1083*
Brand Names Lasix®
Synonyms Frusemide
Generic Available Yes
Therapeutic Category Diuretic, Loop
Use Management of edema associated with congestive heart failure and hepatic or renal disease; used alone or in combination with antihypertensives in treatment of hypertension
Contraindications Hypersensitivity to furosemide or any component; allergy to sulfonamides may result in cross-sensitivity to furosemide
Warnings Loop diuretics are potent diuretics; excess amounts can lead to profound diuresis with fluid and electrolyte loss; close medical supervision and dose evaluation is required, particularly in the elderly
Adverse Reactions
  Cardiovascular: Hypotension
  Central nervous system: Dizziness
  Dermatologic: Urticaria, rash, photosensitivity
  Endocrine & metabolic: Hypokalemia, hyponatremia, hypochloremia, alkalosis, dehydration, hypercalciuria, hyperuricemia
  Gastrointestinal: Pancreatitis, nausea, diarrhea

Genitourinary: Prerenal azotemia
Hematologic: Agranulocytosis, anemia, thrombocytopenia
Otic: Potential ototoxicity
Renal: Nephrocalcinosis, interstitial nephritis

Overdosage Symptoms of overdose include electrolyte depletion, volume depletion, hypotension, dehydration, circulatory collapse

Toxicology Following GI decontamination, treatment is supportive; hypotension responds to fluids and Trendelenburg position; replace electrolytes as necessary

Drug Interactions
Decreased effect: Indomethacin, other NSAIDs
Increased hypotensive effect: Other antihypertensives
Increased level of lithium
Increased risk of ototoxicity: Aminoglycosides, other loop diuretics, vancomycin
When given with digoxin, diuretic-induced hypokalemia increases the risk of digoxin toxicity

Stability Protect from light; do not dispense discolored tablets or injection; I.V. infusion solution mixed in NS or D₅W solution is stable for 24 hours at room temperature

Mechanism of Action Inhibits reabsorption of sodium and chloride in the ascending loop of Henle and distal renal tubule, interfering with the chloride-binding cotransport system, thus causing increased excretion of water, sodium, chloride, magnesium, and calcium

Pharmacodynamics
Oral:
Onset of action: Diuresis begins within 30-60 minutes
Peak effect: Within 1-2 hours
Duration: 6-8 hours
I.V.:
Onset of action: Diuresis starts in 5 minutes
Peak effect: Reduced and delayed in the elderly as compared to younger adults
Duration: 2 hours

Pharmacokinetics
Absorption: Oral: 60% to 67%
Protein binding: >90%
Elimination: In the elderly, total clearance is decreased and dependent on renal function

Usual Dosage Oral, I.M., I.V.:
Geriatrics: Initial: 20 mg/day, increase slowly to desired response
Adults: 20-80 mg/day in divided doses every 6-12 hours up to 600 mg/day
Acute renal failure: Up to 100 mg/day may be necessary to initiate desired response
Dosing adjustment/comments in hepatic disease: Diminished natriuretic effect with increased sensitivity to hypokalemia and volume depletion in cirrhosis; monitor effects, particularly with high doses

Administration For continuous infusion, maximum rate of administration is 4 mg/minute (see Stability)

Monitoring Parameters Blood pressure both standing and sitting/supine, serum electrolytes, renal function, I & O, weight; in high doses monitor auditory function

Reference Range Therapeutic: 1-2 µg/mL (SI: 3-6 µmol/L)

Test Interactions Increased ammonia (B), increased amylase (S), increased glucose, increased uric acid (S); decreased calcium (S), decreased chloride (S), decreased magnesium, decreased sodium (S)

Patient Information May be taken with food or milk; get up slowly from a lying or sitting position to minimize dizziness, lightheadedness or fainting; also use extra care when exercising, standing for long periods of time and during hot weather; take in the morning; may cause increased sensitivity to sunlight

Nursing Implications I.V. injections should be given slowly over 1-2 minutes; replace parenteral therapy with oral therapy as soon as possible; for continuous infusion in patients with severely impaired renal function, do not exceed 4 mg/minute; be alert to complaints about hearing difficulty; check the patient for orthostasis (see Monitoring Parameters)

Additional Information Injection contains 0.162 mEq of sodium per mL; do not use solutions that are yellow in color

Standard diluent: Dose/50 mL D₅W
Minimum volume: 50 mL D₅W
(Continued)

Furosemide (Continued)

Special Geriatric Considerations Severe loss of sodium and/or increase in BUN can cause confusion. For any change in mental status in patients on furosemide, monitor electrolytes and renal function (see Pharmacodynamics and Pharmacokinetics).

Dosage Forms
Injection: 10 mg/mL (2 mL, 4 mL, 5 mL, 6 mL, 8 mL, 10 mL, 12 mL)
Solution, oral: 10 mg/mL (60 mL, 120 mL); 40 mg/5 mL (5 mL, 10 mL, 500 mL)
Tablet: 20 mg, 40 mg, 80 mg

References
Chaudhry AY, Bing RF, Castleden CM, et al, "The Effect of Aging on the Response to Frusemide in Normal Subjects," *Eur J Clin Pharmacol*, 1984, 27(3):303-6.

Mühlberg W, "Pharmacokinetics of Diuretics in Geriatric Patients," *Arch Gerontol Geriatr*, 1989, 9(3):283-90.

Murray MD, Haag, KM, Black PK, et al, "Variable Furosemide Absorption and Poor Predictability of Response in Elderly Patients," *Pharmacotherapy*, 1997, 17(1):98-106.

Furoxone® *see Furazolidone on page 416*

Gabapentin (GA ba pen tin)

Related Information
Antiepileptic Drug Interactions Comparison *on page 1022*

Brand Names Neurontin®

Generic Available No

Therapeutic Category Anticonvulsant, Miscellaneous

Use Adjunct for treatment of drug-refractory partial and secondarily generalized seizures

Unlabeled use: Treatment of chronic pain; restless legs syndrome (RLS)

Contraindications Hypersensitivity to the drug or any component or preparation

Warnings Gabapentin may be associated with a slight incidence (0.6%) of status epilepticus and sudden deaths (0.0038 deaths/patient year); rat studies demonstrated an association with pancreatic adenocarcinoma in male rats; clinical implication unknown

Precautions Routine monitoring not needed (see Reference Range)

Adverse Reactions
Cardiovascular: Syncope, peripheral edema
Central nervous system: Somnolence, dizziness, ataxia, fatigue, nervousness, dysarthria, amnesia, depression, anxiety, hallucinations, psychosis, paranoia, hyperkinesia
Dermatologic: Pruritus
Gastrointestinal: Dyspepsia, dryness of mouth/throat, constipation
Genitourinary: Impotence
Hematologic: Leukopenia
Neuromuscular & skeletal: Back pain, myalgia, paresthesia
Ocular: Diplopia, amblyopia, nystagmus
Respiratory: Rhinitis, bronchospasm
Miscellaneous: Hiccups

Overdosage Symptoms of overdose include ataxia, ptosis, sedation, excitation, dyspnea, diplopia, lethargy, diarrhea, slurred speech

Toxicology Treatment: Hemodialysis can be performed since it is dialyzable; administer give general supportive care

Drug Interactions
Antacids reduce the bioavailability of gabapentin by 20%
Cimetidine may decrease clearance of gabapentin

Mechanism of Action Exact mechanism of action is not known, but does have properties in common with other anticonvulsants; although structurally related to GABA, it does not interact with GABA receptors

Pharmacokinetics
Absorption: ~60%
Half-life: 5-7 hours in normal renal function; increases with decreasing creatinine clearance; must have dose adjusted (see Usual Dosage)

Usual Dosage Geriatric and Adults: Oral: 900-1800 mg/day administered in 3 divided doses; therapy is initiated with a rapid titration, beginning with 300 mg on day 1, 300 mg twice daily on day 2, and 300 mg 3 times/day on day 3; dose is then titrated as needed up to 1800 mg/day; doses up to 2400-3600 mg/day have been used safely

Dosing adjustment in renal impairment:
Cl_{cr} >60 mL/minute: Administer 1200 mg/day

Cl_{cr} 30-60 mL/minute: Administer 600 mg/day
Cl_{cr} 15-30 mL/minute: Administer 300 mg/day
Cl_{cr} <15 mL/minute: Administer 150 mg/day
Hemodialysis: 200-300 mg after each 4-hour dialysis following a loading dose of 300-400 mg

Reference Range Minimum effective serum concentration may be 2 µg/mL; **routine monitoring of drug levels is not required even with concomitant drug therapy**

Patient Information Take only as prescribed; may cause dizziness, somnolence, and other symptoms and signs of CNS depression; do not operate machinery or drive a car until you have experience with the drug; may be administered without regard to meals

Nursing Implications Note dosage must be adjusted for renal function and elderly often have reduced renal function (see Adverse Reactions and Overdosage)

Special Geriatric Considerations No clinical studies to specifically evaluate this drug in elderly have been performed; however, in premarketing studies, patients >65 years of age did not demonstrate any difference in side effect profiles from younger adults; since gabapentin is eliminated renally, dose **must** be adjusted for creatinine clearance in the elderly patient

Dosage Forms Capsule: 100 mg, 300 mg, 400 mg

References
Adler CH, "Treatment of Restless Legs Syndrome With Gabapentin," *Clin Neuropharmacol*, 1997, 20(2):148-51.

Gabitril® *see* Tiagabine *on page 919*

Gamastan® *see* Immune Globulin *on page 482*

Gamimune® N *see* Immune Globulin *on page 482*

Gamma Benzene Hexachloride *see* Lindane *on page 538*

Gammagard® *see* Immune Globulin *on page 482*

Gamma Globulin *see* Immune Globulin *on page 482*

Gammar® *see* Immune Globulin *on page 482*

Gammar®-IV *see* Immune Globulin *on page 482*

Ganciclovir (gan SYE kloe veer)

Related Information
I.V. Medication Recommendations *on page 1080*

Brand Names Cytovene®; Vitrasert®

Synonyms DHPG Sodium; GCV Sodium; Nordeoxyguanosine

Generic Available No

Therapeutic Category Antiviral Agent, Parenteral

Use CMV retinitis treatment of immunocompromised individuals, including patients with acquired immunodeficiency syndrome; treatment of CMV pneumonia in marrow transplant recipients, promising results have been achieved in AIDS patients and organ transplant recipients with CMV colitis, pneumonitis, and multiorgan involvement; attenuation of CMV infection in transplant patients

Contraindications Absolute neutrophil count <500/mm³; platelet count <25,000/mm³; known hypersensitivity to ganciclovir or acyclovir

Warnings Dosage adjustment or interruption of ganciclovir therapy may be necessary in patients with neutropenia and/or thrombocytopenia and patients with impaired renal function. Ganciclovir may adversely affect spermatogenesis and fertility; due to its mutagenic potential, contraceptive precautions for female and male patients need to be followed during and for at least 90 days after therapy with the drug; take care to administer only into veins with good blood flow.

Adverse Reactions
Cardiovascular: Edema, arrhythmias, hypertension
Central nervous system: Headache, seizure, confusion, nervousness, dizziness, hallucinations, coma, fever, encephalopathy, malaise
Dermatologic: Rash, urticaria
Gastrointestinal: Nausea, vomiting, diarrhea
Hematologic: Neutropenia, thrombocytopenia, leukopenia, anemia, eosinophilia
Hepatic: Elevation in liver function tests
Local: Phlebitis
Ocular: Retinal detachment
Renal: Hematuria, increased BUN and serum creatinine
Respiratory: Dyspnea
(Continued)

Ganciclovir *(Continued)*

Overdosage Symptoms of overdose include neutropenia, vomiting, hypersalivation, bloody diarrhea, cytopenia, testicular atrophy

Toxicology Hemodialysis removes 50% of drug; hydration may be of some benefit

Drug Interactions

Increased effect/toxicity with probenecid, imipenem/cilastatin

Increased toxicity in rapidly dividing cells with cytotoxic drugs; increased hematologic toxicity with zidovudine

Stability Reconstituted solution is stable for 12 hours at room temperature; **do not refrigerate**; reconstitute with sterile water **not** bacteriostatic water because parabens may cause precipitation

Mechanism of Action Ganciclovir is phosphorylated to a substrate which competitively inhibits the binding of deoxyguanosine triphosphate to DNA polymerase resulting in inhibition of viral DNA synthesis

Pharmacokinetics

Protein binding: 1% to 2%

Half-life: 1.7-5.8 hours; increases with impaired renal function

Elimination: Majority (94% to 99%) is excreted as unchanged drug in urine

Usual Dosage Slow I.V. infusion (dosing is based on total body weight):

Geriatrics and Adults:

Induction therapy: 5 mg/kg/dose every 12 hours for 14-21 days followed by maintenance therapy; do not use oral dosing for induction

Maintenance therapy: 5 mg/kg/day as a single daily dose for 7 days/week or 6 mg/kg/day for 5 days/week

Dosing interval in renal impairment: See tables and adjust dosing as indicated

Oral Ganciclovir Dose in Renal Impairment

Creatinine Clearance (mL/min)	Ganciclovir Doses
≥70	1000 mg tid or 500 mg q3h, 6 times/d
50-69	1500 mg qd or 500 mg tid
25-49	1000 mg qd or 500 mg bid
10-24	500 mg qd
<10	500 mg 3 times/wk, following hemodialysis

I.V. Ganciclovir Dose in Renal Impairment

Cl_{cr} (mL/min)	Induction dose (mg/kg)	Dosing Interval (hours)	Maintenance Dose (mg/kg)	Dosing Interval (hours)
≥70	5	12	5	24
50-69	2.5	12	2.5	24
25-49	2.5	24	1.25	24
10-24	1.25	24	0.625	24
<10	1.25	3 times/wk, following hemodialysis	0.625	3 times/wk, following hemodialysis

Monitoring Parameters CBC with differential and platelet count, serum creatinine, ophthalmologic exams

Patient Information Ganciclovir is not a cure for CMV retinitis; regular ophthalmologic examinations should be done; close monitoring of blood counts should be done while on therapy and dosage adjustments may need to be made

Nursing Implications Must be prepared in vertical flow hood; use chemotherapy precautions during administration; discard appropriately

Additional Information Sodium content of 500 mg vial: 46 mg

Special Geriatric Considerations Adjust dose based upon renal function (see Usual Dosage)

Dosage Forms

Capsule: 250 mg

Powder for injection, lyophilized: 500 mg (10 mL)

Gantanol® *see* Sulfamethoxazole *on page 876*

Gantrisin® *see* Sulfisoxazole *on page 880*

Garamycin® Injection *see* Gentamicin *on next page*

Garamycin® Ophthalmic *see* Gentamicin *on next page*

Garamycin® Topical *see* Gentamicin *on next page*

Gas-Ban DS® [OTC] *see* Aluminum Hydroxide, Magnesium Hydroxide, and Simethicone *on page 44*

Gastrocrom® Oral *see* Cromolyn Sodium *on page 255*

Gastrosed™ *see* Hyoscyamine *on page 471*

Gas-X® [OTC] *see* Simethicone *on page 856*

Gaviscon®-2 [OTC] *see* Aluminum Hydroxide, Magnesium Trisilicate, Sodium Bicarbonate, and Alginic Acid *on page 46*

Gaviscon® Extra Strength Relief Formula [OTC] *see* Aluminum Hydroxide, Magnesium Trisilicate, Sodium Bicarbonate, and Alginic Acid *on page 46*

G-CSF *see* Filgrastim *on page 381*

GCV Sodium *see* Ganciclovir *on page 419*

Gee Gee® [OTC] *see* Guaifenesin *on page 437*

Gel Kam® *see* Fluoride *on page 392*

Gel-Tin® [OTC] *see* Fluoride *on page 392*

Gelusil® [OTC] *see* Aluminum Hydroxide, Magnesium Hydroxide, and Simethicone *on page 44*

Gemcor® *see* Gemfibrozil *on this page*

Gemfibrozil (jem FI broe zil)

Brand Names Gemcor®; Lopid®

Synonyms CI-719

Generic Available No

Therapeutic Category Antilipemic Agent

Use Hypertriglyceridemia in types IV and V hyperlipidemia for patients who are at greater risk for pancreatitis and who have not responded to dietary intervention; reduction of coronary heart disease in type IIb patients who have low HDL cholesterol, increased LDL cholesterol, and decreased triglycerides

Contraindications Renal or hepatic dysfunction, primary biliary cirrhosis, gallbladder disease, hypersensitivity to gemfibrozil or any component

Precautions Estrogen therapy may increase triglycerides, consider this if appropriate before prescribing

Adverse Reactions

Central nervous system: Headache, dizziness, drowsiness, somnolence, fatigue, mental depression

Dermatologic: Eczema and rash, alopecia, angioedema

Gastrointestinal: Abdominal pain, weight loss, cholelithiasis have been reported, nausea, vomiting, diarrhea, constipation, dyspepsia, dysgeusia and flatulence occur less frequently

Genitourinary: Impotence and decreased male fertility

Hematologic: Anemia, leukopenia, thrombocytopenia

Neuromuscular & skeletal: Paresthesia

Ocular: Blurred vision

Miscellaneous: Lupus-like syndrome

Drug Interactions May potentiate the effects of warfarin; concomitant use with lovastatin or other HMG-CoA reductase inhibitors may lead to rhabdomyolysis

Mechanism of Action The exact mechanism of action of gemfibrozil is unknown, however, several theories exist regarding the VLDL effect; it can inhibit lipolysis and decrease subsequent hepatic fatty acid uptake as well as inhibit hepatic secretion of VLDL; together these actions decrease serum VLDL concentration; increases HDL cholesterol; the mechanism behind HDL elevation is currently unknown

Pharmacokinetics

Absorption: Oral: Well absorbed

Protein binding: 99%; a portion of the drug undergoes enterohepatic recycling

Metabolism: In the liver by oxidation to 2 inactive metabolites

Half-life: 1.4 hours

Time to peak serum concentration: Within 1-2 hours

Elimination: In urine (70%) primarily as glucuronide conjugate; some enterohepatic recycling

Usual Dosage Geriatrics and Adults: Oral: 1200 mg/day in 2 divided doses, 30 minutes before breakfast and supper

Monitoring Parameters Fractionated cholesterol and triglycerides; CBC; liver function tests; blood glucose, especially in diabetics

(Continued)

Gemfibrozil *(Continued)*

Test Interactions Decreased glucose, increased LFTs, decreased hemoglobin or hematocrit, WBC, platelets; positive ANA

Patient Information May cause dizziness or blurred vision, medication may cause abdominal or epigastric pain, diarrhea, nausea, or vomiting; notify physician if these become pronounced; take before meals

Nursing Implications See Monitoring Parameters

Additional Information If no appreciable triglyceride or cholesterol lowering effect occurs after 3 months, the drug should be discontinued

Special Geriatric Considerations Gemfibrozil is the drug of choice for the treatment of hypertriglyceridemia and hypoalphaproteinemia in the elderly; it is usually well tolerated; myositis may be more common in patients with poor renal function. The definition of and, therefore, when to treat hyperlipidemia in the elderly is a controversial issue. The National Cholesterol Education Program recommends that all adults 20 years of age and older maintain a plasma cholesterol <200 mg/dL. By this definition, 60% of all elderly would be considered to have a borderline high (200-239 mg/dL) or high (≥240 mg/dL) plasma cholesterol. However, plasma cholesterol has been shown to be a less reliable predictor of coronary heart disease in the elderly. Therefore, it is the authors' belief that pharmacologic treatment be reserved for those who are unable to obtain a desirable plasma cholesterol concentration by diet alone and for whom the benefits of treatment are believed to outweigh the potential adverse effects, drug interactions, and cost of treatment.

Dosage Forms Tablet: 600 mg

Genabid® *see* Papaverine *on page 714*

Genac® Tablet [OTC] *see* Triprolidine and Pseudoephedrine *on page 966*

Genagesic® *see* Propoxyphene and Acetaminophen *on page 796*

Genahist® Oral *see* Diphenhydramine *on page 302*

Genapap® [OTC] *see* Acetaminophen *on page 16*

Genasoft® Plus [OTC] *see* Docusate and Casanthranol *on page 313*

Genaspor® [OTC] *see* Tolnaftate *on page 939*

Genatap® Elixir [OTC] *see* Brompheniramine and Phenylpropanolamine *on page 130*

Genatuss® [OTC] *see* Guaifenesin *on page 437*

Genatuss DM® [OTC] *see* Guaifenesin and Dextromethorphan *on page 439*

Gencalc® 600 [OTC] *see* Calcium Salts (Oral) *on page 152*

Geneye® Ophthalmic [OTC] *see* Tetrahydrozoline *on page 901*

Gen-K® *see* Potassium Chloride *on page 763*

Genoptic® Ophthalmic *see* Gentamicin *on this page*

Genoptic® S.O.P. Ophthalmic *see* Gentamicin *on this page*

Genpril® [OTC] *see* Ibuprofen *on page 475*

Gentacidin® Ophthalmic *see* Gentamicin *on this page*

Gentak® Ophthalmic *see* Gentamicin *on this page*

Gentamicin *(jen ta MYE sin)*

Related Information

Aminoglycoside Dosing Guidelines *on page 1009*
Cephalosporins, Aminoglycosides, Macrolides, & Quinolones *on page 1014*
I.V. Medication Recommendations *on page 1080*
Prednisolone *on page 774*
Prevention of Bacterial Endocarditis *on page 1062*
Serum Drug Concentrations Commonly Monitored: Guidelines *on page 1114*

Brand Names Garamycin® Injection; Garamycin® Ophthalmic; Garamycin® Topical; Genoptic® Ophthalmic; Genoptic® S.O.P. Ophthalmic; Gentacidin® Ophthalmic; Gentak® Ophthalmic; G-myticin® Topical; Jenamicin® Injection

Therapeutic Category Antibacterial, Topical; Antibiotic, Aminoglycoside; Antibiotic, Ophthalmic; Antibiotic, Topical

Use Treatment of susceptible bacterial infections, normally gram-negative organisms including *Pseudomonas*, *Proteus*, *Serratia*, treatment of bone infections, CNS infections, respiratory tract infections, skin and soft tissue infections, as well as abdominal and urinary tract infections, endocarditis, and septicemia

Contraindications Hypersensitivity to gentamicin or other aminoglycosides

Warnings
Not intended for long-term therapy due to toxic hazards associated with extended administration; pre-existing renal insufficiency, vestibular or cochlear impairment, myasthenia gravis, hypocalcemia, conditions which depress neuromuscular transmission

Parenteral aminoglycosides are associated with significant nephrotoxicity or ototoxicity; the ototoxicity is directly proportional to the amount of drug given and the duration of treatment; tinnitus or vertigo are indications of vestibular injury and impending irreversible bilateral deafness; nephrotoxicity is associated with trough concentrations >2 µg/mL and is usually reversible

Precautions Use with caution in patients with renal impairment; pre-existing auditory or vestibular impairment; and in patients with neuromuscular disorders; dosage modification required in patients with impaired renal function

Adverse Reactions
Dermatologic: Rash, skin itching, photosensitivity
Gastrointestinal: Diarrhea, pseudomembranous colitis
Neuromuscular & skeletal: Neuromuscular blockade
Ocular: Lacrimation, itching, edema of the eyelids, keratitis
Otic: Ototoxicity
Renal: Nephrotoxicity (high trough levels)

Overdosage Symptoms of overdose include ototoxicity, nephrotoxicity, and neuromuscular toxicity

Toxicology The treatment of choice following a single acute overdose appears to be the maintenance of good urine output of at least 3 mL/kg/hour. Dialysis is of questionable value in the enhancement of aminoglycoside elimination. If required, hemodialysis is preferred over peritoneal dialysis in patients with normal renal function. Careful hydration may be all that is required to promote diuresis and therefore the enhancement of the drug's elimination. Chelation with penicillins is experimental.

Drug Interactions Penicillins, cephalosporins, amphotericin B, loop diuretics may increase nephrotoxic potential; neuromuscular blocking agents may increase neuromuscular blockade

Stability I.V. infusion solutions mixed in NS or D_5W solution are stable for 24 hours at room temperature; incompatible with penicillins

Mechanism of Action Interferes with bacterial protein synthesis by binding to 30S and 50S ribosomal subunits resulting in a defective bacterial cell membrane

Pharmacokinetics
Distribution: V_d: Increased by edema, ascites, fluid overload; decreased in patients with dehydration
Adults: 0.2-0.3 L/kg
Protein binding: <30%
Half-life: Adults: 1.5-3 hours; with anuria: 36-70 hours
Time to peak serum concentration:
I.M.: Within 30-90 minutes
I.V.: 30 minutes after a 30-minute I.V. infusion
Elimination: Clearance is directly related to renal function, eliminated almost completely by glomerular filtration of unchanged drug with excretion into the urine
The pharmacokinetics of the aminoglycosides are heterogeneous in the elderly; it is best to assume that clearance is reduced and half-life prolonged in the elderly, while volume of distribution is usually unchanged. The establishment of each patient's pharmacokinetic parameters is important for proper dosing in order to achieve optimal therapeutic benefit and minimize the risk of toxicity.

Usual Dosage Individualization is critical because of the low therapeutic index. Use of ideal body weight (IBW) for determining the mg/kg/dose appears to be more accurate than dosing on the basis of total body weight (TBW). In morbid obesity, dosage requirement may best be estimated using a dosing weight of IBW + 0.4 (TBW - IBW). Initial and periodic peak and trough plasma drug concentration should be determined, particularly in critically ill patients with serious infections or in disease states known to significantly alter aminoglycoside pharmacokinetics (eg, cystic fibrosis, burns, or major surgery).
Dosage should be based on an estimate of ideal body weight. All patients receiving I.M. or I.V. dosing should receive 1.5-2 mg/kg based on ideal body weight as a loading dose regardless of renal function, then administer 3-5 mg/kg in 3 divided doses or as indicated by adjustment for renal function.
Geriatrics and Adults:
Intrathecal: 4-8 mg/day
(Continued)

Gentamicin (Continued)

I.M., I.V.: 1-5 mg/kg/day in 1-2 divided doses

Once daily or extended interval: I.V.: 5-7 mg/kg/dose given every 24, 36, or 48 hours depending on Cl_{cr} (see Dosing Adjustment in Renal Impairment) (see Special Geriatric Considerations)

Dosing adjustment in renal impairment: 2 mg/kg (2-3 serum concentration measurements should be obtained after the initial dose to measure the half-life in order to determine the frequency of subsequent doses)

Cl_{cr} ≥60 mL/minute: Administer every 24 hours

Cl_{cr} 40-59 mL/minute: Administer every 36 hours

Cl_{cr} 20-39 mL/minute: Administer every 48 hours

Cl_{cr} <20 mL/minute: Individualize dose

Dosing adjustment/comments in hepatic disease: Monitor plasma concentrations

Dialyzable (50% to 100%)

Some patients may require larger or more frequent doses (eg, every 6 hours) if serum concentrations document the need (ie, cystic fibrosis or febrile granulocytopenic patients)

2-3 serum concentration measurements should be obtained after the initial dose to measure the half-life in order to determine the frequency of subsequent doses

Topical: Apply 1-4 times/day to affected area

Ophthalmic:

Solution: Instill 1-2 drops every 2-4 hours

Ointment: Instill ½" (1.25 cm) 2-3 times/day to every 3-4 hours

Monitoring Parameters Urinalysis, urine output, BUN, serum creatinine; hearing should be tested before, during, and after treatment; particularly in those at risk for ototoxicity or who will be receiving prolonged therapy (>2 weeks). Obtain peak levels 30 minutes after the end of a 30-minute infusion; trough levels are drawn within 30 minutes before the next dose.

Reference Range

Therapeutic:

Peak: 4-8 µg/mL (SI: 8-17 µmol/L)

Trough: <2 µg/mL (SI: 4 µmol/L) (peak depends in part on the minimal inhibitory concentration of drug against organism being treated)

Once daily or extended interval: Trough: <0.5 µg/mL

Toxic:

Peak: >12 µg/mL (SI: >21 µmol/L)

Trough: >2 µg/mL (SI: >8.4 µmol/L)

Test Interactions Increased protein; decreased magnesium; increased BUN, AST, GPT, alk phos, serum creatinine; decreased potassium, sodium, calcium

Patient Information Report any dizziness or sensations of ringing or fullness in ears; do not touch ophthalmics to eye; use no other eye drops within 5-10 minutes of instilling ophthalmic

Nursing Implications When injected into the muscles of paralyzed patients the results are different than in normal patients, slower absorption and lower peak concentrations probably due to poor circulation in the atrophic muscles, suggest I.V. route; aminoglycoside levels measured in blood taken from Silastic® central catheters can sometime give falsely high readings. Give other antibiotic drugs at least 1 hour before or after gentamicin. Hearing should be tested before, during, and after treatment.

Special Geriatric Considerations The aminoglycosides are important therapeutic interventions for infections due to susceptible organisms and as empiric therapy in seriously ill patients. Their use is not without risk of toxicity, however, these risks can be minimized if initial dosing is adjusted for estimated renal function and appropriate monitoring performed. High dose, once daily aminoglycosides have been advocated as an alternative to traditional dosing regimens. Once daily or extended interval dosing is as effective and may be safer than traditional dosing. The interval must be adjusted for renal function. See Pharmacokinetics and Usual Dosage.

Dosage Forms

Gentamicin sulfate:

Cream, topical (Garamycin®, G-myticin®): 0.1% (15 g)

Infusion, in D_5W: 60 mg, 80 mg, 100 mg

Infusion, in NS: 40 mg, 60 mg, 80 mg, 90 mg, 100 mg, 120 mg

Injection: 40 mg/mL (1 mL, 1.5 mL, 2 mL)

Pediatric: 10 mg/mL (2 mL)

Intrathecal, preservative free (Garamycin®): 2 mg/mL (2 mL)

Ointment:
  Ophthalmic: 0.3% [3 mg/g] (3.5 g)
      Garamycin®, Genoptic® S.O.P., Gentacidin®, Gentak®: 0.3% [3 mg/g] (3.5 g)
    Topical (Garamycin®, G-myticin®): 0.1% (15 g)
  Solution, ophthalmic: 0.3% (5 mL, 15 mL)
    Garamycin®, Genoptic®, Gentacidin®, Gentak®: 0.3% (1 mL, 5 mL, 15 mL)

References

Matzke GR, Jameson JJ, and Halstenson CE, "Gentamicin Disposition in Young and Elderly Patients With Various Degrees of Renal Function," *J Clin Pharmacol*, 1987, 27(3):216-20.

Nicolau DP, Freeman CD, Belliveau PP, et al, "Experience With a Once-Daily Aminoglycoside Program Administered to 2184 Adult Patients," *Antimicrob Agents Chemother*, 1995, 39(3):650-5.

Preston SL and Briceland LL, "Single Daily Dosing of Aminoglycosides," *Pharmacotherapy*, 1995, 15(3):297-316.

Zaske DE, Irvine P, Strand LM, et al, "Wide Interpatient Variations in Gentamicin Dose Requirements for Geriatric Patients," *JAMA*, 1982, 248(23):3122-6.

Gentamicin and Prednisolone see Prednisolone and Gentamicin on page 776

Gen-XENE® see Clorazepate on page 241

Geocillin® see Carbenicillin on page 163

German Measles Vaccine see Rubella Virus Vaccine, Live on page 841

Germinal® see Ergoloid Mesylates on page 342

GG see Guaifenesin on page 437

GG-Cen® [OTC] see Guaifenesin on page 437

Glaucoma Drug Therapy Comparison see page 1032

Glaucon® see Epinephrine on page 336

GlaucTabs® see Methazolamide on page 600

Glibenclamide see Glyburide on page 428

Glimepiride (GLYE me pye ride)

Related Information
  Antacid Drug Interactions on page 1096

Brand Names Amaryl®

Therapeutic Category Antidiabetic Agent; Hypoglycemic Agent, Oral; Sulfonylurea Agent

Use Management of noninsulin-dependent diabetes mellitus; used alone or in combination with insulin

Contraindications Hypersensitivity to glimepiride or any component, other sulfonamides; patients with diabetic ketoacidosis

Warnings Use with caution in patients with impaired renal function, debilitated or malnourished patients, and patients with adrenal, pituitary, or hepatic insufficiency

Adverse Reactions
  Central nervous system: Dizziness, headache
  Dermatologic: Allergic skin reactions
  Endocrine & metabolic: Hypoglycemia, hyponatremia
  Gastrointestinal: Nausea, vomiting, gastrointestinal pain, diarrhea
  Neuromuscular & skeletal: Weakness
  Ocular: Changes in accommodation, blurred vision

Overdosage Hypoglycemia, loss of consciousness or neurologic findings

Toxicology Intoxications with sulfonylureas can cause hypoglycemia and are best managed with glucose administration (oral for milder hypoglycemia or by injection in more severe forms)

Drug Interactions
  Decreased hypoglycemic effects: Thiazides and other diuretics, phenothiazines, estrogens, phenytoin, sympathomimetics, corticosteroids, thyroid products, oral contraceptives, nicotinic acid, INH, beta-blockers
  May reduce effects of warfarin
  Increased hypoglycemic effects: NSAIDs, salicylates, sulfonamides, chloramphenicol, coumarins, probenecid, MAO inhibitors, beta-blockers, miconazole (theoretical)

Mechanism of Action Stimulates insulin release from the functioning pancreatic beta cells; extrapancreatic effects may include increased sensitivity of peripheral tissues to insulin

Pharmacodynamics Maximum glucose lowering effect: 2-3 hours postdose; glucose lowering effect is maintained over 24 hours

Pharmacokinetics The pharmacokinetics of glimepiride are not altered by aging
  Absorption: 100%
(Continued)

Glimepiride *(Continued)*

Protein binding: >99.5%

Metabolism: Oxidative biotransformation to two metabolites; cyclohex-ylhydroxymethyl derivative by cytochrome P-4502C9 which has $\frac{1}{3}$ the activity of parent compound; the other metabolite is inactive

Half-life: 5-9.2 hours

Elimination: 60% in urine, ≥80% as metabolites; 40% in feces, 70% as metabolites

Usual Dosage Geriatrics and Adults: Oral: Initial: 1-2 mg once daily, administered with breakfast or the first main meal; usual maintenance dose: 1-4 mg once daily; maximum dose: 8 mg once daily; increase dose by 1-2 mg every 1-2 weeks based on blood glucose level

Dosing adjustment in renal impairment: 1 mg once daily and titrate to effect

Monitoring Parameters Fasting blood glucose, hemoglobin A_{1c}, fructosamine

Reference Range Fasting blood glucose: Geriatrics: 100-150 mg/dL; Adults: 80-140 mg/dL

Patient Information Take with breakfast or first main meal; seek counseling by someone experienced in diabetes education about the signs and symptoms of hyper- and hypoglycemia, exercise, and diet, blood glucose monitoring, and other related topics; eat regularly, do not skip meals; carry quick source of sugar; wear medical alert bracelet

Nursing Implications Monitor for signs and symptoms of hypoglycemia; patients who are anorexic or NPO may need to have their dose held to avoid hypoglycemia

Special Geriatric Considerations Rapid and prolonged hypoglycemia (>12 hours) despite hypertonic glucose injections have been reported; age, hepatic, and renal impairment are independent risk factors for hypoglycemia; dosage titration should be made at weekly intervals. How "tightly" a geriatric patient's blood glucose should be controlled is controversial; however, a fasting blood sugar <150 mg/dL is now an acceptable end point. Such a decision should be based on the patient's functional and cognitive status, how well they recognize hypoglycemic or hyperglycemic symptoms, and how to respond to them and their other disease states.

Dosage Forms Tablet: 1 mg, 2 mg, 4 mg

Glipizide *(GLIP i zide)*

Related Information

Antacid Drug Interactions *on page 1096*

Brand Names Glucotrol®; Glucotrol® XL

Synonyms Glydiazinamide

Generic Available No

Therapeutic Category Antidiabetic Agent; Hypoglycemic Agent, Oral; Sulfonylurea Agent

Use Management of noninsulin-dependent diabetes mellitus (type II)

Contraindications Hypersensitivity to glipizide or any component, other sulfonamides, type 1 diabetes mellitus

Warnings Use with caution in patients with severe hepatic disease

Precautions Avoid alcohol and alcohol-containing products

Adverse Reactions

Cardiovascular: Edema

Central nervous system: Headache, dizziness

Dermatologic: Rash, urticaria, photosensitivity

Endocrine & metabolic: Hypoglycemia, hyponatremia

Gastrointestinal: Anorexia, nausea, vomiting, diarrhea, heartburn

Hematologic: Blood dyscrasias

Hepatic: Jaundice

Renal: Diuretic effect

Overdosage Symptoms of overdose include low blood sugar, tingling of lips and tongue, nausea, yawning, confusion, agitation, tachycardia, sweating, convulsions, stupor, and coma

Toxicology Intoxications with sulfonylureas can cause hypoglycemia and are best managed with glucose administration (oral for milder hypoglycemia or by injection in more severe forms)

Drug Interactions

Increased effect: H_2 antagonists, anticoagulants, androgens, fluconazole, salicylates, gemfibrozil, sulfonamides, tricyclic antidepressants, probenecid, MAO inhibitors, methyldopa, digitalis glycosides, urinary acidifiers

Decreased effect: Beta-blockers, cholestyramines, hydantoins, rifampin, thiazide diuretics, urinary alkalines, charcoal

Mechanism of Action Stimulates insulin release from the pancreatic beta cells; reduces glucose output from the liver; insulin sensitivity is increased at peripheral target sites

Pharmacodynamics

Onset of action: Oral: Maximal blood glucose reductions occur within 1.5-2 hours

Duration of action: 12-24 hours

Pharmacokinetics

Protein binding: 92% to 99% nonionic; has been reported to be as low as 64% in elderly diabetics

Metabolism: In the liver with metabolites (91% to 97%)

Half-life: 2-4 hours

Elimination: In urine (60% to 80%) and feces (11%)

Usual Dosage

Oral (allow several days between dose titrations):

Geriatrics: Initial: 2.5-5 mg/day; increase by 2.5-5 mg/day every 1-2 weeks; maximum daily dose: 40 mg

Adults: 2.5-40 mg/day; doses >15-20 mg/day can be divided and given twice daily, but it does not appear necessary; maximum daily dose: 40 mg

Dosing adjustment/comments in renal impairment: Cl_{cr} <10 mL/minute: Some investigators recommend not using

Dosing adjustment in hepatic impairment: Initial dosage should be 2.5 mg/day

Monitoring Parameters Fasting blood glucose, hemoglobin A_{1c}, fructosamine

Reference Range Glucose: Geriatrics: 100-150 mg/dL; Adults: 80-140 mg/dL

Test Interactions Decreased prothrombin time, decreased sodium (S)

Patient Information Patients must be counseled by someone experienced in diabetes education about the signs and symptoms of hyper- and hypoglycemia, exercise and diet, blood glucose monitoring, and other related topics; eat regularly, do not skip meals; carry quick source of sugar; medical alert bracelet

Nursing Implications Monitor for signs and symptoms of hypoglycemia; administer 30 minutes before meals to avoid erratic absorption

Special Geriatric Considerations Glipizide is a useful agent since there are few drug interactions and elimination of the active drug is not dependent upon renal function. How "tightly" a geriatric patient's blood glucose should be controlled is controversial; however, a fasting blood sugar of <150 mg/dL is now an acceptable end point. Such a decision should be based on the patient's functional and cognitive status, how well they recognize hypoglycemic or hyperglycemic symptoms, and how to respond to them and their other disease states.

Dosage Forms

Tablet: 5 mg, 10 mg

Tablet, extended release: 5 mg, 10 mg

References

Brodows RG, "Benefits and Risks With Glyburide and Glipizide in Elderly NIDDM Patients," *Diabetes Care*, 1992, 15(1):75-80.

Kradjan WA, Kobayashi KA, Bauer LA, et al, "Glipizide Pharmacokinetics: Effects of Age, Diabetes, and Multiple Dosing," *J Clin Pharmacol*, 1989, 29(12):1121-7.

Kradjan WA, Takenchi KY, Opeim KE, et al, "Pharmacokinetics and Pharmacodynamics of Glipizide After Once-Daily and Divided Doses," *Pharmacotherapy*, 1995, 15(4):465-71.

Rosenstock J, Corrao PJ, Goldberg RB, et al, "Diabetes Control in the Elderly: A Randomized, Comparative Study of Glyburide Versus Glipizide in Noninsulin Dependent Diabetes Mellitus," *Clin Ther*, 1993, 15(6):1031-40.

Glucagon (GLOO ka gon)

Related Information

I.V. Push Recommended Guidelines *on page 1083*

Generic Available No

Therapeutic Category Antihypoglycemic Agent

Use Hypoglycemia; diagnostic aid in the radiologic examination of GI tract when a hypotonic state is needed; used with some success as a cardiac stimulant in management of severe cases of beta-adrenergic blocking agent overdosage

Contraindications Hypersensitivity to glucagon or any component

Warnings Use with caution in patients with a history of insulinoma and/or pheochromocytoma

(Continued)

Glucagon *(Continued)*

Adverse Reactions
Gastrointestinal: Nausea, vomiting
Miscellaneous: Hypersensitivity reactions

Overdosage Symptoms of overdose include hypokalemia, nausea, vomiting

Drug Interactions Increased toxicity: Oral anticoagulant - hypoprothrombinemic effects may be increased possibly with bleeding

Stability After reconstitution, use immediately; may be kept at 5°C for up to 48 hours if necessary

Mechanism of Action Stimulates adenylate cyclase to produce increased cyclic AMP, which promotes hepatic glycogenolysis and gluconeogenesis, causing a raise in blood glucose levels

Pharmacokinetics
Metabolism: In the liver with some inactivation occurring in the kidneys and plasma
Half-life, plasma: 3-10 minutes

Usual Dosage Geriatrics and Adults:
Hypoglycemia or insulin shock therapy: I.M., I.V., S.C.: 0.5-1 mg, may repeat in 20 minutes as needed
Diagnostic aid: I.M., I.V.: 0.25-2 mg 10 minutes prior to procedure

Administration Reconstitute powder for injection by adding 1 or 10 mL of sterile diluent to a vial containing 1 or 10 units of the drug, respectively, to provide solutions containing 1 mg of glucagon/mL; if dose to be administered is <2 mg of the drug, use only the diluent provided by the manufacturer; if >2 mg, use sterile water for injection; use immediately after reconstitution

Monitoring Parameters Blood pressure, blood glucose

Patient Information Instruct a close associate on how to prepare and administer as a treatment for insulin shock

Nursing Implications See Administration and Usual Dosage

Additional Information 1 unit = 1 mg

Special Geriatric Considerations No specific recommendations needed; use as indicated in Usual Dosage

Dosage Forms Powder for injection, lyophilized: 1 mg [1 unit]; 10 mg [10 units]

Glucophage® *see Metformin on page 597*
Glucotrol® *see Glipizide on page 426*
Glucotrol® XL *see Glipizide on page 426*
Glyate® [OTC] *see Guaifenesin on page 437*
Glybenclamide *see Glyburide on this page*
Glybenzcyclamide *see Glyburide on this page*

Glyburide *(GLYE byoor ide)*

Related Information
Antacid Drug Interactions *on page 1096*

Brand Names DiaβetaÂ®; Glynase™ PresTab™; Micronase®

Synonyms Glibenclamide; Glybenclamide; Glybenzcyclamide

Generic Available No

Therapeutic Category Antidiabetic Agent; Hypoglycemic Agent, Oral; Sulfonylurea Agent

Use Management of noninsulin-dependent diabetes mellitus (type II)

Contraindications Hypersensitivity to glyburide or any component, or other sulfonamides; type 1 diabetes mellitus

Precautions Use with caution in patients with renal and hepatic impairment

Adverse Reactions
Dermatologic: Pruritus, rash, photosensitivity
Endocrine & metabolic: Hypoglycemia
Gastrointestinal: Nausea, epigastric fullness, heartburn, constipation, diarrhea, anorexia
Genitourinary: Nocturia
Hematologic: Leukopenia, thrombocytopenia, hemolytic anemia
Hepatic: Cholestatic jaundice
Neuromuscular & skeletal: Arthralgia, paresthesia
Renal: Diuretic effect

Overdosage Symptoms of overdose include low blood sugar, tingling of lips and tongue, nausea, yawning, confusion, agitation, tachycardia, sweating, convulsions, stupor, and coma

Toxicology Intoxications with sulfonylureas can cause hypoglycemia and are best managed with glucose administration (oral for milder hypoglycemia or by injection in more severe forms)

Drug Interactions

Decreased effect: Thiazides and beta-blockers may decrease effectiveness of glyburide

Increased effect: Increased hypoglycemia with phenylbutazone, oral antico-agulants, hydantoins, salicylates, NSAIDs, MAO inhibitors

Increased toxicity: Increased disulfiram reactions with alcohol

Mechanism of Action Stimulates insulin release from the pancreatic beta cells; reduces glucose output from the liver; insulin sensitivity is increased at peripheral target sites

Pharmacodynamics

Insulin levels in the serum begin to increase within 15-60 minutes after a single oral dose and persist for up to 24 hours

Duration of action: 18 hours

Pharmacokinetics

Protein binding: 99% ionic/nonionic

Metabolism: To one moderately active and several inactive metabolites

Half-life: 5-16 hours, may be prolonged with renal insufficiency

Time to peak serum concentration: Oral: Within 2-4 hours

Usual Dosage Oral: Doses >10 mg/day should be divided

Geriatrics: Initial: 1.25-2.5 mg/day, increase by 1.25-2.5 mg/day every 1-3 weeks; maximum daily dose: 20 mg/day

Adults: 1.25-5 mg to start then 1.25-20 mg maintenance dose/day divided in 1-2 doses

Glynase™ PresTab™: Initial: 0.75-3 mg/day, increase by 1.5 mg/day in weekly intervals, maximum: 12 mg/day

Monitoring Parameters Fasting blood glucose, hemoglobin A_{1c}, fructosamine

Reference Range Fasting blood glucose: Geriatrics: 100-150 mg/dL; Adults: 80-140 mg/dL

Test Interactions Decreased prothrombin time, decreased sodium (S)

Patient Information Patients must be counseled by someone experienced in diabetes education about the signs and symptoms of hyper- and hypogly-cemia, exercise and diet, blood glucose monitoring, and other related topics; eat regularly, do not skip meals; carry quick source of sugar; medical alert bracelet

Nursing Implications Monitor for signs and symptoms of hypoglycemia; patients who are anorexic or NPO may need to have their dose held to avoid hypoglycemia

Special Geriatric Considerations Rapid and prolonged hypoglycemia (>12 hours) despite hypertonic glucose injections have been reported; age, hepatic, and renal impairment are independent risk factors for hypoglycemia; dosage titration should be made at weekly intervals. How "tightly" a geriatric patient's blood glucose should be controlled is controversial; however, a fasting blood sugar <150 mg/dL is now an acceptable end point. Such a decision should be based on the patient's functional and cognitive status, how well they recognize hypoglycemic or hyperglycemic symptoms, and how to respond to them and their other disease states. Use with caution in elderly with renal insufficiency.

Dosage Forms

Tablet (Diaβeta®, Micronase®): 1.25 mg, 2.5 mg, 5 mg

Tablet, micronized (Glynase™ PresTab™): 1.5 mg, 3 mg, 6 mg

References

Brodowa RG, "Benefits and Risks With Glyburide and Glipizide in Elderly NIDDM Patients," *Diabetes Care*, 1992, 15(1):75-80.

Rosenstock J, Corrao PJ, Goldberg RB, et al, "Diabetes Control in the Elderly: A Randomized, Comparative Study of Glyburide Versus Glipizide in Noninsulin-Dependent Diabetes Mellitus," *Clin Ther*, 1993, 15(6):1031-40.

Sonnenblick M and Shilo S, "Glibenclamide Induced Prolonged Hypoglycaemia," *Age Ageing*, 1986, 15:185-9.

Glycerin (GLIS er in)

Brand Names Fleet® Babylax® Rectal [OTC]; Ophthalgan® Ophthalmic; Osmoglyn® Ophthalmic; Sani-Supp® Suppository [OTC]

Synonyms Glycerol

Generic Available Yes

Therapeutic Category Laxative, Hyperosmolar

(Continued)

Glycerin *(Continued)*

Use Constipation; reduction of intraocular pressure; reduction of corneal edema; glycerin has been administered orally to reduce intracranial pressure acutely

Contraindications Known hypersensitivity to glycerin, anuria, acute pulmonary edema, severe dehydration

Warnings Use oral glycerin with caution in patients with cardiac, renal, or hepatic disease and in diabetics

Adverse Reactions
Central nervous system: Dizziness, headache
Endocrine & metabolic: Hyperglycemia
Gastrointestinal: Diarrhea, nausea, tenesmus, vomiting
Local: Pain, rectal irritation, cramping pain
Miscellaneous: Thirst

Stability Protect from heat; freezing should be avoided

Mechanism of Action Osmotic dehydrating agent which increases osmotic pressure; draws fluid into colon and thus stimulates evacuation

Pharmacodynamics
Onset of action:
For glycerin suppository: 15-30 minutes
In decreasing IOP: Within 10-30 minutes
Peak effects: Following oral absorption, within 60-90 minutes
Duration of action: 4-8 hours; increased intracranial pressure decreases within 10-60 minutes following an oral dose with a duration of action around 2-3 hours

Pharmacokinetics
Absorbed:
Oral: Well absorbed
Rectal: Poor
Metabolism: Primarily in the liver with 20% metabolized in the kidney
Half-life: 30-45 minutes
Elimination: Only a small percentage of drug is excreted unchanged in urine

Usual Dosage Geriatrics and Adults:
Constipation: Rectal: 1 suppository as needed
Reduction of intraocular pressure: Oral: 1-1.8 g/kg 1 to 1½ hours preoperatively; additional doses may be administered at 5-hour intervals
Reduction of corneal edema: Ophthalmic: Instill 1-2 drops in eye(s) every 3-4 hours
Reduction of intracranial pressure: Oral: 1.5 g/kg/day divided every 4 hours; dose of 1 g/kg/dose every 6 hours has also been used

Administration Apply topical anesthetic before instilling ophthalmic drops

Patient Information Do not use if experiencing abdominal pain, nausea, or vomiting

Nursing Implications See Administration

Additional Information Suppository needs to melt to provide laxative effect

Special Geriatric Considerations The primary use of glycerin in the elderly is as a laxative, although it is not recommended as a first-line treatment

Dosage Forms
Solution:
Ophthalmic, sterile (Ophthalgan®): Glycerin with chlorobutanol 0.55% (7.5 mL)
Oral (lime flavor)(Osmoglyn®): 50% (220 mL)
Rectal (Fleet Babylax®): 4 mL/applicator (6s)
Suppository, rectal (Sani-Supp®): Glycerin with sodium stearate (infant and adult sizes)

References
Heinemeyer G, "Clinical Pharmacokinetic Considerations in the Treatment of Increased Intracranial Pressure," *Clin Pharmacokinet*, 1987, 13(1):1-25.
Rottenberg DA, Hurwitz BJ, and Posner JB, "The Effect of Oral Glycerol on Intraventricular Pressure in Man," *Neurology*, 1977, 27(7):600-8.

Glycerol *see* Glycerin *on previous page*
Glycerol Guaiacolate *see* Guaifenesin *on page 437*
Glyceryl Trinitrate *see* Nitroglycerin *on page 677*

Glycopyrrolate *(glye koe PYE roe late)*
Brand Names Robinul®; Robinul® Forte
Synonyms Glycopyrronium Bromide
Generic Available Yes

Therapeutic Category Anticholinergic Agent; Antispasmodic Agent, Gastro-intestinal

Use Adjunct in treatment of peptic ulcer disease; inhibit salivation and excessive secretions of the respiratory tract preoperatively; reversal of neuromuscular blockade; control of upper airway secretions

Contraindications Narrow-angle glaucoma, acute hemorrhage, tachycardia, hypersensitivity to glycopyrrolate or any component; ulcerative colitis, obstructive uropathy

Warnings Blondes and patients with Down syndrome may be hypersensitive to antimuscarinic effects

Precautions Use with caution in the elderly, autonomic neuropathy, glaucoma, hepatic disease, ulcerative colitis, hiatal hernia with reflux esophagitis, renal disease, prostatic hypertrophy, congestive heart failure, coronary artery disease, arrhythmias, or hypertension

Adverse Reactions
Cardiovascular: Tachycardia, palpitations
Central nervous system: Fatigue, delirium, restlessness, headache (the elderly are at increased risk for confusion and hallucinations, ataxia)
Dermatologic: Dry hot skin
Gastrointestinal: Impaired GI motility, xerostomia
Genitourinary: Urinary hesitancy/retention
Neuromuscular & skeletal: Tremors
Ocular: Mydriasis, blurred vision

Overdosage Symptoms of overdose include blurred vision, urinary retention, tachycardia, absent bowel sounds

Toxicology Anticholinergic toxicity is caused by strong binding of the drug to cholinergic receptors. Cholinesterase inhibitors reduce acetylcholinesterase, the enzyme that breaks down acetylcholine and thereby allows acetylcholine to accumulate and compete for receptor binding with the offending anticholinergic. For anticholinergic overdose with severe life-threatening symptoms, physostigmine 1-2 mg S.C. or I.V., slowly may be given to reverse these effects.

Drug Interactions
Decreased effect of levodopa (decreased absorption)
Increased toxicity (central anticholinergic syndrome): Narcotic analgesics, phenothiazines, and other antipsychotics, tricyclic antidepressants, some antihistamines, quinidine, disopyramide
Antagonistic effect: Tacrine, donepezil

Stability Unstable at pH >6

Mechanism of Action Blocks the action of acetylcholine at parasympathetic sites in smooth muscle, secretory glands and the CNS

Pharmacodynamics
Onset of action:
Oral: Within 50 minutes
I.M.: 20-40 minutes
I.V.: 10-15 minutes
Peak effect: Oral: Within 1 hour

Pharmacokinetics
Absorption: Oral: Poor and erratic
Bioavailability: ~10%

Usual Dosage Geriatrics and Adults:
Reverse neuromuscular blockade: I.V.: 0.2 mg for each 1 mg of neostigmine or 5 mg of pyridostigmine administered
Peptic ulcer:
Oral: 1-2 mg 2-3 times/day
I.M., I.V.: 0.1-0.2 mg 3-4 times/day
Preoperative: I.M.: 4 mcg/kg 30-60 minutes before procedure

Administration For I.V. administration, glycopyrrolate may also be administered via the tubing of a running I.V. infusion of a compatible solution

Monitoring Parameters Pulse, anticholinergic effects

Patient Information Maintain good oral hygiene habits, because lack of saliva may increase chance of cavities. Observe caution while driving or performing other tasks requiring alertness, as may cause drowsiness, dizziness, or blurred vision. Notify physician if skin rash, flushing or eye pain occurs; or if difficulty in urinating, constipation or sensitivity to light becomes severe or persists.

Nursing Implications Monitor for anticholinergic effects

Additional Information Because of its bothersome and potentially dangerous side effects, glycopyrrolate is rarely used for the treatment of peptic ulcer disease

(Continued)

Glycopyrrolate *(Continued)*

Special Geriatric Considerations Anticholinergic agents are generally not well tolerated in the elderly and their use should be avoided when possible (see Precautions and Adverse Reactions)

Dosage Forms
Glycopyrrolate bromide:
Injection: 0.2 mg/mL (1 mL, 2 mL, 5 mL, 20 mL)
Robinul®: 0.2 mg/mL (1 mL, 2 mL, 5 mL, 20 mL)
Tablet:
Robinul®: 1 mg
Robinul® Forte: 2 mg

Glycopyrronium Bromide *see* Glycopyrrolate *on page 430*

Glycotuss® [OTC] *see* Guaifenesin *on page 437*

Glycotuss-dM® [OTC] *see* Guaifenesin and Dextromethorphan *on page 439*

Glydiazinamide *see* Glipizide *on page 426*

Glynase™ PresTab™ *see* Glyburide *on page 428*

Gly-Oxide® Oral [OTC] *see* Carbamide Peroxide *on page 162*

Glytuss® [OTC] *see* Guaifenesin *on page 437*

G-myticin® Topical *see* Gentamicin *on page 422*

Gold Sodium Thiomalate *(gold SOW dee um thye oh MAL ate)*

Brand Names Aurolate®; Myochrysine®

Therapeutic Category Gold Compound

Use Adjunctive treatment in adult active rheumatoid arthritis; alternative or adjunct in treatment of pemphigus; for psoriatic patients who do not respond to NSAIDs

Contraindications Severe hepatic or renal dysfunction; hypersensitivity to gold compounds or any component; systemic lupus erythematosus; history of blood dyscrasias; congestive heart failure, exfoliative dermatitis, colitis

Warnings Explain the possibility of adverse reactions before initiating therapy; signs of gold toxicity include: decrease in hemoglobin, leukopenia, granulocytes and platelets; proteinuria, hematuria, pruritus, stomatitis, persistent diarrhea, rash, metallic taste; diabetes mellitus and congestive heart failure should be in control before initiating therapy; use cautiously in patients with a history of blood dyscrasias, bone marrow suppression, inflammatory bowel disease, allergic hemolytic anemias, drug allergy, or hypersensitivity, skin rash, history of renal or liver disease, uncontrolled hypertension, or compromised cerebral or cardiovascular circulation. Therapy should be discontinued if platelet count falls to <100,000/mm^3, WBC to <4000, or <1500 granulocytes/mm^3.

Precautions Frequent monitoring of patients for signs and symptoms of toxicity will prevent serious adverse reactions; must not be injected I.V.; use with caution in patients with impaired renal or hepatic function; NSAIDs and corticosteroids may be discontinued over time after initiating gold therapy; do not use with penicillamine, antimalarials, immunosuppressives, other than corticosteroids; for mild or minor adverse reactions, hold therapy until reaction resolves then may resume therapy of reduced doses; moderate to severe reaction require discontinuation of gold therapy

Adverse Reactions
Cardiovascular: Flushing
Central nervous system: Dizziness, confusion, fever, hallucinations, seizures, syncope, headache
Dermatologic: Dermatitis, alopecia, pruritus, gray-to-blue pigmentation
Gastrointestinal: Stomatitis, metallic taste, nausea, vomiting, abdominal cramps, abdominal pain, constipation, flatulence, dyspepsia, melena, GI bleeding, mouth ulcers, dysgeusia, dysphagia
Genitourinary: Vaginitis
Hematologic: Leukopenia, thrombocytopenia, eosinophilia
Hepatic: Hepatitis, increased LFTs, jaundice
Neuromuscular & skeletal: Weakness
Ocular: Iritis, corneal ulcers, deposits of gold
Renal: Hematuria, proteinuria, nephrotic syndrome, glomerulitis
Respiratory: Bronchitis, interstitial pneumonitis, fibrosis
Miscellaneous: Diaphoresis

Overdosage Symptoms of overdose include hematuria, proteinuria, fever, nausea, vomiting, diarrhea

Toxicology For mild gold poisoning, dimercaprol 2.5 mg/kg 4 times/day for 2 days or for more severe forms of gold intoxication, dimercaprol 3-5 mg/kg every 4 hours for 2 days, should be initiated. Then after 2 days, the initial dose should be repeated twice daily on the third day, and once daily thereafter for 10 days. Other chelating agents have been used with some success.

Drug Interactions Penicillamine, antimalarials, cytotoxic drugs, or immunosuppressive agents, phenylbutazone, oxyphenbutazone

Stability Should not be used if solution is darker than pale yellow

Mechanism of Action The exact mechanism of action of gold is unknown; gold is taken up by macrophages which result in inhibition of phagocytosis and lysosomal membrane stabilization; other actions observed are decreased serum rheumatoid factor and alterations in immunoglobulins. Additionally, complement activation is decreased, prostaglandin synthesis is inhibited and lysosomal enzyme activity is decreased.

Pharmacodynamics Gold injections may result in decreased morning stiffness in 1-2 months; significant benefit may not be noted for 3-6 months

Pharmacokinetics
Protein binding: 95% to 99%
Half-life: 3-27 days (single dose); 14-40 days (third dose); up to 168 days (11th dose)
Time to peak serum concentrations: I.M.: Within 2-6 hours
Elimination: Majority (60% to 90%) is excreted in urine with smaller amounts (10% to 40%) excreted in feces (via bile)

Usual Dosage Geriatrics and Adults: I.M. (gluteal muscle preferable): 10 mg first week; 25 mg second week; then 25-50 mg/week until 1 g cumulative dose has been given. If improvement occurs without adverse reactions, administer 25-50 mg every week for 2-20 weeks; then every 3-4 weeks if patient is stable; may give maintenance 25-50 mg I.M. every 3-4 weeks indefinitely; if no response after cumulative dose of 1 g, discontinue therapy

Monitoring Parameters Each visit, the patient should have urinalysis, CBC with platelets initially; then every 6 months on maintenance therapy; monitor for other adverse reactions (see Adverse Reactions)

Reference Range Gold: Normal: 0-0.1 µg/mL (SI: 0-0.0064 µmol/L); Therapeutic: 1-3 µg/mL (SI: 0.06-0.18 µmol/L); urine <0.1 µg/24 hours

Patient Information Minimize exposure to sunlight; report any signs of toxicity to physician (ie, pruritus, rash, sore mouth, indigestion, metallic taste); joint pain may take 1-2 months to start to subside

Nursing Implications Therapy should be discontinued if platelet count falls <100,000/mm^3; deep I.M. injection into the upper outer quadrant of the gluteal region; addition of 0.1 mL of 1% lidocaine to each injection may reduce the discomfort with injection; vial should be thoroughly shaken before withdrawing a dose; explain the possibility of adverse reactions before initiating therapy; advise patients to report any symptoms of toxicity; monitor serum concentration, CBC, platelets, urine protein (see Adverse Reactions)

Special Geriatric Considerations Tolerance to gold decreases with advanced age; use cautiously only after traditional therapy and other disease modifying antirheumatic drugs (DMARDs) have been attempted

Dosage Forms Injection: 25 mg/mL (1 mL); 50 mg/mL (1 mL, 10 mL); contains 50% gold

Gordofilm® Liquid see Salicylic Acid on page 845

Granisetron (gra NI se tron)

Brand Names Kytril® Injection

Therapeutic Category Antiemetic; Serotonin Antagonist, Antiemetic

Use Prophylaxis and treatment of chemotherapy-related nausea and emesis; may be prescribed for patients who are refractory to or have severe adverse reactions to standard antiemetic therapy. Granisetron may be prescribed for young patients (ie, <45 years of age who are more likely to develop extrapyramidal reactions to high-dose metoclopramide) who are to receive highly emetogenic chemotherapeutic agents as listed:

Agents with high emetogenic potential (>90%) (dose/m^2):
Carmustine ≥200 mg
Cisplatin ≥75 mg
Cyclophosphamide ≥1000 mg
Cytarabine ≥1000 mg
Dacarbazine ≥500 mg
Ifosfamide ≥1000 mg
Lomustine ≥60 mg
Mechlorethamine
Pentostatin
Streptozocin

(Continued)

Granisetron *(Continued)*

or two agents classified as having high or moderately high emetogenic potential as listed:

Agents with moderately high emetogenic potential (60% to 90%) (dose/m²):
Carmustine <200 mg
Cisplatin <75 mg
Cyclophosphamide 1000 mg
Cytarabine 250-1000 mg
Dacarbazine <500 mg
Doxorubicin ≥75 mg
Ifosfamide
Lomustine <60 mg
Methotrexate ≥250 mg
Mitomycin
Mitoxantrone
Procarbazine

Granisetron should not be prescribed for chemotherapeutic agents with a low emetogenic potential (eg, bleomycin, busulfan, cyclophosphamide <1000 mg, etoposide, 5-fluorouracil, vinblastine, vincristine)

Contraindications Previous hypersensitivity to granisetron

Warnings Use with caution in patients with liver disease; hepatocellular carcinomas and adenomas were induced in rats at doses 400 times recommended for use in humans (see Special Geriatric Considerations)

Adverse Reactions
Cardiovascular: Transient blood pressure changes, sinus bradycardia, atrial fibrillation, A-V block, ventricular ectopy
Central nervous system: Headache, somnolence, agitation, fever, extrapyramidal effects
Dermatologic: Rash
Endocrine & metabolic: Hot flashes
Gastrointestinal: Constipation, diarrhea, dysgeusia
Hepatic: Increased LFTs (AST, ALT)
Neuromuscular & skeletal: Weakness
Miscellaneous: Anaphylactic reactions

Overdosage Doses up to 38.5 mg have been reported without symptoms or slight headache

Toxicology No specific antidote; administer general supportive care

Drug Interactions Drugs which inhibit clearance by cytochrome P-450 system may change clearance of granisetron; induction may occur as well and decrease half-life of granisetron

Stability Stable when mixed in NS or D_5W for 24 hours at room temperature; protect from light; do not freeze vials

Mechanism of Action Selective $5-HT_3$ receptor antagonist, blocking serotonin, both peripherally on vagal nerve terminals and centrally in the chemoreceptor trigger zone

Pharmacodynamics
Onset of action: Commonly controls emesis within 1-3 minutes of administration
Duration: Effects generally last no more than 24 hours maximum

Pharmacokinetics
Distribution: V_d: 2-3 L/kg (range: 0.85-10 L/kg); widely distributed throughout the body
Metabolism: Substrate CYP3A4
Half-life:
Cancer patients: 10-12 hours (range: 1-31 hours)
Healthy volunteers: 3-4 hours
Elimination: Primarily hepatic, 8% to 15% of a dose is excreted unchanged in urine within 48 hours

Usual Dosage Geriatrics and Adults:
Oral or extemporaneously prepared liquid: 1 mg twice daily on days receiving chemotherapy (see Additional Information)
I.V.: 10 mcg/kg for 1-3 doses; doses should be administered as a single IVPB over 5 minutes to 1 hour, given just prior to chemotherapy (15-60 minutes before) and only on days when receiving chemotherapy
As intervention therapy for breakthrough nausea and vomiting, during the first 24 hours following chemotherapy, 2 or 3 repeat infusions (same dose) have been administered, separated by at least 10 minutes

Dosing interval in renal impairment: Creatinine clearance values have no relationship to granisetron clearance

Administration As a general precaution, do not mix in solution with other medications

Monitoring Parameters Monitor for control of nausea and vomiting

Nursing Implications Doses should be given at least 15-60 minutes prior to initiation of chemotherapy

Additional Information Injection: 1 mg/mL as free base (1.12 mg/mL as HCl salt); 1 mL vial

Extemporaneously prepared liquid: To prepare oral liquid, pulverize twelve 1 mg tablets and suspend in 30 mL of distilled water; qs this mixture to 60 mL with cherry syrup; stable for 14 days at room temperature or refrigerated

Special Geriatric Considerations Clinical trials with patients older than 65 years of age are limited; however, data indicate that safety and efficacy are similar to that observed in younger adults; no adjustment in dose necessary for elderly

Dosage Forms

Injection, preservative free: 1 mg/mL (1 mL)

Tablet: 1 mg

References

Quercia RA, Zhang JH, Fan C, et al, "Stability of Granisetron (Kytril®) in an Extemporaneously Prepared Oral Liquid," *International Pharmaceutical Abstracts*, 1996, May 15, Vol 33.

Granulex *see* Trypsin, Balsam Peru, and Castor Oil *on page 971*

Granulocyte Colony Stimulating Factor *see* Filgrastim *on page 381*

Grepafloxacin (grep a FLOX a sin)

Related Information

Antacid Drug Interactions *on page 1096*

Brand Names Raxar®

Therapeutic Category Antibiotic, Quinolone

Use Treatment of acute bacterial exacerbations of chronic bronchitis caused by *Haemophilus influenzae*, *Streptococcus pneumoniae*, or *Moxaxella catarrhalis*; community-acquired pneumonia caused by *Mycoplasma pneumoniae* or the organisms previously mentioned; uncomplicated gonorrhea caused by *Neisseria gonorrhoeae*, and nongonococcal cervicitis and urethritis caused by *Chlamydia trachomatis*

Contraindications Hypersensitivity to grepafloxacin; patients with hepatic failure; given concomitantly with class I and III antiarrhythmics or bepridil due to the potential risk of cardiac arrhythmias (including torsade de pointes)

Adverse Reactions

Cardiovascular: Prolonged QTc interval

Central nervous system: Dizziness, headache

Dermatological: Rash, photosensitivity

Gastrointestinal: Taste disturbance, nausea, diarrhea

Neuromuscular & skeletal: Tendon rupture, tendonitis reported with other quinolones

Overdosage Empty stomach by inducing vomiting or by gastric lavage; observe patient and provide supportive treatment; maintain adequate hydration and electrolyte balance; EKG monitoring is recommended because of QTc interval prolongation; unknown if removed by hemodialysis or peritoneal dialysis

Drug Interactions Divalent cations (iron, zinc, magnesium, calcium, aluminum) and sucralfate decrease absorption if taken within 4 hours; decreased theophylline clearance; may increase the effects of caffeine; effects on CYP3A4 are unknown

Mechanism of Action Inhibits enzymatic activity by DNA gyrase

Pharmacokinetics

Absorption: Rapid, with or without food

Metabolism: Hepatic CYP1A2

Half-life: 15 hours

Time to peak: 2-3 hours

Elimination: Primarily biliary

Note: In the elderly, T_{max} is prolonged, AUC increased, and 24-hour urinary recovery diminished compared to young adults

Usual Dosage Geriatrics and Adults: Oral:

Acute exacerbation of chronic bronchitis: 400-600 mg once daily for 10 days

Community-acquired pneumonia: 600 mg once daily for 10 days

Gonorrhea: Single 400 mg dose

Nongonococcal urethritis: 400 mg once daily for 7 days

Monitoring Parameters Serum theophylline concentrations when theophylline and grepafloxacin are used concurrently

(Continued)

Grepafloxacin *(Continued)*

Patient Information Complete full course of therapy; avoid antacids for 4 hours pre- and post dose; may take with or without meals; notify physician if rash occurs; avoid excessive sunlight or ultraviolet light exposure

Nursing Implications Hold antacids for 4 hours before and after administering

Special Geriatric Considerations Dose adjustment is not necessary when renal function is impaired; not for urinary tract infection (see Usual Dosage and Pharmacokinetics)

Dosage Forms Tablet: 200 mg

References

Kozawa O, Uematsu T, Matsuno H, et al, "Comparative Study of Pharmacokinetics of Two New Fluoroquinolones, Belofloxacin and Grepafloxacin, in Elderly Subjects," *Antimicrob Agents Chemother*, 1996, 40(12):2824-8.

Wagstaff AJ and Balfour JA, "Grepafloxacin," *Drugs*, 1997, 53(5):817-24.

Grifulvin® V *see* Griseofulvin *on this page*

Grisactin® *see* Griseofulvin *on this page*

Grisactin® Ultra *see* Griseofulvin *on this page*

Griseofulvin *(gri see oh FUL vin)*

Brand Names Fulvicin® P/G; Fulvicin-U/F®; Grifulvin® V; Grisactin®; Grisactin® Ultra; Gris-PEG®

Generic Available No

Therapeutic Category Antifungal Agent, Systemic

Use Treatment of susceptible tinea infections of the skin, hair, and nails

Contraindications Hypersensitivity to griseofulvin or any component; severe liver disease, porphyria (interferes with porphyrin metabolism)

Warnings During long-term therapy, periodic assessment of hepatic, renal, and hematopoietic functions should be performed; avoid exposure to intense sunlight to prevent photosensitivity reactions; hypersensitivity cross-reaction between penicillins and griseofulvin is possible

Adverse Reactions

Central nervous system: Fatigue, confusion, impaired judgment, insomnia, headache, incoordination

Dermatologic: Rash, urticaria, photosensitivity

Gastrointestinal: Nausea, vomiting, diarrhea

Hematologic: Leukopenia, granulocytopenia

Hepatic: Hepatotoxicity

Neuromuscular & skeletal: Paresthesia

Renal: Proteinuria

Miscellaneous: Lupus-like syndrome

Overdosage Symptoms of overdose include lethargy, vertigo, blurred vision, nausea, vomiting, diarrhea

Toxicology Following GI decontamination, supportive care only

Drug Interactions

Decreased effect of anticoagulants, oral contraceptives; decreased effect/levels with barbiturates

Disulfiram-like reaction with alcohol

Mechanism of Action Inhibits fungal cell mitosis at metaphase; binds to human keratin making it resistant to fungal invasion

Pharmacokinetics

Absorption: Ultramicrosize griseofulvin is almost complete; absorption of microsize griseofulvin is variable (25% to 70% of an oral dose); absorption is enhanced by ingestion of a fatty meal

Distribution: Deposited in varying concentrations in the keratin layer of the skin, hair, and nails; only a very small fraction is distributed in the body fluids and tissues

Metabolism: Extensive in the liver

Half-life: 9-22 hours

Time to peak serum concentration: ~4 hours

Elimination: <1% excreted unchanged in urine; also excreted in feces and perspiration

Usual Dosage

Geriatrics and Adults: Oral:

Microsize: 500-1000 mg/day in single or divided doses

Ultramicrosize: 330-375 mg/day in single or divided doses; doses up to 750 mg/day have been used for infections more difficult to eradicate such as tinea unguium and tinea pedis

Duration of therapy depends on the site of infection:
Tinea corporis: 2-4 weeks
Tinea capitis: 4-6 weeks or longer
Tinea pedis: 4-8 weeks
Tinea unguium: 4-6 months

Monitoring Parameters Periodic renal, hepatic, and hematopoietic function tests

Test Interactions False-positive urinary VMA levels

Patient Information Avoid exposure to sunlight, take with fatty meal; if patient gets headache, it usually goes away with continued therapy; may cause dizziness, drowsiness, and impair judgment

Additional Information
Microsize: Fulvicin-U/F®, Grifulvin V, Grisactin®
Ultramicrosize: Fulvicin® P/G, Grisactin® Ultra, Gris-PEG®; GI absorption of ultramicrosize is ~1.5 times that of microsize

Special Geriatric Considerations No specific changes in dosing are needed (see Usual Dosage)

Dosage Forms
Microsize:
Capsule (Grisactin®): 125 mg, 250 mg
Suspension, oral (Grifulvin® V): 125 mg/5 mL with alcohol 0.2% (120 mL)
Tablet:
Fulvicin-U/F®, Grifulvin® V: 250 mg
Fulvicin-U/F®, Grifulvin® V, Grisactin-500®: 500 mg
Ultramicrosize:
Tablet:
Fulvicin® P/G: 165 mg, 330 mg
Fulvicin® P/G, Grisactin® Ultra, Gris-PEG®: 125 mg, 250 mg
Grisactin® Ultra: 330 mg

Gris-PEG® see Griseofulvin *on previous page*

Guaifenesin (gwye FEN e sin)

Brand Names Anti-Tuss® Expectorant [OTC]; Breonesin® [OTC]; Diabetic Tussin EX® [OTC]; Duratuss-G®; Fenesin™; Gee Gee® [OTC]; Genatuss® [OTC]; GG-Cen® [OTC]; Glyate® [OTC]; Glycotuss® [OTC]; Glytuss® [OTC]; Guaifenex LA®; GuaiCough® Expectorant [OTC]; Guiatuss® [OTC]; Halotussin® [OTC]; Humibid® L.A.; Humibid® Sprinkle; Hytuss® [OTC]; Hytuss-2X® [OTC]; Liquibid®; Malotuss® [OTC]; Medi-Tuss® [OTC]; Monafed®; Muco-Fen-LA®; Mytussin® [OTC]; Naldecon® Senior EX [OTC]; Organidin® NR; Pneumomist®; Respa-GF®; Robitussin® [OTC]; Scot-Tussin® [OTC]; Siltussin® [OTC]; Sinumist®-SR Capsulets®; Touro Ex® [OTC]; Tusibron® [OTC]; Uni-tussin® [OTC]

Synonyms GG; Glycerol Guaiacolate

Generic Available Yes

Therapeutic Category Expectorant

Use Symptomatic relief of respiratory conditions characterized by a dry, nonproductive cough and in the presence of mucous in the respiratory tract

Contraindications Hypersensitivity to guaifenesin or any component

Warnings Should not be used for persistent or chronic coughs

Adverse Reactions
Central nervous system: Drowsiness, headache
Dermatologic: Rash
Gastrointestinal: Nausea, vomiting, stomach pain

Overdosage Symptoms of overdose include vomiting

Toxicology Treatment is supportive

Stability Protect from light

Mechanism of Action Thought to act as an expectorant by irritating the gastric mucosa and stimulating respiratory tract secretions, thereby increasing respiratory fluid volumes and decreasing phlegm viscosity

Pharmacokinetics
Absorption: Well absorbed from the GI tract
Metabolism: Undergoes hepatic metabolism (60%)
Elimination: Renal excretion of changed and unchanged drug

Usual Dosage Geriatrics and Adults: Oral: 100-400 mg (5-20 mL) every 4 hours to a maximum of 2.4 g/day (60 mL/day)

Monitoring Parameters Cough, sputum consistency and volume

Test Interactions Decreased uric acid (S)

(Continued)

Guaifenesin *(Continued)*

Patient Information Take with a large quantity of fluid to ensure proper action; if cough persists for more than 1 week, is recumbent, or is accompanied by fever, rash or persistent headache, physician should be consulted

Nursing Implications Administer with large quantity of water to ensure proper action; some products contain alcohol

Additional Information Should not be used for persistent or chronic cough such as that occurring with smoking, asthma, chronic bronchitis, or emphysema or for cough associated with excessive phlegm. There is a lack of convincing studies to document the efficacy of guaifenesin. Guaifenesin is available in various combinations. These include phenylpropanolamine; pseudoephedrine; dextromethorphan; codeine; pseudoephedrine and codeine; phenylpropanolamine and dextromethorphan.

Special Geriatric Considerations See Additional Information

Dosage Forms
Capsule: 200 mg
Capsule, sustained release: 300 mg
Liquid: 200 mg/5 mL (118 mL)
Syrup: 100 mg/5 mL (120 mL, 240 mL, 473 mL, 946 mL)
Tablet: 100 mg, 200 mg
Tablet, sustained release: 600 mg

Guaifenesin and Codeine *(gwye FEN e sin & KOE deen)*

Related Information
Codeine *on page 246*
Guaifenesin *on previous page*

Brand Names Brontex® Liquid; Brontex® Tablet; Cheracol®; Guaituss AC®; Guiatussin® with Codeine; Mytussin® AC; Robafen® AC; Robitussin® A-C; Tussi-Organidin® NR

Synonyms Codeine and Guaifenesin

Generic Available Yes

Therapeutic Category Antitussive; Cough Preparation; Expectorant

Use Temporary control of cough due to minor throat and bronchial irritation

Restrictions C-III (Tablet); C-V (Liquid)

Contraindications Hypersensitivity to guaifenesin, codeine or any component

Warnings Should not be used for chronic productive coughs

Precautions Use with caution in patients who have undergone thoracotomies or laparotomies

Adverse Reactions
Codeine:
Cardiovascular: Palpitations, hypotension, bradycardia, peripheral vasodilation
Central nervous system: CNS depression, increased intracranial pressure
Dermatologic: Pruritus
Endocrine & metabolic: Antidiuretic hormone release
Gastrointestinal: Nausea, vomiting, constipation
Ocular: Miosis
Respiratory: Respiratory depression
Miscellaneous: Physical and psychological dependence with prolonged use, biliary or urinary tract spasm, histamine release
Guaifenesin:
Central nervous system: Drowsiness, headache
Dermatologic: Rash
Gastrointestinal: Nausea, vomiting, stomach pain

Overdosage Symptoms of overdose include lethargy, coma, respiratory depression

Toxicology Naloxone 2 mg I.V. with repeat administration as necessary up to a total of 10 mg

Drug Interactions Increased toxicity: Opiate agonists, general anesthetics, tranquilizers, sedatives, hypnotics, TCAs, MAO inhibitors, alcohol, CNS depressants

Usual Dosage Geriatrics and Adults: Oral: 10 mL every 6-8 hours or one tablet every 6 hours

Monitoring Parameters Cough, sputum consistency and volume, mental status, respiratory status

Patient Information Take with a large quantity of fluid to ensure proper action. May cause drowsiness; avoid CNS depressants and alcohol; do not use for chronic or persistent coughs

Nursing Implications Administer with a large quantity of fluid (see Monitoring Parameters)

Special Geriatric Considerations The elderly may be more sensitive to the CNS depressant effects of codeine; monitor closely for excessive sedation

Dosage Forms

Liquid [C-V] (Brontex®): Guaifenesin 75 mg and codeine phosphate 2.5 mg per 5 mL

Syrup [C-V] (Cheracol®, Guaituss AC®, Guiatussin® with Codeine, Mytussin® AC, Robafen® AC, Robitussin® A-C, Tussi-Organidin® NR): Guaifenesin 100 mg and codeine phosphate 10 mg per 5 mL (60 mL, 120 mL, 480 mL)

Tablet [C-III] (Brontex®): Guaifenesin 300 mg and codeine phosphate 10 mg

Guaifenesin and Dextromethorphan

(gwye FEN e sin & deks troe meth OR fan)

Brand Names Benylin® Expectorant [OTC]; Cheracol® D [OTC]; Clear Tussin® 30; Contac® Cough Formula Liquid [OTC]; Diabetic Tussin DM® [OTC]; Extra Action Cough Syrup [OTC]; Fenesin DM®; Genatuss DM® [OTC]; Glycotuss-dM® [OTC]; Guaifenex DM®; GuiaCough® [OTC]; Guiatuss-DM® [OTC]; Halotussin®-DM [OTC]; Humibid® DM [OTC]; Iobid DM® [OTC]; Kolephrin® GG/DM [OTC]; Monafed® DM; Muco-Fen-DM®; Mytussin® DM [OTC]; Naldecon® Senior DX [OTC]; Phanatuss® Cough Syrup [OTC]; Phenadex® Senior [OTC]; Respa-DM®; Rhinosyn-DMX® [OTC]; Robafen DM® [OTC]; Robitussin®-DM [OTC]; Safe Tussin® 30 [OTC]; Scot-Tussin® Senior Clear [OTC]; Siltussin DM® [OTC]; Synacol® CF [OTC]; Syracol-CF® [OTC]; Tolu-Sed® DM [OTC]; Tusibron-DM® [OTC]; Tuss-DM® [OTC]; Tussi-Organidin® DM NR; Unitussin® DM [OTC]; Vicks® 44E [OTC]; Vicks® Pediatric Formula 44E [OTC]

Synonyms Dextromethorphan and Guaifenesin

Generic Available Yes

Therapeutic Category Antitussive; Cough Preparation; Expectorant

Use Temporary control of cough due to minor throat and bronchial irritation

Contraindications Hypersensitivity to guaifenesin, dextromethorphan or any component; patients receiving monoamine oxidase inhibitors

Warnings Should not be used for chronic or persistent coughs

Precautions Some products contain tartrazine dye (FD & C yellow No 5); others contain aspartame which breaks down to phenylalanine; labels should be checked carefully if these substances are to be avoided

Adverse Reactions

Central nervous system: Drowsiness, headache

Dermatologic: Rash

Gastrointestinal: Nausea, vomiting, constipation

Overdosage Symptoms of overdose include nausea, vomiting, drowsiness, dizziness, blurred vision, nystagmus, ataxia, shallow respiration, urinary retention, stupor, coma, hallucinations

Toxicology CNS depression in overdose may be reversed by naloxone

Drug Interactions

Monoamine oxidase inhibitors, selegiline; coadministration of MAO inhibitors and dextromethorphan has caused hypotension, hyperpyrexia, and coma

Increased toxicity: CNS depressants, alcohol

Stability Protect from light

Usual Dosage Geriatrics and Adults: Oral: 10 mL every 6-8 hours

Monitoring Parameters Cough, sputum consistency and volume, mental status

Patient Information Take with a large quantity of fluid to ensure proper action; if cough persists for more than 1 week, is recumbent, or is accompanied by fever, rash or persistent headache, physician should be consulted; may cause drowsiness; avoid CNS depressants and alcohol

Nursing Implications Administer with a large quantity of fluid (see Monitoring Parameters)

Additional Information Should not be used for persistent or chronic cough such as that occurring with smoking, asthma, chronic bronchitis, or emphysema or for cough associated with excessive phlegm

Special Geriatric Considerations See Warnings and Additional Information

Dosage Forms

Syrup:

Benylin® Expectorant: Guaifenesin 100 mg and dextromethorphan hydrobromide 5 mg per 5 mL (118 mL, 236 mL)

Cheracol® D, Clear Tussin® 30, Genatuss DM®, Mytussin® DM, Robitussin®-DM, Siltussin DM®, Tolu-Sed® DM, Tussi-Organidin® DM NR:

(Continued)

Guaifenesin and Dextromethorphan *(Continued)*

Guaifenesin 100 mg and dextromethorphan hydrobromide 10 mg per 5 mL (5 mL, 10 mL, 120 mL, 240 mL, 360 mL, 480 mL, 3780 mL)

Contac® Cough Formula Liquid: Guaifenesin 67 mg and dextromethorphan hydrobromide 10 mg per 5 mL (120 mL)

Extra Action Cough Syrup, GuiaCough®, Guiatuss DM®, Halotussin® DM, Rhinosyn-DMX®, Tusbron-DM®, Uni-Tussin® DM: Guaifenesin 100 mg and dextromethorphan hydrobromide 15 mg per 5 mL (120 mL, 240 mL, 480 mL)

Kolephrin® GG/DM: Guaifenesin 150 mg and dextromethorphan hydrobromide 10 mg per 5 mL (120 mL)

Naldecon® Senior DX: Guaifenesin 200 mg and dextromethorphan hydrobromide 15 mg per 5 mL (118 mL, 480 mL)

Phanatuss®: Guaifenesin 85 mg and dextromethorphan hydrobromide 10 mg per 5 mL

Vicks® 44E: Guaifenesin 66.7 mg and dextromethorphan hydrobromide 6.7 mg per 5 mL

Tablet:

Extended release

Guaifenex DM®, Iobid DM®, Fenesin DM®, Humibid® DM, Respa-DM®: Guaifenesin 600 mg and dextromethorphan hydrobromide 30 mg

Glycotuss-dM®: Guaifenesin 100 mg and dextromethorphan hydrobromide 10 mg

Queltuss®: Guaifenesin 100 mg and dextromethorphan hydrobromide 15 mg

Syracol-CF®: Guaifenesin 200 mg and dextromethorphan hydrobromide 15 mg

Tuss-DM®: Guaifenesin 200 mg and dextromethorphan hydrobromide 10 mg

Guaifenex DM® *see* Guaifenesin and Dextromethorphan *on previous page*
Guaifenex LA® *see* Guaifenesin *on page 437*
Guaituss AC® *see* Guaifenesin and Codeine *on page 438*

Guanabenz (GWAHN a benz)

Brand Names Wytensin®
Generic Available No
Therapeutic Category Alpha-Adrenergic Agonist
Use Management of hypertension
Contraindications Hypersensitivity to guanabenz or any component
Precautions Do not abruptly discontinue this medication; use with caution in patients with severe coronary insufficiency, recent myocardial infarction, severe renal or hepatic impairment
Adverse Reactions
Central nervous system: Drowsiness, dizziness, headache
Gastrointestinal: Xerostomia
Neuromuscular & skeletal: Weakness
Overdosage Symptoms of overdose include CNS depression, hypothermia, apnea, lethargy, diarrhea, hypotension, bradycardia
Toxicology Treatment is primarily supportive and symptomatic. Hypotension usually responds to I.V. fluids or Trendelenburg positioning. If unresponsive to these measures the use of a parenteral vasoconstrictor may be required (eg, norepinephrine 0.1-0.2 mcg/kg/minute titrated to response). Naloxone may be utilized in treating the hypotension, CNS depression and/or apnea and should be given I.V. 0.4-2 mg, with repeats as needed. Atropine 15 mcg/kg I.V. or I.M. may be needed for symptomatic bradycardia.
Drug Interactions
Decreased hypotensive effect of guanabenz with tricyclic antidepressants
Increased effect: Other hypotensive agents
Mechanism of Action Stimulates alpha$_2$-adrenoreceptors in the brain stem, thus activating an inhibitory neuron, resulting in reduced sympathetic outflow, producing a decrease in vasomotor tone and heart rate
Pharmacodynamics Onset of antihypertensive effect: Within 60 minutes
Pharmacokinetics
Absorption: Oral: ~75% administration
Metabolism: Extensive
Half-life: 7-10 hours
Elimination: <1% of dose excreted as unchanged drug in urine
Usual Dosage Oral:
Geriatrics: Initial: 4 mg once daily, increase every 1-2 weeks

Adults: Initial: 4 mg twice daily, increase by 4-8 mg/day every 1-2 weeks; usual dosage range: 4-32 mg twice daily

Monitoring Parameters Blood pressure, standing and sitting/supine

Test Interactions Increased sodium (S)

Patient Information May cause drowsiness; rise from sitting/lying position carefully, may cause dizziness; do not discontinue without notifying physician

Nursing Implications Monitor for orthostasis; do not abruptly discontinue

Additional Information Guanabenz is considered an alternate to clonidine; it causes less sodium retention than clonidine or methyldopa

Special Geriatric Considerations Because of its CNS adverse effects, guanabenz is not considered a drug of choice for the treatment of hypertension in the elderly.

Dosage Forms Tablet, as acetate: 4 mg, 8 mg

Guanadrel (GWAHN a drel)

Brand Names Hylorel®

Generic Available No

Therapeutic Category Alpha-Adrenergic Blocking Agent, Oral

Use Management of hypertension usually combined with a diuretic

Contraindications Known hypersensitivity to guanadrel, pheochromocytoma, congestive heart failure, patients taking MAO inhibitors

Warnings Use cautiously in asthmatic patients; orthostatic hypotension occurs frequently

Precautions Salt and water retention may occur; use cautiously in patients with peptic ulcers

Adverse Reactions

Cardiovascular: Orthostatic hypotension, palpitations, chest pain, peripheral edema

Central nervous system: Fatigue, dizziness, faintness, headache, drowsiness

Gastrointestinal: Diarrhea, increased bowel movements

Genitourinary: Ejaculation disturbances, nocturia

Neuromuscular & skeletal: Weakness

Ocular: Blurred vision

Respiratory: Shortness of breath on exertion

Overdosage Symptoms of overdose include hypotension, blurred vision, dizziness, syncope

Toxicology Treatment is primarily supportive and symptomatic. Hypotension usually responds to I.V. fluids or Trendelenburg positioning. If unresponsive to these measures the use of a parenteral vasoconstrictor may be required (eg, norepinephrine 0.1-0.2 mcg/kg/minute titrated to response).

Drug Interactions

Decreased effect with tricyclic antidepressants, indirect-acting amines (ephedrine, phenylpropanolamine), phenothiazines

Increased toxicity of direct-acting amines (epinephrine, norepinephrine)

Increased effect: Beta-blockers, vasodilators

Mechanism of Action Acts as a false neurotransmitter that blocks the adrenergic actions of norepinephrine; it displaces norepinephrine from its presynaptic storage granules and thus exposes it to degradation; it thereby produces a reduction in total peripheral resistance and therefore blood pressure

Pharmacodynamics

Peak effect: Within 4-6 hours

Duration of action: 4-14 hours

Pharmacokinetics

Absorption: Oral: Rapid

Distribution: Hydrophilic and, therefore, does not cross the blood-brain barrier

Protein binding: 20%

Half-life:

Initial: 1-4 hours

Terminal: 5-45 hours

Time to peak serum concentration: Within 1.5-2 hours

Elimination: Biphasic; excreted in urine 40% as unchanged drug

Usual Dosage

Geriatrics: Initial: 5 mg once daily

Adults: Initial: 10 mg/day (5 mg twice daily); adjust dosage until blood pressure is controlled, usual dosage: 20-75 mg/day, given twice daily

Dosing interval in renal impairment:

Cl_{cr} 10-50 mL/minute: Administer every 12-24 hours

Cl_{cr} <10 mL/minute: Administer every 24-48 hours

Monitoring Parameters Blood pressure, standing and sitting/supine

(Continued)

Guanadrel *(Continued)*

Test Interactions Increased sodium (S)

Patient Information Change positions slowly; do not take any over-the-counter or prescription cold medications without consulting your physician

Nursing Implications Monitor for orthostasis

Additional Information Considered an alternative to guanethidine

Special Geriatric Considerations Because of its CNS adverse effects and high incidence of orthostasis, guanadrel is not considered a drug of choice for the treatment of hypertension in the elderly; if used, adjust dose for renal function in elderly

Dosage Forms Tablet, as sulfate: 10 mg, 25 mg

Guanethidine *(gwahn ETH i deen)*

Brand Names Ismelin®

Generic Available Yes

Therapeutic Category Alpha-Adrenergic Blocking Agent, Oral

Use Treatment of moderate to severe hypertension

Contraindications Pheochromocytoma, MAO inhibitors, hypersensitivity to guanethidine or any component

Warnings Should be withdrawn 2 weeks prior to surgery to decrease chance of vascular collapse and cardiac arrest during anesthesia

Precautions Orthostatic hypotension can occur frequently; avoid the use of guanethidine in the elderly; use with caution in patients with CHF, asthma, or peptic ulcer disease

Adverse Reactions
Cardiovascular: Orthostatic hypotension, edema, syncope
Central nervous system: Dizziness, headache
Gastrointestinal: Diarrhea, increased bowel movements, xerostomia
Genitourinary: Nocturia, ejaculation disturbances
Neuromuscular & skeletal: Weakness
Ocular: Blurred vision
Respiratory: Shortness of breath

Overdosage Symptoms of overdose include hypotension, blurred vision, dizziness, syncope

Toxicology Hypotension usually responds to I.V. fluids or Trendelenburg positioning. If unresponsive to these measures the use of a parenteral vasoconstrictor may be required (eg, norepinephrine 0.1-0.2 mcg/kg/minute titrated to response). Treatment is primarily supportive and symptomatic.

Drug Interactions
Decreased effect with tricyclic antidepressants, indirect-acting amines (ephedrine, phenylpropanolamine), phenothiazines, MAO inhibitors
Increased toxicity of direct-acting amines (epinephrine, norepinephrine)

Mechanism of Action Acts as a false neurotransmitter that blocks the adrenergic actions of norepinephrine; it displaces norepinephrine from its presynaptic storage granules and thus exposes it to degradation; it thereby produces a reduction in total peripheral resistance and therefore blood pressure

Pharmacodynamics
Onset of action: Within 0.5-2 hours
Peak antihypertensive effect: Within 6-8 hours
Duration: 24-48 hours

Pharmacokinetics
Absorption: Oral: Irregular (3% to 55)
Metabolism: Hepatic to inactive metabolites, followed by 25% to 60% of a dose
Half-life: 5-10 days
Elimination: Unchanged in urine, small amounts also appear in feces

Usual Dosage Oral:
Geriatrics: Initial: 5 mg once daily
Adults: Initial: 10 mg; increase by 10-25 mg every 5-7 days; usual dose: 25-50 mg once daily

Monitoring Parameters Blood pressure, standing and sitting/supine

Test Interactions Increased sodium (S); decreased catecholamines (U)

Patient Information May cause drowsiness; rise from sitting/lying carefully, may cause dizziness; do not take any OTC or prescription cough or cold medication without consulting physician

Nursing Implications Tablet may be crushed; monitor for orthostasis

Special Geriatric Considerations Because of its CNS adverse effects and high incidence of orthostatic hypotension, guanethidine is not considered a drug of choice for treatment of hypertension in the elderly.

Dosage Forms Tablet, as monosulfate: 10 mg, 25 mg

Guanfacine (GWAHN fa seen)
Brand Names Tenex®
Generic Available No
Therapeutic Category Alpha-Adrenergic Agonist
Use Management of hypertension
Contraindications Hypersensitivity to guanfacine or any component
Precautions Use with caution in patients with severe coronary insufficiency, recent myocardial infarction, severe renal or hepatic impairment
Adverse Reactions
    Central nervous system: Drowsiness, dizziness, headache
    Gastrointestinal: Nausea, xerostomia, constipation
    Neuromuscular & skeletal: Leg cramps, weakness
    Respiratory: Dyspnea
Overdosage Symptoms of overdose include CNS depression, hypothermia, apnea, lethargy, diarrhea, hypotension, bradycardia
Toxicology Treatment is primarily supportive and symptomatic. Hypotension usually responds to I.V. fluids or Trendelenburg positioning. If unresponsive to these measures the use of a parenteral vasoconstrictor may be required (eg, norepinephrine 0.1-0.2 mcg/kg/minute titrated to response). Naloxone may be utilized in treating the hypotension, CNS depression and/or apnea and should be given I.V. 0.4-2 mg, with repeats as needed. Atropine 15 mcg/kg I.V. or I.M. may be needed for symptomatic bradycardia.
Drug Interactions
    Decreased hypotensive effect of guanfacine with tricyclic antidepressants
    Increased effect: Other hypotensive agents
Mechanism of Action Acts as a false neurotransmitter that blocks the adrenergic actions of norepinephrine; it displaces norepinephrine form its presynaptic storage granules and thus exposes it to degradation; it thereby produces a reduction in total peripheral resistance and therefore blood pressure
Pharmacodynamics
    Peak effect: Within 8-11 hours
    Duration: 24 hours
Pharmacokinetics
    Protein binding: 20% to 30%
    Metabolism: In the liver to glucuronide and sulfate metabolites
    Bioavailability: 80% to 100%
    Half-life: 17 hours
    Time to peak serum concentration: Oral: 1-4 hours
    Elimination: Renal excretion of changed and unchanged drug (30%)
Usual Dosage Geriatrics and Adults: 1 mg usually at bedtime, may increase if needed; 1 mg/day is most common dose; adverse reactions increase with doses >3 mg/day
Monitoring Parameters Blood pressure, standing and sitting/supine
Patient Information May cause drowsiness, dizziness; do not discontinue this medication without consulting your physician; take at bedtime
Nursing Implications Administer dose at bedtime; observe for orthostasis
Additional Information Usually given with a thiazide diuretic
Special Geriatric Considerations Because of adverse effects such as CNS depression, dry mouth, and constipation, guanfacine may not be considered a drug of choice in the elderly.
Dosage Forms Tablet, as hydrochloride: 1 mg

GuiaCough® [OTC] *see* Guaifenesin and Dextromethorphan *on page 439*
GuiaCough® Expectorant [OTC] *see* Guaifenesin *on page 437*
Guiatuss® [OTC] *see* Guaifenesin *on page 437*
Guiatuss-DM® [OTC] *see* Guaifenesin and Dextromethorphan *on page 439*
Guiatussin® with Codeine *see* Guaifenesin and Codeine *on page 438*
G-well® *see* Lindane *on page 538*
Gynecort® [OTC] *see* Hydrocortisone *on page 462*
Gyne-Lotrimin® [OTC] *see* Clotrimazole *on page 242*
Gynogen L.A.® Injection *see* Estradiol *on page 350*
Habitrol™ Patch *see* Nicotine *on page 669*

Halazepam (hal AZ e pam)
Related Information
    Antacid Drug Interactions *on page 1096*
    Anxiolytic/Hypnotic Use in Long-Term Care Facilities *on page 1099*
(Continued)

Halazepam *(Continued)*

Benzodiazepines Comparison *on page 1024*
Federal OBRA Regulations Recommended Maximum Doses - Anxiolytics *on page 1057*
Federal OBRA Regulations Recommended Maximum Doses - Hypnotics *on page 1057*

Brand Names Paxipam®

Generic Available No

Therapeutic Category Antianxiety Agent; Benzodiazepine

Use Management of anxiety disorders; short-term relief of the symptoms of anxiety

Restrictions C-IV

Contraindications Hypersensitivity to halazepam or any component, cross-sensitivity with other benzodiazepines may exist; avoid using in patients with pre-existing CNS depression, severe uncontrolled pain, or narrow-angle glaucoma

Warnings May cause drug dependency; avoid abrupt discontinuance in patients with prolonged therapy or seizure disorders

Precautions Use with caution in patients with a history of drug dependence

Adverse Reactions
Central nervous system: Drowsiness, confusion, dizziness, ataxia, amnesia, slurred speech, paradoxical excitement or rage
Neuromuscular & skeletal: Impaired coordination
Ocular: Blurred vision, diplopia
Respiratory: Decrease in respiratory rate, apnea, laryngospasm
Miscellaneous: Physical and psychological dependence with prolonged use cardiac arrest

Overdosage Symptoms of overdose include somnolence, confusion, coma, and diminished reflexes

Toxicology Treatment for benzodiazepine overdose is supportive; rarely is mechanical ventilation required; flumazenil has been shown to selectively block the binding of benzodiazepines to CNS receptors, resulting in a reversal of benzodiazepine-induced sedation; however, its use may not alter the course of overdose

Drug Interactions
Decreased effect: Benzodiazepines may decrease the effect of levodopa
Decreased metabolism: Cimetidine, fluoxetine
Increased metabolism: Rifampin
Increased toxicity: CNS depressants, alcohol

Mechanism of Action Benzodiazepines appear to potentiate the effects of GABA and other inhibitory neurotransmitters by binding to specific benzodiazepine-receptor sites in various areas of the CNS

Pharmacodynamics
Onset of action: 2-3 hours
Studies have shown that the elderly are more sensitive to the effects of benzodiazepines as compared to younger adults

Pharmacokinetics
Half-life:
Parent: 14 hours
Active metabolite (desmethyldiazepam): 50-100 hours
Peak serum concentration: 1-3 hours
Elimination: <1% excreted unchanged in urine

Usual Dosage Oral:
Geriatrics: 20 mg 1-2 times/day
Adults: 20-40 mg 3 or 4 times/day

Monitoring Parameters Respiratory, cardiovascular and mental status, symptoms of anxiety

Patient Information Avoid alcohol and other CNS depressants; may cause drowsiness; avoid activities needing good psychomotor coordination until CNS effects are known; may cause physical or psychological dependence; avoid abrupt discontinuation after prolonged use

Nursing Implications Assist patient with ambulation, monitor for alertness

Additional Information Halazepam offers no significant advantage over other benzodiazepines

Special Geriatric Considerations Much of halazepam's pharmacologic activity can be attributed to its long-acting metabolite, desmethyldiazepam; updated interpretive guidelines issued by the Health Care Financing Administration discourage the use of this agent in elderly residents of long-term care facilities. Long-acting benzodiazepines have been associated with falls in the elderly; therefore, halazepam is not considered a drug of choice (see Pharmacodynamics).

Dosage Forms Tablet: 20 mg, 40 mg

Halcinonide (hal SIN oh nide)

Related Information

Corticosteroids Comparison, Topical *on page 1030*

Brand Names Halog®; Halog®-E

Generic Available No

Therapeutic Category Corticosteroid, Topical (Very High Potency)

Use Relief of the inflammatory and pruritic manifestations of corticosteroid-responsive dermatoses (very high potency topical corticosteroid)

Contraindications Viral, fungal, or tubercular skin lesions, known hypersensitivity to halcinonide or any component

Precautions Systemic absorption of topical corticosteroids has produced reversible HPA axis suppression. This is more likely to occur when the preparation is used on large surfaces or denuded areas for prolonged periods of time or with an occlusive dressing.

Adverse Reactions

Dermatologic: Acne, hypopigmentation, allergic dermatitis, maceration of the skin, skin atrophy, striae, miliaria, telangiectasia

Endocrine & metabolic: HPA suppression, Cushing's syndrome, growth retardation

Local: Burning, itching, irritation, dryness, folliculitis, hypertrichosis

Miscellaneous: Secondary infection

Mechanism of Action Topical corticosteroids have anti-inflammatory, antipruritic, vasoconstrictive, and antiproliferative actions

Pharmacokinetics Absorption: Percutaneous absorption varies by location of topical application and the use of occlusive dressings

Usual Dosage Geriatrics and Adults: Topical: Apply sparingly 2-3 times/day

Monitoring Parameters Relief of symptoms

Patient Information Use only as prescribed and for no longer than the period prescribed; apply sparingly in a thin film and rub in lightly; avoid contact with eyes; notify physician if condition persists or worsens

Nursing Implications Apply sparingly, do not use on open or weeping lesion

Additional Information Considered a very high potency steroid; avoid use on face

Special Geriatric Considerations Due to age-related changes in skin, limit use of topical glucocorticosteroids (see Precautions)

Dosage Forms

Cream (Halog®): 0.025% (15 g, 60 g, 240 g); 0.1% (15 g, 30 g, 60 g, 240 g)

Cream, emollient base (Halog®-E) : 0.1% (15 g, 30 g, 60 g)

Ointment, topical (Halog®): 0.1% (15 g, 30 g, 60 g, 240 g)

Solution (Halog®): 0.1% (20 mL, 60 mL)

Halcion® *see* Triazolam *on page 952*

Haldol® *see* Haloperidol *on next page*

Haldol® Decanoate *see* Haloperidol *on next page*

Halenol® [OTC] *see* Acetaminophen *on page 16*

Haley's M-O® [OTC] *see* Magnesium Hydroxide and Mineral Oil Emulsion *on page 565*

Halfprin® 81® [OTC] *see* Aspirin *on page 84*

Halobetasol (hal oh BAY ta sol)

Related Information

Corticosteroids Comparison, Topical *on page 1030*

Brand Names Ultravate™

Generic Available No

Therapeutic Category Corticosteroid, Topical (Super High Potency)

Use Short-term relief (<2 weeks) of inflammatory and pruritic manifestations of corticosteroid-response dermatoses [super high potency topical corticosteroid]

Contraindications Hypersensitivity to halobetasol or any component; viral, fungal, or tubercular skin lesions

Precautions Systemic absorption of topical corticosteroids has produced reversible HPA axis suppression. This is more likely to occur when the preparation is used on large surfaces or denuded areas for prolonged periods of time or with an occlusive dressing. Should not be used for longer than 2 weeks; should not be used on the face, axillae, or groin.

(Continued)

445

Halobetasol *(Continued)*

Adverse Reactions

Dermatologic: Acne, hypopigmentation, allergic dermatitis, maceration of the skin, skin atrophy, striae, miliaria, telangiectasia

Endocrine & metabolic: HPA suppression, Cushing's syndrome, growth retardation

Local: Burning, itching, irritation, dryness, folliculitis, hypertrichosis

Miscellaneous: Secondary infection

Mechanism of Action Topical corticosteroids have anti-inflammatory, antipruritic, vasoconstrictive, and antiproliferative actions

Pharmacokinetics Absorption: Percutaneous absorption varies by location of topical application and the use of occlusive dressings

Usual Dosage Geriatrics and Adults: Topical: Apply in thin layer once or twice daily; treatment should not exceed 2 consecutive weeks and total dosage should not exceed 50 g/week

Monitoring Parameters Relief of symptoms

Patient Information Use only as prescribed and for no longer than the period prescribed; apply sparingly in a thin film and rub in lightly; avoid contact with eyes; notify physician if condition persists or worsens; do not use longer than 2 weeks

Nursing Implications Apply sparingly; do not use on open or weeping lesions

Additional Information Considered a super high potency steroid; avoid use on face

Special Geriatric Considerations Due to age-related changes in skin, limit use of topical glucocorticosteroids (see Precautions)

Dosage Forms

Halobetasol propionate:

Cream: 0.05% (15 g, 45 g)

Ointment, topical: 0.05% (15 g, 45 g)

Halog® *see Halcinonide on previous page*

Halog®-E *see Halcinonide on previous page*

Haloperidol *(ha loe PER i dole)*

Related Information

Antipsychotic Agents Comparison *on page 1023*

Antipsychotic Medication Guidelines *on page 1076*

Federal OBRA Regulations Recommended Maximum Doses - Antipsychotics *on page 1056*

I.V. Push Recommended Guidelines *on page 1083*

Brand Names Haldol®; Haldol® Decanoate

Generic Available Yes

Therapeutic Category Antiemetic; Antipsychotic Agent; Neuroleptic Agent

Use Management of psychotic disorders; nonpsychotic symptoms associated with dementia in elderly, Tourette's syndrome, Huntington's chorea (see Special Geriatric Considerations)

Unlabeled uses: Antiemetic (small doses), phencyclidine psychosis

Contraindications Hypersensitivity to haloperidol or any component; narrow-angle glaucoma, bone marrow suppression, CNS depression, severe liver or cardiac disease, subcortical brain damage; circulatory collapse; severe hypotension or hypertension

Warnings

Tardive dyskinesia: Prevalence rate may be 40% in elderly; elderly women especially at risk; embarrassment from dyskinesias may lead to greater social isolation; development of the syndrome and the irreversible nature are proportional to duration and total cumulative dose over time. May be reversible if diagnosed early in therapy; intermittent use of antipsychotics (not proven use) helps decrease total cumulative dose.

EPS: Extrapyramidal reactions are more common in elderly with up to 50% developing these reactions after age 60. These reactions may be more common in dementia patients. Drug-induced **Parkinson's syndrome** occurs often. Discontinuation usually resolves symptoms but may take weeks to months (12+) to clear. **Akathisia** is the most common EPS reaction in elderly. The symptoms of motor restlessness are difficult to diagnose in demented elderly; increased nervousness, assertiveness, restlessness with constant movement may indicate this adverse event. Consider decreasing dose if antipsychotic to treat as well as diagnose problem; usually see this reaction within 2-3 months of initiating antipsychotic drug.

Anticholinergic effects: These side effects most common with low potency antipsychotics (eg, thioridazine, chlorpromazine). CNS toxicity occurs more frequently and severely in elderly; increased confusion, memory loss, psychotic behavior, and agitation frequently occur as a consequence of anticholinergic effects to antipsychotic agents. Peripheral anticholinergic action troublesome to elderly; most peripheral anticholinergic effects last only 2-3 weeks (see Adverse Reactions).

Orthostatic hypotension: More common with low potency agents (eg, thioridazine, chlorpromazine, and clozapine) but of concern with all antipsychotic agents; orthostasis due to alpha-receptor blockade by antipsychotic agents. Elderly present many risk factors for orthostatic hypotension: blunted baroreceptor reflexes, decreased vascular tone, decreased vascular volume, and possible presence of cardiac diseases which result in decreased cardiac output.

Sedation: Common side effect with antipsychotic therapy; should not be used as a hypnotic unless insomnia is associated with target behavior symptoms treated with antipsychotic medications (see Special Geriatric Considerations). Anecdotal reports suggesting antipsychotic sedation in nonpsychotic patients is extremely unpleasant due to feelings of depersonalization, derealization, and dysphoria. Due to the long duration of action with antipsychotic drugs, these reactions may last up to 24 hours and result in decreased daytime function.

Cardiac toxicity: Life-threatening arrhythmias have occurred at therapeutic doses of antipsychotics. Thioridazine more commonly demonstrates EKG changes than other antipsychotics; suggested to use high potency antipsychotic agents (ie, haloperidol) in patients with cardiac conduction defects.

Precautions Watch for hypotension when administering I.M. or I.V.; use with caution in patients with cardiovascular disease, seizures, and Parkinson's disease; benefits of therapy must be weighed against risks of therapy; decanoate form should never be given I.V.

Adverse Reactions

Anticholinergic: Xerostomia (problem for denture user), urinary retention, constipation, adynamic ileus, overflow incontinence, blurred vision

Cardiovascular: Hypotension (especially orthostatic), tachycardia, arrhythmias, abnormal T waves with prolonged ventricular repolarization, EKG changes

Central nervous system: Sedation, drowsiness, restlessness, anxiety, extrapyramidal reactions, dystonic reactions, pseudoparkinsonian signs and symptoms, tardive dyskinesia, neuroleptic malignant syndrome, seizures, altered central temperature regulation

Dermatologic: Photosensitivity (rare)

Endocrine & metabolic: Amenorrhea, galactorrhea, gynecomastia,

Gastrointestinal: Constipation, adynamic ileus, GI upset, xerostomia (problem for denture user), weight gain

Genitourinary: Urinary retention, overflow incontinence, priapism, sexual dysfunction (up to 60%)

Hematologic: Agranulocytosis, leukopenia (usually in patients with large doses for prolonged periods)

Hepatic: Cholestatic jaundice

Ocular: Blurred vision, retinal pigmentation, decreased visual acuity (may be irreversible)

Overdosage Symptoms of overdose include deep sleep, coma, extrapyramidal symptoms, abnormal involuntary muscle movements, hypotension or hypertension; agitation, restlessness, fever, hypothermia or hyperthermia, seizures, cardiac arrhythmias, EKG changes

Toxicology Following initiation of essential overdose management, toxic symptom treatment and supportive treatment should be initiated. Hypotension usually responds to I.V. fluids or Trendelenburg positioning. If unresponsive to these measures the use of a parenteral inotrope may be required (eg, norepinephrine 0.1-0.2 mcg/kg/minute titrated to response). Do not use epinephrine. Seizures commonly respond to diazepam (I.V. 5-10 mg bolus in adults every 15 minutes if needed up to a total of 30 mg) or to phenytoin or phenobarbital. Also critical cardiac arrhythmias often respond to I.V. phenytoin (15 mg/kg up to 1 g), while other antiarrhythmics can be used. Neuroleptics often cause extrapyramidal symptoms (eg, dystonic reactions) requiring management with diphenhydramine 1-2 mg/kg up to a maximum of 50 mg I.M. or I.V. slow push followed by a maintenance dose for 48-72 hours. When these reactions are unresponsive to diphenhydramine, benztropine mesylate (Continued)

Haloperidol *(Continued)*

I.V. 1-2 mg may be effective. These agents are generally effective within 2-5 minutes.

Drug Interactions

Concurrent use with lithium has occasionally caused acute encephalopathy-like syndrome

Carbamazepine, barbiturates, phenytoin may decrease serum concentration of haloperidol

Fluoxetine reported to have EPS when administered with haloperidol

Guanethidine's hypotensive effect is decreased with haloperidol

Lithium administration with haloperidol may increase disorientation

Methyldopa may increase antipsychotic effect or cause psychosis with haloperidol

Propranolol administered with haloperidol may increase hypotensive effect of propranolol

Tricyclic antidepressants may have serum concentrations increased with concomitant administration with haloperidol

Stability Protect oral dosage forms from light

Mechanism of Action Blocks postsynaptic mesolimbic dopaminergic D_1 and D_2 receptors in the brain; exhibits a strong alpha-adrenergic blocking and anticholinergic effect, depresses the release of hypothalamic and hypophyseal hormones; believed to depress the reticular activating system thus affecting basal metabolism, body temperature, wakefulness, vasomotor tone, and emesis

Pharmacodynamics

Onset of action: I.M.: Within 1 hour following administration

Peak serum concentrations: Oral: Occur in 2-4 hours

Decanoate form: Duration of action: ~3 weeks

Pharmacokinetics

Absorption: Oral: May be affected by the inherent anticholinergic action on the gastrointestinal tissue causing variable absorption. Absorption from tablets is erratic with less variation seen with solutions. These agents are widely distributed in tissues with CNS concentrations exceeding that of plasma due to their lipophilic characteristics.

Protein binding: 90%; antipsychotic agents are bound 90% to 99% to plasma proteins; highly bound to brain and lung tissue and other tissues with a high blood perfusion

Metabolism: Metabolized in the liver to inactive compounds; substrate and inhibitor CYP2D6

Half-life: 20 hours

Elimination half-life: Antipsychotic range: 20-40 hours which may be extended in elderly due to decline in oxidative hepatic reactions (phase I) with age

Elimination: 33% to 40% excreted in the urine within 5 days; an additional 15% is excreted in the feces; elimination occurs through hepatic metabolism (oxidation) where numerous active metabolites are produced; active metabolites excreted in urine

The biologic effect of a single dose persists for 24 hours. When the patient has accommodated to initial side effects (sedation), once daily dosing is possible due to the long half-life of antipsychotics.

Steady-state plasma concentrations are achieved in 4-7 days; therefore, if possible, do not make dose adjustments more than once in a 7-day period. Due to the long half-lives of antipsychotics, as needed (prn) use is ineffective since repeated doses are necessary to achieve therapeutic tissue concentrations in the CNS.

Usual Dosage

Geriatrics (nonpsychotic patient; dementia behavior): Initial: 0.25-0.5 mg 1-2 times/day; increase dose at 4- to 7-day intervals by 0.25-0.5 mg/day; increase dosing intervals (bid, tid, etc) as necessary to control response or side effects; maximum daily dose: 4 mg; gradual increases (titration) may prevent some side effects or decrease their severity

Adults (do not administer I.V.):

Oral: 0.5-5 mg 2-3 times/day; usual maximum: 100 mg/day

I.M. (as lactate): 2-5 mg every 4-8 hours as needed

I.M. (as decanoate): Initial: 10-15 times the daily oral dose administered at 4-week intervals

Not dialyzable (0% to 5%)

Monitoring Parameters Orthostatic blood pressures; tremors, gait changes, abnormal movement in trunk, neck, buccal area, or extremities; monitor target behaviors for which the agent is given

Reference Range Therapeutic: 5-20 ng/mL (SI: 10-30 nmol/L) (psychotic disorders - less for Tourette's and mania); Toxic: >42 µg/mL (SI: >84 nmol/L). Therapeutic levels are controversial; dosed by response most commonly.

Test Interactions Decreased cholesterol (S)

Patient Information Oral concentrate must be diluted in 2-4 oz of liquid (water, fruit juice, carbonated drinks, milk, or pudding); do not take antacid within 1 hour of taking drug; avoid alcohol; avoid excess sun exposure (use sun block); may cause drowsiness, rise slowly from recumbent position; use of supportive stockings may help prevent orthostatic hypotension

Nursing Implications Dilute oral concentrate with water or juice before administration; avoid skin contact with oral suspension or solution; may cause contact dermatitis; monitor orthostatic blood pressures 3-5 days after initiation of therapy or a dose increase; observe for tremor and abnormal movement or posturing (extrapyramidal symptoms)

Special Geriatric Considerations See Warnings.

Many elderly patients receive antipsychotic medications for inappropriate nonpsychotic behavior. Before initiating antipsychotic medication, the clinician should investigate any possible reversible cause; any stress or stress from any disease can cause acute "confusion" or worsening of baseline nonpsychotic behavior. Most commonly acute changes in behavior are due to increases in drug dose or addition of new drug to regimen; fluid electrolyte loss; infections; and changes in environment.

Any changes in disease status in any organ system can result in behavior changes.

In the treatment of agitated, demented, elderly patients, authors of meta-analysis of controlled trials of the response to the traditional antipsychotics (phenothiazines, butyrophenones) in controlling agitation have concluded that the use of neuroleptics results in a response rate of 18%. Clearly neuroleptic therapy for behavior control should be limited with frequent attempts to withdraw the agent given for behavior control.

Dosage Forms
Injection, as decanoate: 50 mg/mL (1 mL, 5 mL); 100 mg/mL (1 mL, 5 mL)
Haloperidol lactate:
Concentrate, oral: 2 mg/mL (5 mL, 10 mL, 15 mL, 120 mL, 240 mL)
Injection: 5 mg/mL (1 mL, 2 mL, 2.5 mL, 10 mL)
Tablet: 0.5 mg, 1 mg, 2 mg, 5 mg, 10 mg, 20 mg

References
Peabody CA, Warner MD, Whiteford HA, et al, "Neuroleptics and the Elderly," *J Am Geriatr Soc,* 1987, 35(3):233-8.
Risse SC and Barnes R, "Pharmacologic Treatment of Agitation Associated With Dementia," *J Am Geriatr Soc,* 1986, 34(5):368-76.
Saltz BL, Woerner MG, Kane JM, et al, "Prospective Study of Tardive Dyskinesia Incidence in the Elderly," *JAMA,* 1991, 266(17):2402-6.
Seifert RD, "Therapeutic Drug Monitoring: Psychotropic Drugs," *J Pharm Pract,* 1984, 6:403-16.

Halotussin® [OTC] *see* Guaifenesin *on page 437*

Halotussin®-DM [OTC] *see* Guaifenesin and Dextromethorphan *on page 439*

Haltran® [OTC] *see* Ibuprofen *on page 475*

Havrix® *see* Hepatitis A Vaccine *on page 451*

HBIG *see* Hepatitis B Immune Globulin *on page 452*

H-BIG® *see* Hepatitis B Immune Globulin *on page 452*

25-HCC *see* Calcifediol *on page 139*

HCTZ *see* Hydrochlorothiazide *on page 458*

HDCV *see* Rabies Virus Vaccine *on page 819*

Heavy Mineral Oil *see* Mineral Oil *on page 628*

Hemocyte® [OTC] *see* Ferrous Fumarate *on page 376*

Hemril-HC® Uniserts® *see* Hydrocortisone *on page 462*

Heparin (HEP a rin)
Related Information
I.V. Medication Recommendations *on page 1080*
I.V. Push Recommended Guidelines *on page 1083*
Brand Names Hep-Lock®
Synonyms Heparin Lock Flush
Generic Available Yes
Therapeutic Category Anticoagulant
Use Prophylaxis and treatment of thromboembolic disorders
Contraindications Hypersensitivity to heparin or any component; severe thrombocytopenia, subacute bacterial endocarditis, suspected intracranial (Continued)

449

Heparin *(Continued)*

hemorrhage, shock, severe hypotension, uncontrollable bleeding (unless secondary to disseminated intravascular coagulation)

Warnings Some preparations contain sulfite which may cause allergic reactions.

Precautions Use with caution as hemorrhage may occur; risk factors for hemorrhage include I.M. injections, peptic ulcer disease, intermittent I.V. injections (vs continuous I.V. infusion), increased capillary permeability, severe renal, hepatic, or biliary disease, and indwelling catheters

Adverse Reactions

Central nervous system: Fever, headache, chills

Dermatologic: Urticaria

Gastrointestinal: Nausea, vomiting

Hematologic: Hemorrhage, thrombocytopenia

Hepatic: Elevation of liver enzymes

Local: Irritation, ulceration, cutaneous necrosis has been rarely reported with deep S.C. injections

Neuromuscular & skeletal: Osteoporosis

Overdosage Symptoms of overdose include hemorrhage, nose bleeds, hematuria, and melena are signs of overdose

Toxicology Antidote is protamine; 1 mg neutralized 90 units of heparin

Drug Interactions

Decreased effect with digoxin, TCN, nicotine, antihistamines, I.V. NTG

Increased toxicity with NSAIDs, ASA, dipyridamole, dextran, hydroxychloroquine, clopidogrel

Stability Stable at room temperature; protect from freezing

Mechanism of Action Potentiates the action of antithrombin III and thereby inactivates thrombin (as well as activated coagulation factors IX, X, XI, XII, and plasmin) and prevents the conversion of fibrinogen to fibrin; heparin also stimulates release of lipoprotein lipase (lipoprotein lipase hydrolyzes triglycerides to glycerol and free fatty acids)

Pharmacodynamics

Onset of action:

S.C.: Anticoagulation occurs within 20-30 minutes

I.V.: Immediate

Duration of action: Dose-dependent

Pharmacokinetics

Absorption: Oral, rectal, S.C., I.M.: Erratic

Metabolism: Believed to be partially metabolized in the reticuloendothelial system

Half-life: Mean: 90 minutes with range: 30 minutes to 3 hours (half-life affected by obesity, renal function, hepatic function, malignancy, presence of pulmonary embolism, and infections), half-life is dose-dependent

Elimination: Hepatic metabolism is followed by renal excretion, small amount excreted unchanged in urine

Usual Dosage Note: For full-dose heparin (ie, nonlow-dose), the dose should be titrated according to PTT results. For anticoagulation, an APTT 1.5-2.5 times normal is usually desired. APTT is usually measured prior to heparin therapy, 6-8 hours after initiation of a continuous infusion (following a loading dose), and 6-8 hours after changes in the infusion rate; increase or decrease infusion by 2-4 units/kg/hour dependent on PTT. Continuous I.V. infusion is preferred vs I.V. intermittent injections. For intermittent I.V. injections, PTT is measured 3.5-4 hours after I.V. injection.

Geriatrics and Adults:

Prophylaxis (low-dose heparin): S.C.: 5000 units every 8-12 hours

Intermittent I.V.: Initial: 10,000 units, then 50-70 units/kg (5000-10,000 units) every 4-6 hours

I.V. infusion: Initial: 75-100 units/kg, then 15 units/kg/hour with dose adjusted according to PTT results; usual range: 10-30 units/kg/hour

Administration Do not administer I.M. due to pain, irritation, and hematoma formation

Monitoring Parameters PTT, platelets, hemoglobin, hematocrit, and signs of bleeding

Reference Range Therapeutic: 0.3-0.5 units/mL

Test Interactions Increased thyroxine (S) (competitive protein binding methods)

Nursing Implications See Administration

Additional Information Heparin does not possess fibrinolytic activity and, therefore, cannot lyse established thrombi; discontinue heparin if hemorrhage occurs; severe hemorrhage or overdosage may require protamine; monitor platelet counts, signs of bleeding, PTT.

When using daily flushes of heparin to maintain patency of single and double lumen central catheters. Capped PVC catheters and peripheral heparin locks require flushing more frequently (eg, every 6-8 hours). Volume of heparin flush is usually similar to volume of catheter (or slightly greater) or may be standardized according to specific hospital's policy (eg, 2-5 mL/flush). Dose of heparin flush used should not approach therapeutic per kg dose. Additional flushes should be given when stagnant blood is observed in catheter, after catheter is used for drug or blood administration, and after blood withdrawal from catheter.

Heparin 1 unit/mL (final concentration) may be added to TPN solutions, both central and peripheral. (Addition of heparin to peripheral TPN has been shown to increase duration of line patency.)

Arterial lines are heparinized with a final concentration of 1 unit/mL.

Special Geriatric Considerations In the clinical setting, age has not been shown to be a reliable predictor of a patient's anticoagulant response to heparin. However, it is common for older patients to have a "standard" response for the first 24-48 hours after a loading dose (5000 units) and a maintenance infusion of 800-1000 units/hour. After this period, they then have an exaggerated response (ie, elevated PTT), requiring a lower infusion rate. Hence, monitor closely during this period of therapy. Older women are more likely to have bleeding complications and osteoporosis may be a problem when used >3 months or total daily dose exceeds 30,000 units.

Dosage Forms See table.

Heparin Sodium (Porcine Intestinal Mucosa)

Strength (units/mL)	Availability			
	MDV (mL)	SDV (mL)	UD (mL)	Hep Lock (mL)
10				1, 2, 2.5, 3, 5, 10, 30
100				1, 2, 2.5, 3, 5, 10, 30
1000	5, 10, 30	1	1, 2	
2500		1		
5000	10	1	0.5, 1	
7500		1		
10,000	4, 5, 10	1	1	
15,000		1		
20,000	2, 5, 10	1	1	
40,000	5	1		

MDV = multiple dose vials.

SDV = single dose vials (ampuls).

UD = unit dose.

Hep lock = heparin lock flush solution.

References

Bohannon AD and Lyles KW, "Drug-Induced Bone Disease," *Clin Geriatr Med*, 1994, 10(4):611-23.

Bull BS, Korpman RA, Huse WM, et al, "Heparin Therapy During Extracorporeal Circulation. I. Problems Inherent in Existing Heparin Protocols," *J Thorac Cardiovasc Surg*, 1975, 69(5):674-84.

Jick H, Slone D, Borda IT, et al, "Efficacy and Toxicity of Heparin in Relation to Age and Sex," *N Engl J Med*, 1968, 279(6):284-6.

Heparin Lock Flush *see* Heparin *on page 449*

Hepatitis A Vaccine (hep a TYE tis aye vak SEEN)

Related Information

Immunization Guidelines *on page 1058*

Brand Names Havrix®

Therapeutic Category Vaccine, Inactivated Virus

Use For populations desiring protection against hepatitis A or for populations at high risk of exposure to hepatitis A virus (travelers to developing countries, household and sexual contacts of persons infected with hepatitis A), child day care employees, illicit drug users, male homosexuals, institutional workers (eg, institutions for the mentally and physically handicapped persons, prisons, (Continued)

Hepatitis A Vaccine (Continued)

etc), and healthcare workers who may be exposed to hepatitis A virus (eg, laboratory employees); protection lasts for approximately 15 years

Contraindications Hypersensitivity to any component of hepatitis A vaccine

Warnings Use caution in patients with serious active infection, cardiovascular disease, or pulmonary disorders; treatment for anaphylactic reactions should be immediately available

Adverse Reactions

Central nervous system: Headache, fatigue, fever (rare), Guillain-Barré syndrome, seizures, dizziness, encephalopathy, somnolence (rare), insomnia, vertigo

Dermatologic: Rash, urticaria, pruritus, angioedema (rare), erythema multi-forme, hyperhydrosis

Gastrointestinal: Anorexia, nausea, diarrhea, abdominal pain, vomiting

Hepatic: Transient liver function test abnormalities

Local: Cutaneous reactions at the injection site (pain, soreness, tenderness, edema, warmth, and redness), lymphadenopathy

Neuromuscular & skeletal: Arthralgia, myalgia, paresthesia, elevated CPK

Respiratory: Pharyngitis, dyspnea (rare)

Miscellaneous: Anaphylaxis/anaphylactoid reactions

Drug Interactions No interference of immunogenicity was reported when mixed with hepatitis B vaccine; no known interference when given with other vaccines (see Additional Information)

Mechanism of Action As an inactivated virus vaccine, hepatitis A vaccine offers active immunization against hepatitis A virus infection at an effective immune response rate in up to 99% of subjects

Usual Dosage Geriatrics and Adults: 1 mL (1440 units), with a booster dose at 6-12 months

Administration Inject I.M. into the deltoid muscle, if possible; do not administer I.V., S.C., or intradermally

Monitoring Parameters Liver function tests

Reference Range Seroconversion for Havrix®: Antibody >20 mIU/mL

Patient Information Inform patients of side effects; explain need for booster; patients should report side effects lasting longer than 24 hours

Nursing Implications Shake vial or syringe well before withdrawing or injecting; discard if suspension does not appear as an opaque, uniform suspension; do not administer S.C. or I.V.

Additional Information Some investigators suggest simultaneous or sequential administration of inactivated hepatitis A vaccine and immune globulin for postexposure protection, especially for travelers requiring rapid immunization, although a slight decrease in vaccine immunogenicity may be observed with this technique; if concomitant administration with other vaccines or IgG is anticipated, administer at different sites or injections with separate syringes

Special Geriatric Considerations There is no specific data to suggest dosing is different than it is for younger adults

Dosage Forms Injection: 360 ELISA units/0.5 mL (0.5 mL); 1440 ELISA units/mL (1 mL)

References
Bancroft WH, "Hepatitis A Vaccine," N Engl J Med, 1992, 327(7):453-7.
Lemon SM, "Inactivated Hepatitis A Vaccines," JAMA, 1994, 271(17):1363-4.

Hepatitis B Immune Globulin

(hep a TYE tis bee i MYUN GLOB yoo lin)

Related Information

Immunization Guidelines on page 1058

Brand Names H-BIG®; Hep-B-Gammagee®; HyperHep®

Synonyms HBIG

Therapeutic Category Immune Globulin

Use Provide passive immunity to hepatitis B infection to those individuals exposed

Contraindications Hypersensitivity to hepatitis B immune globulin or any component; allergies to gamma globulin or anti-immunoglobulin antibodies; allergies to thimerosal; IgA deficiency; I.M. injections in patients with thrombocytopenia or coagulation disorders

Warnings Do not administer I.V., hypersensitivity reaction; should have epinephrine 1:1000 available to treat anaphylactic reactions; anaphylactic reactions rarely occur

Precautions Skin testing should not be performed due to misinterpretation of positive reaction

Adverse Reactions
Cardiovascular: Local edema
Central nervous system: Dizziness, malaise
Dermatologic: Urticaria, rash, angioedema
Local: Pain, tenderness, erythema
Neuromuscular & skeletal: Arthralgia
Miscellaneous: Rarely anaphylaxis

Drug Interactions Live virus vaccines

Stability Refrigerate at 2°C to 8°C (36°F to 46°F); do not freeze

Mechanism of Action Solution of immunoglobulin containing high titer of antibody to hepatitis B surface antigen (HB$_s$Ag)

Usual Dosage Geriatrics and Adults: I.M.: 0.06 mL/kg; usual dose: 3-5 mL for postexposure prophylaxis

Patient Information Be aware of adverse effects

Nursing Implications I.M. injection only; to prevent injury from injection care should be taken when giving to patients with thrombocytopenia or bleeding disorders; do not administer I.V.

Additional Information Hepatitis B immune globulin is not indicated for treatment of active hepatitis B infections and is ineffective in the treatment of chronic active hepatitis B infection; administration of HBIG preceding or concomitantly with hepatitis B vaccine does not interfere with the immune response to vaccine; the two together provide more rapid protective antibodies to hepatitis B than when vaccine is used alone; rapid levels may be necessary in certain settings

Special Geriatric Considerations No data available to suggest different dosing in elderly than in younger adults

Dosage Forms Injection: 0.5 mL, 1 mL, 4 mL, 5 mL

Hepatitis B Inactivated Virus Vaccine (plasma derived) see Hepatitis B Vaccine on this page

Hepatitis B Inactivated Virus Vaccine (recombinant DNA) see Hepatitis B Vaccine on this page

Hepatitis B Vaccine (hep a TYE tis bee vak SEEN)
Related Information
Immunization Guidelines on page 1058
Brand Names Engerix-B®; Recombivax HB®
Synonyms Hepatitis B Inactivated Virus Vaccine (plasma derived); Hepatitis B Inactivated Virus Vaccine (recombinant DNA)
Therapeutic Category Vaccine, Inactivated Virus
Use Immunization against infection caused by all known subtypes of hepatitis B virus in individuals considered at high risk of potential exposure to hepatitis B virus or HB$_s$Ag-positive materials
Contraindications Hypersensitivity to yeast, hepatitis B vaccine, or any component
Warnings Acute hypersensitivity reaction (have epinephrine 1:1000 available); immunosuppressed patients may require larger doses; vaccine will not prevent disease if infected at time of vaccination
Precautions Not recommended for patients on hemodialysis or hematology/oncology patients; caution in patients with thrombocytopenia or bleeding disorders; delay vaccination in patients with active, serious infections; use caution in patients with compromised cardiopulmonary disease

Adverse Reactions
Cardiovascular: Syncope, flushing, hypotension, tachycardia, palpitations
Central nervous system: Headache, fever, dizziness, vertigo, lightheadedness, somnolence, insomnia, irritability, agitation, fatigue, migraine headache, Bell's palsy, chills, malaise
Dermatologic: Rash, angioedema, urticaria, petechiae, purpura, pruritus
Gastrointestinal: Nausea, vomiting, abdominal cramps, dyspepsia, anorexia, diarrhea
Hematologic: Thrombocytopenia
Hepatic: Abnormal LFTs
Local: Soreness (erythema, edema), induration, pain, tenderness
Neuromuscular & skeletal: Arthralgia, myalgia, neck and shoulder pain, neck stiffness, generalized aches, weakness, paresthesia
Ocular: Visual disturbances
Respiratory: Cough, bronchospasm, URI, pharyngitis, rhinitis
Miscellaneous: Herpes zoster
(Continued)

Hepatitis B Vaccine *(Continued)*

Drug Interactions Immunosuppressive agents

Stability Refrigerate, do not freeze

Usual Dosage Geriatrics and Adults: I.M., S.C.: 1 mL (20 mcg), repeat in 1 month and 6 months following initial injection; booster: 1 mL (20 mcg). **Note:** The second dose **must** be given at 1 month (±1 day) exactly. This will decrease the chance of not developing a positive response (titer). The third dose is not as "time critical" for response.

Monitoring Parameters Measure serum antibody titers

Reference Range Maintain >10 mIU/mL

Patient Information Inform patient of adverse effects

Nursing Implications I.M. injection preferred; S.C. can be used if patient cannot be given I.M. injection

Additional Information Recombivax HB® is a recombinant vaccine derived from HB$_s$Ag produced in yeast cells

Special Geriatric Considerations Institutionalized elderly may be at risk for hepatitis B such as from human bites; in these cases, administer HBIG 0.06 mL/kg I.M. and administer hepatitis B vaccine I.M. at a separate site within 7 days of exposure; administer second and third dose at 1 and 6 months; no dose adjustments for age is necessary; some studies demonstrate a lower antibody titer in elderly as compared to young adults

Dosage Forms
Injection:
Engerix-B®: Hepatitis B surface antigen 20 mcg/mL
Heptavax-B®: Hepatitis B surface antigen 20 mcg/mL (3 mL)
Recombivax HB®: Hepatitis B surface antigen 10 mcg/mL (3 mL)

References
Gardner P and Schaffner W, "Immunization of Adults," *N Engl J Med*, 1993, 328(17):1252-8.

Hep-B-Gammagee® *see* Hepatitis B Immune Globulin *on page 452*

Hep-Lock® *see* Heparin *on page 449*

Heptalac® *see* Lactulose *on page 523*

Herplex® Ophthalmic *see* Idoxuridine *on page 478*

Hexachlorocyclohexane *see* Lindane *on page 538*

Hexadrol® *see* Dexamethasone *on page 274*

Hexadrol® Phosphate *see* Dexamethasone *on page 274*

Hibiclens® Topical [OTC] *see* Chlorhexidine Gluconate *on page 206*

Hibistat® Topical [OTC] *see* Chlorhexidine Gluconate *on page 206*

Hi-Cor-1.0® *see* Hydrocortisone *on page 462*

Hi-Cor-2.5® *see* Hydrocortisone *on page 462*

Hiprex® *see* Methenamine *on page 601*

Hismanal® *see* Astemizole *on page 87*

Histerone® Injection *see* Testosterone *on page 895*

Hi-Vegi-Lip® *see* Pancreatin *on page 711*

Hold® DM [OTC] *see* Dextromethorphan *on page 278*

Homatropine *(hoe MA troe peen)*

Brand Names AK-Homatropine® Ophthalmic; Isopto® Homatropine Ophthalmic

Generic Available Yes

Therapeutic Category Anticholinergic Agent, Ophthalmic; Ophthalmic Agent, Mydriatic

Use Producing cycloplegia and mydriasis for refraction; treatment of acute inflammatory conditions of the uveal tract

Contraindications Narrow-angle glaucoma, acute hemorrhage or hypersensitivity to the drug or any component in the formulation

Precautions Use with caution in patients with hypertension, cardiac disease, or increased intraocular pressure

Adverse Reactions
Cardiovascular: Vascular congestion, edema (local)
Central nervous system: Drowsiness, delirium, cognitive impairment
Dermatologic: Exudate, eczematoid dermatitis
Local: Stinging
Ocular: Follicular conjunctivitis, blurred vision, increased intraocular pressure, photophobia

Overdosage Symptoms of overdose include blurred vision, urinary retention, tachycardia

Toxicology Anticholinergic toxicity is caused by strong binding of the drug to cholinergic receptors. Cholinesterase inhibitors reduce acetylcholinesterase, the enzyme that breaks down acetylcholine and thereby allows acetylcholine to accumulate and compete for receptor binding with the offending anticholinergic. For anticholinergic overdose with severe life-threatening symptoms, physostigmine 1-2 mg S.C. or I.V., slowly may be given to reverse these effects.

Stability Protect from light

Mechanism of Action Blocks response of iris sphincter muscle and the accommodative muscle of the ciliary body to cholinergic stimulation resulting in dilation and loss of accommodation

Pharmacodynamics
Onset of action: Following ophthalmic instillation, accommodation and pupil effects occur within 30-90 minutes
Duration: Mydriasis persists for 6-24 hours or more and cycloplegia lasts for 10-48 hours

Usual Dosage Geriatrics and Adults:
Mydriasis and cycloplegia for refraction: Instill 1-2 drops of 2% solution or 1 drop of 5% solution before the procedure; repeat at 5- to 10-minute intervals as needed
Uveitis: Instill 1-2 drops 2-3 times/day up to every 3-4 hours as needed

Administration Finger pressure should be applied to lacrimal sac for 1-2 minutes after instillation to decrease risk of absorption and systemic reactions

Patient Information If irritation persists or increases, discontinue use; may cause blurred vision and sensitivity to bright light

Nursing Implications See Administration

Special Geriatric Considerations See Adverse Reactions

Dosage Forms Solution, ophthalmic, as hydrobromide: 2% (1 mL, 5 mL, 15 mL); 5% (1 mL, 2 mL, 5 mL, 15 mL)

References
Barker DB and Solomon DA, "The Potential for Mental Status Changes Associated With Systemic Absorption of Anticholinergic Ophthalmic Medications: Concerns in the Elderly," *DICP Ann Pharmacother*, 1990, 24(9):847-50.

Humalog® *see* Insulin Preparations *on page 488*

Human Diploid Cell Cultures Rabies Vaccine *see* Rabies Virus Vaccine *on page 819*

Human Diploid Cell Cultures Rabies Vaccine (Intradermal use) *see* Rabies Virus Vaccine *on page 819*

Humibid® DM [OTC] *see* Guaifenesin and Dextromethorphan *on page 439*

Humibid® L.A. *see* Guaifenesin *on page 437*

Humibid® Sprinkle *see* Guaifenesin *on page 437*

HuMist® Nasal Mist [OTC] *see* Sodium Chloride *on page 860*

Humulin® 50/50 *see* Insulin Preparations *on page 488*

Humulin® 70/30 *see* Insulin Preparations *on page 488*

Humulin® L *see* Insulin Preparations *on page 488*

Humulin® N *see* Insulin Preparations *on page 488*

Humulin® R *see* Insulin Preparations *on page 488*

Humulin® U *see* Insulin Preparations *on page 488*

Hyaluronidase (hye al yoor ON i dase)

Brand Names Wydase® Injection

Generic Available No

Therapeutic Category Antidote, Extravasation

Use Increase the dispersion and absorption of other drugs; increase rate of absorption of parenteral fluids given by hypodermoclysis; enhance diffusion of locally irritating or toxic drugs in the management of I.V. extravasation

Contraindications Hypersensitivity to hyaluronidase or any component; do not inject in or around infected, inflamed, or cancerous areas

Warnings Drug infiltrates in which hyaluronidase is contraindicated: dopamine, alpha agonists

Precautions An intradermal skin test for sensitivity should be performed before actual administration using 0.02 mL of hyaluronidase

Adverse Reactions Allergic reactions are rare, isolated cases of anaphylactic-like reactions have occurred

Overdosage Symptoms of overdose include urticaria, erythema, chills, nausea, vomiting, dizziness, tachycardia, hypotension

Toxicology Treatment is supportive
(Continued)

Hyaluronidase *(Continued)*

Drug Interactions Decreased effect: Salicylates, cortisone, ACTH, estrogens, antihistamines

Stability Reconstituted hyaluronidase solution remains stable for only 24 hours when stored in the refrigerator; do not use discolored solutions

Mechanism of Action Modifies the permeability of connective tissue through hydrolysis of hyaluronic acid, one of the chief ingredients of tissue cement which offers resistance to diffusion of liquids through tissues

Pharmacodynamics

Onset of action by S.C. or intradermal routes for the treatment of extravasation: Immediate

Duration: 24-48 hours

Usual Dosage Geriatrics and Adults:

Absorption and dispersion of drugs: 150 units is added to the vehicle containing the drug

Hypodermoclysis: 1 mL (150 units) is added to 1000 mL of infusion fluid and 0.5 mL (75 units) is injected into each clysis site at the initiation of the infusion

Monitoring Parameters Fluid status, electrolytes

Nursing Implications Administer hyaluronidase within the first few minutes to 1 hour after the extravasation is recognized; do not administer I.V.

Additional Information The USP hyaluronidase unit is equivalent to the turbidity-reducing (TR) unit and the International Unit; each unit is defined as being the activity contained in 100 mcg of the International Standard Preparation

Special Geriatric Considerations The most common use of hyaluronidase in the elderly is in hypodermoclysis. Hypodermoclysis is very useful in dehydrated patients in whom oral intake is minimal and I.V. access is a problem.

Dosage Forms

Injection:

Lyophilized: 150 units/mL (1 mL, 10 mL)

Stabilized: 150 units/mL (1 mL, 10 mL)

References

Berger EY, "Nutrition by Hypodermoclysis," *J Am Geriatr Soc*, 1984, 32(3):199-203.

Lipschitz S, Campbell AJ, Roberts MS, et al, "Subcutaneous Fluid Administration in Elderly Subjects: Validation of an Underused Technique," *J Am Geriatr Soc*, 1991, 39(1):6-9.

Hycort® *see Hydrocortisone on page 462*

Hydergine® *see Ergoloid Mesylates on page 342*

Hydergine® LC *see Ergoloid Mesylates on page 342*

Hydralazine *(hye DRAL a zeen)*

Brand Names Apresoline®

Generic Available Yes

Therapeutic Category Vasodilator

Use Management of moderate to severe hypertension, congestive heart failure

Contraindications Hypersensitivity to hydralazine or any component, dissecting aortic aneurysm, mitral valve rheumatic heart disease, known or suspected coronary artery disease

Warnings Monitor blood pressure closely with I.V. use; some formulations may contain tartrazines or sulfites

Precautions Discontinue hydralazine in patients who develop SLE-like syndrome or positive ANA. Use with caution in patients with severe renal disease or cerebral vascular accidents.

Adverse Reactions

Cardiovascular: Palpitations, flushing, tachycardia, dizziness, edema, rarely orthostatic hypotension

Central nervous system: Headache

Gastrointestinal: Anorexia, nausea, vomiting, diarrhea

Neuromuscular & skeletal: Weakness, peripheral neuritis

Miscellaneous: SLE-like syndrome (fever, rash, arthralgias, malaise, positive ANA, positive LE cells); this may occur in patients on high doses (>200 mg/day) and prolonged therapy

Note: Because of blunted baroreceptor response, the elderly are less likely to experience reflex tachycardia; this puts them at greater risk for orthostatic hypotension

Overdosage Symptoms of overdose include hypotension, tachycardia, shock

Toxicology Hypotension usually responds to I.V. fluids or Trendelenburg positioning. If unresponsive to these measures the use of a parenteral vasoconstrictor may be required (eg, norepinephrine 0.1-0.2 mcg/kg/minute titrated to response). Treatment is primarily supportive and symptomatic.

Drug Interactions
Decreased effect: Indomethacin
Increased effect: MAO inhibitors, other hypotensive agents

Stability Changes color after contact with a metal filter; do not store intact ampuls in refrigerator

Mechanism of Action Direct vasodilation of arterioles (with little effect on veins) with decreased systemic resistance

Pharmacodynamics
Onset of action:
Oral: 20-30 minutes
I.V.: 5-20 minutes
Duration:
Oral: 6-8 hours
I.V.: 2-4 hours

Pharmacokinetics
Metabolism: Oral: Large first-pass effect
Bioavailability: 30% to 50%; enhanced by the concurrent ingestion of food

Usual Dosage
Geriatrics: Oral: Initial: 10 mg 2-3 times/day, increase by 10-25 mg/day every 2-5 days
Adults:
Oral: Initial: 10 mg 4 times/day, increase by 10-25 mg/dose every 2-5 days to maximum of 300 mg/day
I.M., I.V.: Hypertensive initial: 10-20 mg/dose every 4-6 hours as needed, may increase to 40 mg/dose; change to oral therapy as soon as possible

Monitoring Parameters Blood pressure, standing and sitting/supine

Test Interactions Increased calcium (S)

Patient Information Report flu-like symptoms, rise from sitting/lying carefully, may cause dizziness; take with meals

Nursing Implications Monitor blood pressure closely with I.V. use

Additional Information Has also been used to treat primary pulmonary hypertension. Slow acetylators, patients with decreased renal function and patients receiving >200 mg/day (chronically) are at higher risk for SLE. Titrate dosage to patient's response. Usually administered with diuretic and a beta-blocker to counteract side effects of sodium and water retention and reflex tachycardia although the beta-blocker may not be necessary in the elderly.

Special Geriatric Considerations See Adverse Reactions and Usual Dosage

Dosage Forms
Hydralazine hydrochloride:
Injection: 20 mg/mL (1 mL)
Tablet: 10 mg, 25 mg, 50 mg, 100 mg

References
Birkenhager WH, "Choosing the Optimum Therapy for Older Hypertensive Patients," *Drugs Aging*, 1991, 1(1):36-47.
Sproat TT and Lopez LM, "Hypertension," *Therapeutics in the Elderly*, 2nd ed, Delauente JC, Stewart RB, eds, Cincinnati, OH: Harvey Whitney Books, 1995, 228-46.

Hydralazine and Hydrochlorothiazide
(hye DRAL a zeen & hye droe klor oh THYE a zide)

Related Information
Hydralazine *on previous page*
Hydrochlorothiazide *on next page*

Brand Names Apresazide®; Hydrazide®; Hy-Zide®

Synonyms Hydrochlorothiazide and Hydralazine

Generic Available Yes

Therapeutic Category Antihypertensive, Combination

Special Geriatric Considerations Combination products are not recommended for first-line treatment and divided doses of diuretics may increase the incidence of nocturia in the elderly

Dosage Forms Tablet: Hydralazine hydrochloride 50 mg and hydrochlorothiazide 50 mg; hydralazine hydrochloride 100 mg and hydrochlorothiazide 50 mg; hydralazine hydrochloride 25 mg and hydrochlorothiazide 25 mg; hydralazine hydrochloride 25 mg and hydrochlorothiazide 15 mg

Hydramyn® Syrup [OTC] *see* Diphenhydramine *on page 302*

Hydrate® Injection *see* Dimenhydrinate *on page 300*

Hydrazide® *see* Hydralazine and Hydrochlorothiazide *on previous page*

Hydrea® *see* Hydroxyurea *on page 468*

Hydrobexan® *see* Hydroxocobalamin *on page 466*

Hydrocet® *see* Hydrocodone and Acetaminophen *on page 461*

Hydrochlorothiazide (hye droe klor oh THYE a zide)

Brand Names Esidrix®; Ezide®; HydroDIURIL®; Hydro-Par®; Oretic®

Synonyms HCTZ

Generic Available Yes: Tablet

Therapeutic Category Diuretic, Thiazide

Use Management of mild to moderate hypertension; treatment of edema in congestive heart failure and nephrotic syndrome

Contraindications Anuria, renal decompensation, hypersensitivity to hydrochlorothiazide or any component, cross-sensitivity with other thiazides and sulfonamide derivatives

Precautions Hypokalemia, renal disease, hepatic disease, gout, lupus erythematosus, diabetes mellitus; use with caution in severe renal diseases; ineffective in patients with Cl_{cr} <30 mL/minute

Adverse Reactions
Cardiovascular: Hypotension
Central nervous system: Drowsiness
Dermatologic: Rash, photosensitivity
Endocrine & metabolic: Hypokalemia, hyponatremia, hyperglycemia
Gastrointestinal: Nausea, vomiting, anorexia
Genitourinary: Prerenal azotemia
Hematologic: Aplastic anemia, hemolytic anemia, leukopenia, agranulocytosis, thrombocytopenia (all rare)
Hepatic: Hepatitis
Neuromuscular & skeletal: Paresthesia
Renal: Polyuria

Overdosage Symptoms of overdose include electrolyte depletion, volume depletion, hypotension, dehydration, circulatory collapse

Toxicology Following GI decontamination, treatment is supportive; hypotension responds to fluids and Trendelenburg position

Drug Interactions
Decreased effect: NSAIDs; decreased effect of oral hypoglycemics; decreased absorption with cholestyramine and colestipol
Increased effect with loop diuretics and other antihypertensives
Increased toxicity/levels of lithium; when given with digoxin, diuretic-induced hypokalemia increases the risk of digoxin toxicity

Mechanism of Action Inhibits sodium reabsorption in the distal tubules causing increased excretion of sodium and water as well as potassium and hydrogen ions

Pharmacodynamics
Peak effects require 4 hours while diuresis can continue for 6-12 hours
Onset of diuretic action: Oral: Within 2 hours
Duration of action: 6-12 hours

Pharmacokinetics Absorption: Oral: ~60% to 80%

Usual Dosage Oral:
Geriatrics: Initial: 12.5-25 mg once daily; minimal increase in response and more electrolyte disturbances are seen with doses >50 mg/day
Adults: 25-100 mg/day in 1-2 doses; maximum: 200 mg/day

Monitoring Parameters Blood pressure (both standing and sitting/supine), serum electrolytes, renal function, weight, I & O

Test Interactions Increased ammonia (B), increased amylase (S), increased calcium (S), increased chloride (S), increased cholesterol (S), increased glucose, increased uric acid (S); decreased chloride (S), decreased magnesium, decreased potassium (S), decreased sodium (S). Tyramine and phentolamine tests, histamine tests for pheochromocytoma.

Patient Information May be taken with food or milk; take early in day to avoid nocturia; take the last dose of multiple doses no later than 6 PM unless instructed otherwise. A few people who take this medication become more sensitive to sunlight and may experience skin rash, redness, itching or severe sunburn, especially if sun block SPF ≥15 is not used on exposed skin areas.

Nursing Implications Check patient for orthostasis (see Monitoring Parameters)

Additional Information Effect of drug may be decreased when used every day

Special Geriatric Considerations Hydrochlorothiazide is not effective in patients with a Cl_{cr} <30 mL/minute, therefore, it may not be a useful agent in many elderly patients (see Usual Dosage)

Dosage Forms
Solution:
Oral: 50 mg/5 mL (5 mL, 500 mL)
Oral, concentrate: 100 mg/mL (30 mL)
Tablet: 25 mg, 50 mg, 100 mg

Hydrochlorothiazide and Amiloride *see* Amiloride and Hydrochlorothiazide *on page 54*

Hydrochlorothiazide and Hydralazine *see* Hydralazine and Hydrochlorothiazide *on page 457*

Hydrochlorothiazide and Methyldopa *see* Methyldopa and Hydrochlorothiazide *on page 609*

Hydrochlorothiazide and Reserpine
(hye droe klor oh THYE a zide & re SER peen)

Related Information
Hydrochlorothiazide *on previous page*
Reserpine *on page 825*

Brand Names Hydropres®; Hydro-Serp®; Hydroserpine®

Synonyms Reserpine and Hydrochlorothiazide

Generic Available Yes

Therapeutic Category Antihypertensive, Combination

Special Geriatric Considerations Combination products are not recommended for first-line treatment and divided doses of diuretics may increase the incidence of nocturia in the elderly

Dosage Forms
Tablet:
25: Hydrochlorothiazide 25 mg and reserpine 0.125 mg
50: Hydrochlorothiazide 50 mg and reserpine 0.125 mg

Hydrochlorothiazide and Spironolactone
(hye droe klor oh THYE a zide & speer on oh LAK tone)

Related Information
Hydrochlorothiazide *on previous page*
Spironolactone *on page 869*

Brand Names Alazide®; Aldactazide®; Spironazide®; Spirozide®

Synonyms Spironolactone and Hydrochlorothiazide

Generic Available Yes

Therapeutic Category Antihypertensive, Combination; Diuretic, Combination

Use Management of mild to moderate hypertension; treatment of edema in congestive heart failure and nephrotic syndrome; cirrhosis of the liver accompanied by edema or ascites

Contraindications Anuria, hyperkalemia, renal or hepatic failure, hypersensitivity to hydrochlorothiazide, spironolactone, or any component

Warnings This fixed combination is not indicated for initial therapy of hypertension; therapy requires titration to the individual patient, if dosage so determined represents this fixed combination, its use may be more convenient; has been shown to be tumorigenic in toxicity studies using rats at 25 to 250 times the usual human dose

Adverse Reactions
Cardiovascular: Hypotension
Central nervous system: Lethargy, headache
Dermatologic: Rash
Endocrine & metabolic: Hyperkalemia, gynecomastia, hyperchloremic metabolic acidosis, dehydration, hyponatremia
Gastrointestinal: Anorexia, nausea, vomiting, diarrhea

Overdosage Symptoms of overdose include drowsiness, confusion, clinical signs of dehydration and electrolyte imbalance

Toxicology Ingestion of large amounts of potassium-sparing diuretics may result in life-threatening hyperkalemia. This can be treated with I.V. glucose (dextrose 25% in water), with concurrent I.V. sodium bicarbonate (1 mEq/kg up to 44 mEq/dose), and 0.2-0.5 units of rapid-acting insulin per gram of glucose. If needed, Kayexalate® oral or rectal solutions in sorbitol may also be useful.
(Continued)

Hydrochlorothiazide and Spironolactone *(Continued)*

Drug Interactions
Increased risk of hyperkalemia if given with other potassium-sparing diuretics, potassium supplements, or ACE inhibitors

NSAIDs may reduce therapeutic effect

Usual Dosage Oral:
Geriatrics: Initial: 1 tablet/day, increase as necessary

Adults: 1-8 tablets of Aldactazide®-25 (1-4 tablets of Aldactazide®-50) in 1-2 divided doses

Monitoring Parameters Blood pressure, serum electrolytes, renal function, weight, I & O

Test Interactions Plasma and urinary cortisol levels

Patient Information Take in the morning; take the last dose of multiple doses before 6 PM unless instructed otherwise; may cause increased sensitivity to sunlight; avoid excessive ingestion of foods high in potassium or use of salt substitutes

Nursing Implications May interfere with digoxin serum assays; monitor for signs of hyperkalemia (see Monitoring Parameters)

Additional Information See individual components for full prescribing information

Special Geriatric Considerations The efficacy of hydrochlorothiazide is limited in patients with a Cl_{cr} <30 mL/minute; monitor serum potassium (see Warnings)

Dosage Forms
Tablet:

25/25: Hydrochlorothiazide 25 mg and spironolactone 25 mg

50/50: Hydrochlorothiazide 50 mg and spironolactone 50 mg

Hydrochlorothiazide and Triamterene
(hye droe klor oh THYE a zide & trye AM ter een)

Related Information
Hydrochlorothiazide *on page 458*

Triamterene *on page 951*

Brand Names Dyazide®; Maxzide®

Synonyms Triamterene and Hydrochlorothiazide

Generic Available Yes (Dyazide® strength only)

Therapeutic Category Diuretic, Combination

Use Management of mild to moderate hypertension; treatment of edema in congestive heart failure and nephrotic syndrome

Contraindications Anuria, hyperkalemia, renal, or hepatic failure, hypersensitivity to hydrochlorothiazide, triamterene or any component; concurrent use of potassium supplements

Warnings This fixed combination is not indicated for initial therapy of hypertension; therapy requires titration to the individual patient; if dosage so determined represents this fixed combination, its use may be more convenient

Adverse Reactions
Cardiovascular: Hypotension

Central nervous system: Dizziness, headache

Endocrine & metabolic: Electrolyte disturbances

Gastrointestinal: Nausea, vomiting

Overdosage Symptoms of overdose include drowsiness, confusion, clinical signs of dehydration and electrolyte imbalance

Toxicology Ingestion of large amounts of potassium-sparing diuretics may result in life-threatening hyperkalemia. This can be treated with I.V. glucose (dextrose 25% in water), with concurrent I.V. sodium bicarbonate (1 mEq/kg up to 44 mEq/dose), and 0.2-0.5 units of rapid-acting insulin per gram of glucose. If needed, Kayexalate® oral or rectal solutions in sorbitol may also be useful.

Drug Interactions
Increased risk of hyperkalemia if given with other potassium-sparing diuretics, potassium supplements, or ACE inhibitors

NSAIDs may reduce therapeutic effect

Increased levels of amantadine have been reported with the concomitant administration of HCTZ and triamterene

Drug/Food Interactions Avoid excessive ingestions of foods high in potassium or use of salt substitutes

Stability Protect from light

Usual Dosage Oral:
Geriatrics:
Dyazide®: Initial: 1 capsule/day or every other day
Maxzide®-25: Initial: 1 capsule/day or every other day
Adults:
Dyazide®, Maxzide®-25: 1-2 capsules twice daily after meals
Maxzide®: 1 capsule/day

Monitoring Parameters Blood pressure, serum electrolytes, renal function, weight, I & O

Test Interactions Serum creatinine and BUN, bentiromide test, fluorescent measurement of quinidine

Patient Information Take in the morning with meals or milk; may cause increased sensitivity to sunlight; avoid excessive ingestion of foods high in potassium or use of salt substitutes

Nursing Implications Monitor for signs of hyperkalemia (see Monitoring Parameters)

Additional Information Dyazide® and Maxzide® are not bioequivalent. *One product should not be substituted for the other.* Retitration and appropriate changes in dosage may be necessary if patients are to be transferred from one dosage form to the other. Serum potassium concentrations do not necessarily indicate the true body potassium concentration. A rise in plasma pH or an increase in the circulating levels of insulin or epinephrine may cause a decrease in plasma potassium concentration and an increase in the intracellular potassium concentration.

Special Geriatric Considerations The efficacy of hydrochlorothiazide is limited in patients with Cl$_{cr}$ <30 mL/minute; monitor serum potassium (see Warnings and Additional Information)

Dosage Forms
Capsule (Dyazide®): Hydrochlorothiazide 25 mg and triamterene 37.5 mg
Tablet:
Maxzide®-25: Hydrochlorothiazide 25 mg and triamterene 37.5 mg
Maxzide®: Hydrochlorothiazide 50 mg and triamterene 75 mg

Hydrocil® [OTC] *see* Psyllium *on page 804*

Hydro Cobex® *see* Hydroxocobalamin *on page 466*

Hydrocodone and Acetaminophen
(hye droe KOE done & a seet a MIN oh fen)

Related Information
Narcotic Agonist Comparative Pharmacology *on page 1036*
Pharmacokinetics of Narcotic Agonist Analgesics *on page 1037*

Brand Names Anexsia®; Anodynos-DHC®; Bancap HC®; Co-Gesic®; Dolacet®; DuoCet™; Duradyne DHC®; Hydrocet®; Hydrogesic®; Hy-Phen®; Lorcet®; Lorcet®-HD; Lorcet® Plus; Lortab®; Margesic® H; Medipain 5®; Norcet®; Stagesic®; T-Gesic®; Vicodin®; Vicodin® ES; Vicodin® HP; Zydone®

Synonyms Acetaminophen and Hydrocodone

Generic Available Yes

Therapeutic Category Analgesic, Narcotic

Use Relief of moderate to severe pain; antitussive (hydrocodone)

Restrictions C-III

Contraindications CNS depression, hypersensitivity to hydrocodone, acetaminophen or any component; severe respiratory depression

Warnings Some tablets contain sulfites which may cause allergic reactions

Precautions Use with caution in patients with hypersensitivity reactions to other phenanthrene derivative opioid agonists (morphine, codeine, hydromorphone, oxycodone, oxymorphone, levorphanol)

Adverse Reactions
Cardiovascular: Hypotension, bradycardia, peripheral vasodilation
Central nervous system: CNS depression, drowsiness, dizziness, sedation, confusion, increased intracranial pressure
Endocrine & metabolic: Antidiuretic hormone release
Gastrointestinal: Nausea, vomiting, constipation
Ocular: Miosis
Respiratory: Respiratory depression
Miscellaneous: Physical and psychological dependence with prolonged use, biliary or urinary tract spasm, histamine release

Overdosage Symptoms of overdose include hepatic necrosis, blood dyscrasias, respiratory depression

Toxicology Treatment of an overdose includes support of the patient's airway, establishment of an I.V. line and administration of naloxone 2 mg I.V. with
(Continued)

Hydrocodone and Acetaminophen *(Continued)*

repeat administration as necessary. Mucomyst® (acetylcysteine) 140 mg/kg orally (loading) followed by 70 mg/kg (maintenance) every 4 hours for 17 doses. Therapy should be initiated based upon laboratory analysis suggesting high probability of hepatotoxic potential.

Drug Interactions
Decreased effect with phenothiazines
Increased effect with dextroamphetamine
Increased toxicity with CNS depressants, TCAs

Mechanism of Action
Hydrocodone: Binds to opiate receptors in the CNS, causing inhibition of ascending pain pathways, altering the perception of and response to pain; causes cough supression by direct central action in the medulla; produces generalized CNS depression
Acetaminophen: See individual agent

Pharmacodynamics
Onset of action: Oral: Narcotic analgesia occurs within 10-20 minutes following administration
Duration: 3-6 hours; enhanced analgesia has been seen in elderly patients on therapeutic doses of narcotics; duration of action may be increased in the elderly

Pharmacokinetics
Metabolism: In the liver
Half-life: 3.8 hours
Elimination: In urine

Usual Dosage Doses should be titrated to appropriate analgesic effect
Geriatrics: 2.5-5 mg of the hydrocodone component every 4-6 hours; do not exceed 4 g/day of acetaminophen
Adults: 1-2 tablets or capsules every 4-6 hours

Monitoring Parameters Pain relief, respiratory and mental status, blood pressure

Patient Information May cause drowsiness; avoid alcoholic beverages; do not exceed recommended dose

Nursing Implications Observe patient for excessive sedation, respiratory depression

Special Geriatric Considerations The elderly may be particularly susceptible to the CNS depressant action (sedation, confusion) and constipating effects of narcotics; if 1 tablet/dose is used, it may be useful to add an additional 325 mg of acetaminophen to maximize analgesic effect (see Adverse Reactions and Pharmacodynamics)

Dosage Forms
Capsule: Hydrocodone bitartrate 5 mg and acetaminophen 500 mg
Solution: Hydrocodone bitartrate 2.5 mg and acetaminophen 167 mg per 5 mL (480 mL)
Tablet: Hydrocodone bitartrate 2.5 mg and acetaminophen 500 mg; hydrocodone bitartrate 5 mg and acetaminophen 500 mg; hydrocodone bitartrate 7.5 mg and acetaminophen 500 mg

Hydrocort® *see* Hydrocortisone *on this page*

Hydrocortisone *(hye droe KOR ti sone)*

Related Information
Antacid Drug Interactions *on page 1096*
Corticosteroids Comparison, Systemic *on page 1029*
Corticosteroids Comparison, Topical *on page 1030*
I.V. Push Recommended Guidelines *on page 1083*

Brand Names Aeroseb-HC®; A-hydroCort®; Ala-Cort®; Ala-Scalp®; Anucort-HC® Suppository; Anuprep HC® Suppository; Anusol® HC-1 [OTC]; Anusol® HC-2.5% [OTC]; Anusol-HC® Suppository; Caldecort®; Caldecort® Anti-Itch Spray; Clocort® Maximum Strength; CortaGel® [OTC]; Cortaid® Maximum Strength [OTC]; Cortaid® with Aloe [OTC]; Cort-Dome®; Cortef®; Cortef® Feminine Itch; Cortenema®; Cortifoam®; Cortizone®-5 [OTC]; Cortizone®-10 [OTC]; Delcort®; Dermacort®; Dermarest Dricort®; DermiCort®; Dermolate® [OTC]; Dermtex® HC with Aloe; Eldecort®; Eldcort®; Gynecort® [OTC]; Hemril-HC® Uniserts®; Hi-Cor-1.0®; Hi-Cor-2.5®; Hycort®; Hydrocort®; Hydrocortone® Acetate; Hydrocortone® Phosphate; HydroSKIN®; Hydro-Tex® [OTC]; Hytone®; LactiCare-HC®; Lanacort® [OTC]; Locoid®; Nutracort®; Orabase® HCA; Penecort®; Procort® [OTC]; Proctocort™; Scalpicin®; Solu-Cortef®; S-T Cort®; Synacort®; Tegrin®-HC [OTC]; U-Cort™; Westcort®

Synonyms Compound F; Cortisol

Generic Available Yes

Therapeutic Category Adrenal Corticosteroid; Anti-inflammatory Agent; Corticosteroid, Rectal; Corticosteroid, Systemic; Corticosteroid, Topical (Low Potency); Corticosteroid, Topical (Medium Potency)

Use Management of adrenocortical insufficiency; relief of inflammation of corticosteroid-responsive dermatoses; adjunctive treatment of ulcerative colitis

Contraindications Serious infections, except septic shock or tuberculous meningitis; known hypersensitivity to hydrocortisone; viral, fungal, or tubercular skin lesions

Warnings Acute adrenal insufficiency may occur with abrupt withdrawal after long-term therapy or with stress

Precautions Use with caution in patients with hyperthyroidism, cirrhosis, nonspecific ulcerative colitis, hypertension, osteoporosis, thromboembolic tendencies, congestive heart failure, convulsive disorders, myasthenia gravis, thrombophlebitis, peptic ulcer, diabetes

Adverse Reactions

Cardiovascular: Hypertension, edema, accelerated atherogenesis

Central nervous system: Euphoria, insomnia, headache, vertigo, seizures, psychoses, pseudotumor cerebri

Dermatologic: Acne, dermatitis, skin atrophy, impaired wound healing, hirsutism, striae, miliaria, telangiectasia

Endocrine & metabolic: Hypokalemia, hyperglycemia, Cushing's syndrome, alkalosis, pituitary-adrenal, hot flashes, postmenopausal bleeding, axis suppression, glucose intolerance

Gastrointestinal: Peptic ulcer, pancreatitis, nausea, vomiting

Neuromuscular & skeletal: Osteoporosis, fractures, aseptic necrosis of femoral and humeral heads, steroid myopathy

Ocular: Cataracts, glaucoma

Miscellaneous: Immunosuppression

Toxicology When consumed in excessive quantities for prolonged periods, systemic hypercorticism and adrenal suppression may occur; in those cases, discontinuation and withdrawal of the corticosteroid should be done judiciously

Drug Interactions

Steroids decrease the effect of anticholinesterases, isoniazid, salicylates, insulin, oral hypoglycemics

Decreased effect: Barbiturates, phenytoin, rifampin

Increased effect (hypokalemia) of potassium-depleting diuretics

Increased risk of digoxin toxicity (due to hypokalemia)

Increased effect: Estrogens, ketoconazole

Mechanism of Action Decreases inflammation by suppression of migration of polymorphonuclear leukocytes and reversal of increased capillary permeability

Pharmacokinetics

Absorption: Rapid by all routes, except rectally

Metabolism: In the liver and excreted renally, mainly as 17-hydroxysteroids and 17-ketosteroids; substrate CYP3A4

Half-life: Biologic: 8-12 hours

Usual Dosage

Acute adrenal insufficiency: Geriatrics and Adults: I.M., I.V., S.C.: 15-240 mg every 12 hours of hydrocortisone phosphate

Anti-inflammatory or immunosuppressive:

Geriatrics: Use lowest effective dose

Adults: Oral, I.M., S.C., I.V.: 15-240 mg every 12 hours

Shock: Geriatrics and Adults: I.M., I.V.: 500 mg to 2 g every 2-6 hours (succinate)

Geriatrics and Adults:

Rectal: Apply 1 application 1-2 times/day for 2-3 weeks

Topical: Apply to affected area 3-4 times/day

Monitoring Parameters Blood pressure, blood glucose, electrolytes, weight, symptoms of fluid retention

Reference Range Therapeutic: AM: 5-25 µg/dL (SI: 138-690 nmol/L); PM: 2-9 µg/dL (SI: 55-248 nmol/L) depending on test, assay

Test Interactions Increased amylase (S), chloride (S), increased cholesterol (S), increased glucose, increased protein, increased sodium (S); decreased calcium (S), decreased chloride (S), decreased potassium (S), decreased thyroxine (S)

Patient Information Notify surgeon or dentist before surgical repair; may cause GI upset; take with food or milk; notify physician if any sign of infection occurs; avoid abrupt withdrawal when on long-term oral therapy; carry an

(Continued)

Hydrocortisone *(Continued)*

identification card or bracelet advising that you are on steroids; do not use topical products on broken skin

Nursing Implications Administer with meals to decrease GI upset; apply sparingly

Additional Information

Hydrocortisone: Cortone® tablet, Hydrocortone®

Hydrocortisone acetate: Hydrocortone® acetate injection

Hydrocortisone cypionate: Cortef® suspension

Hydrocortisone sodium phosphate: Hydrocortone® phosphate injection

Hydrocortisone sodium succinate: A-hydroCort® injection, Solu-Cortef® injection

Special Geriatric Considerations Because of the risk of adverse effects, systemic corticosteroids should be used cautiously in the elderly, in the smallest possible dose, and for the shortest possible time.

Dosage Forms

Aerosol, topical: 0.53 mg/1 sec spray (58 g)

Cream, as acetate: 0.5% (15 g, 30 g); 1% (30 g, 120 g)

Cream, as butyrate: 0.1% (15 g, 45 g, 60 g)

Cream:

Rectal: 1% (30 g with applicator)

Topical: 0.25% (30 g); 0.5% (15 g, 30 g, 120 g, 454 g); 1% (15 g, 20 g, 30 g, 120 g, 454 g); 2.5% (20 g, 30 g, 60 g, 454 g)

Topical, as valerate: 0.2% (15 g, 45 g, 60 g)

Enema: 100 mg/60 mL each unit (7 units/box)

Foam, rectal, as acetate: 10% (20 g)

Injection, as acetate: 25 mg/mL (3 mL, 10 mL); 50 mg/mL (5 mL, 10 mL)

Injection, as sodium phosphate: 50 mg/mL (2 mL, 10 mL)

Injection, as succinate: 100 mg, 250 mg, 500 mg

Injection, as sodium succinate: 100 mg, 250 mg, 500 mg, 1000 mg

Lotion: 0.25% (30 mL, 120 mL); 0.5% (30 mL, 60 mL, 120 mL); 1% (30 mL, 60 mL, 120 mL); 2.5% (60 mL, 120 mL)

Lotion, as acetate: 0.5% (30 mL)

Ointment, as acetate: 0.5% (15 g); 1% (30 g)

Ointment, as butyrate: 0.1% (15 g, 45 g)

Ointment:

Topical: 0.5% (30 g)

Topical, as valerate: 0.2% (15 g, 45 g, 60 g)

Paste, oral topical, as acetate: 0.5%

Suppository, as acetate: 25 mg

Suspension, as cypionate, oral: 10 mg/5 mL (120 mL)

Tablet: 5 mg, 10 mg, 20 mg

Hydrocortone® Acetate *see* Hydrocortisone *on page 462*

Hydrocortone® Phosphate *see* Hydrocortisone *on page 462*

Hydro-Crysti-12® *see* Hydroxocobalamin *on page 466*

HydroDIURIL® *see* Hydrochlorothiazide *on page 458*

Hydrogesic® *see* Hydrocodone and Acetaminophen *on page 461*

Hydromagnesium Aluminate *see* Magaldrate *on page 560*

Hydromorphone *(hye droe MOR fone)*

Related Information

I.V. Push Recommended Guidelines *on page 1083*

Narcotic Agonist Comparative Pharmacology *on page 1036*

Pharmacokinetics of Narcotic Agonist Analgesics *on page 1037*

Brand Names Dilaudid®; Dilaudid-5®; Dilaudid-HP®; HydroStat IR®

Synonyms Dihydromorphinone

Generic Available Yes

Therapeutic Category Analgesic, Narcotic; Antitussive

Use Management of moderate to severe pain; antitussive at lower doses

Restrictions C-II

Contraindications Hypersensitivity to hydromorphone or any component

Warnings Injection contains benzyl alcohol

Precautions Tablet and cough syrup contain tartrazine which may cause allergic reactions; hydromorphone shares toxic potential of opiate agonists, and precaution of opiate agonist therapy should be observed; extreme caution should be taken to avoid confusing the highly concentrated injection with the less concentrated injectable product. Use caution in postoperative and pulmonary patients since hydromorphone can suppress the cough reflex.

Use caution in impaired hepatic and/or renal function, and in patients allergic to other phenanthrene opiates

Adverse Reactions

Cardiovascular: Palpitations, hypotension, bradycardia, peripheral vasodilation

Central nervous system: CNS depression

Dermatologic: Pruritus

Endocrine & metabolic: Antidiuretic hormone release

Gastrointestinal: Nausea, vomiting, constipation

Ocular: Miosis

Respiratory: Respiratory depression

Miscellaneous: Increased intracranial pressure, physical and psychological dependence, histamine release, biliary or urinary tract spasm

Overdosage Symptoms of overdose include CNS depression, respiratory depression, miosis, apnea, pulmonary edema

Toxicology Maintain airway, establish I.V. line and administer naloxone 2 mg I.V. with repeat administration as necessary up to a total of 10 mg

Drug Interactions Increased toxicity: CNS depressants, phenothiazines, tricyclic antidepressants

Stability Protect tablets from light; do not store intact ampuls in refrigerator; a slightly yellowish discoloration has not been associated with a loss of potency; not compatible with alkalies, bromides and iodides

Mechanism of Action Binds to opiate receptors in the CNS, causing inhibition of ascending pain pathways, altering the perception of and response to pain; causes cough supression by direct central action in the medulla; produces generalized CNS depression

Pharmacodynamics

Onset of action: Oral: Following administration, analgesic effects occur within 15-30 minutes

Peak effects: Within 30-90 minutes

Duration: 4-5 hours; enhanced analgesia has been seen in elderly patients on therapeutic doses of narcotics; duration of action may be increased in the elderly

Pharmacokinetics

Metabolism: Primarily in the liver

Bioavailability: 62%

Half-life: 1-3 hours

Elimination: In urine principally as glucuronide conjugates

Usual Dosage Doses should be titrated to appropriate analgesic effects; when changing routes of administration, note that oral doses are less than half as effective as parenteral doses (may be only 20% as effective)

Pain:
  Geriatrics: Oral: 1-2 mg every 4-6 hours
  Adults:
    Oral, I.M., I.V., S.C.: 1-4 mg/dose every 4-6 hours as needed; usual adult dose: 2 mg/dose
    Rectal: 3 mg every 6-8 hours
  Antitussive: Geriatrics and Adults: Oral: 1 mg every 3-4 hours as needed

Monitoring Parameters Pain relief, respiratory and mental status, blood pressure

Test Interactions Increased aminotransferase [ALT (SGPT)/AST (SGOT)] (S)

Patient Information May cause drowsiness; avoid the use of alcohol and other CNS depressants

Nursing Implications Observe patient for oversedation, respiratory depression

Additional Information Equianalgesic doses: Morphine 10 mg I.M. = hydromorphone 1.5 mg I.M.

Special Geriatric Considerations The elderly may be particularly susceptible to the CNS depressant and constipating effects of the narcotics (see Pharmacodynamics)

Dosage Forms

Hydromorphone hydrochloride:
  Injection: 1 mg/mL (1 mL); 2 mg/mL (1 mL, 20 mL); 3 mg/mL (1 mL); 4 mg/mL (1 mL); 10 mg/mL (1 mL, 2 mL, 5 mL)
  Suppository, rectal: 3 mg
  Syrup: Hydromorphone hydrochloride 1 mg and guaifenesin 100 mg/5 mL (450 mL)
  Tablet: 1 mg, 2 mg, 3 mg, 4 mg

(Continued)

Hydromorphone *(Continued)*

References
Ferrell BA, "Pain Management in Elderly People," *J Am Geriatr Soc,* 1991, 39(1):64-73.
Kaiko RF, Wallenstein SL, Rogers AG, et al, "Narcotics in the Elderly," *Med Clin North Am,* 1982, 66(5):1079-89.

Hydro-Par® *see* Hydrochlorothiazide *on page 458*

Hydropres® *see* Hydrochlorothiazide and Reserpine *on page 459*

Hydro-Serp® *see* Hydrochlorothiazide and Reserpine *on page 459*

Hydroserpine® *see* Hydrochlorothiazide and Reserpine *on page 459*

HydroSKIN® *see* Hydrocortisone *on page 462*

HydroStat IR® *see* Hydromorphone *on page 464*

Hydro-Tex® [OTC] *see* Hydrocortisone *on page 462*

Hydroxocobalamin (hye droks oh koe BAL a min)

Brand Names Hydrobexan®; Hydro Cobex®; Hydro-Crysti-12®; LA-12®

Synonyms Vitamin B_{12}

Generic Available No

Therapeutic Category Vitamin, Water Soluble

Use Treatment of pernicious anemia, vitamin B_{12} deficiency, increased B_{12} requirements due to thyrotoxicosis, hemorrhage, malignancy, liver or kidney disease, GI dysfunction, or surgery (see Additional Information)

Unlabeled use: Treatment and prevention of cyanide toxicity from sodium nitroprusside

Contraindications Hypersensitivity to cyanocobalamin or any component, cobalt; patients with hereditary optic nerve atrophy

Warnings Some products contain benzoyl alcohol; an intradermal test dose should be performed for hypersensitivity; use only if oral supplementation not possible or when treating pernicious anemia

Precautions Folate doses exceeding 10 mcg/day may produce hematologic response in patients with folate deficiency. Indiscriminate folate use may mask the true diagnosis of pernicious anemia. Single deficiency is rare (except multiple deficiencies). Doses of folate >0.1 mg/day may reverse vitamin B_{12} hematologic abnormalities; however, the neurologic manifestations will not be treated or prevented, and irreversible neurologic damage will ensue; B_{12} deficiency masks signs of polycythemia vera; vegetarian diets may result in B_{12} deficiency; pernicious anemia occurs more often in gastric carcinoma than in general population.

Adverse Reactions
Cardiovascular: Peripheral vascular thrombosis
Dermatologic: Itching, urticaria
Gastrointestinal: Diarrhea
Miscellaneous: Anaphylaxis

Toxicology Excess vitamin B_{12} is excreted in urine; toxic doses are not known

Drug Interactions
Aminosalicylic acid may reduce therapeutic action of vitamin B_{12}
Chloramphenicol may decrease the hematologic effect of vitamin B_{12} in patients with pernicious anemia
Colchicine and prolonged alcohol (>2 weeks) use may decrease absorption of vitamin B_{12}

Stability Clear pink to red solutions are stable at room temperature; protect from light; incompatible with chlorpromazine, phytonadione, prochlorperazine, warfarin, ascorbic acid, dextrose, heavy metals, oxidizing or reducing agents; avoid freezing

Mechanism of Action Coenzyme for various metabolic functions, including fat and carbohydrate metabolism and protein synthesis, used in cell replication, hematopoiesis, and myelin synthesis

Pharmacokinetics
Absorption: From the terminal ileum in the presence of calcium; for absorption to occur, gastric "intrinsic factor" must be present to transfer the compound across the intestinal mucosa
Protein binding: Following absorption, bound to transcobalamin II (the major transport protein) and converted in the tissues to active coenzymes methylcobalamin and deoxyadenosylcobalamin; principally stored in the liver, also stored in the kidneys and adrenals. Hydroxocobalamin (vitamin B_{12a}) is bound highly to protein and is retained in the body longer than cyanocobalamin, but offers no clinical advantage.

Usual Dosage Vitamin B_{12} deficiency: I.M. only: Geriatrics and Adults: 30 mcg/day for 5-10 days, followed by 100-200 mcg/month

Administration Administer I.M. only; may require coadministration of folic acid

Monitoring Parameters Monitor CBC if monocytic anemia is present at initiation

Reference Range Normal range of serum B_{12} is 150-750 pg/mL; this represents 0.1% of total body content. Metabolic requirements are 2-5 µg/day; years of deficiency required before hematologic and neurologic signs and symptoms are seen. Most commercial methods have in the past undergone modification. The lower limit of normal (critical to the diagnosis of B_{12} deficiency/pernicious anemia) has not been firmly established. Clinical correlation and multiple test documentation of the etiology of macrocytic anemia is advised. Occasional patients with significant neuropsychiatric abnormalities may have no hematologic abnormalities and normal serum cobalamin concentrations, 200 pg/mL (SI: >150 pmol/L), or more commonly between 100-200 pg/mL (SI: 75-150 pmol/L).

Test Interactions Methotrexate, pyrimethamine, and most antibiotics interfere with microbiologic assays

Patient Information Therapy is required throughout life; do not take folic acid instead of B_{12} to prevent anemia

Nursing Implications I.M. is the preferred route of administration; oral therapy is markedly inferior to parenteral therapy; monitor potassium concentrations during early therapy; folate therapy may be necessary in first month B_{12} replacement

Additional Information Hydroxocobalamin is more highly bound to protein and is therefore retained longer in the body than is cyanocobalamin. No demonstrated advantage over cyanocobalamin; however, reports on antibody formation to the hydroxocobalamin-transcobalamin II complex have led to clinicians preferring to use cyanocobalamin.

Special Geriatric Considerations There exists evidence that people, particularly elderly whose serum cobalamin concentrations <300 pg/mL, should receive replacement parenteral therapy; this recommendation is based upon neuropsychiatric disorders and cardiovascular disorders associated with lower sodium cobalamin concentrations

Dosage Forms Injection: 1000 mcg/mL (10 mL, 30 mL)

References

Cottrell JE, Casthely P, Brodie JD, et al, "Prevention of Nitroprusside-Induced Cyanide Toxicity With Hydroxocobalamin," *N Engl J Med*, 1978, 298(15):809-11.

Curry SC, Connor DA, and Raschke RA, "Effect of the Cyanide Antidote Hydroxocobalamin on Commonly Ordered Serum Chemistry Studies," *Ann Emerg Med*, 1994, 24(1):65-7.

Holland MA and Kozlowski LM, "Clinical Features and Management of Cyanide Poisoning," *Clin Pharm*, 1986, 5(9):737-41.

Kayser SR and Kurisu S, "Hydroxocobalamin in Nitroprusside Induced Cyanide Toxicity," *Drug Intell Clin Pharm*, 1986, 20:365-6.

Lindenbaum J, Healton EB, Savage DG, et al, "Neuropsychiatric Disorders Caused by Cobalamin Deficiency in the Absence of Anemia or Macrocytosis," *N Engl J Med*, 1988, 318(26):1720-8.

Olszewski AJ, Szostak WB, Bialkowska M, et al, "Reduction of Plasma Lipid and Homocysteine Levels by Pyridoxine, Folate, Cobalamin, Choline, Riboflavin, and Troxerutin in Atherosclerosis," *Atherosclerosis*, 1989, 75(1):1-6.

Regland B, Gottfries CG, and Lindstedt G, "Dementia Patients With Low Serum Cobalamin Concentration: Relationship to Atrophic Gastritis," *Aging Milano*, 1992, 4(1):35-41.

Hydroxycarbamide *see* Hydroxyurea *on next page*

Hydroxychloroquine (hye droks ee KLOR oh kwin)

Brand Names Plaquenil®

Generic Available No

Therapeutic Category Antimalarial Agent

Use Suppresses and treats acute attacks of malaria; treatment of systemic lupus erythematosus and rheumatoid arthritis

Contraindications Retinal or visual field changes attributable to 4-aminoquinolines; hypersensitivity to hydroxychloroquine, 4-aminoquinoline derivatives, or any component

Warnings Use with caution in patients with hepatic disease, G-6-PD deficiency, psoriasis, and porphyria; perform baseline and periodic (6 months) ophthalmologic examinations; test periodically for muscle weakness

Adverse Reactions

Central nervous system: Insomnia, nervousness, nightmares, psychosis, ataxia, headache, confusion, agitation

Dermatologic: Lichenoid dermatitis, bleaching of the hair, pruritus

Gastrointestinal: GI irritation, anorexia, nausea, vomiting

Hematologic: Bone marrow suppression

Neuromuscular & skeletal: Muscle weakness

Ocular: Visual field defects, blindness, retinitis

(Continued)

Hydroxychloroquine *(Continued)*

Overdosage Symptoms of overdose include headache, drowsiness, visual changes, cardiovascular collapse, and seizures followed by respiratory and cardiac arrest

Toxicology Treatment is symptomatic; activated charcoal will bind the drug following GI decontamination; urinary alkalinization will enhance renal elimination; seizures can be treated with diazepam 0.01 mg/kg; shock and hypotension should be treated with fluids and pressors if needed

Drug Interactions Increased digoxin serum concentration

Mechanism of Action Interferes with digestive vacuole function within sensitive malarial parasites by increasing the pH and interfering with lysosomal degradation of hemoglobin; inhibits locomotion of neutrophils and chemotaxis of eosinophils; impairs complement-dependent antigen-antibody reactions

Pharmacokinetics

Absorption: Oral: Complete

Protein binding: 55%

Metabolism: In the liver

Elimination: Metabolites and unchanged drug slowly excreted in urine, may be enhanced by urinary acidification

Usual Dosage Geriatrics and Adults: Oral:

Chemoprophylaxis of malaria: 2 tablets weekly on same day each week; begin 2 weeks before exposure; continue for 4-6 weeks after leaving endemic area

Acute attack: 4 tablets first dose day 1; 2 tablets in 6 hours day 1; 2 tablets in 1 dose day 2; and 2 tablets in 1 dose on day 3

Rheumatoid arthritis: 2-3 tablets/day to start taken with food or milk; usually after 4-12 weeks dose should be reduced by ½ and a maintenance dose of 1-2 tablets/day given (see Additional Information)

Lupus erythematosus: 2 tablets every day or twice daily for several weeks depending on response; 1-2 tablets/day for prolonged maintenance therapy

Monitoring Parameters Ophthalmologic exam, CBC

Patient Information Take with food or milk; complete full course of therapy; wear sunglasses in bright sunlight; notify physician if blurring or other vision changes, ringing in the ears, or hearing loss occurs; may cause nausea, vomiting, diarrhea, loss of appetite, stomach pain, and muscle weakness; should this remain for a prolonged period, report to your physician

Nursing Implications Periodic blood counts and eye examinations are recommended when patient is on chronic therapy; administer with food or milk

Additional Information If long-term use of drug is contemplated, it is recommended to have a complete eye examination performed prior to therapy and at periodic intervals (eg, 6 months)

Special Geriatric Considerations No specific recommendations for dosing (see Monitoring Parameters and Adverse Reactions)

Dosage Forms Tablet, as sulfate: 200 mg [base 155 mg]

25-Hydroxycholecalciferol *see* Calcifediol *on page 139*
Hydroxyethylcellulose *see* Artificial Tears *on page 82*

Hydroxyurea *(hye droks ee yoor EE a)*

Brand Names Hydrea®

Synonyms Hydroxycarbamide

Generic Available No

Therapeutic Category Antineoplastic Agent, Miscellaneous

Use CML in chronic phase; radiosensitizing agent in the treatment of primary brain tumors; head and neck tumors; uterine cervix and nonsmall-cell lung cancer; psoriasis; sickle cell anemia and other hemoglobinopathies; hematologic conditions such as essential thrombocytemia, polycythemia vera, hypereosinophilia, and hyperleukocytosis due to acute leukemia. Has shown activity against renal cell cancer, malignant melanoma, ovarian cancer, head and neck cancer, and prostate cancer.

Contraindications Severe anemia, severe bone marrow suppression; WBC <2500/mm^3 or platelet count <100,000/mm^3; hypersensitivity to hydroxyurea

Warnings The U.S. Food and Drug Administration (FDA) currently recommends that procedures for proper handling and disposal of antineoplastic agents be considered. Use with caution in patients with renal impairment, in patients who have received prior irradiation therapy, and in the elderly.

Precautions Patient who has received irradiation may experience postirradiation erythema; bone marrow suppression is a common side effect; self-limiting megaloblastic erythropoiesis seen commonly upon initiation of hydroxyurea; use with caution in renal impairment and in elderly

Adverse Reactions

Central nervous system: Dizziness, disorientation, hallucinations, seizures, headache

Dermatologic: Maculopapular rash, facial erythema

Endocrine & metabolic: Hyperuricemia

Gastrointestinal: Nausea, vomiting, diarrhea, constipation, anorexia, stomatitis

Hematologic: Myelosuppression, megaloblastic anemia, thrombocytopenia

Hepatic: Elevation of hepatic enzymes

Renal: Dysuria, transient renal tubule dysfunction with increased BUN, serum creatinine, and uric acid

Overdosage
Symptoms of overdose include myelosuppression, facial swelling, hallucinations, disorientation

Toxicology
General supportive care; discontinue drug; consider transfusion of specific blood components

Drug Interactions
Increased toxicity: Fluorouracil: The potential for neurotoxicity may be increased with concomitant administration

Stability
Store capsules at room temperature; capsules may be opened and emptied into water (will not dissolve completely)

Mechanism of Action
Interferes with synthesis of DNA, during the S phase of cell division, without interfering with RNA synthesis; inhibits ribonucleoside diphosphate reductase, preventing conversion of ribonucleotides to deoxyribonucleotides; cell-cycle specific for the S phase and may hold other cells in the G_1 phase of the cell cycle.

Pharmacokinetics

Absorption: Readily from GI tract ($\geq 80\%$)

Distribution: Readily crosses the blood-brain barrier; well distributed into intestine, brain, lung, and kidney tissues

Metabolism: In the liver

Half-life: 3-4 hours

Time to peak serum concentration: Within 2 hours

Elimination: Renal excretion of urea (metabolite) and respiratory excretion of CO_2 (metabolic end product); 50% of the drug is excreted unchanged in urine

Usual Dosage
Oral (refer to individual protocols):

Geriatrics and Adults: Dose should always be titrated to patient response and WBC counts. Usual oral doses range from 10-30 mg/kg/day or 500-3000 mg/day; if WBC count falls to <2500 cells/mm^3, or the platelet count to <100,000/mm^3, therapy should be stopped for at least 3 days and resumed when values rise toward normal

Solid tumors: Intermittent therapy: 80 mg/kg as a single dose every third day; continuous therapy: 20-30 mg/kg/day given as a single dose/day

Concomitant therapy with irradiation: 80 mg/kg as a single dose every third day starting at least 7 days before initiation of irradiation

Resistant chronic myelocytic leukemia: 20-30 mg/kg/day as a single daily dose

Dosing adjustment in renal impairment:

Cl_{cr} 10-50 mL/minute: Administer 50% of normal dose

Cl_{cr} <10 mL/minute: Administer 20% of normal dose

Monitoring Parameters
CBC with differential, platelets, hemoglobin, renal function and liver function tests, serum uric acid

Patient Information
Contents of capsule may be emptied into a glass of water if taken immediately; inform the physician if you develop fever, sore throat, bruising, or bleeding; may cause drowsiness, constipation, and loss of hair

Nursing Implications
See Monitoring Parameters

Additional Information

Myelosuppressive effects:

WBC: Moderate

Platelets: Moderate

Onset (days): 7

Nadir (days): 10

Recovery (days): 21

Special Geriatric Considerations
Elderly may be more sensitive to the effects of this drug; advance dose slowly and adjust dose for renal function with careful monitoring

Dosage Forms
Capsule: 500 mg

25-Hydroxyvitamin D₃ *see* Calcifediol *on page 139*

Hydroxyzine (hye DROKS i zeen)
Related Information
Anxiolytic/Hypnotic Use in Long-Term Care Facilities *on page 1099*
Federal OBRA Regulations Recommended Maximum Doses - Hypnotics *on page 1057*
Brand Names Anxanil®; Atarax®; Atozine®; Durrax®; E-Vista®; Hy-Pam®; Hyzine-50®; Neucalm®; Quiess®; Rezine®; Vamate®; Vistacon-50®; Vistaquel®; Vistaril®; Vistazine®
Generic Available Yes
Therapeutic Category Antianxiety Agent; Antiemetic; Antihistamine; Sedative
Use Treatment of anxiety, as a preoperative sedative, an antipruritic, an antiemetic, and in alcohol withdrawal symptoms
Contraindications Hypersensitivity to hydroxyzine or any component
Warnings Subcutaneous, intra-arterial and I.V. administration **not** recommended since thrombosis and digital gangrene can occur; extravasation can result in sterile abscess and marked tissue induration
Precautions Should be used with caution in patients with narrow-angle glaucoma, prostatic hypertrophy, and bladder neck obstruction; should also be used with caution in patients with asthma or COPD
Adverse Reactions
Cardiovascular: Hypotension
Central nervous system: Drowsiness, dizziness, headache, confusion (especially in the elderly), ataxia
Gastrointestinal: Xerostomia
Local: Pain at injection site
Neuromuscular & skeletal: Weakness
Miscellaneous: Anticholinergic effects (dry eyes, blurred vision, constipation, urinary retention)
Overdosage Symptoms of overdose include seizures, sedation, hypotension, confusion
Toxicology There is no specific treatment for an antihistamine overdose, however, most of its clinical toxicity is due to anticholinergic effects. Cholinesterase inhibitors may be useful by reducing acetylcholinesterase. For anticholinergic overdose with severe life-threatening symptoms, physostigmine 1-2 mg I.V., slowly may be given to reverse these effects.
Drug Interactions
Decreased effect of epinephrine (decreased vasopressor effect)
Increased effect/toxicity: CNS depressants, anticholinergics
Stability Protect from light
Mechanism of Action Competes with histamine for H_1-receptor sites on effector cells in the gastrointestinal tract, blood vessels, and respiratory tract
Pharmacodynamics Onset of action: Within 15-30 minutes; one study found enhanced suppression of H_1-receptor activity in the elderly as compared to younger adults
Pharmacokinetics
Absorption: Oral: Rapid
Distribution: V_d: Increased in elderly
Metabolism: Exact metabolic fate is unknown
Half-life: 3-7 hours; increased in elderly
Time to peak serum concentration: Within 2 hours and lingers for 4-6 hours
Usual Dosage
Geriatrics: Management of pruritus: 10 mg 3-4 times/day; increase to 25 mg 3-4 times/day if necessary
Adults:
Antiemetic: I.M.: 25-100 mg/dose every 4-6 hours as needed
Anxiety: Oral: 25-100 mg 4 times/day; maximum: 600 mg/day
Preoperative sedation:
Oral: 50-100 mg
I.M.: 25-100 mg
Management of pruritus: Oral: 25 mg 3-4 times/day
Monitoring Parameters Relief of symptoms, mental status, blood pressure
Patient Information Will cause drowsiness, avoid alcohol and other CNS depressants, avoid driving and other hazardous tasks until the CNS effects are known
Nursing Implications S.C., intra-arterial, and I.V. administration **not** recommended since thrombosis and digital gangrene can occur; extravasation can result in sterile abscess and marked tissue induration; provide safety

measures (ie, side rails, night light, and call button); remove smoking materials from area; supervise ambulation

Additional Information
Hydroxyzine hydrochloride: Anxanil®, Atarax®, E-Vista®, Hydroxacen®, Quiess®, Vistaril® injection, Vistazine®
Hydroxyzine pamoate: Hy-Pam®, Vistaril® capsule and suspension

Special Geriatric Considerations Anticholinergic effects are not well tolerated in the elderly and frequently result in bowel, bladder, and mental status changes (ie, constipation, confusion, and urinary retention). Hydroxyzine may be useful as a short-term antipruritic, but it is not recommended for use as a sedative or anxiolytic in the elderly. Interpretive guidelines issued by the Health Care Financing Administration (HCFA) discourage the use of hydroxyzine as a sedative or anxiolytic in long-term care facilities.

Dosage Forms
Hydroxyzine hydrochloride:
Injection: 50 mg/mL (1 mL, 2 mL, 10 mL)
Syrup: 10 mg/5 mL (120 mL, 480 mL, 4000 mL)
Tablet: 10 mg, 25 mg, 50 mg, 100 mg
Hydroxyzine pamoate:
Capsule: 25 mg, 50 mg, 100 mg
Suspension: 25 mg/5 mL (120 mL, 480 mL)

References
Simons KJ, Watson WT, Chen XY, et al, "Pharmacokinetic and Pharmacodynamic Studies of the H_1-Receptor Antagonist Hydroxyzine in the Elderly," *Clin Pharmacol Ther*, 1989, 45(1):9-14.

Hygroton® *see* Chlorthalidone *on page 217*
Hylorel® *see* Guanadrel *on page 441*
Hyoscine *see* Scopolamine *on page 850*

Hyoscyamine (hye oh SYE a meen)

Brand Names Anaspaz®; A-Spas® S/L; Cystospaz®; Cystospaz-M®; Donnamar®; ED-SPAZ®; Gastrosed™; Levbid®; Levsin®; Levsinex®; Levsin/SL®

Synonyms l-Hyoscyamine Sulfate

Generic Available No

Therapeutic Category Anticholinergic Agent; Antispasmodic Agent, Gastrointestinal

Use GI tract disorders caused by spasm, adjunctive therapy for peptic ulcers, preoperative medication
Unlabeled use: Urinary incontinence

Contraindications Narrow-angle glaucoma, obstructive uropathy, obstructive GI tract disease, myasthenia gravis, known hypersensitivity to belladonna alkaloids

Precautions Use with caution in hot weather or during exercise. Elderly patients frequently develop increased sensitivity and require strict dosage regulation - side effects may be more severe in elderly patients with atherosclerotic changes. Use with caution in patients with tachycardia, cardiac arrhythmias, hypertension, hypotension, prostatic hypertrophy (especially in the elderly) or any tendency toward urinary retention, liver or kidney disorders and obstructive disease of the GI or GU tract. May exacerbate mental symptoms and precipitate a toxic psychosis when used to treat extrapyramidal reactions resulting from phenothiazines. When given in large doses or to susceptible patients, may cause weakness and inability to move particular muscle groups. Anticholinergic agents can aggravate tardive dyskinesia caused by neuroleptic agents.

Adverse Reactions
Cardiovascular: Tachycardia, palpitations
Central nervous system: Fatigue, delirium, restlessness, headache, ataxia, confusion (the elderly are at increased risk for confusion and hallucinations)
Dermatologic: Dry hot skin
Gastrointestinal: Impaired GI motility, constipation, xerostomia
Genitourinary: Urinary retention
Neuromuscular & skeletal: Tremors
Ocular: Mydriasis, blurred vision, dry eyes

Overdosage Symptoms of overdose include dilated, unreactive pupils; blurred vision; hot, dry flushed skin; dryness of mucous membranes; difficulty in swallowing, foul breath, diminished or absent bowel sounds, urinary retention, tachycardia, hyperthermia, hypertension, increased respiratory rate

Toxicology Anticholinergic toxicity is caused by strong binding of the drug to cholinergic receptors. Cholinesterase inhibitors reduce acetylcholinesterase, the enzyme that breaks down acetylcholine and thereby allows acetylcholine

(Continued)

471

Hyoscyamine *(Continued)*

to accumulate and compete for receptor binding with the offending anticholinergic. For anticholinergic overdose with severe life-threatening symptoms, physostigmine 1-2 mg S.C. or I.V., slowly may be given to reverse these effects.

Drug Interactions
Decreased effect: Metoclopramide, cisapride
Increased toxicity: Amantadine, phenothiazines, tricyclic antidepressants, other anticholinergic agents
Antagonistic effect: Tacrine, donepezil

Mechanism of Action Blocks the action of acetylcholine at parasympathetic sites in smooth muscle, secretory glands and the CNS; increases cardiac output, dries secretions, antagonizes histamine and serotonin

Pharmacodynamics
Onset of action: Within 2-3 minutes
Duration: 4-6 hours

Pharmacokinetics
Absorption: Oral: Absorbed well
Protein binding: 50%
Metabolism: In the liver
Half-life: 13% to 38%
Elimination: In urine

Usual Dosage Geriatrics and Adults:
Oral, S.L.: 0.125-0.25 mg 3-4 times/day before meals or food and at bedtime; 0.375-0.75 mg (timed release) every 12 hours
I.M., I.V., S.C.: 0.25-0.5 mg every 6 hours

Monitoring Parameters Pulse, anticholinergic effects, urine output, GI symptoms

Patient Information Take 30-60 minutes before a meal; maintain good oral hygiene habits, because lack of saliva may increase chance of cavities. Observe caution while driving or performing other tasks requiring alertness, as may cause drowsiness, dizziness, or blurred vision. Notify physician if skin rash, flushing or eye pain occurs; or if difficulty in urinating, constipation or sensitivity to light becomes severe or persists.

Nursing Implications Monitor patient for anticholinergic effects

Special Geriatric Considerations Avoid long-term use; the potential for toxic reactions is higher than the potential benefit, elderly are particularly prone to CNS side effects of anticholinergics (ie, confusion, delirium, hallucinations). Side effects often occur before clinical response is obtained (see Precautions).

Dosage Forms
Hyoscyamine sulfate:
Capsule, timed release (Cystospaz-M®, Levsinex®): 0.375 mg
Elixir (Levsin®): 0.125 mg/5 mL with alcohol 20% (480 mL)
Injection (Levsin®): 0.5 mg/mL (1 mL, 10 mL)
Solution, oral (Gastrosed™, Levsin®): 0.125 mg/mL (15 mL)
Tablet:
Anaspaz®, Gastrosed™, Levsin®, Neoquess®: 0.125 mg
Cystospaz®: 0.15 mg

Hyoscyamine, Atropine, Scopolamine, and Phenobarbital

(hye oh SYE a meen, A troe peen, skoe POL a meen & fee noe BAR bi tal)

Brand Names Barbidonna®; Barophen®; Donnapine®; Donna-Sed®; Donnatal®; Donphen®; Hyosophen®; Kinesed®; Malatal®; Relaxadon®; Spaslin®; Spasmolin®; Spasmophen®; Spasquid®; Susano®

Generic Available Yes

Therapeutic Category Anticholinergic Agent; Antispasmodic Agent, Gastrointestinal

Use Adjunct in the treatment of peptic ulcer disease, irritable bowel, spastic colitis, spastic bladder, and renal colic

Contraindications Hypersensitivity to hyoscyamine, atropine, scopolamine, phenobarbital, or any component; narrow-angle glaucoma, tachycardia, GI and GU obstruction, myasthenia gravis

Precautions Use with caution in patients with hepatic or renal disease, hyperthyroidism, cardiovascular disease, hypertension, prostatic hypertrophy, autonomic neuropathy

Adverse Reactions

Cardiovascular: Tachycardia, palpitations, hypotension

Central nervous system: Fatigue, delirium, restlessness, drowsiness, headache, ataxia, confusion, impairment of judgment and coordination

Dermatologic: Dry hot skin, skin rash

Gastrointestinal: Impaired GI motility, xerostomia, constipation

Genitourinary: Urinary hesitancy/retention

Neuromuscular & skeletal: Tremors

Ocular: Mydriasis, blurred vision, dry eyes

Respiratory: Respiratory depression

Overdosage Symptoms of overdose include unsteady gait, slurred speech, confusion, hypotension, respiratory collapse, dilated unreactive pupils, hot or flushed skin, diminished bowel sounds, urinary retention

Toxicology Anticholinergic toxicity is caused by strong binding of the drug to cholinergic receptors. Cholinesterase inhibitors reduce acetylcholinesterase, the enzyme that breaks down acetylcholine and thereby allows acetylcholine to accumulate and compete for receptor binding with the offending anticholinergic. For anticholinergic overdose with severe life-threatening symptoms, physostigmine 1-2 mg S.C. or I.V., slowly may be given to reverse these effects.

Drug Interactions

Decreased effect with antacids; decreased effect of anticoagulants, metoclopramide, cisapride

Increased effect/toxicity with CNS depressants, alcohol, amantadine, anticholinergics, narcotic analgesics, type I antiarrhythmics, antihistamines, phenothiazines, TCAs

Antagonistic effect: Tacrine, donepezil

Mechanism of Action Belladonna alkaloids inhibit muscarinic actions of acetylcholine at postganglionic receptor sites which decreases hypermotility and hypersecretory state of the gastrointestinal tract.

Pharmacokinetics Absorption: Well absorbed from GI tract

Usual Dosage Geriatrics and Adults: Oral: 1-2 capsules or tablets 3-4 times/day; or 1 Donnatal® Extentab® in sustained release form every 12 hours; or 5-10 mL elixir 3-4 times/day or every 8 hours

Patient Information Maintain good oral hygiene habits, because lack of saliva may increase chance of cavities. Observe caution while driving or performing other tasks requiring alertness, as may cause drowsiness, dizziness, or blurred vision. Notify physician if skin rash, flushing or eye pain occurs; or if difficulty in urinating, constipation or sensitivity to light becomes severe or persists. Do not attempt tasks requiring mental alertness or physical coordination until you know the effects of the drug. Swallow extended release tablet whole, do not crush or chew.

Nursing Implications Do not crush extended release tablets

Special Geriatric Considerations Because of the anticholinergic effects of this product, it is not recommended for use in the elderly (see Contraindications, Precautions, Adverse Reactions)

Dosage Forms

Elixir: Hyoscyamine sulfate 0.1037 mg, atropine sulfate 0.0194 mg, scopolamine hydrobromide 0.0065 mg and phenobarbital 16.2 mg per 5 mL (120 mL, 480 mL, 4000 mL)

Tablet: Hyoscyamine sulfate 0.1037 mg, atropine sulfate 0.0194 mg, scopolamine hydrobromide 0.0065 mg and phenobarbital 16.2 mg

Tablet:

Chewable: Hyoscyamine hydrobromide 0.12 mg, atropine sulfate 0.12 mg, scopolamine hydrobromide 0.12 mg and phenobarbital 16 mg

Long-acting: Hyoscyamine sulfate 0.3111 mg, atropine sulfate 0.0582 mg, scopolamine hydrobromide 0.0195 mg and phenobarbital 48.6 mg

Hyoscyamine, Atropine, Scopolamine, Kaolin, Pectin, and Opium

(hye oh SYE a meen, A troe peen, skoe POL a meen, KAY oh lin, PEK tin, & OH pee um)

Brand Names Donnapectolin-PG®; Kapectolin PG®

Therapeutic Category Antidiarrheal

Use Treatment of diarrhea; also used in gastritis, enteritis, colitis, acute gastrointestinal upsets, and nausea which may accompany these conditions

Restrictions C-V

Contraindications Advanced renal or hepatic disease, narrow-angle glaucoma, known hypersensitivity to belladonna alkaloids, kaolin, pectin or opium, (Continued)

Hyoscyamine, Atropine, Scopolamine, Kaolin, Pectin, and Opium (Continued)

myocardial ischemia, tachycardia, gastrointestinal obstruction, paralytic ileus, intestinal atony (elderly), severe ulcerative colitis, toxic megacolon, obstructive uropathy, myasthenia gravis, asthma; pseudomembranous colitis (Clostridium difficile infections)

Warnings Drug dependence; incomplete intestinal obstruction (eg, ileostomy, colostomy) may present with diarrhea, thus needing evaluation before administering; sudden withdrawal of large doses of scopolamine in Parkinson's disease may precipitate malaise, vomiting, salivation, and sweating; heat prostration may occur in high environmental temperatures; gastric ulcer (delayed emptying time); anticholinergic psychosis; elderly may exhibit agitation, confusion, short-term memory loss, hallucinations, delirium with anticholinergic medications

Precautions Use with caution in geriatric patients (see Warnings); hazardous tasks (driving, etc); glaucoma (narrow-angle), ileus, hiatal hernia with reflux, prostatic hypertrophy, cardiac arrhythmias, congestive heart failure, hypertension, COPD, hyperthyroidism, and anatomic neuropathy

Adverse Reactions

Cardiovascular: Bradycardia (low-dose atropine), tachycardia (high dose), flushing, palpitations

Central nervous system: Confusion, insomnia, excitement, headache, drowsiness, hallucinations, delirium, nervousness

Gastrointestinal: Nausea, vomiting, heartburn, constipation, bloating, ileus, xerostomia, dysgeusia

Genitourinary: Urinary retention, impotence

Ocular: Photophobia, dilated pupils, blurred vision, increased IOP

Overdosage Symptoms of overdose include dry mouth, thirst, vomiting, abdominal distention, difficulty swallowing, muscular weakness, CNS stimulation, delirium, drowsiness, anxiety, stupor, confusion, hallucinations, seizures, psychotic behavior, tachycardia, rapid respiration, hypertension or hypotension, respiratory depression, urinary urgency, blurred vision, dilated pupils, flushed hot dry skin

Toxicology Anticholinergic toxicity is caused by strong binding of the drug to cholinergic receptors. Cholinesterase inhibitors reduce acetylcholinesterase, the enzyme that breaks down acetylcholine and thereby allows acetylcholine to accumulate and compete for receptor binding with the offending anticholinergic. For anticholinergic overdose with severe life-threatening symptoms, physostigmine 1-2 mg S.C. or I.V., slowly may be given to reverse these effects. Induce emesis or perform gastric lavage and administer charcoal slurry; administer supportive care. Diazepam, chloral hydrate are used to treat CNS stimulation.

Drug Interactions

Amantadine may enhance anticholinergic effects

Pharmacologic effects of atenolol may be increased; pharmacologic effects of digoxin may be enhanced

Phenothiazines may have decreased antipsychotic action but increased anticholinergic effects (additive)

Antidepressants (TCAs) may have increased anticholinergic effects (additive)

May increase anticholinergic effects of any drug with anticholinergic action

Decreased effect with tacrine, metoclopramide, cisapride

Mechanism of Action Belladonna alkaloids inhibit muscarinic actions of acetylcholine at postganglionic receptor sites which decreases hypermotility and hypersecretory state of the gastrointestinal tract. Opium delays transit of intraluminal contents, increases gut capacity, increases sphincter tone, stimulates fluid movement across gut mucosa, relieves tenesmus and pain.

Pharmacokinetics Atropine stimulates CNS; scopolamine is a CNS depressant

Absorption: Oral: Belladonna alkaloids are rapidly absorbed

Distribution: Readily crosses blood-brain barrier

Half-life: Atropine: 2.5 hours

Elimination: 94% of dose eliminated renally in 24 hours

Usual Dosage Geriatrics and Adults: Initial: 30 mL (1 fluid oz) followed by 15-30 mL after each loose stool (do not exceed 120 mL in 12 hours); use lower dose recommendations initially before increasing dose to 30 mL after each loose stool

Monitoring Parameters Monitor stool frequency, consistency; heart rate, signs of CNS toxicity; bladder dysfunction and respiratory rate with multiple doses, dehydration, fluid/electrolyte loss

Patient Information Shake well before using; do not exceed recommended doses; report failure to respond to physician

Nursing Implications See Warnings, Precautions, Monitoring Parameters, and Special Geriatric Considerations

Additional Information Hyoscyamine is dialyzable but is ineffective for atropine

Special Geriatric Considerations Elderly are particularly prone to CNS side effects to anticholinergics (ie, confusion, delirium, hallucinations). The use of this product is discouraged in elderly since systemic side effects often occur before clinical response obtained for GI problem.

Dosage Forms Suspension, oral: Hyoscyamine sulfate 0.1037 mg, atropine sulfate 0.0194 mg, scopolamine hydrobromide 0.0065 mg, kaolin 6 g, pectin 142.8 mg, and powdered opium 24 mg per 30 mL with alcohol 5%

Hyosophen® *see* Hyoscyamine, Atropine, Scopolamine, and Phenobarbital *on page 472*

Hy-Pam® *see* Hydroxyzine *on page 470*

Hyperab® *see* Rabies Immune Globulin (Human) *on page 818*

HyperHep® *see* Hepatitis B Immune Globulin *on page 452*

Hyper-Tet® *see* Tetanus Immune Globulin, Human *on page 897*

Hy-Phen® *see* Hydrocodone and Acetaminophen *on page 461*

HypoTears® Ophthalmic Ointment [OTC] *see* Ocular Lubricant *on page 688*

HypoTears PF Solution [OTC] *see* Artificial Tears *on page 82*

HypoTears Solution [OTC] *see* Artificial Tears *on page 82*

Hyrexin-50® Injection *see* Diphenhydramine *on page 302*

Hytakerol® *see* Dihydrotachysterol *on page 296*

Hytone® *see* Hydrocortisone *on page 462*

Hytrin® *see* Terazosin *on page 890*

Hytuss® [OTC] *see* Guaifenesin *on page 437*

Hytuss-2X® [OTC] *see* Guaifenesin *on page 437*

Hyzaar® *see* Losartan *on page 553*

Hy-Zide® *see* Hydralazine and Hydrochlorothiazide *on page 457*

Hyzine-50® *see* Hydroxyzine *on page 470*

Ibidomide Hydrochloride *see* Labetalol *on page 520*

Ibuprin® [OTC] *see* Ibuprofen *on this page*

Ibuprofen (eye byoo PROE fen)

Brand Names Aches-N-Pain® [OTC]; Advil® [OTC]; Children's Advil® Oral Suspension [OTC]; Children's Motrin® Oral Suspension [OTC]; Excedrin® IB [OTC]; Genpril® [OTC]; Haltran® [OTC]; Ibuprin® [OTC]; Ibuprohm® [OTC]; Ibu-Tab®; Junior Strength Motrin® [OTC]; Medipren® [OTC]; Menadol® [OTC]; Midol® 200 [OTC]; Motrin®; Motrin® IB [OTC]; Nuprin® [OTC]; Pamprin IB® [OTC]; PediaProfen™; Rufen®; Saleto-200® [OTC]; Saleto-400®; Trendar® [OTC]; Uni-Pro® [OTC]

Synonyms *p*-Isobutylhydratropic Acid

Generic Available Yes: Tablet

Therapeutic Category Analgesic, Non-narcotic; Anti-inflammatory Agent; Antipyretic; Nonsteroidal Anti-inflammatory Agent (NSAID), Oral

Use Inflammatory diseases and rheumatoid disorders including rheumatoid arthritis; mild to moderate pain; fever; gout; osteoarthritis; sunburn, ankylosing spondylitis, acute migraine headache

Contraindications Hypersensitivity to ibuprofen, any component, aspirin or other nonsteroidal anti-inflammatory drugs (NSAIDs)

Warnings GI toxicity (bleeding, ulceration, perforation); CNS effects may occur (headaches, confusion, depression); cross-sensitivity with aspirin and other NSAIDs exists; hypersensitivity, anaphylactoid reactions (intermittent tolmetin use more often); renal function decline, acute renal insufficiency, interstitial nephritis, dysuria, cystitis, hematuria, nephrotic syndrome, hyperkalemia in acute renal insufficiency, hyponatremia, papillary necrosis, hepatic function impairment; elderly have increased risk for adverse reactions to NSAIDs (see Special Geriatric Considerations)

Precautions Use with caution in patients with congestive heart failure, hypertension, decreased renal or hepatic function, history of GI disease (bleeding or ulcers), or those receiving anticoagulants; perform ophthalmologic evaluation for those who develop eye complaints during therapy (blurred vision, diminished vision, changes in color vision, retinal changes); NSAIDs may mask signs/symptoms of infections; photosensitivity reported
(Continued)

Ibuprofen (Continued)

Adverse Reactions

Cardiovascular: Congestive heart failure, angina, hypertension, hypotension, arrhythmias, edema

Central nervous system: Headache, drowsiness, vertigo, dizziness, fatigue, hallucinations, confusion, depression, emotional lability, psychotic behavior, pyrexia

Dermatologic: Rash, urticaria, angioedema, Stevens-Johnson syndrome, exfoliative dermatitis, bruising, petechiae, purpura

Endocrine & metabolic: Hyperglycemia, hypoglycemia, hyperkalemia, gynecomastia, hyponatremia, fluid retention

Gastrointestinal: Dyspepsia, heartburn, nausea, diarrhea, constipation, flatulence, stomatitis, vomiting, abdominal pain, peptic ulcer, GI bleeding, GI perforation, gingival ulcers, pancreatitis, proctitis, paralytic ulcers, colitis, anorexia, weight loss, dry mucous membranes

Genitourinary: Impotence, azotemia

Hematologic: Neutropenia, anemia, agranulocytosis, bone marrow suppression, hemolytic anemia, hemorrhage, inhibition of platelet aggregation

Hepatic: Hepatitis, elevated LFTs, cholestatic jaundice

Neuromuscular & skeletal: Involuntary muscle movements, muscle weakness, tremors, weakness

Ocular: Vision changes

Otic: Tinnitus

Renal: Dysuria, polyuria, pyuria, oliguria, anuria, acute renal failure

Respiratory: Exacerbation of asthma, dyspnea

Miscellaneous: Thirst, diaphoresis

Overdosage
Symptoms include drowsiness, lethargy, disorientation, confusion, dizziness, numbness, paresthesia, nausea, vomiting, gastric irritation, abdominal pain, headache, tinnitus, sweating, blurred vision, muscle twitching, seizures, coma, acute renal failure, increased BUN and serum creatinine, hypotension, tachycardia, and metabolic acidosis

Toxicology
Management of a nonsteroidal anti-inflammatory agent (NSAID) intoxication is primarily supportive and symptomatic. Fluid therapy is commonly effective in managing the hypotension that may occur following an acute NSAID overdose, except when this is due to an acute blood loss. Seizures tend to be very short-lived and often do not require drug treatment although recurrent seizures should be treated with I.V. diazepam. Since many of the NSAIDs undergo enterohepatic cycling, multiple doses of charcoal may be needed to reduce the potential for delayed toxicities. NSAIDs are highly bound to plasma proteins, therefore hemodialysis and peritoneal dialysis are not useful.

Drug Interactions
May increase digoxin, methotrexate, and lithium serum concentrations

Aspirin and other salicylates may decrease NSAID serum concentrations

Other NSAIDs may increase adverse GI effects

Increased prothrombin time with anticoagulants

Decreased antihypertensive effects of ACE inhibitors, beta-blockers, and thiazide diuretics

Increased response to sympathomimetics

Probenecid may increase toxicity of NSAIDs by increase in serum concentrations

Effects of loop diuretics may be decreased

May enhance azotemia in elderly receiving loop diuretics; may increase risk for renal insufficiency when used with diuretics

Mechanism of Action
Inhibits prostaglandin synthesis, acts on the hypothalamus heat-regulating center to reduce fever, blocks prostaglandin synthetase action which prevents formation of the platelet-aggregating substance thromboxane A_2; decreases pain receptor sensitivity. Other proposed mechanisms of action are lysosomal stabilization, inhibition of kinin and leukotriene production, alteration of chemotactic factors, and inhibition of neutrophil activation. This latter mechanism may be the most significant pharmacologic action to reduce inflammation.

Pharmacodynamics
Onset of analgesia: 30 minutes to 1 hour

Duration: 4-6 hours

Onset of anti-inflammatory: Up to 7 days

Peak action: 1-2 weeks

Pharmacokinetics
Absorption: Oral: Rapid, 85%

Protein binding: 90% to 99%

Metabolism: In the liver by oxidation; substrate CYP2C9

Half-life: 2-4 hours

Time to peak serum concentration: Within 1-2 hours

Elimination: In urine (1% as free drug); some biliary excretion occurs

Usual Dosage Geriatrics and Adults: Oral:

Inflammatory disease: 400-800 mg/dose 3-4 times/day; maximum dose: 3.2 g/day

Pain/fever: 200-400 mg/dose every 4-6 hours; maximum daily dose: 1.2 g

Monitoring Parameters Monitor response (pain, range of motion, grip strength, mobility, ADL function), inflammation; observe for weight gain, edema; monitor renal function; observe for bleeding, bruising; evaluate gastrointestinal effects (abdominal pain, bleeding, dyspepsia); mental confusion, disorientation, CBC, serum, creatinine, BUN, liver function tests

Reference Range Plasma concentrations >200 µg/mL may be associated with severe toxicity

Test Interactions Increased chloride (S), increased sodium (S)

Patient Information Serious gastrointestinal bleeding can occur as well as ulceration and perforation. Pain may or may not be present. Avoid aspirin and aspirin-containing products while taking this medication. If gastric upset occurs, take with food, milk, or antacid. If gastric adverse effects persist, contact physician. May cause drowsiness, dizziness, blurred vision, and confusion. Use caution when performing tasks which require alertness (eg, driving). Do not take for more than 3 days for fever or 10 days for pain without physician's advice.

Nursing Implications See Patient Information, Overdosage, Monitoring Parameters, and Special Geriatric Considerations

Additional Information There are no clinical guidelines to predict which NSAID will give response in a particular patient. Trials with each must be initiated until response determined. Consider dose, patient convenience, and cost.

Special Geriatric Considerations Elderly are a high-risk population for adverse effects from nonsteroidal anti-inflammatory agents. As much as 60% of elderly can develop peptic ulceration and/or hemorrhage asymptomatically. The concomitant use of H_2 blockers, omeprazole, and sucralfate is not effective as prophylaxis with the exception of NSAID-induced duodenal ulcers which may be prevented by the use of ranitidine. Misoprostol and proton pump inhibitors are the only agents proven to help prevent the development of NSAID-induced ulcers. Also, concomitant disease and drug use contribute to the risk for GI adverse effects. Use lowest effective dose for shortest period possible. Consider renal function decline with age. Use of NSAIDs can compromise existing renal function especially when Cl_{cr} is ≤30 mL/minute. Tinnitus may be a difficult and unreliable indication of toxicity due to age-related hearing loss or eighth cranial nerve damage. CNS adverse effects such as confusion, agitation, and hallucination are generally seen in overdose or high dose situations, but elderly may demonstrate these adverse effects at lower doses than younger adults.

Dosage Forms

Suspension: 100 mg/5 mL (120 mL)

Tablet: 300 mg, 400 mg, 600 mg, 800 mg

Tablet, chewable: 50 mg, 100 mg

Tablet [OTC]: 200 mg

References

Brooks PM, Day RO, "Nonsteroidal Anti-inflammatory Drugs - Differences and Similarities," *N Engl J Med*, 1991, 324(24):1716-25.

Clinch D, Banerjee AK, Ostick G, "Absence of Abdominal Pain in Elderly Patients With Peptic Ulcer," *Age Ageing*, 1984, 13(2):120-3.

Clive DM, Stoff JS, "Renal Syndromes Associated With Nonsteroidal Anti-inflammatory Drugs," *N Engl J Med*, 1984, 310(9):563-72.

Graham DY, "Prevention of Gastroduodenal Injury Induced by Chronic Nonsteroidal Anti-inflammatory Drug Therapy," *Gastroenterology*, 1989, 96(2 Pt 2 Suppl):675-81.

Gurwitz JH, Avorn J, Ross-Degnan D, et al, "Nonsteroidal Anti-Inflammatory Drug-Associated Azotemia in the Very Old," *JAMA*, 1990, 264(4):471-5.

Hawkey CJ, Karrasch JA, Szczepaski L, et al, "Omeprazole Compared With Misoprostrol for Ulcers Associated With Nonsteroidal Anti-inflammatory Drugs," *N Engl J Med*, 1998, 338(11):727-34.

Knodel LC, "Preventing NSAID-Induced Ulcers: The Role of Misoprostol," *Consult Pharm*, 1989, 4:37-41.

Pounder R, "Silent Peptic Ulceration: Deadly Silence or Golden Silence?" *Gastroenterology*, 1989, 96:(2 Pt 2 Suppl)626-31.

Yeomans ND, Tulassay Z, Juhasz L, et al, "A Comparison of Omeprazole With Ranitidine for Ulcers Associated With Nonsteroidal Anti-inflammatory Drugs," *N Engl J Med*, 1998, 338(11):719-26.

Ibuprohm® [OTC] *see* Ibuprofen *on page 475*

Ibu-Tab® *see* Ibuprofen *on page 475*

Idoxuridine (eye doks YOOR i deen)
Brand Names Herplex® Ophthalmic
Synonyms IDU; IUDR
Generic Available No
Therapeutic Category Antiviral Agent, Ophthalmic
Use Treatment of herpes simplex keratitis
Contraindications Hypersensitivity to idoxuridine or any component; concurrent use in patients receiving corticosteroids with superficial dendritic keratitis
Warnings Use with caution in patients with corneal ulceration or patients receiving corticosteroid applications; if no response in epithelial infections within 14 days, consider a second form of therapy
Adverse Reactions
Local: Irritation, pruritus, pain, inflammation
Ocular: Corneal clouding, photophobia, small punctate defects on the corneal epithelium, mild edema of the eyelids and cornea, follicular conjunctivitis; ointment may produce a temporary visual haze
Toxicology Due to frequent dosing, small defects on the epithelium may result. Mutagenic and cytotoxic and should be considered as being potentially carcinogenic; no treatment is indicated for accidental ingestion
Drug Interactions Increased toxicity (initiation): Do not coadminister with boric acid containing solutions
Stability Store in tight, light-resistant containers at 2\°C to 8°C until dispensed; do not mix with other medications; solution must be refrigerated
Mechanism of Action Incorporated into viral DNA in place of thymidine resulting in mutations and inhibition of viral replication
Pharmacokinetics
Absorption: Ophthalmic: Poor following instillation; tissue uptake is a function of cellular metabolism, which is inhibited by high concentrations of the drug (absorption decreases as the concentration of drug increases)
Metabolism: To iodouracil, uracil, and iodide
Elimination: Unchanged drug and metabolites excreted in urine
Usual Dosage Geriatrics and Adults: Ophthalmic:
Solution: Instill 1 drop in eye(s) every hour during day and every 2 hours at night, continue until definite improvement is noted, then reduce daytime dose to 1 drop every 2 hours and every 4 hours at night; continue for 5-7 days after healing appears complete
Patient Information May cause sensitivity to bright light; minimize by wearing sunglasses; notify physician if improvement is not seen in 7-8 days, if condition worsens, or if pain, decreased vision, itching, or swelling of the eye occur; do not exceed recommended dose
Nursing Implications Idoxuridine solution should not be mixed with other medications (see Patient Information)
Special Geriatric Considerations Assess patient's ability to self-administer (see Adverse Reactions)
Dosage Forms Solution, ophthalmic: 0.1% (15 mL)

IDU *see* Idoxuridine *on this page*
IFLrA *see* Interferon Alfa-2a *on page 490*
IG *see* Immune Globulin *on page 482*
IGIM *see* Immune Globulin *on page 482*
Ilosone® **Oral** *see* Erythromycin *on page 344*
Ilotycin® **Ophthalmic** *see* Erythromycin, Topical *on page 347*
Ilozyme® *see* Pancrelipase *on page 712*
Imdur™ *see* Isosorbide Mononitrate *on page 505*
I-Methasone® *see* Dexamethasone *on page 274*
Imipemide *see* Imipenem and Cilastatin *on this page*

Imipenem and Cilastatin (i mi PEN em & sye la STAT in)
Related Information
I.V. Medication Recommendations *on page 1080*
Penicillins, Penicillin-Related Antibiotics, & Other Antibiotics *on page 1010*
Brand Names Primaxin®
Synonyms Imipemide
Generic Available No
Therapeutic Category Antibiotic, Miscellaneous
Use Treatment of documented multidrug resistant gram-negative infection due to organisms proven or suspected to be susceptible to imipenem/cilastatin;

treatment of multiple organism infection in which other agents have an insufficient spectrum of activity or are contraindicated due to toxic potential

Contraindications Hypersensitivity to imipenem/cilastatin or any component

Warnings Prolonged use may result in superinfection; patients with CNS abnormalities at increased risk for seizures

Precautions Dosage adjustment required in patients with impaired renal function; use with caution in patients with penicillin or cephalosporin allergy

Adverse Reactions

Cardiovascular: Hypotension, palpitations

Central nervous system: Seizures

Dermatologic: Rash

Gastrointestinal: Nausea, vomiting, diarrhea, pseudomembranous colitis

Hematologic: Neutropenia, eosinophilia, positive Coombs' test

Local: Pain at injection site, phlebitis

Miscellaneous: Emergence of resistant strains of *P. aeruginosa*

Toxicology Discontinue the drug; many beta-lactam-containing antibiotics have the potential to cause neuromuscular hyperirritability or convulsive seizures; hemodialysis may be helpful to aid in the removal of the drug from the blood, otherwise most treatment is supportive or symptom directed. Diazepam 0.01 mg/kg can be used for seizures.

Drug Interactions Probenecid (minimal increase in imipenem plasma concentration), ganciclovir (may increase risk for seizures)

Stability Stable for 10 hours at room temperature following reconstitution with 100 mL of 0.9% sodium chloride injection; up to 48 hours when refrigerated at 5°C. If reconstituted with 5% or 10% dextrose injection, 5% dextrose and sodium bicarbonate, 5% dextrose and 0.9% sodium chloride, is stable for 4 hours at room temperature and 24 hours when refrigerated.

Mechanism of Action Inhibits cell wall synthesis by binding to penicillin-binding proteins on the bacterial outer membrane; cilastatin prevents renal metabolism of imipenem by competitive inhibition of dehydropeptidase along the brush border of the proximal renal tubules

Pharmacokinetics

Protein binding: Cilastatin is 40% plasma protein bound

Metabolism:

Imipenem: Metabolized in the kidney by dehydropeptidase

Cilastatin: Partially metabolized in the kidneys

Half-life (both): 60 minutes, extended with renal insufficiency

Elimination: When imipenem is given with cilastatin, urinary excretion of unchanged imipenem increases to 70%

Cilastatin: 70% to 80% of a dose is excreted unchanged in the urine

Half-life and V_d (L/kg) have been reported to be increased and decreased, respectively, in the older adult compared to younger adults

Usual Dosage Geriatrics and Adults (dosage recommendation based on imipenem component):

I.M.: 500 mg or 750 mg every 12 hours depending on the severity of infection

I.V.:

Serious infection: 2-4 g/day in divided doses every 6 hours

Mild to moderate infection: 1-2 g/day in divided doses every 6 hours

Dosing adjustment in renal impairment:

Cl_{cr} <30-70 mL/minute/1.73 m²: Reduced dose

Moderately dialyzable (20% to 50%). See table.

Creatinine Clearance mL/min/1.73 m²	Frequency	% Decrease in Daily Maximum Dose
30-70	q6h	50
20-30	q8h	63
5-20	q12h	75

Administration Not for direct infusion; vial contents must be transferred to 100 mL of infusion solution; final concentration should not exceed 5 mg/mL; infuse over 30-60 minutes; watch for convulsions; I.M. preparation is for I.M. use only, I.V. preparation is for I.V. use only

Monitoring Parameters Signs and symptoms of infection; mental status, WBC, periodic renal, hepatic, and hematologic function tests

Test Interactions Interferes with urinary glucose determination using Clinitest®

Nursing Implications Do not mix with or physically add to other antibiotics; however, may administer concomitantly; do not interchange I.M. and I.V. products (see Administration)

(Continued)

Imipenem and Cilastatin *(Continued)*

Additional Information Sodium content of 1 g: 3.2 mEq

Special Geriatric Considerations Imipenem/cilastatin's role is limited to the treatment of infections caused by susceptible multiresistant organism(s) and in patients whose bacterial infection(s) have failed to respond to other appropriate antimicrobials; many of the seizures attributed to imipenem/cilastatin were in elderly patients; dose must be adjusted for creatinine clearance

Dosage Forms

Powder for injection I.V.: Imipenem 250 mg and cilastatin 250 mg (13 mL); imipenem 500 mg and cilastatin 500 mg (13 mL)

Primaxin® I.M.: Imipenem 500 mg and cilastatin 500 mg; imipenem 750 mg and cilastatin 750 mg

References

Finch RG, Craddock C, Kelly J, et al, "Pharmacokinetic Studies of Imipenem/Cilastatin in Elderly Patients," *J Antimicrob Chemother*, 1986, 18(Suppl E):103-7.

Toon S, Hopkins KJ, Garstang FM, et al, "Pharmacokinetics of Imipenem and Cilastatin After Their Simultaneous Administration to the Elderly," *Br J Clin Pharmacol*, 1987, 23(2):143-9.

Yoshikawa TT, "Antimicrobial Therapy for the Elderly Patient," *J Am Geriatr Soc*, 1990, 38(12):1353-72.

Imipramine *(im IP ra meen)*

Related Information

Antidepressant Agents Comparison *on page 1021*
Antidepressant Medication Guidelines *on page 1075*
Federal OBRA Regulations Recommended Maximum Doses - Antidepressants *on page 1056*
Serum Drug Concentrations Commonly Monitored: Guidelines *on page 1114*

Brand Names Janimine®; Tofranil®; Tofranil-PM®

Generic Available Yes: Tablet

Therapeutic Category Antidepressant, Tricyclic

Use Treatment of various forms of depression, often in conjunction with psychotherapy

Unlabeled use: Neurogenic pain, urinary incontinence, panic disorder

Contraindications Hypersensitivity to imipramine (cross-sensitivity with other tricyclics may occur); patients receiving MAO inhibitors within past 14 days; narrow-angle glaucoma

Warnings To avoid cholinergic crisis do not discontinue abruptly in patients receiving long-term high dose therapy; some oral preparations contain tartrazine and injection contains sulfites both of which can cause allergic reactions

Precautions Use with caution in patients with cardiovascular disease, conduction disturbances, seizure disorders, urinary retention, bipolar illness, renal or hepatic impairment, hyperthyroidism or those receiving thyroid replacement; an EKG prior to the start of therapy is advised

Adverse Reactions Less sedation and anticholinergic effects than amitriptyline

Cardiovascular: Arrhythmias, hypotension

Central nervous system: Drowsiness, sedation, confusion, delirium, dizziness, fatigue, anxiety, nervousness, sleep disorders, seizures

Dermatologic: Rash, photosensitivity

Gastrointestinal: Nausea, vomiting, constipation, xerostomia

Genitourinary: Urinary retention

Hematologic: Blood dyscrasias

Hepatic: Hepatitis, cholestatic jaundice

Neuromuscular & skeletal: Weakness

Ocular: Blurred vision, increased intraocular pressure

Miscellaneous: Has been associated with falls, hypersensitivity reactions

Overdosage Symptoms of overdose include confusion, hallucinations, seizure, constipation, cyanosis, tachycardia

Toxicology Following initiation of essential overdose management, toxic symptoms should be treated. Ventricular arrhythmias often respond to phenytoin 15-20 mg/kg with concurrent systemic alkalinization (sodium bicarbonate 0.5-2 mEq/kg I.V.). Arrhythmias unresponsive to this therapy may respond to lidocaine 1 mg/kg I.V. followed by a titrated infusion. Physostigmine (1-2 mg I.V. slowly) may be indicated in reversing cardiac arrhythmias that are due to vagal blockade or for anticholinergic effects. Seizures usually respond to diazepam I.V. boluses (5-10 mg, up to 30 mg). If seizures are unresponsive or recur, phenytoin or phenobarbital may be required.

Drug Interactions

May decrease or reverse effects of guanethidine and clonidine; may increase effects of CNS depressants, adrenergic agents, dicumarol, and anticholinergic agents

With MAO inhibitors, hyperpyrexia, tachycardia, hypertension, seizures and death may occur; similar interactions as with other tricyclics may occur

Cimetidine, fluoxetine, methylphenidate, and haloperidol may decrease the metabolism and/or increase TCA levels; phenobarbital may increase TCA metabolism

Stability Solutions stable at a pH of 4-5; turns yellowish or reddish on exposure to light. Slight discoloration does not affect potency; marked discoloration is associated with loss of potency. Capsules stable for 3 years following date of manufacture

Mechanism of Action Traditionally believed to increase the synaptic concentration of serotonin and/or norepinephrine in the central nervous system by inhibition of their reuptake by the presynaptic neuronal membrane. However, additional receptor effects have been found including desensitization of adenyl cyclase, down regulation of beta-adrenergic receptors, and down regulation of serotonin receptors. In urinary incontinence, imipramine is used for its anticholinergic effect and its direct beta-adrenergic stimulation of the bladder.

Pharmacodynamics Maximum antidepressant effects usually occur after ≥2 weeks; 5-HT >NE

Pharmacokinetics

Absorption: Oral: Well absorbed

Metabolism: In the liver by microsomal enzymes to desipramine (active) and other metabolites; significant first-pass metabolism; substrate CYP2D6, 2C9, 2C19, and 3A4; metabolism may be decreased in older patients

Half-life: 6-18 hours; mean half-life: ~24 hours

Elimination: In urine

Plasma concentrations and half-life are positively associated with age; utility of serum concentration monitoring is controversial

Usual Dosage

Geriatrics: Initial: 10-25 mg at bedtime; increase by 10-25 mg every 3 days for inpatients and weekly for outpatients if tolerated; average daily dose to achieve a therapeutic concentration: 100 mg/day (range: 50-150 mg)

Urinary incontinence (urge or mixed type): 10-50 mg at bedtime or twice daily

Adults:

Oral: Initial: 25 mg 3-4 times/day, increase dose gradually, total dose may be given at bedtime; maximum: 300 mg/day

I.M.: Initial: Up to 100 mg/day in divided doses; change to oral as soon as possible

Monitoring Parameters Improvement of depressive symptoms; blood pressure, pulse; may need to use serum concentrations to help monitor response

Reference Range Therapeutic: Imipramine and desipramine 150-250 ng/mL (SI: 530-890 nmol/L); desipramine 150-300 ng/mL (SI: 560-1125 nmol/L); Toxic: >500 ng/mL (SI: 446-893 nmol/L)

Test Interactions Elevated glucose

Patient Information May require 2-4 weeks to achieve desired effect; avoid alcohol ingestion; do not discontinue medication abruptly; may cause urine to turn blue-green; may cause drowsiness, constipation, blurred vision; use water or hard candy for dry mouth; rise slowly to avoid dizziness

Nursing Implications Monitor blood pressure and pulse rate prior to and during initial therapy; evaluate mental status; monitor weight, may increase appetite; offer patient water or hard candy for dry mouth

Additional Information

Imipramine hydrochloride: Tofranil®, Janimine®

Imipramine pamoate: Tofranil-PM®

Special Geriatric Considerations Orthostatic hypotension is a concern with this agent, especially in patients taking other medications that may affect blood pressure; may precipitate arrhythmias in predisposed patients; may aggravate seizures; a less anticholinergic antidepressant may be a better choice. Data from a clinical trial comparing fluoxetine to tricyclics suggest that fluoxetine is significantly less effective than nortriptyline in hospitalized elderly patients with unipolar major affective disorder, especially those with melancholia and concurrent cardiovascular diseases.

Dosage Forms

Imipramine hydrochloride:

Injection: 12.5 mg/mL (2 mL)

(Continued)

Imipramine *(Continued)*

Tablet: 10 mg, 25 mg, 50 mg
Capsule, as pamoate: 75 mg, 100 mg, 125 mg, 150 mg

References
Nies A, Robinson DS, Friedman MS, et al, "Relationship Between Age and Tricyclic Antidepressant Plasma Levels," *Am J Psychiatry*, 1977, 134:790-3.
Roose SP, Glassman AH, Attia E, et al, "Comparative Efficacy of Selective Serotonin Reuptake Inhibitors and Tricyclics in the Treatment of Melancholia," *Am J Psychiatry*, 1994, 151(12):1735-9.

Imitrex® *see* Sumatriptan Succinate *on page 883*

Immune Globulin (i MYUN GLOB yoo lin)

Related Information
Immunization Guidelines *on page 1058*
Brand Names Gamastan®; Gamimune® N; Gammagard®; Gammar®; Gammar®-IV; Iveegam®; Sandoglobulin®; Venoglobulin®-I
Synonyms Gamma Globulin; IG; IGIM; Immune Serum Globulin; ISG
Therapeutic Category Immune Globulin
Use Immunodeficiency syndrome; idiopathic thrombocytopenia purpura; B-cell chronic lymphocytic leukemia; prophylaxis against hepatitis A, measles, varicella, and possibly rubella and immunoglobulin deficiency; Kawasaki syndrome
Contraindications Thrombocytopenia or coagulation disorder, hypersensitivity to immune globulin, thimerosal, IgA deficiency
Warnings Do not administer I.V. except specific formulations of immune globulin I.V., hypersensitivity reactions should have epinephrine 1:1000 available for anaphylactic reactions; anaphylactic reaction more common with I.V. administration
Precautions Skin testing should not be performed; easy to misinterpret a positive reaction
Adverse Reactions
Cardiovascular: Chest tightness
Central nervous system: Lethargy, fever, chills
Dermatologic: Urticaria, angioedema
Gastrointestinal: Vomiting, nausea
Local: Tenderness, induration, erythema
Neuromuscular & skeletal: Myalgia, muscle stiffness
Renal: Nephrotic syndrome
Miscellaneous: Rarely hypersensitivity reactions
Drug Interactions Live virus vaccines
Stability Keep in refrigerator; do not freeze
Mechanism of Action Provides passive immunity by increasing the antibody titer and antigen-antibody reaction potential
Pharmacodynamics Duration of immune effects: Usually 3-4 weeks
Pharmacokinetics
Half-life: 21-23 days
Time to peak:
I.M.: Peak antibody serum concentration occur within 2-5 days
I.V.: Provides immediate antibody levels
Usual Dosage
I.M.:
Hepatitis A: 0.02 mL/kg
Travel into endemic areas:
1-3 months: 0.02 mL/kg
>3 months: 0.06 mL/kg; repeat every 4-6 months
IgG deficiency: 1.3 mL/kg then 0.66 mL/kg in 3-4 weeks
Measles: 0.25 mL/kg
Rubella: 0.55 mL/kg, within 72 hours of exposure
Varicella: 0.6-1.2 mL/kg
I.V.:
Immunodeficiency syndrome:
Sandoglobulin®: 200 mg/kg once monthly; may be increased to 300 mg/kg if prior dose insufficient; rate: 0.5-1 mL/minute for 15-30 minutes, increase to 1.5-2.5 mL/minute
Gammagard®: 200-400 mg/kg once monthly; rate: 0.5 mL/kg/hour
Gammar®-IV: 100-200 mg/kg every 3-4 weeks; rate: 0.01 mL/kg/minute; increase to 0.02 mL/kg/minute after 15-30 minutes, then, if tolerated 0.03-0.06 mL/kg/hour

Venoglobulin®-I: 200 mg/kg once monthly; increase to 300-400 mg/kg if response is insufficient; rate: 0.01-0.02 mL/kg/minute for 30 minutes; if tolerated, increase rate to 0.04 mL/kg/minute

Gamimune® N: 100-200 mg/kg once monthly; may increase to 400 mg/kg if insufficient response; rate: 0.01-0.02 mL/kg/minute for 30 minutes; if tolerated, increase to 0.08 mL/kg/minute

Iveegam®: 200 mg/kg once monthly; doses up to 800 mg/kg have been tolerated; rate: 1-2 mL/minute

Idiopathic thrombocytopenia purpura:

Sandoglobulin®: 400 mg/kg day for 2-5 days

Gammagard®: 1000 mg/kg/day up to 3 doses on alternate days; monitor response by platelet counts

Venoglobulin®-I: 500 mg/kg/day for 2-7 days; maintenance (platelet counts <30,000/mm³): 500-2000 mg/kg as a single dose at 1- to 2-week intervals; monitor platelets

Gamimune® N: 400 mg/kg/day for 5 days

B-cell CLL: Gammagard®: 400 mg/kg as a single dose every 3-4 weeks

Monitoring Parameters I.V. may cause hypotension; monitor for anaphylaxis, platelet counts, serum IgG concentration

Reference Range Serum IgG: 300 mg/dL

Test Interactions Skin tests should **not** be done

Nursing Implications Intramuscular injection only; do not mix with other medications; skin testing should not be performed as local irritation can occur and be misinterpreted as a positive reaction

Additional Information Epidemiologic and laboratory data indicate that current IMIG products do not have a discernible risk of transmitting HIV

Special Geriatric Considerations No special recommendations are made for elderly, doses are same as recommended for younger adults

Dosage Forms

Injection:

I.M.: 165±15 mg (protein)/mL (2 mL, 10 mL)

I.V.: 0.5 g, 1 g, 2.5 g, 3 g, 5 g, 6 g, 10 g; 5% (10 mL, 50 mL, 100 mL)

Immune Serum Globulin *see* Immune Globulin *on previous page*

Immunization Guidelines *see page 1058*

Imodium® *see* Loperamide *on page 548*

Imodium® A-D [OTC] *see* Loperamide *on page 548*

Imogam® *see* Rabies Immune Globulin (Human) *on page 818*

Imovax® Rabies I.D. Vaccine *see* Rabies Virus Vaccine *on page 819*

Imovax® Rabies Vaccine *see* Rabies Virus Vaccine *on page 819*

Imuran® *see* Azathioprine *on page 98*

I-Naphline® Ophthalmic *see* Naphazoline *on page 653*

Inapsine® *see* Droperidol *on page 324*

Indapamide (in DAP a mide)

Brand Names Lozol®

Generic Available No

Therapeutic Category Diuretic, Miscellaneous

Use Management of mild to moderate hypertension; treatment of edema in congestive heart failure and nephrotic syndrome

Contraindications Hypersensitivity to indapamide or any component

Adverse Reactions

Cardiovascular: Arrhythmia, weak pulse, hypotension

Central nervous system: Mood changes, numbness or tingling in hands, feet or lips

Dermatologic: Photosensitivity

Gastrointestinal: Xerostomia

Endocrine & metabolic: Hypokalemia, hyponatremia, hyperglycemia

Neuromuscular & skeletal: Muscle cramps, myalgia, unusual weakness

Respiratory: Shortness of breath

Miscellaneous: Increased thirst

Overdosage Symptoms of overdose include electrolyte depletion, volume depletion, hypotension, dehydration, circulatory collapse

Toxicology Following GI decontamination, treatment is supportive; hypotension responds to fluids and Trendelenburg position

Drug Interactions

Decreased effect of oral hypoglycemics; decreased absorption with cholestyramine and colestipol

Increased effect with loop diuretics and other antihypertensives

(Continued)

Indapamide *(Continued)*

Increased toxicity/levels of lithium; when given with digoxin, diuretic-induced hypokalaemia increases the risk of digoxin toxicity

Mechanism of Action Enhances sodium, chloride and water excretion by interfering with the transport of sodium ions across the renal tubular epithelium; diuretic effect is localized at the proximal segment of the distal tubule of the nephron; it does not appear to have significant effect on glomerular filtration rate nor renal blood flow; differs chemically from the thiazide

Pharmacokinetics

Absorption: Oral: Completely from GI tract

Protein binding: 71% to 79%

Metabolism: Extensive in the liver

Half-life: 14-18 hours

Time to peak serum concentration: 2-2.5 hours

Elimination: ~60% of dose excreted in urine within 48 hours, about 16% to 23% excreted via bile into feces

Usual Dosage Geriatrics and Adults: Oral:

Hypertension: 1.25 mg/day; if no response after 4 weeks, increase to 2.5 mg/day; maximum dose: 5 mg **Note:** There is little therapeutic benefit to increasing the dose to >5 mg/day; there is, however, an increased risk of electrolyte disturbances

Congestive heart failure: 2.5 mg/day; if no response after 1 week, increase to 5 mg

Monitoring Parameters Blood pressure (both standing and sitting/supine), serum electrolytes, renal function, weight, I & O

Test Interactions Increased ammonia (B), increased amylase (S), increased calcium (S), increased cholesterol (S), increased glucose, increased uric acid (S); decreased chloride (S), decreased magnesium, decreased potassium (S), decreased sodium (S)

Patient Information Take early in the day to avoid nocturia. May cause photosensitivity; use a sun block with an SPF of 15 or more.

Nursing Implications Check for orthostasis (see Monitoring Parameters)

Additional Information Indapamide offers no specific advantage over thiazides except it is effective in patients with impaired renal function (Cl_{cr} <30 mL/minute)

Special Geriatric Considerations Thiazide diuretics lose efficacy when Cl_{cr} is <30-35 mL/minute; many elderly may have Cl_{cr} below this limit; calculate Cl_{cr} for elderly before initiating therapy; indapamide has the advantage over thiazide diuretics in that it is effective when Cl_{cr} is <30 mL/minute (see Additional Information)

Dosage Forms Tablet: 1.25 mg, 2.5 mg

Inderal® *see* Propranolol *on page 797*

Inderal® LA *see* Propranolol *on page 797*

Inderide® *see* Propranolol and Hydrochlorothiazide *on page 799*

Indochron E-R® *see* Indomethacin *on this page*

Indocin® *see* Indomethacin *on this page*

Indocin® I.V. *see* Indomethacin *on this page*

Indocin® SR *see* Indomethacin *on this page*

Indometacin *see* Indomethacin *on this page*

Indomethacin *(in doe METH a sin)*

Related Information

Antacid Drug Interactions *on page 1096*

Brand Names Indochron E-R®; Indocin®; Indocin® I.V.; Indocin® SR

Synonyms Indometacin; Indomethacin Sodium Trihydrate

Generic Available Yes

Therapeutic Category Analgesic, Non-narcotic; Anti-inflammatory Agent; Antipyretic; Nonsteroidal Anti-inflammatory Agent (NSAID), Oral

Use Management of inflammatory diseases and rheumatoid disorders; moderate pain; acute gouty arthritis; ankylosing spondylitis, osteoporosis, tendonitis, bursitis, acute painful shoulder, sunburn, migraine, headache prophylaxis, cluster headache

Contraindications Hypersensitivity to indomethacin, any component, aspirin, or other nonsteroidal anti-inflammatory drugs (NSAIDs); active GI bleeding, ulcer disease; impaired renal function, IVH, active bleeding, thrombocytopenia

Warnings GI toxicity (bleeding, ulceration, perforation); CNS effects may occur (headaches, confusion, depression); hypersensitivity, anaphylactoid reactions (intermittent tolmetin use more often); renal function decline, acute renal insufficiency, interstitial nephritis, dysuria, cystitis, hematuria, nephrotic syndrome, hyperkalemia in acute renal insufficiency, hyponatremia, papillary necrosis, hepatic function impairment; elderly have increased risk for adverse reactions to NSAIDs (see Special Geriatric Considerations)

Precautions Use with caution in patients with congestive heart failure, hypertension, decreased renal or hepatic function, history of GI disease (bleeding or ulcers), or those receiving anticoagulants; perform ophthalmologic evaluation for those who develop eye complaints during therapy (blurred vision, diminished vision, changes in color vision, retinal changes); NSAIDs may mask signs/symptoms of infections; photosensitivity reported

Adverse Reactions Elderly have high incidence of confusion and other adverse reactions (see Special Geriatric Considerations)

Cardiovascular: Headache, hypertension, edema

Central nervous system: Somnolence, vertigo, fatigue, depression, confusion, dizziness

Dermatologic: Rash

Endocrine & metabolic: Hyperkalemia, dilutional hyponatremia (I.V.), hypoglycemia (I.V.)

Gastrointestinal: Nausea, vomiting, diarrhea, constipation, flatulence, anorexia, epigastric pain, abdominal pain, anorexia, GI bleeding, ulcers, gingival ulcers, proctitis

Genitourinary: Cystitis

Hematologic: Hemolytic anemia, bone marrow suppression, agranulocytosis, thrombocytopenia, inhibition of platelet aggregation

Hepatic: Hepatitis, cholestatic jaundice

Ocular: Papillary necrosis, perforation, corneal opacities

Otic: Tinnitus

Renal: Dysuria, hematuria, nephrotic syndrome, oliguria, renal failure

Miscellaneous: Hypersensitivity reactions

Overdosage Symptoms include drowsiness, lethargy, disorientation, confusion, dizziness, numbness, paresthesia, nausea, vomiting, gastric irritation, abdominal pain, headache, tinnitus, sweating, blurred vision, muscle twitching, seizures, coma, acute renal failure, increased BUN and serum creatinine, hypotension, tachycardia, and metabolic acidosis

Toxicology Management of a nonsteroidal anti-inflammatory agent (NSAID) intoxication is primarily supportive and symptomatic. Fluid therapy is commonly effective in managing the hypotension that may occur following an acute NSAID overdose, except when this is due to an acute blood loss. Seizures tend to be very short-lived and often do not require drug treatment although recurrent seizures should be treated with I.V. diazepam. Since many of the NSAIDs undergo enterohepatic cycling, multiple doses of charcoal may be needed to reduce the potential for delayed toxicities.

Drug Interactions

Indomethacin may increase serum concentrations of digoxin, methotrexate, lithium, and aminoglycosides

May increase nephrotoxicity of cyclosporine

May decrease antihypertensive and diuretic effects of furosemide and thiazides

Effects of loop diuretics may decrease

May increase serum K^+ with potassium-sparing diuretics

May decrease antihypertensive effects of beta-blockers, hydralazine and captopril

Aspirin or other salicylates may decrease and probenecid may increase indomethacin serum concentrations

Concomitant administration with dipyridamole may cause enhance water retention

Indomethacin may increase bioavailability of penicillamine; coadministration with phenylpropanolamine may increase blood pressure

Other NSAIDs may increase GI adverse effects

May increase or enhance azotemia in elderly receiving loop diuretics

Stability Protect from light; not stable in alkaline solution; reconstitute just prior to administration; discard any unused portion; do not use preservative containing diluents for reconstitution

Mechanism of Action Inhibits prostaglandin synthesis, acts on the hypothalamus heat-regulating center to reduce fever, blocks prostaglandin synthetase action which prevents formation of the platelet-aggregating substance thromboxane A_2; decreases pain receptor sensitivity. Other proposed mechanisms of action are lysosomal stabilization, inhibition of kinin and leukotriene (Continued)

Indomethacin *(Continued)*

production, alteration of chemotactic factors, and inhibition of neutrophil activation. This latter mechanism may be the most significant pharmacologic action to reduce inflammation.

Pharmacodynamics

Onset of action: Within 30 minutes

Duration: 4-6 hours

Onset of anti-inflammatory action: Within 7 days

Peak effect: 1-2 weeks

Pharmacokinetics

Absorption: Promptly and extensively

Distribution: V_d: 0.34-1.57 L/kg

Protein binding: 90%

Metabolism: In the liver with significant enterohepatic recycling; substrate CYP2C9

Half-life: 4-6 hours

Time to peak serum concentration: Oral: Within 1-2 hours; sustained release: 2-4 hours

Elimination: In urine principally as glucuronide conjugates

Usual Dosage Geriatrics and Adults: 25-50 mg/dose 2-3 times/day; maximum dose: 200 mg/day; extended release capsule should be given on a 1-2 times/day schedule; maximum dose for sustained release is 150 mg/day; best to start elderly on 25 mg dose given 2-3 times/day

Monitoring Parameters Monitor response (pain, range of motion, grip strength, mobility, ADL function), inflammation; observe for weight gain, edema; monitor renal function; observe for bleeding, bruising; evaluate gastrointestinal effects (abdominal pain, bleeding, dyspepsia); mental confusion, disorientation, CBC, serum, creatinine, BUN, liver function tests

Test Interactions Positive Coombs' [direct]

Patient Information Extended release capsules must be swallowed intact. Serious gastrointestinal bleeding can occur as well as ulceration and perforation. Pain may or may not be present. Avoid aspirin and aspirin-containing products while taking this medication. If gastric upset occurs, take with food, milk, or antacid. If gastric adverse effects persist, contact physician. May cause drowsiness, dizziness, blurred vision, and confusion. Use caution when performing tasks which require alertness (eg, driving). Do not take for more than 3 days for fever or 10 days for pain without physician advice.

Nursing Implications Extended release capsules must be swallowed intact (see Overdosage, Monitoring Parameters, Patient Information, and Special Geriatric Considerations)

Additional Information There are no clinical guidelines to predict which NSAID will give response in a particular patient; trials with each must be initiated until response determined; consider dose, patient convenience, and cost

Special Geriatric Considerations Elderly are a high-risk population for adverse effects from nonsteroidal anti-inflammatory agents. As much as 60% of elderly can develop peptic ulceration and/or hemorrhage asymptomatically. The concomitant use of H_2 blockers, omeprazole, and sucralfate is not effective as prophylaxis with the exception of NSAID-induced duodenal ulcers which may be prevented by the use of ranitidine. Misoprostol and proton pump inhibitors are the only agents proven to help prevent the development of NSAID-induced ulcers. Also, concomitant disease and drug use contribute to the risk for GI adverse effects. Use lowest effective dose for shortest period possible. Consider renal function decline with age. Use of NSAIDs can compromise existing renal function especially when Cl_{cr} is ≤30 mL/minute. Tinnitus may be a difficult and unreliable indication of toxicity due to age-related hearing loss or eighth cranial nerve damage. CNS adverse effects such as confusion, agitation, and hallucination are generally seen in overdose or high dose situations, but elderly may demonstrate these adverse effects at lower doses than younger adults. Indomethacin frequently causes confusion at recommended doses in the elderly.

Dosage Forms

Capsule: 25 mg, 50 mg

Capsule, sustained release: 75 mg

Suppository: 50 mg

Suspension, oral: 25 mg/5 mL (5 mL, 10 mL, 237 mL, 500 mL)

References

Brooks PM, Day RO, "Nonsteroidal Anti-inflammatory Drugs - Differences and Similarities," *N Engl J Med*, 1991, 324(24):1716-25.

Clinch D, Banerjee AK, Ostick G, "Absence of Abdominal Pain in Elderly Patients With Peptic Ulcer," *Age Ageing*, 1984, 13:120-3.

Clive DM, Stoff JS, "Renal Syndromes Associated With Nonsteroidal Anti-inflammatory Drugs," *N Engl J Med*, 1984, 310(9):563-72.

Graham DY, "Prevention of Gastroduodenal Injury Induced by Chronic Nonsteroidal Anti-inflammatory Drug Therapy," *Gastroenterology*, 1989, 96(2 Pt 2 Suppl):675-81.

Gurwitz JH, Avorn J, Ross-Degnan D, et al, "Nonsteroidal Anti-Inflammatory Drug-Associated Azotemia in the Very Old," *JAMA*, 1990, 264(4):471-5.

Hawkey CJ, Karrasch JA, Szczepaski L, et al, "Omeprazole Compared With Misoprostrol for Ulcers Associated With Nonsteroidal Anti-inflammatory Drugs," *N Engl J Med*, 1998, 338(11):727-34.

Knodel LC, "Preventing NSAID-Induced Ulcers: The Role of Misoprostol," *Consult Pharm*, 1989, 4:37-41.

Pounder R, "Silent Peptic Ulceration: Deadly Silence or Golden Silence?" *Gastroenterology*, 1989, 96(2 Pt 2 Suppl):626-31.

Yeomans ND, Tulassay Z, Juhasz L, et al, "A Comparison of Omeprazole With Ranitidine for Ulcers Associated With Nonsteroidal Anti-inflammatory Drugs," *N Engl J Med*, 1998, 338(11):719-26.

Indomethacin Sodium Trihydrate *see Indomethacin on page 484*

InFed™ Injection *see Iron Dextran Complex on page 497*

Inflamase® Forte Ophthalmic *see Prednisolone on page 774*

Inflamase® Mild Ophthalmic *see Prednisolone on page 774*

Influenza Virus Vaccine (in floo EN za VYE rus vak SEEN)

Related Information
Immunization Guidelines *on page 1058*

Brand Names Flu-Imune®; Fluogen®; Fluzone®

Synonyms Influenza Virus Vaccine (inactivated whole-virus); Influenza Virus Vaccine (purified surface antigen); Influenza Virus Vaccine (split-virus)

Therapeutic Category Vaccine, Inactivated Virus

Use Provide active immunity to influenza virus strains contained in the vaccine; for high risk persons, previous year vaccines should not be to prevent present year influenza

Those at risk for influenza injection:

Persons ≥65 years of age

Institutionalized patients

Persons of any age with chronic disorders of pulmonary and/or cardiovascular system

Persons who have required medical follow-up following hospitalization for other chronic diseases such as diabetes, renal disease, immunodepressive disorders, etc

Travelers, especially those at risk (above)

Contraindications Persons with allergy history to eggs or egg products, chicken, chicken feathers or chicken dander, hypersensitivity to thimerosal, influenza virus vaccine or any component, presence of acute respiratory disease or other active infections or illnesses, delay immunization in a patient with an active neurological disorder

Warnings Hypersensitivity reaction (have epinephrine 1:1000 available); immunosuppressed patients may fail to develop protective antibody titers (amantadine may be given as a supplement)

Precautions Antigenic response may not be as great as expected in patients receiving immunosuppressive drug; hypersensitivity reactions may occur; because of potential for febrile reactions, risks and benefits must be carefully considered in patients with history of febrile convulsions; influenza vaccines from previous seasons must not be used; patients with sulfite sensitivity may be affected by this product; concurrent administration of other vaccines (pneumococcal) is acceptable as long as other vaccines are given at a different site; seroconversion does not develop in all persons receiving vaccine; Guillain-Barré syndrome (1978-81 years had the highest incidence of GBS); temporary neurologic disorders

Adverse Reactions Side effects are minor and uneventful in those few who develop them; most reactions occur within 6-12 hours and may last 1-2 days

Central nervous system: Malaise, fever, Guillain-Barré syndrome
Dermatologic: Urticaria, angioedema
Local: Local soreness
Neuromuscular & skeletal: Myalgia rarely
Respiratory: Asthma
Miscellaneous: Rarely anaphylactoid reactions, allergic reactions

Drug Interactions Immunosuppressive agents, theophylline, anticoagulants, phenytoin; do not administer within seven days after administration of diphtheria and tetanus toxoids and pertussis vaccine adsorbed (DTP)

Stability Refrigerate at 2°C to 8°C (36°F to 46°F); do not freeze

(Continued)

Influenza Virus Vaccine *(Continued)*

Usual Dosage Geriatrics and Adults: I.M.: 0.5 mL each year of appropriate vaccine for the year, one dose is all that is necessary; administer in late fall to allow maximum titers to develop by peak epidemic periods usually occurring in early December

Reference Range Less than a fourfold increase in titer; >1:10 IgG and IgM

Patient Information Be aware of possible adverse effects

Nursing Implications Inspect for particulate matter and discoloration prior to administration; for I.M. administration only

Additional Information Pharmacy will stock the formulations(s) standardized according to the USPHS requirements for the season. Influenza vaccines from previous seasons must not be used.

Special Geriatric Considerations Limited data on elderly exists due to ethical considerations precluding use of placebo and differences in studies and vaccines; 80% develop a 1:40 HA titer, 70% are completely protected, 90% protected from death; amantadine may be used to prophylax against influenza type A in the following situations:

High-risk institutionalized patients, both vaccinated and unvaccinated

Epidemic environment

Supplement vaccine in those who may have inadequate response (immunosuppressed)

Those who refuse vaccine

Those hypersensitive to vaccine or its components

Amantadine dose must be adjusted for renal failure, see Amantadine monograph; administer for 2 weeks in vaccinated patients and 6-12 weeks in unvaccinated patients

Dosage Forms

Injection:

Split-virus (Fluogen®; Fluzone®): 0.5 mL, 5 mL

Whole-virus (Fluzone®): 5 mL

References

Bentley DW, "Vaccinations," *Clin Geriatr Med*, 1992, 8(4):745-60.

Gardner P and Schaffner W, "Immunization of Adults," *N Engl J Med*, 1993, 328(17):1252-8.

Influenza Virus Vaccine (inactivated whole-virus) *see* Influenza Virus Vaccine *on previous page*

Influenza Virus Vaccine (purified surface antigen) *see* Influenza Virus Vaccine *on previous page*

Influenza Virus Vaccine (split-virus) *see* Influenza Virus Vaccine *on previous page*

Infumorph™ Injection *see* Morphine Sulfate *on page 640*

Inhaled Medications Comparison *see page 1034*

Inocor® *see* Amrinone *on page 76*

Insulin Preparations (IN su lin prep a RAY shuns)

Related Information

I.V. Push Recommended Guidelines *on page 1083*

Brand Names Humalog®; Humulin® 50/50; Humulin® 70/30; Humulin® L; Humulin® N; Humulin® R; Humulin® U; Lente® Iletin® I; Lente® Iletin® II; Lente® Insulin; Lente® L; Novolin® 70/30; Novolin® L; Novolin® N; Novolin® R; NPH Iletin® I; NPH Insulin; NPH-N; Pork NPH Iletin® II; Pork Regular Iletin® II; Regular (Concentrated) Iletin® II U-500; Regular Iletin® I; Regular Insulin; Regular Purified Pork Insulin; Velosulin® Human

Synonyms Lente®; NPH; Semilente®; Ultralente®

Therapeutic Category Antidiabetic Agent

Use Treatment of insulin-dependent diabetes mellitus, also noninsulin-dependent diabetes mellitus unresponsive to treatment with diet and/or oral hypoglycemics; acute management of hyperkalemia; to assure proper utilization of glucose and reduce glucosuria in nondiabetic patients receiving parenteral nutrition whose glucosuria cannot be adequately controlled with infusion rate adjustments or those who require assistance in achieving optimal caloric intakes

Warnings Any change of insulin should be made cautiously; changing manufacturers, type and/or method of manufacture, may result in the need for a change of dosage; human insulin differs from animal-source insulin

Precautions Any change of insulin should be made cautiously; changing manufacturers, type and/or method of manufacture, may result in the need for a change of dosage; human insulin differs from animal-source insulin

Adverse Reactions

Cardiovascular: Palpitations, tachycardia, local edema

Central nervous system: Fatigue, mental confusion, loss of consciousness, headache

Dermatologic: Urticaria

Endocrine & metabolic: Hypoglycemia, hypothermia

Gastrointestinal: Hunger, nausea, numbness of mouth

Local: Itching, redness, stinging, or warmth at injection site, atrophy or hypertrophy of S.C. fat tissue

Neuromuscular & skeletal: Muscle weakness, tremors, paresthesia

Ocular: Transient presbyopia or blurred vision

Miscellaneous: Diaphoresis, anaphylaxis, pallor

Overdosage Symptoms of overdose include tachycardia, anxiety, hunger, tremors, pallor, headache, motor dysfunction, speech disturbances, sweating, palpitations

Drug Interactions See table.

Drug Interactions With Insulin Injection

Decrease Hypoglycemic Effect of Insulin	Increase Hypoglycemic Effect of Insulin
Contraceptives, oral	Alcohol
Corticosteroids	Alpha blockers
Dextrothyroxine	Anabolic steroids
Diltiazem	Beta-blockers*
Dobutamine	Clofibrate
Epinephrine	Fenfluramine
Smoking	Guanethidine
Thiazide diuretics	MAO inhibitors
Thyroid hormone	Pentamidine
Niacin	Phenylbutazone
	Salicylates
	Sulfinpyrazone
	Tetracyclines

*Nonselective beta-blockers may delay recovery from hypoglycemic episodes and mask signs/symptoms of hypoglycemia. Cardioselective agents may be alternatives.

Stability Bottle in use is stable at room temperature up to 1 month; cold (freezing) causes more damage to insulin than room temperatures up to 100°F; avoid direct sunlight; cold injections should be avoided

Mechanism of Action Replacement therapy for persons unable to produce the hormone naturally or in insufficient amounts to maintain glycemic control

Pharmacodynamics Onset and duration of hypoglycemic effects depend upon preparation administered; see table.

Preparation	Onset of Action	Peak	Duration
Lispro	15 min	45 min	3 h
Regular	30 min	2.5-5 h	5-8 h
Semilente®	1-2 h	3-10 h	10-16 h
Lente®	2.5 h	7-15 h	18-23 h
NPH	90 min	4-12 h	24 h
Humulin® U	4-8 h	10-30 h	>36 h
70/30	30 min		24 h
Isophane/Regular	6	4-8 h	

Usual Dosage

Geriatrics and Adults: Dose requires continuous medical supervision; only regular insulin may be given I.V. The daily dose should be divided up depending upon the product used and the patient's response (eg, regular insulin every 4-6 hours); see table; NPH insulin every 12-24 hours.

Adults: S.C.: 0.5-1 unit/kg/day

Dosing adjustment in renal impairment (regular):

Cl_{cr} 10-50 mL/minute: Administer at 75% of normal dose

Cl_{cr} <10 mL/minute: Administer at 25% to 50% of normal dose; monitor blood glucose closely

Monitoring Parameters Plasma or finger stick blood glucose concentrations; hemoglobin A_{1c} (glycosylated Hgb) fructosamine

(Continued)

Insulin Preparations *(Continued)*

Reference Range Therapeutic, serum (fasting): 5-20 µU/mL (SI: 35-145 pmol/L)

Test Interactions Increased catecholamines (U); decreased potassium (S)

Patient Information Do not change insulins without physician's approval; know signs and symptoms of hyperglycemia and hypoglycemia and how to respond to them; reinforce proper use and storage; assess patient's ability to drawing and self inject dose, and to accurately perform home blood glucose (fingerstick) monitoring; insulin lispro should be given just before a meal

Nursing Implications Patients using human insulin may be less likely to recognize hypoglycemia than if they use uses pork insulin, patients on pork insulin that have low blood sugar exhibit hunger and sweating; insulin lispro should be given just before a meal

Special Geriatric Considerations How "tightly" a geriatric patient's blood glucose should be controlled is controversial; however, a fasting blood sugar of <150 mg/dL is now an acceptable end point. Such a decision should be based on the patient's functional and cognitive status, how well they recognize hypoglycemic or hyperglycemic symptoms and how to respond to them and their other disease states; patients who are unable to accurately draw up their dose will need assistance such as prefilled syringes. Initial doses may require considerations for renal function in elderly with dosing adjusted subsequently based on blood glucose monitoring (see Patient Information).

Dosage Forms All insulins are 100 units/mL (10 mL) except where indicated:

RAPID-ACTING:

Insulin lispro rDNA origin: Humalog® [*Lilly*] (1.5 mL, 10 mL)

Insulin Injection (Regular Insulin)

  Beef and pork: Regular Iletin® I [*Lilly*]

  Human:

    rDNA: Humulin® R [*Lilly*], Novolin® R [*Novo Nordisk*]

    Semisynthetic: Velosulin® Human [*Novo Nordisk*]

  Pork: Regular Insulin [*Novo Nordisk*]

  Purified pork:

    Pork Regular Iletin® II [*Lilly*], Regular Purified Pork Insulin [*Novo Nordisk*]

    Regular (Concentrated) Iletin® II U-500 (*Lilly*): 500 units/mL

INTERMEDIATE-ACTING:

Insulin Zinc Suspension (Lente®)

  Beef and pork: Lente® Iletin® I [*Lilly*]

  Human, rDNA: Humulin® L [*Lilly*], Novolin® L [*Novo Nordisk*]

  Purified pork: Lente® Iletin® II [*Lilly*], Lente® L [*Novo Nordisk*]

Isophane Insulin Suspension (NPH)

  Beef and pork: NPH Iletin® I [*Lilly*]

  Human, rDNA: Humulin® N [*Lilly*], Novolin® N [*Novo Nordisk*]

  Purified pork: Pork NPH Iletin® II [*Lilly*], NPH-N [*Novo Nordisk*]

LONG-ACTING:

Insulin zinc suspension, extended (Ultralente®)

  Human, rDNA: Humulin® U [Lilly]

COMBINATIONS:

Isophane Insulin Suspension and Insulin Injection

  Isophane insulin suspension (50%) and insulin injection (50%) human (rDNA): Humulin® 50/50 [*Lilly*]

  Isophane insulin suspension (70%) and insulin injection (30%) human (rDNA): Humulin® 70/30 [*Lilly*], Novolin® 70/30 [*Novo Nordisk*]

References

Nathan DM, "Insulin Treatment in the Elderly Diabetic Patient," *Clin Geriatr Med*, 1990, 6(4):923-31.

Morley JE and Perry HM 3d, "The Management of Diabetes Mellitus in Older Individuals," *Drugs*, 1991, 41(4):548-65.

Intal® Inhalation Capsule *see* Cromolyn Sodium *on page 255*

Intal® Nebulizer Solution *see* Cromolyn Sodium *on page 255*

Intal® Oral Inhaler *see* Cromolyn Sodium *on page 255*

Interferon Alfa-2a (in ter FEER on AL fa too aye)

Brand Names Roferon-A®

Synonyms IFLrA; rIFN-A

Generic Available No

Therapeutic Category Biological Response Modulator; Interferon

Use FDA approved: Patients >18 years of age: Hairy cell leukemia, AIDS-related Kaposi's sarcoma, chronic phase of Philadelphia chromosome positive CML

Unlabeled use: A number of neoplastic diseases have been treated including bladder cancers, carcinoid tumor, cutaneous T-cell lymphoma, non-Hodgkin's lymphoma, essential thrombocytopenia, acute leukemias, cervical carcinoma, CLL, Hodgkin's disease, malignant melanoma, malignant gliomas, multiple myeloma, mycosis fungoides, nasopharyngeal carcinoma, osteosarcoma, ovarian carcinoma, renal carcinoma; viral infections including chronic non-A, non-B hepatitis, condyloma acuminatum, cytomegaloviruses, herpes keratoconjunctivitis, cutaneous warts, herpes simplex, papillomavirus, rhinoviruses, varicella zoster, hepatitis B, HIV infection (slow progression)

Contraindications Hypersensitivity to alfa-2a interferon or any component of the product

Warnings The U.S. Food and Drug Administration (FDA) currently recommends that procedures for proper handling and disposal of antineoplastic agents be considered. Use with caution in patients with seizure disorders, brain metastases, compromised CNS, multiple sclerosis, and patients with pre-existing cardiac disease, severe renal or hepatic impairment, or myelosuppression. Higher doses in the elderly or in malignancies other than hairy cell leukemia may result in severe obtundation. Depression, suicidal ideation, suicidal attempts and suicides have been reported in association with this drug. Patients should be informed of these potential adverse effects and be instructed to report any depression or ideas of suicide to the prescribing physician immediately. Monitor patients closely for depression and consider discontinuing therapy. Although dose reduction or cessation of therapy may lead to resolution or depressive symptoms, depression may persist and suicides have occurred after withdrawal of therapy.

Other warnings: GI hemorrhage; use cautiously in patients with severe renal or hepatic disease, seizure disorders, myelosuppressive or compromised CNS function, and any patient with cardiac disease; CNS reactions, leukopenia, elevated LFTs, anemia, renal/hepatic impairment.

Precautions Prior to therapy, obtain baseline hemoglobin, platelets, granulocytes, hair cells and bone marrow hairy cells, if applicable, and liver function tests; monitor CBC and LFTs periodically (monthly); monitor cause of disease and if no response is seen within 6 months, discontinue therapy; obtain an EKG for those with cardiac disease (see Warnings before initiating therapy)

Adverse Reactions The majority of adverse reactions are reversible with dose reduction or discontinuation of therapy; continue or reinitiate therapy cautiously with close monitoring (see Warnings and Precautions)

Cardiovascular: Chest pain, hypertension, edema, palpitations, arrhythmias, hypotension, syncope, flushing

Central nervous system: Depression, sleep disturbance, anxiety, lethargy, confusion, involuntary movements, vertigo, forgetfulness, ataxia, seizures, aphasia, amnesia, fever, fatigue, chills

Dermatologic: Petechiae, alopecia, rash, pruritus, dry skin, urticaria, bruising

Endocrine & metabolic: Hypothyroidism, hypertriglyceridemia, uric acid levels (increased), hypocalcemia, hyperphosphatemia

Gastrointestinal: Anorexia, nausea, vomiting, diarrhea, abdominal pain, throat irritation, constipation, flatulence, dysgeusia, gingival bleeding, weight loss

Hematologic: Leukopenia, neutropenia, thrombocytopenia, anemia, LFT increase, LDH increase

Local: Thrombophlebitis

Neuromuscular & skeletal: Paresthesia, numbness, tremor, weakness, myalgia, back pain, arthralgia

Ocular: Visual disturbance

Renal: Proteinuria, increased serum creatinine, BUN elevated,

Respiratory: Cough, rhinorrhea, sinusitis, inflammation of oropharynx, dyspnea, chest congestion, bronchospasm, epistaxis

Miscellaneous: Diaphoresis

Overdosage Signs and symptoms of overdose include depression, obtundation, flu-like symptoms, myelosuppression, other CNS abnormalities

Toxicology General supportive care

Drug Interactions

Increased effect:

Cimetidine: May augment the antitumor effects of interferon in melanoma

Theophylline: Clearance has been reported to be decreased in patients receiving interferon

(Continued)

Interferon Alfa-2a *(Continued)*

Drugs which are neurotoxic, hematotoxic, or cardiotoxic may be enhanced by administration of interferon alfa-2a

Increased toxicity: Vinblastine: Enhances interferon toxicity in several patients; increased incidence of paresthesia has also been noted

Stability Refrigerate (2°C to 8°C/36°F to 46°F); do not freeze; do not shake; after reconstitution, the solution is stable for 24 hours at room temperature and for 1 month when refrigerated

Mechanism of Action Inhibits cellular growth, alters the state of cellular differentiation, interferes with oncogene expression, alters cell surface antigen expression, increases phagocytic activity of macrophages and augments cytotoxicity of lymphocytes for target cells

Pharmacokinetics

Absorption: Filtered and absorbed at the renal tubule

Distribution: The V_d of interferon is 31 L; but has been noted to be much greater (370-720 L) in leukemia patients receiving continuous infusion IFN; IFN does not penetrate the CSF

Metabolism: Alfa interferons are filtered through the glomeruli; majority of dose thought to be metabolized by proteolytic degradation during tubular reabsorption

Bioavailability:

I.M.: 83%

S.C.: 90%

Half-life: Elimination: 4-8 hours (mean: 5 hours)

Time to peak serum concentration: I.M., S.C.: ~6-8 hours

Usual Dosage Refer to individual protocols

Geriatrics and Adults: I.M., S.C.:

Hairy cell leukemia:

Induction: 3 million units/day for 16-24 weeks.

Maintenance: 3 million units 3 times/week (may be treated for up to 20 consecutive weeks)

AIDS-related Kaposi's sarcoma:

Induction: 36 million units/day for 10-12 weeks

Maintenance: 36 million units 3 times/week (may begin with dose escalation from 3-9-18 million units each day over 3 consecutive days followed by 36 million units/day for the remainder of the 10-12 weeks of induction)

Chronic myelogenous leukemia:

Induction: I.M., S.C.: 9 million units daily; experience has demonstrated better tolerance if dosages are titrated upward over the first week; 3 million units for day 1-3, 6 million units for days 4-6, then 9 million units daily thereafter

Maintenance: Has not been determined to date

If severe adverse reactions occur, modify dosage (50% reduction) or temporarily discontinue therapy until adverse reactions abate

Administration S.C. administration is suggested for those who are at risk for bleeding or are thrombocytopenic (platelets <50,000/mm³); rotate S.C. injection site; patient should be well hydrated

Monitoring Parameters Baseline chest x-ray, EKG, CBC with differential, liver function tests, electrolytes, platelets, weight; patients with pre-existing cardiac abnormalities, or in advanced stages of cancer should have EKGs taken before and during treatment

Reference Range Peak serum concentration following an I.V. dose of 36 million units: 10,400-17,470 pg/mL

Test Interactions Increased AST, increased ALT, decreased WBC, decreased Hg, decreased platelets, increased alkaline phosphatase, increased creatinine (S), increased BUN

Patient Information Possible mental status changes may occur while on therapy; report to physician any persistent or severe sore throat, fever, fatigue, unusual bleeding, or bruising; do not operate heavy machinery while on therapy since changes in mental status may occur

Nursing Implications Do not freeze or shake solution; a flu-like syndrome (fever, chills) occurs in the majority of patients 2-6 hours after a dose; pretreatment with nonsteroidal anti-inflammatory drug (NSAID) or acetaminophen can decrease fever and its severity and alleviate headache

Additional Information Indications and dosage regimens are specific for a particular brand of interferon; other brands of interferon (ie, Intron® A) have different indications and dosage guidelines; do not change brands of interferon as changes in dosage may result

Special Geriatric Considerations No specific data available for the elderly; however, pay close attention to Warnings and Precautions

Dosage Forms
Injection: 3 million units/mL (1 mL); 6 million units/mL (3 mL); 9 million units/mL (1 mL); 36 million units/mL (1 mL)
Powder for injection: 6 million units/mL when reconstituted

Interferon Beta-1b (in ter FEER on BAY ta won bee)

Brand Names Betaseron®

Synonyms rIFN-b

Therapeutic Category Interferon

Use Reduces the frequency of clinical exacerbations in ambulatory patients with relapsing-remitting multiple sclerosis (MS)

Unlabeled use: Treatment in AIDS, AIDS-related Kaposi's sarcoma, acute non-A/non-B hepatitis; renal cell carcinoma (metastatic), malignant melanoma; cutaneous T-cell lymphoma

Contraindications Hypersensitivity to *E. coli*-derived products, recombinant interferon beta, or albumin

Warnings Depression and suicidal tendency, anxiety, myelosuppression, confusion, depersonalization, emotional lability

Precautions Patients must be instructed on safe use; baseline laboratory tests are recommended periodically throughout treatment (ie, every 3 months); recommended laboratory tests include CBC with differential, platelets, liver function tests

Adverse Reactions Due to the pivotal position of interferon in the immune system, toxicities can affect nearly every organ system; injection site reactions, injection site necrosis, flu-like symptoms, menstrual disorders, depression (with suicidal ideations), somnolence, palpitations, peripheral vascular disorders, hypertension, blood dyscrasias, dyspnea, laryngitis, cystitis, gastrointestinal complaints, photosensitization

Stability Use within 3 hours of reconstitution; store at 2°C to 8°C (36°F to 46°F); discard any unused portions

Mechanism of Action Interferon beta-1b differs from naturally occurring human protein by a single amino acid substitution and the lack of carbohydrate side chains; alters the expression and response to surface antigens and can enhance immune cell activities. Properties of interferon beta-1b that modify biologic responses are mediated by cell surface receptor interactions; mechanism in the treatment of MS is unknown.

Pharmacokinetics Limited data due to small doses used
Time to peak serum concentration: 1-8 hours
Bioavailability: 50%
Half-life: 8 minutes to 4.3 hours

Usual Dosage Geriatrics and Adults: S.C.: 0.25 mg (8 million units) every other day

Administration Inject 1 mL S.C. with a 27-gauge needle; may be injected into arms, thighs, hips, and abdomen

Monitoring Parameters Hemoglobin, liver function, and blood chemistries; stop therapy if absolute neutrophil count (ANC) drops below 750/mm³; may restart therapy at half-dose when ANC returns to >750/mm³; if LFTs increase to 10 times upper limit of normal or bilirubin increased more than 5 times the upper limit of normal, therapy should be stopped; restart half-dose when return to normal

Patient Information Patients must be instructed in aseptic technique when injecting themselves, proper disposal of needles and syringes; injection site may develop a reaction, but this does not dictate the stopping of therapy; flu-like symptoms may occur but the use of aspirin or acetaminophen will relieve the symptoms; warn about depression, feelings of suicide, and photosensitivity; report changes in mental state to physician; use sun block to prevent photosensitivity reactions

Nursing Implications Patient should be informed of possible side effects, especially depression and suicidal ideations; flu-like symptoms such as chills, fever, malaise, sweating, and myalgia are common (see Monitoring Parameters)

Additional Information May be available only in small supplies; for information on availability and distribution, call the patient information line at 800-580-3837

Special Geriatric Considerations No specific recommendations necessary for use in the elderly; monitor for CNS adverse effects which may be significant in elderly (see Warnings)

Dosage Forms Powder for injection, lyophilized: 0.3 mg [9.6 million units]

Intropin® Injection *see* Dopamine *on page 316*
Iobid DM® *see* Guaifenesin and Dextromethorphan *on page 439*

Iodoquinol (eye oh doe KWIN ole)

Brand Names Yodoxin®
Synonyms Diiodohydroxyquin
Therapeutic Category Amebicide
Use Treatment of acute and chronic intestinal amebiasis; asymptomatic cyst passers; *Blastocystis hominis* infections
Contraindications Known hypersensitivity to iodine or iodoquinol; hepatic or renal damage; pre-existing optic neuropathy
Warnings Optic neuritis, optic atrophy, and peripheral neuropathy have occurred following prolonged use; avoid long-term therapy
Precautions Use with caution in patients with thyroid disease or neurological disorders
Adverse Reactions
   Central nervous system: Agitation, retrograde amnesia, fever, headache
   Dermatologic: Anal pruritus, rash, acne
   Endocrine & metabolic: Enlargement of the thyroid
   Gastrointestinal: Nausea, vomiting, diarrhea, gastritis
   Neuromuscular & skeletal: Peripheral neuropathy, weakness
   Ocular: Optic neuritis, optic atrophy, visual impairment
Overdosage Symptoms of overdose include vomiting, diarrhea, abdominal pain, metallic taste, delirium, stupor, collapse, coma
Mechanism of Action Contact amebicide that works in the lumen of the intestine by an unknown mechanism
Pharmacokinetics
   Absorption: Oral: Poor and irregular
   Metabolism: In the liver
   Elimination: High percentage of dose excreted in feces
Usual Dosage Geriatrics and Adults: Oral: 650 mg 3 times/day after meals for 20 days; not to exceed 2 g/day
Administration Tablets may be crushed and mixed with applesauce or chocolate syrup
Test Interactions May increase protein-bound serum iodine concentrations reflecting a decrease in iodine 131 uptake; false-positive ferric chloride test for phenylketonuria
Patient Information Complete full course of therapy; may cause nausea, vomiting, or diarrhea
Nursing Implications See Administration
Special Geriatric Considerations No special considerations for the elderly, however, this agent is no longer a drug of choice; use only if other therapy is contraindicated or has failed. Due to optic nerve damage, use cautiously in the elderly.
Dosage Forms
   Powder: 25 g
   Tablet: 210 mg, 650 mg

Iopidine® *see* Apraclonidine *on page 78*

Ipecac Syrup (IP e kak SIR up)

Generic Available Yes
Therapeutic Category Antidote, Emetic
Use Treatment of acute oral drug overdosage and in certain poisonings
Contraindications Do not use in unconscious patients, patients with absent gag reflex; ingestion of strong bases or acids, volatile oils; seizures
Warnings Do not confuse ipecac syrup with ipecac fluid extract, which is 14 times more potent; use with caution in patients with cardiovascular disease and bulimics
Precautions May be ineffective in overdoses of antiemetics; may be cardiotoxic if not vomited and allowed to be absorbed
Adverse Reactions
   Cardiovascular: Cardiotoxicity
   Central nervous system: Lethargy
   Gastrointestinal: Protracted vomiting, diarrhea
   Neuromuscular & skeletal: Myopathy
Overdosage Symptoms of overdose include diarrhea, persistent vomiting, hypotension, atrial fibrillation
Toxicology Activated charcoal to absorb ipecac or perform gastric lavage; support cardiovascular system by symptomatic care

Drug Interactions
Decreased effect with activated charcoal, milk, carbonated beverages
Increased toxicity of phenothiazines (chlorpromazine has been associated with serious dystonic reactions)

Mechanism of Action Irritates the gastric mucosa and stimulates the medullary chemoreceptor trigger zone to induce vomiting

Pharmacodynamics
Onset of emesis: Within 15-30 minutes
Duration: 20-25 minutes; can last longer, 60 minutes in some cases

Usual Dosage Geriatrics and Adults: Oral: 15-30 mL followed by 200-300 mL of water; repeat dose one time if vomiting does not occur within 20 minutes; if vomiting does not occur after second dose, perform gastric lavage

Patient Information Call the Poison Center before administering. Patients should be kept active and moving following administration of ipecac; follow dose with 8 oz of water following initial episode; if vomiting, no food or liquids should be ingested for 1 hour.

Nursing Implications Do **not** administer to unconscious patients; patients should be kept active and moving following administration of ipecac; if vomiting does not occur after second dose, gastric lavage may be considered to remove ingested substance

Additional Information See Patient Information; Nursing Implications

Special Geriatric Considerations See Precautions and Adverse Reactions

Dosage Forms
Syrup:
OTC: 70 mg/mL, 1.5% alcohol (15 mL, 30 mL)
Prescription: 70 mg/mL, 2% alcohol (30 mL, pints, gallons; UD 15 mL & 30 mL)

I-Phrine® Ophthalmic Solution see Phenylephrine on page 740

IPOL™ see Poliovirus Vaccine, Inactivated on page 761

Ipratropium (i pra TROE pee um)

Related Information
Asthma Guidelines on page 1040
Inhaled Medications Comparison on page 1034

Brand Names Atrovent®

Generic Available No

Therapeutic Category Anticholinergic Agent; Bronchodilator

Use Anticholinergic bronchodilator used for the prevention of bronchospasm associated with COPD, bronchitis, and emphysema
Nasal spray: Perennial rhinitis (0.03%); common cold (0.06%)

Contraindications Hypersensitivity to atropine or its derivatives

Warnings Not indicated for the initial treatment of acute episodes of bronchospasm

Precautions Use with caution in patients with narrow-angle glaucoma, prostatic hypertrophy or bladder neck obstruction

Adverse Reactions Note: Ipratropium is poorly absorbed from the lung, so systemic effects are rare

Cardiovascular: Palpitations
Central nervous system: Nervousness, dizziness, fatigue, headache
Dermatologic: Rash
Gastrointestinal: Nausea, xerostomia; dry mouth with nasal spray
Ocular: Blurred vision
Respiratory: Cough; epistaxis, nasal dryness, nasal congestion with nasal spray

Overdosage Symptoms of overdose include dry mouth, drying of respiratory secretions, cough, nausea, GI distress, blurred vision or impaired visual accommodation, headache, nervousness

Toxicology Acute overdosage with ipratropium by inhalation is unlikely since it is so poorly absorbed. However, if poisoning occurs it can be treated like any other anticholinergic toxicity. An anticholinergic overdose with severe life-threatening symptoms, may be treated with physostigmine 1-2 mg S.C. or I.V., slowly.

Mechanism of Action Blocks the action of acetylcholine at parasympathetic sites in bronchial smooth muscle causing bronchodilation

Pharmacodynamics
Onset of action: Bronchodilation begins 1-3 minutes after administration with a maximal effect occurring within 1.5-2 hours
Duration: 4-6 hours
(Continued)

495

Ipratropium *(Continued)*

Pharmacokinetics
Absorption: Inhalation: Not readily absorbed into the systemic circulation from the surface of the lung or from GI tract
Distribution: 15% of dose reaches the lower airways

Usual Dosage Geriatrics and Adults:
Inhalation: 2 inhalations 4 times/day up to 12 inhalations/24 hours
Nebulization: 500 mcg 3-4 times/day
Nasal spray: 0.03%: 2 sprays 2 or 3 times/day; 0.06%: 2 sprays 3 or 4 times/day; safety and efficacy of use beyond 4 days in patients with the common cold have not been established
See also Additional Information

Monitoring Parameters Pulmonary function tests

Patient Information Temporary blurred vision may occur if sprayed into eyes. Follow instructions for use accompanying the product. Close eyes when administering ipratropium; wait at least one full minute between inhalations. Nasal spray: Initial pump priming requires 7 actuations. Do not interchange oral and nasal products.

Nursing Implications Teach patients how to use the inhaler; shake inhaler before administering

Additional Information Some patients may require higher doses (4-8 inhalations/dose); ipratropium solution may be mixed with albuterol solution if used within 1 hour

Special Geriatric Considerations Older patients may find it difficult to use the metered dose inhaler. A spacer device may be useful. Ipratropium has not been specifically studied in the elderly, but it is poorly absorbed from the airways and appears to be safe in this population.

Dosage Forms
Ipratropium bromide: solution:
Inhalation: 18 mcg/actuation (14 g)
Nasal spray: 0.03% (30 mL); 0.06% (15 mL)
Nebulizing: 0.02% (2.5 mL)

References
Hughes DT, "The Use of Anticholinergic Drugs in Nocturnal Asthma," *Postgrad Med J*, 1987, 63(Suppl 1):47-51.

Iproveratril Hydrochloride *see* Verapamil *on page 986*

IPV *see* Poliovirus Vaccine, Inactivated *on page 761*

Irbesartan *(ir be SAR tan)*

Brand Names Avapro®

Generic Available No

Therapeutic Category Angiotensin II Antagonists

Use Treatment of hypertension alone or in combination with other antihypertensives

Unlabeled use: Heart failure; studies are evaluating irbesartan in reducing the rates of progression of renal disease and adverse clinical sequelae of hypertension in diabetes nephropathy in type 2 diabetes mellitus

Contraindications Hypersensitivity to irbesartan or any components; severe hepatic insufficiency, biliary cirrhosis or biliary obstruction, primary hyperaldosteronism, bilateral renal artery stenosis

Warnings Use extreme caution with concurrent administration of potassium-sparing diuretics or potassium supplements, in patients with mild-moderate hepatic dysfunction (adjust dose), in those who may be sodium/water depleted (eg, on high-dose diuretics), and in the elderly; avoid use in patients with congestive heart failure, unilateral renal artery stenosis, aortic/mitral valve stenosis, coronary artery disease, or hypertrophic cardiomyopathy

Precautions Elevations of liver function tests frequently occur, including serum bilirubin; serum creatinine and BUN may be increased; decreases in hemoglobin and hematocrit (>20%); serum potassium increases of greater than 20% observed in 4% of patients

Adverse Reactions Similar incidence to placebo; independent of race, age, and gender

Cardiovascular: Edema, chest pain, tachycardia
Central nervous system: Headache, dizziness, drowsiness, ataxia, insomnia, fatigue, anxiety/nervousness
Dermatologic: Rash
Endocrine & metabolic: Decreased libido
Gastrointestinal: Diarrhea, abdominal pain, nausea, abnormal taste, dyspepsia, heartburn

Hematologic: Neutropenia, anemia

Hepatic: Increased LFTs

Neuromuscular & skeletal: Arthralgia, pain, muscle cramps, myalgia

Renal: Polyuria, increased creatinine

Respiratory: Cough, upper respiratory infection, rhinitis, sinusitis, nasal congestion, pharyngitis

Overdosage Symptoms include hypotension and tachycardia; bradycardia due to vagal response

Toxicology Treatment is symptomatic (eg, fluids) and supportive

Drug Interactions

Decreased effect: Phenobarbital, ketoconazole, troleandomycin

Increased effect: Cimetidine

Drug/Food Interactions Food does not affect absorption/bioavailability

Mechanism of Action Irbesartan is an angiotensin receptor antagonist. It displaces angiotensin II from the AT_1 receptor and produces its blood pressure lowering effects by antagonizing AT_1-induced vasoconstriction, aldosterone release, catecholamine release, arginine vasopressin release, water intake, and hypertrophic responses. This action results in more efficient blockade of the cardiovascular effects of angiotensin II and fewer side effects than the ACE inhibitors.

Pharmacokinetics

Distribution: 53-93 L

Protein binding: 90%

Metabolism: Metabolized in the liver (CYP2C9); <20% metabolites

Bioavailability: 60% to 80%

Half-life: 11-15 hours

Time to peak concentration: 1.5-2 hours

Elimination: Urine unchanged ~20%; recovered in feces ~80%

Usual Dosage Adults: Oral: 150 mg once daily with or without food; patients may be titrated to 300 mg once daily (see Additional Information)

Monitoring Parameters Baseline and periodic electrolyte panels, renal and liver function tests, urinalysis; symptoms of hypotension or hypersensitivity; monitor blood pressure and pulse

Patient Information Do not stop taking this medication unless instructed by a physician; take a missed dose as soon as possible unless it is almost time for your next dose; call your physician immediately if you have symptoms of allergy or develop side effects including headache and dizziness

Nursing Implications Monitor initial doses for hypotension; stress need for adequate fluid intake (see Warnings and Precautions)

Additional Information Addition of a diuretic gives an additive effect. For patients who have an adequate response to 300 mg, no gain in antihypertensive effect can be seen by increasing dose beyond 300 mg/day. Consider adding a diuretic or other antihypertensive.

Special Geriatric Considerations No dosage adjustment is necessary when initiating angiotensin II receptor antagonists in elderly. In clinical studies, no differences between younger adults and elderly were demonstrated.

Dosage Forms Tablet: 75 mg, 150 mg, 300 mg

References

Munger MA and Furniss SM, "Angiotensin II Receptor Blockers: Novel Therapy for Heart Failure?" *Pharmacotherapy*, 1996, 16(2 Pt 2):59S-68S.

Ircon® **[OTC]** *see Ferrous Fumarate on page 376*

Iron Dextran Complex (EYE ern DEKS tran KOM pleks)

Related Information

Antacid Drug Interactions *on page 1096*

I.V. Medication Recommendations *on page 1080*

I.V. Push Recommended Guidelines *on page 1083*

Brand Names Dexferrum® Injection; InFed™ Injection

Generic Available Yes

Therapeutic Category Iron Salt

Use Treatment of microcytic hypochromic anemia resulting from iron deficiency in whom oral administration is infeasible or ineffective

Contraindications Hypersensitivity to iron dextran; all anemias that are not involved with iron deficiency; hemochromatosis, hemolytic anemia

Warnings Deaths associated with parenteral administration following anaphylactic-type reactions have been reported; use only in patients where the iron deficient state is not amenable to oral iron therapy; I.M. injections have been reported to be carcinogenic in rats and mice

(Continued)

Iron Dextran Complex *(Continued)*

Precautions Use with caution in patients with history of asthma, hepatic impairment rheumatoid arthritis; epinephrine should be immediately available to treat hypersensitivity reactions

Adverse Reactions
Cardiovascular: Cardiovascular collapse, hypotension
Central nervous system: Dizziness, fever, headache, chills
Dermatologic: Urticaria
Gastrointestinal: Nausea, metallic taste
Hematologic: Leukocytosis
Local: Pain, staining of skin at the site of I.M. injection, phlebitis, flushing
Neuromuscular & skeletal: Arthralgia
Respiratory: Respiratory difficulty
Miscellaneous: Lymphadenopathy, diaphoresis

Overdosage Symptoms of overdose include lethargy, tarry stools, hypotension, acidosis, pulmonary edema, hyperthermia, convulsions, tachycardia, enlargement of lymph nodes

Toxicology Although rare, if a severe iron overdose (when the serum iron concentration exceeds the total iron-binding capacity) occurs, it may be treated with deferoxamine. Deferoxamine may be administered I.V. (80 mg/kg over 24 hours) or I.M. (40-90 mg/kg every 8 hours). Hypersensitivity reactions should be treated with 0.5 mL of a 1:1000 solution of epinephrine given I.M. or S.C.

Drug Interactions Decreased effect with chloramphenicol

Stability Commercial injection should be stored at room temperature; stability of parenteral admixture at room temperature (25°C): 3 months

Mechanism of Action The released iron, from the plasma, eventually replenishes the depleted iron stores in the bone marrow where it is incorporated into hemoglobin

Pharmacokinetics
Absorption: I.M.: Prompt, 50% to 90% absorbed, balance slowly absorbed over months
Elimination: By reticuloendothelial system and excreted in urine and feces (via bile)

Usual Dosage Geriatrics and Adults: A 0.5 mL test dose should be given prior to starting iron dextran therapy

Total replacement dosage of iron dextran (mg) = (0.3) (weight in lbs) (100 - 100 x Hgb divided by 14.8)

I.V.: This dose can be given in its entirety after a minimum 1-hour waiting period has elapsed after the test dose. Individual daily doses of ≤2 mL can be given I.V. or I.M. until the cumulative total dose necessary for replacement has been reached.

Administration Use Z-track technique for I.M. administration (deep into the upper outer quadrant of buttock); may be administered I.V. bolus at rate ≤50 mg/minute or diluted in 250-1000 mL NS and infused over 1-6 hours

Monitoring Parameters Hemoglobin, hematocrit, ferritin, reticulocyte count

Reference Range Therapeutic: Male: 75-175 µg/dL (SI: 13.4-31.3 µmol/L); Female: 65-165 µg/dL (SI: 11.6-29.5 µmol/L); ranges may vary by laboratory

Test Interactions Increased serum iron concentration for 3 weeks

Patient Information Report any unusual systemic or local reactions to your physician; pain on administration

Nursing Implications See Administration

Additional Information Avoid iron injection if oral intake is feasible; a test dose of 0.5 mL I.V. or I.M. should be given to observe for adverse reactions

Special Geriatric Considerations Anemia in the elderly is most often caused by "anemia of chronic disease", a result of aging effect in bone marrow, or associated with inflammation rather than blood loss. Iron stores are usually normal or increased, with a serum ferritin >50 ng/mL and a decreased total iron binding capacity. Hence, the anemia is not secondary to iron deficiency but the inability of the reticuloendothelial system to use available iron stores. I.V. administration of iron dextran is often preferred over I.M. in the elderly secondary to a decreased muscle mass and the need for daily injections.

Dosage Forms Injection: 50 mg/mL (2 mL, 5 mL, 10 mL)

References
Lipschitz DA, "The Anemia of Chronic Disease," *J Am Geriatr Soc*, 1990, 38(11):1258-64.

ISD *see* Isosorbide Dinitrate *on page 503*

ISDN *see* Isosorbide Dinitrate *on page 503*

ISG *see* Immune Globulin *on page 482*

Ismelin® *see* Guanethidine *on page 442*

ISMN *see* Isosorbide Mononitrate *on page 505*

ISMO™ *see* Isosorbide Mononitrate *on page 505*

Ismotic® *see* Isosorbide *on page 502*

Isobamate *see* Carisoprodol *on page 165*

Isoetharine (eye soe ETH a reen)

Related Information
Asthma Guidelines *on page 1040*
Inhaled Medications Comparison *on page 1034*

Brand Names Arm-a-Med® Isoetharine; Beta-2®; Bronkometer®; Bronkosol®; Dey-Lute® Isoetharine

Generic Available Yes

Therapeutic Category Adrenergic Agonist Agent; Bronchodilator

Use Bronchodilator in bronchial asthma and for reversible bronchospasm occurring with bronchitis and emphysema

Contraindications Known hypersensitivity to isoetharine

Warnings Isoetharine hydrochloride solution contains sulfites which may cause allergic reactions in some patients. Use caution in patients with unstable vasomotor symptoms, diabetes, hyperthyroidism, prostatic hypertrophy, or a history of seizures. Also use caution in the elderly and those patients with cardiovascular disorders such as coronary artery disease, arrhythmias, and hypertension.

Precautions Excessive or prolonged use may result in decreased effectiveness

Adverse Reactions
Cardiovascular: Tachycardia, hypertension
Central nervous system: Anxiety, dizziness, restlessness, excitement, headache
Gastrointestinal: Nausea, vomiting
Neuromuscular & skeletal: Tremors (may be more common in the elderly), weakness

Overdosage Symptoms of overdose include nausea, vomiting, hypertension, tremors

Toxicology In cases of overdose, supportive therapy should be instituted, and prudent use of a cardioselective beta-adrenergic blocker (eg, atenolol or metoprolol) should be considered, keeping in mind the potential for induction of bronchoconstriction in an asthmatic individual. Dialysis has not been shown to be of value in the treatment of an overdose with this agent.

Drug Interactions
Decreased effect with beta-blockers
Increased toxicity with other sympathomimetics (eg, epinephrine)

Stability Do not use if solution is discolored or a precipitation is present; compatible with sterile water, 0:45% NaCl, and 0.9% NaCl

Mechanism of Action Relaxes bronchial smooth muscle by action on beta$_2$-receptors with little effect on heart rate

Pharmacodynamics
Peak effect: Inhalation: Within 5-15 minutes
Duration: 1-4 hours

Pharmacokinetics
Metabolism: In many tissues including the liver and lungs
Elimination: Primarily (90%) as metabolites

Usual Dosage Treatments are usually not repeated more often than every 4 hours, except in severe cases

Geriatrics and Adults:
Aerosol nebulizer: 1-2 inhalations every 4 hours as needed
Hand nebulizer: 3-7 inhalations undiluted every 4 hours as needed

Monitoring Parameters Pulmonary function, blood pressure, pulse

Patient Information Follow instructions for use of nebulizer

Nursing Implications Monitor lung sounds, blood pressure, pulse; instruct patient on use of nebulizer

Additional Information
Isoetharine hydrochloride: Arm-a-Med® isoetharine, Beta-2®, Bronkosol®, Dey-Lute® isoetharine
Isoetharine mesylate: Bronkometer®
Isoetharine has a shorter duration of action than other beta$_2$ selective agonists; therefore, it is usually not considered a first-line drug of choice
(Continued)

Isoetharine *(Continued)*

Special Geriatric Considerations The elderly may find it useful to utilize a spacer device when using a metered dose inhaler (see Additional Information)

Dosage Forms
Aerosol, oral, as mesylate: 340 mcg/metered spray
Solution, inhalation, as hydrochloride: 0.062% (4 mL); 0.08% (3.5 mL); 0.1% (2.5 mL, 5 mL); 0.125% (4 mL); 0.167% (3 mL); 0.17% (3 mL); 0.2% (2.5 mL); 0.25% (2 mL, 3.5 mL); 0.5% (0.5 mL); 1% (0.5 mL, 0.25 mL, 10 mL, 14 mL, 30 mL)

Isoniazid *(eye soe NYE a zid)*

Related Information
Antacid Drug Interactions *on page 1096*

Brand Names Laniazid® Oral; Nydrazid® Injection

Synonyms Isonicotinic Acid Hydrazide

Generic Available Yes

Therapeutic Category Antitubercular Agent

Use Treatment of susceptible tuberculosis infections and prophylactically to those individuals exposed to tuberculosis

Contraindications Acute liver disease; hypersensitivity to isoniazid or any component; previous history of hepatic damage during isoniazid therapy

Warnings Severe and sometimes fatal hepatitis may occur or develop even after many months of treatment; patients must report any prodromal symptoms of hepatitis, such as fatigue, weakness, malaise, anorexia, nausea, or vomiting

Precautions Use with caution in patients with renal impairment and chronic liver disease

Adverse Reactions
Central nervous system: Seizure, stupor, dizziness, psychosis, fever, ataxia, depression
Dermatologic: Skin eruptions
Endocrine & metabolic: Hyperglycemia
Gastrointestinal: Nausea, vomiting, epigastric distress
Hematologic: Blood dyscrasias
Hepatic: Hepatitis, elevated liver transaminase levels
Neuromuscular & skeletal: Hyper-reflexia, peripheral neuritis
Ocular: Optic neuritis
Otic: Tinnitus

Overdosage Symptoms of overdose include nausea, vomiting, slurred speech, dizziness, blurred vision, hallucinations, stupor, coma, intractable seizures

Toxicology Because of the severe morbidity and high mortality rates with isoniazid overdose, patients who are asymptomatic after an overdose, should be monitored for 4-6 hours. Pyridoxine has been shown to be effective in the treatment of intoxication, especially when seizures occur. Pyridoxine I.V. is administered on a milligram to milligram dose. If the amount of isoniazid ingested is unknown, 5 g of pyridoxine should be given over 3-5 minutes and may be followed by an additional 5 g in 30 minutes.

Drug Interactions
Inhibits the metabolism and increased toxicity of phenytoin, carbamazepine, primidone, warfarin, diazepam (and other hepatically metabolized benzodiazepines), prednisone, disulfiram
Decreased effect/levels of isoniazid with aluminum salts

Stability Protect oral dosage forms from light

Mechanism of Action Unknown, but may include the inhibition of myocolic acid synthesis resulting in disruption of the bacterial cell wall

Pharmacokinetics
Absorption: Oral, I.M.: Rapid and complete
Distribution: Into all body tissues and fluids including the CSF
Protein binding: 10% to 15%
Metabolism: By the liver with decay rate determined genetically by acetylation phenotype; substrate and inducer CYP2E1, inhibitor CYP1A2
Half-life:
Fast acetylators: 30-100 minutes
Slow acetylators: 2-5 hours; half-life may be prolonged in patients with impaired hepatic function or severe renal impairment
Time to peak serum concentration: Oral: Within 1-2 hours; rate of absorption can be slowed when administered with food

Elimination: In urine (75% to 95%), feces, and saliva

Usual Dosage Oral, I.M.:
Geriatrics and Adults: 5 mg/kg/day given daily (usual dose: 300 mg)
Disseminated disease: 10 mg/kg/day in 1-2 divided doses
Prophylaxis: 300 mg/day given daily
American Thoracic Society and CDC currently recommend twice weekly therapy as part of a short-course regimen (6-9 months) which follows 1-2 months of daily treatment for uncomplicated pulmonary tuberculosis in compliant patients
Geriatrics and Adults: 15 mg/kg/dose (up to 900 mg) twice weekly
Dialyzable (50% to 100%)

Monitoring Parameters Monitor transaminase concentrations at baseline 1, 3, 6, and 9 months

Reference Range Therapeutic: 1-7 µg/mL (SI: 7-51 µmol/L); Toxic: 20-710 µg/mL (SI: 146-5176 µmol/L)

Test Interactions False-positive urinary glucose with Clinitest®

Patient Information Report any prodromal symptoms of hepatitis (fatigue, weakness, nausea, vomiting, dark urine, or yellowing of eyes) or any burning, tingling, or numbness in the extremities

Nursing Implications Monitor monthly for signs or symptoms of active disease, hepatitis, or other adverse effects

Additional Information Pyridoxine should be given concomitantly in persons with conditions in which neuropathy is common (eg, diabetes, alcoholism, malnutrition)

Special Geriatric Considerations Age has not been shown to affect the pharmacokinetics of INH since acetylation phenotype determines clearance and half-life, acetylation rate does not change significantly with age; most strains of *M. tuberculosis* found the elderly should be susceptible to INH since most acquired their initial infection prior to INH's introduction

Dosage Forms
Injection: 100 mg/mL (10 mL)
Syrup: 50 mg/5 mL (473 mL)
Tablet: 50 mg, 100 mg, 300 mg

References
Bass JB Jr, Farer LS, Hopewell PC, et al, "Treatment of Tuberculosis and Tuberculosis Infection in Adults and Children," *Am J Respir Crit Care Med*, 1994, 149(5):1359-74.
Kergueris MF, Bourin M, and Larousse C, "Pharmacokinetics of Isoniazid: Influence of Age," *Eur J Clin Pharmacol*, 1986, 30(3):335-40.
Van Scoy RE and Wilkowske CJ, "Antituberculous Agents: Isoniazid, Rifampin, Streptomycin, Ethambutol, and Pyrazinamide," *Mayo Clin Proc*, 1983, 58(4):233-40.
Yoshikawa TT, "Tuberculosis in Aging Adults," *J Am Geriatr Soc*, 1992, 40(2):178-87.

Isonicotinic Acid Hydrazide *see Isoniazid on previous page*

Isonipecaine Hydrochloride *see Meperidine on page 584*

Isoprenaline Hydrochloride *see Isoproterenol on this page*

Isoproterenol (eye soe proe TER e nole)

Related Information
Asthma Guidelines *on page 1040*
Inhaled Medications Comparison *on page 1034*

Brand Names Arm-a-Med® Isoproterenol; Dey-Dose® Isoproterenol; Dispos-a-Med® Isoproterenol; Isuprel®; Medihaler-Iso®; Norisodrine®

Synonyms Isoprenaline Hydrochloride

Generic Available Yes

Therapeutic Category Adrenergic Agonist Agent; Bronchodilator

Use Asthma or COPD (reversible airway obstruction); A-V nodal block; hemodynamically compromised bradyarrhythmias or atropine-resistant brady-arrhythmias, temporary use in third degree A-V block until pacemaker insertion; low cardiac output; vasoconstrictive shock states

Contraindications Angina, pre-existing cardiac arrhythmias (ventricular); tachycardia or A-V block caused by cardiac glycoside intoxication; allergy to sulfites or isoproterenol or other sympathomimetic amines

Warnings Use with caution in congestive heart failure, ischemia, or aortic stenosis

Precautions Geriatric patients, diabetics, renal or cardiovascular disease, hyperthyroidism

Adverse Reactions
Cardiovascular: Hypertension, tachycardia, palpitations, arrhythmias
Central nervous system: Nervousness, restlessness, anxiety, dizziness, headache
Gastrointestinal: Nausea, vomiting
(Continued)

Isoproterenol *(Continued)*

Neuromuscular & skeletal: Tremors

Overdosage Symptoms of overdose include nausea, vomiting, hypertension, tremors

Toxicology In cases of overdose, supportive therapy should be instituted, and prudent use of a cardioselective beta-adrenergic blocker (eg, atenolol or metoprolol) should be considered, keeping in mind the potential for induction of bronchoconstriction in an asthmatic individual. Dialysis has not been shown to be of value in the treatment of an overdose with this agent.

Drug Interactions Increased toxicity: Sympathomimetic agents, general anesthetics

Stability Do not use discolored solutions; limit exposure to heat, light, or air; incompatible with alkaline solutions

Stability of parenteral admixture at room temperature (25°C): 24 hours
Stability of parenteral admixture at refrigeration temperature (4°C): 24 hours

Mechanism of Action Relaxes bronchial smooth muscle by action on beta$_2$-receptors; causes increased heart rate and contractility by action on beta$_1$-receptors

Pharmacokinetics

Metabolism: By conjugation in many tissues including the liver and lungs
Half-life: 2.5-5 minutes
Time to peak serum concentration: Oral: Within 1-2 hours
Elimination: In urine principally as sulfate conjugates

Usual Dosage Geriatrics and Adults:

Bronchodilation, metered dose inhaler: 1-2 inhalations 4-6 times/day
Hand bulb nebulizer: 5-15 inhalations of a 1:200 solution up to 5 times/day
Glosset: S.L.: 10-20 mg every 3-4 hours as needed up to 60 mg/day
A-V nodal block: I.V. infusion: 2-20 mcg/minute

Monitoring Parameters Pulmonary function, blood pressure, pulse

Patient Information Follow instructions accompanying inhaler; do not exceed recommended doses

Nursing Implications Instruct patient on how to use inhaler or nebulizer

Additional Information Isoproterenol is not a drug of first choice in the chronic treatment of asthma because of its beta$_1$ effects

Special Geriatric Considerations The elderly may find it useful to utilize a spacer device when using a metered dose inhaler (see Additional Information)

Dosage Forms

Isoproterenol hydrochloride:
Inhalation: 0.5% (1 mL, 10 mL); 1% (1 mL, 10 mL)
Inhalation, aerosol: 0.25% (15 mL, 22.5 mL)
Injection: 0.2 mg/mL (1 mL, 5 mL, 10 mL)
Tablet (Glosset), sublingual: 10 mg, 15 mg

Isoptin® *see* Verapamil *on page 986*

Isoptin® SR *see* Verapamil *on page 986*

Isopto® Atropine *see* Atropine *on page 92*

Isopto® Carbachol Ophthalmic *see* Carbachol *on page 159*

Isopto® Carpine Ophthalmic *see* Pilocarpine *on page 748*

Isopto® Cetamide® Ophthalmic *see* Sulfacetamide Sodium *on page 874*

Isopto® Cetapred® Ophthalmic *see* Sulfacetamide Sodium and Prednisolone *on page 875*

Isopto® Frin Ophthalmic Solution *see* Phenylephrine *on page 740*

Isopto® Homatropine Ophthalmic *see* Homatropine *on page 454*

Isopto® Hyoscine Ophthalmic *see* Scopolamine *on page 850*

Isopto® Plain Solution [OTC] *see* Artificial Tears *on page 82*

Isopto® Tears Solution [OTC] *see* Artificial Tears *on page 82*

Isordil® *see* Isosorbide Dinitrate *on next page*

Isosorbide *(eye soe SOR bide)*

Brand Names Ismotic®

Generic Available No

Therapeutic Category Diuretic, Osmotic; Ophthalmic Agent, Osmotic

Use Short-term emergency treatment of acute angle-closure glaucoma and short-term reduction of intraocular pressure prior to and following intraocular surgery; may be used to interrupt an acute glaucoma attack; preferred agent when need to avoid nausea and vomiting

Contraindications Severe renal disease, anuria, severe dehydration, acute pulmonary edema, severe cardiac decompensation, known hypersensitivity to isosorbide

Warnings Maintain fluid/electrolyte balance with multiple doses; monitor urinary output; if urinary output declines, need to review clinical status

Precautions Use with caution in patients with impending pulmonary edema, and in the elderly; hypernatremia and dehydration may begin to occur after 72 hours of continuous administration; use is not recommended in patients with anuria, severe dehydration

Adverse Reactions
Cardiovascular: Syncope
Central nervous system: Headache, confusion, disorientation, lethargy, vertigo, dizziness, lightheadedness, irritability
Dermatologic: Rash
Endocrine & metabolic: Hypernatremia, hyperosmolarity
Gastrointestinal: Nausea, vomiting, abdominal/gastric discomfort (infrequently)
Miscellaneous: Hiccups

Overdosage Symptoms of overdose include dehydration, hypotension, hypernatremia

Toxicology General supportive care; fluid administration, electrolyte balance, discontinue agent

Mechanism of Action Elevate osmolarity of glomerular filtrate to hinder the tubular resorption of water and increase excretion of sodium and chloride to result in diuresis; creates an osmotic gradient between plasma and ocular fluids

Pharmacodynamics
Onset of action: Within 10-30 minutes
Peak action: 1-1.5 hours
Duration: 5-6 hours

Pharmacokinetics
Distribution: In total body water
Metabolism: Not metabolized
Half-life: 5-9.5 hours
Elimination: By glomerular filtration (see Mechanism of Action)

Usual Dosage Geriatrics and Adults: Oral: Initial: 1.5 g/kg with a usual range of 1-3 g/kg 2-4 times/day

Monitoring Parameters Monitor for signs of dehydration, blood pressure, renal output, intraocular pressure reduction

Nursing Implications Palatability may be improved if poured over ice and sipped

Additional Information Each 220 mL contains isosorbide 100 g, sodium 4.6 mEq and potassium 0.9 mEq; hypernatremia and dehydration may begin to occur after 72 hours of continuous administration; palatability may be improved by sipping over cracked ice

Special Geriatric Considerations Use cautiously due to the elderly's predisposition to dehydration and the fact that they frequently have concomitant diseases which may be aggravated by the use of isosorbide (see Contraindications and Precautions)

Dosage Forms Solution: 45% (100 g/220 mL)

Isosorbide Dinitrate (eye soe SOR bide dye NYE trate)

Brand Names Dilatrate®-SR; Isordil®; Sorbitrate®
Synonyms ISD; ISDN
Generic Available Yes
Therapeutic Category Antianginal Agent; Nitrate; Vasodilator, Coronary
Use Prevention and treatment of angina pectoris; for congestive heart failure; to relieve pain, dysphagia, and spasm in esophageal spasm with GE reflux

Contraindications Severe anemia, closed-angle glaucoma, postural hypotension, cerebral hemorrhage, head trauma, early MI (sublingual), hypersensitivity to isosorbide dinitrate or any component

Warnings Do not crush or chew sublingual dosage form; do not crush chewable tablets before administration; use with caution in patients with hypovolemia, glaucoma, increased intracranial pressure, hypotension

Precautions Increased intracranial pressure; may increase intraocular pressure in patients with glaucoma; use caution in dehydrated or volume depleted patients; hypotension may accompany paradoxial bradycardia with increased anginal pain; do not use sustained-release products in patients with GI hypermotility or malabsorption syndrome; do not stop use abruptly to avoid

(Continued)

Isosorbide Dinitrate *(Continued)*

withdrawal reactions (angina); must gradually reduce daily doses to withdraw; tolerance to vascular effects of nitrates has been demonstrated (see Usual Dosage for recommendation to minimize development of tolerance)

Adverse Reactions

Cardiovascular: Postural hypotension, syncope, cutaneous flushing of head, neck, and clavicular area, tachycardia, rebound hypertension, arrhythmias, atrial fibrillation, paradoxial bradycardia with angina

Central nervous system: Dizziness, vertigo, headache, restlessness, weakness, anxiety, agitation, confusion, nervousness, insomnia, hypokinesia, hypoasthesia, nightmares, malaise

Dermatologic: Rash, flushing, pruritus, exfoliative dermatitis

Gastrointestinal: Nausea, abdominal pain, GI upset, diarrhea, tenesmus

Genitourinary: Dysuria, frequency, impotence

Neuromuscular & skeletal: Arthralgia, muscle twitching, neck pain

Ocular: Diplopia

Respiratory: Bronchitis and pneumonia reported

Miscellaneous: Diaphoresis, edema, tooth pain

Overdosage Symptoms of overdose include hypotension, throbbing headache, palpitations, visual disturbances, flushing, perspiring skin, vertigo, diaphoresis, dizziness, syncope, nausea, vomiting, anorexia, dyspnea, heart block, confusion, fever, paralysis

Toxicology Formation of methemoglobinemia is dose-related and unusual in normal doses; high levels can cause signs and symptoms of hypoxemia; treatment consists of placing patient in recumbent position and administer fluids; alpha-adrenergic vasopressors may be required; treat methemoglobinemia with oxygen and methylene blue at a dose of 1-2 mg/kg I.V. slowly

Drug Interactions May antagonize the anticoagulant effect of heparin; alcohol increases hypotension; aspirin increases serum nitrate concentration; calcium channel blockers increase hypotension; dihydroergotamine antagonizes nitrate effect by increasing standing systolic blood pressure

Mechanism of Action Stimulation of intracellular cyclic-GMP results in vascular smooth muscle relaxation of both arterial and venous vasculature. Increased venous pooling decreases left ventricular pressure (preload) and arterial dilatation decreases arterial resistance (afterload). Therefore, this reduces cardiac oxygen demand by decreasing left ventricular pressure and systemic vascular resistance by dilating arteries. Additionally, coronary artery dilation improves collateral flow to ischemic regions; esophageal smooth muscle is relaxed via the same mechanism.

Pharmacodynamics See table.

Dosage Form	Onset of Action	Duration
Sublingual tablet	2-10 min	1-2 h
Chewable tablet	3 min	0.5-2 h
Oral tablet	45-60 min	4-6 h
Sustained release tablet	30 min	6-12 h

Pharmacokinetics

Metabolism: Extensive in the liver to conjugated metabolites, including isosorbide 5-mononitrate (active) and 2-mononitrate (active)

Half-life:

Parent: 1-4 hours

5-mononitrate: 4 hours

Elimination: In urine and feces

Usual Dosage

Geriatrics (administer lowest recommended daily dose initially and titrate upward) and Adults:

Oral: 5-30 mg 3-4 times/day or 40 mg every 6-12 hours in sustained-released dosage form

Chewable: 5-10 mg every 2-3 hours

Sublingual: 2.5-10 mg every 4-6 hours

Tolerance to nitrate effects develops with chronic exposure. Dose escalation does not overcome this effect. Tolerance can only be overcome by short periods of nitrate absence from the body. Short periods (10-12 hours) of nitrate withdrawal help minimize tolerance. General recommendations are to take the last dose of short-acting agents no later than 7 PM; administer 2-3 times/day rather than 4 times/day. Sustained release preparations could be administered at times to allow a 15- to 17-hour interval between first and last daily dose. Example: Administer sustained release at 8 AM and 2 PM for a twice daily regimen.

Monitoring Parameters Monitor number of anginal episodes, orthostatic blood pressures; a decrease of 15 mm Hg pressure systolic and/or 10 mm Hg diastolic or an increase in heart rate of 10 beats/minute from baseline (no drug) indicates approximate maximal cardiodynamic effects to nitrates and end point for dosing

Test Interactions Decreased cholesterol (S)

Patient Information Dispense drug in easy-to-open container; do not chew or crush sublingual or sustained-release dosage form; do not change brands without consulting your pharmacist or physician; patient should be instructed to take sublingual and chewable tablets while sitting down; any angina that persists for more than 20 minutes should be evaluated by a physician immediately

Nursing Implications Do not crush sustained release or sublingual drug product; monitor blood pressure reduction for maximal effect and orthostatic hypotension

Special Geriatric Considerations The first dose of nitrates (sublingual, chewable, oral) should be taken in a physician's office to observe for maximal cardiovascular dynamic effects (see Monitoring Parameters) and adverse effects (orthostatic blood pressure drop, headache). The use of nitrates for angina may occasionally promote reflux esophagitis. This may require dose adjustments or changing therapeutic agents to correct this adverse effect (see Precautions and Contraindications).

Dosage Forms
Capsule, sustained release: 40 mg
Tablet:
  Chewable: 5 mg, 10 mg
  Oral: 5 mg, 10 mg, 20 mg, 30 mg, 40 mg
  Sublingual: 2.5 mg, 5 mg, 10 mg
  Sustained release: 40 mg

References
Flaherty JT, "Hemodynamic Attenuation and the Nitrate-Free Interval: Alternative Dosing Strategies for Transdermal Nitroglycerin," *Am J Cardiol*, 1985, 56(17):321-71.
Parker JO, "Eccentric Dosing With Isosorbide-5-Mononitrate in Angina Pectoris," *Am J Cardiol*, 1993, 72(12):871-6.
Parker JO, Fanell B, Lahey KA, et al, "Effect of Intervals Between Doses on the Development to Tolerance to Isosorbide Dinitrate," *N Engl J Med*, 1987, 316(23):1440-4.

Isosorbide Mononitrate (EYE soe sor bide mon oh NYE trate)

Brand Names Imdur™; ISMO™; Monoket®

Synonyms ISMN

Generic Available No

Therapeutic Category Antianginal Agent; Nitrate; Vasodilator, Coronary

Use Long-acting metabolite of the vasodilator isosorbide dinitrate used for the prophylactic treatment of angina pectoris

Contraindications Contraindicated due to potential increases in intracranial pressure in patients with head trauma or cerebral hemorrhage; hypersensitivity or idiosyncrasy to nitrates

Warnings Postural hypotension, transient episodes of weakness, dizziness, or syncope may occur even with small doses; alcohol accentuates these effects; tolerance and cross-tolerance to nitrate antianginal and hemodynamic effects may occur during prolonged isosorbide mononitrate therapy; (minimized by using the smallest effective dose, by alternating coronary vasodilators or offering drug-free intervals of as little as 12 hours). Excessive doses may result in severe headache, blurred vision, or dry mouth; increased anginal symptoms may be a result of dosage increases.

Precautions Increased intracranial pressure; may increase intraocular pressure in patients with glaucoma; use caution in dehydrated or volume depleted patients; hypotension may accompany paradoxial bradycardia with increased anginal pain; do not use sustained-release products in patients with GI hypermotility or malabsorption syndrome; do not stop use abruptly to avoid withdrawal reactions (angina); must gradually reduce daily doses to withdraw; tolerance to vascular effects of nitrates has been demonstrated (see Usual Dosage for recommendation to minimize development of tolerance)

Adverse Reactions
Cardiovascular: Angina pectoris, arrhythmias, atrial fibrillation, hypotension, palpitations, postural hypotension, premature ventricular contractions, supraventricular tachycardia, syncope, edema
Central nervous system: Malaise, agitation, anxiety, confusion, hypoesthesia, insomnia, nervousness, nightmares, headache
(Continued)

Isosorbide Mononitrate *(Continued)*

Dermatologic: Pruritus, rash

Gastrointestinal: Abdominal pain, diarrhea, dyspepsia, tenesmus, increased appetite, dizziness, nausea, vomiting

Genitourinary: Impotence, polyuria, dysuria

Hematologic: Methemoglobinemia (rarely)

Neuromuscular & skeletal: Neck stiffness, rigors, arthralgia, dyscoordination, weakness

Ocular: Blurred vision, diplopia

Respiratory: Bronchitis, pneumonia, upper respiratory tract infection

Miscellaneous: Tooth disorder, cold sweat

Overdosage Symptoms of overdose include hypotension, dry mouth, increased anginal symptoms, throbbing headache, palpitations, visual disturbances (blurred vision), vertigo, tachycardia, methemoglobinemia, flushing, diaphoresis, dizziness, syncope, nausea, vomiting, anorexia, dyspnea, heart block, confusion, fever, metabolic acidosis, coma

Toxicology High levels or methemoglobinemia can cause signs and symptoms of hypoxemia; treatment consists of placing patient in recumbent position and administering fluids; alpha-adrenergic vasopressors may be required; treat methemoglobinemia with oxygen and methylene blue at a dose of 1-2 mg/kg I.V. slowly.

Drug Interactions May antagonize the anticoagulant effect of heparin; alcohol increases hypotension; aspirin increases serum nitrate concentration; calcium channel blockers increase hypotension; dihydroergotamine antagonizes nitrate effect by increasing standing systolic blood pressure

Stability Tablets should be stored in a tight container at room temperature of 15°C to 30°C (59°F to 86°F)

Mechanism of Action Prevailing mechanism of action for nitroglycerin (and other nitrates) is systemic venodilation through stimulation of intracellular cyclic-GMP, thus, decreasing preload as measured by pulmonary capillary wedge pressure and left ventricular end diastolic volume and pressure; the average reduction in LVEDV is 25% at rest, with a corresponding increase in ejection fractions of 50% to 60%. This effect improves congestive symptoms in heart failure and improves the myocardial perfusion gradient in patients with coronary artery disease.

Pharmacokinetics

Absorption: Oral: Nearly complete and low intersubject variability in its pharmacokinetic parameters and plasma concentrations

Metabolism: Metabolite of isosorbide dinitrate

Half-life: Mononitrate: ~4 hours (8 times that of dinitrate)

Usual Dosage Geriatrics (start with lowest recommended dose) and Adults: Oral:

Regular tablet: 5-10 mg twice daily with the two doses given 7 hours apart (eg, 8 AM and 3 PM) to decrease tolerance development; then titrate to 10 mg twice daily in first 2-3 days

Extended release tablet (Imdur™): Initial: 30-60 mg given in morning as a single dose; titrate upward as needed, giving at least 3 days between increases; maximum daily single dose: 240 mg

Dosing adjustment in renal impairment: Not necessary for elderly or patients with altered renal or hepatic function

Tolerance to nitrate effects develops with chronic exposure. Dose escalation does not overcome this effect. Tolerance can only be overcome by short periods of nitrate absence from the body. Short periods (10-12 hours) of nitrate withdrawal help minimize tolerance. General recommendations are to take the last dose of short-acting agents no later than 7 PM; administer 2-3 times/day rather than 4 times/day. Sustained release preparations could be administered at times to allow a 15- to 17-hour interval between first and last daily dose. Example: Administer sustained release at 8 AM and 2 PM for a twice daily regimen.

Administration Do not administer around-the-clock

Monitoring Parameters Monitor number of anginal episodes, orthostatic blood pressures; a decrease of 15 mm Hg pressure systolic and/or 10 mm Hg diastolic or an increase in heart rate of 10 beats/minute from baseline (no drug) indicates approximate maximal cardiodynamic effects to nitrates and end point for dosing

Test Interactions Decreased cholesterol(s)

Patient Information Dispense drug in easy-to-open container; do not change brands without consulting pharmacist or physician; keep tablets or capsules tightly closed in original container; extended release tablets should not be chewed or crushed and should be swallowed together with a half-glassful of fluid; the antianginal efficacy of tablets can be maintained by carefully following the prescribed schedule of dosing (2 doses taken 7 hours apart); headaches are sometimes a marker of the activity of the drug; any angina that persists for more than 20 minutes should be evaluated by a physician immediately

Nursing Implications Do not crush; 10 to 12-hour nitrate-free interval is needed each day to prevent or reduce tolerance

Special Geriatric Considerations The first dose of nitrates (sublingual, chewable, oral) should be taken in a physician's office to observe for maximal cardiovascular dynamic effects (see Monitoring Parameters) and adverse effects (orthostatic blood pressure drop, headache). The use of nitrates for angina may occasionally promote reflux esophagitis. This may require dose adjustments or changing therapeutic agents to correct this adverse effect (see Precautions and Contraindications).

Dosage Forms
Tablet (Ismo™, Monoket®): 10 mg, 20 mg
Tablet, extended release (Imdur™): 30 mg, 60 mg, 120 mg

References
Flaherty JT, "Hemodynamic Attenuation and the Nitrate Dose-Free Interval: Alternative Dosing Strategies for Transdermal Nitroglycerin," *Am J Cardiol*, 1985, 56(17):321-71.
Parker JO, "Eccentric Dosing With Isosorbide-5-Mononitrate in Angina Pectoris," *Am J Cardiol*, 1993, 72(12):871-6.
Parker JO, Fanell B, Lahey KA, et al, "Effect of Intervals Between Doses on the Development to Tolerance to Isosorbide Dinitrate," *N Engl J Med*, 1987, 316(23):1440-4.

Isoxsuprine (eye SOKS syoo preen)

Brand Names Vasodilan®

Generic Available Yes

Therapeutic Category Vasodilator

Use Considered "possibly effective" for treatment of peripheral vascular diseases, such as arteriosclerosis obliterans and Raynaud's disease

Contraindications Presence of arterial bleeding

Warnings May cause hypotension in elderly

Precautions See Warnings

Adverse Reactions
Cardiovascular: Hypotension, tachycardia, chest pain
Central nervous system: Dizziness
Dermatologic: Rash
Gastrointestinal: Nausea, vomiting, diarrhea, abdominal distress
Neuromuscular & skeletal: Weakness

Overdosage Symptoms of overdose include hypotension, flushing

Toxicology Vasodilation mediated second to alpha-adrenergic stimulation or direct smooth muscle effects; treat with I.V. fluids, alpha-adrenergic pressors may be required

Drug Interactions May enhance effects of other vasodilators/hypotensive agents; use with caution in elderly

Mechanism of Action In studies on normal human subjects, isoxsuprine increases muscle blood flow but skin blood flow is usually unaffected. Isoxsuprine was originally thought to increase muscle blood flow by beta-receptor stimulations. Since beta-receptor blocking drugs do not antagonize its vascular effects, isoxsuprine probably has a direct action on vascular smooth muscle. Isoxsuprine was shown to inhibit prostaglandin synthetase at high serum concentrations; with low concentrations there was an increase in the P-G synthesis. At high doses blood viscosity is lowered and platelet aggregation is inhibited.

Pharmacokinetics
Absorption: Nearly completely
Metabolism: Partially conjugated in the liver
Serum half-life: 1.25 hours mean
Time to peak serum concentration: Oral, I.M.: Within 1 hour
Elimination: Primarily in urine

Usual Dosage Oral: Geriatrics and Adults: 10-20 mg 3-4 times/day; start with lower dose in elderly due to potential hypotension

Monitoring Parameters Monitor orthostatic blood pressure

Patient Information May cause skin rash; discontinue use if rash occurs; arise slowly from prolonged sitting or lying

Nursing Implications See Monitoring Parameters and Patient Information

Special Geriatric Considerations Vasodilators have been used to treat dementia upon the premise that dementia is secondary to a cerebral blood

(Continued)

Isoxsuprine *(Continued)*

flow insufficiency. The hypothesis is that if blood flow could be increased, cognitive function would be increased. This hypothesis is no longer valid. The use of vasodilators for cognitive dysfunction is not recommended or proven by appropriate scientific study.

Dosage Forms Tablet, as hydrochloride: 10 mg, 20 mg

References

Erwin WG, "Senile Dementia of the Alzheimer Type," *Clin Pharm*, 1984, 3:497-504.

Higbee MD, "Noncholinergic Approaches to Treating Senile Dementia of the Alzheimer's Type," *Consult Pharm*, 1992, 7(6):635-41.

Waters C, "Cognitive Enhancing Agents: Current Status in the Treatment of Alzheimer's Disease," *Can J Neurol Sci*, 1988, 15:249-56.

Yesavage JA, Tinklenberg JR, Hollister LE, et al, "Vasodilators in Senile Dementias: A Review of the Literature," *Arch Gen Psychiatry*, 1979, 36:220-3.

Isradipine (iz RA di peen)

Related Information

Calcium Channel Blocking Agents Comparison *on page 1027*

Brand Names DynaCirc®

Generic Available No

Therapeutic Category Calcium Channel Blocker

Use Management of hypertension, alone or concurrently with thiazide-type diuretics

Contraindications Sinus bradycardia; advanced heart block; ventricular tachycardia; cardiogenic shock, hypotension, congestive heart failure; hypersensitivity to isradipine or any component, hypersensitivity to calcium channel blockers and adenosine; atrial fibrillation or flutter associated with accessory conduction pathways; not to be given within a few hours of I.V. beta-blocking agents

Warnings Hypotension, congestive heart failure, cardiac conduction defects, PVCs, idiopathic hypertrophic subaortic stenosis; may cause platelet inhibition; do not abruptly withdraw (chest pain); hepatic dysfunction, increased angina; increased intracranial pressure with cranial tumors; elderly may have greater hypotensive effect

The FDA's Cardiovascular and Renal Drug Advisory Committee reviewed current data regarding the risk of heart attacks in patients treated with calcium channel blockers and determined that as a class, the calcium channel antagonists are safe; however, they warned that short-acting nifedipine could increase the risk of myocardial infarction in some patients. The committee was in agreement with a statement issued September, 1995 by the National Heart Lung, and Blood Institute of the National Institute of Health, that warned that short-acting nifedipine should be used with great caution especially at higher doses.

Precautions Sick sinus syndrome, severe left ventricular dysfunction, congestive heart failure, hepatic impairment, hypertrophic cardiomyopathy (especially obstructive); concomitant therapy with beta-blockers or digoxin, edema

Adverse Reactions

Cardiovascular: Atrial and ventricular fibrillation, TIAs, stroke, flushing, hypotension, palpitations, A-V block, congestive heart failure, myocardial infarction, tachycardia, abnormal EKG, peripheral edema

Central nervous system: Fatigue, lethargy, dizziness, lightheadedness, drowsiness, disturbed sleep, psychotic symptoms, equilibrium dysfunction, headache, insomnia

Dermatologic: Rash, pruritus

Gastrointestinal: Nausea, vomiting, diarrhea, constipation, abdominal pain, xerostomia

Genitourinary: Urinary incontinence

Hematologic: Leukopenia

Neuromuscular & skeletal: Numbness, leg and feet cramps, weakness, paresthesia

Ocular: Blurred vision

Renal: Polyuria, nocturia

Respiratory: Throat discomfort, shortness of breath, cough

Miscellaneous: Diaphoresis, gingival swelling and inflammation

Overdosage Symptoms of overdose include heartblock, hypotension, asystole, nausea, weakness, dizziness, drowsiness, confusion, and slurred speech; profound bradycardia and occasionally hyperglycemia

Toxicology Ipecac-induced emesis can hypothetically worsen calcium antagonist toxicity since it can produce vagal stimulation. The potential for seizures precipitously following acute ingestion of large doses of a calcium antagonist may also contraindicate the use of ipecac. Supportive and symptomatic treatment, including I.V. fluids and Trendelenburg positioning, should be initiated as intoxication may cause hypotension. Although calcium (calcium chloride I.V. 1-2 g over 5-10 minutes with repeats as needed) has been used as an "antidote" for acute intoxications, there is limited experience to support its routine use and should be reserved for those cases where definite signs of myocardial depression are evident. Heart block may respond to isoproterenol, glucagon, atropine and/or calcium, although a temporary pacemaker may be required.

Drug Interactions Beta-blockers increased cardiac and A-V conduction depression; fentanyl increased volume requirements and hypotension; although the drug is new, other drug interactions not reported to the same degree as older agents; however, should be suspect of any drug interaction reported with other calcium channel blockers

Mechanism of Action Inhibits calcium ion from entering the "slow channels" or select voltage sensitive areas of vascular smooth muscle and myocardium during depolarization; produces a relaxation of coronary vascular smooth muscle and coronary vasodilation; increases myocardial oxygen delivery in patients with vasospastic angina

Pharmacodynamics
Onset of action: 2 hours
Peak effect: 2-4 weeks

Pharmacokinetics
Absorption: Oral: 90% to 95%
Protein binding: 95%
Metabolism: In the liver
Bioavailability: Absolute due to first-pass elimination 15% to 24%
Half-life: 8 hours
Time to peak serum concentration: 1-1.5 hours
Elimination: Renal excretion by metabolites (cyclic lactone and monoacids)

Usual Dosage Geriatrics and Adults: 2.5 mg twice daily; antihypertensive response seen in 2-3 hours; maximal response in 2-4 weeks; increase dose at 2- to 4-week intervals at 2.5-5 mg increments; usual dose range: 5-20 mg/day. **Note:** Most patients show no improvement with doses >10 mg/day except adverse reaction rate increases; therefore, maximal dose in elderly should be 10 mg/day.

Monitoring Parameters Heart rate, blood pressure, signs and symptoms of congestive heart failure

Patient Information Notify physician if you experience irregular heartbeat, shortness of breath, swelling, constipation, nausea, hypotension, or dizziness; do not stop or interrupt therapy without physician advice

Nursing Implications Do not crush sustained release capsules (see Warnings, Precautions, Monitoring Parameters, and Special Geriatric Considerations)

Additional Information Only approved indication is hypertension, but may be used for congestive heart failure; similar to nifedipine in actions, except for fewer side effects

Special Geriatric Considerations Elderly may experience a greater hypotensive response; constipation may be more of a problem in elderly; calcium channel blockers are no more effective in elderly than other therapies; however, they do not cause significant CNS effects which is an advantage over some antihypertensive agents (see Note in Usual Dosage)

Dosage Forms Capsule: 2.5 mg, 5 mg

Isuprel® *see* Isoproterenol *on page 501*

Itraconazole (i tra KOE na zole)

Brand Names Sporanox®
Generic Available No
Therapeutic Category Antifungal Agent, Systemic
Use Treatment of susceptible fungal infections in immunocompromised and nonimmunocompromised patients including blastomycosis and histoplasmosis; onychomycosis
Contraindications Known hypersensitivity to itraconazole or other azoles; concurrent use with terfenadine, astemizole, or cisapride
Warnings Coadministration with terfenadine is contraindicated; rare cases of serious cardiovascular adverse event, including death, ventricular tachycardia and torsade de pointes have been observed due to increased terfenadine concentrations induced by itraconazole; patients who develop abnormal liver function tests during itraconazole therapy should be monitored closely for the
(Continued)

Itraconazole *(Continued)*

development of more severe hepatic injury; if clinical signs and symptoms consistent with liver disease develop that may be attributable to itraconazole, itraconazole should be discontinued

Adverse Reactions
Cardiovascular: Hypertension
Central nervous system: Headache, dizziness, insomnia
Dermatologic: Skin rash, exfoliative skin disorders
Endocrine & metabolic: Hypokalemia, adrenal insufficiency, gynecomastia, breast pain (male)
Gastrointestinal: Nausea, vomiting, diarrhea, abdominal pain, anorexia, flatulence
Genitourinary: Impotence
Hepatic: Elevated AST, ALT, or alkaline phosphatase

Toxicology Overdoses are well tolerated; supportive measures and gastric decontamination with ipecac or sodium bicarbonate lavage should be employed; not removed by dialysis

Drug Interactions
Decreased effect: Rifampin, isoniazid, phenytoin, H_2 antagonists, and omeprazole, antacids, phenobarbital, carbamazepine
Increased effect: May increase cyclosporine (when high doses used), digoxin and phenytoin levels, increase effect of warfarin and sulfonylureas
Increased toxicity of astemizole, terfenadine, and cisapride (cardiotoxicity)

Pharmacokinetics
Absorption: Rapid and complete
Protein binding: >99%
Metabolism: Hepatic, >97%; inhibitor CYP3A4
Elimination: 85% renally excreted, 40% as inactive metabolites

Usual Dosage
Geriatrics and Adults: Oral: 200 mg once daily, if no obvious improvement or there is evidence of progressive fungal disease, increase the dose in 100 mg increments to a maximum of 400 mg/day
Onychomycosis: 200 mg once daily for 12 weeks
Life-threatening: Loading dose: 200 mg 3 times/day (600 mg/day) should be given for the first 3 days

Administration Doses >200 mg/day are given in 2 divided doses; do not administer with antacids

Monitoring Parameters Signs and symptoms of infection, baseline LFTs, recheck LFTs if therapy is to go beyond 2 weeks (see Drug Interactions)

Patient Information Take with food; do not take with antacids

Nursing Implications See Administration

Special Geriatric Considerations No specific data for elderly; use does not require alteration in dose or dose intervals

Dosage Forms
Capsule: 100 mg
Solution, oral: 100 mg/10 mL (150 mL)

I-Tropine® *see Atropine on page 92*

IUDR *see Idoxuridine on page 478*

Iveegam® *see Immune Globulin on page 482*

I.V. Medication Recommendations *see page 1080*

I.V. Push Recommended Guidelines *see page 1083*

Janimine® *see Imipramine on page 480*

Jenamicin® Injection *see Gentamicin on page 422*

Junior Strength Motrin® [OTC] *see Ibuprofen on page 475*

Just Tears® Solution [OTC] *see Artificial Tears on page 82*

K+ 10® *see Potassium Chloride on page 763*

Kabikinase® *see Streptokinase on page 870*

Kadian® Capsule *see Morphine Sulfate on page 640*

Kalcinate® *see Calcium Gluconate (Parenteral) on page 149*

Kanamycin *(kan a MYE sin)*

Related Information
Aminoglycoside Dosing Guidelines *on page 1009*

Brand Names Kantrex®

Therapeutic Category Antibiotic, Aminoglycoside

Use Treatment of susceptible bacterial infection including gram-negative aerobes, gram-positive *Bacillus* as well as some mycobacteria

Oral: Preoperative bowel preparation in the prophylaxis of infections and adjunctive treatment of hepatic coma (oral kanamycin is not indicated in the treatment of systemic infections)

Parenteral: Rarely used in antibiotic irrigations during surgery

Contraindications Hypersensitivity to kanamycin or any component

Warnings Aminoglycosides are associated with significant nephrotoxicity or ototoxicity; the ototoxicity is directly proportional to the amount of drug given and the duration of treatment. Tinnitus or vertigo are indications of vestibular injury and impending bilateral irreversible damage; renal damage is usually reversible. Elderly patients with pre-existing tinnitus or vertigo or known subclinical deafness, those receiving other ototoxic drugs, or those receiving >15 g kanamycin sulfate should be observed very carefully for eighth nerve damage.

Adverse Reactions

Central nervous system: Neuromuscular blockade

Dermatologic: Rash, photosensitivity

Hematologic: Granulocytopenia, agranulocytosis, thrombocytopenia

Otic: Ototoxicity (auditory and vestibular)

Renal: Nephrotoxicity

Overdosage Symptoms of overdose include ototoxicity, nephrotoxicity, and neuromuscular toxicity

Toxicology The treatment of choice following a single acute overdose appears to be the maintenance of good urine output of at least 3 mL/kg/hour. Dialysis is of questionable value in the enhancement of aminoglycoside elimination. If required, hemodialysis is preferred over peritoneal dialysis in patients with normal renal function. Careful hydration may be all that is required to promote diuresis and therefore the enhancement of the drug's elimination.

Drug Interactions

Increased/prolonged effect of depolarizing and nondepolarizing neuromuscular blocking agents

Increased toxicity: Concurrent use of amphotericin may increase nephrotoxicity

Stability Darkening of vials does not indicate loss of potency

Mechanism of Action Interferes with protein synthesis in bacterial cell by binding to ribosomal subunit

Pharmacokinetics

Distribution: V_d: 0.19 L/kg

Half-life: 2-4 hours, increases in anuria to 80 hours; in older adults the mean half-life has been reported to be longer, 2.5 hours in 50-70 years of age and 4.7 hours in 70-90 years of age; the plasma half-life and V_d have also been reported to be increased in elderly bedridden patients

Time to peak serum concentration: I.M.: Within 1-2 hours

Elimination: Entirely in the kidney, principally by glomerular filtration

Usual Dosage

Geriatrics: I.M., I.V.: Initial dose should be 5-7.5 mg/kg based on ideal body weight (except in obese patients); maintenance dose and interval should be adjusted for estimated renal function; dosing interval in most older patients is every 12-24 hours (see Dosing Adjustment in Renal Impairment)

Adults:

Infections: 15 mg/kg/day in divided doses every 8-12 hours

Preoperative intestinal antisepsis: Oral: 1 g every 4-6 hours for 36-72 hours

Dosing adjustment in renal impairment: It is best to adjust therapy by appropriate serum assays; if not possible, reduce dose interval: dose interval (hour) = serum creatinine (mg/dL) x 9

Dialyzable (50% to 100%)

Administration Dilute to 100-200 mL and infuse over 30 minutes; I.M. doses should be given in a large muscle mass (ie, gluteus maximus)

Monitoring Parameters Serum creatinine and BUN every 2-3 days; peak and trough concentrations; hearing

Reference Range

Therapeutic:

Peak: 25-35 µg/mL (SI: 52-72 µmol/L)

Trough: 4-8 µg/mL (SI: 8-16 µmol/L)

Toxic:

Peak: >35 µg/mL (SI: >72 µmol/L)

Trough: >10 µg/mL (SI: >21 µmol/L)

Test Interactions Increased ammonia (B), protein; decreased magnesium

Nursing Implications Aminoglycoside levels in blood taken from Silastic® central catheters can sometime give falsely high readings. Give around-the-
(Continued)

Kanamycin *(Continued)*

clock rather than 4 times/day, 3 times/day, etc (ie, 12-6-12-6, not 9-1-5-9) to promote less variation in peak and trough serum concentrations; modify dosage in patients with renal impairment (see Administration).

Special Geriatric Considerations Kanamycin is not a drug of choice in the elderly since the elderly may have increased adverse effects (renal) (see Warnings, Pharmacokinetics, and Usual Dosage)

Dosage Forms

Kanamycin sulfate:
Capsule: 500 mg
Injection: 1 g/3 mL

References

Kristensen M, Molholm HJ, Kampmann J, et al, "Letter: Drug Elimination and Renal Function," *J Clin Pharmacol*, 1974, 14(5-6):307-8.

Yasuhara H, Kobayashi S, Sakamoto K, et al, "Pharmacokinetics of Amikacin and Cephalothin in Bedridden Elderly Patients," *J Clin Pharmacol*, 1982, 22:403-9.

Kantrex® *see* Kanamycin *on page 510*

Kaochlor® *see* Potassium Chloride *on page 763*

Kaochlor® SF *see* Potassium Chloride *on page 763*

Kaodene® [OTC] *see* Kaolin and Pectin *on this page*

Kaolin and Pectin (KAY oh lin & PEK tin)

Brand Names Kaodene® [OTC]; Kao-Spen® [OTC]; Kapectolin® [OTC]

Synonyms Pectin and Kaolin

Therapeutic Category Antidiarrheal

Use Treatment of uncomplicated diarrhea

Restrictions See Warnings and Precautions

Contraindications Hypersensitivity to kaolin or pectin; fecal impaction, ileus

Warnings Do not use with diarrhea associated with toxigenic bacteria or pseudomembranous colitis

Precautions Use with caution in patients >60 years of age; presence of high fever; do not use in patients predisposed to fecal impaction

Adverse Reactions Gastrointestinal: Constipation, fecal impaction

Overdosage May cause bowel impaction and obstruction

Drug Interactions Oral lincomycin and oral digoxin

Mechanism of Action Controls diarrhea because of its adsorbent action

Usual Dosage Geriatrics and Adults: Oral: 60-120 mL after each loose stool

Monitoring Parameters Monitor for reduction of stools per day and increased consistency; monitor for signs of fluid and electrolyte loss

Patient Information If diarrhea is not controlled in 48 hours, contact a physician

Nursing Implications Shake well before giving

Special Geriatric Considerations Elderly often present bowel impaction with diarrhea. The use of adsorbents in the face of fecal impaction could aggravate this serious condition. Also, diarrhea causes fluid/electrolyte loss which elderly do not tolerate well. Use of adsorbents can cause further loss of fluid/electrolytes.

Dosage Forms Suspension, oral: Kaolin 975 mg and pectin 22 mg per 5 mL

Kaolin and Pectin With Opium

(KAY oh lin & PEK tin with OH pee um)

Brand Names Parepectolin®

Therapeutic Category Antidiarrheal

Use Symptomatic relief of diarrhea

Restrictions C-V

Contraindications Should not be used to treat diarrhea (opium) caused by poisons, toxins, or infectious agents until GI tract has been cleared of causative agent; do not use in patients with hypersensitivity to opium or morphine derivatives

Warnings Do not use with diarrhea associated with toxigenic bacteria or pseudomembranous colitis

Precautions Use with caution in geriatric patients predisposed to fecal impaction/intestinal obstruction; use with caution in patients >60 years of age, presence of high fever

Adverse Reactions Gastrointestinal: Constipation, fecal impaction

Overdosage Symptoms of overdose include constipation, bowel obstruction, fecal impaction; opium absorption may cause signs of narcotic drug use (confusion, lethargy, hypotension, drowsiness, sedation)

Drug Interactions Chloroquine, digoxin, lincomycin, CNS depressants, anticholinergic drugs, disulfiram, MAO inhibitors, metronidazole, procarbazine

Mechanism of Action Opium reduces intestinal motility, relieves tenesmus, cramps, and colic pain secondary to diarrhea. Kaolin and pectin act by adsorbent action.

Pharmacokinetics Absorption: Opium is absorbed from GI tract; kaolin and pectin are not absorbed

Usual Dosage Geriatrics and Adults: Oral: 15-30 mL with each loose bowel movement, not to exceed 120 mL in 12 hours

Patient Information If diarrhea is not controlled in 48 hours, contact a physician

Nursing Implications Monitor for signs of opium (narcotic) action (see Overdosage); shake well before giving

Special Geriatric Considerations Elderly often present with bowel impaction and diarrhea. The use of adsorbents in the face of fecal impaction could aggravate this serious condition. Also, diarrhea causes fluid/electrolyte loss which elderly do not tolerate well. Use of adsorbents can cause further loss of fluid/electrolytes. The use of this product in elderly is discouraged due to side effect potential and lack of clinical efficacy for disease process.

Dosage Forms Suspension: Kaolin 5.5 g, pectin 162 mg and opium 15 mg per 30 mL = 3.7 mL paregoric (240 mL)

Kaon® *see* Potassium Gluconate *on page 765*

Kaon-Cl® *see* Potassium Chloride *on page 763*

Kaon Cl-10® *see* Potassium Chloride *on page 763*

Kaopectate® Advanced Formula [OTC] *see* Attapulgite *on page 94*

Kaopectate® II [OTC] *see* Loperamide *on page 548*

Kaopectate® Maximum Strength Caplets *see* Attapulgite *on page 94*

Kao-Spen® [OTC] *see* Kaolin and Pectin *on previous page*

Kapectolin® [OTC] *see* Kaolin and Pectin *on previous page*

Kapectolin PG® *see* Hyoscyamine, Atropine, Scopolamine, Kaolin, Pectin, and Opium *on page 473*

Karidium® *see* Fluoride *on page 392*

Karigel® *see* Fluoride *on page 392*

Karigel®-N *see* Fluoride *on page 392*

Kasof® [OTC] *see* Docusate *on page 312*

Kato® *see* Potassium Chloride *on page 763*

Kaybovite-1000® *see* Cyanocobalamin *on page 257*

Kay Ciel® *see* Potassium Chloride *on page 763*

Kayexalate® *see* Sodium Polystyrene Sulfonate *on page 864*

Kaylixir® *see* Potassium Gluconate *on page 765*

K+ Care® *see* Potassium Chloride *on page 763*

KCl *see* Potassium Chloride *on page 763*

K-Dur® 10 *see* Potassium Chloride *on page 763*

K-Dur® 20 *see* Potassium Chloride *on page 763*

Keflex® *see* Cephalexin *on page 194*

Keflin® *see* Cephalothin *on page 195*

Keftab® *see* Cephalexin *on page 194*

Kefurox® Injection *see* Cefuroxime *on page 193*

Kefzol® *see* Cefazolin *on page 175*

Kemadrin® *see* Procyclidine *on page 785*

Kenacort® *see* Triamcinolone *on page 949*

Kenaject-40® *see* Triamcinolone *on page 949*

Kenalog® *see* Triamcinolone *on page 949*

Kenalog-10® *see* Triamcinolone *on page 949*

Kenalog-40® *see* Triamcinolone *on page 949*

Kenalog® H *see* Triamcinolone *on page 949*

Kenalog® in Orabase® *see* Triamcinolone *on page 949*

Kenonel® *see* Triamcinolone *on page 949*

Keoxifene Hydrochloride *see* Raloxifene *on page 820*

Kerlone® Oral *see* Betaxolol *on page 116*

Ketoconazole (kee toe KOE na zole)

Related Information

Antacid Drug Interactions *on page 1096*

Brand Names Nizoral®

(Continued)

Ketoconazole *(Continued)*

Therapeutic Category Antifungal Agent, Systemic; Antifungal Agent, Topical

Use Treatment of susceptible fungal infections, including candidiasis, oral thrush, blastomycosis, histoplasmosis, paracoccidioidomycosis, chronic mucocutaneous candidiasis, as well as certain recalcitrant cutaneous dermatophytoses; used topically for treatment of tinea corporis, tinea cruris, tinea versicolor, and cutaneous candidiasis

Investigational use: Advanced prostate cancer

Contraindications Hypersensitivity to ketoconazole or any component; CNS fungal infections (due to poor CNS penetration); concurrent use of terfenadine, astemizole, or cisapride

Warnings Has been associated with hepatotoxicity, including some fatalities; perform periodic liver function tests; high doses of ketoconazole may depress adrenocortical function

Precautions Gastric acidity is necessary for the dissolution and absorption of ketoconazole; use with caution in patients with impaired hepatic function; lowers serum testosterone at dose of 800 mg/day and abolishes them at doses of 1600 mg/day (see Drug Interactions)

Adverse Reactions

Central nervous system: Severe depression, suicidal tendencies (rare), dizziness, somnolence, fever

Dermatologic: Pruritus, rash

Endocrine & metabolic: Adrenal cortical insufficiency, gynecomastia

Gastrointestinal: Nausea, vomiting, abdominal discomfort, GI bleeding, diarrhea

Genitourinary: Impotence

Hematologic: Thrombocytopenia, leukopenia, hemolytic anemia

Hepatic: Hepatotoxicity

Local: Irritation, stinging

Ocular: Photophobia

Overdosage Symptoms of overdose include dizziness, headache, nausea, vomiting, diarrhea; institute supportive measures (ie, gastric lavage with sodium bicarbonate)

Drug Interactions

Drugs that decrease absorption (raise gastric pH) such as antacids, H_2-receptor blockers

Drugs that decreased serum concentrations of ketoconazole include rifampin, isoniazid, phenytoin, phenobarbital, carbamazepine

Drug concentrations that are increased by ketoconazole include phenytoin, cyclosporine, theophylline, terfenadine, warfarin, astemizole, cisapride

Mechanism of Action Alters the permeability of the cell wall; inhibits biosynthesis of triglycerides and phospholipids by fungi; inhibits several fungal enzymes that results in a build-up of toxic concentrations of hydrogen peroxide

Pharmacokinetics

Absorption: Oral: Rapid (~75%)

Distribution: Minimal into the CNS

Protein binding: 93% to 96%

Metabolism: Partially in the liver by enzymes to inactive compounds; substrate and inhibitor CYP3A4

Bioavailability: Decreases as pH of the gastric contents increase

Half-life, biphasic:

Initial: 2 hours

Terminal: 8 hours

Time to peak serum concentration: Within 1-2 hours

Elimination: Primarily in feces (57%) with smaller amounts excreted in urine (13%)

Usual Dosage Geriatrics and Adults:

Oral: 200-400 mg/day as a single daily dose for 1-2 weeks for candidiasis and 6 weeks for other mycoses

Shampoo: Apply twice weekly for 4 weeks with at least 3 days between each shampoo

Topical: Rub gently into the affected area 1-2 times/day

Not dialyzable (0% to 5%)

Administration Administer 2 hours prior to antacids or H_2-receptor antagonists (give with cola drink) to prevent decreased absorption due to the high pH of gastric contents

Monitoring Parameters Signs and symptoms of infection, baseline LFTs; recheck if therapy is to go beyond 2 weeks; serum concentration and subjective response (see Drug Interactions)

Reference Range Therapeutic: Peak: 1-4 mg/L; Trough: ≤1 mg/L

Patient Information Cream is for topical application to the skin only; avoid contact with the eye; avoid taking antacids or H_2 antagonists at the same time as ketoconazole; may cause headache, dizziness or drowsiness, observe caution when driving or operating machinery; notify physician of GI side effects or if dark urine or pale stools occur

Nursing Implications See Administration and Monitoring Parameters

Special Geriatric Considerations No specific recommendations for the elderly (see Usual Dosage and Monitoring Parameters)

Dosage Forms
Cream: 2% (15 g, 30 g, 60 g)
Shampoo: 2% (120 mL)
Tablet: 200 mg

Ketoprofen (kee toe PROE fen)

Brand Names Actron® [OTC]; Orudis®; Orudis® KT [OTC]; Oruvail®

Generic Available No

Therapeutic Category Analgesic, Non-narcotic; Anti-inflammatory Agent; Antipyretic; Nonsteroidal Anti-inflammatory Agent (NSAID), Oral

Use Acute or long-term treatment of rheumatoid arthritis and osteoarthritis; mild to moderate pain, sunburn, migraine headache prophylaxis

Contraindications Known hypersensitivity to ketoprofen or other NSAIDs/aspirin

Warnings GI toxicity (bleeding, ulceration, perforation); CNS effects may occur (headaches, confusion, depression); hypersensitivity, anaphylactoid reactions (intermittent tolmetin use more often); renal function decline, acute renal insufficiency, interstitial nephritis, dysuria, cystitis, hematuria, nephrotic syndrome, hyperkalemia in acute renal insufficiency, hyponatremia, papillary necrosis, hepatic function impairment; elderly have increased risk for adverse reactions to NSAIDs (see Special Geriatric Considerations)

Precautions Use with caution in patients with congestive heart failure, hypertension, decreased renal or hepatic function, history of GI disease (bleeding or ulcers), or those receiving anticoagulants; perform ophthalmologic evaluation for those who develop eye complaints during therapy (blurred vision, diminished vision, changes in color vision, retinal changes); NSAIDs may mask signs/symptoms of infections; photosensitivity reported

Adverse Reactions
Cardiovascular: Congestive heart failure, angina, hypertension, hypotension, arrhythmias, edema
Central nervous system: Headache, drowsiness, vertigo, dizziness, fatigue, hallucinations, confusion, depression, emotional lability, psychotic behavior, pyrexia
Dermatologic: Rash, urticaria, angioedema, Stevens-Johnson syndrome, exfoliative dermatitis, bruising, petechiae, purpura
Endocrine & metabolic: Hyperglycemia, hypoglycemia, hyperkalemia, gynecomastia, hyponatremia, fluid retention
Gastrointestinal: Dyspepsia, heartburn, nausea, diarrhea, constipation, flatulence, stomatitis, vomiting, abdominal pain, peptic ulcer, GI bleeding, GI perforation, gingival ulcers, pancreatitis, proctitis, paralytic ulcers, colitis, anorexia, weight loss, dry mucous membranes
Genitourinary: Impotence, azotemia
Hematologic: Neutropenia, anemia, agranulocytosis, bone marrow suppression, hemolytic anemia, hemorrhage, inhibition of platelet aggregation
Hepatic: Hepatitis, elevated LFTs, cholestatic jaundice
Neuromuscular & skeletal: Involuntary muscle movements, muscle weakness, tremors, weakness
Ocular: Vision changes
Otic: Tinnitus
Renal: Dysuria, polyuria, pyuria, oliguria, anuria, acute renal failure
Respiratory: Exacerbation of asthma, dyspnea
Miscellaneous: Thirst, diaphoresis

Overdosage Symptoms include drowsiness, lethargy, disorientation, confusion, dizziness, numbness, paresthesia, nausea, vomiting, gastric irritation, abdominal pain, headache, tinnitus, sweating, blurred vision, muscle twitching, seizures, coma, acute renal failure, increased BUN and serum creatinine, hypotension, tachycardia, and metabolic acidosis
(Continued)

Ketoprofen (Continued)

Toxicology Management of a nonsteroidal anti-inflammatory agent (NSAID) intoxication is primarily supportive and symptomatic. Fluid therapy is commonly effective in managing the hypotension that may occur following an acute NSAID overdose, except when this is due to an acute blood loss. Seizures tend to be very short-lived and often do not require drug treatment although recurrent seizures should be treated with I.V. diazepam. Since many of the NSAIDs undergo enterohepatic cycling, multiple doses of charcoal may be needed to reduce the potential for delayed toxicities.

Drug Interactions
May increase digoxin, methotrexate, and lithium serum concentrations
Aspirin or other salicylates may decrease NSAID serum concentrations
Other NSAIDs may increase adverse GI effects
Increased prothrombin time with anticoagulants
Decreased antihypertensive effects of ACE inhibitors, beta-blockers, and thiazide diuretics
Effects of loop diuretics may decrease
Increased response to sympathomimetics
Probenecid may increase toxicity of NSAIDs by increase in serum concentrations
Diuretics increase risk of acute renal insufficiency
Azotemia may be enhanced in elderly receiving loop diuretics

Mechanism of Action Inhibits prostaglandin synthesis, acts on the hypothalamus heat-regulating center to reduce fever, blocks prostaglandin synthetase action which prevents formation of the platelet-aggregating substance thromboxane A_2; decreases pain receptor sensitivity. Other proposed mechanisms of action are lysosomal stabilization, inhibition of kinin and leukotriene production, alteration of chemotactic factors, and inhibition of neutrophil activation. This latter mechanism may be the most significant pharmacologic action to reduce inflammation.

Pharmacokinetics
Absorption: Almost completely
Protein binding: >90%
Metabolism: In the liver
Half-life: 1-4 hours
Time to peak serum concentration: Oral: Within 0.5-2 hours
Elimination: Renal excretion (60% to 75% of a dose), primarily as glucuronide conjugates

Usual Dosage Oral:
Geriatrics: Initial: 25-50 mg 3-4 times/day; increase up to 150-300 mg/day (maximum daily dose: 300 mg)
Adults: 50-75 mg 3-4 times/day up to 300 mg/day (maximum)

Monitoring Parameters Monitor response (pain, range of motion, grip strength, mobility, ADL function), inflammation; observe for weight gain, edema; monitor renal function; observe for bleeding, bruising; evaluate gastrointestinal effects (abdominal pain, bleeding, dyspepsia); mental confusion, disorientation, CBC, serum, creatinine, BUN, liver function tests

Test Interactions Increased chloride (S), increased sodium (S)

Patient Information Serious gastrointestinal bleeding can occur as well as ulceration and perforation. Pain may or may not be present. Avoid aspirin and aspirin-containing products while taking this medication. If gastric upset occurs, take with food, milk, or antacid. If gastric adverse effects persist, contact physician. May cause drowsiness, dizziness, blurred vision, and confusion. Use caution when performing tasks which require alertness (eg, driving). Do not take for more than 3 days for fever or 10 days for pain without physician advice.

Nursing Implications See Overdosage, Monitoring Parameters, Patient Information, and Special Geriatric Considerations

Additional Information Dose must be lowest recommended in renal insufficiency. There are no clinical guidelines to predict which NSAID will give response in a particular patient. Trials with each must be initiated until response determined. Consider dose, patient convenience, and cost.

Special Geriatric Considerations Elderly are a high-risk population for adverse effects from nonsteroidal anti-inflammatory agents. As much as 60% of elderly can develop peptic ulceration and/or hemorrhage asymptomatically. The concomitant use of H_2 blockers, omeprazole, and sucralfate is not effective as prophylaxis with the exception of NSAID-induced duodenal ulcers which may be prevented by the use of ranitidine. Misoprostol and proton pump inhibitors are the only agents proven to help prevent the development of NSAID-induced ulcers. Also, concomitant disease and drug use contribute to the risk for GI adverse effects. Use lowest effective dose for shortest period possible. Consider renal function decline with age. Use of NSAIDs can compromise existing renal function especially when Cl_{cr} is ≤30 mL/minute. Tinnitus may be a difficult and unreliable indication of toxicity due to age-related hearing loss or eighth cranial nerve damage. CNS adverse effects such as confusion, agitation, and hallucination are generally seen in overdose or high dose situations, but elderly may demonstrate these adverse effects at lower doses than younger adults.

Dosage Forms
Capsule:
Orudis®: 25 mg, 50 mg, 75 mg
Actron®, Orudis® KT [OTC]: 12.5 mg
Capsule, extended release (Oruvail®): 100 mg, 200 mg

References
Brooks PM, Day RO, "Nonsteroidal Anti-inflammatory Drugs - Differences and Similarities," *N Engl J Med*, 1991, 324(24):1716-25.

Clinch D, Banerjee AK, Ostick G, "Absence of Abdominal Pain in Elderly Patients With Peptic Ulcer," *Age Ageing*, 1984, 13:120-3.

Clive DM, Stoff JS, "Renal Syndromes Associated With Nonsteroidal Anti-inflammatory Drugs," *N Engl J Med*, 1984, 310(9):563-72.

Graham DY, "Prevention of Gastroduodenal Injury Induced by Chronic Nonsteroidal Anti-inflammatory Drug Therapy," *Gastroenterology*, 1989, 96(2 Pt 2 Suppl):675-81.

Gurwitz JH, Avorn J, Ross-Degnan D, et al, "Nonsteroidal Anti-Inflammatory Drug-Associated Azotemia in the Very Old," *JAMA*, 1990, 264(4):471-5.

Hawkey CJ, Karrasch JA, Szczepaski L, et al, "Omeprazole Compared With Misoprostrol for Ulcers Associated With Nonsteroidal Anti-inflammatory Drugs," *N Engl J Med*, 1998, 338(11):727-34.

Knodel LC, "Preventing NSAID-Induced Ulcers: The Role of Misoprostol," *Consult Pharm*, 1989, 4:37-41.

Pounder R, "Silent Peptic Ulceration: Deadly Silence or Golden Silence?" *Gastroenterology*, 1989, 96(2 Pt 2 Suppl):626-31.

Yeomans ND, Tulassay Z, Juhasz L, et al, "A Comparison of Omeprazole With Ranitidine for Ulcers Associated With Nonsteroidal Anti-inflammatory Drugs," *N Engl J Med*, 1998, 338(11):719-26.

Ketorolac Tromethamine (KEE toe role ak troe METH a meen)
Related Information
I.V. Push Recommended Guidelines *on page 1083*
Brand Names Acular® Ophthalmic; Toradol® Injection; Toradol® Oral
Generic Available No
Therapeutic Category Analgesic, Non-narcotic; Anti-inflammatory Agent; Anti-inflammatory Agent, Ophthalmic; Antipyretic; Nonsteroidal Anti-inflammatory Agent (NSAID), Ophthalmic; Nonsteroidal Anti-inflammatory Agent (NSAID), Oral; Nonsteroidal Anti-inflammatory Agent (NSAID), Parenteral
Use
Oral: Limited duration, as needed, for management of pain
I.M.: Short-term management of pain, up to 5 days
Ophthalmic: Relief of ocular itching secondary to seasonal allergic conjunctivitis
Contraindications In patients who have developed nasal polyps, angioedema, or bronchospastic reactions to other NSAIDs; hypersensitivity to ketorolac or any component of the products used
Warnings The use of ketorolac at recommended doses for more than 5 days is associated with an increased frequency and severity of adverse events; cross-sensitivity to aspirin and other NSAIDs exists; GI toxicity (bleeding, ulceration, perforation); CNS effects may occur (headaches, confusion, depression); hypersensitivity, anaphylactoid reactions (intermittent tolmetin use more often); renal function decline, acute renal insufficiency, interstitial nephritis, dysuria, cystitis, hematuria, nephrotic syndrome, hyperkalemia in acute renal insufficiency, hyponatremia, papillary necrosis, hepatic function impairment; elderly have increased risk for adverse reactions to NSAIDs (see Special Geriatric Considerations)

Note: Ophthalmic solution: Use caution if patients wears soft contact lenses; eye irritation, redness, and burning reported; also systemic absorption may lead to adverse effects (ie, bleeding)

Precautions Use extra caution and reduce dosages in the elderly because it is cleared renally somewhat slower and the elderly are also more sensitive to the renal effects of NSAIDs; use with caution in patients with congestive heart failure, hypertension, decreased renal or hepatic function, history of GI disease (bleeding or ulcers), or those receiving anticoagulants; perform ophthalmologic evaluation for those who develop eye complaints during therapy (blurred vision, diminished vision, changes in color vision, retinal
(Continued)

Ketorolac Tromethamine *(Continued)*

changes); NSAIDs may mask signs/symptoms of infections; photosensitivity reported

Adverse Reactions

Cardiovascular: Congestive heart failure, angina, hypertension, hypotension, arrhythmias, edema

Central nervous system: Headache, drowsiness, vertigo, dizziness, fatigue, hallucinations, confusion, depression, emotional lability, psychotic behavior, pyrexia

Dermatologic: Rash, urticaria, angioedema, Stevens-Johnson syndrome, exfoliative dermatitis, bruising, petechiae, purpura

Endocrine & metabolic: Hyperglycemia, hypoglycemia, hyperkalemia, gynecomastia, hyponatremia, fluid retention

Gastrointestinal: Dyspepsia, heartburn, nausea, diarrhea, constipation, pain, flatulence, anorexia, stomatitis, vomiting, abdominal pain, peptic ulcer, GI bleeding, GI perforation, gingival ulcers, pancreatitis, proctitis, paralytic ulcers, colitis, weight loss, dry mucous membranes

Genitourinary: Impotence, azotemia

Hematologic: Postoperative hematomas, wound bleeding (with I.M.), neutropenia, anemia, agranulocytosis, bone marrow suppression, hemolytic anemia, hemorrhage, inhibition of platelet aggregation

Hepatic: Hepatitis, elevated LFTs, cholestatic jaundice

Local: Pain at injection site

Neuromuscular & skeletal: Involuntary muscle movements, muscle weakness, tremors, weakness

Ocular: Vision changes, burning, redness, irritation, stinging and burning is transient (40%); allergic reactions (3%), superficial keratitis, ocular infections

Otic: Tinnitus

Renal: Dysuria, polyuria, pyuria, oliguria, anuria, renal impairment, acute renal failure

Respiratory: Exacerbation of asthma, dyspnea

Miscellaneous: Thirst, diaphoresis

Overdosage Symptoms include drowsiness, lethargy, disorientation, confusion, dizziness, numbness, paresthesia, nausea, vomiting, gastric irritation, abdominal pain, headache, tinnitus, sweating, blurred vision, muscle twitching, seizures, coma, acute renal failure, increased BUN and serum creatinine, hypotension, tachycardia, and metabolic acidosis

Toxicology Management of a nonsteroidal anti-inflammatory drug (NSAID) intoxication is primarily supportive and symptomatic. Fluid therapy is commonly effective in managing the hypotension that may occur following an acute NSAID overdose, except when this is due to an acute blood loss. Seizures tend to be very short-lived and often do not require drug treatment although recurrent seizures should be treated with I.V. diazepam. Since many of the NSAIDs undergo enterohepatic cycling, multiple doses of charcoal may be needed to reduce the potential for delayed toxicities; NSAIDs are highly bound to plasma proteins; therefore, hemodialysis and peritoneal dialysis are not useful; if ocular solution is ingested, dilute with oral fluids.

Drug Interactions

Cyclosporine; may increase digoxin, methotrexate, and lithium serum concentrations

Aspirin or other salicylates may decrease NSAID serum concentrations

Other nonsteroidal anti-inflammatories may increase adverse GI effects

Increased prothrombin time with anticoagulants

Decreased antihypertensive effects of ACE inhibitors, beta-blockers, and thiazide diuretics

Effects of loop diuretics may be decreased

Increased response to sympathomimetics

Probenecid may increase toxicity of NSAIDs by increase in serum concentrations

Diuretics increase risk of acute renal insufficiency

Azotemia may be increased in elderly receiving loop diuretics

Stability Protect from light

Mechanism of Action Inhibits prostaglandin synthesis by decreasing the activity of the enzyme, cyclo-oxygenase, which results in decreased formation of prostaglandin precursors; acts on the hypothalamus heat-regulating center to reduce fever, blocks prostaglandin synthetase action which prevents formation of the platelet-aggregating substance thromboxane A_2; decreases pain receptor sensitivity. Other proposed mechanisms of action are lysosomal stabilization, inhibition of kinin and leukotriene production, alteration of chemotactic factors, and inhibition of neutrophil activation. This latter mechanism may be the most significant pharmacologic action to reduce inflammation. Prostaglandins appear to have a role in the miotic response produced during ocular surgery by constricting the iris sphincter independently of cholinergic response. Ketorolac inhibits the miosis induced during the course of surgery. In animals, prostaglandins are mediators of intraocular inflammation; prostaglandins produce disruption of the blood-aqueous humor barrier, increased vascular permeability, vasodilation, leukocytosis, and increased intraocular pressure (IOP).

Pharmacodynamics
Onset of action: I.M.: Within 10 minutes
Peak effect: Within 75-150 minutes
Duration of action: 6-8 hours

Pharmacokinetics
Absorption: Oral: Well absorbed
Protein binding: 99%
Metabolism: In the liver
Half-life: 2-8 hours, half-life is increased 30% to 50% in elderly
Time to peak serum concentration: Within 30-60 minutes
Elimination: Renal excretion, 61% appearing in urine as unchanged drug

Usual Dosage
Geriatrics and Adults:
  Oral: 10 mg every 4-6 hours as needed for limited-duration treatment of pain; do not use chronic doses of 10 mg 4 times/day; maximum daily dose: 40 mg
  I.M., I.V.: <50 kg: 30 mg loading dose then 15 mg every 6 hours; maximum dose in the first 24 hours: 150 mg with 120 mg/24 hours thereafter; elderly (≥65 years of age) should be dosed upon the limits for those <50 kg; limit duration of use to 5 days
  Ophthalmic: Instill 1 drop (0.25 mg) 4 times/day; efficacy has not been proved beyond 1 week of therapy
Adults >50 kg: I.M.: 30-60 mg loading dose then 15-30 mg every 6 hours
Transition from parenteral to oral dosing: Limit maximum dose on day of transition to 120 mg including oral dose; subsequent oral dose should not exceed 40 mg/day

Monitoring Parameters Monitor response (pain, range of motion, grip strength, mobility, ADL function), inflammation; observe for weight gain, edema; monitor renal function (creatinine, BUN); observe for bleeding, bruising; evaluate gastrointestinal effects (abdominal pain, bleeding, dyspepsia); mental confusion, disorientation, CBC, serum, liver function tests

Reference Range Serum concentration: Therapeutic: 0.3-5 µg/mL; Toxic: >5 µg/mL

Test Interactions Increases chloride (S), sodium (S), bleeding time

Patient Information Serious gastrointestinal bleeding can occur as well as ulceration and perforation. Pain may or may not be present. Avoid aspirin and aspirin-containing products while taking this medication. If gastric upset occurs, take with food, milk, or antacid. If gastric adverse effects persist, contact physician. May cause drowsiness, dizziness, blurred vision, and confusion. Use caution when performing tasks which require alertness (eg, driving). Do not take for more than 3 days for fever or 10 days for pain without physician's advice.

Nursing Implications See Overdosage, Monitoring Parameters, Patient Information, and Special Geriatric Considerations

Additional Information First parenteral NSAID for analgesia; 30 mg provides the analgesia comparable to 12 mg of morphine or 100 mg of meperidine; pain relief usually begins within 10 minutes; there are no clinical guidelines to predict which NSAID will give response in a particular patient. Trials with each must be initiated until response determined. Consider dose, patient convenience, and cost.

Special Geriatric Considerations Ketorolac is cleared more slowly in the elderly. It is recommended to use lower doses in elderly. The elderly are a high-risk population for adverse effects from nonsteroidal anti-inflammatory agents. As much as 60% of elderly can develop peptic ulceration and/or hemorrhage asymptomatically. The concomitant use of H₂ blockers, omeprazole, and sucralfate is not effective as prophylaxis with the exception of NSAID-induced duodenal ulcers which may be prevented by the use of ranitidine. Misoprostol and proton pump inhibitors are the only agents proven to help prevent the development of NSAID-induced ulcers. Also, concomitant disease and drug use contribute to the risk for GI adverse effects. Use lowest effective dose for shortest period possible. Consider renal function decline (Continued)

Ketorolac Tromethamine *(Continued)*

with age. Use of NSAIDs can compromise existing renal function especially when Cl$_{cr}$ is ≤30 mL/minute. Tinnitus may be a difficult and unreliable indication of toxicity due to age-related hearing loss or eighth cranial nerve damage. CNS adverse effects such as confusion, agitation, and hallucination are generally seen in overdose or high dose situations, but elderly may demonstrate these adverse effects at lower doses than younger adults (see Pharmacokinetics).

Dosage Forms

Injection, single dose syringes: 15 mg, 30 mg, 60 mg

Solution, ophthalmic: 0.5% (5 mL)

Tablet: 10 mg

References

Brooks PM, Day RO, "Nonsteroidal Anti-inflammatory Drugs - Differences and Similarities," *N Engl J Med*, 1991, 324(24):1716-25.

Clinch D, Banerjee AK, Ostick G, "Absence of Abdominal Pain in Elderly Patients With Peptic Ulcer," *Age Ageing*, 1984, 13:120-3.

Clive DM, Stoff JS, "Renal Syndromes Associated With Nonsteroidal Anti-inflammatory Drugs," *N Engl J Med*, 1984, 310(9):563-72.

Graham DY, "Prevention of Gastroduodenal Injury Induced by Chronic Nonsteroidal Anti-inflammatory Drug Therapy," *Gastroenterology*, 1989, 96(2 Pt 2 Suppl):675-81.

Hawkey CJ, Karrasch JA, Szczepaski L, et al, "Omeprazole Compared With Misoprostrol for Ulcers Associated With Nonsteroidal Anti-inflammatory Drugs," *N Engl J Med*, 1998, 338(11):727-34.

Jallad NS, Garg DC, Martinez JJ, et al, "Pharmacokinetics of Single-Dose Oral and Intramuscular Ketorolac Tromethamine in the Young and Elderly," *J Clin Pharmacol*, 1990, 30(1):76-81.

Knodel LC, "Preventing NSAID-Induced Ulcers: The Role of Misoprostol," *Consult Pharm*, 1989, 4:37-41.

Pounder R, "Silent Peptic Ulceration: Deadly Silence or Golden Silence?" *Gastroenterology*, 1989, 96(2 Pt 2 Suppl):626-31.

Yeomans ND, Tulassay Z, Juhasz L, et al, "A Comparison of Omeprazole With Ranitidine for Ulcers Associated With Nonsteroidal Anti-inflammatory Drugs," *N Engl J Med*, 1998, 338(11):719-26.

Key-Pred® Injection *see* Prednisolone *on page 774*

Key-Pred-SP® Injection *see* Prednisolone *on page 774*

K-G® *see* Potassium Gluconate *on page 765*

Kinesed® *see* Hyoscyamine, Atropine, Scopolamine, and Phenobarbital *on page 472*

K-Lease® *see* Potassium Chloride *on page 763*

Klonopin™ *see* Clonazepam *on page 237*

K-Lor™ *see* Potassium Chloride *on page 763*

Klor-Con® *see* Potassium Chloride *on page 763*

Klor-Con® 8 *see* Potassium Chloride *on page 763*

Klor-Con® 10 *see* Potassium Chloride *on page 763*

Klor-Con/25® *see* Potassium Chloride *on page 763*

Kloromin® [OTC] *see* Chlorpheniramine *on page 208*

Klorvess® *see* Potassium Chloride *on page 763*

Klotrix® *see* Potassium Chloride *on page 763*

K-Lyte/Cl® *see* Potassium Chloride *on page 763*

K-Norm® *see* Potassium Chloride *on page 763*

Kolephrin® GG/DM [OTC] *see* Guaifenesin and Dextromethorphan *on page 439*

Konakion® *see* Phytonadione *on page 747*

Kondon's Nasal® [OTC] *see* Ephedrine *on page 335*

Kondremul® [OTC] *see* Mineral Oil *on page 628*

Konsyl® [OTC] *see* Psyllium *on page 804*

Konsyl-D® [OTC] *see* Psyllium *on page 804*

K-Phos® Neutral *see* Potassium Phosphate and Sodium Phosphate *on page 767*

K-Phos® Original *see* Potassium Acid Phosphate *on page 762*

K-Tab® *see* Potassium Chloride *on page 763*

Ku-Zyme® HP *see* Pancrelipase *on page 712*

Kytril® Injection *see* Granisetron *on page 433*

L-3-Hydroxytyrosine *see* Levodopa *on page 530*

LA-12® *see* Hydroxocobalamin *on page 466*

Labetalol *(la BET a lole)*

Related Information

Beta-Blockers Comparison *on page 1026*

I.V. Push Recommended Guidelines *on page 1083*

Brand Names Normodyne®; Trandate®

Synonyms Ibidomide Hydrochloride

Generic Available No

Therapeutic Category Alpha-/Beta- Adrenergic Blocker; Beta-Adrenergic Blocker

Use Treatment of mild to severe hypertension; I.V. for hypertensive emergencies

Contraindications Asthma, cardiogenic shock, uncompensated congestive heart failure, bradycardia, pulmonary edema, or heart block

Warnings Orthostatic hypotension may occur with I.V. administration; patient should remain supine during and for up to 3 hours after I.V. administration; abrupt withdrawal of labetalol should be avoided; withdraw over a 1- to 2-week period

Precautions Paradoxical increase in blood pressure has been reported with treatment of pheochromocytoma or clonidine withdrawal syndrome; use with extreme caution in patients with hyper-reactive airway disease, congestive heart failure, diabetes mellitus, hepatic dysfunction

Adverse Reactions

Cardiovascular: Orthostatic hypotension especially with I.V. administration, edema, congestive heart failure, A-V conduction disturbances, bradycardia

Central nervous system: Drowsiness, fatigue, dizziness, behavior disorders, headache

Dermatologic: Tingling in scalp or skin (transient with initiation of therapy), rash

Gastrointestinal: Nausea, xerostomia

Genitourinary: Sexual dysfunction, urinary problems

Neuromuscular & skeletal: Reversible myopathy, paresthesia

Respiratory: Bronchospasm, nasal congestion

Overdosage Symptoms of overdose include hypotension, bradycardia, bronchospasm

Toxicology Sympathomimetics (eg, epinephrine or dopamine), glucagon or a pacemaker can be used to treat the toxic bradycardia, asystole, and/or hypotension. Initially, fluids may be the best treatment for toxic hypotension. Patients should remain supine; serum glucose and potassium should be measured. Use supportive measures: lavage, syrup of ipecac. I.V. glucose should be administered for hypoglycemia; seizures may be treated with phenytoin or diazepam intravenously; continuous monitoring of blood pressure and EKG is necessary. If PVCs occur, treat with lidocaine or phenytoin; avoid quinidine, procainamide, and disopyramide since these agents further depress myocardial function. Bronchospasm can be treated with theophylline on beta$_2$ agonists (epinephrine).

Drug Interactions

Decreased effect of beta-adrenergic agonists

Increased effect: Cimetidine, other hypotensives

Increased toxicity: Halothane (with I.V. labetalol)

Labetalol effects are decreased (enzyme induction): Rifampin

Labetalol effects increase (enzyme inhibitor): Ritonavir, fluoxetine, paroxetine, sertraline, and mibefradil

Stability Stable in D_5W, saline for 24 hours; incompatible with alkaline solutions; use only solutions that are clear or slightly yellow; may cause a precipitate if exposed to alkaline admixture

Stability of parenteral admixture at room temperature (25°C) and refrigeration temperature (4°C): 24 hours

Mechanism of Action Blocks alpha$_1$-, beta$_1$- and beta$_2$-adrenergic receptor sites; elevated renins are reduced

Pharmacodynamics

Onset of action:

Oral: 20 minutes to 2 hours; maximum: 1-4 hours

I.V.: 2-5 minutes; maximum: 5-15 minutes

Duration:

Oral: 8-24 hours (dose-dependent)

I.V.: 2-4 hours

Pharmacokinetics

Distribution: V_d: Adults: 3-16 L/kg, mean: 9.4 L/kg; moderately lipid soluble, therefore, it can enter the CNS

Protein binding: 50%

Metabolism: Extensive first-pass effect; metabolized in liver primarily via glucuronide conjugation; substrate CYP2D6

Bioavailability: Oral: 25%; increased bioavailability with liver disease, in elderly, and with concurrent cimetidine

(Continued)

Labetalol *(Continued)*

Half-life: 6-8 hours

Elimination: In elderly, total body clearance of labetalol is decreased; <5% excreted in urine unchanged

Usual Dosage

Geriatrics: Oral: Initial: 100 mg 1-2 times/day increasing as needed

Adults:

Oral: Initial: 100 mg twice daily, may increase as needed every 2-3 days by 100 mg until desired response is obtained; usual dose: 200-400 mg twice daily; not to exceed 2.4 g/day

I.V.: 20 mg or 1-2 mg/kg whichever is lower, IVP over 2 minutes, may administer 40-80 mg at 10-minute intervals, up to 300 mg total dose

I.V. infusion: Initial: 2 mg/minute; titrate to response

Monitoring Parameters Blood pressure, standing and sitting/supine, pulse, mental status; if used in a diabetic patient, monitor glucose carefully; if used in patients with COPD, monitor pulmonary function

Test Interactions False-positive urine catecholamines, VMA if measured by fluorometric or photometric methods; use HPLC or specific catecholamine radioenzymatic technique

Patient Information Do not stop medication without consulting physician; may mask signs and symptoms of hypoglycemia in diabetic patients; sweating will still be present

Special Geriatric Considerations Due to alterations in the beta-adrenergic autonomic nervous system, beta-adrenergic blockade may result in less hemodynamic response than seen in younger adults. Studies indicate that despite decreased sensitivity to the chronotropic effects of beta blockade with age, there appears to be an increased myocardial sensitivity to the negative inotropic effect during stress (ie, exercise). Controlled trials have shown the overall response rate for propranolol to be only 20% to 50% in elderly populations. Therefore, all beta-adrenergic blocking drugs may result in a decreased response as compared to younger adults.

Dosage Forms

Labetalol hydrochloride:

Injection: 5 mg/mL (20 mL, 40 mL, 60 mL)

Tablet: 100 mg, 200 mg, 300 mg

Lacril® Ophthalmic Solution [OTC] *see* Artificial Tears *on page 82*

Lacri-Lube® NP Ophthalmic Ointment [OTC] *see* Ocular Lubricant *on page 688*

Lacri-Lube® S.O.P. Ophthalmic Ointment [OTC] *see* Ocular Lubricant *on page 688*

LactiCare-HC® *see* Hydrocortisone *on page 462*

Lactinex® [OTC] *see Lactobacillus acidophilus* and *Lactobacillus bulgaricus* on this page

Lactobacillus acidophilus and *Lactobacillus bulgaricus*

(lak toe ba SIL us as i DOF fil us & lak toe ba SIL us bul GAR i cus)

Brand Names Bacid® [OTC]; Lactinex® [OTC]; More-Dophilus® [OTC]

Generic Available No

Therapeutic Category Antidiarrheal

Use Dietary supplement

Unlabeled use: Treatment of uncomplicated diarrhea particularly that is caused by antibiotic therapy; re-establishes normal physiologic and bacterial flora of the intestinal tract (see Warnings)

Contraindications Allergy to milk or lactose

Warnings Discontinue if high fever present; the FDA has determined that these agents are not generally recognized as safe and effective as antidiarrheal agents

Adverse Reactions Gastrointestinal: Intestinal flatus

Stability Store in the refrigerator (capsules and granules) (see Additional Information)

Mechanism of Action Creates an environment unfavorable to potentially pathogenic fungi or bacteria through the production of lactic acid, and favors establishment of an aciduric flora, thereby suppressing the growth of pathogenic microorganisms; helps re-establish normal intestinal flora

Pharmacokinetics

Absorption: Oral: Not absorbed

Distribution: Locally, primarily in the colon

Elimination: In feces

Usual Dosage Geriatrics and Adults: Oral:

Capsules: 2 capsules 2-4 times/day

Granules: 1 packet added to or taken with cereal, food, milk, fruit juice, or water, 3-4 times/day

Powder: 1/4 to 1 teaspoonful 1-3 times/day with liquid

Tablet, chewable: 4 tablets 3-4 times/day; may follow each dose with a small amount of milk, fruit juice, or water

See Additional Information

Administration See Usual Dosage

Monitoring Parameters Monitor for decrease in frequency of stool and increased mass of stool

Patient Information Refrigerate; granules may be added to or taken with cereal, food, milk, fruit juice, or water

Nursing Implications Granules may be added to or given with cereal, food, milk, fruit juice, or water

Additional Information Pro-Bionate®, Superdophilus® and Lactinex®, mixed *L. acidophilus* and *L. bulgaricus*, More-Dophilus® can be stored at room temperature

Special Geriatric Considerations No specific recommendations due to age; keep in mind that elderly suffer significantly with fluid and electrolyte loss (lethargy, confusion, etc) and diarrhea should be aggressively treated

Dosage Forms

Capsule: 50s, 100s

Granules: 1 g/packet (12 packets/box)

Powder: 12 oz

Tablet, chewable: 50s

Lactulose (LAK tyoo lose)

Brand Names Cephulac®; Cholac®; Chronulac®; Constilac®; Constulose®; Duphalac®; Enulose®; Evalose®; Heptalac®; Lactulose PSE®

Therapeutic Category Ammonium Detoxicant; Laxative

Use Adjunct in the prevention and treatment of portal-systemic encephalopathy; treatment of chronic constipation

Contraindications Patients with galactosemia

Warnings Use cautiously in patients undergoing electrocautery procedures due to the accumulation of H_2 gas which may explode when ignited by electrical spark. This complication has not been reported with lactulose; patients should have bowel cleansing done with a nonfermentable agent.

Precautions Use with caution in patients with diabetes mellitus since lactulose contains small amounts of galactose and lactose; monitor periodically for electrolyte imbalance when lactulose is used >6 months or in patients predisposed to electrolyte abnormalities; patients receiving lactulose and an oral anti-infective agent should be monitored for possible inadequate response to lactulose; use with concomitant laxative in initial treatment of portal-systemic encephalopathy may result in early loose stools, incorrectly indicating adequate dose of lactulose

Adverse Reactions

Cardiovascular: Hypotension

Gastrointestinal: Cramping (20%), flatulence, abdominal discomfort, diarrhea, nausea, vomiting

Endocrine & metabolic: Dehydration, electrolyte loss

Overdosage Symptoms of overdose include potassium depletion; manifests by abdominal pain and diarrhea

Drug Interactions Oral neomycin, other antibiotics, laxatives, antacids

Stability Keep solution at room temperature to reduce viscosity; discard solution if cloudy or very dark

Mechanism of Action Prevents absorption of ammonia in colon as a result of bacterial degradation into low molecular weight organic acids which decrease the pH; produces an osmotic effect in the colon with resultant distention promoting peristalsis

Pharmacokinetics

Absorption: Oral: Not absorbed appreciably, this is desirable since the intended site of action is within the colon; requires colonic flora for primary drug activation

Metabolism: By colonic flora to lactic acid and acetic acid

Elimination: Primarily in feces and urine (~3%)

(Continued)

Lactulose *(Continued)*

Usual Dosage Geriatrics and Adults:

Oral:

Acute episodes of portal systemic encephalopathy: 30-45 mL at 1- to 2-hour intervals until laxative effect observed

Laxative: 15-30 mL 1-2 times/day

Chronic therapy: 30-45 mL/dose 3-4 times/day; titrate dose to produce 2-3 soft stools daily

Rectal: 300 mL diluted with 700 mL of water or normal saline, and given via a rectal balloon catheter and retained for 30-60 minutes; may administer every 4-6 hours

Monitoring Parameters Monitor for number of stools per day, dehydration, hypotension; measure serum electrolytes with long-term use; monitor serum ammonia concentrations when treating hepatic encephalopathy

Test Interactions Decreased ammonia (B)

Patient Information Lactulose can be taken "as is" or diluted with water, fruit juice or milk, or taken in a food; laxative results may not occur for 24-48 hours; take with a full glass of water

Nursing Implications Dilute lactulose in water, usually 60-120 mL, prior to administering through a gastric or feeding tube; monitor serum ammonia in hepatic disease (see Monitoring Parameters)

Additional Information Diarrhea indicates overdosage and responds to dose reduction

Special Geriatric Considerations Elderly are more likely to show CNS signs of dehydration and electrolyte loss than younger adults. Therefore, monitor closely for fluid and electrolyte loss with chronic use. Sorbitol is equally effective as a laxative and less expensive. However, sorbitol **cannot be substituted** in the treatment of hepatic encephalopathy.

Dosage Forms Syrup: 10 g/15 mL (15 mL, 30 mL, 237 mL, 473 mL, 946 mL, 1890 mL)

References

Lederle FA, Busch DL, Mattox KM, et al, "Cost-Effective Treatment of Constipation in the Elderly: A Randomized Double-Blind Comparison of Sorbitol and Lactulose," *Am J Med*, 1990, 89(5):597-601.

Lactulose PSE® *see Lactulose on previous page*

Lamictal® *see Lamotrigine on this page*

Lamisil® Oral *see Terbinafine, Oral on page 891*

Lamisil® Topical *see Terbinafine, Topical on page 893*

Lamotrigine *(la MOE tri jeen)*

Related Information

♪ Antiepileptic Drug Interactions Comparison *on page 1022*

Brand Names Lamictal®

Synonyms BW-430C; LTG

Generic Available No

Therapeutic Category Anticonvulsant, Miscellaneous

Use Adjunctive treatment of partial seizures

Unlabeled use: Generalized tonic-clonic seizures in adults, absence, atypical absence, and myoclonic seizures

Contraindications Hypersensitivity to lamotrigine or any of its components

Warnings Dermatologic: Rash develops in ~10% of patients; rash usually occurs in first 4-6 weeks of therapy; occurs more often in patients receiving valproic acid; Stevens-Johnson syndrome, toxic epidermal necrolysis, and angioedema have been reported (0.3% of rashes)

Sudden death is rare (0.0035 deaths/patient year); withdrawal seizures occur when AED is abruptly discontinued. Status epilepticus reported with the use of lamotrigine (7/2343). Multiorgan failure and hepatic failure have been reported. Renal/hepatic dysfunction requires dose reductions and close monitoring.

Precautions No accepted plasma concentration values have been established for therapeutic effect or toxicity. Use with caution in patients with hepatic failure, renal dysfunction, or drugs (AEDs) affecting lamotrigine clearance. Photosensitivity may occur; patients should take precaution. Since lamotrigine binds to melanin, periodic eye examinations are advised with long-term use. The efficacy of using lamotrigine with valproic acid as a two-drug regimen is not recommended due to a lack of data.

Adverse Reactions

Cardiovascular: Atrial fibrillation, hypertension, myocardial infarction, hypotension (<0.1%)

Central nervous system: Dizziness, sedation, ataxia, insomnia, depression, anxiety, irritability, speech disorder, memory decrease, headache, migraine

Dermatologic: Hypersensitivity rash, angioedema, Stevens-Johnson syndrome

Gastrointestinal: Nausea, vomiting, dyspepsia, gingival hyperplasia, stomatitis, gastritis

Neuromuscular & skeletal: Tremors, arthralgia, back pain, chest pain, myalgia

Ocular: Nystagmus, diplopia, blurred vision

Renal: Hematuria

Respiratory: Rhinitis

Overdosage Signs and symptoms of overdose include coma, dizziness, headache, and somnolence

Toxicology Treatment of overdosage is general supportive care; monitor vital signs, induce emesis if indicated, however, the drug is rapidly absorbed; uncertain if hemodialysis is effective

Drug Interactions

Lamotrigine serum concentrations are decreased by carbamazepine, phenobarbital, primidone, and phenytoin

Increased serum concentrations of carbamazepine epoxide

Lamotrigine serum concentrations increased by valproic acid (twofold)

Lamotrigine decreases valproic acid serum concentrations

Mechanism of Action Exact mechanism of action is unknown; may stabilize neuronal membranes by inhibiting sodium channels and, thereby, inhibits release of glutamine, an excitatory amino acid; has a weak inhibitory effect on serotonin 5-HT$_3$ receptors

Pharmacokinetics

Distribution: V$_d$: 1.1 L/kg

Protein binding: 55%

Metabolism: Hepatic and renal

Half-life: 24 hours; increases to 59 hours with concomitant valproic acid therapy; decreases with concomitant phenytoin or carbamazepine therapy to 15 hours

Elimination: Hepatic and renal

Elderly: In a single dose study the pharmacokinetics of lamotrigine were similar to those of young adults

Usual Dosage Geriatrics and Adults: Initial:

When administered with other antiepileptic agents **except** valproic acid: 50 mg once daily for 2 weeks; then 50 mg twice daily for 2 weeks; then increase to maintenance dose of 300-500 mg/day in 2 divided doses by 100 mg/day/week

When administered with valproic acid: 25 mg every other day for 2 weeks; 25 mg daily for 2 weeks; then increase to a maintenance dose of 100-150 mg/day in 2 divided doses per day by increasing daily dose by 25-50 mg/day every 1-2 weeks

Monitoring Parameters Monitor for therapeutic response and for adverse reactions; no established therapeutic serum concentrations

Reference Range Therapeutic: 2-4 mcg/mL

Patient Information Rash should be reported immediately to physician; patients should be warned of photosensitivity and take precautions (ie, sunscreen use, sunglasses, protective clothing, avoiding sunlight)

Nursing Implications See Precautions and Patient Information

Additional Information Low water solubility

Special Geriatric Considerations No pharmacokinetic differences noted between young adults and elderly; use with caution in elderly with significant renal decline

Dosage Forms Tablet: 25 mg, 100 mg, 150 mg, 200 mg

Lamprene® see Clofazimine on page 234

Lanacort® [OTC] see Hydrocortisone on page 462

Laniazid® Oral see Isoniazid on page 500

Lanophyllin® see Theophylline on page 902

Lanoxicaps® see Digoxin on page 292

Lanoxin® see Digoxin on page 292

Lansoprazole (lan SOE pra zole)

Related Information

Regimens Used to Treat *Helicobacter pylori* and Ulcers on page 1033

Brand Names Prevacid®

Therapeutic Category Gastric Acid Secretion Inhibitor

(Continued)

Lansoprazole (Continued)

Use Treatment (4 weeks) for healing and symptom relief of duodenal ulcer; short-term (8 weeks) treatment for erosive esophagitis, and long-term treatment of pathological hypersecretory conditions (including Zollinger-Ellison syndrome); maintenance of healed erosive esophagitis

Contraindications Hypersensitivity to this agent or any of its components

Warnings Due to animal (mice/rat) data suggesting long-term use causing dose-related enterochromaffin-like cell hyperplasia, maintenance therapy for duodenal ulcer disease and erosive esophagitis is not recommended despite some human data of use over 1 year without evidence of such hyperplasia. Further data needed before maintenance therapy can be recommended.

Precautions Symptomatic relief of symptoms of peptic ulcer disease does not preclude the presence of gastric neoplastic disease; must rule out by examination, especially in elderly

Adverse Reactions Lansoprazole is well tolerated; the most common side effect is diarrhea (dose-related: 3.6% to 7.4%)

Cardiovascular: Syncope, hypertension, hypotension, palpitations, shock, angina pectoris, myocardial infarction, edema

Central nervous system: Headache, confusion, anxiety, apathy, amnesia, depression, dizziness, hallucinations, nervousness, stroke, malaise, agitation, hostility

Dermatologic: Acne, rash, pruritus, urticaria, alopecia

Endocrine & metabolic: Decreased libido, hypoglycemia, hyperglycemia, diabetes mellitus, goiter, gout, gynecomastia, breast tenderness

Gastrointestinal: Diarrhea, abdominal pain, nausea, melena, constipation, xerostomia, flatulence, gastroenteritis, esophageal ulcer, hematemesis, rectal hemorrhage, stomatitis, tenesmus, fecal color changes, dyspepsia, dysphagia, anorexia, increased appetite, weight gain, halitosis

Genitourinary: Impotence

Hematologic: Anemia, hemolysis

Neuromuscular & skeletal: Paresthesia, weakness

Renal: Hematuria, albuminuria

Respiratory: Asthma, bronchitis, cough, epistaxis, hemoptysis, dyspnea

Miscellaneous: Hiccups, flu syndrome

Overdosage Only one report of an overdose; no adverse reactions observed; lansoprazole is not removed by hemodialysis

Drug Interactions Lansoprazole, when administered with theophylline, **increases** serum theophylline 10% (usually clinically insignificant); sucralfate **decreases** (30%) lansoprazole's absorption

Mechanism of Action Lansoprazole inhibits (H^+, K^+)-ATPase enzyme system in gastric parietal cells, thus decreases acid secretion by blocking final step in acid production (proton pump inhibitor). This action is dose-related and inhibits both basal and stimulated gastric acid secretion.

Pharmacodynamics

Onset of action: Following multiple daily dosing: 1 hour at 30 mg dose and 1-2 hours after 15 mg dose

Duration of action: 2-4 days required for gastric pH to return to normal after multiple daily dosing

Pharmacokinetics

Absorption: Rapidly and extensively absorbed in small intestine

Protein binding: 97% to plasma proteins

Metabolism: Extensively metabolized in the liver by the cytochrome P-450 system in CYP 3A and CYP 2C19 isoenzyme functions

Bioavailability: >80%; food decreases peak concentration (C_{max}) and AUC by 50%

Half-life: 1.5 hours

Time to peak: ~1.7 hours

Elimination: Metabolites excreted primarily through biliary-fecal elimination

Usual Dosage Geriatrics and Adults:

Duodenal ulcer: 15 mg/day for 4 weeks

Erosive esophagitis: 30 mg/day for up to 8 weeks; if healing is not complete after 8 weeks, an additional 8-week course is indicated

Hypersecretory diseases: Recommended starting dose: 60 mg/day; adjust dose as clinically necessary to control symptoms and treat as long as clinically indicated (some patients with Zollinger-Ellison syndrome have been treated for over 4 years). Daily total doses >120 mg should be given in divided doses (doses of 90 mg twice daily have been used).

Monitoring Parameters Symptoms of peptic ulcer disease, occult blood; use of gastroscopy is preferred

Test Interactions Abnormal LFTs, RBCs, WBCs, and platelets reported; also increases in creatinine, lipids, eosinophils, and electrolyte changes reported; false increase in gastrin

Patient Information Take before eating; capsules should not be crushed or chewed; swallow capsules whole

Nursing Implications Do not crush; patients should swallow whole; may take with antacids; capsules can be opened and given with applesauce or via a feeding tube

Special Geriatric Considerations The clearance of lansoprazole is decreased in elderly, however, the half-life is only increased by 50% to 100%. This still results in a short half-life and no accumulation is seen in elderly. The rate of healing and side effects is similar to younger adults; no dosage adjustment is necessary.

Dosage Forms Capsule, delayed release: 15 mg, 30 mg

Larodopa® see Levodopa on page 530
Lasix® see Furosemide on page 416

Latanoprost (la TAN oh prost)
Brand Names Xalatan®

Therapeutic Category Prostaglandin, Ophthalmic

Use Reduction of elevated intraocular pressure in patients with open-angle glaucoma and ocular hypertension who are intolerant of the other IOP lowering medications or insufficiently responsive (failed to achieve target IOP determined after multiple measurements over time) to another IOP lowering medication

Contraindications Hypersensitivity to any component of product

Warnings Latanoprost may gradually change eye color, increasing the amount of brown pigment in the iris by increasing the number of melanosomes in melanocytes. The long-term effects on the melanocytes and the consequences of potential injury to the melanocytes or deposition of pigment granules to other areas of the eye is currently unknown. Patients should be examined regularly, and depending on the clinical situation, treatment may be stopped if increased pigmentation ensues.

There have been reports of bacterial keratitis associated with the use of multiple-dose containers of topical ophthalmic products. Do not administer while wearing contact lenses.

Adverse Reactions
Cardiovascular: Chest pain, angina pectoris
Dermatologic: Rash, allergic skin reaction
Neuromuscular & skeletal: Myalgia, arthralgia, back pain
Ocular: Blurred vision, burning and stinging, conjunctival hyperemia, foreign body sensation, itching, increased pigmentation of the iris, punctate epithelial keratopathy, dry eye, excessive tearing, eye pain, lid crusting, lid edema, lid erythema, lid discomfort/pain, photophobia, conjunctivitis, diplopia, discharge from the eye, retinal artery embolus, retinal detachment, vitreous hemorrhage from diabetic retinopathy
Respiratory: Upper respiratory tract infection, cold, flu

Overdosage Symptoms include ocular irritation and conjunctival or episcleral hyperemia treatment should be symptomatic

Drug Interactions Decreased effect: *In vitro* studies have shown that precipitation occurs when eye drops containing thimerosal are mixed with latanoprost. If such drugs are used, administer with an interval of at least 5 minutes between applications

Stability Protect from light; store intact bottles under refrigeration (2°C to 8°C/36°F to 46°F). Once opened, the container may be stored at room temperature up to 25°C (77°F) for 6 weeks.

Mechanism of Action Latanoprost is a prostaglandin F_2-alpha analog believed to reduce intraocular pressure by increasing the outflow of the aqueous humor

Pharmacodynamics
Onset of effect: 3-4 hours
Maximum effect: 8-12 hours

Pharmacokinetics
Absorption: Through the cornea where the isopropyl ester prodrug is hydrolyzed by esterases to the biologically active acid. Peak concentration in the aqueous humor is reached in 2 hours after topical administration.
Distribution: V_d: 0.16 L/kg
Half-life: 17 minutes (prodrug ester)
Metabolism: Primarily metabolized by the liver via fatty acid beta-oxidation
(Continued)

Latanoprost *(Continued)*

Elimination: After hepatic metabolism, the metabolites are mainly eliminated via the kidneys

Usual Dosage Geriatrics and Adults: Ophthalmic: Instill 1 drop in the affected eye(s) once daily in the evening; do not exceed the once daily dosage because it has been shown that more frequent administration may decrease the IOP lowering effect

Administration If more than one topical ophthalmic drug is being used, administer the drugs at least 5 minutes apart

Monitoring Parameters Intraocular pressure, funduscopic exam, visual field testing

Patient Information Inform patients about the possibility of iris color change because of an increase of the brown pigment and resultant cosmetically different eye coloration that may occur. Iris pigmentation changes may be more noticeable in patients with green-brown, blue/gray-brown, or yellow-brown irises.

Do not touch the tip of the dropper to eye or any other surface.

If any ocular reactions occur, such as conjunctivitis or lid reactions, immediately report to eye specialist.

Latanoprost contains benzalkonium chloride, which may be absorbed by contact lenses. Remove contact lenses prior to administration of the solution. Lenses may be reinserted 15 minutes following latanoprost administration.

If more than one topical ophthalmic drug is being used, administer the drugs at least 5 minutes apart.

Nursing Implications Teach patient proper instillation technique (see Patient Information)

Special Geriatric Considerations Evaluate patient's ability to self-administer eye drop

Dosage Forms Solution, ophthalmic: 0.005% (2.5 mL)

References
Patel SS and Spencer CM, "Latanoprost: A Review of Its Pharmacological Properties, Clinical Efficacy and Tolerability in the Management of Primary Open-Angle Glaucoma and Ocular Hypertension," *Drugs Aging*, 1996, 9(5):363-78.

l-Bunolol Hydrochloride *see* Levobunolol *on next page*

L-Deprenyl *see* Selegiline *on page 851*

L-Dopa *see* Levodopa *on page 530*

Ledercillin® VK *see* Penicillin V Potassium *on page 725*

Lente® *see* Insulin Preparations *on page 488*

Lente® Iletin® I *see* Insulin Preparations *on page 488*

Lente® Iletin® II *see* Insulin Preparations *on page 488*

Lente® Insulin *see* Insulin Preparations *on page 488*

Lente® L *see* Insulin Preparations *on page 488*

Lescol® *see* Fluvastatin *on page 405*

Leukeran® *see* Chlorambucil *on page 202*

Leuprolide Acetate *(loo PROE lide AS e tate)*

Brand Names Lupron®; Lupron Depot®; Lupron Depot-Ped™

Generic Available No

Therapeutic Category Antineoplastic Agent, Hormone (Gonadotropin Hormone-Releasing Antigen); Gonadotropin Releasing Hormone Analog

Use Palliative treatment of advanced prostate carcinoma, endometriosis
Unlabeled use: Treatment of breast, ovarian, and endometrial cancer; prostatic hypertrophy; leiomyoma uteri

Contraindications Hypersensitivity to leuprolide; gonadotropin-releasing hormone (GnRH); GnRH agonists analogs; undiagnosed abnormal vaginal bleeding

Warnings Tumor flare and bone pain may occur at initiation of therapy; transient weakness and paresthesia of lower limbs, hematuria, and urinary tract obstruction in first week of therapy; animal studies have shown dose-related benign pituitary hyperplasia and benign pituitary adenomas after 2 years of use

Precautions Use with caution in patients hypersensitive to benzyl alcohol; after 6 months use of Depot® leuprolide, vertebral bone density decreased (average 13.5%)

Adverse Reactions
Cardiovascular: Edema, cardiac arrhythmias, EKG changes, elevated blood pressure, hypotension, angina

Central nervous system: Dizziness, lethargy, insomnia, headache, nervousness

Dermatologic: Rash, hair growth

Endocrine & metabolic: Estrogenic effects (gynecomastia, breast tenderness), decreased testicular size, hot flashes

Gastrointestinal: Nausea, vomiting, diarrhea, GI bleed, anorexia, peptic ulcer

Genitourinary: Urinary urgency/frequency, bladder spasm, impotence, decreased libido

Hematologic: Decreased hemoglobin and hematocrit

Neuromuscular & skeletal: Myalgia, pain, bone loss, pelvic fibrosis, paresthesia

Ocular: Blurred vision

Respiratory: Dyspnea, cough, pneumonia, hemoptysis

Miscellaneous: Diaphoresis

Overdosage Animal (rats) data: Dyspnea, decreased activity, injection site irritation

Toxicology General supportive care; decrease dose

Stability Store unopened vials in refrigerator, vial in use can be kept at room temperature for several months with minimal loss of potency; upon reconstitution, the suspension is stable for 24 hours, however the product does not contain a preservative

Mechanism of Action Continuous daily administration results in suppression of ovarian and testicular steroidogenesis due to decreased levels of LH and FSH with subsequent decrease in testosterone (males) and estrogen (females) levels

Pharmacokinetics Serum testosterone concentrations first increase within 3 days of therapy, then decrease after 2-4 weeks with continued therapy; requires parenteral administration since it is rapidly destroyed within the GI tract

Bioavailability: Not bioavailable if given orally; bioavailability of S.C. and I.V. doses is comparable

Half-life: 3-4.25 hours

Elimination: Not well defined

Usual Dosage Geriatrics and Adults:

Advanced prostatic carcinoma:

I.M. (suspension): 7.5 mg/dose given monthly (28-33)

S.C.: 1 mg/day

Endometriosis: I.M. (Depot®): 3.75 mg/month

Monitoring Parameters Serum concentrations of testosterone, acid phosphatase; bone density in high-risk patients (osteoporosis, use of Depot® leuprolide)

Patient Information Patient must be taught aseptic technique and S.C. injection technique. Rotate S.C. injection sites frequently. Disease flare (increased bone pain, urinary retention) can briefly occur with initiation of therapy. Store vials under refrigeration but do not freeze. Do not discontinue medication without physician's advice.

Nursing Implications When administering the Depot® form, do not use needles smaller than 22-gauge; reconstitute only with diluent provided; must teach patient injection technique; rotate S.C. injection site frequently (see Monitoring Parameters)

Special Geriatric Considerations Leuprolide has the advantage of not increasing risk of atherosclerotic vascular disease, causing swelling of breasts, fluid retention, and thromboembolism as compared to estrogen therapy

Dosage Forms

Leuprorelin acetate:

Injection: 5 mg/mL (2.8 mL)

Powder for injection (Depot-Ped™): 7.5 mg, 11.25 mg, 15 mg

Suspension, Depot®: 3.75 mg/mL; 7.5 mg/mL

Levaquin® *see* Levofloxacin *on page 532*

Levatol® *see* Penbutolol *on page 717*

Levbid® *see* Hyoscyamine *on page 471*

Levobunolol (lee voe BYOO noe lole)

Related Information

Glaucoma Drug Therapy Comparison *on page 1032*

Brand Names AKBeta®; Betagan® Liquifilm®

Synonyms *l*-Bunolol Hydrochloride

Generic Available No

(Continued)

Levobunolol *(Continued)*

Therapeutic Category Beta-Adrenergic Blocker, Ophthalmic

Use Lower intraocular pressure in chronic open-angle glaucoma or ocular hypertension

Contraindications Known hypersensitivity to levobunolol; bronchial asthma, severe COPD, sinus bradycardia, second or third degree A-V block; cardiac failure, cardiogenic shock

Precautions Use with caution in patients with congestive heart failure, diabetes mellitus, hyperthyroidism, cerebral insufficiency due to systemic absorption

Adverse Reactions
Cardiovascular: Bradycardia, arrhythmia, hypotension
Central nervous system: Dizziness, headache
Dermatologic: Skin rash
Local: Stinging, burning, erythema, itching, alopecia
Ocular: Blepharoconjunctivitis, decreased visual acuity, conjunctivitis, keratitis
Respiratory: Bronchospasm

Overdosage Symptoms of overdose include bradycardia, hypotension, bronchospasm

Toxicology Flush eye(s) with water or normal saline

Drug Interactions Systemic beta-adrenergic blocking agents; ophthalmic epinephrine (increased blood pressure/loss of IOP effect), quinidine (sinus bradycardia), verapamil (bradycardia and asystole have been reported)

Mechanism of Action A nonselective beta-adrenergic blocking agent that most likely lowers intraocular pressure by reducing aqueous humor production and possibly increasing the outflow of aqueous humor

Pharmacodynamics
Onset of action: Following ophthalmic instillation decreases in intraocular pressure (IOP) can be noted within 1 hour
Peak effects: Within 2-6 hours; reductions in IOP can last from 1-7 days

Pharmacokinetics Elimination not well defined

Usual Dosage Geriatrics and Adults: Instill 1 drop in eye(s) 1-2 times/day

Administration Apply finger pressure over nasolacrimal duct to decrease systemic absorption

Monitoring Parameters Intraocular pressure, heart rate, funduscopic exam, visual field testing

Patient Information May sting on instillation, do not touch dropper to eye; visual acuity may be decreased after administration; night vision may be decreased; distance vision may be altered; apply finger pressure between the bridge of the nose and corner of the eye to decrease systemic absorption; assess patient's or caregiver's ability to administer

Nursing Implications See Administration

Additional Information Contains metabisulfite

Special Geriatric Considerations Because systemic absorption does occur with ophthalmic administration, the elderly with other disease states or syndromes that may be affected by a beta-blocker (CHF, COPD, etc) should be monitored closely

Dosage Forms Solution, ophthalmic, as hydrochloride: 0.25% (5 mL, 10 mL, 15 mL); 0.5% (2 mL, 5 mL, 10 mL, 15 mL)

Levodopa *(lee voe DOE pa)*

Related Information
Antacid Drug Interactions *on page 1096*

Brand Names Dopar®; Larodopa®

Synonyms *L*-3-Hydroxytyrosine; *L*-Dopa

Generic Available No

Therapeutic Category Anti-Parkinson's Agent

Dosage Forms
Capsule: 100 mg, 250 mg, 500 mg
Tablet: 100 mg, 250 mg, 500 mg

Levodopa and Carbidopa *(lee voe DOE pa & kar bi DOE pa)*

Brand Names Sinemet®

Synonyms Carbidopa and Levodopa

Generic Available No

Therapeutic Category Anti-Parkinson's Agent

Use Treatment of parkinsonian syndrome

Unlabeled use: Restless legs syndrome

Contraindications Narrow-angle glaucoma, MAO inhibitors, hypersensitivity to levodopa, carbidopa, or any component; do not use in patients with malignant melanoma or undiagnosed skin lesions

Precautions Use with caution in patients with history of myocardial infarction, arrhythmias, asthma, wide-angle glaucoma, peptic ulcer disease; sudden discontinuation of levodopa may cause a worsening of Parkinson's disease

Adverse Reactions

Cardiovascular: Orthostatic hypotension, palpitations, cardiac arrhythmias

Central nervous system: Memory loss, nervousness, anxiety, insomnia, fatigue, hallucinations, ataxia, confusion

Gastrointestinal: Nausea, vomiting, GI bleeding, xerostomia

Neuromuscular & skeletal: Dystonic movements, "on-off"

Ocular: Blurred vision

Overdosage Symptoms of overdose include palpitations, arrhythmias, hypotension

Toxicology Treatment is supportive; initiate gastric lavage, administer I.V. fluids judiciously and monitor EKG

Drug Interactions

Decreased effect: Phenytoin, benzodiazepines, tricyclic antidepressants, phenothiazines, haloperidol, reserpine, methyldopa

Increased effect: Antacids

Increased toxicity: Nonselective MAO inhibitors

Mechanism of Action Parkinson's symptoms are due to a lack of striatal dopamine; levodopa circulates in the plasma to the blood-brain-barrier (BBB), where it crosses, to be converted by striatal enzymes to dopamine; carbidopa inhibits the peripheral plasma breakdown of levodopa by inhibiting its decarboxylation, and thereby increases available levodopa at the BBB

Pharmacodynamics Peak effect: Oral: Within 1-2 hours after administration; may take 2-3 weeks to see the full therapeutic effect

Pharmacokinetics

Carbidopa:

Absorption: Oral: 40% to 70%

Protein binding: 36%

Half-life: 1-2 hours

Elimination: Excreted unchanged

Levodopa:

Absorption: May be decreased if given with a high protein meal

Half-life: 1.2-2.3 hours

Elimination: Primarily in urine (80%) as dopamine, norepinephrine, and homovanillic acid

Usual Dosage Oral (see Additional Information):

Geriatrics: Initial: 25/100 twice daily, increase as necessary; Sinemet® CR may be used as initial therapy

Adults: Initial: 25/100 2-4 times/day, increase as necessary to a maximum of 200/2000 mg/day

Conversion from Sinemet® to Sinemet® CR (50/200): (Sinemet® [total daily dose of levodopa] / Sinemet® CR)

300-400 mg / 1 tablet twice daily

500-600 mg / 1½ tablets twice daily or one 3 times/day

700-800 mg / 4 tablets in 3 or more divided doses

900-1000 mg / 5 tablets in 3 or more divided doses

Intervals between doses of Sinemet® CR should be 4-8 hours while awake

Monitoring Parameters Blood pressure, standing and sitting/supine; symptoms of parkinsonism, dyskinesias, mental status

Test Interactions False-positive reaction for urinary glucose with Clinitest®; false-negative reaction using Clinistix®; false-positive urine ketones with Acetest®, Ketostix®, Labstix®

Patient Information Take on an empty stomach if possible; if GI distress occurs, take with meals; rise carefully from lying or sitting position; do not crush or chew sustained release product

Nursing Implications Space doses evenly over the waking hours; do not crush sustained release product

Additional Information 50-100 mg/day of carbidopa is needed to block the peripheral conversion of levodopa to dopamine. "On-off" can be managed by giving smaller, more frequent doses of Sinemet® or adding a dopamine agonist or selegiline; when adding a new agent, doses of Sinemet® should usually be decreased. To avoid fluctuations in levodopa absorption, avoid giving with high protein meals. After a daily levodopa dose of 600-800 mg is (Continued)

Levodopa and Carbidopa *(Continued)*

reached, some experts recommend adding a dopamine agonist to the regimen, rather than increasing the levodopa dose.

Special Geriatric Considerations The elderly may be more sensitive to the CNS effects of levodopa

Dosage Forms
Tablet:
Sinemet®-10/100: Carbidopa 10 mg and levodopa 100 mg
Sinemet®-25/100: Carbidopa 25 mg and levodopa 100 mg
Sinemet®-25/250: Carbidopa 25 mg and levodopa 250 mg
Sinemet® CR: Carbidopa 25 mg and levodopa 100 mg
Sinemet® CR: Carbidopa 50 mg and levodopa 200 mg

References
Koller WC, Silver DE, and Lieberman A, "An Algorithm for the Management of Parkinson's Disease," *Neurology*, 1994, 44(12 Suppl 10):S1-52.
Stern MB, "Contemporary Approaches to the Pharmacotherapeutic Management of Parkinson's Disease: An Overview," *Neurology*, 1997, 49(1 Suppl 1):S2-9.
Walker SW, Fina A, and Kryger MH, "L-Dopa/Carbidopa for Nocturnal Movement Disorders in Uremia," *Sleep*, 1996, 19(3):214-8.

Levo-Dromoran® *see Levorphanol on next page*

Levofloxacin *(lee voe FLOKS a sin)*

Related Information
Antacid Drug Interactions *on page 1096*
I.V. Medication Recommendations *on page 1080*

Brand Names Levaquin®

Therapeutic Category Antibiotic, Quinolone

Use Acute maxillary sinusitis due to *S. pneumoniae*, *H. influenzae*, or *M. catarrhalis*; also for acute bacterial exacerbation of chronic bronchitis and community-acquired pneumonia due to *S. aureus*, *S. pneumoniae*, *H. influenzae*, *H. parainfluenzae*, or *M. catarrhalis*, *C. pneumoniae*, *L. pneumophila*, or *M. pneumoniae*; may be used for uncomplicated skin and skin structure infection (due to *S. aureus* or *S. pyogenes*) and complicated urinary tract infection due to gram-negative enterobacteriae, including acute pyelonephritis (caused by *E. coli*); although clinical efficacy has been similar between levofloxacin and ofloxacin, levofloxacin is more potent and may be given in lower doses

Contraindications Hypersensitivity to levofloxacin, any component, or other quinolones; pregnancy, lactation

Warnings Not recommended in children <18 years of age; other quinolones have caused transient arthropathy in children; CNS stimulation may occur (tremor, restlessness, confusion, and very rarely hallucinations or seizures); use with caution in patients with known or suspected CNS disorders or renal dysfunction; prolonged use may result in superinfection; if an allergic reaction (itching, urticaria, dyspnea, pharyngeal or facial edema, loss of consciousness, tingling, cardiovascular collapse) occurs, discontinue the drug immediately; use caution to avoid possible photosensitivity reactions during and for several days following fluoroquinolone therapy; pseudomembranous colitis may occur and should be considered in patients who present with diarrhea

Adverse Reactions
Central nervous system: Dizziness, headache, insomnia
Dermatologic: Rash
Gastrointestinal: Nausea, vomiting, increased transaminases
Hematologic: Leukopenia, thrombocytopenia
Neuromuscular & skeletal: Tremor, arthralgia

Overdosage Symptoms of overdose include acute renal failure, seizures

Toxicology Treatment should include GI decontamination and supportive care; not removed by peritoneal or hemodialysis

Drug Interactions
Decreased effect: Decreased absorption with antacids containing aluminum, magnesium, and/or calcium (by up to 98% if given at the same time); phenytoin serum concentration may be reduced by quinolones; antineoplastic agents may also decrease serum concentration of fluoroquinolones
Increased toxicity/serum concentration: Quinolones cause increased levels of caffeine, warfarin, azlocillin, cyclosporine, and theophylline (one study indicates no effect on theophylline metabolism); azlocillin, cimetidine, and probenecid increases quinolone levels; an increased incidence of seizures may occur with foscarnet

Stability Stable for 72 hours when diluted to 5 mg/mL in a compatible I.V. fluid and stored at room temperature; stable for 14 days when stored at room temperature; stable for 6 months when frozen, do not refreeze; do not thaw in microwave or by bath immersion; **incompatible** with mannitol and sodium bicarbonate

Mechanism of Action As the S (-) enantiomer of the fluoroquinolone, ofloxacin, levofloxacin, inhibits DNA-gyrase in susceptible organisms; inhibits relaxation of supercoiled DNA and promotes breakage of double-stranded DNA

Pharmacokinetics
Absorption: Well absorbed
Distribution: V_d: 1.25 L/kg; CSF concentrations ~15% of serum concentration; high concentrations are achieved in prostate and gynecological tissues, sinus, breast milk, and saliva
Protein binding: 50%
Metabolism: Hepatic, minimal
Half-life: 6 hours
Bioavailability: 100%
Time to peak serum concentration: 1 hour
Elimination: Most excreted unchanged in urine

Usual Dosage Geriatrics and Adults: Oral, I.V. (infuse I.V. solution over 60 minutes):
Acute bacterial exacerbation of chronic bronchitis: 500 mg every 24 hours for at least 7 days
Community acquired pneumonia: 500 mg every 24 hours for 7-14 days
Acute maxillary sinusitis: 500 mg every 24 hours for 10-14 days
Uncomplicated skin infections: 500 mg every 24 hours for 7-10 days
Complicated urinary tract infections include acute pyelonephritis: 250 mg every 24 hours for 10 days
Dosing adjustment in renal impairment:
Cl_{cr} 20-49 mL/minute: Administer 250 mg every 24 hours (initial: 500 mg)
Cl_{cr} 10-19 mL/minute: Administer 250 mg every 48 hours (initial: 500 mg for most infections; 250 mg for renal infections)
Hemodialysis/CAPD: 250 mg every 48 hours (initial: 500 mg)

Monitoring Parameters Evaluation of organ system functions (renal, hepatic, ophthalmologic, and hematopoietic) is recommended periodically during therapy; the possibility of crystalluria should be assessed; WBC and signs of infection

Patient Information May be taken with or without food; drink plenty of fluids; avoid exposure to direct sunlight during therapy and for several days following; do not take antacids within 4 hours before or 2 hours after dosing; contact your physician immediately if signs of allergy occur; do not discontinue therapy until your course has been completed; take a missed dose as soon as possible, unless it is almost time for your next dose.

Nursing Implications Infuse I.V. solutions over 60 minutes

Special Geriatric Considerations Expanded spectra and once daily dosing; adjust dose for renal function (see Usual Dosage)

Dosage Forms
Infusion, in D_5W: 5 mg/mL (50 mL, 100 mL)
Injection: 25 mg/mL (20 mL)
Tablet: 250 mg, 500 mg

Levorphanol (lee VOR fa nole)

Related Information
Narcotic Agonist Comparative Pharmacology *on page 1036*
Pharmacokinetics of Narcotic Agonist Analgesics *on page 1037*

Brand Names Levo-Dromoran®
Synonyms Levorphan Tartrate
Generic Available No
Therapeutic Category Analgesic, Narcotic
Use Relief of moderate to severe pain; also used parenterally for preoperative sedation and an adjunct to nitrous oxide/oxygen anesthesia
Restrictions C-II
Contraindications Hypersensitivity to levorphanol or any component
Warnings Levorphanol is not usually recommended for use in the elderly because of its long half-life and, therefore, its tendency to accumulate
Precautions Levorphanol tartrate shares the toxic potentials of opiate agonists, and usual precautions of opiate agonist therapy should be observed
Adverse Reactions
Cardiovascular: Palpitations, hypotension, bradycardia, peripheral vasodilation
(Continued)

Levorphanol *(Continued)*

Central nervous system: CNS depression, drowsiness, sedation, increased intracranial pressure

Dermatologic: Pruritus

Endocrine & metabolic: Antidiuretic hormone release

Gastrointestinal: Nausea, vomiting, constipation

Genitourinary: Urinary retention

Ocular: Miosis

Respiratory: Respiratory depression

Miscellaneous: Physical and psychological dependence, biliary or urinary tract spasm, histamine release

Overdosage Symptoms of overdose include CNS depression, respiratory depression, miosis, apnea, pulmonary edema, convulsions

Toxicology Naloxone 2 mg I.V. with repeat administration as necessary up to a total of 10 mg

Drug Interactions Increased toxicity: CNS depressants

Stability Store at room temperature, protect from freezing

Mechanism of Action Binds to opiate receptors in the CNS, causing inhibition of ascending pain pathways, altering the perception of and response to pain; produces generalized CNS depression

Pharmacodynamics

Onset of action: Oral: 10-60 minutes

Duration: 6-8 hours; enhanced analgesia has been seen in elderly patients on therapeutic dose of narcotics; duration of action may be increased in the elderly

Pharmacokinetics

Metabolism: In the liver

Half-life: 11 hours

Elimination: In urine as glucuronide

Usual Dosage Geriatrics and Adults: Oral, S.C.: 2 mg, up to 3 mg if necessary every 12 hours

Monitoring Parameters Pain relief, respiratory and mental status, blood pressure

Patient Information May cause drowsiness; avoid alcoholic beverages

Nursing Implications Observe patient for oversedation, respiratory depression

Additional Information 2 mg levorphanol I.M. produces analgesia comparable to that produced by 10 mg of morphine I.M.

Special Geriatric Considerations The elderly may be particularly susceptible to the CNS depressant and constipating effects of narcotics (see Pharmacodynamics, Warnings)

Dosage Forms

Levorphanol tartrate:

Injection: 2 mg/mL (1 mL, 10 mL)

Injection (PCA syringe): 0.1 mg/mL (30 mL, 60 mL)

Tablet: 2 mg

Levorphan Tartrate *see* Levorphanol *on previous page*

Levo-T™ *see* Levothyroxine *on this page*

Levothroid® *see* Levothyroxine *on this page*

Levothyroxine *(lee voe thye ROKS een)*

Related Information

I.V. Push Recommended Guidelines *on page 1083*

Brand Names Eltroxin®; Levo-T™; Levothroid®; Levoxyl™; Synthroid®

Synonyms *L*-Thyroxine Sodium; T_4

Generic Available Yes

Therapeutic Category Thyroid Hormone; Thyroid Product

Use Replacement or supplemental therapy in hypothyroidism; pituitary TSH suppressants (thyroid nodules, thyroiditis, multinodular goiter, thyroid cancer), thyrotoxicosis, diagnostic suppression tests

Contraindications Recent myocardial infarction or thyrotoxicosis, uncomplicated by hypothyroidism; uncorrected adrenal insufficiency, hypersensitivity to active or extraneous constituents

Warnings Ineffective for weight reduction; high doses may produce serious or even life-threatening toxic effects particularly when used with some anorectic drugs; use cautiously in patients with pre-existing cardiovascular disease (angina, CHD), elderly since they may be more likely to have compromised cardiovascular functions

Precautions Patients with angina pectoris or other cardiovascular disease; adrenal insufficiency, myxedema, diabetes mellitus and insipidus may have symptoms exaggerated or aggravated; thyroid replacement requires periodic assessment of thyroid status. Chronic hypothyroidism predisposes patients to coronary artery disease.

Adverse Reactions

Cardiovascular: Palpitations, tachycardia, cardiac arrhythmias

Central nervous system: Nervousness, tachycardia, cardiac, headache arrhythmias, insomnia, fever

Dermatologic: Alopecia

Endocrine & metabolic: Excessive bone loss with overtreatment (excess thyroid replacement)

Gastrointestinal: Weight loss, increased appetite, diarrhea, abdominal cramps, vomiting

Neuromuscular & skeletal: Tremors

Miscellaneous: Diaphoresis, heat intolerance

Overdosage Chronic excessive use results in signs and symptoms of hyperthyroidism, weight loss, nervousness, sweating, tachycardia, insomnia, heat intolerance, palpitations, vomiting, psychosis, fever, seizures, angina, arrhythmias, and congestive heart failure in those predisposed

Toxicology Reduce dose or temporarily discontinue therapy; normal hypothalamic-pituitary-thyroid axis will return to normal in 6-8 weeks; serum T_4 levels do not correlate well with toxicity; in massive acute ingestion, reduce GI absorption, administer general supportive care; treat congestive heart failure with digitalis glycosides; excessive adrenergic activity (tachycardia) require propranolol 1-3 mg I.V. over 10 minutes or 80-160 mg orally/day; fever may be treated with acetaminophen

Drug Interactions

Cholestyramine and colestipol decrease the effect of orally administered thyroid replacement

Estrogens increase TBG, thereby decreasing effect of thyroid replacement

Anticoagulants may increase action

Beta-blocker effect is decreased when patients become euthyroid

Serum digitalis concentrations are reduced in hyperthyroidism or when hypothyroid patients are converted to a euthyroid state

Theophylline levels decrease when hypothyroid patients converted to a euthyroid state

Stability Protect tablets from light; do not mix I.V. solution with other I.V. infusion solutions; reconstituted solutions should be used immediately and any unused portions discarded

Mechanism of Action Exact mechanism of action is unknown; however, it is believed the thyroid hormone exerts its many metabolic effects through control of DNA transcription and protein synthesis; involved in normal metabolism, growth, and development; promotes gluconeogenesis, increases utilization and mobilization of glycogen stores and stimulates protein synthesis, increases basal metabolic rate

Pharmacodynamics

Onset of action:

Oral: Therapeutic effects require 3-5 days

I.V.: Within 6-8 hours, with maximum effect within 24 hours; 4-6 weeks may be required to see maximal effect for each dose

Pharmacokinetics

Absorption: Oral: Erratic, 48% to 79%; T_3 is 95% absorbed

Distribution: 80% of T_3 is derived from monodeiodination of T_4 in the periphery (liver, kidneys, other tissues)

Half-life: 6-7 days for T_4 and 1-2 days for T_3

Time to peak serum concentrations: Within 2-4 hours

Elimination: As conjugated forms in feces, bile

Usual Dosage Geriatrics and Adults: Dosage should be individualized and response monitored both clinically and with appropriate laboratory (TSH, T_4) (see Additional Information)

Oral: 12.5-25 mcg/day to start, then increase by 25-50 mcg/day at intervals of 2-4 weeks; average adult dose: 100-200 mcg/day; many elderly can be safely initiated on 25 mcg/day

I.M., I.V.: 50% of oral dose

Myxedema coma or stupor: I.V.: 200-500 mcg one time, then 100-300 mcg the next day if necessary; normal T_4 levels achieved in 24 hours; T_3 normalizes in 3 days; maintenance: 0.05-1 mg/day; begin oral therapy as soon as patient is stabilized

Thyroid suppression therapy: 2.6 mcg/kg/day for 7-10 days

(Continued)

Levothyroxine (Continued)

Monitoring Parameters T_4, TSH, heart rate, blood pressure, clinical signs of hypo- and hyperthyroidism; TSH is the most reliable guide for evaluating adequacy of thyroid replacement dosage. TSH may be elevated during the first few months of thyroid replacement despite patients being clinically euthyroid. In cases where T_4 remains low and TSH is within normal limits, an evaluation of "free" (unbound) T_4 is needed to evaluate further increase in dosage

Reference Range

TSH: 0.4-10 (for those ≥80 years) mIU/L

T_4: 4-12 µg/dL (SI: 51-154 nmol/L)

T_3 (RIA) (total T_3): 80-230 ng/dL (SI: 1.2-3.5 nmol/L)

T_4 free (Free T_4): 0.7-1.8 ng/dL (SI: 9-23 pmol/L)

Test Interactions Increased calcium (S); many drugs may have effects on thyroid function tests; para-aminosalicylic acid, aminoglutethimide, amiodarone, barbiturates, carbamazepine, chloral hydrate, clofibrate, colestipol, corticosteroids, danazol, diazepam, estrogens, ethionamide, fluorouracil, I.V. heparin, insulin, lithium, methadone, methimazole, mitotane, nitroprusside, oxyphenbutazone, phenylbutazone, PTU, perphenazine, phenytoin, propranolol, salicylates, sulfonylureas, and thiazides

Patient Information Do not change brands without physician's knowledge; report immediately to physician any chest pain, increased pulse, palpitations, heat intolerance, excessive sweating; do not stop use without physician's advice; replacement therapy will be for life; take as a single dose before breakfast

Nursing Implications I.V. form must be prepared immediately prior to administration; dilute 200 mcg/mL vial with 2 mL of 0.9% sodium chloride injection and shake well until a clear solution is obtained; should not be admixed with other solutions (see Monitoring Parameters, Reference Range, Warnings, and Special Geriatric Considerations)

Additional Information Levothroid® tablets contain lactose. To convert doses: Levothyroxine 0.05-0.06 mg is equivalent to 60 mg thyroid USP; 60 mg thyroglobulin; 4.5 mg thyroid strong; 1 grain (60 mg) liotrix.

Special Geriatric Considerations The elderly do not have a change in serum thyroxine associated with aging; however, plasma T_3 concentrations are decreased 25% to 40% in the elderly. There is not a compensatory rise in thyrotropin suggesting that lower T_3 is not reacted upon as a deficiency by the pituitary. This indicates a slightly lower than normal dosage of thyroid hormone replacement is usually sufficient in older patients than in younger adult patients. TSH must be monitored since insufficient thyroid replacement (elevated TSH) is a risk for coronary artery disease and excessive replacement (low TSH) may cause signs of hyperthyroidism and excessive bone loss. Some clinicians suggest levothyroxine is the drug of choice for replacement therapy (see Usual Dosage and Overdosage).

Dosage Forms

Levothyroxine sodium:

Powder for injection, lyophilized: 200 mcg/vial (6 mL, 10 mL); 500 mcg/vial (6 mL, 10 mL)

Tablet: 25 mcg, 50 mcg, 75 mcg, 88 mcg, 100 mcg, 112 mcg, 125 mcg, 150 mcg, 175 mcg, 200 mcg, 300 mcg

References

Helfand M and Crapo LM, "Monitoring Therapy in Patients Taking Levothyroxine," *Ann Intern Med*, 1990, 113(6):450-4.

Johnson DG and Campbell S, "Hormonal and Metabolic Agents," *Geriatric Pharmacology*, Bressler R and Katz MD, eds, New York, NY: McGraw-Hill, 1993, 427-50.

Sanders LR, "Pituitary, Thyroid, Adrenal and Parathyroid Diseases in the Elderly," *Geriatric Medicine*, 1990, 475-87.

Sawin CT, Geller A, Hershman JM, et al, "The Aging Thyroid. The Use of Thyroid Hormone in Older Persons," *JAMA*, 1989, 261(18):2653-5.

Watts NB, "Use of a Sensitive Thyrotropin Assay for Monitoring Treatment With Levothyroxine," *Arch Intern Med*, 1989, 149(2):309-12.

Lidex-E® *see* Fluocinonide *on page 392*

Lidocaine (LYE doe kane)
Related Information
Serum Drug Concentrations Commonly Monitored: Guidelines *on page 1114*
Brand Names
Anestacon®; Dermaflex® Gel; Dilocaine®; Dr Scholl's® Cracked Heel Relief Cream [OTC]; Duo-Trach®; LidoPen® Auto-Injector; Nervocaine®; Octocaine®; Solarcaine® Aloe Extra Burn Relief [OTC]; Xylocaine®; Zilactin-L® [OTC]
Synonyms
Lignocaine Hydrochloride
Generic Available
Yes
Therapeutic Category
Antiarrhythmic Agent, Class I-B; Local Anesthetic, Injectable; Local Anesthetic, Topical
Use
Local anesthetic and acute treatment of ventricular arrhythmias from myocardial infarction, cardiac manipulation, digitalis intoxication
Contraindications
Known hypersensitivity to amide-type local anesthetics; patients with Adams-Stokes syndrome or with severe degree of S-A, A-V, or intraventricular heart block (without a pacemaker); Wolff-Parkinson-White syndrome
Warnings
Do not use preparations containing preservatives for spinal or epidural (including caudal) anesthesia
Precautions
Hepatic disease, heart failure, marked hypoxia, severe respiratory depression, hypovolemia or shock; incomplete heart block or bradycardia, atrial fibrillation
Adverse Reactions
Cardiovascular: Bradycardia, hypotension, heart block, arrhythmias, cardiovascular collapse

Central nervous system: Lethargy, coma, agitation, slurred speech, seizures, anxiety, euphoria, hallucinations, lightheadedness, nervousness, drowsiness, confusion

Gastrointestinal: Nausea, vomiting

Neuromuscular & skeletal: Twitching, tremors, paresthesia

Ocular: Blurred vision, diplopia

Otic: Tinnitus

Respiratory: Depression or arrest
Overdosage
Symptoms of overdose include convulsions, respiratory failure, bradycardia, hypotension, cardiovascular collapse, euphoria, tinnitus
Toxicology
Treatment is primarily symptomatic and supportive. Termination of anesthesia by pneumatic tourniquet inflation should be attempted when the agent is administered by infiltration or regional injection. Seizures commonly respond to diazepam, while hypotension responds to I.V. fluids and Trendelenburg positioning. Bradyarrhythmias (when the heart rate is <60) can be treated with I.V., I.M., or S.C. atropine 15 mcg/kg. With the development of metabolic acidosis, I.V. sodium bicarbonate 0.5-2 mEq/kg and ventilatory assistance should be instituted. Methemoglobinemia should be treated with methylene blue 1-2 mg/kg in a 1% sterile aqueous solution I.V. push over 4-6 minutes repeated up to a total dose of 7 mg/kg.
Drug Interactions
Concomitant cimetidine or propranolol may result in increased serum concentrations of lidocaine with resultant toxicity

Procainamide may have enhanced pharmacologic action on myocardium

Succinylcholine may have prolonged neuromuscular blockade
Stability
I.V. infusion solutions admixed in D_5W are stable for a minimum of 24 hours
Mechanism of Action
Class IB antiarrhythmic; suppresses automaticity of conduction tissue, by increasing electrical stimulation threshold of ventricle, HIS-Purkinje system, and spontaneous depolarization of the ventricles during diastole by a direct action on the tissues; blocks both the initiation and conduction of nerve impulses by decreasing the neuronal membrane's permeability to sodium ions which results in inhibition of depolarization with resultant blockade of conduction
Pharmacodynamics
Onset of action (single bolus dose): 45-90 seconds

Duration: 10-20 minutes
Pharmacokinetics
Distribution: V_d alterable by many patient factors, decreased in congestive heart failure and liver disease

Protein binding: 60% to 80%; binds to alpha$_1$-acid glycoprotein

(Continued)

Lidocaine *(Continued)*

Metabolism: 90% metabolized in liver; substrate CYP3A4; active metabolites monoethylglycinexylidide (MEGX) and glycinexylidide (GX) can accumulate and may cause CNS toxicity

Half-life: Biphasic:
Alpha: 7-30 minutes
Beta: Terminal: Adults: 1.5-2 hours

Usual Dosage Geriatrics and Adults:

Topical: Apply to affected area as needed; maximum: 3 mg/kg/dose; do not repeat within 2 hours

Injectable local anesthetic: Varies with procedure, degree of anesthesia needed, vascularity of tissue, duration of anesthesia required, and physical condition of patient; maximum: 4.5 mg/kg/dose; do not repeat within 2 hours

Antiarrhythmic:
I.M.: 300 mg may be repeated in 1-1.5 hours
I.V.: 50-100 mg bolus over 2-3 minutes; may repeat in 5-10 minutes up to 200-300 mg in a 1-hour period; continuous infusion of 20-50 mcg/kg/minute or 1-4 mg/minute; decrease the dose in patients with congestive heart failure, shock, or hepatic disease

Not dialyzable (0% to 5%)

Monitoring Parameters EKG, blood pressure, pulse, paresthesias

Reference Range Therapeutic: 1.5-4.0 µg/mL (SI: 6.4-17.1 µmol/L), up to 6.0 µg/mL (SI: 25.6 µmol/L) if necessary; Toxic: >8 µg/mL (SI: >34.2 µmol/L)

Nursing Implications Local thrombophlebitis may occur in patients receiving prolonged I.V. infusions; pain with I.M. injection

Special Geriatric Considerations Due to decreases in phase I metabolism and possibly decrease in splanchnic perfusion with age, there may be a decreased clearance or increased half-life in elderly and increased risk for CNS side effects and cardiac effects

Dosage Forms

Lidocaine hydrochloride:
Cream: 2% (56 g)
Injection: 0.5% [5 mg/mL] (50 mL); 1% [10 mg/mL] (2 mL, 5 mL, 10 mL, 20 mL, 30 mL, 50 mL); 1.5% [15 mg/mL] (20 mL); 2% [20 mg/mL] (2 mL, 5 mL, 10 mL, 20 mL, 30 mL, 50 mL); 4% [40 mg/mL] (5 mL); 10% [100 mg/mL] (10 mL); 20% [200 mg/mL] (10 mL, 20 mL)
Injection:
I.M. use: 10% [100 mg/mL] (3 mL, 5 mL)
Direct I.V.: 1% [10 mg/mL] (5 mL, 10 mL); 20 mg/mL (5 mL)
I.V. admixture, preservative free: 4% [40 mg/mL] (25 mL, 30 mL); 10% [100 mg/mL] (10 mL); 20% [200 mg/mL] (5 mL, 10 mL)
I.V. infusion, in D_5W: 0.2% [2 mg/mL] (500 mL); 0.4% [4 mg/mL] (250 mL, 500 mL, 1000 mL); 0.8% [8 mg/mL] (250 mL, 500 mL)
Gel, topical: 2% (30 mL); 2.5% (15 mL)
Liquid, topical: 2.5% (7.5 mL)
Liquid, viscous: 2% (20 mL, 100 mL)
Ointment, topical: 2.5% [OTC], 5% (35 g)
Solution, topical: 2% (15 mL, 240 mL); 4% (50 mL)

LidoPen® Auto-Injector *see Lidocaine on previous page*

Lignocaine Hydrochloride *see Lidocaine on previous page*

Lindane *(LIN dane)*

Brand Names G-well®; Scabene®

Synonyms Benzene Hexachloride; Gamma Benzene Hexachloride; Hexachlorocyclohexane

Generic Available Yes

Therapeutic Category Antiparasitic Agent, Topical; Pediculocide; Scabicidal Agent; Shampoos

Use Treatment of scabies and pediculosis

Contraindications Hypersensitivity to lindane or any component; acutely inflamed skin or raw, weeping surfaces

Warnings Avoid contact with the face, eyes, mucous membranes, and urethral meatus

Precautions Use with caution in patients with existing seizure disorder

Adverse Reactions Seizures have been reported in geriatric patients 4-5 days after application; serum concentration 1 week after application higher than expected; skin and adipose tissue may act as repositories

Central nervous system: Dizziness, restlessness, ataxia, seizures, headache

Dermatologic: Eczematous eruptions, contact dermatitis
Gastrointestinal: Nausea, vomiting
Hematologic: Aplastic anemia
Hepatic: Hepatitis
Renal: Hematuria
Respiratory: Pulmonary edema

Overdosage Symptoms of overdose include vomiting, restlessness, ataxia, seizures, arrhythmia, pulmonary edema, hematuria, hepatitis

Toxicology Absorbed through skin and mucous membranes and GI tract, has occasionally caused serious CNS, hepatic and renal toxicity when used excessively for prolonged periods, or when accidental ingestion has occurred; diazepam 0.01 mg/kg can be used to control seizures

Drug Interactions Oil based hair dressing may increase toxic potential

Mechanism of Action Directly absorbed by parasites and ova through the exoskeleton; stimulates the nervous system resulting in seizures and death of parasitic arthropods

Pharmacokinetics
Absorption: Up to 13% systemically; stored in body fat
Metabolism: By the liver
Elimination: In urine and feces

Usual Dosage Geriatrics and Adults: Topical:
Scabies: Apply a thin layer of lotion and massage it on skin from the neck to the toes. For adults, bathe and remove the drug after 8-12 hours
Pediculosis: 15-30 mL of shampoo is applied and lathered for 4-5 minutes; rinse hair thoroughly and comb with a fine tooth comb to remove nits; repeat treatment in 7 days if lice or nits are still present

Patient Information For topical use only; do not apply to face; avoid getting in eyes, do not bathe prior to application

Nursing Implications Drug should not be administered orally; apply with rubber gloves

Special Geriatric Considerations Because of the potential for systemic absorption and CNS side effects, lindane should be used with caution; not considered a drug of first choice; consider permethrin or crotamiton agent first

Dosage Forms
Cream: 1% (60 g, 454 g)
Lotion: 1% (60 mL, 473 mL, 4000 mL)
Shampoo: 1% (60 mL, 473 mL, 4000 mL)

Lioresal® see Baclofen on page 104

Liothyronine (lye oh THYE roe neen)

Brand Names Cytomel® Oral; Triostat™ Injection
Synonyms Sodium L-Triiodothyronine; T₃ Sodium
Generic Available Yes
Therapeutic Category Thyroid Product
Use Replacement or supplemental therapy in hypothyroidism, management of nontoxic goiter, chronic lymphocytic thyroiditis, as an adjunct in thyrotoxicosis and as a diagnostic aid
Unlabeled use: Augmentation therapy with an antidepressant

Contraindications Recent myocardial infarction or thyrotoxicosis, uncomplicated by hypothyroidism; uncorrected adrenal insufficiency, hypersensitivity to active or extraneous constituents

Warnings Ineffective for weight reduction; high doses may produce serious or even life-threatening toxic effects particularly when used with some anorectic drugs; use cautiously in patients with pre-existing cardiovascular disease (angina, CHD), elderly since they may be more likely to have compromised cardiovascular function

Precautions Patients with angina pectoris or other cardiovascular disease; adrenal insufficiency, myxedema, diabetes mellitus and insipidus may have symptoms exaggerated or aggravated; thyroid replacement requires periodic assessment of thyroid status. Chronic hypothyroidism predisposes patients to coronary artery disease.

Adverse Reactions
Cardiovascular: Palpitations, tachycardia, cardiac arrhythmias
Central nervous system: Nervousness, headache, insomnia, fever
Dermatologic: Alopecia
Endocrine & metabolic: Excessive bone loss with overtreatment (excess thyroid replacement)
Gastrointestinal: Weight loss, increased appetite, diarrhea, abdominal cramps, vomiting
(Continued)

Liothyronine *(Continued)*

Neuromuscular & skeletal: Tremors
Miscellaneous: Diaphoresis, heat intolerance

Overdosage Chronic excessive use results in signs and symptoms of hyper-thyroidism, weight loss, nervousness, sweating, tachycardia, insomnia, heat intolerance, palpitations, vomiting, psychosis, fever, seizures, angina, arrhythmias, and congestive heart failure in those predisposed

Toxicology Reduce dose or temporarily discontinue therapy; normal hypothalamic-pituitary-thyroid axis will return to normal in 6-8 weeks; serum T_4 levels do not correlate well with toxicity; in massive acute ingestion, reduce GI absorption, administer general supportive care; treat congestive heart failure with digitalis glycosides; excessive adrenergic activity (tachycardia) require propranolol 1-3 mg I.V. over 10 minutes or 80-160 mg orally/day; fever may be treated with acetaminophen

Drug Interactions

Cholestyramine and colestipol decrease the effect of orally administered thyroid replacement

Estrogens increase TBG, thereby decreasing effect of thyroid replacement

Anticoagulants may increase action

Beta-blocker effect is decreased when patients become euthyroid

Serum digitalis concentrations are reduced in hyperthyroidism or when hypothyroid patients are converted to a euthyroid state

Theophylline concentrations decrease when hypothyroid patients converted to a euthyroid state

Stability Store between 2°C to 8°C (36°F to 46°F)

Mechanism of Action The primary active compound is T_3 (triiodothyronine), which may be converted from T_4 (thyroxine) and then circulates throughout the body to influence growth and maturation of various tissues; exact mechanism of action is unknown; however, it is believed the thyroid hormone exerts its many metabolic effects through control of DNA transcription and protein synthesis; involved in normal metabolism, growth, and development; promotes gluconeogenesis, increases utilization and mobilization of glycogen stores, and stimulates protein synthesis, increases basal metabolic rate

Pharmacodynamics

Onset of effects: Within 24-72 hours
Duration: 72 hours

Pharmacokinetics

Absorption: Oral: Well absorbed, ~85% to 90%
Metabolism: Liver metabolism to inactive conjugated compounds
Half-life: 1-2 days
Elimination: In urine

Usual Dosage See Additional Information

Hypothyroidism:

Geriatrics: Initial: 5 mcg/day, increase dose 5 mcg/day every 1-2 weeks; usual maintenance dose: 25-75 mcg/day in divided doses

Adults: Initial: 25 mcg/day; increase by 12.5-25 mcg/day at 1- to 2-week intervals; administer in divided doses

Nontoxic goiter: 5 mcg/day, increase by 5-10 mcg/day at 1- to 2-week intervals; use 5 mcg increments in elderly

T_3 suppression test: 75-100 mcg/day for 7 days; use lowest dose for elderly

Myxedema: 5 mcg/day; increase 5-10 mcg/day at 1- to 2-week intervals; usual maintenance dose: 50-100 mcg/day; use 5 mcg increments in elderly

Monitoring Parameters T_4, TSH, heart rate, blood pressure, clinical signs of hypo- and hyperthyroidism; TSH is the most reliable guide for evaluating adequacy of thyroid replacement dosage. TSH may be elevated during the first few months of thyroid replacement despite patients being clinically euthyroid. In cases where T_4 remains low and TSH is within normal limits, an evaluation of "free" (unbound) T_4 is needed to evaluate further increase in dosage (see Special Geriatric Considerations).

Reference Range Free T_3, Serum: 250-390 pg/dL; TSH: 0.4-10 (for those ≥80 years of age) mIU/L

Test Interactions Increased calcium (S); many drugs may have effects on thyroid function tests; para-aminosalicylic acid, aminoglutethimide, amiodarone, barbiturates, carbamazepine, chloral hydrate, clofibrate, colestipol, corticosteroids, danazol, diazepam, estrogens, ethionamide, fluorouracil, I.V. heparin, insulin, lithium, methadone, methimazole, mitotane, nitroprusside, oxyphenbutazone, phenylbutazone, PTU, perphenazine, phenytoin, propranolol, salicylates, sulfonylureas, and thiazides

Patient Information Do not change brands without physician's knowledge; report immediately to physician any chest pain, increased pulse, palpitations, heat intolerances, excessive sweating; do not stop use without physician's advice; replacement therapy will be for life; take as a single dose before breakfast

Nursing Implications See Monitoring Parameters, Reference Range, Warnings, and Special Geriatric Considerations

Additional Information Short duration action permits fast dosage changes or diminishes toxicity rapidly; the rapid onset and dissipation of action make this a difficult agent to use in those likely to have adverse effects to thyroid such as elderly; if rapid correction of thyroid is needed, T_3 is preferred but use cautiously and with lower recommended doses. 15-37.5 mcg is equivalent to 0.05-0.06 mg levothyroxine; 60 mg thyroid USP; 45 mg Thyroid Strong®, and 60 mg thyroglobulin

Special Geriatric Considerations Elderly do not have a change in serum thyroxine associated with aging; however, plasma T_3 concentrations are decreased 25% to 40% in elderly. There is not a compensatory rise in thyrotropin suggesting that lower T_3 is not reacted upon as a deficiency by the pituitary. This indicates a slightly lower than normal dosage of thyroid hormone replacement is usually sufficient in older patients than in younger adult patients. TSH must be monitored since insufficient thyroid replacement (elevated TSH) is a risk for coronary artery disease and excessive replacement (low TSH) may cause signs of hyperthyroidism and excessive bone loss (see Usual Dosage and Overdosage).

Dosage Forms
Liothyronine sodium:
Injection: 10 mcg/mL (1 mL)
Tablet: 5 mcg, 25 mcg, 50 mcg

References
Helfand M and Crapo LM, "Monitoring Therapy in Patients Taking Levothyroxine," *Ann Intern Med*, 1990, 113(6):450-4.

Johnson DG and Campbell S, "Hormonal and Metabolic Agents," *Geriatric Pharmacology*, Bressler R and Katz MD, eds, New York, NY: McGraw-Hill, 1993, 427-50.

Sanders LR, "Pituitary, Thyroid, Adrenal and Parathyroid Diseases in the Elderly," *Geriatric Medicine*, 1990, 475-87.

Sawin CT, Geller A, Hershman JM, et al, "The Aging Thyroid. The Use of Thyroid Hormone in Older Persons," *JAMA*, 1989, 261(18):2653-5.

Watts NB, "Use of a Sensitive Thyrotropin Assay for Monitoring Treatment With Levothyroxine," *Arch Intern Med*, 1989, 149(2):309-12.

Liotrix (LYE oh triks)

Brand Names Thyrolar®

Synonyms T_3/T_4 Liotrix

Therapeutic Category Thyroid Hormone

Use Replacement or supplemental therapy in hypothyroidism and thyroid cancer

Contraindications Hypersensitivity to liotrix or any component; recent myocardial infarction or thyrotoxicosis, uncomplicated by hypothyroidism; uncorrected adrenal insufficiency, hypersensitivity to active or extraneous constituents

Warnings Ineffective for weight reduction; high doses may produce serious or even life-threatening toxic effects particularly when used with some anorectic drugs; use cautiously in patients with pre-existing cardiovascular disease (angina, CHD), elderly since they may be more likely to have compromised cardiovascular function

Precautions Patients with angina pectoris or other cardiovascular disease; adrenal insufficiency, myxedema, diabetes mellitus and insipidus may have symptoms exaggerated or aggravated; thyroid replacement requires periodic assessment of thyroid status; TSH is the most reliable guide for evaluating adequacy of thyroid replacement dosage. Chronic hypothyroidism predisposes patients to coronary artery disease.

Adverse Reactions
Cardiovascular: Palpitations, tachycardia, cardiac arrhythmias
Central nervous system: Nervousness, headache, insomnia, fever
Dermatologic: Alopecia
Endocrine & metabolic: Excessive bone loss with overtreatment (excess thyroid replacement)
Gastrointestinal: Weight loss, increased appetite, diarrhea, abdominal cramps, vomiting
Neuromuscular & skeletal: Tremors
Miscellaneous: Diaphoresis, heat intolerance
(Continued)

Liotrix (Continued)

Overdosage Chronic excessive use results in signs and symptoms of hyperthyroidism, weight loss, nervousness, sweating, tachycardia, insomnia, heat intolerance, palpitations, vomiting, psychosis, fever, seizures, angina, arrhythmias, and congestive heart failure in those predisposed

Toxicology Reduce dose or temporarily discontinue therapy; normal hypothalamic-pituitary-thyroid axis will return to normal in 6-8 weeks; serum T_4 levels do not correlate well with toxicity; in massive acute ingestion, reduce GI absorption, administer general supportive care; treat congestive heart failure with digitalis glycosides; excessive adrenergic activity (tachycardia) require propranolol 1-3 mg I.V. over 10 minutes or 80-160 mg orally/day; fever may be treated with acetaminophen

Drug Interactions

Cholestyramine and colestipol decrease the effect of orally administered thyroid replacement

Estrogens increase TBG, thereby decreasing effect of thyroid replacement

Anticoagulants may increase action

Beta-blocker effect is decreased when patients become euthyroid

Serum digitalis concentrations are reduced in hyperthyroidism or when hypothyroid patients are converted to a euthyroid state

Theophylline concentrations decrease when hypothyroid patients converted to a euthyroid state

Mechanism of Action Liotrix is uniform mixture of synthetic T_4 and T_3 in 4:1 ratio; exact mechanism of action is unknown; however, it is believed the thyroid hormone exerts its many metabolic effects through control of DNA transcription and protein synthesis; involved in normal metabolism, growth, and development; promotes gluconeogenesis, increases utilization and mobilization of glycogen stores and stimulates protein synthesis, increases basal metabolic rate

Pharmacokinetics

Absorption: 50% to 95% from GI tract

Metabolism: Partially in liver, kidneys, and intestines

Half-life: 6-7 days

Time to peak: 12-48 hours

Elimination: In feces and bile as conjugated metabolites

Usual Dosage See Additional Information

Geriatrics: Initial: 15 mg, adjust dose at 2- to 4-week intervals in increments of 15 mg

Adults: Initial: 15-30 mg, adjust dose at 2- to 4-week intervals in increments of 15 mg

Usual maintenance dose: 60-120 mg/day

Thyroid cancer: Doses will be larger than usual maintenance dose

Monitoring Parameters T_4, TSH, heart rate, blood pressure, clinical signs of hypo- and hyperthyroidism; TSH is the most reliable guide for evaluating adequacy of thyroid replacement dosage. TSH may be elevated during the first few months of thyroid replacement despite patients being clinically euthyroid. In cases where T_4 remains low and TSH is within normal limits, an evaluation of "free" (unbound) T_4 is needed to evaluate further increase in dosage (see Special Geriatric Considerations).

Reference Range

TSH: 0.4-10 (for those ≥80 years) mIU/L

T_4: 4-12 µg/dL (SI: 51-154 nmol/L)

T_3 (RIA) (total T_3): 80-230 ng/dL (SI: 1.2-3.5 nmol/L)

T_4 free (Free T_4): 0.7-1.8 ng/dL (SI: 9-23 pmol/L)

Test Interactions Increased calcium (S); many drugs may have effects on thyroid function tests; para-aminosalicylic acid, aminoglutethimide, amiodarone, barbiturates, carbamazepine, chloral hydrate, clofibrate, colestipol, corticosteroids, danazol, diazepam, estrogens, ethionamide, fluorouracil, I.V. heparin, insulin, lithium, methadone, methimazole, mitotane, nitroprusside, oxyphenbutazone, phenylbutazone, PTU, perphenazine, phenytoin, propranolol, salicylates, sulfonylureas, and thiazides

Patient Information Do not change brands without physician's knowledge; report immediately to physician any chest pain, increased pulse, palpitations, heat intolerances, excessive sweating; do not stop use without physician's advice; replacement therapy will be for life; take as a single dose before breakfast

Nursing Implications See Warnings, Monitoring Parameters, Reference Range, and Special Geriatric Considerations

Additional Information Since T_3 is produced by monodeiodination of T_4 in peripheral tissues (80%) and since elderly have decreased T_3 (25% to 40%), little advantage to this product exists and cost is not justified; no advantage over synthetic levothyroxine sodium; 1 grain (60 mg) liotrix is equivalent to 0.05-0.06 mg levothyroxine; 60 mg thyroid USP and thyroglobulin; and 45 mg of Thyroid Strong®

Special Geriatric Considerations Elderly do not have a change in serum thyroxine associated with aging; however, plasma T_3 concentrations are decreased 25% to 40% in elderly. There is not a compensatory rise in thyrotropin suggesting that lower T_3 is not reacted upon as a deficiency by the pituitary. This indicates a slightly lower than normal dosage of thyroid hormone replacement is usually sufficient in older patients than in younger adult patients. TSH must be monitored since insufficient thyroid replacement (elevated TSH) is a risk for coronary artery disease and excessive replacement (low TSH) may cause signs of hyperthyroidism and excessive bone loss (see Usual Dosage and Overdosage).

Dosage Forms Tablet: 30 mg, 60 mg, 120 mg, 180 mg (thyroid equivalent)

References

Helfand M and Crapo LM, "Monitoring Therapy in Patients Taking Levothyroxine," *Ann Intern Med*, 1990, 113(6):450-4.

Johnson DG and Campbell S, "Hormonal and Metabolic Agents," *Geriatric Pharmacology*, Bressler R and Katz MD, eds, New York, NY: McGraw-Hill, 1993, 427-50.

Sanders LR, "Pituitary, Thyroid, Adrenal and Parathyroid Diseases in the Elderly," *Geriatric Medicine*, 1990, 475-87.

Sawin CT, Geller A, Hershman JM, et al, "The Aging Thyroid. The Use of Thyroid Hormone in Older Persons," *JAMA*, 1989, 261(18):2653-5.

Watts NB, "Use of a Sensitive Thyrotropin Assay for Monitoring Treatment With Levothyroxine," *Arch Intern Med*, 1989, 149(2):309-12.

Lipancreatin *see* Pancrelipase *on page 712*

Lipitor® *see* Atorvastatin *on page 91*

Liquibid® *see* Guaifenesin *on page 437*

Liquid Paraffin *see* Mineral Oil *on page 628*

Liquid Pred® *see* Prednisone *on page 776*

Liquifilm® Forte Solution [OTC] *see* Artificial Tears *on page 82*

Liquifilm® Tears Solution [OTC] *see* Artificial Tears *on page 82*

Liquiprin® [OTC] *see* Acetaminophen *on page 16*

Lisinopril (lyse IN oh pril)

Related Information

ACE Inhibitors Comparison *on page 1019*

Brand Names Prinivil®; Zestril®

Generic Available No

Therapeutic Category Angiotensin-Converting Enzyme (ACE) Inhibitors

Use Treatment of hypertension, either alone or in combination with other antihypertensive agents; adjunctive therapy in treatment of systolic congestive heart failure

Contraindications Hypersensitivity to lisinopril or any component or any ACE inhibitor

Warnings Neutropenia, agranulocytosis, angioedema, decreased renal function (hypertension, renal artery stenosis, congestive heart failure), hepatic dysfunction (elimination, activation), proteinuria, first-dose hypotension (hypovolemia, CHF, dehydrated patients at risk, eg, diuretic use, elderly), elderly (due to renal function changes)

Precautions Use with caution and modify dosage in patients with renal impairment; use with caution in patients with collagen vascular disease, congestive heart failure, hypovolemia, valvular stenosis, hyperkalemia (>5.7 mEq/L), anesthesia

Adverse Reactions

Cardiovascular: Hypotension, tachycardia, arrhythmias, orthostatic blood pressure changes, angina, palpitations, chest pain, syncope, myocardial infarction, CVA, flushing, peripheral edema

Central nervous system: Nervousness, depression, confusion, somnolence, fatigue, dizziness, headache, insomnia, malaise, vertigo, fever

Dermatologic: Rash, pruritus, urticaria, angioedema

Endocrine & metabolic: Hyperkalemia

Gastrointestinal: Pancreatitis, constipation, anorexia, nausea, vomiting, diarrhea, abdominal pain, xerostomia, dysgeusia, dyspepsia, flatulence, pancreatitis, ageusia

Genitourinary: Impotence, decreased libido, azotemia (progressive)

Hematologic: Anemia, neutropenia, agranulocytosis

Hepatic: Hepatitis, hepatocellular/cholestatic jaundice

(Continued)

Lisinopril *(Continued)*

Neuromuscular & skeletal: Myalgia, arthralgia, muscle cramps, arthritis, paresthesia, weakness

Ocular: Blurred vision

Renal: Oliguria, proteinuria, increased BUN, serum creatinine

Respiratory: Chronic cough (nonproductive, persistent; more often in women and seen in 15% to 30% of patients), asthma, bronchitis, bronchospasm, dyspnea, sinusitis

Miscellaneous: Diaphoresis

Overdosage Symptoms of overdose include hypotension

Toxicology Following initiation of essential overdose management, toxic symptom treatment and supportive treatment should be initiated. Hypotension usually responds to I.V. fluids or Trendelenburg positioning. If unresponsive to these measures, the use of a parenteral inotrope may be required (eg, norepinephrine 0.1-0.2 mcg/kg/minute titrated to response). Seizures commonly respond to diazepam (I.V. 5-10 mg bolus in adults every 15 minutes if needed up to a total of 30 mg) or to phenytoin or phenobarbital.

Drug Interactions

ACE inhibitors (captopril) and potassium-sparing diuretics may cause additive hyperkalemic effect

ACE inhibitors (captopril) and indomethacin or nonsteroidal anti-inflammatory agents may cause reduced antihypertensive response to ACE inhibitors

Allopurinol and ACE inhibitors (captopril) may cause neutropenia

Antacids and ACE inhibitors may decrease absorption of ACE inhibitors

Phenothiazines and ACE inhibitors may increase ACE inhibitor effect

Probenecid and ACE inhibitors (captopril) may increase ACE inhibitors (captopril) levels

Rifampin and ACE inhibitors (enalapril) may decrease ACE inhibitor effect

Digoxin and ACE inhibitors may increase serum digoxin concentrations

Lithium and ACE inhibitors may increase lithium serum concentration

Tetracycline and ACE inhibitors (quinapril) may decrease tetracycline absorption (up to 37%)

Capsaicin may enhance or cause cough associated with ACE inhibitors

Food decreases captopril absorption; rate, but not extent, of ramipril and fosinopril is reduced by concomitant administration with food; food does not reduce absorption of enalapril, lisinopril, or benazepril

Mechanism of Action Competitive inhibitor of angiotensin-converting enzyme (ACE); prevents conversion of angiotensin I to angiotensin II, a potent vasoconstrictor; results in lower levels of angiotensin II which causes an increase in plasma renin activity and a reduction in aldosterone secretion; a CNS mechanism may also be involved in hypotensive effect as angiotensin II increases adrenergic outflow from CNS; vasoactive kallikreins may be decreased in conversion to active hormones by ACE inhibitors, thus reducing blood pressure

Pharmacodynamics Oral:

Onset of action: Within 1 hour

Peak effects: Within 6 hours

Duration: 24 hours

Pharmacokinetics

Absorption: Oral: Well absorbed

Protein binding: 25%

Half-life: 11-12 hours

Time to peak concentration: 6-7 hours; unaffected by food

Elimination: Almost entirely in urine as unchanged drug (100%)

Usual Dosage

Geriatrics: Initial: 2.5-5 mg/day; increase doses 2.5-5 mg/day at 1- to 2-week intervals; maximum daily dose: 40 mg

Adults: Initial: 10 mg/day; increase doses 5-10 mg/day at 1- to 2-week intervals; maximum daily dose: 40 mg

Congestive heart failure: Initial: 2.5-5 mg/day; titrate dose slowly over several weeks to a "target dose" of 20 mg once daily; do not exceed 20 mg/day

Patients taking diuretics should have them discontinued 2-3 days prior to initiating lisinopril if possible; restart diuretic after blood pressure is stable if needed; in patients with hyponatremia (<130 mEq/L), start dose at 2.5 mg/day

Dosing adjustment in renal impairment: Cl_{cr} <30 mL/minute: Drug is eliminated (100%) renally; start doses at lowest recommended dose (2.5 mg) and adjust dose at 1- to 2-week intervals based upon blood pressure response; titrate dose until blood pressure is controlled or a maximum dose of 40 mg/day is attained

Monitoring Parameters Serum potassium concentration, BUN, serum creatinine, WBC

Test Interactions Increased potassium (S); increased serum creatinine/BUN

Patient Information Do not stop therapy except under prescriber advice; notify physician if you develop sore throat, fever, swelling of hands, feet, face, eyes, lips, and tongue; difficult breathing, irregular heartbeats, chest pains, or cough. May cause dizziness, fainting, and lightheadedness, especially in first week of therapy, sit and stand up slowly; may cause changes in taste or rash; do not add a salt substitute (potassium) without advice of physician.

Nursing Implications Watch for hypotensive effect within 1-3 hours of first dose or new higher dose (see Precautions, Warnings, Monitoring Parameters, and Special Geriatric Considerations)

Special Geriatric Considerations Due to frequent decreases in glomerular filtration (also creatinine clearance) with aging, elderly patients may have exaggerated responses to ACE inhibitors; differences in clinical response due to hepatic changes are not observed. ACE inhibitors may be preferred agents in elderly patients with congestive heart failure and diabetes mellitus. Diabetic proteinuria is reduced and insulin sensitivity is enhanced. In general, the side effect profile is favorable in elderly and causes little or no CNS confusion; use lowest dose recommendations initially.

Dosage Forms Tablet: 2.5 mg, 5 mg, 10 mg, 20 mg, 40 mg

References

Konstam MA, Drakup K, Baker DW, et al, "Heart Failure: Evaluation and Care of Patients With Left Ventricular Systolic Dysfunction," *Clinical Practice Guideline No 11*, Rockville, MD: Agency for Health Care Policy and Research, Public Health Service, U.S. Department of Health and Human Services, 1994.

McAreavey D and Robertson JIS, "Angiotensin Converting Enzyme Inhibitors and Moderate Hypertension," *Drugs*, 1990, 40(3):326-45.

Williams JF, Bristow MR, Fowler MB, et al, "Guidelines for the Evaluation and Management of Heart Failure: Report of the American College of Cardiology/American Heart Association Task Force on Practice Guidelines (Committee on Evaluation and Management of Heart Failure)," *J Am Coll Cardiol*, 1995, 26:1376-8.

Listermint® with Fluoride [OTC] *see* Fluoride on page 392

Lithane® *see* Lithium on this page

Lithium (LITH ee um)

Related Information

Antacid Drug Interactions on page 1096

Serum Drug Concentrations Commonly Monitored: Guidelines on page 1114

Brand Names Eskalith®; Lithane®; Lithobid®; Lithonate®; Lithotabs®

Generic Available Yes

Therapeutic Category Antimanic Agent

Use Treatment of manic episodes in bipolar disorders; prevention of subsequent manic episodes

Contraindications Hypersensitivity to lithium or any component; severe cardiovascular or renal disease

Warnings Lithium toxicity is closely related to serum concentration and can occur at therapeutic doses; serum lithium determinations are required to monitor therapy; concomitant use of lithium with thiazide diuretics may decrease renal excretion and enhance lithium toxicity; lithium dosage may need to be reduced by 30%

Precautions Use with caution in patients with cardiovascular or thyroid disease

Adverse Reactions

Cardiovascular: Arrhythmias, sinus node dysfunction

Central nervous system: Sedation, confusion, somnolence, seizures, fatigue, headache, vertigo

Dermatologic: Rash

Endocrine & metabolic: Nephrogenic diabetes insipidus (thirst, polyuria, polydipsia), goiter, hypothyroidism

Gastrointestinal: Nausea, diarrhea, vomiting, xerostomia

Hematologic: Leukocytosis

Neuromuscular & skeletal: Muscle hyperirritability (twitching, fasciculations), tremors, muscle weakness

Overdosage Symptoms of overdose include sedation, confusion, tremors, joint pain, visual changes, seizures, coma

Toxicology There is no specific antidote for lithium poisoning. In the acute ingestion, following initiation of essential overdose management, correction of fluid and electrolyte imbalances should be commenced. Activated charcoal (Continued)

Lithium *(Continued)*

may not be effective in adsorbing lithium but is not harmful if used. Theophylline, mannitol and urea have all been shown to decrease serum lithium concentration by enhancing its elimination, but hemodialysis is the treatment of choice for severe intoxications.

Drug Interactions
Decreased effect with xanthines (eg, theophylline, caffeine)
Increased effect/toxicity of CNS depressants, iodide salts (increased hypothyroid effect), neuromuscular blockers
Increased toxicity with thiazide diuretics, NSAIDs, haloperidol, phenothiazines (neurotoxicity), carbamazepine, fluoxetine, ACE inhibitors

Mechanism of Action Alters cation transport across cell membrane in nerve and muscle cells and influences reuptake of serotonin and/or norepinephrine

Pharmacokinetics
Distribution: Adults:
V_d: Initial: 0.3-0.4 L/kg
V_{dss}: 0.7-1 L/kg
Half-life: Terminal: 18-24 hours, can increase to more than 36 hours in elderly or patients with renal impairment
Time to peak serum concentration: Oral: Within 0.5-2 hours following absorption (nonsustained release product)
Elimination: 90% to 98% of dose excreted in urine as unchanged drug; other excretory routes include feces (1%) and sweat (4% to 5%)

Usual Dosage Monitor serum concentrations and clinical response (efficacy and toxicity) to determine proper dose. Total daily dose will be decreased in patients with renal impairment. Oral:

Geriatrics: Initial dose: 300 mg twice daily, increase weekly in increments of 300 mg/day, monitoring levels; rarely need to go >900-1200 mg/day
Adults: 300 mg 3-4 times/day; usual maximum maintenance dose: 2.4 g/day
Dosing adjustment in renal impairment:
Cl_{cr} 10-50 mL/minute: Administer 50% to 75% of normal dose
Cl_{cr} <10 mL/minute: Administer 25% to 50% of normal dose
Dialyzable (50% to 100%)

Monitoring Parameters Lithium serum concentrations, fluid status, serum electrolytes, renal function

Reference Range Therapeutic: 0.6-1.2 mEq/L (SI: 0.6-1.2 mmol/L), for acute mania; 0.8-1 mEq/L (SI: 0.8-1 mmol/L) for protection against future episodes in most patients with bipolar disorder. A higher rate of relapse is described in subjects who are maintained below 0.4 mEq/L (SI: 0.4 mmol/L), geriatric patients can usually be maintained at the lower end of the therapeutic range (0.6-0.8 mEq/L); Toxic: >2 mEq/L (SI: >2 mmol/L).

Test Interactions Increased calcium (S), glucose, magnesium, potassium (S); decreased thyroxine (S)

Patient Information Avoid tasks requiring psychomotor coordination until the CNS effects are known, blood level monitoring is required to determine the proper dose; maintain a steady salt and fluid intake especially during the summer months; do not crush or chew slow or controlled release tablets, swallow whole; take with meals

Nursing Implications Administer with meals to decrease GI upset, encourage adequate fluid intake, monitor for signs of toxicity; do not crush slow or controlled release tablets

Additional Information Lithium levels should be obtained 12 hours after the last dose of the day; 5 mL of lithium citrate syrup contains 8 mEq of lithium and is approximately equivalent to 300 mg of lithium carbonate
Lithium citrate: Cibalith-S®
Lithium carbonate: Eskalith®, Lithane®, Lithobid®, Lithonate®, Lithotabs®

Special Geriatric Considerations Some elderly patients may be extremely sensitive to the effects of lithium; initial doses need to be adjusted for renal function in elderly; thereafter, adjust doses based upon serum concentrations and response (see Usual Dosage and Reference Range)

Dosage Forms
Lithium carbonate:
Capsule: 150 mg, 300 mg, 600 mg
Tablet: 300 mg
Tablet:
Controlled release: 450 mg
Slow release: 300 mg
Syrup, as citrate: 300 mg/5 mL (5 mL, 10 mL, 480 mL)

References
Foster JF, Gershell WJ, and Goldfarb AI, "Lithium Treatment in the Elderly. I. Clinical Usage," *J Gerontol*, 1977, 32(3):299-302.

Hicks R, Dysken MW, Davis JM, et al, "The Pharmacokinetics of Psychotropic Medication in the Elderly: A Review," *J Clin Psychiatry*, 1981, 42(10):374-85.

Lithobid® *see* Lithium *on page 545*

Lithonate® *see* Lithium *on page 545*

Lithotabs® *see* Lithium *on page 545*

8-L-Lysine Vasopressin *see* Lypressin *on page 559*

Locoid® *see* Hydrocortisone *on page 462*

Lodine® *see* Etodolac *on page 363*

Lodine® XL *see* Etodolac *on page 363*

Lodosyn® *see* Carbidopa *on page 164*

Lodoxamide Tromethamine
(loe DOKS a mide troe METH a meen)

Brand Names Alomide® Ophthalmic

Therapeutic Category Ophthalmic Agent, Miscellaneous

Use Treatment of vernal keratoconjunctivitis, vernal conjunctivitis, and vernal keratitis

Contraindications Hypersensitivity to any component of product

Warnings Not for injection; not for use in patients wearing soft contact lenses during treatment

Adverse Reactions
Central nervous system: Headache, dizziness, somnolence
Dermatologic: Rash
Gastrointestinal: Nausea, stomach discomfort
Ocular: Blurred vision, corneal erosion/ulcer, eye pain, corneal abrasion, blepharitis; transient burning, stinging, discomfort
Respiratory: Sneezing, dry nose

Overdosage Symptoms of overdose include feeling of warmth, headache, dizziness, fatigue, sweating, nausea, and loose stools following oral administration

Toxicology Consider emesis in the event of accidental ingestion

Mechanism of Action Mast cell stabilizer that inhibits the *in vivo* type I immediate hypersensitivity reaction to increase cutaneous vascular permeability associated with IgE and antigen-mediated reactions

Pharmacokinetics Absorption: Topical: Very small and undetectable

Usual Dosage Geriatrics and Adults: Instill 1-2 drops in eye(s) 4 times/day for up to 3 months

Patient Information May sting or burn upon instillation; do not touch dropper to the eye

Special Geriatric Considerations Assure the patient or caregiver can adequately administer ophthalmic medication

Dosage Forms Solution, ophthalmic: 0.1% (10 mL)

Lofene® *see* Diphenoxylate and Atropine *on page 303*

Logen® *see* Diphenoxylate and Atropine *on page 303*

Lomanate® *see* Diphenoxylate and Atropine *on page 303*

Lomefloxacin (loe me FLOKS a sin)

Related Information
Antacid Drug Interactions *on page 1096*
Cephalosporins, Aminoglycosides, Macrolides, & Quinolones *on page 1014*

Brand Names Maxaquin®

Therapeutic Category Antibiotic, Quinolone

Use Quinolone antibiotic for skin and skin structure, lower respiratory and urinary tract infections, and sexually transmitted diseases; prophylaxis preoperatively to transurethral procedures

Contraindications Hypersensitivity to lomefloxacin or other members of the quinolone group such as nalidixic acid, oxolinic acid, cinoxacin, norfloxacin, and ciprofloxacin

Warnings Use with caution in patients with epilepsy or other CNS diseases which could predispose them to seizures

Adverse Reactions
Cardiovascular: Hyper- and hypotension, syncope, bradycardia, tachycardia, arrhythmias, angina, cardiac failure, flushing, facial edema
Central nervous system: Fatigue, malaise, seizures, vertigo, headache, dizziness, coma
(Continued)

Lomefloxacin (Continued)

Dermatologic: Rash, photosensitivity

Gastrointestinal: Abdominal pain, nausea, vomiting, flatulence, constipation, tongue discoloration, dysgeusia, diarrhea, xerostomia, pseudomembranous colitis

Genitourinary: Micturition disorder

Hematologic: Thrombocytopenia purpura

Neuromuscular & skeletal: Tremors, gout, myalgia, leg cramps, hyperkinesia, paresthesia

Renal: Dysuria, hematuria, anuria

Respiratory: Dyspnea

Miscellaneous: Flu-like symptoms, decreased heat tolerance, diaphoresis

Overdosage Symptoms of overdose include acute renal failure, seizures

Toxicology GI decontamination and supportive care; diazepam for seizures; not removed by peritoneal or hemodialysis

Drug Interactions

Decreased effect: Bismuth subsalicylate, antacids (aluminum, magnesium), iron salts, zinc salts, sucralfate

Increased levels: Probenecid, cimetidine

Increased levels/effect/toxicity: Warfarin, cyclosporine, NSAIDs (increased seizures)

Mechanism of Action Exerts a broad spectrum antimicrobial effect. The primary target of the fluoroquinolones is DNA gyrase (topoisomerase II), an essential bacterial enzyme that maintains the superhelical structure of DNA. DNA gyrase is required for DNA replication and transcription, DNA repair, recombination, and transposition.

Pharmacokinetics

Absorption: Well absorbed

Distribution: V_d: 2.4-3.5 L/kg

Protein binding: 20%

Half-life, elimination: 5-7.5 hours; prolonged to a mean of 12.7 hours in middle age and elderly patients

Elimination: Primarily unchanged in urine

Usual Dosage Geriatrics and Adults: Oral: 400 mg once daily for 10-14 days

Dosing adjustment in renal impairment: Cl_{cr} >10 but <40 mL/minute/1.73 m^2: Administer 400 mg first dose, followed by 200 mg/day for a total of 10-14 days

Monitoring Parameters Signs and symptoms of infection, WBC, mental status

Patient Information Take 1 hour before or 2 hours after meals

Nursing Implications See Warnings and Adverse Reactions

Special Geriatric Considerations Dosage adjustment not necessary in patients with normal renal function; otherwise follow dosage guidelines in renal impairment; age-associated increase in half-life and decrease in clearance thought to be secondary to age-related changes in renal function

Dosage Forms Tablet, as hydrochloride: 400 mg

References

Kovarik JM, Hoepelman AI, Smit JM, et al, "Steady-State Pharmacokinetics and Sputum Penetration of Lomefloxacin in Patients With Chronic Obstructive Pulmonary Disease and Acute Respiratory Tract Infections," Antimicrob Agents Chemother, 1992, 36(11):2458-61.

Lomodix® see Diphenoxylate and Atropine on page 303

Lomotil® see Diphenoxylate and Atropine on page 303

Loniten® see Minoxidil on page 630

Lonox® see Diphenoxylate and Atropine on page 303

Loperamide (loe PER a mide)

Brand Names Diar-aid® [OTC]; Imodium®; Imodium® A-D [OTC]; Kaopectate® II [OTC]; Pepto® Diarrhea Control [OTC]

Therapeutic Category Antidiarrheal

Use Treatment of acute diarrhea and chronic diarrhea associated with inflammatory bowel disease; decrease the volume of ileostomy discharge

Unlabeled use: Treatment of traveler's diarrhea in combination with trimethoprim-sulfamethoxazole (3 days of therapy)

Contraindications Hypersensitivity to loperamide or any component; patients who must avoid constipation; diarrhea resulting from some infections; patients with pseudomembranous colitis; bloody diarrhea

Warnings Should not be used if diarrhea accompanied by high fever, blood in stool, liver disease; may induce toxic megacolon in patients with acute ulcerative colitis; discontinue use in ulcerative colitis if abdominal distention occurs

Precautions Large first-pass metabolism, use with caution in hepatic dysfunction; if clinical improvement is not seen in 48 hours, discontinue use

Adverse Reactions

Central nervous system: Sedation, fatigue, dizziness, drowsiness

Dermatologic: Rash

Gastrointestinal: Nausea, vomiting, constipation, abdominal cramping, xerostomia, abdominal distention

Overdosage Symptoms of overdose include CNS depression, constipation, GI irritation, nausea, vomiting; overdosage is noted when daily doses approximate 60 mg of loperamide

Toxicology Treatment of overdose: Gastric lavage followed by 100 g activated charcoal through a nasogastric tube. Monitor for signs of CNS depression. If they occur, administer naloxone 2 mg I.V.; repeat as necessary. Loperamide has a short duration of action (1-3 hours).

Drug Interactions CNS depressants (antidepressants, antipsychotics, hypnotics, anxiolytics, alcohol) may be enhanced in action

Mechanism of Action Acts directly on intestinal muscles to inhibit peristalsis and prolongs transit time enhancing fluid and electrolyte movement through intestinal mucosa; reduces fecal volume, increases viscosity, and diminishes fluid and electrolyte loss; demonstrates antisecretory activity; exhibits peripheral action

Pharmacodynamics Onset of action: Oral: Occurs within 30-60 minutes

Pharmacokinetics

Absorption: Oral: <40%

Protein binding: 97%

Metabolism: Hepatic metabolism (>50%) to inactive compounds

Half-life: 7-14 hours

Elimination: Fecal and urinary (1%) excretion of metabolites and unchanged drug (30% to 40%)

Usual Dosage Geriatrics and Adults: Oral: Initial: 4 mg (2 capsules), followed by 2 mg after each loose stool, up to 16 mg/day (8 capsules) (see Additional Information)

Monitoring Parameters Monitor stool frequency and consistency; observe for toxicity with use more than 48 hours

Patient Information Do not take more than 8 capsules/80 mL in 24 hours; may cause drowsiness; use caution when driving; may cause dry mouth; notify physician if diarrhea persists or abdominal distention occurs; if diarrhea does not subside in 2-3 days, consult physician when buying without physician's advice.

Nursing Implications Therapy for chronic diarrhea should not exceed 10 days; if diarrhea persists longer than 48 hours for acute diarrhea, etiology should be examined; monitor stool frequency and consistency

Additional Information If clinical improvement is not achieved after 16 mg/day for 10 days, control is unlikely with further use. Continue use if diet or other treatment does not control. Imodium® 2 mg capsules are legend.

Special Geriatric Considerations Elderly are particularly sensitive to fluid and electrolyte loss. This generally results in lethargy, weakness, and confusion. Repletion and maintenance of electrolytes and water are essential in the treatment of diarrhea. Drug therapy must be limited in order to avoid toxicity with this agent.

Dosage Forms

Loperamide hydrochloride:

Caplet: 2 mg

Capsule: 2 mg

Liquid, oral: 1 mg/5 mL (60 mL, 90 mL, 120 mL)

Tablet: 2 mg

Lopid® *see* Gemfibrozil *on page 421*

Lopressor® *see* Metoprolol *on page 619*

Lorabid™ *see* Loracarbef *on this page*

Loracarbef (lor a KAR bef)

Related Information

Cephalosporins, Aminoglycosides, Macrolides, & Quinolones *on page 1014*

Brand Names Lorabid™

Generic Available No

Therapeutic Category Antibiotic, Carbacephem

(Continued)

Loracarbef (Continued)

Use Infections caused by susceptible organisms involving the respiratory tract, acute otitis media, sinusitis, skin and skin structure, bone and joint, and urinary tract and gynecologic

Contraindications Patients with a history of hypersensitivity to loracarbef

Warnings Use with caution in patients with a previous history of hypersensitivity to other cephalosporins; use with caution in patients allergic to other beta-lactams

Adverse Reactions

Cardiovascular: Vasodilation

Central nervous system: Somnolence, nervousness, dizziness, headache

Dermatologic: Skin rashes

Gastrointestinal: Diarrhea, nausea, vomiting, abdominal pain, anorexia, pseudomembranous colitis

Genitourinary: Vaginitis, vaginal moniliasis

Hematologic: Transient thrombocytopenia, leukopenia, eosinophilia

Hepatic: Transient elevations of ALT, AST, and alkaline phosphatase

Renal: Transient elevations of creatinine and BUN

Overdosage Symptoms of overdose include abdominal discomfort, diarrhea

Toxicology Supportive care only

Drug Interactions Increased serum concentration with probenecid

Drug/Food Interactions Decreased bioavailability with food

Stability Suspension may be kept at room temperature for 14 days

Mechanism of Action Inhibits bacterial cell wall synthesis by binding to one or more of the penicillin binding proteins (PBPs); inhibits the final transpeptidation step of peptidoglycan synthesis in bacterial cell walls, thus inhibiting cell wall biosynthesis. It is thought that beta-lactam antibiotics inactivate transpeptidase via acylation of the enzyme with cleavage of the CO-N bond of the beta-lactam ring. Upon exposure to beta-lactam antibiotics, bacteria eventually lyse due to ongoing activity of cell wall autolytic enzymes (autolysins and murein hydrolases) while cell wall assembly is arrested.

Pharmacokinetics

Absorption: Oral: Rapid

Half-life, elimination: ~1 hour

Time to peak serum concentration: Oral: Within 1 hour

Elimination: Plasma clearance: ~200-300 mL/minute

Usual Dosage Oral:

Geriatrics and Adults:

Uncomplicated urinary tract infections: 200 mg once daily for 7 days

Skin and soft tissue: 200-400 mg every 12-24 hours

Upper respiratory tract:

Pharyngitis/tonsillitis: 200 mg every 12 hours for 10 days

Sinusitis: 400 mg every 12 hours for 14 days

Uncomplicated pyelonephritis: 400 mg every 12 hours for 14 days

Dosing comments in renal impairment:

Cl_{cr} ≥50 mL/minute: Administer usual dose

Cl_{cr} 10-49 mL/minute: 50% of usual dose at usual interval

Cl_{cr} <10 mL/minute: Administer usual dose every 3-5 days

Hemodialysis: Doses should be administered after dialysis sessions

Administration Take on an empty stomach

Monitoring Parameters Signs and symptoms of infection, WBC, mental status

Patient Information Take on an empty stomach at least 1 hour before or 2 hours after meals; complete full course of therapy

Nursing Implications See Administration

Special Geriatric Considerations Half-life slightly prolonged with age, presumably due to the reduced creatinine clearance related to aging; adjust dose for renal function (see Usual Dosage)

Dosage Forms

Capsule: 200 mg, 400 mg

Suspension, oral: 100 mg/5 mL (50 mL, 100 mL); 200 mg/5 mL (50 mL, 100 mL)

References

DeSante KA and Zeckel ML, "Pharmacokinetic Profile of Loracarbef," *Am J Med*, 1992, 92(6A):16S-9S.

Loratadine (lor AT a deen)

Brand Names Claritin®

Generic Available No

Therapeutic Category Antihistamine

Use Relief of nasal and non-nasal symptoms of seasonal allergic rhinitis

Contraindications Patients hypersensitive to loratadine or any of its components

Warnings Patients with liver impairment should start with a lower dose (10 mg every other day), since their ability to clear the drug will be reduced

Adverse Reactions
  Central nervous system: Low incidence of fatigue, dizziness, headache, sedation
  No significant anticholinergic effects, though xerostomia has been reported

Overdosage Symptoms of overdose include somnolence, tachycardia, headache

Toxicology No specific antidote is available, treatment is first decontamination, then symptomatic and supportive; loratadine is not eliminated by dialysis

Drug Interactions
  Increased toxicity: Procarbazine, other antihistamines, alcohol
  Increased plasma concentrations of loratadine and its active metabolite with ketoconazole; erythromycin increases the AUC of loratadine and its active metabolite; no change in Q-T$_c$ interval was seen; indinivir, saquinavir, and ritonavir

Mechanism of Action Long-acting tricyclic antihistamine with selective peripheral histamine H$_1$-receptor antagonistic properties

Pharmacokinetics
  Absorption: Rapid
  Metabolism: Extensive to an active metabolite; substrate CYP2D6, 3A4
  Half-life:
    Geriatrics: 18.2 hours (6.7-37 hours)
    Adults: 12-15 hours
  Elimination: In one study, the AUC and peak plasma levels of both loratadine and its active metabolite were approximately 50% higher in elderly patients as compared to younger adults

Usual Dosage Geriatrics and Adults: Oral: 10 mg/day on empty stomach
  Dosing interval in hepatic impairment: 10 mg every other day to start

Monitoring Parameters Relief of symptoms, mental status

Patient Information Drink plenty of water; may cause dry mouth, sedation, drowsiness, and can impair judgment and coordination

Nursing Implications See Monitoring Parameters

Special Geriatric Considerations Loratadine is one of the newer, nonsedating antihistamines; because of its low incidence of side effects, it seems to be a good choice in the elderly. However, there is a wide variation in loratadine half-life reported in the elderly and this should be kept in mind when initiating dosing.

Dosage Forms
  Solution, oral: 1 mg/mL
  Tablet: 10 mg
    Rapid-disintegrating tablets: 10 mg (RediTabs®)

Lorazepam (lor A ze pam)
Related Information
  Antacid Drug Interactions *on page 1096*
  Anxiolytic/Hypnotic Use in Long-Term Care Facilities *on page 1099*
  Benzodiazepines Comparison *on page 1024*
  Federal OBRA Regulations Recommended Maximum Doses - Anxiolytics *on page 1057*
  Federal OBRA Regulations Recommended Maximum Doses - Hypnotics *on page 1057*
  I.V. Push Recommended Guidelines *on page 1083*

Brand Names Ativan®

Generic Available Yes

Therapeutic Category Antianxiety Agent; Benzodiazepine; Hypnotic; Sedative

Use Management of anxiety, status epilepticus, preoperative sedation, and amnesia

Restrictions C-IV

Contraindications Hypersensitivity to lorazepam or any component; there may be a cross-sensitivity with other benzodiazepines; do not use in comatose patients, those with pre-existing CNS depression, narrow-angle glaucoma, severe uncontrolled pain, severe hypotension

Warnings Dilute injection prior to I.V. use with equal volume of compatible diluent (D$_5$W, 0.9% NaCl, sterile water for injection); do **not** inject intra-
(Continued)

Lorazepam *(Continued)*

arterially, arteriospasm and gangrene may occur; injection contains benzyl alcohol 2%, polyethylene glycol and propylene glycol

Precautions Use caution in patients with renal or hepatic impairment, dementia, myasthenia gravis, Parkinson's disease, or a history of drug dependence

Adverse Reactions

Cardiovascular: Cardiac arrest, hypertension or hypotension, bradycardia, circulatory collapse

Central nervous system: Drowsiness, confusion, dizziness, ataxia, amnesia, slurred speech, paradoxical excitement or rage, transitory hallucinations

Gastrointestinal: Constipation, xerostomia, nausea, vomiting

Genitourinary: Urinary incontinence or retention

Local: Phlebitis, pain with injection

Neuromuscular & skeletal: Impaired coordination

Ocular: Blurred vision, diplopia, nystagmus

Respiratory: Decrease in respiratory rate, apnea, laryngospasm

Miscellaneous: Physical and psychological dependence with prolonged use

Overdosage Symptoms of overdose include somnolence, confusion, coma, and diminished reflexes

Toxicology Treatment for benzodiazepine overdose is supportive; rarely is mechanical ventilation required; flumazenil has been shown to selectively block the binding of benzodiazepines to CNS receptors, resulting in a reversal of benzodiazepine-induced sedation; however, its use may not alter the course of overdose

Drug Interactions Increased toxicity: CNS depressants, alcohol

Stability Intact vials should be refrigerated, protect from light; may be stored at room temperature for up to 2 weeks; do not use discolored or precipitate containing solutions

Stability of parenteral admixture at room temperature (25°C): 4 hours

Mechanism of Action Benzodiazepines appear to potentiate the effects of GABA and other inhibitory neurotransmitters by binding to specific benzodiazepine-receptor sites in various areas of the CNS

Pharmacodynamics

Onset of action: I.M.: Hypnosis occurs in ~20-30 minutes

Duration: 6-8 hours

Studies have shown that the elderly are more sensitive to the effects of benzodiazepines as compared to younger adults

Pharmacokinetics

Absorption: Oral, I.M.: Promptly absorbed

Protein binding: 85%; free fraction may be significantly higher in the elderly

Metabolism: In the liver to inactive compounds with urinary excretion and minimal fecal clearance; metabolism is not significantly affected in the elderly

Half-life: 10-16 hours; one study found the half-life in elderly to be 15.9 hours as compared to 14.1 hours in younger adults

Usual Dosage

Anxiety and sedation: Oral:

Geriatrics: Initial: 0.5-1 mg/day in divided doses; initial dose should not exceed 2 mg/day

Adults: 1-10 mg/day in 2-3 divided doses; usual dose: 2-6 mg/day in divided doses

Insomnia: Oral:

Geriatrics: 0.5-1 mg at bedtime

Adults: 2-4 mg at bedtime

Preoperative: Geriatrics and Adults:

I.M.: 0.05 mg/kg administered 2 hours before surgery; maximum: 4 mg/dose

I.V.: 0.044 mg/kg 15-20 minutes before surgery; usual maximum: 2 mg/dose

Operative amnesia: Geriatrics and Adults: I.V.: up to 0.05 mg/kg; maximum: 4 mg/dose

Status epilepticus: Geriatrics and Adults: I.V.: 4 mg/dose given slowly over 2-5 minutes; may repeat in 10-15 minutes; usual maximum dose: 8 mg

Administration See Warnings

Monitoring Parameters Respiratory, cardiovascular and mental status, symptoms of anxiety

Reference Range Therapeutic: 50-240 ng/mL (SI: 156-746 nmol/L)

Test Interactions May increase the results of liver function tests

Patient Information Avoid alcohol and other CNS depressants; may cause drowsiness; avoid activities needing good psychomotor coordination until CNS effects are known; may cause physical or psychological dependence; avoid abrupt discontinuation after prolonged use

Nursing Implications Keep injectable form in the refrigerator; inadvertent intra-arterial injection may produce arteriospasm resulting in gangrene which may require amputation; emergency resuscitative equipment should be available when administering by I.V.; prior to I.V. use, Ativan® injection must be diluted with an equal amount of compatible diluent; injection must be made slowly with repeated aspiration to make sure the injection is not intra-arterial and that perivascular extravasation has not occurred; do not exceed 2 mg/minute, if given faster, lorazepam may cause respiratory depression; provide safety measures (ie, side rails, night light, and call button); remove smoking materials from area; supervise ambulation

Additional Information I.M. lorazepam is rapidly and completely absorbed and, therefore, may be more predictable as compared to I.M. chlordiazepoxide or diazepam

Special Geriatric Considerations Because lorazepam is relatively short-acting with an inactive metabolite, it is a preferred agent to use in elderly patients when a benzodiazepine is indicated (see Pharmacokinetics, Pharmacodynamics, and Usual Dosage)

Dosage Forms
Injection: 2 mg/mL (1 mL, 10 mL); 4 mg/mL (1 mL, 10 mL)
Solution, oral concentrated, alcohol and dye free: 2 mg/mL (30 mL)
Tablet: 0.5 mg, 1 mg, 2 mg

References
Divoll M and Greenblatt DJ, "Effect of Age and Sex on Lorazepam Protein Binding," *J Pharm Pharmacol*, 1982, 34(2):122-3.
Greenblatt DJ, Allen MD, Locniskar A, et al, "Lorazepam Kinetics in the Elderly," *Clin Pharmacol Ther*, 1979, 26(1):103-13.

Lorcet® *see* Hydrocodone and Acetaminophen *on page 461*

Lorcet®-HD *see* Hydrocodone and Acetaminophen *on page 461*

Lorcet® Plus *see* Hydrocodone and Acetaminophen *on page 461*

Lortab® *see* Hydrocodone and Acetaminophen *on page 461*

Losartan (loe SAR tan)

Brand Names Cozaar®; Hyzaar®

Synonyms DuP 753; Losartan and Hydrochlorothiazide; MK594

Therapeutic Category Angiotensin II Antagonists

Use Treatment of hypertension, alone or in combination with other hypertensive medications

Contraindications Hypersensitivity to this product or any of its components

Warnings As with ACE inhibitors, the inhibition of the RAA system may decrease renal function in patients with low perfusion states (eg, CHF, renal failure, and severe reduction with age). ACE inhibitors cause increases in serum creatinine and blood urea nitrogen (BUN) in patients with unilateral or bilateral renal artery stenosis. Losartan may cause similar effects. Patients with intravascular volume depletion (dehydration, diuretics) may experience hypotension; African-American hypertensive patients have a significantly decreased response to losartan than do non-African-American patients which is similar to ACE inhibitors; hepatic impairment results in significant accumulation in losartan (fivefold) and its active metabolite (1.7 times higher) as compared to young adults.

Precautions Use with caution in volume depleted patients since hypotension may be experienced. Correct volume status before initiating losartan; clinically minor increases in serum creatinine and BUN may be seen; clinically insignificant decreases in hematocrit and hemoglobin also noted in studies; elevations in liver enzymes and bilirubin have been reported infrequently.

Adverse Reactions Losartan is well tolerated with reported adverse effects similar to placebo in clinical trials. Adverse drug reactions do not appear to be dose related. Reported side effect rate is low (generally 1% to 3%). No effect in clinical trials on electrolytes, uric acid, triglycerides, glucose, or cholesterol.
Cardiovascular: Flushing
Central nervous system: Anxiety, ataxia, dizziness, insomnia, confusion, depression, memory impairment, nervousness, somnolence, vertigo, abnormal dreams, panic disorder
Dermatologic: Rash, urticaria, pruritus, dermatitis, alopecia, erythema, photosensitivity, dry skin
Gastrointestinal: Diarrhea, constipation, dyspepsia, anorexia, vomiting, flatulence, xerostomia, gastritis, dysgeusia
(Continued)

Losartan *(Continued)*

Genitourinary: Nocturia, polyuria, impotence

Hematologic: Anemia, hemolysis

Neuromuscular & skeletal: Joint edema, muscle cramps, arthralgia, muscle weakness, arthritis, back pain, leg pain, tremors, paresthesia, peripheral neuropathy, musculoskeletal pain, fibromyalgia

Ocular: Burning eyes, blurred vision, conjunctivitis, decreased visual acuity

Otic: Tinnitus

Respiratory: Nasal congestion, cough, sinusitis, dyspnea, bronchitis, epistaxis, upper respiratory infection, rhinitis, lower airway congestion

Miscellaneous: Dental pain

Overdosage Limited data available; symptoms include hypotension, tachycardia, or bradycardia secondary to parasympathetic stimulation

Toxicology Losartan and its active metabolite are not removed by hemodialysis; following initiation of essential overdose management, toxic symptom treatment and supportive treatment should be initiated. Hypotension should respond to I.V. fluids or Trendelenburg positioning. If unresponsive to these measures, the use of a parenteral inotrope may be required (eg, norepinephrine 0.1-0.2 mcg/kg/minute titrated to response). Administer general supportive care.

Drug Interactions Losartan and its active carboxylic acid metabolite are metabolized by the cytochrome P-450 2C9 and 3A4 fractions. Although little data available, practitioners should use caution when giving with drugs metabolized by these fractions. Cimetidine **increases** losartan (18%), but not metabolites; phenobarbital **decreases** losartan and its active carboxylic acid derivative (20%).

Mechanism of Action Losartan is an angiotensin II receptor (type AT_1) antagonist. Losartan, through biotransformation, forms an active carboxylic acid metabolite that is 10-40 times more potent by weight than the parent compound. Both are competitive, reversible antagonists of AT_1 receptors which are associated with cardiovascular homeostasis; neither active substance inhibits ACE. Losartan and its metabolites also decrease aldosterone release. Aldosterone plasma concentrations decrease following losartan administration, but no significant change in potassium serum concentration is usually observed.

Pharmacodynamics

Duration/peak effect: Losartan inhibits pressor effect 85% at peak serum concentrations and maintains a 25% to 40% reduction for 24 hours

Pharmacokinetics

Absorption: Well absorbed from gastrointestinal tract

Distribution: V_d: Losartan: 34 L; active metabolite: 12 L

Metabolism: Significant first-pass metabolism; the carboxylic acid metabolite is active (14%); substrate CYP2C9, 3A4

Bioavailability: 33%

Half-life: Losartan: 2 hours; active metabolite: 6-9 hours

Protein binding: Losartan and its active metabolite are highly bound to albumin; (free fractions 1.3% and 0.2% respectively).

Time to peak serum concentration: 1 hour for losartan; 3-4 hours for active metabolite

Elimination: ~35% of losartan and its metabolites eliminated renally with the remainder excreted in the feces; biliary excretion contributes significantly to elimination. Serum concentrations of losartan are not affected by mild renal impairment (Cl_{cr} as low as 31 mL/minute). Creatinine clearances <30 mL/minute are 50% higher than patients with normal renal function. Plasma concentrations of the active metabolite are not changed with renal impairment.

Usual Dosage Geriatrics and Adults: Oral: 50 mg once daily; patients with possible hypovolemia (eg, dehydration, diuretic therapy) should initiate therapy with 25 mg/day. Patients with hepatic impairment should begin with 25 mg/day. If patients are not controlled throughout a 24-hour period with daily dosing, giving total daily dose in twice-daily regimen may be helpful (see Warnings and Precautions).

Administration See Usual Dosage

Monitoring Parameters Monitor blood pressure and pulse; no clinically important changes seen with laboratory electrolytes, glucose, uric acid, triglycerides, or cholesterol

Patient Information Patients may administer losartan with other medications and food. Compliance is important for full therapeutic effect. Report episodes of hypotension to physician.

Nursing Implications Monitor initial doses for hypotension; stress the need to assure proper fluid intake (see Warnings and Precautions)

Additional Information Advantage of losartan over ACE inhibitors is that losartan does not cause cough; also available in combination with hydrochlorothiazide as Hyzaar®

Special Geriatric Considerations Serum concentrations of losartan and its metabolites are not significantly different and no initial dose adjustment is necessary even in low creatinine clearance states (<30 mL/minute)

Dosage Forms
Tablet, as potassium (Cozaar®): 25 mg, 50 mg
Tablet, combination (Hyzaar®): Losartan 50 mg and hydrochlorothiazide 12.5 mg [potassium 4.24 mg]

References
Brunner HR, Christen Y, Munafo A, et al, "Clinical Experience With Angiotensin II Receptor Antagonists," *Am J Hypertens*, 1992, 5(12 Pt 2):243S-246S.
Gansevoort RT, de Zeeuw D, Shahinfar S, et al, "Effects of the Angiotensin II Antagonist Losartan in Hypertensive Patients With Renal Disease," *J Hypertens Suppl*, 1994, 12(2):S37-S42.
Munger MA and Furniss SM, "Angiotensin II Receptor Blockers: Novel Therapy for Heart Failure?" *Pharmacotherapy*, 1996, 16(2 Pt 2):59S-68S.
Shaw W, Keane W, Sica D, et al, "Safety and Antihypertensive Effects of Losartan (MK-954; DUP753); A New Angiotensin II Receptor Antagonist in Patients With Hypertension and Renal Disease," *Clin Pharmacol Ther*, 1993, 53:140.

Losartan and Hydrochlorothiazide *see* Losartan *on page 553*

Losec® *see* Omeprazole *on page 693*

Lotensin® *see* Benazepril *on page 107*

Lotensin HCT® *see* Benazepril and Hydrochlorothiazide *on page 109*

Lotrimin® *see* Clotrimazole *on page 242*

Lotrimin® AF Cream [OTC] *see* Clotrimazole *on page 242*

Lotrimin® AF Lotion [OTC] *see* Clotrimazole *on page 242*

Lotrimin® AF Powder [OTC] *see* Miconazole *on page 625*

Lotrimin® AF Solution [OTC] *see* Clotrimazole *on page 242*

Lotrimin® AF Spray Liquid [OTC] *see* Miconazole *on page 625*

Lotrimin® AF Spray Powder [OTC] *see* Miconazole *on page 625*

Lovastatin (LOE va sta tin)

Brand Names Mevacor®

Synonyms Mevinolin; Monacolin K

Generic Available No

Therapeutic Category Antilipemic Agent; HMG-CoA Reductase Inhibitor

Use Adjunct to dietary therapy to decrease elevated serum total and LDL cholesterol concentrations in primary hypercholesterolemia

Contraindications Active liver disease or unexplained persistent elevations of LFTs, hypersensitivity to lovastatin or any component

Warnings Musculoskeletal effects include myopathy (myalgia and/or muscle weakness accompanied by markedly elevated CK concentrations), rash and/or pruritus; hepatocellular carcinomas have been found in mice taking in excess of 300 times the recommended dose based on body weight

Precautions May elevate aminotransferases; LFTs should be performed before and every 4- 6 weeks during the first 12-15 months of therapy and periodically thereafter; serum cholesterol and triglyceride concentrations should be determined prior to and regularly during therapy; use with caution in patients who consume large quantities of alcohol

Adverse Reactions
Central nervous system: Headache, dizziness
Dermatologic: Rash, pruritus
Endocrine & metabolic: Gynecomastia
Gastrointestinal: Flatulence, abdominal pain, cramps, diarrhea pancreatitis, constipation, nausea
Hepatic: Increased LFTs
Neuromuscular & skeletal: Myalgia, muscle cramps, myopathy
Ocular: Blurred vision, myositis

Overdosage Few cases have been reported; no patients were symptomatic and all recovered without adverse effects

Drug Interactions Increased anticoagulant effect of warfarin; concurrent use of niacin, gemfibrozil, erythromycin, clarithromycin, troleandomycin, itraconazole, indinavir, nelfinavir, ritonavir, saquinavir, and cyclosporine increases the risk of rhabdomyolysis or myopathy

Mechanism of Action Lovastatin acts by competitively inhibiting 3-hydroxy-3-methylglutaryl-coenzyme A reductase (HMG-Co-A reductase), the enzyme that catalyzes the rate-limiting step in cholesterol biosynthesis

(Continued)

Lovastatin *(Continued)*

Pharmacokinetics
Absorption: Oral, 30%
Metabolism: Substrate CYP3A4
Protein binding: 95%
Half-life: 1.1-1.7 hours
Time to peak serum concentration: Within 2-4 hours while LDL cholesterol concentration reductions require 3 days of therapy
Elimination: ~80% to 85% of dose excreted in feces and 10% in urine following liver hydrolysis

Usual Dosage Oral:
Geriatrics and Adults: Initial: 20 mg with evening meal (for patients with serum cholesterol >300 mg/dL: 40 mg/day initially), then adjust at 4-week intervals to between 20-80 mg/day; maximum dose: 80 mg/day
Patients taking immunosuppressive drugs: Maximum dose: 20 mg/day

Monitoring Parameters Serum cholesterol (total and fractionated), CPK serum concentrations; LFTs before and every 4-6 weeks during the first 12-15 months of therapy and periodically thereafter or LFTs before and every 4-6 weeks during the first 3 months of therapy and then every 6-12 weeks during the next 12 months and periodically thereafter

Test Interactions Increased ALT, AST, CPK, alkaline phosphatase, bilirubin; altered thyroid function tests

Patient Information Promptly report any unexplained muscle pain, tenderness or weakness, especially if accompanied by malaise or fever; follow prescribed diet; take with meals

Nursing Implications Best effect is seen when administered in the evening (see Adverse Reactions, Monitoring Parameters, and Special Geriatric Considerations)

Additional Information For explicit guidelines on the risk factors for CHD and when to treat high blood cholesterol (see References)

Special Geriatric Considerations The definition of and, therefore, when to treat hyperlipidemia in the elderly is a controversial issue. The National Cholesterol Education Program recommends that all adults 20 years of age and older maintain a plasma cholesterol <200 mg/dL. By this definition, 60% of all elderly would be considered to have a borderline high (200-239 mg/dL) or high (≥240 mg/dL) plasma cholesterol. However, plasma cholesterol has been shown to be a less reliable predictor of coronary heart disease in the elderly. Therefore, it is the authors' belief that pharmacologic treatment be reserved for those who are unable to obtain a desirable plasma cholesterol concentration by diet alone and for whom the benefits of treatment are believed to outweigh the potential adverse effects, drug interactions, and cost of treatment.

Dosage Forms Tablet: 10 mg, 20 mg, 40 mg

References
"Summary of the Second Report of the National Cholesterol Education Program (NCEP) Expert Panel on Detection, Evaluation, and Treatment of High Blood Cholesterol in Adults (Adult Treatment Panel II)," *JAMA*, 1993, 269(23):3015-23.

Lovenox® Injection *see* Enoxaparin *on page 334*
Low-Quel® *see* Diphenoxylate and Atropine *on page 303*

Loxapine (LOKS a peen)

Related Information
Antipsychotic Agents Comparison *on page 1023*
Antipsychotic Medication Guidelines *on page 1076*
Federal OBRA Regulations Recommended Maximum Doses - Antipsychotics *on page 1056*

Brand Names Loxitane®
Synonyms Oxilapine Succinate
Generic Available No
Therapeutic Category Antipsychotic Agent; Neuroleptic Agent
Use Management of psychotic disorders; nonpsychotic symptoms associated with dementia in elderly, Tourette's syndrome, Huntington's chorea
Contraindications Hypersensitivity to loxapine or any component, avoid use in patients with narrow-angle glaucoma, bone marrow suppression, severe liver or cardiac disease; severe CNS depression, coma; subcortical brain damage; circulatory collapse, severe hypotension or hypertension

Warnings
Tardive dyskinesia: Prevalence rate may be 40% in elderly; elderly women especially at risk; embarrassment from dyskinesias may lead to greater

social isolation; development of the syndrome and the irreversible nature are proportional to duration and total cumulative dose over time. May be reversible if diagnosed early in therapy; intermittent use of antipsychotics (not proven use) helps decrease total cumulative dose.

EPS: Extrapyramidal reactions are more common in elderly with up to 50% developing these reactions after age 60. These reactions may be more common in dementia patients. Drug-induced **Parkinson's syndrome** occurs often. Discontinuation usually resolves symptoms but may take weeks to months (12+) to clear. **Akathisia** is the most common EPS reaction in elderly. The symptoms of motor restlessness are difficult to diagnose in demented elderly; increased nervousness, assertiveness, restlessness with constant movement may indicate this adverse event. Consider decreasing dose if antipsychotic to treat as well as diagnose problem; usually see this reaction within 2-3 months of initiating antipsychotic drug.

Anticholinergic effects: These side effects most common with low potency antipsychotics (eg, thioridazine, chlorpromazine). CNS toxicity occurs more frequently and severely in elderly; increased confusion, memory loss, psychotic behavior, and agitation frequently occur as a consequence of anticholinergic effects to antipsychotic agents. Peripheral anticholinergic action troublesome to elderly; most peripheral anticholinergic effects last only 2-3 weeks (see Adverse Reactions).

Orthostatic hypotension: More common with low potency agents (eg, thioridazine, chlorpromazine, and clozapine) but of concern with all antipsychotic agents; orthostasis due to alpha-receptor blockade by antipsychotic agents. Elderly present many risk factors for orthostatic hypotension: blunted baroreceptor reflexes, decreased vascular tone, decreased vascular volume, and possible presence of cardiac diseases which result in decreased cardiac output.

Sedation: Common side effect with antipsychotic therapy; should not be used as a hypnotic unless insomnia is associated with target behavior symptoms treated with antipsychotic medications (see Special Geriatric Considerations). Anecdotal reports suggesting antipsychotic sedation in nonpsychotic patients is extremely unpleasant due to feelings of depersonalization, derealization, and dysphoria. Due to the long duration of action with antipsychotic drugs, these reactions may last up to 24 hours and result in decreased daytime function.

Cardiac toxicity: Life-threatening arrhythmias have occurred at therapeutic doses of antipsychotics. Thioridazine more commonly demonstrates EKG changes than other antipsychotics; suggested to use high potency antipsychotic agents (ie, haloperidol) in patients with cardiac conduction defects.

Precautions Use with caution in patients with cardiovascular disease, seizures, and Parkinson's disease; benefits of therapy must be weighed against risks of therapy

Adverse Reactions

Anticholinergic: Xerostomia (problem for denture user), urinary retention, constipation, adynamic ileus, overflow incontinence, blurred vision

Cardiovascular: Hypotension (especially orthostatic), tachycardia, arrhythmias, abnormal T waves with prolonged ventricular repolarization, EKG changes

Central nervous system: Sedation, drowsiness, restlessness, anxiety, extrapyramidal reactions, dystonic reactions, pseudoparkinsonian signs and symptoms, tardive dyskinesia, neuroleptic malignant syndrome, seizures, altered central temperature regulation

Endocrine & metabolic: Amenorrhea, galactorrhea, gynecomastia

Gastrointestinal: Constipation, adynamic ileus, GI upset, xerostomia (problem for denture user), weight gain

Genitourinary: Urinary retention, overflow incontinence, priapism, sexual dysfunction (up to 60%)

Hematologic: Agranulocytosis, leukopenia (usually in patients with large doses for prolonged periods)

Hepatic: Cholestatic jaundice

Ocular: Blurred vision, retinal pigmentation, decreased visual acuity (may be irreversible)

Overdosage Symptoms of overdose include deep sleep, coma, extrapyramidal symptoms, abnormal involuntary muscle movements, hypotension or hypertension; agitation, restlessness, fever, hypothermia or hyperthermia, seizures, cardiac arrhythmias, EKG changes

Toxicology Following initiation of essential overdose management, toxic symptom treatment and supportive treatment should be initiated. Hypotension (Continued)

Loxapine *(Continued)*

usually responds to I.V. fluids or Trendelenburg positioning. If unresponsive to these measures the use of a parenteral inotrope may be required (eg, norepinephrine 0.1-0.2 mcg/kg/minute titrated to response). Do not use epinephrine. Seizures commonly respond to diazepam (I.V. 5-10 mg bolus in adults every 15 minutes if needed up to a total of 30 mg) or to phenytoin or phenobarbital. Also critical cardiac arrhythmias often respond to I.V. phenytoin (15 mg/kg up to 1 g), while other antiarrhythmics can be used. Neuroleptics often cause extrapyramidal symptoms (eg, dystonic reactions) requiring management with diphenhydramine 1-2 mg/kg up to a maximum of 50 mg I.M. or I.V. slow push followed by a maintenance dose for 48-72 hours. When these reactions are unresponsive to diphenhydramine, benztropine mesylate I.V. 1-2 mg may be effective. These agents are generally effective within 2-5 minutes.

Drug Interactions
May increase CNS depression with other CNS depressants
Anticonvulsants (phenytoin, carbamazepine, phenobarbital) may decrease serum concentrations of loxapine
May increase CNS disorientation with lithium

Stability Protect from light; dispense in amber or opaque vials

Mechanism of Action Unclear mechanism of action, thought to be similar to chlorpromazine; blocks postsynaptic mesolimbic dopaminergic D_1 and D_2 receptors in the brain; exhibits a strong alpha-adrenergic blocking and anticholinergic effect, depresses the release of hypothalamic and hypophyseal hormones; believed to depress the reticular activating system thus affecting basal metabolism, body temperature, wakefulness, vasomotor tone, and emesis

Pharmacodynamics
Onset of action: Oral: Within 20-30 minutes
Peak effects: 90-180 minutes
Duration: ~12 hours

Pharmacokinetics
Metabolism: Liver metabolism to glucuronide conjugates
Half-life: Biphasic:
Initial: 5 hours
Terminal: 12-19 hours
Elimination: In urine, and to a smaller degree, the feces within 24 hours

Usual Dosage Oral:
Geriatrics (nonpsychotic patients, dementia behavior): Initial: 5-10 mg 1-2 times/day; increase dose at 4- to 7-day intervals by 5-10 mg/day; increase dosing intervals (twice daily, 3 times/day, etc) as necessary to control response or side effects; maximum daily dose: 125 mg; gradual increases (titration) may prevent some side effects or their severity.
Adults: 10 mg twice daily, increase dose until psychotic symptoms are controlled; usual dose range: 60-100 mg/day in divided doses 2-4 times/day
Not dialyzable (0% to 5%)

Monitoring Parameters Orthostatic blood pressures; tremors, gait changes, abnormal movement in trunk, neck, buccal area, or extremities; monitor target behaviors for which the agent is given

Patient Information Oral concentrate must be diluted in 2-4 oz of liquid (water, fruit juice, carbonated drinks, milk, or pudding); do not take antacid within 1 hour of taking drug; avoid alcohol; avoid excess sun exposure (use sun block); may cause drowsiness, rise slowly from recumbent position; use of supportive stockings may help prevent orthostatic hypotension

Nursing Implications Dilute the oral concentrate with water or juice before administration; avoid skin contact with oral suspension or solution; may cause contact dermatitis; monitor orthostatic blood pressures 3-5 days after initiation of therapy or a dose increase; observe for tremor and abnormal movement or posturing (extrapyramidal symptoms)

Additional Information
Loxapine hydrochloride: Loxitane® C oral concentrate
Loxapine succinate: Loxitane® capsule

Special Geriatric Considerations See Warnings.

Many elderly patients receive antipsychotic medications for inappropriate nonpsychotic behavior. Before initiating antipsychotic medication, the clinician should investigate any possible reversible cause; any stress or stress from any disease can cause acute "confusion" or worsening of baseline nonpsychotic behavior. Most commonly acute changes in behavior are due to increases in drug dose or addition of new drug to regimen; fluid electrolyte loss; infections; and changes in environment.

Any changes in disease status in any organ system can result in behavior changes.

In the treatment of agitated, demented, elderly patients, authors of meta-analysis of controlled trials of the response to the traditional antipsychotics (phenothiazines, butyrophenones) in controlling agitation have concluded that the use of neuroleptics results in a response rate of 18%. Clearly neuroleptic therapy for behavior control should be limited with frequent attempts to withdraw the agent given for behavior control.

Dosage Forms
Capsule, as succinate: 5 mg, 10 mg, 25 mg, 50 mg
Concentrate, oral, as hydrochloride: 25 mg/mL (120 mL dropper bottle)

References
Peabody CA, Warner MD, Whiteford HA, et al, "Neuroleptics and the Elderly," *J Am Geriatr Soc*, 1987, 35(3):233-8.
Risse SC and Barnes R, "Pharmacologic Treatment of Agitation Associated With Dementia," *J Am Geriatr Soc*, 1986, 34(5):368-76.
Saltz BL, Woerner MG, Kane JM, et al, "Prospective Study of Tardive Dyskinesia Incidence in the Elderly," *JAMA*, 1991, 266(17):2402-6.
Seifert RD, "Therapeutic Drug Monitoring: Psychotropic Drugs," *J Pharm Pract*, 1984, 6:403-16.

Loxitane® *see* Loxapine *on page 556*

Lozol® *see* Indapamide *on page 483*

L-PAM *see* Melphalan *on page 582*

L-Sarcolysin *see* Melphalan *on page 582*

LTG *see* Lamotrigine *on page 524*

L-Thyroxine Sodium *see* Levothyroxine *on page 534*

LubriTears® Ophthalmic Ointment [OTC] *see* Ocular Lubricant *on page 688*

LubriTears® Solution [OTC] *see* Artificial Tears *on page 82*

Ludiomil® *see* Maprotiline *on page 569*

Luminal® *see* Phenobarbital *on page 737*

Lupron® *see* Leuprolide Acetate *on page 528*

Lupron Depot® *see* Leuprolide Acetate *on page 528*

Lupron Depot-Ped™ *see* Leuprolide Acetate *on page 528*

Luride® *see* Fluoride *on page 392*

Luride® Lozi-Tab® *see* Fluoride *on page 392*

Luride®-SF Lozi-Tab® *see* Fluoride *on page 392*

Luvox® *see* Fluvoxamine *on page 406*

LY170053 *see* Olanzapine *on page 689*

Lyphocin® *see* Vancomycin *on page 980*

Lypressin (lye PRES in)

Brand Names Diapid®
Synonyms 8-L-Lysine Vasopressin
Generic Available No
Therapeutic Category Antidiuretic Hormone Analog; Pituitary Hormone; Vasopressin Analog
Use Controls or prevents signs and complications of neurogenic diabetes insipidus; postoperative abdominal distention; remove interfering "gas shadows" in abdominal x-rays
Unlabeled use: Manage bleeding esophageal varices
Contraindications Known anaphylaxis or hypersensitivity to lypressin
Warnings Use with caution in patients with coronary artery disease; may cause water intoxication
Precautions Exercise caution when using in patients with heart failure, asthma, seizure disorder, or migraine headaches
Adverse Reactions
Cardiovascular: Chest tightness
Central nervous system: Dizziness, headache, pounding in head
Endocrine & metabolic: Water intoxication
Gastrointestinal: Abdominal cramping, increased bowel movements, nausea, vomiting, flatulence, heartburn
Local: Irritation or burning
Neuromuscular & skeletal: Tremor
Ocular: Conjunctivitis
Respiratory: Coughing, dyspnea, nasal congestion, rhinorrhea, bronchial constriction, nasal pruritus
(Continued)

Lypressin (Continued)

Miscellaneous: Periorbital edema, diaphoresis

Overdosage Symptoms of overdose include drowsiness, headache, confusion, weight gain, hypertension; systemic toxicity is unlikely to occur from the nasal spray but may cause transient fluid retention

Toxicology Temporarily remove drug until polyuria occurs; treat with supportive care; severe water intoxication may require osmotic diuresis

Drug Interactions Increased effect: Chlorpropamide, clofibrate, carbamazepine → prolongation of antidiuretic effects

Mechanism of Action Within renal tubule epithelium, vasopressin increases cyclic adenosine monophosphate (cAMP) which increases water permeability at the renal tubule resulting in decreased urine volume and increased osmolality. Smooth muscle contraction is marked in the renal vascular bed (vasopressor effect); likewise, smooth muscle vasoconstriction is significant in partial and splanchnic vessels. Less vasoconstriction occurs in peripheral, coronary, pulmonary, and cerebral vasculature. Vasopressin causes peristalsis by directly stimulating the smooth muscle in the GI tract.

Pharmacodynamics

Onset of antidiuretic effect: Intranasal spray: Within 0.5-2 hours
Duration: 3-8 hours

Pharmacokinetics

Metabolism: In the liver and kidneys
Half-life: 15-20 minutes
Elimination: Urinary excretion

Usual Dosage Geriatrics and Adults: Instill 1-2 sprays into one or both nostrils whenever frequency of urination increases or significant thirst develops; usual dosage is 1-2 sprays 4 times/day; range: 1 spray/day at bedtime to 10 sprays each nostril every 3-4 hours (see Additional Information)

Monitoring Parameters Urinary frequency

Patient Information To control nocturia, an additional dose may be given at bedtime; notify physician if drowsiness, fatigue, headache, shortness of breath, abdominal cramps, or severe nasal irritation occurs

Nursing Implications Monitor urination frequency

Additional Information Approximately 2 USP posterior pituitary pressor units per spray

Special Geriatric Considerations No specific data available for geriatrics. Given the pathophysiology and treatment response, no specific recommendations are necessary. Treat the elderly as indicated for adults.

Dosage Forms Spray: 0.185 mg/mL (equivalent to 50 USP posterior pituitary units/mL) (8 mL)

Maalox® [OTC] see Aluminum Hydroxide and Magnesium Hydroxide on page 43

Maalox Anti-Gas® [OTC] see Simethicone on page 856

Maalox® Plus [OTC] see Aluminum Hydroxide, Magnesium Hydroxide, and Simethicone on page 44

Maalox® Therapeutic Concentrate [OTC] see Aluminum Hydroxide and Magnesium Hydroxide on page 43

Macrobid® see Nitrofurantoin on page 676

Macrodantin® see Nitrofurantoin on page 676

Magaldrate (MAG al drate)

Brand Names Riopan® [OTC]

Synonyms Hydromagnesium Aluminate

Generic Available Yes

Therapeutic Category Antacid

Use Symptomatic relief of hyperacidity associated with peptic ulcer, gastritis, peptic esophagitis and hiatal hernia

Contraindications Patients with colostomy or an ileostomy, appendicitis, ulcerative colitis, diverticulitis

Warnings Sodium content may be significant for patients with hypertension, renal failure, congestive heart failure; hypermagnesemia may result with renal insufficiency when >50 mEq of magnesium is administered daily; patients with Cl_{cr} <30 mL/minute are at risk for hypermagnesemia

Precautions Aluminum intoxication, osteomalacia, patients with GI hemorrhage; use with caution in patients on low sodium diets (patients with congestive heart failure, edema, hypertension), cirrhosis, and renal failure; magnesium intoxication may occur with renal insufficiency

Adverse Reactions

Endocrine & metabolic: Dehydration or fluid restriction

Gastrointestinal: Constipation, decreased bowel motility, fecal impaction

Miscellaneous: Hemorrhoids

Overdosage

Aluminum: Osteomalacia (bone pain), malaise, weakness, and aluminum intoxication (encephalopathy) may occur in patients with renal insufficiency

Magnesium: CNS depression, confusion, hypotension, muscle weakness, blockage of peripheral neuromuscular transmission; serum >4 mEq/L (4.8 mg/dL): deep tendon reflexes may be depressed; serum ≥10 mEq/L (12 mg/dL): deep tendon reflexes may disappear, respiratory paralysis may occur, heart block may occur

Toxicology Deferoxamine, traditionally used as an iron chelator, has been shown to increase urinary aluminum output. Deferoxamine chelation of aluminum has resulted in improvements of clinical symptoms and bone histology. Deferoxamine, however, remains an experimental treatment for aluminum poisoning and has a significant potential for adverse effects. Hypermagnesemia, toxic symptoms usually present with serum concentration >4 mEq/L; concurrent hypocalcemia, impaired clotting, somnolence, and disappearance of deep tendon reflexes. Serum concentration >12 mEq/L may be fatal, serum concentration ~10 mEq/L may cause complete heart block; I.V. calcium (5-10 mEq) will reverse respiratory depression or heart block; peritoneal dialysis or hemodialysis may be needed.

Drug Interactions

Magnesium and aluminum combination compounds decrease the pharmacologic effect of benzodiazepines, captopril, glucocorticosteroids, fluoroquinolones, H_2 antagonists, hydantoins, iron compounds, ketoconazole, penicillamine, phenothiazines, salicylates, tetracyclines, ticlopidine; concomitant use with sodium polystyrene sulfonate may cause metabolic alkalosis in patients with renal insufficiency

Magnesium and aluminum combination compounds increase the pharmacologic effect of levodopa, quinidine, sulfonylureas, valproic acid

Mechanism of Action Neutralize gastric acid and, therefore, increase pH of the stomach and duodenal bulb; with increased pH >4, the proteolytic activity of pepsin is diminished. Antacids also increase lower esophageal sphincter tone; aluminum ions inhibit gastric emptying by decreasing smooth muscle contraction.

Pharmacodynamics Acid-neutralizing capacity varies from product to product; antacids ingested in a fasting state give reduced acidity for 30 minutes; if ingested 1 hour after meals, reduced acidity may be extended for 3 hours

Usual Dosage Geriatrics and Adults: Oral: 480-1080 mg between meals (1-2 hours after meals) and at bedtime

Monitoring Parameters

Aluminum: Monitor phosphorous levels periodically when patient is on chronic therapy; when used as a phosphate binder, dose to achieve a serum phosphate concentration ≤4 mg/100 mL; observe for complaints or bone pain, malaise, and muscular weakness

Magnesium: Observe for signs of mental confusion and increased somnolence (see Overdosage)

Reference Range

Aluminum: Normal range (serum): 0-6 ng/mL; dialysis patients may attain up to 40 ng/mL without symptoms of toxicity; >100 ng/mL possible CNS toxicity

Magnesium: Normal range (serum): 1.5-2.3 mg/dL (1.25-1.9 mEq/L); toxicity occurs with serum concentrations >4 mEq/L (4.8 mg/dL)

Test Interactions Decreased inorganic phosphorus

Patient Information Chew tablets thoroughly before swallowing with water; notify physician if relief is not obtained or if signs of bleeding from GI tract occur

Nursing Implications Administer 1-2 hours apart from oral drugs; shake suspensions well; observe for constipation, fecal impaction, diarrhea, and hypophosphatemia (see Monitoring Parameters and Reference Range)

Additional Information A chemical entity known as hydroxy magnesium aluminate equivalent to magnesium oxide and aluminum oxide; unlike other magnesium containing antacids, Riopan® is safe to use in renal patients if used cautiously

Special Geriatric Considerations Elderly, due to disease or drug therapy, may be predisposed to diarrhea or constipation. Diarrhea may result in electrolyte imbalance. Decreased renal function (Cl_{cr} <30 mL/minute) may result
(Continued)

Magaldrate *(Continued)*

in toxicity of aluminum or magnesium (see Precautions and Contraindications). Drug interactions must be considered. If possible, administer antacid 1-2 hours apart from other drugs. When treating ulcers, consider buffer capacity (mEq/mL) antacid.

Dosage Forms Suspension, oral: 540 mg/5 mL (360 mL)

References

Gams JG, "Clinical Significance of Magnesium: A Review," *Drug Intell Clin Pharm*, 1987, 21(3):240-6.

Peterson WL, Sturdevant RAL, Franki HD, et al, "Healing of Duodenal Ulcer With an Antacid Regimen," *N Engl J Med*, 1977, 297(7):341-5.

Magaldrate and Simethicone (MAG al drate & sye METH i kone)

Related Information

Magaldrate *on page 560*

Simethicone *on page 856*

Brand Names Riopan Plus® [OTC]

Synonyms Simethicone and Magaldrate

Therapeutic Category Antacid; Antiflatulent

Use Relief of hyperacidity associated with peptic ulcer, gastritis, peptic esophagitis and hiatal hernia which are accompanied by symptoms of gas

Contraindications Patients with colostomy or an ileostomy, appendicitis, ulcerative colitis, diverticulitis

Warnings Sodium content may be significant for patients with hypertension, renal failure, congestive heart failure; hypermagnesemia may result with renal insufficiency when >50 mEq of magnesium is administered daily; patients with Cl_{cr} <30 mL/minute are at risk for hypermagnesemia

Precautions Aluminum intoxication, osteomalacia, patients with GI hemorrhage; use with caution in patients on low sodium diets (patients with congestive heart failure, edema, hypertension), cirrhosis, and renal failure; magnesium intoxication may occur with renal insufficiency

Adverse Reactions

Endocrine & metabolic: Dehydration or fluid restriction

Gastrointestinal: Constipation, decreased bowel motility, fecal impaction

Miscellaneous: Hemorrhoids

Overdosage

Aluminum: Osteomalacia (bone pain), malaise, weakness, and aluminum intoxication (encephalopathy) may occur in patients with renal insufficiency

Magnesium: CNS depression, confusion, hypotension, muscle weakness, blockage of peripheral neuromuscular transmission serum >4 mEq/L (4.8 mg/dL): deep tendon reflexes may be depressed; serum ≥10 mEq/L (12 mg/dL): deep tendon reflexes may disappear, respiratory paralysis may occur, heart block may occur

Toxicology Deferoxamine, traditionally used as an iron chelator, has been shown to increase urinary aluminum output. Deferoxamine chelation of aluminum has resulted in improvements of clinical symptoms and bone histology. Deferoxamine, however, remains an experimental treatment for aluminum poisoning and has a significant potential for adverse effects. Hypermagnesemia, toxic symptoms usually present with serum concentration >4 mEq/L; concurrent hypocalcemia, impaired clotting, somnolence, and disappearance of deep tendon reflexes. Serum concentration >12 mEq/L may be fatal, serum concentration ~10 mEq/L may cause complete heart block; I.V. calcium (5-10 mEq) will reverse respiratory depression or heart block; peritoneal dialysis or hemodialysis may be needed.

Drug Interactions

Magnesium and aluminum combination compounds decrease the pharmacologic effect of benzodiazepines, captopril, glucocorticosteroids, fluoroquinolones, H_2 antagonists, hydantoins, iron compounds, ketoconazole, penicillamine, phenothiazines, salicylates, tetracyclines, ticlopidine; concomitant use with sodium polystyrene sulfonate may cause metabolic alkalosis in patients with renal insufficiency

Magnesium and aluminum combination compounds increase the pharmacologic effect of levodopa, quinidine, sulfonylureas, valproic acid

Mechanism of Action Neutralize gastric acid and, therefore, increase pH of the stomach and duodenal bulb; with increased pH >4, the proteolytic activity of pepsin is diminished. Antacids also increase lower esophageal sphincter tone; aluminum ions inhibit gastric emptying by decreasing smooth muscle contraction.

Pharmacodynamics Acid-neutralizing capacity varies from product to product; antacids ingested in a fasting state give reduced acidity for 30

minutes; if ingested 1 hour after meals, reduced acidity may be extended for 3 hours

Usual Dosage Geriatrics and Adults: Oral: 480-1080 mg between meals (1-2 hours after meals) and at bedtime

Monitoring Parameters

Aluminum: Monitor phosphorous levels periodically when patient is on chronic therapy; when used as a phosphate binder, dose to achieve a serum phosphate concentration ≤4 mg/100 mL; observe for complaints or bone pain, malaise, and muscular weakness

Magnesium: Observe for signs of mental confusion and increased somnolence (see Overdosage)

Reference Range

Aluminum: Normal range (serum): 0-6 ng/mL; dialysis patients may attain up to 40 ng/mL without symptoms of toxicity; >100 ng/mL possible CNS toxicity

Magnesium: Normal range (serum): 1.5-2.3 mg/dL (1.25-1.9 mEq/L); toxicity occurs with serum concentrations >4 mEq/L (4.8 mg/dL)

Test Interactions Decreased inorganic phosphorus

Patient Information Notify physician if relief is not obtained or if signs of bleeding from GI tract occur

Nursing Implications Administer 1-2 hours apart from oral drugs; shake suspensions well; observe for constipation, fecal impaction, diarrhea, and hypophosphatemia (see Monitoring Parameters and Reference Range)

Additional Information A chemical entity known as hydroxy magnesium aluminate equivalent to magnesium oxide and aluminum oxide; unlike other magnesium containing antacids, Riopan® is safe to use in renal patients if used cautiously

Special Geriatric Considerations Elderly, due to disease or drug therapy, may be predisposed to diarrhea or constipation. Diarrhea may result in electrolyte imbalance. Decreased renal function (Cl_{cr} <30 mL/minute) may result in toxicity of aluminum or magnesium (see Precautions and Contraindications). Drug interactions must be considered. If possible, administer antacid 1-2 hours apart from other drugs. When treating ulcers, consider buffer capacity (mEq/mL) antacid.

Dosage Forms Suspension: Magaldrate 480 mg and simethicone 20 mg/5 mL (360 mL)

References

Gams JG, "Clinical Significance of Magnesium: A Review," *Drug Intell Clin Pharm*, 1987, 21(3):240-6.

Peterson WL, Sturdevant RAL, Franki HD, et al, "Healing of Duodenal Ulcer With an Antacid Regimen," *N Engl J Med*, 1977, 297(7):341-5.

Magalox Plus® [OTC] *see* Aluminum Hydroxide, Magnesium Hydroxide, and Simethicone *on page 44*

Magan® *see* Salicylates (Various Salts) *on page 842*

Magnesia Magma *see* Magnesium Hydroxide *on next page*

Magnesium Citrate (mag NEE zhum SIT rate)

Brand Names Evac-Q-Mag® [OTC]

Synonyms Citrate of Magnesia

Generic Available Yes

Therapeutic Category Laxative, Saline

Use Evacuate bowel prior to certain surgical and diagnostic procedures or overdose situations

Contraindications Renal failure, appendicitis, abdominal pain, intestinal impaction, obstruction or perforation, diabetes mellitus, complications in gastrointestinal tract, patients with colostomy, ileostomy, ulcerative colitis or diverticulitis

Warnings Monitor serum magnesium concentration, respiratory rate, deep tendon reflex

Precautions Use with caution in patients with impaired renal function, especially if Cl_{cr} <30 mL/minute (accumulation of magnesium which may lead to magnesium intoxication); use with caution in digitalized patients (may alter cardiac conduction leading to heart block); use with caution in patients with lithium administration; use with caution with neuromuscular blocking agents, CNS depressants

Adverse Reactions

Cardiovascular: Hypotension, heart block

Endocrine & metabolic: Hypermagnesemia

Gastrointestinal: Abdominal cramps, diarrhea, gas formation

Respiratory: Respiratory depression

(Continued)

Magnesium Citrate *(Continued)*

Overdosage Serious, potentially life-threatening electrolyte disturbances may occur with long-term use or overdosage due to diarrhea; hypermagnesemia may occur; CNS depression, confusion, hypotension, muscle weakness, blockage of peripheral neuromuscular transmission; serum >4 mEq/L (4.8 mg/dL): deep tendon reflexes may be depressed; serum ≥10 mEq/L (12 mg/dL): deep tendon reflexes may disappear, respiratory paralysis may occur, heart block may occur; I.V. calcium (5-10 mEq) will reverse respiratory depression or heart block; in extreme cases, peritoneal dialysis or hemodialysis may be required

Toxicology Toxic symptoms usually present with serum concentration >4 mEq/L; concurrent hypocalcemia, impaired clotting, somnolence, and disappearance of deep tendon reflexes; serum concentration >12 mEq/L may be fatal, serum concentration ~10 mEq/L may cause complete heart block

Drug Interactions

Magnesium compounds decrease the pharmacologic effect of benzodiazepines, chloroquine, glucocorticosteroids, digoxin, H_2 antagonists, hydantoins, iron compounds, nitrofurantoin, penicillamine, phenothiazines, tetracyclines, ticlopidine

Magnesium compounds increase the pharmacologic effect of dicumarol, quinidine, sulfonylureas

Mechanism of Action Promotes bowel evacuation by causing osmotic retention of fluid which distends the colon with increased peristaltic activity

Pharmacodynamics Onset of cathartic action: Oral: Within 1-2 hours

Pharmacokinetics

Absorption: Oral: 15% to 30%

Elimination: Renal

Usual Dosage Geriatrics and Adults: Cathartic: Oral: ½ to 1 full bottle (120-240 mL)

Monitoring Parameters See Overdosage

Reference Range Adults: 2.2-2.8 mg/dL ~1.8-2.3 mEq/L

Test Interactions Increased magnesium; decreased protein, calcium (S), decreased potassium (S)

Patient Information Take with a glass of water, fruit juice, or citrus flavored carbonated beverage; report severe abdominal pain to physician

Nursing Implications To increase palatability, manufacturer suggests chilling the solution prior to administration (see Overdosage)

Additional Information 3.85-4.71 mEq of magnesium/5 mL

Special Geriatric Considerations Elderly, due to disease or drug therapy, may be predisposed to diarrhea. Diarrhea may result in electrolyte imbalance. Decreased renal function (Cl_{cr} <30 mL/minute) may result in toxicity; monitor for toxicity and Cl_{cr} <30 mL/minute (see Precautions and Contraindications).

Dosage Forms Solution: 300 mL

References

Chernow B, Smith J, Rainey TG, et al, "Hypomagnesemia: Implications for the Critical Care Specialist," *Crit Care Med*, 1982, 10(3):193-6.

Gams JG, "Clinical Significance of Magnesium: A Review," *Drug Intell Clin Pharm*, 1987, 21(3):240-6.

Magnesium Hydroxide *(mag NEE zhum hye DROKS ide)*

Brand Names Phillips'® Milk of Magnesia [OTC]

Synonyms Magnesia Magma; Milk of Magnesia; MOM

Generic Available Yes

Therapeutic Category Antacid; Laxative, Saline; Magnesium Salt

Use Short-term treatment of occasional constipation and symptoms of hyperacidity

Contraindications Patients with colostomy or an ileostomy, intestinal obstruction, fecal impaction, renal failure, appendicitis; heart block, myocardial damage, serious renal impairment, hepatitis, and Addison's disease

Warnings Hypermagnesemia and toxicity may occur due to decreased renal clearance (Cl_{cr} <30 mL/minute) of absorbed magnesium; monitor serum magnesium concentration, respiratory rate, deep tendon reflex, renal function when $MgSO_4$ is administered parenterally

Precautions Use with caution in patients with impaired renal function (accumulation of magnesium which may lead to magnesium intoxication); use with caution in digitalized patients (may alter cardiac conduction leading to heart block); use with caution with neuromuscular blocking agents, lithium administration

Adverse Reactions
Cardiovascular: Hypotension
Endocrine & metabolic: Hypermagnesemia
Gastrointestinal: Diarrhea, abdominal cramps
Neuromuscular & skeletal: Muscle weakness
Respiratory: Respiratory depression

Overdosage May cause severe diarrhea, CNS depression, confusion, hypotension, muscle weakness, blockage of peripheral neuromuscular transmission; serum >4 mEq/L (4.8 mg/dL): deep tendon reflexes may be depressed; serum ≥10 mEq/L (12 mg/dL): deep tendon reflexes may disappear, respiratory paralysis may occur, heart block may occur; I.V. calcium (5-10 mEq) will reverse respiratory depression or heart block; in extreme cases, peritoneal dialysis or hemodialysis may be required

Toxicology Toxic symptoms usually present with serum concentration >4 mEq/L; concurrent hypocalcemia, impaired clotting, somnolence, and disappearance of deep tendon reflexes; serum concentration >12 mEq/L may be fatal, serum concentration ~10 mEq/L may cause complete heart block

Drug Interactions
Magnesium compounds decrease the pharmacologic effect of benzodiazepines, chloroquine, glucocorticosteroids, digoxin, H_2 antagonists, hydantoins, iron compounds, nitrofurantoin, penicillamine, phenothiazines, tetracyclines, ticlopidine
Magnesium compounds increase the pharmacologic effect of dicumarol, quinidine, sulfonylureas

Mechanism of Action Promotes bowel evacuation by causing osmotic retention of fluid which distends the colon with increased peristaltic activity; reacts with hydrochloric acid in stomach to form magnesium chloride

Pharmacodynamics Onset of laxative action: Within 4-8 hours

Pharmacokinetics
Absorption: Absorbed magnesium ions (up to 30%)
Elimination: Usually by kidneys, unabsorbed drug is excreted in feces

Usual Dosage Oral:
Geriatrics: Laxative: 30 mL/day
Adults:
Laxative: 30-60 mL/day or in divided doses
Antacid: 5-15 mL as needed

Monitoring Parameters See Overdosage

Reference Range Adults: 2.2-2.8 mg/dL ~1.8-2.3 mEq/L

Test Interactions Increased magnesium; decreased protein, calcium (S), decreased potassium (S)

Patient Information Dilute dose in water or juice, shake well; chew tablets well

Nursing Implications MOM concentrate is 3 times as potent as regular strength product; monitor for toxicity in patients with decreased renal function (see Special Geriatric Considerations)

Additional Information 1.05 g magnesium = ~87 mEq magnesium/30 mL

Special Geriatric Considerations Elderly, due to disease or drug therapy, may be predisposed to diarrhea. Diarrhea may result in electrolyte imbalance. Decreased renal function (Cl_{cr} <30 mL/minute) may result in toxicity; monitor for toxicity (see Precautions and Contraindications).

Dosage Forms
Liquid: 390 mg/5 mL (10 mL, 15 mL, 20 mL, 30 mL, 100 mL, 120 mL, 180 mL, 360 mL, 720 mL)
Suspension, oral: 2.5 g/30 mL (10 mL, 15 mL, 30 mL)
Tablet: 300 mg, 600 mg

References
Chernow B, Smith J, Rainey TG, et al, "Hypomagnesemia: Implications for the Critical Care Specialist," *Crit Care Med*, 1982, 10(3):193-6.
Gams JG, "Clinical Significance of Magnesium: A Review," *Drug Intell Clin Pharm*, 1987, 21(3):240-6.

Magnesium Hydroxide and Aluminum Hydroxide *see* Aluminum Hydroxide and Magnesium Hydroxide *on page 43*

Magnesium Hydroxide and Mineral Oil Emulsion
(mag NEE zhum hye DROKS ide & MIN er al oyl e MUL shun)
Related Information
Magnesium Hydroxide *on previous page*
Mineral Oil *on page 628*
Brand Names Haley's M-O® [OTC]
Synonyms MOM/Mineral Oil Emulsion
(Continued)

Magnesium Hydroxide and Mineral Oil Emulsion
(Continued)

Generic Available No

Therapeutic Category Laxative, Lubricant; Laxative, Saline

Use Short-term treatment of occasional constipation

Contraindications Patients with colostomy or an ileostomy, intestinal obstruction, fecal impaction, renal failure, appendicitis; heart block, myocardial damage, serious renal impairment, hepatitis, and Addison's disease

Warnings Hypermagnesemia and toxicity may occur due to decreased renal clearance (Cl_{cr} <30 mL/minute) of absorbed magnesium; monitor serum magnesium concentration, respiratory rate, deep tendon reflex

Precautions Use with caution in patients with impaired renal function (accumulation of magnesium which may lead to magnesium intoxication); use with caution in digitalized patients (may alter cardiac conduction leading to heart block); use with caution with neuromuscular blocking agents, lithium administration (see Special Geriatric Considerations)

Adverse Reactions
Cardiovascular: Hypotension
Endocrine & metabolic: Hypermagnesemia
Gastrointestinal: Diarrhea, abdominal cramps
Neuromuscular & skeletal: Muscle weakness
Respiratory: Respiratory depression

Overdosage May cause severe diarrhea and fluid and electrolyte imbalance, hypermagnesemia

Toxicology Toxic symptoms usually present with serum concentration >4 mEq/L; concurrent hypocalcemia, impaired clotting, somnolence, and disappearance of deep tendon reflexes; serum concentration >12 mEq/L may be fatal, serum concentration ~10 mEq/L may cause complete heart block

Drug Interactions
Magnesium compounds decrease the pharmacologic effect of benzodiazepines, chloroquine, glucocorticosteroids, digoxin, H_2 antagonists, hydantoins, iron compounds, nitrofurantoin, penicillamine, phenothiazines, tetracyclines, ticlopidine
Magnesium compounds increase the pharmacologic effect of dicumarol, quinidine, sulfonylureas

Mechanism of Action Promotes bowel evacuation by causing osmotic retention of fluid which distends colon and therefore increases peristaltic action. Mineral oil retards colonic absorption of fecal water and softens stool

Pharmacodynamics Onset of action: 4-8 hours

Pharmacokinetics
Absorption: Absorbed magnesium ions (up to 30%)
Elimination: Usually by kidneys, unabsorbed drug is excreted in feces

Usual Dosage Geriatrics and Adults: Oral: 5-45 mL at bedtime

Monitoring Parameters See Overdosage

Reference Range Adults: 2.2-2.8 mg/dL ~1.8-2.3 mEq/L

Test Interactions Increased magnesium; decreased protein

Patient Information Shake well; take with full glass of water; report persistent diarrhea or abdominal pains with incidence of blood in stool or vomit

Nursing Implications See Overdosage

Special Geriatric Considerations The use of mineral oil products may be hazardous in elderly with conditions predisposing them to aspiration. Elderly, due to disease or drug therapy, may be predisposed to diarrhea. Diarrhea may result in electrolyte imbalance. Decreased renal function (Cl_{cr} <30 mL/minute) may result in toxicity from magnesium absorption; monitor for toxicity (see Precautions and Contraindications).

Dosage Forms Suspension: Equivalent to magnesium hydroxide 24 mL/mineral oil emulsion (30 mL unit dose)

References
Chernow B, Smith J, Rainey TG, et al, "Hypomagnesemia: Implications for the Critical Care Specialist," *Crit Care Med*, 1982, 10(3):193-6.
Gams JG, "Clinical Significance of Magnesium: A Review," *Drug Intell Clin Pharm*, 1987, 21(3):240-6.

Magnesium Oxide (mag NEE zhum OKS ide)
Brand Names Maox®

Therapeutic Category Antacid

Use Short-term treatment of occasional constipation and symptoms of hyperacidity; treat or prevent hypomagnesemia

Contraindications Patients with colostomy or an ileostomy, appendicitis, ulcerative colitis, diverticulitis; heart block, myocardial damage, serious renal impairment, hepatitis, and Addison's disease

Warnings Hypermagnesemia and toxicity may occur due to decreased renal clearance (Cl_{cr} <30 mL/minute) of absorbed magnesium; monitor serum magnesium concentration, respiratory rate, deep tendon reflex

Precautions Use with caution in patients with impaired renal function (accumulation of magnesium which may lead to magnesium intoxication); use with caution in digitalized patients (may alter cardiac conduction leading to heart block); use with caution in patients with lithium administration

Adverse Reactions

Cardiovascular: Hypotension, EKG changes

Central nervous system: Mental depression, coma

Gastrointestinal: Nausea, vomiting

Respiratory: Respiratory depression

Overdosage May cause diarrhea, severe electrolyte imbalance, and hypermagnesemia, CNS depression, confusion, hypotension, muscle weakness, blockage of peripheral neuromuscular transmission serum >4 mEq/L (4.8 mg/dL): deep tendon reflexes may be depressed; serum ≥10 mEq/L (12 mg/dL): deep tendon reflexes may disappear, respiratory paralysis may occur, heart block may occur; intravenous calcium (5-10 mEq) will reverse respiratory depression or heart block; in extreme cases, peritoneal dialysis or hemodialysis may be required

Toxicology Toxic symptoms usually present with serum concentration >4 mEq/L; concurrent hypocalcemia, impaired clotting, somnolence, and disappearance of deep tendon reflexes; serum concentration >12 mEq/L may be fatal, serum concentration ~10 mEq/L may cause complete heart block

Drug Interactions

Magnesium compounds decrease the pharmacologic effect of benzodiazepines, chloroquine, glucocorticosteroids, digoxin, H_2 antagonists, hydantoins, iron compounds, nitrofurantoin, penicillamine, phenothiazines, tetracyclines, ticlopidine

Magnesium compounds increase the pharmacologic effect of dicumarol, quinidine, sulfonylureas

Mechanism of Action Promotes bowel evacuation by causing osmotic retention of fluid which distends the colon with increased peristaltic activity when taken orally

Pharmacokinetics

Absorption: Absorbed magnesium is rapidly eliminated by the kidneys (see Special Geriatric Considerations)

Elimination: Primarily excreted in feces

Usual Dosage Geriatrics and Adults: Oral:

Antacid: 140 mg to 1.5 g with water or milk 3-4 times/day after meals and at bedtime

Laxative: 2-4 g with full glass of water; cathartic action occurs within 1-2 hours

Monitoring Parameters See Overdosage

Reference Range Adults: 2.2-2.8 mg/dL ~1.8-2.3 mEq/L

Test Interactions Increased magnesium; decreased protein, calcium (S), decreased potassium (S)

Patient Information Chew tablets before swallowing; take with full glass of water; notify physician if relief not obtained or if any signs of bleeding occur (black tarry stools, "coffee ground" vomit)

Nursing Implications Monitor for diarrhea and signs of hypermagnesemia (see Overdosage)

Special Geriatric Considerations Elderly, due to disease or drug therapy, may be predisposed to diarrhea. Diarrhea may result in electrolyte imbalance. Decreased renal function (Cl_{cr} <30 mL/minute) may result in toxicity; monitor for toxicity (see Precautions and Contraindications).

Dosage Forms

Capsule: 140 mg

Tablet: 400 mg, 420 mg, 500 mg

References

Chernow B, Smith J, Rainey TG, et al, "Hypomagnesemia: Implications for the Critical Care Specialist," *Crit Care Med*, 1982, 10(3):193-6.

Gams JG, "Clinical Significance of Magnesium: A Review," *Drug Intell Clin Pharm*, 1987, 21(3):240-6.

Magnesium Salicylate *see* Salicylates (Various Salts) *on page 842*

Magnesium Salts (Various Salts) (mag NEE zhum salts)

Brand Names Almora® [OTC]; Epsom Salt [OTC]; Magonate® [OTC]; Mg-plus® [OTC]; Slow-Mag® [OTC]

Generic Available Yes

Therapeutic Category Anticonvulsant, Miscellaneous; Electrolyte Supplement, Parenteral; Laxative, Saline; Magnesium Salt

Use Treatment and prevention of hypomagnesemia; short-term treatment of constipation

Restrictions See Precautions and Contraindications

Contraindications Heart block, myocardial damage, serious renal impairment, hepatitis and Addison's disease

Warnings Monitor serum magnesium concentration, respiratory rate, deep tendon reflex, renal function when $MgSO_4$ is administered parenterally

Precautions Use with caution in patients with impaired renal function, especially when Cl_{cr} <30 mL/minute (accumulation of magnesium which may lead to magnesium intoxication); use with caution in digitalized patients (may alter cardiac conduction leading to heart block); use with caution with neuromuscular blocking agents, lithium administration

Adverse Reactions
Serum magnesium concentrations >3 mg/dL:
  Central nervous system: Depressed CNS, blocked peripheral neuromuscular transmission leading to anticonvulsant effects
  Gastrointestinal: Diarrhea
Serum magnesium concentrations >5 mg/dL:
  Cardiovascular: Flushing
  Central nervous system: Somnolence
Serum magnesium concentrations >12.5 mg/dL:
  Cardiovascular: Complete heart block
  Respiratory: Respiratory paralysis

Overdosage Symptoms of overdose include CNS depression, confusion, hypotension, muscle weakness, blockage of peripheral neuromuscular transmission serum >4 mEq/L (4.8 mg/dL): deep tendon reflexes may be depressed; serum ≥10 mEq/L (12 mg/dL): deep tendon reflexes may disappear, respiratory paralysis may occur, heart block may occur; I.V. calcium (5-10 mEq) will reverse respiratory depression or heart block; in extreme cases, peritoneal dialysis or hemodialysis may be required

Toxicology Toxic symptoms usually present with serum concentration >4 mEq/L; concurrent hypocalcemia, impaired clotting, somnolence, and disappearance of deep tendon reflexes; serum concentration >12 mEq/L may be fatal; serum concentration ~10 mEq/L may cause complete heart block

Drug Interactions
Magnesium compounds decrease the pharmacologic effect of benzodiazepines, chloroquine, glucocorticosteroids, digoxin, H_2 antagonists, hydantoins, iron compounds, nitrofurantoin, penicillamine, phenothiazines, tetracyclines, ticlopidine
Magnesium compounds increase the pharmacologic effect of dicumarol, quinidine, sulfonylureas

Stability Refrigeration of intact ampuls may result in precipitation or crystallization; stability of parenteral admixture at room temperature (25°C): 60 days

Mechanism of Action Promotes bowel evacuation by causing osmotic retention of fluid which distends the colon with increased peristaltic activity when taken orally; parenterally, decreases acetylcholine in motor nerve terminals and acts on myocardium by slowing rate of S-A node impulse formation and prolonging conduction time

Pharmacodynamics
Onset of action:
  Oral: Within 1-2 hours
  I.M.: Within 60 minutes
  I.V.: Immediately
Duration:
  I.M.: 3-4 hours
  I.V.: 30 minutes

Pharmacokinetics
Absorption: Absorbed magnesium is rapidly eliminated by the kidneys (see Special Geriatric Considerations)
Elimination: Primarily excreted in feces

Usual Dosage Dose represented as $MgSO_4$ unless stated otherwise
Hypomagnesemia: Geriatrics and Adults:
  Oral: 3 g every 6 hours for 4 doses as needed

I.M., I.V.: 1 g every 6 hours for 4 doses or 250 mg/kg over a 4-hour period; for severe hypomagnesemia: 8-12 g MgSO₄/day in divided doses has been used

Hypomagnesemia with hypovolemia: Oral: 200-400 mg/day in divided doses

Cathartic: Geriatrics and Adults: Oral: 10-30 g

Dietary supplement: 50-500 mg/day in divided doses; gluconate: 27-54 mg (magnesium) 2-3 times/day

Hyperalimentation: 8-24 mEq/day

Recommended daily allowance: Adults:
Male: 350-400 mg/day
Female: 280-300 mg/day

Monitoring Parameters See Overdosage

Reference Range Adults: 2.2-2.8 mg/dL ~1.8-2.3 mEq/L

Test Interactions Increased magnesium; decreased protein, calcium (S), decreased potassium (S)

Patient Information Take in divided doses; report diarrhea (>5 stools/day) or changes in mental function to physician, nurse, or pharmacist

Nursing Implications Monitor blood pressure when administering MgSO₄ I.V.; serum magnesium concentrations should be monitored to avoid overdose; monitor for diarrhea, hypotension, CNS confusion

Additional Information 1 g magnesium = 8.3 mEq (41.1 mmol); see individual agents for magnesium content per dose

Special Geriatric Considerations Elderly, due to disease or drug therapy, may be predisposed to diarrhea. Diarrhea may result in electrolyte imbalance. Decreased renal function (Cl_cr <30 mL/minute) may result in toxicity; monitor for toxicity.

Dosage Forms

Granules, as sulfate: ~40 mEq magnesium/5 g (240 g)

Injection, as sulfate: 10% = 0.8 mEq/mL (2 mL, 10 mL, 20 mL, 30 mL, 50 mL); 20% = 1.97 mEq/mL (2 mL, 10 mL, 20 mL, 30 mL, 50 mL); 50% = 4 mEq/mL (2 mL, 10 mL, 20 mL, 30 mL, 50 mL)

Liquid, as sulfate: 54 mg/5 mL; gluconate: 54 mg/5 mL (gluconate has 27 mg magnesium)

Tablet, as various salts: 140 mg, 400 mg, 500 mg

References

Chernow B, Smith J, Rainey TG, et al, "Hypomagnesemia: Implications for the Critical Care Specialist," *Crit Care Med*, 1982, 10(3):193-6.

Gams JG, "Clinical Significance of Magnesium: A Review," *Drug Intell Clin Pharm*, 1987, 21(3):240-6.

Magonate® [OTC] *see* Magnesium Salts (Various Salts) *on previous page*

Maigret-50 *see* Phenylpropanolamine *on page 741*

Malatal® *see* Hyoscyamine, Atropine, Scopolamine, and Phenobarbital *on page 472*

Mallamint® [OTC] *see* Calcium Salts (Oral) *on page 152*

Mallazine® Eye Drops [OTC] *see* Tetrahydrozoline *on page 901*

Malotuss® [OTC] *see* Guaifenesin *on page 437*

Mandol® *see* Cefamandole *on page 174*

Mantoux *see* Tuberculin Purified Protein Derivative *on page 971*

Maox® *see* Magnesium Oxide *on page 566*

Mapap® [OTC] *see* Acetaminophen *on page 16*

Maprotiline (ma PROE ti leen)

Related Information

Antidepressant Agents Comparison *on page 1021*

Antidepressant Medication Guidelines *on page 1075*

Federal OBRA Regulations Recommended Maximum Doses - Antidepressants *on page 1056*

Brand Names Ludiomil®

Generic Available No

Therapeutic Category Antidepressant, Tetracyclic

Use Treatment of depression and anxiety associated with depression

Contraindications Narrow-angle glaucoma, hypersensitivity to maprotiline or any component

Warnings To avoid cholinergic crisis do not discontinue abruptly in patients receiving high doses chronically

Precautions Use with caution in patients with cardiac conduction disturbances, history of hyperthyroidism; an EKG prior to starting therapy is advised

(Continued)

Maprotiline (Continued)

Adverse Reactions
Cardiovascular: Stroke, heart block, tachycardia, orthostatic hypotension

Central nervous system: Seizures, sedation, confusion

Dermatologic: Rash

Gastrointestinal: Constipation, increased appetite, weight gain, extreme xerostomia, weight loss, nausea, vomiting

Genitourinary: Urinary retention, swollen testicles

Neuromuscular & skeletal: Tremors

Ocular: Blurred vision, increased intraocular pressure

Otic: Tinnitus

Overdosage
Symptoms of overdose include agitation, confusion, hallucinations, urinary retention, hypothermia, hypotension, tachycardia

Toxicology
Following initiation of essential overdose management, toxic symptoms should be treated. Ventricular arrhythmias often respond to phenytoin 15-20 mg/kg with concurrent systemic alkalinization (sodium bicarbonate 0.5-2 mEq/kg I.V.). Arrhythmias unresponsive to this therapy may respond to lidocaine 1 mg/kg I.V. followed by a titrated infusion. Physostigmine (1-2 mg I.V. slowly) may be indicated in reversing cardiac arrhythmias that are due to vagal blockade or for anticholinergic effects. Seizures usually respond to diazepam I.V. boluses (5-10 mg, up to 30 mg). If seizures are unresponsive or recur, phenytoin or phenobarbital may be required.

Drug Interactions
Decreased effect of clonidine and guanethidine; decreased effect with barbiturates, phenytoin, carbamazepines

Increased effect/toxicity of CNS depressants, MAO inhibitors (hyperpyretic crisis), anticholinergics, sympathomimetics, thyroid (increased cardiotoxicity), phenothiazines (seizures), benzodiazepines

Mechanism of Action
Traditionally believed to increase the synaptic concentration of norepinephrine in the central nervous system by inhibition of their reuptake by the presynaptic neuronal membrane. However, additional receptor effects have been found including desensitization of adenyl cyclase, down regulation of beta-adrenergic receptors, and down regulation of serotonin receptors.

Pharmacodynamics
Onset of therapeutic effects: May take 1-3 weeks before effects are seen; norepinephrine only

Pharmacokinetics
Absorption: Oral: Slow

Protein binding: 88%

Metabolism: Metabolized in the liver to active and inactive compounds; substrate CYP2D6

Half-life: 21-25 hours

Time to peak serum concentration: Within 12 hours

Elimination: In urine (70%) and feces (30%)

Geriatrics: After a single 125 mg oral dose in 5 subjects between 75-83 years of age 50% of the dose was absorbed, the average time to peak was 7 hours, and the average elimination half-life was 31.5 hours

Usual Dosage
Oral:

Geriatrics: Initial: 25 mg at bedtime, increase by 25 mg every 3 days for inpatients and weekly for outpatients if tolerated; usual maintenance dose: 50-75 mg/day, higher doses may be necessary in nonresponders

Adults: 75 mg/day to start, increase by 25 mg every 2 weeks up to 150-225 mg/day; given in 3 divided doses or in a single daily dose

Monitoring Parameters
Sleep, appetite, mood, somatic complaints, mental status, weight, blood pressure and heart rate, urine flow/output

Reference Range
Therapeutic: 200-600 ng/mL (SI: 721-2163 nmol/L); not well established

Patient Information
Do not drink alcoholic beverages, may cause drowsiness, dry mouth, constipation, blurred vision; rise slowly to avoid dizziness

Nursing Implications
Offer patient sugarless hard candy for dry mouth (see Monitoring Parameters)

Special Geriatric Considerations
Use with caution due to sedation and anticholinergic effects (confusion, constipation, difficulty urinating, dry mouth) (see Pharmacokinetics and Usual Dosage)

Dosage Forms
Tablet, as hydrochloride: 25 mg, 50 mg, 75 mg

References
Hrdina PD, Rovei V, Henry JF, et al, "Comparison of Single-Dose Pharmacokinetics of Imipramine and Maprotiline in the Elderly," *Psychopharmacology*, 1980, 70(1):29-34.

Maranox® [OTC] see Acetaminophen on page 16

Marbaxin® *see* Methocarbamol *on page 604*

Marcillin® *see* Ampicillin *on page 73*

Marezine® **[OTC]** *see* Cyclizine *on page 258*

Margesic® **H** *see* Hydrocodone and Acetaminophen *on page 461*

Marmine® **Injection** *see* Dimenhydrinate *on page 300*

Marmine® **Oral [OTC]** *see* Dimenhydrinate *on page 300*

Marthritic® *see* Salsalate *on page 847*

Mavik® *see* Trandolapril *on page 944*

Maxair™ **Autohaler**™ *see* Pirbuterol *on page 756*

Maxair™ **Inhaler** *see* Pirbuterol *on page 756*

Maxaquin® *see* Lomefloxacin *on page 547*

Maxidex® *see* Dexamethasone *on page 274*

Maximum Strength Desenex® **Antifungal Cream [OTC]** *see* Miconazole *on page 625*

Maximum Strength Nytol® **[OTC]** *see* Diphenhydramine *on page 302*

Maxipime® *see* Cefepime *on page 177*

Maxitrol® *see* Neomycin, Polymyxin B, and Dexamethasone *on page 661*

Maxivate® *see* Betamethasone *on page 114*

Maxolon® *see* Metoclopramide *on page 616*

Maxzide® *see* Hydrochlorothiazide and Triamterene *on page 460*

Measles and Rubella Vaccines, Combined
(MEE zels & roo BEL a vak SEENS, kom BINED)

Related Information
Immunization Guidelines *on page 1058*

Brand Names M-R-VAX® II

Synonyms Rubella and Measles Vaccines, Combined

Generic Available No

Therapeutic Category Vaccine

Use Simultaneous immunization against measles and rubella

Contraindications Immune deficiency condition

Warnings Immunocompromised persons; history of anaphylactic reaction following receipt of neomycin; do not administer concurrently with ISG

Precautions Hypersensitivity to either component, eggs, or chicken feathers; temporarily may depress tuberculin skin testing, do not vaccinate for at least 3 months following blood transfusion or immune serum globulin

Adverse Reactions All serious adverse reactions must be reported to the FDA

Central nervous system: Fever <100°F, fever between 100°F and 103°F, fever >103°F (prolonged), malaise, headache, fatigue, convulsions, encephalitis, confusion, severe headache

Dermatologic: Urticaria, rash, local erythema, itching, reddening of skin (especially around ears and eyes)

Gastrointestinal: Sore throat, vomiting

Hematologic: Thrombocytopenic purpura

Local: Burning at injection site, local tenderness

Neuromuscular & skeletal: Arthralgia, stiff neck

Ocular: Diplopia, optic neuritis

Respiratory: Dyspnea

Miscellaneous: Allergic reaction (delayed type), lymphadenopathy, hypersensitivity

Drug Interactions Whole blood, immune globulin, immunosuppressive drugs should not be given within 1 month of other live virus vaccines except monovalent or trivalent polio vaccine; may temporarily depress tuberculin skin test sensitivity; decreased effect when immune globulin is given within 3 months and with concurrent use of corticosteroids and other immunosuppressant agents

Stability Refrigerate prior to use (2°C to 8°C); use as soon as possible; discard if not used within 8 hours of reconstitution; protect from light

Usual Dosage Geriatrics and Adults: S.C.: Inject 0.5 mL into outer aspect of upper arm; no routine booster for rubella (see Additional Information)

Administration Not for I.V. administration

Monitoring Parameters Monitor site of injection and for adverse reactions

Patient Information Patients should be instructed about common side effects and told to report any unusual or serious effects to physician

Measles vaccine:
A rash may occur from 1-2 weeks after receiving the measles vaccine
(Continued)

Measles and Rubella Vaccines, Combined *(Continued)*

A fever after receiving the first vaccination of the measles vaccine may occur; fever occurs less often after a second injection

Rubella vaccine:

Swelling of the lymph glands in the neck or a rash that lasts 1-2 days; this could happen 1-2 weeks after receiving the rubella vaccine

Mild pain or stiffness in the joints that may last up to 3 days; this could occur from 1-3 weeks after vaccination, and may be encountered in 25 out of 100 adults vaccinated. Women have this side effect more than men up to 40 women out of every 100. Rarely, pain or stiffness can last for months or longer and can be fluctuant.

Painful swelling of the joints (arthritis) occurs in 10 out of 100 adults who receive the rubella vaccine.

Pain or numbness, or "pins and needles" feeling in the hands and feet that lasts for a short time; happens rarely

Nursing Implications Vaccine should not be given I.V.; S.C. injection preferred with a 25-gauge ⅝" needle; federal law requires that the date of administration, the vaccine manufacturer, lot number of vaccine, and the administering person's name, title and address be entered into the patient's permanent medical record

Additional Information Federal law requires that the date of administration, the vaccine manufacturer, lot number of vaccine, and the administering person's name, title and address be entered into the patient's permanent medical record

Adults born before 1957 are generally considered to be immune to measles; all born in or after 1957 without documentation of live vaccine on or after first birthday, physician-diagnosed measles, or laboratory evidence of immunity should be vaccinated with two doses separated by or less than 1 month. For those previously vaccinated with one dose of measles vaccine, revaccination is indicated for healthcare workers at time of employment, and for travelers to endemic areas. Guidelines for rubella vaccination are the same with the exception of birth year. All adults should be vaccinated against rubella. A booster dose of rubella vaccine is not necessary. MMR is the vaccine of choice if recipients are likely to be susceptible to mumps as well as measles and rubella.

Special Geriatric Considerations Most adults and elderly are immune to measles (rubeola) and it is not necessary to vaccinate; if no history of measles exposure or patient is from an isolated community where measles is not endemic, vaccination may be required; testing may be indicated; may need to test for rubella; vaccinate those traveling into endemic areas with no evidence of immunity; no dose restriction necessary

Dosage Forms Injection: 1000 TCID$_{50}$ each of live attenuated measles virus vaccine and live rubella virus vaccine

References

Gardner P and Schaffner W, "Immunization of Adults," *N Engl J Med*, 1993, 328(17):1252-8.

Measles, Mumps, and Rubella Vaccines, Combined

(MEE zels, mumpz & roo BEL a vak SEENS, kom BINED)

Related Information

Immunization Guidelines *on page 1058*

Brand Names M-M-R® II

Synonyms MMR; Mumps, Measles and Rubella Vaccines, Combined; Rubella, Measles and Mumps Vaccines, Combined

Generic Available No

Therapeutic Category Vaccine

Use Measles, mumps, and rubella prophylaxis in adults born after 1956 with no evidence of immunity to measles or mumps

Contraindications Blood dyscrasias; cancers affecting the bone marrow or lymphatic systems; known hypersensitivity to measles, mumps, and rubella vaccine; known hypersensitivity to neomycin; acute infections and respiratory illness; known hypersensitivity to eggs, chicken, or chicken feathers; severely immunocompromised persons

Warnings

MMR vaccine should not be given within 3 months of immune globulin or whole blood

Have epinephrine available during and after administration

MMR vaccine should not be administered to severely immunocompromised persons

Severely immunocompromised patients and symptomatic HIV-infected patients who are exposed to measles should receive immune globulin, regardless of prior vaccination status

The immunogenicity of measles virus vaccine is decreased if vaccine is administered <6 months after immune globulin

Precautions Hypersensitivity to any component, eggs, chicken feathers, neomycin; may temporarily suppress tuberculin skin testing; do not vaccinate for at least 3 months following blood transfusions or immune serum globulin

Adverse Reactions All serious adverse reactions must be reported to the FDA

Central nervous system: Seizures, malaise, fever
Dermatologic: Transient rash, tenderness, erythema, edema
Gastrointestinal: Sore throat
Miscellaneous: Allergic reactions

Drug Interactions Decreased effect when immune globulin is given within 3 months and with concurrent use of corticosteroids and other immunosuppressant agents; decreased effect with concurrent infection, immunoglobulin within 1 month, other live vaccines with the exception of attenuated measles, rubella, or polio

Stability Refrigerate, protect from light prior to reconstitution; use as soon as possible; discard 8 hours after reconstitution

Usual Dosage Geriatrics and Adults: 0.5 mL; requires two doses; second dose in no less than 30 days (see Additional Information)

Administration Not for I.V. administration; administer in outer aspect of the upper arm with a 25-gauge ⅝" needle

Monitoring Parameters Monitor site of injection and for systemic side effects

Test Interactions Temporary suppression of TB skin test reactivity with onset approximately 3 days after administration

Patient Information Inform patients of common adverse effects and to report serious or unusual side effects

Measles vaccine:
A rash may occur from 1-2 weeks after receiving the measles vaccine
A fever ≥103°F after receiving the first measles vaccine; fever occurs less often after a second injection.

Mumps vaccine: A little swelling of the glands in the cheeks and under the jaw that lasts for a few days; this could happen from 1-2 weeks after the mumps vaccine; happens rarely

Rubella vaccine: Swelling of the lymph glands in the neck or a rash that lasts 1-2 days

Mild pain or stiffness in the joints that may last up to 3 days; happens in 25 out of 100 adults who are vaccinated. Women have this side effect more than men in up to 40 women out of every 100. Rarely, pain or stiffness can last for months or longer.

Painful swelling of the joints (arthritis) happens 10 out of 100 adults which usually lasts a few days to a week. Rarely, this swelling has been reported to last longer.

Pain or numbness, or "pins and needles" feeling in the hands and feet that lasts for a short time; happens rarely

Nursing Implications Inject in outer aspect of upper arm with a 25-gauge ⅝" needle

Additional Information Live, attenuated vaccine. Federal law requires that the date of administration, the vaccine manufacturer, lot number of vaccine, and the administering person's name, title and address be entered into the patient's permanent medical record

Adults born before 1957 are generally considered to be immune to measles and mumps; all born in or after 1957 without documentation of live vaccine on or after first birthday, physician-diagnosed measles or mumps, or laboratory evidence of immunity should be vaccine with two doses separated by no less than 1 month; for those previously vaccinated with one dose of measles vaccine, revaccination is indicated healthcare workers at time of employment, and for travelers to endemic areas. Guidelines for rubella vaccination are the same with the exception of birth year; all adults should be vaccinated against rubella. Booster doses of mumps and rubella are not necessary.

Special Geriatric Considerations Most adults and elderly are immune to measles (rubeola) and it is not necessary to vaccinate; if no history of measles exposure or patient is from an isolated community where measles is not endemic, vaccination may be required; testing may be indicated; may
(Continued)

573

Measles, Mumps, and Rubella Vaccines, Combined
(Continued)

need to test for rubella; vaccinate those traveling into endemic areas with no evidence of immunity; no dose restriction necessary

Dosage Forms Injection: 1000 $TCID_{50}$ each of measles virus vaccine and rubella virus vaccine, 5000 $TCID_{50}$ mumps virus vaccine

References
Plichta AM, "Immunization: Protecting Older Patients From Infectious Disease," *Geriatrics*, 1996, 51(9):47-52.

Measles Virus Vaccine, Live (MEE zels VYE rus vak SEEN, live)
Related Information
Immunization Guidelines *on page 1058*

Brand Names Attenuvax®

Synonyms More Attenuated Enders Strain; Rubeola Vaccine

Therapeutic Category Vaccine, Live Virus

Use Immunization against measles (rubeola) in persons ≥15 months of age and adults in isolated communities where measles is not endemic

Contraindications Known hypersensitivity to eggs, known hypersensitivity to neomycin, acute respiratory infections, activated tuberculosis, immunosuppressed patients (drug induced or disease)

Warnings Do not administer with ISG concurrently

Precautions History of febrile seizures, hypersensitivity reactions may occur if sensitive to eggs, chickens, chicken feathers; do not administer with other live vaccines; may depress tuberculin skin testing temporarily

Adverse Reactions
Cardiovascular: Headache, local edema
Central nervous system: Fever, rarely encephalitis
Dermatologic: Rarely urticaria
Hematologic: Thrombocytopenia
Local: Burning or stinging, induration, erythema
Respiratory: Sore throat, coryza
Miscellaneous: Lymphadenopathy

Drug Interactions Whole blood, immune globulin, immunosuppressive drugs, should not be given within 1 month of other live virus vaccines except monovalent or trivalent polio vaccine; may temporarily depress tuberculin skin test sensitivity

Stability Refrigerate at 2°C to 8°C (36°F to 46°F); discard if left at room temperature for over 8 hours

Mechanism of Action 97% respond; antibody levels last 8 years

Usual Dosage Geriatrics and Adults: S.C.: Administer entire volume of reconstituted vaccine in outer aspect of the upper arm

Monitoring Parameters Monitor for side effects

Nursing Implications Vaccine should not be given I.V.; S.C. injection preferred with a 25-gauge ⁵⁄₈" needle; federal law requires that the date of administration, the vaccine manufacturer, lot number of vaccine, and the administering person's name, title and address be entered into the patient's permanent medical record

Special Geriatric Considerations Generally not recommended for adults since most have become immune; if from an isolated community where measles is not endemic, may require vaccination; no dose reduction is necessary

Dosage Forms Injection: 1000 $TCID_{50}$ per dose

References
Gardner P and Schaffner W, "Immunization of Adults," *N Engl J Med*, 1993, 328(17):1252-8.

Measurin® [OTC] *see* Aspirin *on page 84*

Mebaral® *see* Mephobarbital *on page 586*

Meclizine (MEK li zeen)
Brand Names Antivert®; Antrizine®; Bonine® [OTC]; Dizmiss® [OTC]; Dramamine® II [OTC]; Meni-D®; Nico-Vert® [OTC]; Ru-Vert-M®; Vergon® [OTC]

Synonyms Meclizine Hydrochloride

Generic Available Yes

Therapeutic Category Antiemetic; Antihistamine

Use Prevention and treatment of nausea, vomiting, and dizziness of motion sickness; management of vertigo with diseases affecting the vestibular system (only "possibly" effective)

Contraindications Hypersensitivity to meclizine, cyclizine, or any component

Precautions Use with caution in patients with angle-closure glaucoma, prostatic hypertrophy, or GI obstruction; elderly may be at risk for anticholinergic side effects such as glaucoma, constipation, urinary retention, confusion

Adverse Reactions

Cardiovascular: Palpitations, tachycardia, hypotension

Central nervous system: Drowsiness, fatigue, restlessness, excitation, insomnia, confusion, euphoria, vertigo, visual hallucinations, auditory hallucinations

Dermatologic: Rash, urticaria

Gastrointestinal: Xerostomia, anorexia, nausea, vomiting, diarrhea, constipation

Genitourinary: Polyuria, urinary retention, dysuria

Ocular: Blurred vision, diplopia

Otic: Tinnitus

Respiratory: Dry nose

Overdosage Symptoms of overdose include excitation alternating with drowsiness, respiratory depression, hallucinations

Toxicology There is no specific treatment for an antihistamine overdose, however, most of its clinical toxicity is due to anticholinergic effects. Cholinesterase inhibitors may be useful by reducing acetylcholinesterase. Acetylcholinesterase inhibitors include physostigmine, neostigmine, pyridostigmine, and edrophonium. For anticholinergic overdose with severe life-threatening symptoms, physostigmine 1-2 mg I.V., slowly may be given to reverse these effects.

Drug Interactions May enhance anticholinergic action of drugs with anticholinergic pharmacologic action (see Adverse Reactions)

Mechanism of Action Has antiemetic, anticholinergic, and antihistaminic activity; has central anticholinergic action by blocking chemoreceptor trigger zone; decreases excitability of the middle ear labyrinth and blocks conduction in the middle ear vestibular-cerebellar pathways

Pharmacodynamics

Onset of action: Oral: Within 30-60 minutes

Duration: 8-24 hours

Pharmacokinetics

Metabolism: Reportedly in the liver

Half-life: 6 hours

Elimination: As metabolites in urine and as unchanged drug in feces

Usual Dosage Geriatrics and Adults: Oral:

Motion sickness: 12.5-25 mg initially 1 hour before travel, repeat dose every 12-24 hours if needed; doses up to 50 mg may be needed

Vertigo: 25-100 mg/day in divided doses

Monitoring Parameters Monitor for CNS anticholinergic side effects in elderly, relief of symptoms

Patient Information May impair ability to perform hazardous tasks; may cause drowsiness; may cause dry mouth, constipation, difficulty urinating, dry eyes

Nursing Implications See Precautions and Special Geriatric Considerations

Special Geriatric Considerations Due to anticholinergic action, use lowest dose in divided doses to avoid side effects and their inconvenience; limit use if possible; may cause confusion or aggravate symptoms of confusion in those with dementia; if vertigo does not respond in 1-2 weeks, it is advised to discontinue use

Dosage Forms

Meclizine hydrochloride:

Capsule: 25 mg

Tablet: 12.5 mg, 25 mg, 50 mg

Tablet, chewable; 25 mg

Meclofenamate (me kloe fen AM ate)

Brand Names Meclomen®

Generic Available Yes

Therapeutic Category Analgesic, Non-narcotic; Anti-inflammatory Agent; Antipyretic; Nonsteroidal Anti-inflammatory Agent (NSAID), Oral

Use Treatment of inflammatory disorders such as rheumatoid arthritis, mild to moderate pain, osteoarthritis, pain of sunburn, migraine headaches (acute)

Contraindications Active GI bleeding, ulcer disease, hypersensitivity to meclofenamate or other NSAIDs

Warnings GI toxicity (bleeding, ulceration, perforation); CNS effects may occur (headaches, confusion, depression); hypersensitivity, anaphylactoid reactions (intermittent tolmetin use more often); renal function decline, acute

(Continued)

Meclofenamate *(Continued)*

renal insufficiency, interstitial nephritis, dysuria, cystitis, hematuria, nephrotic syndrome, hyperkalemia in acute renal insufficiency, hyponatremia, papillary necrosis, hepatic function impairment; elderly have increased risk for adverse reactions to NSAIDs (see Special Geriatric Considerations)

Precautions Use with caution in patients with congestive heart failure, hypertension, decreased renal or hepatic function, history of GI disease (bleeding or ulcers), or those receiving anticoagulants; perform ophthalmologic evaluation for those who develop eye complaints during therapy (blurred vision, diminished vision, changes in color vision, retinal changes); NSAIDs may mask signs/symptoms of infections; photosensitivity reported

Adverse Reactions

Cardiovascular: Congestive heart failure, angina, hypertension, hypotension, arrhythmias, edema

Central nervous system: Headache, drowsiness, vertigo, dizziness, fatigue, hallucinations, confusion, depression, emotional lability, psychotic behavior, pyrexia

Dermatologic: Rash, urticaria, angioedema, Stevens-Johnson syndrome, exfoliative dermatitis, bruising, petechiae, purpura

Endocrine & metabolic: Hyperglycemia, hypoglycemia, hyperkalemia, gynecomastia, hyponatremia, fluid retention

Gastrointestinal: Dyspepsia, heartburn, nausea, diarrhea, constipation, flatulence, stomatitis, vomiting, abdominal pain, peptic ulcer, GI bleeding, GI perforation, gingival ulcers, pancreatitis, proctitis, paralytic ulcers, colitis, anorexia, weight loss, dry mucous membranes

Genitourinary: Impotence, azotemia

Hematologic: Neutropenia, anemia, agranulocytosis, bone marrow suppression, hemolytic anemia, hemorrhage, inhibition of platelet aggregation

Hepatic: Hepatitis, elevated LFTs, cholestatic jaundice

Neuromuscular & skeletal: Involuntary muscle movements, muscle weakness, tremors, weakness

Ocular: Vision changes

Otic: Tinnitus

Renal: Dysuria, polyuria, pyuria, oliguria, anuria, acute renal failure

Respiratory: Exacerbation of asthma, dyspnea

Miscellaneous: Thirst, diaphoresis

Overdosage Symptoms of overdose include drowsiness, lethargy, disorientation, confusion, dizziness, numbness, paresthesia, nausea, vomiting, gastric irritation, abdominal pain, headache, tinnitus, sweating, blurred vision, muscle twitching, seizures, coma, acute renal failure, increased BUN and serum creatinine, hypotension, tachycardia, and metabolic acidosis

Toxicology Management of a nonsteroidal anti-inflammatory agent (NSAID) intoxication is primarily supportive and symptomatic. Fluid therapy is commonly effective in managing the hypotension that may occur following an acute NSAID overdose, except when this is due to an acute blood loss. Seizures tend to be very short-lived and often do not require drug treatment although recurrent seizures should be treated with I.V. diazepam. Since many of the NSAIDs undergo enterohepatic cycling, multiple doses of charcoal may be needed to reduce the potential for delayed toxicities. Dialysis may be required to correct serious azotemia/electrolyte shift.

Drug Interactions

May increase digoxin, methotrexate, and lithium serum concentrations

Aspirin or other salicylates may decrease NSAID serum concentrations

Other NSAIDs may increase adverse GI effects

Increased prothrombin time with anticoagulants

Decreased antihypertensive effects of ACE inhibitors, beta-blockers, and thiazide diuretics

Increased response to sympathomimetics

Probenecid may increase toxicity of NSAIDs by increase in serum concentrations

Effects of loop diuretics may decrease

Diuretics may increase the risk of acute renal insufficiency

Azotemia may be increased in elderly receiving loop diuretics

Mechanism of Action Inhibits prostaglandin synthesis, acts on the hypothalamus heat-regulating center to reduce fever, blocks prostaglandin synthetase action which prevents formation of the platelet-aggregating substance thromboxane A_2; decreases pain receptor sensitivity. Other proposed mechanisms of action are lysosomal stabilization, inhibition of kinin and leukotriene production, alteration of chemotactic factors, and inhibition of neutrophil activation. This latter mechanism may be the most significant pharmacologic action to reduce inflammation.

Pharmacodynamics
Onset of analgesia: 30 minutes to 1 hour
Duration of action: 2-4 hours
Onset of anti-inflammatory action: 3-4 days
Peak effect: 2-3 weeks

Pharmacokinetics
Protein binding: 99%
Half-life: 2-3.3 hours
Time to peak serum concentration: Oral: Within 30-90 minutes
Elimination: Principally in urine and in feces as glucuronide conjugates

Usual Dosage Geriatrics and Adults: Oral: Initial:
Mild to moderate pain. 50 mg every 4-6 hours; increases to 100 mg may be required; maximum dose: 400 mg (see Additional Information)
Rheumatoid arthritis and osteoarthritis: 50 mg every 4-6 hours; increase, over weeks, to 200-400 mg/day in 3-4 divided doses; do not exceed 400 mg/day; maximal benefit for any dose may not be seen for 2-3 weeks (see Additional Information)

Monitoring Parameters
Monitor response (pain, range of motion, grip strength, mobility, ADL function), inflammation; observe for weight gain, edema; monitor renal function; observe for bleeding, bruising; evaluate gastrointestinal effects (abdominal pain, bleeding, dyspepsia); mental confusion, disorientation, CBC, serum, creatinine, BUN, liver function tests

Test Interactions
Increased chloride (S), increased sodium (S)

Patient Information
Serious gastrointestinal bleeding can occur as well as ulceration and perforation. Pain may or may not be present. Avoid aspirin and aspirin-containing products while taking this medication. If gastric upset occurs, take with food, milk, or antacid. If gastric adverse effects persist, contact physician. May cause drowsiness, dizziness, blurred vision, and confusion. Use caution when performing tasks which require alertness (eg, driving). Do not take for more than 3 days for fever or 10 days for pain without physician advice.

Nursing Implications
See Overdosage, Monitoring Parameters, Patient Information, and Special Geriatric Considerations

Additional Information
There are no clinical guidelines to predict which NSAID will give response in a particular patient. Trials with each must be initiated until response determined. If diarrhea develops, reduce dose or discontinue use of meclofenamate for a short time (until diarrhea stops). Some patients are not able to tolerate further use. Consider dose, patient convenience, and cost.

Special Geriatric Considerations
Elderly are a high-risk population for adverse effects from nonsteroidal anti-inflammatory agents. As much as 60% of elderly can develop peptic ulceration and/or hemorrhage asymptomatically. The concomitant use of H_2 blockers, omeprazole, and sucralfate is not effective as prophylaxis with the exception of NSAID-induced duodenal ulcers which may be prevented by the use of ranitidine. Misoprostol and proton pump inhibitors are the only agents proven to help prevent the development of NSAID-induced ulcers. Also, concomitant disease and drug use contribute to the risk for GI adverse effects. Use lowest effective dose for shortest period possible. Consider renal function decline with age. Use of NSAIDs can compromise existing renal function especially when Cl_{cr} is ≤30 mL/minute. Tinnitus may be a difficult and unreliable indication of toxicity due to age-related hearing loss or eighth cranial nerve damage. CNS adverse effects such as confusion, agitation, and hallucination are generally seen in overdose or high dose situations, but elderly may demonstrate these adverse effects at lower doses than younger adults.

Dosage Forms Capsule, as sodium: 50 mg, 100 mg

References
Brooks PM, Day RO, "Nonsteroidal Anti-inflammatory Drugs - Differences and Similarities," *N Engl J Med*, 1991, 324(24):1716-25.

Clinch D, Banerjee AK, Ostick G, "Absence of Abdominal Pain in Elderly Patients With Peptic Ulcer," *Age Ageing*, 1984, 13:120-3.

Clive DM, Stoff JS, "Renal Syndromes Associated With Nonsteroidal Anti-inflammatory Drugs," *N Engl J Med*, 1984, 310(9):563-72.

Graham DY, "Prevention of Gastroduodenal Injury Induced by Chronic Nonsteroidal Anti-inflammatory Drug Therapy," *Gastroenterology*, 1989, 96(2 Pt 2 Suppl):675-81.

Gurwitz JH, Avorn J, Ross-Degnan D, et al, "Nonsteroidal Anti-Inflammatory Drug-Associated Azotemia in the Very Old," *JAMA*, 1990, 264(4):471-5.

(Continued)

Meclofenamate *(Continued)*

Hawkey CJ, Karrasch JA, Szczepaski L, et al, "Omeprazole Compared With Misoprostrol for Ulcers Associated With Nonsteroidal Anti-inflammatory Drugs," *N Engl J Med*, 1998, 338(11):727-34.

Knodel LC, "Preventing NSAID-Induced Ulcers: The Role of Misoprostol," *Consult Pharm*, 1989, 4:37-41.

Pounder R, "Silent Peptic Ulceration: Deadly Silence or Golden Silence?" *Gastroenterology*, 1989, 96(2 Pt 2 Suppl):626-31.

Yeomans ND, Tulassay Z, Juhasz L, et al, "A Comparison of Omeprazole With Ranitidine for Ulcers Associated With Nonsteroidal Anti-inflammatory Drugs," *N Engl J Med*, 1998, 338(11):719-26.

Meclomen® *see Meclofenamate on page 575*

Meclozine Hydrochloride *see Meclizine on page 574*

Medihaler-Iso® *see Isoproterenol on page 501*

Medipain 5® *see Hydrocodone and Acetaminophen on page 461*

Mediplast® Plaster [OTC] *see Salicylic Acid on page 845*

Medipren® [OTC] *see Ibuprofen on page 475*

Medi-Tuss® [OTC] *see Guaifenesin on page 437*

Medralone® Injection *see Methylprednisolone on page 611*

Medrol® Oral *see Methylprednisolone on page 611*

Medroxyprogesterone Acetate

(me DROKS ee proe JES te rone AS e tate)

Brand Names Amen® Oral; Curretab® Oral; Cycrin® Oral; Depo-Provera® Injection; Provera® Oral

Synonyms Acetoxymethylprogesterone; Methylacetoxyprogesterone

Therapeutic Category Contraceptive, Progestin Only; Progestin

Use Endometrial carcinoma or renal carcinoma as well as secondary amenorrhea or abnormal uterine bleeding due to hormonal imbalance

Unlabeled use: Treatment of menopausal symptoms, to stimulate respiration in obstructive sleep apnea, and to induce endometrial shedding in postmenopausal women taking estrogens

Contraindications Thrombophlebitis; hypersensitivity to medroxyprogesterone or any component; cerebral apoplexy, undiagnosed vaginal bleeding, liver dysfunction

Precautions Use with caution in patients with depression, diabetes, epilepsy, asthma, migraines, renal or cardiac dysfunction; pretreatment exams should include Pap smear, physical exam of breasts and pelvic areas. May increase serum cholesterol, LDL, decrease HDL and triglycerides

Adverse Reactions

Cardiovascular: Edema, thromboembolic disorders

Central nervous system: Depression, dizziness, nervousness

Dermatologic: Melasma, chloasma, urticaria, acne

Endocrine & metabolic: Breakthrough bleeding, breast tenderness

Gastrointestinal: Weight gain

Hepatic: Cholestatic jaundice

Toxicology Toxicity is unlikely following single exposures of excessive doses, and supportive treatment is adequate in most cases

Drug Interactions Aminoglutethimide may decrease the effects by increasing hepatic metabolism

Mechanism of Action Inhibits secretion of pituitary gonadotropins, which prevents follicular maturation and ovulation, stimulates growth of mammary tissue, and transform proliferative endometrium into secretory endometrium

Pharmacokinetics

Absorption: I.M.: Slow

Metabolism: Oral: In the liver

Elimination: In urine and feces

Usual Dosage Geriatrics and Adults: Oral:

Accompanying postmenopausal estrogen therapy, postmenopausal: 2.5-10 mg the last 10-13 days of estrogen dosing each month or 2.5-5 mg daily

Abnormal uterine bleeding: 5-10 mg for 5-10 days starting on day 16 or 21 of cycle

Endometrial or renal carcinoma: I.M.: 400-1000 mg/week

Monitoring Parameters In diabetics, glucose tolerance may be decreased

Test Interactions Altered thyroid and liver function tests

Patient Information Take this medicine only as directed; do not take more of it and do not take it for a longer period of time; drug will induce menstrual bleeding in women with an intact uterus; when taken daily with estrogen, spotting will occur for the first 6-12 months of therapy; take with food if GI upset occurs

Nursing Implications Patients should receive a copy of the patient labeling for the drug

Special Geriatric Considerations See Usual Dosage and Patient Information

Dosage Forms

Injection, suspension: 100 mg/mL (5 mL); 150 mg/mL (1 mL); 400 mg/mL (1 mL, 2.5 mL, 10 mL)

Tablet: 2.5 mg, 5 mg, 10 mg

Mefenamic Acid (me fe NAM ik AS id)

Brand Names Ponstel®

Generic Available No

Therapeutic Category Analgesic, Non-narcotic; Anti-inflammatory Agent; Antipyretic; Nonsteroidal Anti-inflammatory Agent (NSAID), Oral

Use Short-term relief of mild to moderate pain, sunburn, migraine headache (acute)

Contraindications Known hypersensitivity to mefenamic acid or other NSAIDs

Warnings GI toxicity (bleeding, ulceration, perforation); CNS effects may occur (headaches, confusion, depression); hypersensitivity, anaphylactoid reactions (intermittent tolmetin use more often); renal function decline, acute renal insufficiency, interstitial nephritis, dysuria, cystitis, hematuria, nephrotic syndrome, hyperkalemia in acute renal insufficiency, hyponatremia, papillary necrosis, hepatic function impairment; elderly have increased risk for adverse reactions to NSAIDs (see Special Geriatric Considerations)

Precautions Use with caution in patients with congestive heart failure, hypertension, decreased renal or hepatic function, history of GI disease (bleeding or ulcers), or those receiving anticoagulants; perform ophthalmologic evaluation for those who develop eye complaints during therapy (blurred vision, diminished vision, changes in color vision, retinal changes); NSAIDs may mask signs/symptoms of infections; photosensitivity reported

Adverse Reactions

Cardiovascular: Congestive heart failure, angina, hypertension, hypotension, arrhythmias, edema

Central nervous system: Headache, drowsiness, vertigo, dizziness, fatigue, hallucinations, confusion, depression, emotional lability, psychotic behavior, pyrexia

Dermatologic: Rash, urticaria, angioedema, Stevens-Johnson syndrome, exfoliative dermatitis, bruising, petechiae, purpura

Endocrine & metabolic: Hyperglycemia, hypoglycemia, hyperkalemia, gynecomastia, hyponatremia, fluid retention

Gastrointestinal: Dyspepsia, heartburn, nausea, diarrhea, constipation, flatulence, stomatitis, vomiting, abdominal pain, peptic ulcer, GI bleeding, GI perforation, gingival ulcers, pancreatitis, proctitis, paralytic ulcers, colitis, anorexia, weight loss, dry mucous membranes

Genitourinary: Impotence, azotemia

Hematologic: Neutropenia, anemia, agranulocytosis, bone marrow suppression, hemolytic anemia, hemorrhage, inhibition of platelet aggregation

Hepatic: Hepatitis, elevated LFTs, cholestatic jaundice

Neuromuscular & skeletal: Involuntary muscle movements, muscle weakness, tremors, weakness

Ocular: Vision changes

Otic: Tinnitus

Renal: Dysuria, polyuria, pyuria, oliguria, anuria, acute renal failure

Respiratory: Exacerbation of asthma, dyspnea

Miscellaneous: Thirst, diaphoresis

Overdosage Symptoms include drowsiness, lethargy, disorientation, confusion, dizziness, numbness, paresthesia, nausea, vomiting, gastric irritation, abdominal pain, headache, tinnitus, sweating, blurred vision, muscle twitching, seizures, coma, acute renal failure, increased BUN and serum creatinine, hypotension, tachycardia, and metabolic acidosis

Toxicology Management of a nonsteroidal anti-inflammatory agent (NSAID) intoxication is primarily supportive and symptomatic. Fluid therapy is commonly effective in managing the hypotension that may occur following an acute NSAID overdose, except when this is due to an acute blood loss. Seizures tend to be very short-lived and often do not require drug treatment although recurrent seizures should be treated with I.V. diazepam. Since many of the NSAIDs undergo enterohepatic cycling, multiple doses of charcoal may be needed to reduce the potential for delayed toxicities.

(Continued)

Mefenamic Acid *(Continued)*

Drug Interactions
May increase digoxin, methotrexate, and lithium serum concentrations
Aspirin or other salicylates may decrease NSAID serum concentrations
Other NSAIDs may increase adverse GI effects
Increased prothrombin time with anticoagulants
Decreased antihypertensive effects of ACE inhibitors, beta-blockers, and thiazide diuretics
Increased response to sympathomimetics
Probenecid may increase toxicity of NSAIDs by increase in serum concentrations
Effects of loop diuretics may decrease
Diuretics may increase the risk of acute renal insufficiency
Azotemia may be increased in elderly receiving loop diuretics

Mechanism of Action Inhibits prostaglandin synthesis, acts on the hypothalamus heat-regulating center to reduce fever, blocks prostaglandin synthetase action which prevents formation of the platelet-aggregating substance thromboxane A_2; decreases pain receptor sensitivity. Other proposed mechanisms of action are lysosomal stabilization, inhibition of kinin and leukotriene production, alteration of chemotactic factors, and inhibition of neutrophil activation. This latter mechanism may be the most significant pharmacologic action to reduce inflammation.

Pharmacodynamics
Peak effect: Oral: Within 2-4 hours
Duration: Up to 6 hours

Pharmacokinetics
Protein binding: High (>90%)
Metabolism: Conjugated in the liver; substrate CYP2C9
Half-life: 3.5 hours
Elimination: In urine (50%) and feces as unchanged drug and metabolites

Usual Dosage Geriatrics and Adults: Oral: 500 mg to start then 250 mg every 6 hours as needed; maximum therapy: 1 week; maximum dose: 1000 mg/day (see Additional Information)

Monitoring Parameters Monitor for pain relief, gastric adverse effects, bleeding, confusion; renal function

Test Interactions Increased chloride (S), increased sodium (S), positive Coombs' [direct]

Patient Information Serious gastrointestinal bleeding can occur as well as ulceration and perforation. Pain may or may not be present. Avoid aspirin and aspirin-containing products while taking this medication. If gastric upset occurs, take with food, milk, or antacid. If gastric adverse effects persist, contact physician. May cause drowsiness, dizziness, blurred vision, and confusion. Use caution when performing tasks which require alertness (eg, driving). Do not take for more than 3 days for fever or 10 days for pain without physician advice.

Nursing Implications See Overdosage, Monitoring Parameters, Patient Information, and Special Geriatric Considerations

Additional Information There are no clinical guidelines to predict which NSAID will give response in a particular patient. Trials with each must be initiated until response determined. If diarrhea develops, reduce dose or discontinue use of mefenamic acid for a short time (until diarrhea stops). Some patients may be unable to tolerate further use. Consider dose, patient convenience, and cost.

Special Geriatric Considerations Elderly are a high-risk population for adverse effects from nonsteroidal anti-inflammatory agents. As much as 60% of elderly can develop peptic ulceration and/or hemorrhage asymptomatically. The concomitant use of H_2 blockers, omeprazole, and sucralfate is not effective as prophylaxis with the exception of NSAID-induced duodenal ulcers which may be prevented by the use of ranitidine. Misoprostol and proton pump inhibitors are the only agents proven to help prevent the development of NSAID-induced ulcers. Also, concomitant disease and drug use contribute to the risk for GI adverse effects. Use lowest effective dose for shortest period possible. Consider renal function decline with age. Use of NSAIDs can compromise existing renal function especially when Cl_{cr} is ≤30 mL/minute. Tinnitus may be a difficult and unreliable indication of toxicity due to age-related hearing loss or eighth cranial nerve damage. CNS adverse effects such as confusion, agitation, and hallucination are generally seen in overdose or high dose situations, but elderly may demonstrate these adverse effects at lower doses than younger adults.

Dosage Forms Capsule: 250 mg

References

Brooks PM, Day RO, "Nonsteroidal Anti-inflammatory Drugs - Differences and Similarities," *N Engl J Med*, 1991, 324(24):1716-25.

Clinch D, Banerjee AK, Ostick G, "Absence of Abdominal Pain in Elderly Patients With Peptic Ulcer," *Age Ageing*, 1984, 13:120-3.

Clive DM, Stoff JS, "Renal Syndromes Associated With Nonsteroidal Anti-inflammatory Drugs," *N Engl J Med*, 1984, 310(9):563-72.

Graham DY, "Prevention of Gastroduodenal Injury Induced by Chronic Nonsteroidal Anti-inflammatory Drug Therapy," *Gastroenterology*, 1989, 96(2 Pt 2 Suppl):675-81.

Gurwitz JH, Avorn J, Ross-Degnan D, et al, "Nonsteroidal Anti-Inflammatory Drug-Associated Azotemia in the Very Old," *JAMA*, 1990, 264(4):471-5.

Hawkey CJ, Karrasch JA, Szczepaski L, et al, "Omeprazole Compared With Misoprostrol for Ulcers Associated With Nonsteroidal Anti-inflammatory Drugs," *N Engl J Med*, 1998, 338(11):727-34.

Knodel LC, "Preventing NSAID-Induced Ulcers: The Role of Misoprostol," *Consult Pharm*, 1989, 4:37-41.

Pounder R, "Silent Peptic Ulceration: Deadly Silence or Golden Silence?" *Gastroenterology*, 1989, 96(2 Pt 2 Suppl):626-31.

Yeomans ND, Tulassay Z, Juhasz L, et al, "A Comparison of Omeprazole With Ranitidine for Ulcers Associated With Nonsteroidal Anti-inflammatory Drugs," *N Engl J Med*, 1998, 338(11):719-26.

Mefoxin® see Cefoxitin *on page 184*

Megace® see Megestrol Acetate *on this page*

Megestrol Acetate (me JES trole AS e tate)

Brand Names Megace®

Generic Available Yes

Therapeutic Category Antineoplastic Agent, Hormone (Gonadotropin Hormone-Releasing Antigen); Progestin

Use Palliative treatment of breast and endometrial carcinomas

Unlabeled use: Appetite stimulation and promotion of weight gain in cachexia

Contraindications Hypersensitivity to megestrol or any component

Warnings The use in other types of neoplastic disease is not recommended.

Precautions Use with caution in patients with a history of thrombophlebitis

Adverse Reactions
Cardiovascular: Edema
Central nervous system: Carpal tunnel syndrome
Dermatologic: Alopecia, rash
Endocrine & metabolic: Vaginal bleeding and discharge, hyperglycemia
Gastrointestinal: Weight gain, nausea, vomiting
Local: Deep vein thrombophlebitis
Respiratory: Hyperpnea, dyspnea, pulmonary embolism
Miscellaneous: Tumor flare

Mechanism of Action Megestrol is an antineoplastic progestin thought to act through an antileutenizing effect mediated via the pituitary

Pharmacokinetics
Absorption: Oral: Well absorbed
Metabolism: Completely in the liver to free steroids and glucuronide conjugates
Time to peak serum concentration: Oral: Within 1-3 hours

Usual Dosage Geriatrics and Adults: Oral:
Breast carcinoma: 40 mg 4 times/day
Endometrial carcinoma: 40-320 mg/day in divided doses
Use for 2 continuous months to determine efficacy; maximum doses used have been up to 800 mg/day

Monitoring Parameters Monitor for tumor response; observe for signs of thromboembolic phenomena

Patient Information Report any calf pain, difficulty breathing, or vaginal bleeding to physician; may cause abdominal pain, headache, nausea, vomiting, breast tenderness; notify physician if these persist

Nursing Implications Monitor for thromboembolism (see Adverse Reactions)

Special Geriatric Considerations Elderly females may have vaginal bleeding or discharge and need to be forewarned of this side effect and inconvenience. No specific changes in dose are required for elderly. Megestrol has been used in the treatment of the failure to thrive syndrome in cachectic elderly in addition to proper nutrition.

Dosage Forms
Suspension, oral: 40 mg/mL with alcohol 0.06% (240 mL)
Tablet: 20 mg, 40 mg

Mellaril® see Thioridazine *on page 910*

Mellaril-S® *see* Thioridazine *on page 910*

Melphalan (MEL fa lan)
Brand Names Alkeran®
Synonyms L-PAM; L-Sarcolysin; Phenylalanine Mustard
Generic Available No
Therapeutic Category Antineoplastic Agent, Alkylating Agent (Nitrogen Mustard)
Use Palliative treatment of multiple myeloma and nonresectable epithelial ovarian carcinoma; neuroblastoma, rhabdomyosarcoma; breast cancer; limb perfusion in malignant melanoma
Contraindications Hypersensitivity to melphalan or any component; severe bone marrow suppression; patients whose disease was resistant to prior therapy
Warnings The U.S. Food and Drug Administration (FDA) currently recommends that procedures for proper handling and disposal for antineoplastic agents be considered. Is potentially mutagenic, carcinogenic, and teratogenic; produces amenorrhea.
Precautions Reduce dosage or discontinue therapy if total leukocyte count is <3000/mm³ or platelet count is <100,000/mm³; use with caution in patients with bone marrow suppression and impaired renal function
Adverse Reactions
Cardiovascular: Vasculitis
Dermatologic: Alopecia, rash, pruritus, vesiculation of skin
Endocrine & metabolic: Leukopenia, thrombocytopenia, anemia, agranulocytosis, hemolytic anemia
Gastrointestinal: Nausea, vomiting, diarrhea, stomatitis
Genitourinary: Bladder irritation, hemorrhagic cystitis
Local: Burning and discomfort at injection site
Respiratory: Pulmonary fibrosis
Overdosage Symptoms of overdose include hypocalcemia, pulmonary fibrosis
Toxicology General supportive measures; monitor CBC 3-6 weeks; transfusions as needed; no known antidote available
Drug Interactions Cyclosporine
Stability Store at room temperature; protect from light; do not refrigerate; use within 1 hour of reconstitution; dispense in glass
Mechanism of Action Alkylating agent that inhibits DNA and RNA synthesis via formation of carbonium ions; cross-links strands of DNA
Pharmacokinetics
Absorption: Oral: Variable and incomplete
Half-life: Terminal: 90 minutes
Time to peak serum concentration: Within 2 hours; food interferes with absorption
Elimination: 10% to 15% of dose excreted unchanged in urine; after oral administration, 20% to 50% is excreted in stool
Usual Dosage
Oral (refer to individual protocols):
Geriatrics: See adult dose; no specific recommendations for creatinine clearance changes with age
Adults:
Multiple myeloma: 6 mg/m²/day for 5 days, repeat every 6 weeks, or 0.1 mg/kg/day for 2-3 weeks; maintenance dose: 2-4 mg/day when bone marrow has recovered (see Precautions)
Ovarian carcinoma: 0.2 mg/kg/day for 5 days, repeat in 4-5 weeks
I.V. (refer to individual protocols):
Adults: Multiple myeloma: 16 mg/m² administered at 2-week intervals for 4 doses, then repeat monthly as per protocol for multiple myeloma
Monitoring Parameters Observe for signs of infection or bleeding (see Precautions)
Test Interactions False-positive Coombs' test [direct]
Patient Information Any signs of infection, easy bruising or bleeding, shortness of breath, or painful or burning urination should be brought to physician's attention. Nausea, vomiting, or hair loss sometimes occur
Nursing Implications Protect tablets from light; monitor WBCs and platelets; observe for infections and bleeding (see Warnings and Additional Information)

Additional Information
Myelosuppressive effects:
WBC: Moderate
Platelets: Moderate
Onset (days): 7
Nadir (days): 10-18
Recovery (days): 42-50

Special Geriatric Considerations Toxicity to immunosuppressives is increased in elderly. Start with lowest recommended adult doses. Signs of infection, such as fever and WBC rise, may not occur; lethargy and confusion may be more prominent signs of infection.

Dosage Forms
Powder for injection: 50 mg
Tablet: 2 mg

References
Hutchins LF and Lipschitz DA, "Cancer, Clinical Pharmacology, and Aging," *Clin Geriatr Med*, 1987, 3(3):483-503.

Kaplan HG, "Use of Cancer Chemotherapy in the Elderly," *Drug Treatment in the Elderly*, Vestal RE, ed, Boston, MA: ADIS Health Science Press, 1984, 338-49.

Menadol® [OTC] *see* Ibuprofen *on page 475*

Meni-D® *see* Meclizine *on page 574*

Meningococcal Polysaccharide Vaccine, Groups A, C, Y, and W-135
(me NIN joe kok al pol i SAK a ride vak SEEN groops aye, see, why & dubl yoo won thur tee fyve)

Related Information
Immunization Guidelines *on page 1058*

Brand Names Menomune®-A/C/Y/W-135

Generic Available No

Therapeutic Category Vaccine, Inactivated Bacteria

Use
Immunization of persons 2 years of age and above in epidemic or endemic areas as might be determined in a population delineated by neighborhood, school, dormitory, or other reasonable boundary. The prevalent serogroup in such a situation should match a serogroup in the vaccine. Individuals at particular high-risk include persons with terminal component complement deficiencies and those with anatomic or functional asplenia.

Travelers visiting areas of a country that are recognized as having hyperendemic or epidemic meningococcal disease

Vaccinations should be considered for household or institutional contacts of persons with meningococcal disease as an adjunct to appropriate antibiotic chemoprophylaxis as well as medical and laboratory personnel at risk of exposure to meningococcal disease

Note: Routine vaccination in the United States is not recommended since meningococcal disease is infrequent and vaccine does not protect from serogroup B which is most prevalent

Contraindications Acute illness

Warnings Patients who undergo splenectomy secondary to trauma or nonlymphoid tumors respond well; however, those asplenic patients with lymphoid tumors who receive either chemotherapy or irradiation respond poorly

Precautions Hypersensitivity: Have epinephrine 1:1000 available at time of vaccination

Adverse Reactions
>10%:
Central nervous system: Pain
Dermatologic: Erythema and induration
Local: Tenderness
1% to 10%: Central nervous system: Headache, malaise, fever, chills

Drug Interactions Decreased effect with administration of immunoglobulin within 1 month

Stability Discard remainder of vaccine within 5 days after reconstitution; store reconstituted vaccine in refrigerator

Mechanism of Action Induces the formation of bactericidal antibodies to meningococcal antigens; the presence of these antibodies is strongly correlated with immunity to meningococcal disease caused by *Neisseria meningitidis* groups A, C, Y and W-135.

Pharmacodynamics
Onset: Antibody levels are achieved within 10-14 days after administration
(Continued)

Meningococcal Polysaccharide Vaccine, Groups A, C, Y, and W-135 (Continued)

Duration: Antibodies against group A and C polysaccharides decline markedly (to prevaccination levels) over the first 3 years following a single dose of vaccine

Usual Dosage One dose S.C. (0.5 mL); the need for booster is unknown

Monitoring Parameters Monitor for side effects, especially local effects at site of injection

Patient Information Inform patients about common side effects; patients should report serious and unusual effects to physician

Nursing Implications Epinephrine 1:1000 should be available to control allergic reaction

Special Geriatric Considerations No specific data; would only recommend for patients traveling to highly endemic areas

Dosage Forms Injection: 10 dose, 50 dose

Menomune®-A/C/Y/W-135 see Meningococcal Polysaccharide Vaccine, Groups A, C, Y, and W-135 on previous page

Meperidine (me PER i deen)
Related Information
I.V. Push Recommended Guidelines on page 1083
Narcotic Agonist Comparative Pharmacology on page 1036
Pharmacokinetics of Narcotic Agonist Analgesics on page 1037

Brand Names Demerol®

Synonyms Isonipecaine Hydrochloride; Pethidine Hydrochloride

Generic Available Yes

Therapeutic Category Analgesic, Narcotic

Use Management of moderate to severe pain; adjunct to anesthesia and preoperative sedation

Restrictions C-II

Contraindications Hypersensitivity to meperidine or any component; patients receiving MAO inhibitors presently or in the past 14 days

Warnings Some preparations contain sulfites which may cause allergic reaction; use with caution in patients with renal failure or seizure disorders or those receiving high dose meperidine: normeperidine (an active metabolite and CNS stimulant) may accumulate and precipitate twitches, tremors, or seizures

Precautions Use with caution in patients with pulmonary, hepatic, or renal disorders; patients with tachycardia, biliary colic, or increased intracranial pressure

Adverse Reactions
Cardiovascular: Palpitations, hypotension, bradycardia, peripheral vasodilation, tachycardia
Central nervous system: CNS depression, dizziness, drowsiness, sedation, increased intracranial pressure
Dermatologic: Pruritus
Endocrine & metabolic: Antidiuretic hormone release
Gastrointestinal: Nausea, vomiting, constipation
Neuromuscular & skeletal: Metabolite normeperidine may precipitate tremors or seizures
Ocular: Miosis
Respiratory: Respiratory depression
Miscellaneous: Physical and psychological dependence, biliary or urinary tract spasm, histamine release

Overdosage Symptoms of overdose include CNS depression, respiratory depression, mydriasis, bradycardia, pulmonary edema, chronic tremors, CNS excitability, seizures

Toxicology Treatment of an overdose includes support of the patient's airway, establishment of an I.V. line and administration of naloxone 2 mg I.V. with repeat administration as necessary up to a total of 10 mg

Drug Interactions
Decreased effect with phenytoin (increased toxicity of meperidine concurrently)
Increased effect/toxicity of isoniazid; increased effect/toxicity with MAO inhibitors (can be fatal), serotonin reuptake inhibitors (eg, fluoxetine), CNS depressants, TCAs, phenothiazines, barbiturates, amphetamines, cimetidine

Stability Protect oral dosage forms from light

Mechanism of Action Binds to opiate receptors in the CNS, causing inhibition of ascending pain pathways, altering the perception of and response to pain; produces generalized CNS depression

Pharmacodynamics
Onset of action:
Oral, S.C., I.M.: Within 10-15 minutes
I.V.: Effects within 5 minutes
Peak effects: Oral, S.C., I.M.: Within 1 hour
Duration: Oral, S.C., I.M.: 2-4 hours
Enhanced analgesia has been seen in elderly patients on therapeutic doses of narcotics; duration of action may be increased in the elderly

Pharmacokinetics
Distribution: V_d: Increased in elderly
Protein binding: 65% to 75%; decreased in elderly
Metabolism: In liver
Bioavailability: ~50% to 60%, increased bioavailability with liver disease
Half-life:
Adults:
Terminal: 2.5-4 hours
Terminal in liver disease: 7-11 hours
Elderly: 7 hours
Normeperidine (active metabolite): 15-30 hours; normeperidine half-life is dependent on renal function and can accumulate with high doses or in patients with decreased renal function
Time to peak serum concentration: Longer in elderly
Elimination: ~5% meperidine eliminated unchanged in urine

Usual Dosage Doses should be titrated to appropriate analgesic effect; when changing route of administration, note that oral doses are about half as effective as parenteral dose.

Geriatrics:
Oral: 50 mg every 4 hours
I.M.: 25 mg every 4 hours
Adults: Oral, I.M., I.V.: S.C.: 50-150 mg/dose every 3-4 hours as needed
Dosing adjustment in renal impairment:
Cl_{cr} 10-50 mL/minute: Administer at 75% of normal dose
Cl_{cr} <10 mL/minute: Administer at 50% of normal dose
Dosing adjustment/comments in hepatic disease: Increased narcotic effect in cirrhosis; reduction in dose more important for oral than I.V. route

Monitoring Parameters Pain relief, respiratory and mental status, blood pressure

Reference Range Therapeutic: 70-500 ng/mL (SI: 283-2020 nmol/L); Toxic: >1000 ng/mL (SI: >4043 nmol/L)

Patient Information Will cause drowsiness; avoid alcoholic beverages

Nursing Implications Observe patient for excessive sedation, CNS depression, seizures; if I.V. administration is required, inject very slowly using a diluted solution

Special Geriatric Considerations Meperidine is not recommended as a drug of first choice for the treatment of chronic pain in the elderly due to the accumulation of its metabolite, normeperidine which leads to serious CNS side effects (eg, tremor, seizures, etc); for acute pain, its use should be limited to 1-2 doses (see Warnings, Adverse Reactions, and Pharmacodynamics)

Dosage Forms
Meperidine hydrochloride:
Injection:
Multiple dose vials: 50 mg/mL (30 mL); 100 mg/mL (20 mL)
Single dose: 10 mg/mL (5 mL, 10 mL, 30 mL); 25 mg/mL (0.5 mL, 1 mL); 50 mg/dose (1 mL); 75 mg/dose (1 mL, 1.5 mL); 100 mg/dose (1 mL)
Syrup: 50 mg/5 mL (500 mL)
Tablet: 50 mg, 100 mg

References
Ferrell BA, "Pain Management in Elderly People," *J Am Geriatr Soc*, 1991, 39(1):64-73.

Mephenytoin (me FEN i toyn)

Brand Names Mesantoin®
Synonyms Methoin; Methylphenylethylhydantoin; Phenantoin
Therapeutic Category Anticonvulsant, Hydantoin
Use Treatment of tonic-clonic and partial seizures in patients who are uncontrolled with less toxic anticonvulsants
Contraindications Hypersensitivity to mephenytoin or any component
(Continued)

Mephenytoin *(Continued)*

Warnings Fatal irreversible aplastic anemia has occurred

Precautions Abrupt withdrawal may precipitate seizures

Adverse Reactions
Central nervous system: Sedation, ataxia, nervousness, mental confusion
Dermatologic: Rash, erythema multiforme, alopecia
Endocrine & metabolic: Nausea, vomiting, insomnia
Gastrointestinal: Weight gain
Hematologic: Neutropenia, leukopenia, thrombocytopenia, agranulocytosis, anemia
Hepatic: Hepatitis
Neuromuscular & skeletal: Tremors
Ocular: Diplopia, photophobia
Miscellaneous: Hodgkin's disease-like syndrome, serum sickness

Overdosage Symptoms of overdose include restlessness, dizziness, drowsiness, nausea, vomiting, nystagmus, ataxia, dysarthria, tremor, slurred speech, hypotension, respiratory depression, coma

Drug Interactions
Increased hydantoin effects (inhibited metabolism) seen with allopurinol, amiodarone, benzodiazepines, chloramphenicol, cimetidine, fluconazole, isoniazid, metronidazole, miconazole, omeprazole, phenacemide, phenylbutazone, succinimides, sulfonamides, trimipramine, valproic acid
The following displace hydantoin anticonvulsants and increase effects: Salicylates, tricyclic antidepressants, valproic acid; other agents increasing effects of hydantoins include ibuprofen, chlorpheniramine, phenothiazines
Decreased effects of hydantoin by increased metabolism with barbiturates, carbamazepine, diazoxide, rifampin, theophylline
Decreased absorption with antacids, sucralfate
Decreased hydantoin effect with folic acid, influenza vaccine, loxapine, nitrofurantoin, pyridoxine

Mechanism of Action Stabilizes neuronal membranes and decreases seizure activity by increasing efflux or decreasing influx of sodium ions across cell membranes in the motor cortex during generation of nerve impulses; prolongs effective refractory period and suppresses ventricular pacemaker automaticity, shortens action potential in the heart

Pharmacodynamics
Onset of action: 30 minutes
Duration of action: 24-48 hours

Pharmacokinetics
Absorption: Oral: Rapid
Metabolism: In the liver; substrate 2C18, 2C19
Half-life: 144 hours
Elimination: In urine

Usual Dosage Adults: Oral: Initial dose: 50-100 mg/day given daily; increase by 50-100 mg at weekly intervals; usual maintenance dose: 200-600 mg/day in 3 divided doses; maximum: 800 mg/day

Reference Range 10-20 µg/mL; **Note:** Some clinicians now recommend 5-20 µg/mL

Test Interactions Increased alkaline phosphatase (S); decreased calcium (S)

Nursing Implications Monitor CBC and platelets

Additional Information Usually listed in combination with other anticonvulsants

Special Geriatric Considerations Elderly may have reduced hepatic clearance due to age decline in phase I metabolism

Dosage Forms Tablet: 100 mg

Mephobarbital *(me foe BAR bi tal)*

Brand Names Mebaral®

Synonyms Methylphenobarbital

Generic Available No

Therapeutic Category Anticonvulsant; Barbiturate; Sedative

Use Sedative; treatment of grand mal and petit mal epilepsy

Restrictions C-IV

Contraindications Hypersensitivity to mephobarbital, other barbiturates, or any component; pre-existing CNS depression; respiratory depression; severe uncontrolled pain; history of porphyria; hepatic impairment, renal disease

Warnings Use with caution in patients with renal impairment, pulmonary insufficiency, or hepatic dysfunction; sometimes used in specific patients who have excessive sedation or hyperexcitability from phenobarbital; abrupt withdrawal may precipitate status epilepticus; use with caution in patients with depression, suicidal threats, or history of drug abuse; use cautiously in patients with pain as signs may be masked by barbiturate; vitamin D requirements may be increased (increased metabolism); renal impairment decreases clearance; hepatic disease may slow clearance; use cautiously in elderly (see Special Geriatric Considerations)

Precautions Use with caution in patients with myxedema or myasthenia gravis; barbiturates may be habit forming; abrupt withdrawal in patients with seizure disorders may precipitate status epilepticus

Adverse Reactions

Cardiovascular: Hypotension, bradycardia, syncope

Central nervous system: Dizziness, lightheadedness, drowsiness, "hangover" effect, confusion, mental depression, unusual excitement, nervousness, faint feeling, headache, insomnia, nightmares, ataxia, hallucinations, vertigo, lethargy

Dermatologic: Rash, exfoliative dermatitis, Stevens-Johnson syndrome, angioedema

Gastrointestinal: Constipation, nausea, vomiting

Hematologic: Agranulocytosis, megaloblastic anemia, thrombocytopenia

Local: Thrombophlebitis

Respiratory: Respiratory depression

Miscellaneous: Dependence

Overdosage Symptoms of overdose include CNS depression, respiratory depression, hypothermia, tachycardia, hypotension

Toxicology Repeated oral doses of activated charcoal significantly reduce the half-life of barbiturates resulting from an enhancement of nonrenal elimination. The usual dose is 30-60 g every 4-6 hours for 3-4 days unless the patient has no bowel movement causing the charcoal to remain in the GI tract. Assure adequate hydration and renal function.

Urinary alkalinization with I.V. sodium bicarbonate also helps to enhance elimination. Hemodialysis or hemoperfusion is of uncertain value. Patients in stage IV coma due to high serum barbiturate concentrations may require charcoal hemoperfusion.

Drug Interactions

Decreased effect: Phenothiazines, haloperidol, quinidine, cyclosporine, TCAs, corticosteroids, theophylline, ethosuximide, warfarin, oral contraceptives, chloramphenicol, griseofulvin, doxycycline, beta-blockers

Increased effect/toxicity: Propoxyphene, benzodiazepines, CNS depressants, valproic acid, methylphenidate, chloramphenicol

Mechanism of Action Increases seizure threshold in the motor cortex; depresses monosynaptic and polysynaptic transmission in the CNS

Pharmacodynamics

Onset of action: 20-60 minutes

Duration: 10-16 hours

Pharmacokinetics

Absorption: Oral: ~50%

Metabolism: By the liver to phenobarbital

Half-life: 34 hours

Elimination: In urine

Usual Dosage Oral:

Epilepsy: Adults: 200-600 mg/day in 2-4 divided doses

Sedation:

Geriatrics: Start with lowest recommended doses for adults (see Additional Information)

Adults: 32-100 mg 3-4 times/day

Dosing adjustment in renal or hepatic impairment: Use with caution and reduce dosages

Reference Range Phenobarbital level should be in the range of 15-40 µg/mL

Test Interactions ↑ alk phos (S), ↑ ammonia (B), ↓ bilirubin (S), ↓ calcium (S)

Patient Information May cause drowsiness, may impair coordination and judgment; do not discontinue abruptly; notify physician of dark urine, pale stools, jaundice, abdominal pain, persistent nausea, and vomiting; do not skip doses

Nursing Implications Observe patient for excessive sedation, respiratory depression; raise bed rails, institute safety precautions, assist with ambulation

Additional Information May use in combination with phenobarbital or phenytoin. When using with phenobarbital, both agents should be started at ½ (Continued)

Mephobarbital *(Continued)*

dose. When mephobarbital is used with phenytoin, the dose of phenytoin must be reduced. Full doses of mephobarbital may be given.

Special Geriatric Considerations Using barbiturates in elderly may induce paradoxical stimulation, cause or aggravate depression and confusion. Due to mephobarbital's long half-life and risk of dependence, it is not a drug of choice in elderly as a sedative/hypnotic. Interpretive guidelines from healthcare financing administrations OBRA regulations discourage the use of barbiturates as sedative/hypnotics in nursing home patients.

Dosage Forms Tablet: 32 mg, 50 mg, 100 mg

References
Pond SM, Olson KR, Osterloh JD, et al, "Randomized Study of the Treatment of Phenobarbital Overdose With Repeated Doses of Activated Charcoal," *JAMA,* 1984, 251(23):3104-8.
Zawada ET, Nappi J, Done G, et al, "Advances in the Hemodialysis Management of Phenobarbital Overdose," *South Med J,* 1983, 76(1):6-8.

Mephyton® *see* Phytonadione *on page 747*

Meprobamate *(me proe BA mate)*

Related Information
Anxiolytic/Hypnotic Use in Long-Term Care Facilities *on page 1099*
Federal OBRA Regulations Recommended Maximum Doses - Anxiolytics *on page 1057*

Brand Names Equanil®; Miltown®; Neuramate®

Generic Available Yes

Therapeutic Category Antianxiety Agent

Use Management of anxiety disorders

Restrictions C-IV

Contraindications Acute intermittent porphyria; hypersensitivity to meprobamate or any component; do not use in a comatose patient or in those with pre-existing CNS depression

Warnings Physical and psychological dependence and abuse may occur; use with caution in patients with renal or hepatic impairment, or with a history of seizures

Precautions Allergic reaction may occur in patients with history of dermatological condition (usually by fourth dose)

Adverse Reactions
Cardiovascular: Palpitations, tachycardia, arrhythmias, syncope
Central nervous system: Drowsiness, ataxia, slurred speech, dizziness
Gastrointestinal: Nausea, vomiting, diarrhea

Overdosage Symptoms of overdose include drowsiness, lethargy, ataxia, coma, hypotension, shock, death

Toxicology Treatment is supportive following attempts to enhance drug elimination. Hypotension should be treated with I.V. fluids and/or Trendelenburg positioning. Dialysis and hemoperfusion have not demonstrated significant reductions in blood drug concentrations.

Drug Interactions Increased toxicity: CNS depressants, alcohol

Mechanism of Action Precise mechanism is not yet clear, but many effects have been ascribed to its central depressant actions

Pharmacodynamics Onset of action: Oral: Following administration sedation occurs within 60 minutes

Pharmacokinetics
Metabolism: Promptly in the liver
Half-life: 10 hours
Elimination: In urine (8% to 20% as unchanged drug) and in feces (10% as metabolites)

Usual Dosage Oral:
Geriatrics (use lowest effective dose): Initial: 200 mg 2-3 times/day
Adults: 400 mg 3-4 times/day, up to 2400 mg/day
Moderately dialyzable (20% to 50%)

Monitoring Parameters Mental status

Reference Range Therapeutic: 6-12 µg/mL (SI: 28-55 µmol/L); Toxic: >60 µg/mL (SI: >275 µmol/L)

Patient Information May cause drowsiness; avoid alcoholic beverages

Nursing Implications Monitor mental status; assist with ambulation

Special Geriatric Considerations Meprobamate is not considered a drug of choice in the elderly because of its potential to cause physical and psychological dependence; interpretive guidelines from the Health Care Financing Administration (HCFA) strongly discourage the use of meprobamate in residents of long-term care facilities

Dosage Forms Tablet: 200 mg, 400 mg

Mepron™ *see* Atovaquone *on page 92*

Mercaptopurine (mer kap toe PYOOR een)
Brand Names Purinethol®
Synonyms 6-Mercaptopurine; 6-MP
Generic Available No
Therapeutic Category Antineoplastic Agent, Antimetabolite; Antineoplastic Agent, Purine
Use Treatment of leukemias, Crohn's disease, ulcerative colitis, other collagen vascular diseases
Contraindications Hypersensitivity to mercaptopurine or any component; severe liver disease; severe bone marrow suppression; patients whose disease showed prior resistance to mercaptopurine or thioguanine
Warnings The U.S. Food and Drug Administration (FDA) currently recommends that procedures for proper handling and disposal of antineoplastic agents be considered. Mercaptopurine may be potentially carcinogenic
Precautions Adjust dosage in patients with renal impairment or hepatic failure; patients who receive allopurinol concurrently should have the mercaptopurine dose reduced $1/3$ to $1/4$ of the usual dose
Adverse Reactions
Dermatologic: Rash
Endocrine & metabolic: Hyperuricemia
Gastrointestinal: Mild nausea or vomiting, diarrhea, stomatitis
Hematologic: Myelosuppression
Hepatic: Hepatotoxicity (occurs most frequently with doses greater than 2.5 mg/kg/day)
Renal: Renal toxicity (oliguria, hematuria)
Miscellaneous: Drug fever
Overdosage Symptoms of overdose include bone marrow suppression, nausea, vomiting, diarrhea, hepatic necrosis, gastroenteritis
Toxicology No known pharmacologic antagonist for mercaptopurine
Drug Interactions Allopurinol may potentiate the effect of bone marrow suppression (inhibits xanthine oxidase); trimethoprim and sulfamethoxazole may enhance bone marrow suppression of mercaptopurine
Mechanism of Action Purine antagonist which inhibits DNA and RNA synthesis through pseudofeedback inhibition of the first step of purine synthesis which disrupts purine biosynthesis of purine nucleotides
Pharmacokinetics
Absorption: Variable and incomplete (16% to 50%)
Protein binding: 19%
Metabolism: Undergoes first-pass metabolism in the GI mucosa and liver; metabolized in the liver to sulfate conjugates, 6-thiouric acid and other inactive compounds
Half-life (adults): 47 minutes
Time to peak concentration: Within 2 hours
Elimination: Prompt excretion in urine
Usual Dosage Oral (refer to individual protocols):
Geriatrics: Due to renal decline with age, start with lower recommended doses for adults
Adults:
Induction: 2.5-5 mg/kg/day or 80-100 mg/m^2/day given once daily
Maintenance: 1.5-2.5 mg/kg/day; calculate doses to nearest 25 mg daily dosage
Monitoring Parameters Monitor leukocyte count and platelets
Test Interactions Increased potassium (S)
Patient Information Do not take with meals; nausea and vomiting are rare with usual doses; report to physician if fever, sore throat, bleeding, bruising, shortness of breath, or painful urination occurs; hair loss occurs sometimes
Nursing Implications Adjust dosage in patients with renal insufficiency to lowest recommended dose; monitor dose response with WBC and platelet counts; observe for signs of infection and bleeding or bruising (see Additional Information)
Additional Information Myelosuppressive effects:
WBC: Moderate
Platelets: Moderate
Onset (days): 7-10
Nadir (days): 14
Recovery (days): 21
(Continued)

Mercaptopurine *(Continued)*

Special Geriatric Considerations Toxicity to immunosuppressives is increased in elderly. Start with lowest recommended adult doses. Signs of infection, such as fever and WBC rise, may not occur. Lethargy and confusion may be more prominent signs of infection.

Dosage Forms Tablet: 50 mg

References

Hutchins LF and Lipschitz DA, "Cancer, Clinical Pharmacology, and Aging," *Clin Geriatr Med*, 1987, 3(3):483-503.

Kaplan HG, "Use of Cancer Chemotherapy in the Elderly," *Drug Treatment in the Elderly*, Vestal RE, ed, Boston, MA: ADIS Health Science Press, 1984, 338-49.

6-Mercaptopurine *see* Mercaptopurine *on previous page*

Meropenem *(mer oh PEN em)*

Brand Names Merrem® I.V.

Generic Available No

Therapeutic Category Antibiotic, Carbapenem

Use Intra-abdominal infections (complicated appendicitis and peritonitis) caused by viridans group streptococci, *E. coli*, *K. pneumoniae*, *P. aeruginosa*, *B. fragilis*, *B. thetaiotamicron*, and *Peptostreptococcus* sp; meropenem has also been used to treat soft tissue infections, febrile neutropenia, and urinary tract infections

Contraindications Patients with known hypersensitivity to meropenem, any component, or other carbapenems (eg, imipenem); patients who have experienced anaphylactic reactions to other beta-lactams

Warnings Pseudomembranous colitis and hypersensitivity reactions have occurred and often require immediate drug discontinuation; thrombocytopenia has been reported in patients with significant renal dysfunction; seizures have occurred in patients with underlying neurologic disorders (less frequent than with Primaxin®); superinfection possible with long courses of therapy

Adverse Reactions

Cardiovascular: Hypotension, heart failure (MI and arrhythmias), tachycardia, hypertension, edema, seizures

Central nervous system: Headache, insomnia, agitation, confusion, hallucinations, depression, seizures, fever

Dermatologic: Rash, pruritus, urticaria

Gastrointestinal: Diarrhea, nausea, vomiting, constipation, oral moniliasis, glossitis, anorexia, flatulence, ileus

Genitourinary: Dysuria, RBCs in urine

Hematologic: Anemia, hypo- and hypercytosis, bleeding events (epistaxis, melena, etc)

Hepatic: Cholestatic jaundice, hepatic failure, increase LFTs

Local: Pain at injection site, phlebitis, thrombophlebitis

Neuromuscular & skeletal: Paresthesia, whole body pain

Renal: Renal failure, elevation of creatinine and BUN

Respiratory: Apnea

Overdosage No cases of acute overdosage are reported which have resulted in symptoms

Toxicology Supportive therapy is recommended; meropenem and metabolite are removable by dialysis

Drug Interactions Increased effect: Probenecid competes with meropenem for active tubular secretion and inhibits the renal excretion of meropenem (half-life increased by 38%)

Stability Store at room temperature; when vials are reconstituted with NaCl/D_5W, they are stable for 2 hours/1 hour at room temperature or for 18 hours/8 hours when refrigerated; when diluted in minibags, they are stable for up to 24 hours refrigerated in NaCl and 6 hours in D_5W

Mechanism of Action Inhibits bacterial cell wall synthesis by binding to several of the penicillin-binding proteins; bactericidal against many gram-positive aerobes and gram-negative aerobes and anaerobes, especially *E. coli*, *P. aeruginosa*, and *S. aureus*; not bactericidal against *L-monocytogenes*; has significant stability against beta-lactamases with the exception of matollo-beta-lactamases; not effective against MRSA; cross-resistance possible with other strains resistant to carbapenems; may act synergistically with aminoglycosides

Pharmacokinetics

Distribution: V_d: ~0.3 L/kg in adults; penetrates well into most body fluids and tissues; CSF concentrations approximate those of the plasma

Protein binding: 2%

Metabolism: Hepatic; metabolizes to open beta-lactam form (inactive); not metabolized by same enzyme as imipenem which results in toxic metabolite

Half-life:

Normal renal function: 1-1.5 hours

Cl_{cr} 30-80 mL/minute: 1.9-3.3 hours

Cl_{cr} 2-30 mL/minute: 3.82-5.7 hours

Time to peak tissue concentration: 1 hour following infusion

Elimination: Renal, ~25% as the inactive metabolite

Usual Dosage I.V.: Geriatrics and Adults: 1 g every 8 hours

Dosing adjustment in renal impairment:

Cl_{cr} 26-50 mL/minute: Administer 1 g every 12 hours

Cl_{cr} 10-25 mL/minute: Administer 500 mg every 12 hours

Cl_{cr} <10 mL/minute: Administer 500 mg every 24 hours

Dialysis: Meropenem and its metabolites are readily dialyzable

Additional Information 1 g of meropenem contains 90.2 mg of sodium as sodium carbonate (3.92 mEq)

Special Geriatric Considerations Adjust dose based on renal function (see Usual Dosage); see Warnings

Dosage Forms

Infusion: 500 mg (100 mL); 1 g (100 mL)

Infusion, ADD-vantage®: 500 mg (15 mL); 1 g (15 mL)

Injection: 25 mg/mL (20 mL); 33.3 mg/mL (30 mL)

References

Ljungberg B and Nilsson-Ehle I, "Pharmacokinetics of Meropenem an Its Metabolites in Young and Elderly Healthy Men," *Antimicrob Agents Chemother,* 1992, 36(7):1437-40.

Wiseman LR, Wagstaff AJ, Brogden RN, et al, "Meropenem. A Review of Its Antibacterial Activity, Pharmacokinetic Properties and Clinical Efficacy," *Drugs,* 1995, 50(1):73-101.

Merrem® I.V. *see Meropenem on previous page*

Meruvax® II *see Rubella Virus Vaccine, Live on page 841*

Mesalamine (me SAL a meen)

Brand Names Asacol® Oral; Pentasa® Oral; Rowasa® Rectal

Synonyms 5-Aminosalicylic Acid; 5-ASA; Fisalamine; Mesalazine

Therapeutic Category 5-Aminosalicylic Acid Derivative; Anti-inflammatory Agent, Rectal

Use Treatment of ulcerative colitis, proctosigmoiditis, and proctitis

Contraindications Known hypersensitivity to mesalamine, sulfites, sulfasalazines, or salicylates

Warnings Reported to produce intolerance or exacerbation of colitis (3%) in some patients; paracolitis reported in some patients when using mesalamine; renal impairment has occurred in some patients

Precautions Pericarditis should be considered in patients with chest pain; pancreatitis should be considered in any patient with new abdominal complaints; sulfite hypersensitivity

Adverse Reactions

Central nervous system: Malaise, dizziness, chills, depression, anxiety, fever

Dermatologic: Rash, pruritus

Gastrointestinal: Abdominal pain, cramps, diarrhea, dyspepsia, eructation, nausea, vomiting, discomfort, headache, flatulence, pancreatitis, xerostomia, tenesmus, dysgeusia

Genitourinary: Urinary urgency, epididymitis

Hematologic: Agranulocytosis, leukopenia

Neuromuscular & skeletal: Peripheral neuropathy, arthralgia, back pain, hypertonia, pain, tremors, weakness

Ocular: Eye pain

Otic: Tinnitus

Renal: Dysuria, hematuria

Respiratory: Pharyngitis, chest pain, asthma exacerbation, rhinitis, sinusitis

Miscellaneous: Lymphadenopathy, flu symptoms

Overdosage Symptoms of overdose include renal function impairment

Toxicology Treat with emesis, gastric lavage, and follow with activated charcoal slurry

Stability Unstable in presence of water or light; once foil has been removed, unopened bottles have an expiration of 1 year following the date of manufacture

Mechanism of Action Mesalamine (5-aminosalicylic acid) is the active component of sulfasalazine; the specific mechanism of action of mesalamine is unknown; however, it is thought that it modulates chemical mediators of the inflammatory response, especially leukotrienes; action appears topical rather than systemic

(Continued)

Mesalamine *(Continued)*

Pharmacokinetics
Absorption: Rectal: ~15%, this is variable and dependent upon retention time, underlying GI disease, and colonic pH

Metabolism: In the liver by acetylation to acetyl-5-aminosalicylic acid (active), and to glucuronide conjugates; intestinal metabolism may also occur

Half-life:
5-ASA: 30-90 minutes
acetyl 5-ASA: 5-10 hours

Time to peak serum concentrations: Within 4-7 hours

Elimination: Most metabolites are excreted in urine with <2% appearing in feces

Usual Dosage Geriatrics and Adults: Adults (usual course of therapy is 3-6 weeks):
Oral:
Capsule: 1 g 4 times/day
Tablet: 800 mg 3 times/day

Retention enema: 60 mL (4 g) at bedtime, retained overnight, approximately 8 hours

Rectal suppository: Insert 1 suppository in rectum twice daily

Some patients may require rectal and oral therapy concurrently

Monitoring Parameters Renal status (serum creatinine); stool frequency; GI symptoms; sigmoidoscopy

Test Interactions Elevations in AST, ALT, alkaline phosphatase, serum creatine, BUN

Patient Information Retain enemas for 8 hours or as long as practical; shake well before administering; (oral) do not chew or break tablets; (suppositories) remove foil wrapper, avoid excessive handling; shake suspension well

Nursing Implications Provide patient with copy of mesalamine administration instructions; monitor renal status and bowel function/status

Special Geriatric Considerations Elderly may have difficulty administering and retaining rectal suppositories. Given renal function decline with aging, monitor serum creatinine often during therapy.

Dosage Forms
Capsule, controlled release (Pentasa®): 250 mg
Suppository, rectal (Rowasa®): 500 mg
Suspension, rectal (Rowasa®): 4 g/60 mL (7s)
Tablet, enteric coated (Asacol®): 400 mg

Mesalazine *see Mesalamine on previous page*

Mesantoin® *see Mephenytoin on page 585*

Mesoridazine *(mez oh RID a zeen)*

Related Information
Antacid Drug Interactions *on page 1096*
Antipsychotic Agents Comparison *on page 1023*
Antipsychotic Medication Guidelines *on page 1076*
Federal OBRA Regulations Recommended Maximum Doses - Antipsychotics *on page 1056*

Brand Names Serentil®

Generic Available No

Therapeutic Category Antipsychotic Agent; Neuroleptic Agent; Phenothiazine Derivative

Use Management of manifestations of psychotic disorders; depressive neurosis; alcohol withdrawal; nausea and vomiting; nonpsychotic symptoms associated with dementia in elderly, Tourette's syndrome; Huntington's chorea; spiromatic torticollis and Reye's syndrome (see Special Geriatric Considerations)

Contraindications Hypersensitivity to mesoridazine or any component, cross-sensitivity with other phenothiazines may exist; avoid use in patients with narrow-angle glaucoma, bone marrow suppression, severe liver or cardiac disease; subcortical brain damage, circulatory collapse, severe hypotension or hypertension

Warnings
Tardive dyskinesia: Prevalence rate may be 40% in elderly; elderly women especially at risk; embarrassment from dyskinesias may lead to greater social isolation; development of the syndrome and the irreversible nature are proportional to duration and total cumulative dose over time. May be reversible if diagnosed early in therapy; intermittent use of antipsychotics (not proven use) helps decrease total cumulative dose.

EPS: Extrapyramidal reactions are more common in elderly with up to 50% developing these reactions after age 60. These reactions may be more common in dementia patients. Drug-induced **Parkinson's syndrome** occurs often. Discontinuation usually resolves symptoms but may take weeks to months (12+) to clear. **Akathisia** is the most common EPS reaction in elderly. The symptoms of motor restlessness are difficult to diagnose in demented elderly; increased nervousness, assertiveness, restlessness with constant movement may indicate this adverse event. Consider decreasing dose if antipsychotic to treat as well as diagnose problem; usually see this reaction within 2-3 months of initiating antipsychotic drug.

Anticholinergic effects: These side effects most common with low potency antipsychotics (eg, thioridazine, chlorpromazine). CNS toxicity occurs more frequently and severely in elderly; increased confusion, memory loss, psychotic behavior, and agitation frequently occur as a consequence of anticholinergic effects to antipsychotic agents. Peripheral anticholinergic action troublesome to elderly; most peripheral anticholinergic effects last only 2-3 weeks (see Adverse Reactions).

Orthostatic hypotension: More common with low potency agents (eg, thioridazine, chlorpromazine, and clozapine) but of concern with all antipsychotic agents; orthostasis due to alpha-receptor blockade by antipsychotic agents. Elderly present many risk factors for orthostatic hypotension: blunted baroreceptor reflexes, decreased vascular tone, decreased vascular volume, and possible presence of cardiac diseases which result in decreased cardiac output.

Sedation: Common side effect with antipsychotic therapy; should not be used as a hypnotic unless insomnia is associated with target behavior symptoms treated with antipsychotic medications (see Special Geriatric Considerations). Anecdotal reports suggesting antipsychotic sedation in nonpsychotic patients is extremely unpleasant due to feelings of depersonalization, derealization, and dysphoria. Due to the long duration of action with antipsychotic drugs, these reactions may last up to 24 hours and result in decreased daytime function.

Cardiac toxicity: Life-threatening arrhythmias have occurred at therapeutic doses of antipsychotics. Thioridazine more commonly demonstrates EKG changes than other antipsychotics; suggested to use high potency antipsychotic agents (ie, haloperidol) in patients with cardiac conduction defects.

Precautions Use with caution in patients with cardiovascular disease, seizures, and Parkinson's disease; benefits of therapy must be weighed against risks of therapy

Adverse Reactions Sedation and anticholinergic effects are more pronounced than extrapyramidal effects

Cardiovascular: Orthostatic hypotension, tachycardia, arrhythmias, abnormal T waves with prolonged ventricular repolarization, EKG changes

Central nervous system: Sedation, drowsiness, restlessness, anxiety, extrapyramidal reactions, pseudoparkinsonian signs and symptoms, tardive dyskinesia, neuroleptic malignant syndrome, seizures, altered central temperature regulation

Dermatologic: Hyperpigmentation, pruritus, rash, photosensitivity

Endocrine & metabolic: Amenorrhea, galactorrhea, gynecomastia

Gastrointestinal: GI upset, xerostomia (problem for denture users), constipation, adynamic ileus, weight gain

Genitourinary: Urinary retention, overflow incontinence, priapism, sexual dysfunction (up to 60%), impotence

Hematologic: Agranulocytosis, leukopenia (usually in patients with large doses for prolonged periods), thrombocytopenia, hemolytic anemia, eosinophilia

Hepatic: Cholestatic jaundice (rare)

Ocular: Retinal pigmentation, blurred vision

Miscellaneous: Anaphylactoid reactions

Overdosage Symptoms of overdose include deep sleep, coma, extrapyramidal symptoms, abnormal involuntary muscle movements, hypotension or hypertension; agitation, restlessness, fever, hypothermia or hyperthermia, seizures, cardiac arrhythmias, EKG changes

Toxicology Following initiation of essential overdose management, toxic symptom treatment and supportive treatment should be initiated. Hypotension usually responds to I.V. fluids or Trendelenburg positioning. If unresponsive to these measures the use of a parenteral inotrope may be required (eg, norepinephrine 0.1-0.2 mcg/kg/minute titrated to response). Do not use epinephrine. Seizures commonly respond to diazepam (I.V. 5-10 mg bolus (Continued)

Mesoridazine *(Continued)*

every 15 minutes if needed up to a total of 30 mg) or to phenytoin or pheno-barbital. Also critical cardiac arrhythmias often respond to I.V. phenytoin (15 mg/kg up to 1 g), while other antiarrhythmics can be used. Neuroleptics often cause extrapyramidal symptoms (eg, dystonic reactions) requiring management with diphenhydramine 1-2 mg/kg up to a maximum of 50 mg I.M. or I.V. slow push followed by a maintenance dose for 48-72 hours. When these reactions are unresponsive to diphenhydramine, benztropine mesylate I.V. 1-2 mg may be effective. These agents are generally effective within 2-5 minutes.

Drug Interactions

Alcohol may increase CNS sedation

Anticholinergic agents may decrease pharmacologic effects; increase anticholinergic side effects; may enhance tardive dyskinesia

Aluminum salts may decrease absorption of phenothiazines

Barbiturates may decrease phenothiazine serum concentrations

Bromocriptine may have decreased efficacy when administered with phenothiazines

Guanethidine's hypotensive effect is decreased by phenothiazines

Lithium administration with phenothiazines may increase disorientation

Meperidine and phenothiazine coadministration increases sedation and hypotension

Methyldopa administration with phenothiazine (trifluoperazine) may significantly increase blood pressure

Norepinephrine, epinephrine have decreased pressor effect when administered with chlorpromazine; therefore, be aware of possible decreased effectiveness or when any phenothiazine is used

Phenytoin serum concentrations may increase or decrease with phenothiazines; tricyclic antidepressants may have increased serum concentrations with concomitant administration with phenothiazines

Propranolol administered with phenothiazines may increase serum concentrations of both drugs

Valproic acid may have increased half-life when administered with phenothiazines (chlorpromazine)

Stability Protect all dosage forms from light, clear or slightly yellow solutions may be used; should be dispensed in amber or opaque vials/bottles. Solutions may be diluted or mixed with fruit juices or other liquids but must be administered immediately after mixing; do not prepare bulk dilutions or store bulk dilutions.

Mechanism of Action Blocks postsynaptic mesolimbic dopaminergic D_1 and D_2 receptors in the brain; exhibits a strong alpha-adrenergic blocking and anticholinergic effect, depresses the release of hypothalamic and hypophyseal hormones; believed to depress the reticular activating system thus affecting basal metabolism, body temperature, wakefulness, vasomotor tone, and emesis

Pharmacokinetics

Absorption: Oral: May be affected by the inherent anticholinergic action on the gastrointestinal tissue causing variable absorption. Absorption from tablets is erratic with less variation seen with solutions. These agents are widely distributed in tissues with CNS concentrations exceeding that of plasma due to their lipophilic characteristics.

Protein binding: Antipsychotic agents are bound 90% to 99% to plasma proteins; highly bound to brain and lung tissue and other tissues with a high blood perfusion

Half-life: Elimination half-lives of antipsychotics range from 20-40 hours which may be extended in elderly due to decline in oxidative hepatic reactions (phase I) with age

Time to peak concentrations: 2-4 hours

Elimination: Excretion occurs through hepatic metabolism (oxidation) where numerous active metabolites are produced; active metabolites excreted in urine

The biologic effect of a single dose persists for 24 hours. When the patient has accommodated to initial side effects (sedation), once daily dosing is possible due to the long half-life of antipsychotics.

Steady-state plasma concentrations are achieved in 4-7 days; therefore, if possible, do not make dose adjustments more than once in a 7-day period. Due to the long half-lives of antipsychotics, as needed (prn) use is ineffective since repeated doses are necessary to achieve therapeutic tissue concentrations in the CNS.

Usual Dosage

Geriatrics (nonpsychotic patients, dementia behavior): Oral: Initial: 10 mg 1-2 times/day; if <10 mg/day desires, consider administering 10 mg every other day (qod); increase dose at 4- to 7-day intervals by 10-25 mg/day; increase dose intervals (bid, tid, etc) as necessary to control response or side effects; maximum daily dose: 250 mg; gradual increases (titration) may prevent some side effects or decrease their severity

Geriatrics and Adults: I.M.: Initial: 25 mg; repeat doses in 30-60 minutes if necessary; dose range: 25-200 mg/day. Elderly usually require less than maximal daily dose.

Adults: Oral: Initial: 25 mg for most patients; may repeat dose in 30-60 minutes, if necessary; usual optimum dosage range: 25-200 mg/day. Concentrate may be diluted just prior to administration with distilled water, acidified tap water, orange or grape juice; do not prepare and store bulk dilutions.

Not dialyzable (0% to 5%)

Monitoring Parameters Orthostatic blood pressures; tremors, gait changes, abnormal movement in trunk, neck, buccal area, or extremities; monitor target behaviors for which the agent is given

Test Interactions Increased cholesterol (S), increased glucose; decreased uric acid (S)

Patient Information Oral concentrate must be diluted in 2-4 oz of liquid (water, fruit juice, carbonated drinks, milk, or pudding); do not take antacid within 1 hour of taking drug; avoid alcohol; avoid excess sun exposure (use sun block); may cause drowsiness, rise slowly from recumbent position; use of supportive stockings may help prevent orthostatic hypotension

Nursing Implications Watch for hypotension when administering I.M. or I.V.; dilute the oral concentrate with water or juice before administration; avoid skin contact with oral solution; may cause contact dermatitis; monitor orthostatic blood pressures 3-5 days after initiation of therapy or a dose increase; observe for tremor and abnormal movement or posturing (extrapyramidal symptoms)

Special Geriatric Considerations See Warnings.

Many elderly patients receive antipsychotic medications for inappropriate nonpsychotic behavior. Before initiating antipsychotic medication, the clinician should investigate any possible reversible cause; any stress or stress from any disease can cause acute "confusion" or worsening of baseline nonpsychotic behavior. Most commonly acute changes in behavior are due to increases in drug dose or addition of new drug to regimen; fluid electrolyte loss; infections; and changes in environment.

Any changes in disease status in any organ system can result in behavior changes.

In the treatment of agitated, demented, elderly patients, authors of meta-analysis of controlled trials of the response to the traditional antipsychotics (phenothiazines, butyrophenones) in controlling agitation have concluded that the use of neuroleptics results in a response rate of 18%. Clearly neuroleptic therapy for behavior control should be limited with frequent attempts to withdraw the agent given for behavior control.

Dosage Forms

Mesoridazine besylate:
Injection: 25 mg/mL (1 mL)
Liquid, oral: 25 mg/mL (118 mL)
Tablet: 10 mg, 25 mg, 50 mg, 100 mg

References

Peabody CA, Warner MD, Whiteford HA, et al, "Neuroleptics and the Elderly," *J Am Geriatr Soc,* 1987, 35(3):233-8.

Risse SC and Barnes R, "Pharmacologic Treatment of Agitation Associated With Dementia," *J Am Geriatr Soc,* 1986, 34(5):368-76.

Saltz BL, Woerner MG, Kane JM, et al, "Prospective Study of Tardive Dyskinesia Incidence in the Elderly," *JAMA,* 1991, 266(17):2402-6.

Seifert RD, "Therapeutic Drug Monitoring: Psychotropic Drugs," *J Pharm Pract,* 1984, 6:403-16.

Mestinon® Injection *see Pyridostigmine on page 806*

Mestinon® Oral *see Pyridostigmine on page 806*

Metacortandralone *see Prednisolone on page 774*

Metamucil® [OTC] *see Psyllium on page 804*

Metamucil® Instant Mix [OTC] *see Psyllium on page 804*

Metandren® *see Methyltestosterone on page 613*

Metaprel® *see Metaproterenol on next page*

Metaproterenol (met a proe TER e nol)

Related Information
Asthma Guidelines *on page 1040*
Inhaled Medications Comparison *on page 1034*

Brand Names Alupent®; Arm-a-Med® Metaproterenol; Dey-Dose® Metaproterenol; Metaprel®; Prometa®

Synonyms Orciprenaline Sulfate

Generic Available Yes (except inhaler)

Therapeutic Category Adrenergic Agonist Agent; Beta$_2$-Adrenergic Agonist Agent; Bronchodilator

Use Bronchodilator in reversible airway obstruction due to asthma or COPD

Contraindications Hypersensitivity to metaproterenol or any component; pre-existing cardiac arrhythmias associated with tachycardia

Warnings Use caution in patients with unstable vasomotor symptoms, diabetes, hyperthyroidism, prostatic hypertrophy, or a history of seizures; also use caution in the elderly and those patients with cardiovascular disorders such as coronary artery disease, arrhythmias, and hypertension.

Precautions Excessive use may result in tolerance; deaths have been reported after excessive use; though the exact cause is unknown, cardiac arrest after a severe asthmatic crisis is suspected

Adverse Reactions
Cardiovascular: Tachycardia, palpitations, elevation or depression of blood pressure
Central nervous system: Nervousness, CNS stimulation, hyperactivity, insomnia
Gastrointestinal: GI upset
Neuromuscular & skeletal: Tremors (may be more common in the elderly)

Overdosage Symptoms of overdose include tremor, dizziness, nervousness, headache, nausea, coughing, seizures, angina, hypertension

Toxicology In cases of overdose, supportive therapy should be instituted, and prudent use of a cardioselective beta-adrenergic blocker (eg, atenolol or metoprolol) should be considered, keeping in mind the potential for induction of bronchoconstriction in an asthmatic individual. Dialysis has not been shown to be of value in the treatment of an overdose with this agent.

Drug Interactions
Decreased therapeutic effect: Beta-adrenergic blockers (eg, propranolol)
Increased therapeutic effect: Inhaled ipratropium may increase duration of bronchodilation, nifedipine may increase FEV-1
Increased toxicity (cardiovascular): MAO inhibitors, tricyclic antidepressants, sympathomimetic agents (eg, amphetamine, dopamine, dobutamine), inhaled anesthetics (eg, enflurane)

Stability Store in tight, light-resistant container

Mechanism of Action Relaxes bronchial smooth muscle by action on beta$_2$-receptors with little effect on heart rate

Pharmacodynamics
Onset of action: Oral: Bronchodilation occurs within 15 minutes; following inhalation these effects occur within 5 minutes
Peak effect: Within 1 hour
Duration of action: Similar (~3-4 hours) regardless of route administered

Pharmacokinetics
Absorption: Oral: 40% from GI tract
Metabolism: In the liver
Elimination: Via kidneys as metabolites

Usual Dosage
Oral:
Geriatrics: Initial: 10 mg 3-4 times/day increasing as necessary up to 20 mg 3-4 times/day
Adults: 20 mg 3-4 times/day
Nebulizer: Geriatrics and Adults: 5-20 breaths of full strength 5% metaproterenol **or** 0.2-0.3 mL of 5% metaproterenol in 2.5-3 mL normal saline nebulized every 4-6 hours (can be given more frequently according to need)
Inhalation, metered dose: Geriatrics and Adults: 2-3 inhalations every 3-4 hours to a maximum of 12 inhalations/day

Monitoring Parameters Pulmonary function, blood pressure, pulse

Patient Information Do not exceed recommended dosage - excessive use may lead to adverse effects or loss of effectiveness. Follow instructions accompanying inhaler. If more than one inhalation per dose is necessary, wait at least 1 full minute between inhalations - second inhalation is best delivered after 10 minutes for Alupent®. May cause nervousness, restlessness, insomnia - if these effects continue after dosage reduction, notify physician. Also notify physician if palpitations, tachycardia, chest pain, muscle tremors, dizziness, headache, flushing, or if breathing difficulty persists.

Nursing Implications Before using, the inhaler must be shaken well; assess lung sounds, pulse, and blood pressure before administration and during peak of medication; observe patient for wheezing after administration, if this occurs, call physician

Additional Information Metaproterenol has more beta$_1$ activity than other sympathomimetics such as albuterol and, therefore, may no longer be the beta agonist of first choice

Special Geriatric Considerations The elderly may find it useful to utilize a spacer device when using a metered dose inhaler. Oral use should be avoided due to the increased incidence of adverse effects (see Additional Information).

Dosage Forms
Metaproterenol sulfate:
Aerosol, oral: 0.65 mg/dose (5 mL, 10 mL)
Solution for inhalation, preservative free: 0.4% [4 mg/mL] (2.5 mL); 0.6% [6 mg/mL] (2.5 mL); 5% [50 mg/mL] (10 mL, 30 mL)
Syrup: 10 mg/5 mL (480 mL)
Tablet: 10 mg, 20 mg

Metformin (met FOR min)

Brand Names Glucophage®

Therapeutic Category Antidiabetic Agent; Hypoglycemic Agent, Oral

Use Treatment of nonketosis-prone patients with noninsulin-dependent diabetes mellitus who have been unable to control their blood glucose with diet and exercise. Metformin has also been used in combination with a sulfonylurea when a sulfonylurea alone, or metformin and diet have not provided adequate glucose control. Limited information is available on the efficacy of the drug in insulin-dependent diabetes mellitus.

Contraindications Renal disease or renal dysfunction (suggested as serum creatinine concentration ≥1.5 mg/dL for men and ≥1.4 mg/dL for women; congestive heart failure requiring pharmacologic treatment); acute or chronic metabolic acidosis, including diabetic ketoacidosis

Warnings Lactic acidosis is a rare but sometimes fatal side effect that is related to accumulation of metformin. Conditions that may affect the elimination of metformin or contribute to an acidotic state should be carefully monitored, including renal function (check renal function at least annually); medications that may affect metformin elimination or cause renal dysfunction; hypoxic states or respiratory insufficiency (shock, myocardial infarction, acute heart failure, etc); situations where food and fluid are restricted or prohibited (eg, surgery, temporarily suspend use for surgical procedures; prolonged nausea or vomiting, etc); concomitant alcohol intake which causes acute hepatic toxicity. Avoid use in hepatic dysfunction and in patients with a history of lactic acidosis. Metformin should not be initiated in patients ≥80 years of age unless measurement of creatinine clearance demonstrates that renal function is not reduced, as these patients are more susceptible to developing lactic acidosis. Patients undergoing radiologic studies involving parenteral iodinated contrast media should have metformin stopped at the time of or prior to the procedure and held for 48 hours afterwards. Metformin should also be held prior to surgery.

Adverse Reactions
Dermatologic: Rash
Endocrine & metabolic: Hypoglycemia (see Toxicology and Drug Interactions), lactic acidosis
Gastrointestinal: Diarrhea, nausea, vomiting, abdominal bloating, anorexia, metallic taste, weight loss
Hematologic: Asymptomatic subnormal serum vitamin B$_{12}$ concentration, with possible anemia
Miscellaneous: Reduction of cholesterol and triglyceride levels

Toxicology
Hypoglycemia has not been observed with ingestions of up to 85 g of metformin, although lactic acidosis has occurred in such circumstances
Hypoglycemia is not caused by this drug, only when used with a hypoglycemic agent is there an increased risk
Metformin is dialyzable with a clearance of up to 170 mL/minute; hemodialysis may be useful for removal of accumulated drug from patients in whom metformin overdosage is suspected

(Continued)

Metformin *(Continued)*

Drug Interactions Increased level with cimetidine due to renal mechanisms; possibly increased level with furosemide, nifedipine, cationic drugs eliminated via renal tubular secretion (amiloride, digoxin, morphine, procainamide, quinidine, quinine, ranitidine, triamterene, trimethoprim, vancomycin); possibly decreased furosemide level; increased effects (hypoglycemia) with concurrent administration of another hypoglycemic agent; iodinated contrast material (see Contraindications)

Mechanism of Action Suppresses hepatic glucose production/glycogenolysis; stimulates insulin-mediated glucose uptake in peripheral tissues (including skeletal muscle and fat); may also increase insulin receptor binding, improve glucose transport across cell membranes, inhibit gastrointestinal absorption of glucose, and increase noninsulin-mediated glucose metabolism in the intestine; does not stimulate pancreatic insulin secretion, nor increase noninsulin-mediated glucose use in the brain, renal medulla, or skin. Additional effects include a reduction of cholesterol and triglyceride levels and weight loss.

Pharmacokinetics
Distribution: V_d: 654 L (mean)
Protein binding: Negligible
Bioavailability: 50% to 60%
Half-life:
　Normal renal function: 1.5 hours
　Renal dysfunction: 4.9 hours
Time to reach steady state: 24-48 hours
Elimination: Unchanged in urine by renal tubular secretion
Dialyzable

Usual Dosage Geriatrics and Adults: Oral:
500 mg: 1 tablet twice daily with morning and evening meals; if necessary, increase dose by 1 tablet every week, up to a 2500 mg/day; doses >2000 mg/day should be given in 3 divided doses with meals
850 mg: 1 tablet daily with the morning meal; if necessary, increase dose by 1 tablet every other week, given in divided doses with meals, up to 2550 mg/day

Monitoring Parameters Urine for glucose and ketones, fasting blood glucose, hemoglobin A_{1c}, and fructosamine. Initial and periodic monitoring of hematologic parameters (eg, hemoglobin/hematocrit and red blood cell indices) and renal function should be performed, at least annually. While megaloblastic anemia has been rarely seen with metformin, if suspected, vitamin B_{12} deficiency should be excluded.

Reference Range Glucose:
Adults: 60-110 mg/dL
Elderly: 100-180 mg/dL

Patient Information May cause lactic acidosis; stop immediately and call physician if unexplained difficulty breathing/rapid breathing, muscle aches, malaise, dizziness or lightheadedness, unexpected stomach discomfort, or unusual sedation occur; avoid excessive alcohol ingestion, either acutely or chronically; take with meals to minimize gastrointestinal symptoms; notify physician if you develop an illness that causes severe vomiting, diarrhea, and/or fever, or if normal fluid intake is significantly reduced

Nursing Implications Patients who are NPO may need to have their dose held to avoid hypoglycemia

Additional Information May be used in combination with oral sulfonylureas if indicated for glycemic control; gradual dose titration should minimize gastrointestinal side effects. This agent does not cause weight gain and may actually decrease adipose tissue mass; may be preferred for obese patients.

Special Geriatric Considerations Limited data suggest that metformin's total body clearance may be decreased and AUC and half-life increased in older patients; presumably due to decreased renal clearance. Metformin has been well tolerated by the elderly but lower doses and frequent monitoring are recommended. In one study of elderly subjects, its effects could not be distinguished from tolbutamide, except for weight loss. Initial dosage is advised to be conservative and renal function assessed prior to start of therapy; one study used doses of 850 mg/day for patients with Cl_{cr} between 30-60 mL/minute with satisfactory results (see Warnings).

Dosage Forms Tablet, as hydrochloride: 500 mg, 850 mg

References
Bailey CJ and Turner RC, "Metformin," *N Engl J Med*, 1996, 334(9):574-9.
Dunn CJ and Peters DH, "Metformin: A Review of Its Pharmacologic Properties and Therapeutic Use in Diabetes Mellitus," *Drugs*, 1995, 49(5):721-49.

Josephkutty S and Potter JM, "Comparison of Tolbutamide and Metformin in Elderly Diabetic Patients," *Diabet Med*, 1990, 7(16):510-4.

Lalau JD, Vermersch A, Hary L, et al, "Type 2 Diabetes in the Elderly: An Assessment of Metformin," *Int J Clin Pharmacol Ther Toxicol*, 1990, 28(8):329-32.

Methadone (METH a done)

Related Information
Narcotic Agonist Comparative Pharmacology *on page 1036*
Pharmacokinetics of Narcotic Agonist Analgesics *on page 1037*

Brand Names Dolophine®

Generic Available Yes

Therapeutic Category Analgesic, Narcotic

Use Management of severe pain, used in narcotic detoxification maintenance programs

Restrictions C-II

Contraindications Hypersensitivity to methadone or any component

Warnings Tablets are to be used only for oral administration and **must not** be used for injection

Precautions Cumulative effect of methadone, dose and frequency should be titrated for optimal response

Adverse Reactions
Cardiovascular: Palpitations, hypotension, bradycardia, peripheral vasodilation

Central nervous system: CNS depression, increased intracranial pressure

Dermatologic: Pruritus

Endocrine & metabolic: Antidiuretic hormone release

Gastrointestinal: Nausea, vomiting, constipation

Ocular: Miosis

Respiratory: Respiratory depression

Miscellaneous: Physical and psychological dependence, histamine release, biliary or urinary tract spasm

Overdosage Symptoms of overdose include respiratory depression, CNS depression, miosis, hypothermia, circulatory collapse, convulsions

Toxicology Naloxone 2 mg I.V. with repeat administration as necessary up to a total of 10 mg

Drug Interactions
Decreased effect with phenytoin, phenobarbital, carbamazepine (increased withdrawal), rifampin (may cause withdrawal), pentazocine (may cause withdrawal)

Increased effect/toxicity with CNS depressants, phenothiazines, TCAs, MAO inhibitors, ritonavir

Mechanism of Action Binds to opiate receptors in the CNS, causing inhibition of ascending pain pathways, altering the perception of and response to pain; produces generalized CNS depression

Pharmacodynamics
Onset of action:
Oral: Within 30-60 minutes
Parenteral: Within 10-20 minutes

Duration: Oral: 6-8 hours; after repeated oral doses, duration of effect increases to 22-48 hours; enhanced analgesia has been seen in elderly patients on therapeutic doses of narcotics; duration of action may be increased in the elderly

Peak effects: Within 1-2 hours

Pharmacokinetics
Protein binding: 80% to 85%

Metabolism: Liver metabolism (N-demethylation); substrate CYP1A2

Half-life:
Elderly: >36 hours
Adults: 15-29 hours, half-life may be prolonged with alkaline pH

Elimination: In urine (<10% as unchanged drug); increased renal excretion with urine pH <6

Usual Dosage Doses should be titrated to appropriate effects:
Geriatrics: Oral, I.M.: 2.5 mg every 8-12 hours

Adults: Analgesia: Oral, I.M., I.V., S.C.: 2.5-10 mg every 3-8 hours as needed, up to 5-20 mg every 6-8 hours

Dosing interval in renal impairment:
Cl_{cr} >50 mL/minute: Administer every 6 hours
Cl_{cr} 10-50 mL/minute: Administer every 8 hours
Cl_{cr} <10 mL/minute: Administer every 8-12 hours

(Continued)

Methadone *(Continued)*

Monitoring Parameters Pain relief, respiratory and mental status, blood pressure

Reference Range Therapeutic: 100-400 ng/mL (SI: 0.32-1.29 µmol/L); Toxic: >2 µg/mL (SI: >6.46 µmol/L)

Test Interactions Increased thyroxine (S), increased aminotransferase [ALT (SGPT)/AST (SGOT)] (S)

Patient Information May cause drowsiness, avoid alcohol and other CNS depressants

Nursing Implications Observe patient for excessive sedation, respiratory depression, implement safety measures, assist with ambulation

Special Geriatric Considerations Because of its long half-life and risk of accumulation, methadone is not considered a drug of first choice in the elderly; the elderly may be particularly susceptible to the CNS depressant and constipating effects of narcotics (see Usual Dosage); adjust dose for renal function

Dosage Forms

Methadone hydrochloride:
Injection: 10 mg/mL (1 mL, 10 mL, 20 mL)
Solution:
Oral: 5 mg/5 mL (5 mL, 500 mL); 10 mg/5 mL (500 mL)
Oral, concentrate: 10 mg,mL (30 mL)
Tablet: 5 mg, 10 mg

References

Ferrell BA, "Pain Management in Elderly People," *J Am Geriatr Soc*, 1991, 39(1):64-73.

Methaminodiazepoxide Hydrochloride *see* Chlordiazepoxide *on page 205*

Methazolamide *(meth a ZOE la mide)*

Related Information

Glaucoma Drug Therapy Comparison *on page 1032*

Brand Names GlaucTabs®; Neptazane®

Generic Available No

Therapeutic Category Carbonic Anhydrase Inhibitor; Diuretic, Carbonic Anhydrase Inhibitor

Use Adjunctive treatment of open-angle or secondary glaucoma; short-term therapy of narrow-angle glaucoma when delay of surgery is desired

Contraindications Marked kidney or liver dysfunction, severe pulmonary obstruction, hypersensitivity to methazolamide or any component

Precautions Sulfonamide-type reactions, melena, anorexia, nausea, vomiting, constipation, hematuria, glycosuria, urinary frequency, renal colic, renal calculi, crystalluria, polyuria, hepatic insufficiency, various CNS effects, transient myopia, bone marrow suppression, thrombocytopenia/purpura, hemolytic anemia, leukopenia, pancytopenia, agranulocytosis, urticaria, pruritus, rash, Stevens-Johnson syndrome, weight loss, fever, acidosis

Adverse Reactions

Central nervous system: Fever, depression, drowsiness, dizziness, malaise
Dermatologic: Rash
Endocrine & metabolic: Hyperchloremic metabolic acidosis, hypokalemia
Gastrointestinal: GI irritation, anorexia
Genitourinary: Polyuria
Hematologic: Bone marrow suppression
Neuromuscular & skeletal: Paresthesia
Renal: Crystalluria, dysuria

Drug Interactions Increased lithium excretion and altered excretion of other drugs by alkalinization of the urine, such as amphetamines, quinidine, procainamide, methenamine, phenobarbital, salicylates; hypokalemia may be compounded with concurrent diuretic use or steroids; primidone absorption may be delayed; digitalis toxicity may occur if hypokalemia is untreated

Mechanism of Action Reversible inhibition of the enzyme carbonic anhydrase resulting in decreased intraocular pressure; noncompetitive inhibition of the enzyme carbonic anhydrase; thought that carbonic anhydrase is located at the luminal border of cells of the proximal tubule. When the enzyme is inhibited, there is an increase in urine volume and a change to an alkaline pH with a subsequent decrease in the excretion of titratable acid and ammonia.

Pharmacodynamics

Onset of action: 2-4 hours
Peak effect: 6-8 hours
Duration: 10-18 hours

Pharmacokinetics
Absorption: Slow from GI tract
Distribution: Well into tissue
Protein binding: ~55%
Half-life: ~14 hours
Elimination: ~25% excreted unchanged in urine

Usual Dosage Geriatrics and Adults: Oral: 50-100 mg 2-3 times/day

Monitoring Parameters Intraocular pressure, serum potassium, serum bicarbonate, serum sodium

Test Interactions Increased chloride (S)

Patient Information Take with food; ability to perform tasks requiring mental alertness and/or physical coordination may be impaired; report numbness or tingling of extremities to physician

Nursing Implications May cause an alteration in taste, especially when drinking carbonated beverages

Special Geriatric Considerations Malaise and complaints of tiredness and myalgia are signs of excessive dosing and acidosis in the elderly

Dosage Forms Tablet: 25 mg, 50 mg

Methenamine (meth EN a meen)

Brand Names Hiprex®; Urex®

Generic Available Yes

Therapeutic Category Antibiotic, Miscellaneous

Use Prophylaxis or suppression of recurrent urinary tract infections; urinary tract discomfort secondary to hypermotility

Contraindications Severe dehydration, renal insufficiency, hepatic insufficiency in patients receiving hippurate salt, hypersensitivity to methenamine or any component

Warnings Doses ≥8 g/day for prolonged periods may lead to bladder irritation, dysuria, and frequent micturition; an acidic urine (pH ≤6) must be present or the drug will not be effective; methenamine mandelate suspensions have a vegetable oil base which if aspirated may result in a lipid pneumonitis

Precautions Patients with liver dysfunction should have periodic liver function tests; gout (precipitation of uric acid crystals in the urine)

Adverse Reactions
Central nervous system: Headache
Dermatologic: Rash, pruritus
Gastrointestinal: Nausea, vomiting, diarrhea, abdominal cramping, anorexia
Genitourinary: Hematuria, bladder irritation
Hepatic: Elevation in AST and ALT
Renal: Dysuria, crystalluria

Toxicology Well tolerated GI decontamination and supportive care

Drug Interactions Sulfonamides (may precipitate); sodium bicarbonate and acetazolamide will decrease effect secondary to alkalinization of urine

Stability Protect from excessive heat

Mechanism of Action Methenamine is hydrolyzed to formaldehyde and ammonia in acidic urine; formaldehyde has nonspecific bactericidal action

Pharmacokinetics
Absorption: Readily from GI tract; 10% to 30% of drug will be hydrolyzed by gastric juices unless it is protected by an enteric coating
Metabolism: ~10% to 25% is metabolized in the liver
Half-life: 3-6 hours
Elimination: Occurs via glomerular filtration and tubular secretion with ~70% to 90% of dose excreted unchanged in urine within 24 hours; a urinary formaldehyde concentration >25 mcg/mL is necessary for antibacterial activity

Usual Dosage Geriatrics and Adults: Oral:
Hippurate: 1 g twice daily
Mandelate: 1 g 4 times/day after meals and at bedtime
Must be accompanied by 1 g of ascorbic acid (vitamin C) 4 times (or more)/day
Note: Studies have shown that 8-12 g of vitamin C are required to acidify urine

Monitoring Parameters Urinalysis, periodic liver function tests in patients, temperature

Test Interactions False increase in catecholamines, vanillylmandelic acid, and 17-hydroxycorticosteroids in urine; false decrease in 5-hydroxyindoleacetic acid

(Continued)

Methenamine *(Continued)*

Patient Information Take with ascorbic acid to acidify urine and avoid intake of alkalinizing agents (sodium bicarbonate, antacids); take with food to minimize GI upset; drink plenty of fluids to ensure adequate urine flow; complete full course of therapy; notify physician of rash or if side effects persist or are bothersome

Nursing Implications Administer around-the-clock to promote less variation in peak and trough serum concentration

Additional Information Hippurate salt should not be used to treat infections outside of the lower urinary tract

Special Geriatric Considerations Methenamine has little, if any, role in the treatment or prevention of infections in patients with indwelling urinary (Foley®) catheters; furthermore, in noncatheterized patients, more effective antibiotics are available for the prevention or treatment of urinary tract infections; the influence of decreased renal function on the pharmacologic effects of methenamine results are unknown (see Warnings)

Dosage Forms
Methenamine mandelate:
Suspension, oral, as mandelate (Mandelamine®): 250 mg/5 mL (coconut flavor), 500 mg/5 mL (cherry flavor)
Tablet, as mandelate, enteric coated (Mandelamine®): 250 mg, 500 mg, 1 g
Tablet, as hippurate (Hiprex®, Urex®): 1 g (Hiprex® contains tartrazine dye)

References
Vainrub B and Musher DM, "Lack of Effect of Methenamine in Suppression of, or Prophylaxis Against, Chronic Urinary Tract Infection," *Antimicrob Agents Chemother,* 1977, 12:625-9.

Methicillin *(meth i SIL in)*

Related Information
I.V. Medication Recommendations *on page 1080*
Penicillins, Penicillin-Related Antibiotics, & Other Antibiotics *on page 1010*

Brand Names Staphcillin®

Synonyms Dimethoxyphenyl Penicillin Sodium; Sodium Methicillin

Therapeutic Category Antibiotic, Penicillin

Use Treatment of susceptible bacterial infections such as osteomyelitis, septicemia, endocarditis, and CNS infections due to penicillinase-producing strains of *Staphylococcus*

Contraindications Known hypersensitivity to methicillin or any penicillin

Precautions Modify dosage in patients with renal impairment; use with caution in cephalosporin allergic patients

Adverse Reactions
Central nervous system: Fever
Dermatologic: Rash
Hematologic: Eosinophilia, anemia leukopenia, neutropenia, thrombocytopenia
Local: Phlebitis
Renal: Nephrotoxicity (interstitial nephritis), hemorrhagic cystitis
Miscellaneous: Serum sickness like reactions

Overdosage Symptoms of overdose include neuromuscular hypersensitivity, seizure

Toxicology Many beta-lactam-containing antibiotics have the potential to cause neuromuscular hyperirritability or convulsive seizures. Hemodialysis may be helpful to aid in the removal of the drug from the blood, otherwise most treatment is supportive or symptom directed.

Drug Interactions Probenecid may increase levels

Stability Reconstituted solution is stable for 24 hours at room temperature and 4 days when refrigerated; discard solutions if it has a distinctive hydrogen sulfide odor and/or color turns to a deep orange; incompatible with aminoglycosides and tetracyclines

Mechanism of Action Interferes with bacterial cell wall synthesis during active multiplication causing cell death and resultant bactericidal activity against susceptible bacteria

Pharmacokinetics
Protein binding: 40%
Half-life: Adults with normal renal function: 0.4-0.5 hours
Time to peak serum concentration:
I.M.: Within 30-60 minutes
I.V. infusion: Within 5 minutes
Elimination: ~60% to 70% of dose is eliminated unchanged in urine within 4 hours, by tubular secretion and glomerular filtration

Usual Dosage Geriatrics and Adults: I.M., I.V.: 4-12 g/day in divided doses every 4-6 hours

> **Dosing interval in renal impairment:** Cl$_{cr}$ <10 mL/minute: Do not exceed 2 g/12 hours
> Not dialyzable (0% to 5%)

Administration Can be administered IVP at a rate not to exceed 200 mg/minute or intermittent infusion over 20-30 minutes; final concentration for administration should not exceed 20 mg/mL

Monitoring Parameters Renal function, signs and symptoms of infection, temperature

Test Interactions Positive Coombs' test [direct]

Nursing Implications See Administration

Special Geriatric Considerations Because of its greater potential for interstitial nephritis, methicillin is not the parenteral antistaphylococcal agent of choice; either nafcillin or oxacillin are preferred alternatives; adjust dose for renal function

Dosage Forms Powder for injection, as sodium: 1 g, 4 g, 6 g, 10 g

Methimazole (meth IM a zole)

Brand Names Tapazole®
Synonyms Thiamazole
Generic Available No
Therapeutic Category Antithyroid Agent
Use Palliative treatment of hyperthyroidism, to return the hyperthyroid patient to a normal metabolic state prior to thyroidectomy, and to control thyrotoxic crisis that may accompany thyroidectomy

Contraindications Hypersensitivity to methimazole or any component

Warnings Use of antithyroid drugs may cause agranulocytosis, thyroid, hyperplasia, thyroid carcinoma

Precautions Use with extreme caution in patients receiving other drugs known to cause agranulocytosis, patients >40 years of age; avoid doses >40 mg/day

Adverse Reactions
Cardiovascular: Edema, cutaneous vasculitis, periarteritis
Central nervous system: Headache, drowsiness, CNS stimulation, depression, neuritis, vertigo, drug fever
Dermatologic: Rash, urticaria, pruritus, exfoliative dermatitis
Gastrointestinal: Nausea, vomiting, ageusia
Hematologic: Aplastic anemia, agranulocytosis, thrombocytopenia, bleeding
Hepatic: Jaundice, hepatitis
Neuromuscular & skeletal: Arthralgia, paresthesia
Renal: Nephritis
Miscellaneous: Lupus-like syndrome

Overdosage Symptoms of overdose include nausea, vomiting, arthralgia, pancytopenia, and signs of hypothyroidism

Toxicology General supportive care; monitor bone marrow response

Stability Protect from light

Mechanism of Action Inhibits the synthesis of thyroid hormones by blocking the oxidation of iodine in the thyroid gland, blocking iodine's ability to combine with tyrosine to form thyroxine and triiodothyronine (T$_3$); does not inactivate circulating T$_4$ and T$_3$

Pharmacodynamics
Onset of action: Oral: Within 30-40 minutes
Duration: 2-4 hours

Pharmacokinetics
Half-life: 4-13 hours
Elimination: Renally with ~12% excreted in urine within 24 hours and remainder metabolized hepatically

Usual Dosage Geriatrics and Adults: Oral: Initial: 15 mg/day (doses best given in divided doses at 8-hour intervals); more severe disease may require doses from 30-60 mg/day; maintenance: 5-15 mg/day

Monitoring Parameters Monitor signs of hypo- and hyperthyroidism, T$_4$, T$_3$, TSH, CBC

Test Interactions Increased prothrombin (S)

Patient Information Take with meals; do not exceed prescribed dosage; take at regular intervals around-the-clock; notify physician or pharmacist if fever, sore throat, unusual bleeding or bruising, headache, or general malaise occurs

Nursing Implications See Warnings, Precautions, Monitoring Parameters, and Special Geriatric Considerations

(Continued)

Methimazole *(Continued)*

Additional Information Periodic blood counts are recommended with chronic therapy (see Warnings)

Special Geriatric Considerations The use of antithyroid thioamides is as effective in elderly as they are in younger adults; however, the expense, potential adverse effects, and inconvenience (compliance, monitoring) make them undesirable. The use of radioiodine due to ease of administration and less concern for long-term side effects and reproduction problems (some older males) makes it a more appropriate therapy.

Dosage Forms Tablet: 5 mg, 10 mg

References
Johnson DG and Campbell S, "Hormonal and Metabolic Agents," *Geriatric Pharmacology*, Bressler R and Katz MD, eds, New York, NY: McGraw-Hill, 1993, 427-50.

Raby C, Lagorce JF, Jambut-Absil AC, et al, "The Mechanism of Action of Synthetic Antithyroid Drugs: Iodine Complexation During Oxidation of Iodide," *Endocrinology*, 1990, 126(3):1683-91.

Methocarbamol *(meth oh KAR ba mole)*

Brand Names Delaxin®; Marbaxin®; Robaxin®; Robomol®

Generic Available Yes

Therapeutic Category Skeletal Muscle Relaxant

Use Treatment of muscle spasm associated with acute painful musculoskeletal conditions; supportive therapy in tetanus

Contraindications Renal impairment (I.V. only), hypersensitivity to methocarbamol or any component

Precautions Do not exceed 3 g/day I.V./I.M. for more than 3 consecutive days except in the treatment of tetanus; use I.V. form cautiously in epileptic patients

Adverse Reactions I.V. only: In excessive doses, renal impairment has occurred due to the polyethylene glycol base

Cardiovascular: Syncope, hypotension, bradycardia
Central nervous system: Lightheadedness, dizziness, drowsiness, seizures (I.V. only)
Gastrointestinal: Nausea
Ocular: Conjunctivitis, blurred vision
Renal: Renal impairment
Respiratory: Nasal congestion (I.V. only)
Miscellaneous: Allergic manifestations

Overdosage Symptoms of overdose include CNS depression, coma

Toxicology Treatment is supportive following attempts to enhance drug elimination. Hypotension should be treated with I.V. fluids and/or Trendelenburg positioning. Dialysis and hemoperfusion and osmotic diuresis have all been useful in reducing serum drug concentrations. The patient should be observed for possible relapses due to incomplete gastric emptying.

Drug Interactions Increased effect/toxicity: Alcohol, CNS depressants

Mechanism of Action Causes skeletal muscle relaxation by reducing the transmission of impulses from the spinal cord to skeletal muscle

Pharmacodynamics Onset of action: Oral: Muscle relaxation reportedly occurs within 30 minutes

Pharmacokinetics
Metabolism: In the liver
Half-life: 1-2 hours
Time to peak serum concentration: ~2 hours
Elimination: Renal

Usual Dosage
Geriatrics: Oral: Initial: 500 mg 4 times/day; titrate to response
Adults: Muscle spasm:
Oral: 1.5 g 4 times/day for 2-3 days, then decrease to 4-4.5 g/day in 3-6 divided doses
I.M., I.V.: 1 g every 8 hours if oral not possible for a maximum of 3 days

Administration
I.M. administration: No more than 500 mg (5 mL)/dose should be injected in each gluteal region
I.V. administration: Infuse over 3-4 hours or administer IVP no faster than 300 mg/minute

Monitoring Parameters Relief of symptoms, mental status; blood pressure, pulse in I.V. administration

Patient Information May cause drowsiness, impair judgment or coordination; avoid alcohol or other CNS depressants; may turn urine brown, black, or green; notify physician of rash, itching, or nasal congestion

Nursing Implications The parenteral form is hypertonic and causes irritation; avoid extravasation. During the infusion, the patient should be recumbent to minimize adverse reactions; patient should remain recumbent for 15 minutes after the end of the infusion (see Administration)

Special Geriatric Considerations There is no specific information on the use of skeletal muscle relaxants in the elderly. Methocarbamol has a short half-life, so it may be considered one of the safer agents in this class.

Dosage Forms
Injection: 100 mg/mL (10 mL)
Tablet: 500 mg, 750 mg

Methoin see Mephenytoin on page 585

Methotrexate (meth oh TREKS ate)
Related Information
Serum Drug Concentrations Commonly Monitored: Guidelines on page 1114
Brand Names Folex® PFS; Rheumatrex®
Synonyms Amethopterin; MTX
Generic Available Yes
Therapeutic Category Antineoplastic Agent, Antimetabolite; Antipsoriatic Agent, Topical
Use Treatment of trophoblastic neoplasms, leukemias, psoriasis, rheumatoid arthritis, osteosarcoma, non-Hodgkin's lymphoma, breast cancer, lung cancer
Contraindications Hypersensitivity to methotrexate or any component; severe renal or hepatic impairment; pre-existing profound bone marrow suppression in patients with psoriasis or rheumatoid arthritis; alcoholism, alcoholic liver disease; AIDS, pre-existing blood dyscrasia
Warnings The U.S. Food and Drug Administration (FDA) currently recommends that procedures for proper handling and disposal of antineoplastic agents be considered. Because of the possibility of severe toxic reactions, fully inform patient of the risks involved; may cause hepatotoxicity, interstitial pneumonitis, fibrosis and cirrhosis, along with marked bone marrow suppression; death from intestinal perforation may occur.
Precautions May cause photosensitivity type reaction; reduce dosage in patients with renal or hepatic impairment, ascites, and pleural effusion; use with caution in patients with peptic ulcer disease, ulcerative colitis, pre-existing bone marrow suppression and immunodeficiency syndrome
Adverse Reactions
Cardiovascular: Vasculitis
Central nervous system: Malaise, fatigue, fever, chills, dizziness, encephalopathy, headaches, seizures, confusion
Dermatologic: Alopecia, rash, photosensitivity, depigmentation or hyperpigmentation of skin
Endocrine & metabolic: Rarely diabetes
Gastrointestinal: Ulcerative stomatitis, nausea, abdominal distress, vomiting, diarrhea, anorexia, stomatitis, enteritis
Hematologic: Leukopenia, myelosuppression, anemia, hemorrhage
Hepatic: Hepatotoxicity
Neuromuscular & skeletal: Rarely arthralgia
Ocular: Blurred vision
Pulmonary: Interstitial pneumonitis, chronic interstitial obstructive pulmonary disease
Renal: Renal failure, cystitis
Respiratory: Pneumonitis
Miscellaneous: Decreased resistance to infection, rarely anaphylaxis
Overdosage Symptoms of overdose include bone marrow suppression, nausea, vomiting, alopecia, melena, diarrhea
Toxicology Antidote: Leucovorin. Leucovorin should be administered as soon as toxicity is seen; administer 10 mg/m^2 orally or parenterally; follow with 10 mg/m^2 orally every 6 hours for 72 hours. After 24 hours following methotrexate administration, if the serum creatinine is ≥50% premethotrexate serum creatinine, increase leucovorin dose to 100 mg/m^2 every 3 hours until serum MTX level is <5 x 10^{-8}M. Hydration and alkalinization may be used to prevent precipitation of MTX or MTX metabolites in the renal tubules. Toxicity in low dose range is negligible, but may present mucositis and mild bone marrow suppression.
Drug Interactions Nonsteroidal anti-inflammatory drugs (NSAIDs) and salicylates (may suppress MTX's clearance), sulfonamides, live virus vaccines, pyrimethamine, phenytoin, 5-FU; probenecid decreased renal elimination of MTX; phenytoin serum concentrations may decrease
(Continued)

Methotrexate *(Continued)*

Stability Store intact vials at room temperature; intrathecal solutions should be diluted immediately prior to use; reconstituted solutions remain stable for 4 weeks at room temperature and 3 months when refrigerated; protect from light

Mechanism of Action An antimetabolite that inhibits DNA synthesis and cell reproduction in cancerous cells; interferes with the conversion of folic acid to tetrahydrofolic acid by binding to the enzyme dihydrofolate reductase; in psoriasis, methotrexate decreases the proliferation rate of epithelial cells

Pharmacokinetics

Absorption: Oral: Rapid; well absorbed orally at low doses (<30 mg/m^2); incomplete absorption after large doses; completely absorbed after I.M. injection

Protein binding: 50%; does not achieve therapeutic concentrations in the CSF; sustained concentrations are retained in the kidney and liver

Half-life: 8-15 hours with high doses (>30 mg/m^2) and 3-10 hours with low doses (<30 mg/m^2)

Time to peak serum concentration:

Oral: Within 1-2 hours

Parenteral: 30-60 minutes

Elimination: Small amounts excreted in feces; primarily excreted in urine (90%) via glomerular filtration and active transport

Usual Dosage Refer to individual protocols

Geriatrics:

Rheumatoid arthritis/psoriasis: Initial: 5 mg once weekly; if nausea occurs, split dose to 2.5 mg every 12 hours for the day of administration; dose may be increased to 7.5 mg/week based upon response; not to exceed 20 mg/week

Neoplastic disease: Refer to specific disease protocols

Adults:

Trophoblastic neoplasms: Oral, I.M.: 15-30 mg/day for 5 days, repeat in 7 days for 3-5 courses; creatinine clearance must be >60 mL/minute before starting therapy

Rheumatoid arthritis: Oral: 7.5 mg once weekly or 2.5 mg every 12 hours for 3 doses/week; not to exceed 20 mg/week

Dosing interval in renal impairment:

Cl$_{cr}$ 10-50 mL/minute: Reduce dose 50%

Cl$_{cr}$ <10 mL/minute: Avoid use

Not dialyzable (0% to 5%)

Geriatrics and Adults: Psoriasis: Oral, I.M., I.V.: Weekly single doses of 10-25 mg until adequate response; do not exceed 30 mg/week; the elderly should be started with low doses (10 mg); divided dose schedule: 2.5 mg every 12 hours for 3 doses; do not exceed 30 mg/week

Monitoring Parameters For prolonged use (especially rheumatoid arthritis, psoriasis); liver biopsies are recommended in patients with a history of cirrhosis or alcohol abuse or if liver function test increase; WBC and platelet counts every 4 weeks; CBC and creatinine, LFTs every 3-4 months; chest x-ray, pulmonary function tests prior to starting therapy; liver biopsies are recommended in patients with a history of cirrhosis or alcohol abuse or if liver function tests increase

Reference Range Therapeutic range is dependent upon therapeutic approach. "High-dose" regimens produce drug levels 10^{-6}M and 10^{-7}M 24-72 hours after drug infusion. Toxic: low-dose therapy: >9.1 ng/mL (SI: >20 nmol/L); high-dose therapy: >454 ng/mL (SI: >1000 nmol/L).

Test Interactions Increased potassium (S)

Patient Information Any signs of infection (fever, chills, sore throat), easy bruising or bleeding, shortness of breath, black tarry stools, yellow discoloration of skin or eyes, bloody or dark urine, joint pain, swelling, or painful or burning urination should be brought to physician's attention. Any signs of pulmonary disease (nonproductive cough, dyspnea) should be reported immediately to the physician. Nausea, vomiting, or hair loss sometimes occur. Food may delay absorption; take on empty stomach; avoid alcohol, prolonged sun exposure; may cause loss of appetite.

Nursing Implications For intrathecal use, mix methotrexate without preservative with Elliott's B solution to concentration no greater than 2 mg/mL (see Patient Information and Monitoring Parameters)

Additional Information

Myelosuppressive effects:

WBC: Mild

Platelets: Moderate
Onset (days): 7
Nadir (days): 10
Recovery (days): 21
Sodium content of 100 mg injection: 20 mg (0.86 mEq)
Sodium content of 100 mg (low sodium) injection: 15 mg (0.65 mEq)

Special Geriatric Considerations Toxicity to methotrexate or any immuno-suppressive is increased in elderly. Must monitor carefully. For rheumatoid arthritis and psoriasis, immunosuppressive therapy should only be used when disease is active and less toxic, traditional therapy is ineffective. Recommended doses should be reduced when initiating therapy in elderly due to possible decreased metabolism, reduced renal function, and presence of interacting diseases and drugs. Adjust dose as needed for renal function (Cl_{cr}).

Dosage Forms
Methotrexate sodium:
Injection: 2.5 mg/mL (2 mL); 25 mg/mL (2 mL, 4 mL, 8 mL, 10 mL)
Injection, preservative free: 25 mg (2 mL, 4 mL, 8 mL, 10 mL)
Powder, for injection: 20 mg, 25 mg, 50 mg, 100 mg, 250 mg, 1 g
Tablet: 2.5 mg
Tablet, dose pack: 2.5 mg (4 cards with 2, 3, 4, 5, or 6 tablets each)

References
Hutchins LF and Lipschitz DA, "Cancer, Clinical Pharmacology, and Aging," *Clin Geriatr Med*, 1987, 3(3):483-503.

Kaplan HG, "Use of Cancer Chemotherapy in the Elderly," *Drug Treatment in the Elderly*, Vestal RE, ed, Boston, MA: ADIS Health Science Press, 1984, 338-49.

Tugwell P, Pincus T, Yocum D, et al, "Combination Therapy With Cyclosporine and Methotrexate in Severe Rheumatoid Arthritis," *N Engl J Med*, 1995, 333(3):137-41.

Methsuximide (meth SUKS i mide)

Brand Names Celontin®

Generic Available No

Therapeutic Category Anticonvulsant, Succinimide

Use Control of absence (petit mal) seizures; useful adjunct in refractory, partial complex (psychomotor) seizures

Contraindications Known hypersensitivity to methsuximide or other succinimides

Warnings Blood dyscrasias have occurred; can cause hepatic and renal dysfunction; may result in drug-induced lupus erythematosus

Precautions Use with caution in patients with hepatic or renal disease; avoid abrupt withdrawal of methsuximide; succinimides may exacerbate grand mal seizures

Adverse Reactions
Central nervous system: Drowsiness, ataxia, dizziness, nervousness, headache, insomnia, lethargy, mental confusion, depression, sleep disturbances, aggressiveness
Dermatologic: Urticaria, pruritic rash, Stevens-Johnson syndrome
Gastrointestinal: Gum hypertrophy, nausea, vomiting, abdominal pain, anorexia, diarrhea, constipation
Genitourinary: Polyuria
Hematologic: Eosinophilia, leukopenia, agranulocytosis, granulocytopenia, bone marrow suppression, pancytopenia, monocytosis
Ocular: Periorbital edema
Miscellaneous: Hiccups

Overdosage Symptoms of overdose include dizziness, ataxia, stupor, coma, confusion, sleepiness, flaccid muscles, shallow respirations, hypotension, nausea, vomiting; chronic overdosage includes skin rash, confusion, ataxia, dizziness, drowsiness, depression, irritability, hepatic dysfunction, hematologic changes, nausea, vomiting, muscular weakness

Toxicology General supportive care; charcoal hemoperfusion and dialysis may be helpful

Drug Interactions Succinimides increase hydantoin serum concentrations, decreased primidone levels and either increased or decreased valproic acid levels

Stability Protect from high temperature

Mechanism of Action Increases the seizure threshold and suppresses paroxysmal spike-and-wave pattern in absence seizures; depresses nerve transmission in the motor cortex

Pharmacokinetics
Methsuximide is rapidly demethylated in the liver to the active metabolite N-desmethylmethsuximide

(Continued)

Methsuximide *(Continued)*

Half-life: 2-4 hours

Time to peak serum concentration: Oral: Within 1-3 hours

Elimination: <1% excreted in urine as unchanged drug

Usual Dosage Geriatrics and Adults: Oral: 300 mg/day for the first week; may increase by 300 mg/day at weekly intervals up to 1.2 g in 2-4 divided doses/day

Monitoring Parameters Monitor serum concentrations, CBC, renal function, LFTs

Reference Range Therapeutic: 10-40 µg/mL (SI: 53-212 µmol/L); Toxic: >40 µg/mL (SI: >212 µmol/L)

Test Interactions Increased alkaline phosphatase (S); decreased calcium (S)

Patient Information May cause drowsiness; periodic blood test monitoring required; if stomach upset occurs, take with food; do not stop medication without physician's advice; notify physician if skin rash, joint pain, fever, sore throat, dizziness, or blurred vision occur

Nursing Implications See Monitoring Parameters

Special Geriatric Considerations No specific data available for the elderly. This drug is rarely used in elderly, however, if it is used for partial complex seizure control, monitor closely (see Monitoring Parameters).

Dosage Forms Capsule: 150 mg, 300 mg

Methylacetoxyprogesterone *see* Medroxyprogesterone Acetate *on page 578*

Methyldopa *(meth il DOE pa)*

Related Information

I.V. Medication Recommendations *on page 1080*

Brand Names Aldomet®

Generic Available Yes

Therapeutic Category Alpha-Adrenergic Agonist; Alpha-Adrenergic Inhibitors, Central

Use Management of moderate to severe hypertension

Contraindications Hypersensitivity to methyldopa or any component; (oral suspension contains benzoic acid and sodium bisulfite; injection contains sodium bisulfite); liver disease, pheochromocytoma

Warnings May rarely produce hemolytic anemia and liver disorders; positive Coombs' test occurs in 10% to 20% of patients; perform periodic CBCs

Precautions Sedation (usually transient) may occur during initial therapy or whenever the dose is increased. Use with caution in patients with previous liver disease or dysfunction, the active metabolites of methyldopa accumulate in uremia. Patients with impaired renal function may respond to smaller doses. Elderly patients may experience syncope (avoid by giving smaller doses). Tolerance may occur usually between the second and third month of therapy. Adding a diuretic or increasing the dosage of methyldopa frequently restores blood pressure control.

Adverse Reactions

Cardiovascular: Orthostatic hypotension, bradycardia, edema

Central nervous system: Drowsiness, sedation, vertigo, headache, depression, memory lapse, fever

Dermatologic: Rash

Endocrine & metabolic: Sodium retention, gynecomastia

Gastrointestinal: Nausea, vomiting, diarrhea, xerostomia, "black" tongue, weight gain

Genitourinary: Sexual dysfunction

Hematologic: Hemolytic anemia, positive Coombs' test, leukopenia

Hepatic: Hepatitis, increased liver enzymes, jaundice, cirrhosis

Neuromuscular & skeletal: Weakness

Respiratory: Nasal congestion

Overdosage Symptoms of overdose include hypotension, sedation, bradycardia, dizziness, constipation or diarrhea, flatus, nausea, vomiting

Toxicology Hypotension usually responds to I.V. fluids or Trendelenburg positioning. If unresponsive to these measures the use of a parenteral vasoconstrictor may be required (eg, norepinephrine 0.1-0.2 mcg/kg/minute titrated to response). Treatment is primarily supportive and symptomatic.

Drug Interactions

Increased effect of tolbutamide, levodopa (and hypotension)

Increased toxicity of lithium, haloperidol (CNS effect), sympathomimetics (hypertension)

Stability Injectable dosage form is most stable at acid to neutral pH; stability of parenteral admixture at room temperature (25°C): 24 hours

Mechanism of Action Metabolized to alpha-methyl norepinephrine which lowers arterial pressure by the stimulation of central inhibitory alpha-adrenergic receptors, false neurotransmission, or reduction of plasma renin activity

Pharmacodynamics
Peak hypotensive effect: Oral, parenteral: Within 3-6 hours
Duration: 12-24 hours

Pharmacokinetics
Protein binding: <15%
Metabolism: Intestinally and in the liver with most (85%) metabolites appearing in urine within 24 hours
Half-life: 75-80 minutes
Elimination: Most (85%) metabolites appearing in urine within 24 hours

Usual Dosage
Geriatrics: Oral: Initial: 125 mg 1-2 times/day; increase by 125 mg every 2-3 days as needed
Adults:
Oral: Initial: 250 mg 2-3 times/day; increase every 2 days as needed; usual dose 500 mg to 2 g/day in 2-4 divided doses; maximum: 3 g/day
I.V.: 250-1000 mg every 6-8 hours
Slightly dialyzable (5% to 20%)

Administration Infuse over 30-60 minutes

Monitoring Parameters Blood pressure (standing and sitting/lying down), weight, symptoms of fluid retention

Reference Range Therapeutic: 1-5 µg/mL (SI: 4.7-23.7 µmol/L); Toxic: >7 µg/mL (SI: >33 µmol/L)

Test Interactions Methyldopa interferes with the following laboratory tests: urinary uric acid, serum creatinine (alkaline picrate method), AST (colorimetric method), and urinary catecholamines (falsely high levels)

Patient Information May cause transient drowsiness; may cause urine discoloration; notify physician of unexplained prolonged general tiredness, fever or jaundice; rise slowly from sitting/lying position

Nursing Implications Transient sedation or depression may be common for first 72 hours of therapy; usually disappears over time

Special Geriatric Considerations Because of its CNS effects, methyldopa is not considered a drug of first choice in the elderly

Dosage Forms
Injection, as methyldopate hydrochloride: 50 mg/mL (5 mL, 10 mL)
Suspension, oral: 250 mg/5 mL (5 mL, 473 mL)
Tablet: 125 mg, 250 mg, 500 mg

Methyldopa and Hydrochlorothiazide
(meth il DOE pa & hye droe klor oh THYE a zide)

Related Information
Hydrochlorothiazide on page 458
Methyldopa on previous page

Brand Names Aldoril®

Synonyms Hydrochlorothiazide and Methyldopa

Generic Available Yes

Therapeutic Category Antihypertensive, Combination

Special Geriatric Considerations Combination products are not recommended for first-line therapy and divided doses of diuretics may increase the incidence of nocturia in the elderly. Because of its CNS effects, methyldopa is not considered a drug of first choice in the elderly.

Dosage Forms
Tablet (Aldoril®):
15: Methyldopa 250 mg and hydrochlorothiazide 15 mg
25: Methyldopa 250 mg and hydrochlorothiazide 25 mg
D30: Methyldopa 500 mg and hydrochlorothiazide 30 mg
D50: Methyldopa 500 mg and hydrochlorothiazide 50 mg

Methylmorphine see Codeine on page 246

Methylphenidate (meth il FEN i date)
Brand Names Ritalin®; Ritalin-SR®

Generic Available Yes

Therapeutic Category Central Nervous System Stimulant, Nonamphetamine

(Continued)

Methylphenidate *(Continued)*

Use Treatment of attention deficit disorder and symptomatic management of narcolepsy

Unlabeled use: Depression in the elderly, poststroke, and cancer patients

Restrictions C-II

Contraindications Hypersensitivity to methylphenidate or any component; glaucoma; motor tics; Tourette's syndrome; patients with marked agitation, tension, and anxiety

Warnings Has high potential for abuse, may lower seizure disorder

Precautions Use with caution in patients with hypertension, seizures

Adverse Reactions

Cardiovascular: Tachycardia, hypertension, hypotension, palpitation, cardiac arrhythmias

Central nervous system: Nervousness, insomnia, dizziness, drowsiness, agitation, movement disorders, precipitation of Tourette's syndrome, and toxic psychosis (rare), visual hallucinations, fever, headache; may produce sedation paradoxically

Dermatologic: Rash

Gastrointestinal: Anorexia, nausea, abdominal pain, weight loss

Hematologic: Thrombocytopenia

Ocular: Visual disturbances (rare)

Respiratory: Shortness of breath

Miscellaneous: Hypersensitivity reactions

Overdosage Symptoms of overdose include vomiting, agitation, tremors, hyperpyrexia, muscle twitching, hallucinations, tachycardia, mydriasis, sweating, palpitations

Toxicology There is no specific antidote for methylphenidate intoxication and the bulk of the treatment is supportive. Hyperactivity and agitation usually respond to reduced sensory input, however with extreme agitation haloperidol (2-5 mg I.M. for adults) may be required. Hyperthermia is best treated with external cooling measures, or when severe or unresponsive, muscle paralysis with pancuronium may be needed. Hypertension is usually transient and generally does not require treatment unless severe. For diastolic blood pressures >110 mm Hg. a nitroprusside infusion should be initiated. Seizures usually respond to diazepam I.V. and/or phenytoin maintenance regimens.

Drug Interactions May increase serum concentrations of tricyclic antidepressants, warfarin, phenytoin, phenobarbital and primidone; MAO inhibitors may potentiate effects of methylphenidate; effects of guanethidine, bretylium may be antagonized by methylphenidate; selegiline possible added stimulant effects

Mechanism of Action Appears to stimulate the cerebral cortex and subcortical structures similar to amphetamines; exact mechanism is not well defined

Pharmacodynamics

Immediate-release tablet:

Peak cerebral stimulation: Within 2 hours

Duration: 3-6 hours

Sustained-release tablet:

Peak effect: Within 4-7 hours

Duration: 8 hours

Pharmacokinetics

Absorption: Slow and incomplete from GI tract

Metabolism: In the liver via hydroxylation to ritolinic acid

Half-life: 2-4 hours

Elimination: In urine as metabolites and unchanged drug with 45% to 50% excreted in feces via bile

Usual Dosage Geriatrics and Adults:

Narcolepsy: 10 mg 2-3 times/day, up to 60 mg/day

Depression: Initial: 2.5 mg every morning before 9 AM; dosage may be increased by 2.5-5 mg every 2-3 days as tolerated until maximum of 20 mg/day; dosage may be divided (ie, 7 AM and 12 noon), but should not be given after noon. Do not use the sustained release product.

Administration Do not crush or allow patient to chew sustained release dosage form; dosing should be completed by 12 noon

Monitoring Parameters Blood pressure, heart rate, signs and symptoms of depression

Patient Information Last daily dose should be given several hours before retiring; notify physician if headache, palpitations, nervousness, dizziness, or skin rash occurs; do not crush or chew sustained release form

Nursing Implications See Administration

Additional Information Discontinue periodically to re-evaluate or if no improvement occurs within 1 month

Special Geriatric Considerations Methylphenidate is often useful in treating elderly patients who are discouraged, withdrawn, apathetic, or disinterested in their activities. In particular, it is useful in patients who are starting a rehabilitation program but have resigned themselves to fail; these patients may not have a major depressive disorder; will not improve memory or cognitive function; use with caution in patients with dementia who may have increased agitation and confusion (see Usual Dosage and Adverse Reactions).

Dosage Forms
Methylphenidate hydrochloride:
Tablet: 5 mg, 10 mg, 20 mg
Tablet, sustained release: 20 mg

References
Emptage RE and Semla TP, "Depression in the Medically Ill Elderly: A Focus on Methylphenidate," *Ann Pharmacother*, 1996, 30(2):151-7.

Lazarus LW, Moberg PJ, Langsley PR, et al, "Methylphenidate and Nortriptyline in the Treatment of Poststroke Depression: A Retrospective Comparison," *Arch Phys Med Rehabil*, 1994, 75(4):403-6.

Wallace AE, Kofoed LL and West AN, "Double-Blind, Placebo-Controlled Trial of Methylphenidate in Older, Depressed, Medically Ill Patients," *Am J Psychiatry*, 1995, 152(6):929-31.

Methylphenobarbital *see* Mephobarbital *on page 586*
Methylphenylethylhydantoin *see* Mephenytoin *on page 585*
Methylphenyl Isoxazolyl Penicillin *see* Oxacillin *on page 698*
Methylphytyl Napthoquinone *see* Phytonadione *on page 747*

Methylprednisolone (meth il pred NIS oh lone)

Related Information
Antacid Drug Interactions *on page 1096*
Asthma Guidelines *on page 1040*
Corticosteroids Comparison, Systemic *on page 1029*
I.V. Push Recommended Guidelines *on page 1083*

Brand Names Adlone® Injection; A-methaPred® Injection; depMedalone® Injection; Depoject® Injection; Depo-Medrol® Injection; Depopred® Injection; D-Med® Injection; Duralone® Injection; Medralone® Injection; Medrol® Oral; M-Prednisol® Injection; Solu-Medrol® Injection

Synonyms 6-α-Methylprednisolone; Methylprednisolone Acetate; Methylprednisolone Sodium Succinate

Generic Available Yes

Therapeutic Category Adrenal Corticosteroid; Anti-inflammatory Agent; Corticosteroid, Systemic

Use Primarily as an anti-inflammatory or immunosuppressant agent in the treatment of a variety of diseases including those of hematologic, allergic, inflammatory, neoplastic, and autoimmune origin

Contraindications Hypersensitivity to methylprednisolone or any component; administration of live virus vaccines; systemic fungal infections

Precautions Use with caution in patients with hypothyroidism, cirrhosis, hypertension, congestive heart failure, nonspecific ulcerative colitis, thromboembolic disorders; patients at increased risk for peptic ulcer disease; gradually taper dose to withdraw therapy

Adverse Reactions
Cardiovascular: Edema, hypertension, accelerated atherogenesis
Central nervous system: Vertigo, seizures, psychoses, pseudotumor cerebri, headache
Dermatologic: Acne, skin atrophy, impaired wound healing
Endocrine & metabolic: Cushing's syndrome, pituitary-adrenal axis suppression, growth suppression, glucose intolerance, hypokalemia, alkalosis, postmenopausal bleeding, hot flashes
Gastrointestinal: Peptic ulcer, nausea, vomiting
Neuromuscular & skeletal: Muscle weakness, osteoporosis, fractures
Ocular: Cataracts, glaucoma

Toxicology When consumed in excessive quantities for prolonged periods, systemic hypercorticism and adrenal suppression may occur; in those cases, discontinuation and withdrawal of the corticosteroid should be done judiciously

Drug Interactions
Steroids decrease the effect of anticholinesterases, isoniazid, salicylates, insulin, oral hypoglycemics
Decreased effect: Barbiturates, phenytoin, rifampin
(Continued)

Methylprednisolone *(Continued)*

Increased effect (hypokalemia) of potassium-depleting diuretics
Increased risk of digoxin toxicity (due to hypokalemia)
Increased effect: Estrogens, ketoconazole

Stability
Stability of parenteral admixture (Solu-Medrol®) at room temperature (25°C): 24 hours
Stability of parenteral admixture (Solu-Medrol®) at refrigeration temperature (4°C): 24 hours

Mechanism of Action Decreases inflammation by suppression of migration of polymorphonuclear leukocytes and reversal of increased capillary permeability

Pharmacodynamics Time to obtain peak effects and the duration of these effects is dependent upon the route of administration; see table.

Route	Peak Effect	Duration
Oral	1-2 h	30-36 h
I.M.	4-8 d	1-4 wk
Intra-articular	1 wk	1-5 wk

Pharmacokinetics A single dose study found a slower methylprednisolone clearance in older volunteers compared to younger ones
Distribution: V_d: 0.7 L/kg
Half-life: 3-3.5 hours

Usual Dosage Only sodium succinate salt may be given I.V.
Geriatrics: Use the lowest effective dose
Adults:
Anti-inflammatory or immunosuppressive: Oral: 2-60 mg/day in 1-4 divided doses to start, followed by gradual reduction in dosage to the lowest possible level consistent with maintaining an adequate clinical response
I.M. (sodium succinate): 10-80 mg/day once daily
I.M. (acetate): 40-120 mg every 1-2 weeks
I.V. (sodium succinate): 10-40 mg over a period of several minutes and repeated I.V. or I.M. at intervals depending on clinical response; when high dosages are needed, administer 30 mg/kg over a period of 10-20 minutes and may be repeated every 4-6 hours not longer than 48-72 hours
Status asthmaticus: I.V. (sodium succinate): Loading dose: 2 mg/kg/dose, then 0.5-1 mg/kg/dose every 6 hours for up to 5 days
Lupus nephritis:
I.V. (sodium succinate): 1 g/day for 3 days
Intra-articular (acetate): 4-80 mg every 1-5 weeks
Intralesional (acetate): 20-60 mg every 1-5 weeks
Note: Alternate day dosing may be attempted in some disease states
Slightly dialyzable (5% to 20%)

Administration Succinate: I.V. push over 1-15 minutes; intermittent infusion over 15-60 minutes; maximum concentration: IVP: 125 mg/mL

Monitoring Parameters Blood pressure, blood glucose, electrolytes, symptoms of fluid retention

Test Interactions Increased amylase (S), chloride (S), increased cholesterol (S), increased glucose, increased protein, increased sodium (S); decreased calcium (S), decreased chloride (S), decreased potassium (S), decreased thyroxine (S)

Patient Information Do not discontinue or decrease the drug without contacting your physician; carry an identification card or bracelet advising that you are on steroids; may take with meals to decrease GI upset; apply topical product sparingly

Nursing Implications Administer with meals to decrease GI upset (see Administration and Usual Dosage)

Additional Information Sodium content of 1 g sodium succinate injection: 2.01 mEq; 53 mg of sodium succinate salt is equivalent to 40 mg of methylprednisolone base
Methylprednisolone acetate: Depo-Medrol®; methylprednisolone sodium succinate: Solu-Medrol®

Special Geriatric Considerations Because of the risk of adverse effects, systemic corticosteroids should be used cautiously in the elderly, in the smallest possible dose, and for the shortest possible time

Dosage Forms

Injection, as acetate: 20 mg/mL (5 mL, 10 mL); 40 mg/mL (1 mL, 5 mL, 10 mL); 80 mg/mL (1 mL, 5 mL)

Injection, as sodium succinate: 40 mg (1 mL, 3 mL); 125 mg (2 mL, 5 mL); 500 mg (1 mL, 4 mL, 8 mL, 20 mL); 1000 mg (1 mL, 8 mL, 50 mL); 2000 mg (30.6 mL)

Tablet: 2 mg, 4 mg, 8 mg, 16 mg, 24 mg, 32 mg

Tablet, dose pack: 4 mg (21s)

References

Tornatore KM, Logue G, Venuto RC, et al, "Pharmacokinetics of Methylprednisolone in Elderly and Young Healthy Males," *J Am Geriatr Soc*, 1994, 42(10):1118-22.

6-α-Methylprednisolone *see* Methylprednisolone *on page 611*

Methylprednisolone Acetate *see* Methylprednisolone *on page 611*

Methylprednisolone Sodium Succinate *see* Methylprednisolone *on page 611*

Methyltestosterone (meth il tes TOS te rone)

Brand Names Android®; Metandren®; Oreton® Methyl; Testred®; Virilon®

Generic Available Yes

Therapeutic Category Androgen

Use

Male: Hypogonadism; delayed puberty; impotence and climacteric symptoms

Female: Palliative treatment of metastatic breast cancer; postpartum breast pain and/or engorgement

Contraindications Hypersensitivity to methyltestosterone or any component, known or suspected carcinoma of the breast or the prostate

Warnings Use with extreme caution in patients with liver or kidney disease or serious heart disease; may accelerate bone maturation without producing compensatory gain in linear growth

Adverse Reactions

Males: Virilism, priapism, prostatic hypertrophy, prostatic carcinoma, impotence, testicular atrophy, gynecomastia (mastodynia possible)

Females: Virilism, menstrual problems (amenorrhea), breast soreness (mastodynia), hirsutism (increase in pubic hair growth)

Cardiovascular: Edema

Central nervous system: Anxiety, sleep apnea syndrome, headache

Dermatologic: Acne

Endocrine & metabolic: Gynecomastia, hypercalcemia, retention of water, sodium, chloride, potassium, calcium, and phosphates, changes in libido, increased serum cholesterol

Gastrointestinal: GI irritation, nausea, vomiting

Hematologic: Leukopenia, polycythemia, suppression of clotting factors II, V, VII, X

Hepatic: Hepatic dysfunction, hepatic necrosis, cholestatic hepatitis

Local: Inflammation at site of injection

Miscellaneous: Hypersensitivity reactions, diaphoresis,

Toxicology Abnormal liver function tests

Drug Interactions Decreased effect: Oral anticoagulant effect or decrease insulin requirements

Mechanism of Action Stimulates receptors in organs and tissues to promote growth and development of male sex organs and maintains secondary sex characteristics in androgen-deficient males

Pharmacokinetics

Absorption: From GI tract and oral mucosa

Metabolism: Hepatic

Elimination: In urine

Usual Dosage Adults (buccal absorption produces twice the androgenic activity of oral tablets):

Male:

Oral: 10-40 mg/day

Buccal: 5-25 mg/day

Female:

Breast pain/engorgement:

Oral: 80 mg/day for 3-5 days

Buccal: 40 mg/day for 3-5 days

Breast cancer:

Oral: 50-200 mg/day

Buccal: 25-100 mg/day

Monitoring Parameters Cholesterol, PSA, electrolyte changes

(Continued)

Methyltestosterone *(Continued)*

Patient Information Men should report overly frequent or persistent penile erections; women should report menstrual irregularities; all patients should report persistent GI distress, diarrhea, or jaundice; buccal tablet should not be chewed or swallowed

Nursing Implications See Adverse Reactions and Monitoring Parameters

Special Geriatric Considerations See Adverse Reactions; since elderly males have prostate changes with age, it would be best to obtain a PSA initially and periodically; retention of sodium and water could be a problem in patients with CHF and hypertension

Dosage Forms
Capsule: 10 mg
Tablet: 10 mg, 25 mg
Tablet, buccal: 5 mg, 10 mg

Methysergide (meth i SER jide)

Brand Names Sansert®

Generic Available No

Therapeutic Category Ergot Alkaloid

Use Prophylaxis of vascular headache; do not use for acute management

Contraindications Peripheral vascular disease, valvular heart disease, severe arteriosclerosis, pulmonary disease, severe hypertension, phlebitis, serious infections, cellulitis of lower extremities, collagen disorders, impaired renal or hepatic function

Warnings Patients receiving long-term therapy may develop retroperitoneal fibrosis, pleuropulmonary fibrosis and fibrotic thickening of the cardiac valves. Fibrosis occurs rarely when therapy is interrupted for 3-4 weeks every 6 months. Use as a prophylactic agent should be considered only in those patients who have severe, uncontrolled, and frequent vascular headache attacks. Use caution in patients with impairment of renal of hepatic function; some products may contain tartrazine.

Precautions This product contains tartrazine which might cause an allergic reaction

Adverse Reactions
Cardiovascular: Postural hypotension, peripheral ischemia, facial flush, peripheral edema, tachycardia, bradycardia
Central nervous system: Insomnia, overstimulation, drowsiness, mild euphoria, lethargy, mental depression, vertigo, unsteadiness, confusion, dizziness, weakness, hyperesthesia, rebound headache may occur if methysergide is discontinued abruptly
Dermatologic: Rash, increased hair loss
Gastrointestinal: Nausea, vomiting, abdominal pain, diarrhea, heartburn, weight gain
Hematologic: Eosinophilia, neutropenia
Neuromuscular & skeletal: Arthralgia, myalgia
Ocular: Visual disturbances
Respiratory: Fibrosis

Overdosage Symptoms of overdose include hyperactivity, spasms in limbs, impaired mental function, impaired circulation

Mechanism of Action A semisynthetic ergotamine congener, however actions appear to differ; methysergide has minimal ergotamine-like oxytocic or vasoconstrictive properties, and has significantly greater serotonin-like properties; its mechanism of action has not been established but inhibits the effects of serotonin by displacing it from receptor pressor sites on the walls of cranial vessels, preserving the vasoconstriction effects of serotonin.

Pharmacodynamics
Onset: Protective effects: 1-2 days
Duration: After discontinuation, effects last 1-2 days

Pharmacokinetics
Metabolism: Undergoes liver metabolism
Half-life, plasma elimination: ~10 hours
Elimination: Not well defined

Usual Dosage Geriatrics and Adults: Oral: 4-8 mg/day with meals; if no improvement is noted after 3 weeks, drug is unlikely to be beneficial; must not be given continuously for longer than 6 months, and a drug-free interval of 3-4 weeks must follow each 6-month course

Patient Information Do not take increased doses per day or for longer time than prescribed; take with meals; may cause drowsiness, impair judgment and coordination; arise slowly from prolonged sitting or lying; notify physician if cold, numbness, painful extremities, chest pain, shortness of breath, or painful urination occurs

Nursing Implications Advise patient to make position changes slowly

Special Geriatric Considerations Use cautiously in elderly, particularly since many elderly have cardiovascular disease which would put them at risk for cardiovascular adverse effects

Dosage Forms Tablet, as maleate: 2 mg

Meticorten® *see* Prednisone *on page 776*

Metimyd® Ophthalmic *see* Sulfacetamide Sodium and Prednisolone *on page 875*

Metipranolol (met i PRAN oh lol)

Related Information
Glaucoma Drug Therapy Comparison *on page 1032*

Brand Names OptiPranolol®

Generic Available No

Therapeutic Category Beta-Adrenergic Blocker, Ophthalmic

Use Treatment of elevated intraocular pressure in patients with chronic open-angle glaucoma

Contraindications Uncompensated congestive heart failure, cardiogenic shock, bradycardia or heart block, bronchial asthma, severe chronic obstructive pulmonary disease or history of asthma; hypersensitivity to beta-blocking agents

Precautions Use with caution in patients with cardiac failure or diabetes mellitus

Adverse Reactions
Cardiovascular: Bradycardia, A-V block, congestive heart failure
Dermatologic: Erythema
Neuromuscular & skeletal: Weakness
Ocular: Conjunctivitis, blepharitis, tearing, itching eyes, keratitis, photophobia, decreased corneal sensitivity, mild ocular stinging and discomfort, eye irritation, blurred vision, browache
Respiratory: Bronchospasm

Overdosage Symptoms of overdose include bradycardia, hypotension, A-V block

Toxicology Sympathomimetics (eg, epinephrine or dopamine), glucagon or a pacemaker can be used to treat the toxic bradycardia, asystole, and/or hypotension; initially, fluids may be the best treatment for toxic hypotension

Drug Interactions Increased toxicity with systemic beta-blockers

Mechanism of Action Reduces intraocular pressure by reducing the production of aqueous humor

Pharmacodynamics
Onset of action: ≤30 minutes
Maximum effects: ~2 hours
Duration of action: Intraocular pressure reduction has persisted for 24 hours following ocular instillation

Pharmacokinetics
Metabolism: Rapid and complete to deacetyl metipranolol, an active metabolite
Half-life, elimination: ~3 hours

Usual Dosage Geriatrics and Adults: Ophthalmic: Instill 1 drop in the affected eye(s) twice daily

Monitoring Parameters Intraocular pressure, funduscopic exam, visual field testing

Patient Information May sting on instillation; do not touch dropper to eye; visual acuity may be decreased after administration; distance vision may be altered; assess patient's or caregiver's ability to administer; apply gentle pressure to lacrimal sac during and immediately following instillation (1 minute) to avoid systemic absorption; stop drug if breathing difficulty occurs

Nursing Implications Monitor for systemic effect of beta-blockade (bradycardia, hypotension, respiratory difficulty); teach proper instillation of eye drops

Special Geriatric Considerations Because systemic absorption occurs with ophthalmic administration, elderly patients with other disease states or syndromes that may be affected by a beta-blocker (ie, CHF, COPD, etc) should be closely monitored.

Dosage Forms Solution, ophthalmic, as hydrochloride: 0.3% (5 mL, 10 mL)

Metoclopramide (met oh kloe PRA mide)

Related Information
I.V. Medication Recommendations *on page 1080*
I.V. Push Recommended Guidelines *on page 1083*

Brand Names Clopra®; Maxolon®; Octamide®; Reglan®

Generic Available Yes

Therapeutic Category Antiemetic

Use Symptomatic treatment of diabetic gastric stasis, hiccups, gastroesophageal reflux; prevention of nausea associated with chemotherapy or post-surgery and facilitates intubation of the small intestine

Contraindications Hypersensitivity to metoclopramide or any component; GI obstruction, perforation or hemorrhage; pheochromocytoma, history of seizure disorder

Warnings Extrapyramidal reactions (0.2% to 1%), depression; may exacerbate seizures in seizure patients

Precautions Use with caution in patients with Parkinson's disease; dosage and/or frequency of administration should be modified in response to degree of renal impairment; hypoglycemia may be precipitated in patients with gastroparesis when insulin is used for glycemic control; may cause drowsiness, therefore use caution performing hazardous tasks (eg, driving)

Adverse Reactions
Cardiovascular: Transient hypertension, hypotension, supraventricular tachycardia, bradycardia
Central nervous system: Drowsiness, fatigue, lassitude, mental depression, suicidal thoughts, restlessness, anxiety, agitation, extrapyramidal reaction, confusion, hallucinations, dizziness, headache, insomnia, Parkinson-like symptoms, tardive dyskinesia, akathisia, seizures, dystonia, neuroleptic malignant syndrome
Dermatologic: Rash, urticaria
Endocrine & metabolic: Nipple tenderness and gynecomastia in males, fluid retention (transient aldosterone increase)
Gastrointestinal: Constipation, diarrhea, nausea, glossal edema
Genitourinary: Impotence, incontinence
Hematologic: Methemoglobinemia, neutropenia, leukopenia, agranulocytosis
Neuromuscular & skeletal: Myoclonus
Ocular: Visual disturbances
Respiratory: Bronchospasm, laryngeal edema

Overdosage Symptoms of overdose include drowsiness, ataxia, extrapyramidal reactions, seizures, disorientation, muscle hypertonia, irritability, and agitation are common

Toxicology Metoclopramide often causes extrapyramidal symptoms (eg, dystonic reactions) requiring management with diphenhydramine 1-2 mg/kg (adults) up to a maximum of 50 mg I.M. or I.V. slow push followed by a maintenance dose for 48-72 hours. When these reactions are unresponsive to diphenhydramine, benztropine mesylate I.V. 1-2 mg (adults) may be effective. These agents are generally effective within 2-5 minutes.

Drug Interactions
Increases rate of absorption of alcohol
May decrease bioavailability of cimetidine (H_2 blockers)
May decrease absorption of digoxin due to increased transit time
Levodopa may decrease effects of metoclopramide on gastrointestinal tract
May increase effect of levodopa in Parkinson's disease
Metoclopramide increases effect of MAO inhibitors
Anticholinergic drugs may decrease effects of metoclopramide

Stability Protection of dilutions do not require light protection if used within 24 hours
Stability of parenteral admixture at room temperature (25°C): 2 days
Stability of parenteral admixture at refrigeration temperature (4°C): 2 days

Mechanism of Action Blocks dopamine receptors in chemoreceptor trigger zone of the CNS; enhances the response to acetylcholine of tissue in upper GI tract causing enhanced motility and accelerated gastric emptying without stimulating secretions

Pharmacodynamics
Onset of action:
Oral: Within 30-60 minutes
I.V.: Within 1-3 minutes
Duration: 1-2 hours, regardless of route administered

Pharmacokinetics
Protein binding: 30%

Half-life: 4-7 (half-life and clearance may be dose-dependent)

Elimination: Primarily as unchanged drug in urine and feces

Usual Dosage

Antiemetic (chemotherapy-induced emesis): Geriatrics and Adults:

I.V.: 1-2 mg/kg/dose every 2-4 hours or (postsurgery); direct I.V. administration should be given slowly over 1-2 minutes

I.M.: 10-20 mg (near end of surgery)

Diabetic gastroparesis:

Geriatrics:

Oral: Initial: 5 mg 30 minutes before meals and at bedtime for 2-8 weeks; increase if necessary to 10 mg doses

I.V.: Initiate at 5 mg over 1-2 minutes; increase to 10 mg if necessary

Adults:

Oral: 10 mg 30 minutes before meals and at bedtime for 2-8 weeks

I.V. (for severe symptoms): 10 mg over 1-2 minutes; 10 days of I.V. therapy may be necessary for best response

Gastroesophageal reflux: Oral:

Geriatrics: 5 mg 4 times/day, 30 minutes before meals and at bedtime; increase dose to 10 mg 4 times/day if no response at lower dose

Adults: 10-15 mg 4 times/day, 30 minutes before meals and at bedtime; single doses of 20 mg are occasionally needed for provoking situations

Postoperative nausea and vomiting: I.M.:

Geriatrics: 5 mg near end of surgery; may repeat dose if necessary

Adults: 10 mg near end of surgery; 20 mg doses can be used

Dosing adjustment in renal impairment: Since elimination is primarily renal, patients with Cl$_{cr}$ <40 mL/minute should have therapy initiated at ½ the recommended **adult** dose (see Additional Information)

Not dialyzable (0% to 5%)

Monitoring Parameters Monitor for dystonic reactions; monitor for signs of hypoglycemia in patients using insulin and those being treated for gastroparesis; monitor for agitation and irritable confusion

Test Interactions Increased aminotransferase [ALT (SGPT)/AST (SGOT)] (S), increased amylase (S)

Patient Information May impair mental alertness or physical coordination; produces drowsiness, dizziness; avoid alcohol, barbiturates or other CNS depressants; take medication 30 minutes before meals; notify physician if any abnormal muscle movements occur

Nursing Implications Parenteral doses of up to 10 mg should be given I.V. push over 1-2 minutes; rapid boluses cause transient anxiety and restlessness followed by drowsiness; higher doses to be given IVPB (see Monitoring Parameters and Special Geriatric Considerations)

Additional Information Infuse over at least 15 minutes. For patients who may need rectal administration, an extemporaneous suppository may be prepared with 5 pulverized tablets in polyethylene glycol. Administer 1 suppository 30-60 minutes before meals and at bedtime; use ½ for elderly.

Special Geriatric Considerations Elderly are more likely to develop tardive dyskinesia syndrome (especially elderly females) reactions than younger adults; use lowest recommended doses initially; must consider renal function (estimate creatinine clearance); it is recommended to do involuntary movement assessments on elderly using this medication at high dose and for long-term therapy (see Usual Dosage)

Dosage Forms

Injection: 5 mg/mL (2 mL, 10 mL, 30 mL, 50 mL, 100 mL)

Syrup, sugar-free: 5 mg/5 mL (10 mL, 480 mL)

Tablet: 5 mg, 10 mg

Metolazone (me TOLE a zone)

Brand Names Mykrox®; Zaroxolyn®

Generic Available No

Therapeutic Category Diuretic, Miscellaneous

Use Management of mild to moderate hypertension; treatment of edema in congestive heart failure and nephrotic syndrome; impaired renal function

Contraindications Hypersensitivity to metolazone or any component; cross-sensitivity with other thiazides and sulfonamides may occur; patients with hepatic coma

Warnings Mykrox® is **not** therapeutically equivalent to Zaroxolyn® and they should not be interchanged for one another

Precautions When metolazone is used in combination with other diuretics, there is an increased risk of azotemia and electrolyte depletion, particularly in the elderly; monitor closely

(Continued)

Metolazone *(Continued)*

Adverse Reactions
Cardiovascular: Palpitations, chest pain, orthostatic hypotension

Central nervous system: Vertigo, headache, chills

Dermatologic: Rash, photosensitivity

Endocrine & metabolic: Hypokalemia, hyponatremia, hypochloremia, metabolic alkalosis, hyperglycemia, hyperuricemia

Gastrointestinal: Abdominal bloating, GI irritation

Genitourinary: Prerenal azotemia

Hematologic: Aplastic anemia, hemolytic anemia, leukopenia, agranulocytosis, thrombocytopenia (all rare)

Renal: Polyuria

Overdosage
Symptoms of overdose include electrolyte depletion, volume depletion, hypotension, dehydration, circulatory collapse

Toxicology
Following GI decontamination, treatment is supportive; hypotension responds to fluids and Trendelenburg position

Drug Interactions
Decreased effect of oral hypoglycemics; decreased absorption with cholestyramine and colestipol

Increased effect with loop diuretics and other antihypertensives

Increased toxicity/levels of lithium; when given with digoxin, diuretic-induced hypokalemia increases the risk of digoxin toxicity

Mechanism of Action
Inhibits sodium reabsorption in the distal tubules causing increased excretion of sodium and water as well as potassium and hydrogen ions; does not substantially decrease glomerular filtration rate or renal plasma flow

Pharmacodynamics
Irrespective of formulation, diuresis occurs within 60 minutes and continues for 12-24 hours

Pharmacokinetics
Absorption: Oral: Incomplete

Protein binding: 95%

Metabolism: Enterohepatic recycled

Bioavailability: Mykrox® reportedly has the highest bioavailability

Half-life: 6-20 hours, renal function dependent

Elimination: 80% to 95% in urine

Usual Dosage
Oral:

Zaroxolyn®:

Geriatrics: Initial: 2.5 mg/day or every other day

Adults:

Edema: 5-20 mg/dose every 24 hours

Hypertension: 2.5-5 mg/dose every 24 hours

Mykrox®: Geriatrics and Adults: 0.5 mg once daily; may increase to 1 mg if response is inadequate; do not use more than 1 mg/day

See Additional Information

Not dialyzable (0% to 5%)

Monitoring Parameters
Blood pressure both standing and sitting/supine, serum electrolytes, renal function, weight, I & O

Test Interactions
Increased ammonia (B), increased amylase (S), increased calcium (S), increased chloride (S), increased cholesterol (S), increased glucose, increased uric acid (S); decreased chloride (S), decreased magnesium, decreased potassium (S), decreased sodium (S)

Patient Information
Take in the morning, may be taken with food or milk; take the last dose of multiple doses no later than 6 PM unless instructed otherwise; may cause increased sensitivity to sunlight

Nursing Implications
Check patient for orthostasis (see Monitoring Parameters)

Additional Information
5 mg is approximately equivalent to 50 mg of hydrochlorothiazide; may be effective in patients with glomerular filtration rate <20 mL/minute; metolazone is often used in combination with a loop diuretic in patients who are unresponsive to the loop diuretic alone

Special Geriatric Considerations
See Precautions, Usual Dosage, and Additional Information

Dosage Forms
Tablet:

Zaroxolyn®: 2.5 mg, 5 mg, 10 mg

Mykrox®: 0.5 mg

Metoprolol (me toe PROE lole)

Related Information
Beta-Blockers Comparison *on page 1026*
I.V. Push Recommended Guidelines *on page 1083*

Brand Names Lopressor®; Toprol XL®

Therapeutic Category Antianginal Agent; Beta-Adrenergic Blocker

Use Treatment of hypertension and angina pectoris; prevention of myocardial infarction (I.V. and immediate-release tablets)

Unlabeled use: Treatment of ventricular arrhythmias, atrial ectopy, migraine prophylaxis, essential tremor, aggressive behavior; diastolic congestive heart failure

Contraindications Hypersensitivity to beta-blocking agents, uncompensated congestive heart failure; cardiogenic shock; bradycardia (heart rate <45 bpm) or heart block; sinus node dysfunction; A-V conduction abnormalities, systolic blood pressure <100 mm Hg; although metoprolol primarily blocks $beta_1$-receptors, high doses can result in $beta_2$-receptor blockage; therefore, use with caution in elderly with bronchospastic lung disease.

Warnings Abrupt withdrawal of beta-blockers may result in an exaggerated cardiac beta-adrenergic responsiveness. Symptomatology has included reports of tachycardia, hypertension, ischemia, angina, myocardial infarction, and sudden death. It is recommended that patients be tapered gradually off of beta-blockers over a 2-week period rather than via abrupt discontinuation.

Precautions Administer to CHF patients with caution; administer with caution to patients with bronchospastic disease, diabetes mellitus, hyperthyroidism, myasthenia gravis, impaired hepatic and renal function decline, and severe peripheral vascular disease. Abrupt withdrawal of the drug should be avoided, drug should be discontinued over 2 weeks.

Adverse Reactions
Cardiovascular: Persistent bradycardia, hypotension, chest pain, edema, heart failure, Raynaud's phenomena
Central nervous system: Fatigue, dizziness, insomnia, lethargy, nightmares, depression, confusion, headache
Gastrointestinal: Constipation, diarrhea, nausea
Genitourinary: Impotence
Miscellaneous: Cold extremities

Overdosage Symptoms of overdose include bradycardia, hypotension, heart failure, bronchospasm (see Toxicology)

Toxicology Sympathomimetics (eg, epinephrine or dopamine), glucagon or a pacemaker can be used to treat the toxic bradycardia, asystole, and/or hypotension. Initially, fluids may be the best treatment for toxic hypotension. Patients should remain supine; serum glucose and potassium should be measured. Use supportive measures: lavage, syrup of ipecac; not significantly removed by dialysis I.V. glucose should be administered for hypoglycemia; seizures may be treated with phenytoin or diazepam intravenously; continuous monitoring of blood pressure and EKG is necessary. If PVCs occur, treat with lidocaine or phenytoin; avoid quinidine, procainamide, and disopyramide since these agents further depress myocardial function. Bronchospasm can be treated with theophylline on $beta_2$ agonists (epinephrine).

Drug Interactions
Pharmacologic action of beta antagonists may be decreased by aluminum compounds, calcium salts, barbiturates, cholestyramine, colestipol, NSAIDs, penicillins (ampicillin), protease inhibitors, rifampin, salicylates, sulfinpyrazone, thyroid hormones; hypoglycemic effect of sulfonylureas may be blunted

Pharmacologic effect of beta antagonists may be enhanced with concomitant use of calcium channel blockers, oral contraceptives, flecainide (bioavailability and effect of flecainide also enhanced), haloperidol (hypotensive effects of both drugs), H_2 antagonists (decreased metabolism), hydralazine (both drugs hypotensive effects increased), loop diuretics (increased serum concentrations of beta-blockers except atenolol), MAO inhibitors, phenothiazines, SSRIs, propafenone, quinidine, quinolones, thioamines; beta-blockers may decrease clearance of acetaminophen; beta-blockers may increase anticoagulant effects of warfarin (propranolol); benzodiazepine effects enhanced by the lipophilic beta-blockers (atenolol does not interact); significant and fatal increases in blood pressure have occurred after decrease in dose or discontinuation of clonidine in patients receiving both clonidine and beta-blockers together (reduce doses of each cautiously with small decreases); peripheral ischemia of ergot alkaloids enhanced by beta-blockers; beta-blockers increase serum concentration of lidocaine; beta-blockers increase hypotensive effect of prazosin

(Continued)

Metoprolol *(Continued)*

Mechanism of Action Competitively blocks beta$_1$-receptors, with little or no effect on beta$_2$-receptors except in high doses; does not exhibit any membrane stabilizing or intrinsic sympathomimetic activity; has moderate lipid solubility, therefore, will penetrate blood-brain barrier

Pharmacodynamics
Peak effects: Oral: Within 1.5-4 hours
Duration: 10-20 hours

Pharmacokinetics
Absorption: 95%
Protein binding: 8%
Metabolism: Significant first-pass metabolism; extensively metabolized in the liver; substrate CYP2D6
Bioavailability: Oral: 40% to 50%
Half-life: 3-4 hours
Elimination: In urine (3% to 10% as unchanged drug)

Usual Dosage
Geriatrics: Initial: 25 mg/day; usual dose range: 25-300 mg/day; increase at 1- to 2-week intervals
  Extended release: 50 mg/day initially as a single dose; increase at 1- to 2-week intervals
Adults:
  Oral: 100-450 mg/day in 1-2 divided doses; increase at 1- to 2-week intervals
    Extended release: 50-100 mg/day as a single dose; increase at 1- to 2-week intervals as necessary; do not exceed 400 mg/day
  I.V.: 5 mg every 2 minutes for 3 doses in early treatment of myocardial infarction

Monitoring Parameters Blood pressure, orthostatic hypotension, heart rate, CNS effects

Test Interactions Increased cholesterol (S), increased glucose

Patient Information Do not discontinue medication abruptly, sudden stopping of medication may precipitate or cause angina; consult pharmacist or physician before taking with other adrenergic drugs (eg, cold medications); notify physician if any of the following symptoms occur: difficult breathing, night cough, swelling of extremities, slow pulse, dizziness, lightheadedness, confusion, depression, skin rash, fever, sore throat, unusual bleeding or bruising; may produce drowsiness, dizziness, lightheadedness, blurred vision, confusion; use with caution while driving or performing tasks requiring alertness; may mask signs of hypoglycemia in diabetics; may be taken without regard to meals

Nursing Implications Monitor hemodynamic status carefully after acute MI, monitor orthostatic blood pressures, apical and peripheral pulse and mental status changes (ie, confusion, depression)

Special Geriatric Considerations Due to alterations in the beta-adrenergic autonomic nervous system, beta-adrenergic blockade may result in less hemodynamic response than seen in younger adults. Studies indicate that despite decreased sensitivity to the chronotropic effects of beta blockade with age, there appears to be an increased myocardial sensitivity to the negative inotropic effect during stress (ie, exercise). Controlled trials have shown the overall response rate for propranolol to be only 20% to 50% in elderly populations. Therefore, all beta-adrenergic blocking drugs may result in a decreased response as compared to younger adults.

Dosage Forms
Metoprolol tartrate:
  Injection: 1 mg/mL (5 mL)
  Tablet: 50 mg, 100 mg
  Tablet, sustained release: 50 mg, 100 mg, 200 mg

References
Aagaard GN, "Treatment of Hypertension in The Elderly," *Drug Treatment in the Elderly*, Vestal RE, ed, Boston, MA: ADIS Health Science Press, 1984, 77.

Metreton® Ophthalmic *see* Prednisolone *on page 774*

MetroGel® Topical *see* Metronidazole *on this page*

MetroGel®-Vaginal *see* Metronidazole *on this page*

Metro I.V.® Injection *see* Metronidazole *on this page*

Metronidazole *(me troe NI da zole)*

Related Information
I.V. Medication Recommendations *on page 1080*

Penicillins, Penicillin-Related Antibiotics, & Other Antibiotics *on page 1010*
Regimens Used to Treat *Helicobacter pylori* and Ulcers *on page 1033*

Brand Names Flagyl® Oral; MetroGel® Topical; MetroGel®-Vaginal; Metro I.V.® Injection; Protostat® Oral

Generic Available Yes

Therapeutic Category Amebicide; Antibiotic, Anaerobic; Antibiotic, Topical; Antiprotozoal

Use Treatment of susceptible anaerobic bacterial and protozoal infections in the following conditions: amebiasis, symptomatic and asymptomatic trichomoniasis; skin and skin structure infections; CNS infections; intra-abdominal infections; systemic anaerobic infections; topically for the treatment of acne rosacea pressure sores; treatment of antibiotic-associated pseudomembranous colitis (AAPC); treatment of peptic ulcers due to *H. pylori*

Contraindications Hypersensitivity to metronidazole or any component

Warnings Has been shown to be carcinogenic in rodents

Precautions Use with caution in patients with liver impairment, blood dyscrasias; reduce dosage in patients with severe liver impairment, CNS disease, and severe renal failure (GFR <10 mL/minute)

Adverse Reactions
Central nervous system: Dizziness, confusion, seizures, headache
Dermatologic: Rash
Endocrine & metabolic: Disulfiram-type reaction with alcohol
Gastrointestinal: Metallic taste, nausea, xerostomia, diarrhea, furry tongue
Hematologic: Leukopenia
Local: Thrombophlebitis
Neuromuscular & skeletal: Peripheral neuropathy

Overdosage Symptoms of overdose include nausea, vomiting, ataxia, seizures, peripheral neuropathy

Drug Interactions
Alcohol (disulfiram-like GI reaction), disulfiram (psychosis and confusion), warfarin and other coumarin derivatives (increased anticoagulant effect)
Metronidazole may decrease the clearance of phenytoin, quinidine, cisapride, and lithium and increase their serum concentrations and half-lives
Phenobarbital may increase metronidazole's metabolism
Cimetidine may decrease metronidazole's metabolism

Stability Reconstituted solution is stable for 96 hours when refrigerated; for I.V. infusion in NS or D_5W and neutralized (with sodium bicarbonate), solution is stable for 24 hours at room temperature; do not refrigerate neutralized solution because a precipitate will occur

Mechanism of Action Reduced to a product which interacts with DNA to cause a loss of helical DNA structure and strand breakage resulting in inhibition of protein synthesis and cell death in susceptible organisms

Pharmacokinetics
Absorption: Oral: Well absorbed
Protein binding: <20%
Metabolism: 30% to 60% in the liver; inhibitor CYP2C9, 3A4
Half-life, normal: 6-8 hours (half-life increases with hepatic impairment)
Time to peak serum concentration: Within 1-2 hours
Elimination: Final excretion via urine (20% as unchanged drug) and feces (6% to 15%).
Following a single 500 mg oral dose, serum concentration and AUCs were increased, total clearance and V_d reduced in subject >70 years compared to younger subjects (20-25 years); the decreased V_d was attributed to a significant decrease in red blood cell binding
Drug is extensively removed by hemodialysis and peritoneal dialysis; dosage adjustment is not necessary for mild to moderate renal insufficiency

Usual Dosage
Geriatrics: Use the lower end of the dosing recommendations for adults; do not administer as single dose as efficacy has not been established
Adults:
Amebiasis: Oral: 500-750 mg every 8 hours
Other parasitic infections: Oral: 250 mg every 8 hours or 2 g as a single dose
Anaerobic infections: Oral, I.V.: 30 mg/kg/day in divided doses every 6 hours; not to exceed 4 g/day
Antibiotic-associated pseudomembranous colitis: Oral: 250-500 mg 3-4 times/day for 10-14 days
Topical: Apply a thin film twice daily to affected areas
Vaginal: One applicatorful in vagina each morning and evening, as needed

(Continued)

Metronidazole *(Continued)*

Dosing interval in renal impairment: No change necessary unless Cl$_{cr}$ <10 mL/minute

Dialyzable (50% to 100%)

Monitoring Parameters Signs and symptoms of infection; diarrhea

Test Interactions May cause falsely decreased AST and ALT levels

Patient Information Urine may be discolored to a dark or reddish-brown; do not take alcohol for at least 24 hours after the last dose; avoid beverage alcohol during therapy; may cause metallic taste; may be taken with food to minimize stomach upset

Nursing Implications Even though metronidazole can be detected in the blood after **topical** application, no antabuse-like reactions have been reported; avoid contact between the drug and aluminum in the infusion set

Additional Information Sodium content of 500 mg (I.V.): 322 mg (14 mEq)

Special Geriatric Considerations See Pharmacokinetics and Usual Dosage

Dosage Forms

Capsule: 375 mg

Gel, topical: 0.75% [7.5 mg/mL] (30 g)

Gel, vaginal: 0.75% (5 g applicator delivering 37.5 mg in 70 g tube)

Injection, ready to use: 5 mg/mL (100 mL)

Powder for injection, as hydrochloride: 500 mg

Tablet: 250 mg, 500 mg

References

Ludwig E, Csiba A, Magyar T, et al, "Age-Associated Pharmacokinetic Changes of Metronidazole," *Int J Clin Pharmacol Ther Toxicol*, 1983, 21(2):87-91.

"Treatment of *Clostridium difficile* Diarrhea," *Med Lett Drugs Ther*, 1989, 31(803):94-5.

Mevacor® *see* Lovastatin *on page 555*

Mevinolin *see* Lovastatin *on page 555*

Mexiletine (MEKS i le teen)

Brand Names Mexitil®

Generic Available No

Therapeutic Category Antiarrhythmic Agent, Class I-B

Use Management of life-threatening ventricular arrhythmias

Unlabeled use: Diabetic neuropathy associated pain and paresthesias

Contraindications Cardiogenic shock, second or third degree heart block, hypersensitivity to mexiletine or any component

Warnings Exercise extreme caution in patients with pre-existing sinus node dysfunction; mexiletine can worsen CHF, bradycardias, and other arrhythmias; mexiletine, like other antiarrhythmic agents, is proarrhythmic; cost studies indicate a trend toward increased mortality with antiarrhythmics in the face of cardiac disease (myocardial infarction); elevation of AST/ALT; hepatic necrosis reported; leukopenia, agranulocytopenia, and thrombocytopenia; seizures; alterations in urinary pH may change urinary excretion; electrolyte disturbances (hypokalemia, hyperkalemia, etc) after drug response

Precautions A-V second or third degree block, sinus node dysfunction, intraventricular conduction abnormalities; follow closely in patients with liver disease, seizure disorder; avoid drugs or diets that greatly alter urinary pH; mexiletine can worsen arrhythmias; hepatic impairment prolongs half-life; elevations of AST; use with caution in patients with severe congestive heart failure, hypotension

Adverse Reactions

Cardiovascular: Edema, palpitations, bradycardia, chest pain, syncope, hypotension, atrial or ventricular arrhythmias

Central nervous system: Dizziness, confusion, lightheadedness, nervousness, fatigue, depression, memory loss, psychosis, seizures, ataxia

Dermatologic: Rash, dry skin

Gastrointestinal: Nausea, vomiting, diarrhea, heartburn, abdominal pain

Genitourinary: Urinary retention

Hematologic: Rarely thrombocytopenia, rarely positive antinuclear antibody

Hepatic: Rarely hepatitis

Neuromuscular & skeletal: Coordination difficulties, arthralgia, tremors, weakness, paresthesia

Ocular: Diplopia, blurred vision

Otic: Tinnitus

Respiratory: Dyspnea

Miscellaneous: Hiccups

Toxicology Utilize general supportive therapy and general poisoning management if necessary; gastric lavage followed by charcoal administration indicated; atropine may be used for mexiletine-induced bradycardia; acidify urine to elimination; hemodialysis does not eliminate

Drug Interactions

Phenobarbital, phenytoin, rifampin, and other hepatic enzyme inducers may lower mexiletine plasma concentrations

Cimetidine, SSRIs, amiodarone, quinidine, ritonavir may increase mexiletine levels

Antacids, narcotics, metoclopramide, or anticholinergics may decrease rate of absorption

Metoclopramide may increase rate of absorption; drugs or diets which affect urine pH can increase or decrease excretion of mexiletine

Theophylline levels increased; caffeine clearance decreased

Mechanism of Action Class IB antiarrhythmic, structurally related to lidocaine, which may cause increase in systemic vascular resistance and decrease in cardiac output; no significant negative inotropic effect; inhibits inward sodium current, decreasing phase O, and effective refractory period

Pharmacodynamics Onset of action: Oral: Within 30 minutes to 2 hours

Pharmacokinetics

Absorption: Elderly have a slightly slower rate of absorption but extent of absorption is the same as young adults

Distribution: V_d: 5-7 L/kg

Protein binding: 50% to 70%

Metabolism: Low first-pass metabolism; inhibitor CYP1A2; substrate CYP2D6

Half-life: Adults: 10-14 hours (average: 14.4 hours elderly, 12 hours in younger adults); increase in half-life with hepatic or heart failure

Time to peak serum concentration: 2-3 hours

Elimination: 10% to 15% excreted unchanged in urine; urinary acidification increases excretion, alkalinization decreases excretion

Usual Dosage Geriatrics and Adults: Oral: Initial: 200 mg every 8 hours (may load with 400 mg if necessary); adjust dose every 2-3 days; usual dose: 200-300 mg every 8 hours; maximum dose: 1.2 g/day (some patients respond to every 12-hour dosing); patients with hepatic impairment or CHF may require dose reduction; when switching from another antiarrhythmic, initiate a 200 mg dose 6-12 hours after stopping former agents, 3-6 hours after stopping procainamide

Monitoring Parameters EKG, blood pressure, pulse, serum concentrations

Reference Range Therapeutic: 0.5-2 µg/mL; Potentially toxic: >2 µg/mL

Test Interactions Abnormal liver function test, positive ANA, thrombocytopenia

Patient Information Take with food; notify physician of side effects such as jaundice, fever, palpitations, dizziness, tremor, heartburn, and sore throat

Nursing Implications Administer around-the-clock rather than 4 times/day, 3 times/day, etc (ie, 12-6-12-6, not 9-1-5-9) to promote less variation in peak and trough serum concentrations

Additional Information I.V. form under investigation

Special Geriatric Considerations No specific changes in dose are necessary (see Pharmacokinetics)

Dosage Forms Capsule: 150 mg, 200 mg, 250 mg

References

Fenster PE and Nolan PE, "Antiarrhythmic Drugs," *Geriatric Pharmacology*, Bressler R and Katz MD, eds, New York, NY: McGraw-Hill, 1993, 6:105-49.

Mexitil® see Mexiletine *on previous page*

Mezlin® see Mezlocillin *on this page*

Mezlocillin (mez loe SIL in)

Related Information

I.V. Medication Recommendations *on page 1080*
Penicillins, Penicillin-Related Antibiotics, & Other Antibiotics *on page 1010*

Brand Names Mezlin®

Therapeutic Category Antibiotic, Penicillin

Use Treatment of infections caused by susceptible gram-negative aerobic bacilli (*Klebsiella*, *Proteus*, *Escherichia coli*, *Enterobacter*, *Pseudomonas aeruginosa*, *Serratia*) involving the skin and skin structure, bone and joint, respiratory tract, urinary tract, gastrointestinal tract, as well as septicemia

Contraindications Hypersensitivity to mezlocillin or any component or penicillins

(Continued)

Mezlocillin *(Continued)*

Warnings If bleeding occurs during therapy, mezlocillin should be discontinued

Precautions Dosage modification required in patients with impaired renal function; use with caution in patients with renal impairment or biliary obstruction; use with caution in patients with cephalosporin allergy

Adverse Reactions

Central nervous system: Seizures, dizziness, fever, headache

Dermatologic: Rash, exfoliative dermatitis

Endocrine & metabolic: Hypokalemia, hypernatremia

Gastrointestinal: Diarrhea

Hematologic: Eosinophilia, hemolytic anemia, neutropenia, leukopenia, thrombocytopenia, prolonged bleeding time, positive Coombs' direct test

Hepatic: Elevated liver enzymes

Local: Thrombophlebitis

Renal: Interstitial nephritis, elevated serum creatinine and BUN

Miscellaneous: Serum sickness-like reaction

Overdosage Symptoms of overdose include neuromuscular hypersensitivity, seizure

Toxicology Many beta-lactam-containing antibiotics have the potential to cause neuromuscular hyperirritability or convulsive seizures. Hemodialysis may be helpful to aid in the removal of the drug from the blood, otherwise most treatment is supportive or symptom directed.

Drug Interactions Aminoglycosides (synergy), probenecid (decreased clearance), vecuronium (prolonged duration of action), heparin (increased risk of bleeding)

Stability Reconstituted solution is stable for 48 hours at room temperature and 7 days when refrigerated; for I.V. infusion in NS or D_5W solution is stable for 48 hours at room temperature, 7 days when refrigerated or 28 days when frozen; after freezing, thawed solution is stable for 48 hours at room temperature or 7 days when refrigerated; if precipitation occurs under refrigeration, warm in water bath (37°C) for 20 minutes and shake well

Mechanism of Action Interferes with bacterial cell wall synthesis during active multiplication causing cell death and resultant bactericidal activity against susceptible bacteria

Pharmacokinetics

Absorption: I.M.: 63%

Distribution: Into bile, heart, peritoneal fluid, sputum, bone; does not cross the blood-brain barrier well unless meninges are inflamed

Protein binding: 30%

Metabolism: Minimal

Half-life: 50-70 minutes (dose dependent), half-life increased in renal impairment

Time to peak serum concentration:

I.M.: Within 45-90 minutes

I.V. infusion: Within 5 minutes

Elimination: Principally as unchanged drug in urine, also excreted via bile

The pharmacokinetics of mezlocillin in the elderly have not been shown to be significantly altered with increased age

Usual Dosage Geriatrics and Adults: I.M., I.V.:

For uncomplicated urinary tract infection: 1.5-2 g every 6 hours; serious infections: 3-4 g every 4-6 hours

Acute, uncomplicated gonococcal urethritis: 1-2 g, plus 1 g probenecid at time of dose or up to 30 minutes before

Dosing interval in renal impairment:

Cl_{cr} 10-30 mL/minute: Administer every 6-8 hours

Cl_{cr} <10 mL/minute: Administer every 8-12 hours

Moderately dialyzable (20% to 50%)

Dosing adjustment in hepatic impairment: Reduce dose by 50%

Monitoring Parameters Signs and symptoms of infection, electrolytes

Test Interactions False-positive direct Coombs'; false-positive urinary protein

Patient Information Notify physician if diarrhea develops within 2 weeks after completion of therapy

Nursing Implications Administer around-the-clock rather than 4 times/day, 3 times/day, etc (ie, 12-6-12-6, not 9-1-5-9) to promote less variation in peak and trough serum concentrations; dosage modification required in patients with impaired renal function; administer I.M. injections in large muscle mass, not more than 2 g/injection. I.M. injections given over 12-15 seconds will be less painful.

Additional Information Minimum volume: 50 mL D$_5$W (concentration should not exceed 1 g/10 mL); sodium content of 1 g: 42.6 mg (1.85 mEq)

Special Geriatric Considerations Mezlocillin and the other antipseudomonal infections should be used in combination with another antibiotic for the treatment of mixed infections or against gram-negative bacilli such as *P. aeruginosa* (ie, with an aminoglycoside); sodium content is the lowest of the penicillins; adjust dose for renal function (see Pharmacokinetics)

Dosage Forms Powder for injection, as sodium: 1 g, 2 g, 3 g, 4 g, 20 g

References

Meyers BR, Mendelson MH, Srulevitch-Chin E, et al, "Pharmacokinetic Properties of Mezlocillin in Ambulatory Elderly Subjects," *J Clin Pharmacol*, 1987, 27(9):678-81.

Yoshikawa TT, "Antimicrobial Therapy for the Elderly Patient," *J Am Geriatr Soc*, 1990, 38(12):1353-72.

Mg-plus® [OTC] see Magnesium Salts (Various Salts) on page 568

Miacalcin® Injection see Calcitonin on page 142

Miacalcin® Nasal Spray see Calcitonin on page 142

Micatin® Topical [OTC] see Miconazole on this page

Miconazole (mi KON a zole)

Brand Names Absorbine® Antifungal Foot Powder [OTC]; Breezee® Mist Antifungal [OTC]; Fungoid® Creme; Fungoid® Tincture; Lotrimin® AF Powder [OTC]; Lotrimin® AF Spray Liquid [OTC]; Lotrimin® AF Spray Powder [OTC]; Maximum Strength Desenex® Antifungal Cream [OTC]; Micatin® Topical [OTC]; Monistat-Derm™ Topical; Monistat i.v.™ Injection; Monistat™ Vaginal; Ony-Clear® Spray; Prescription Strength Desenex® [OTC]; Zeasorb-AF® Powder [OTC]

Generic Available Yes

Therapeutic Category Antifungal Agent, Topical; Antifungal Agent, Vaginal

Use

Topical: Treatment of vulvovaginal candidiasis and a variety of skin and mucous membrane fungal infections

I.V.: Treatment of severe systemic fungal infections and fungal meningitis that are refractory to standard treatment

Contraindications Hypersensitivity to miconazole, fluconazole, ketoconazole, or polyoxyl 35 castor oil or any component

Precautions Administer I.V. with caution to patients with hepatic insufficiency, cardiorespiratory arrest or anaphylaxis, tachycardia, or arrhythmias with too rapid injection

Adverse Reactions

Cardiovascular: Tachycardia (I.V.), arrhythmias (I.V.)

Central nervous system: Arachnoiditis (I.T.), 8th cranial nerve palsy (I.T.), headache

Dermatologic: Maceration, urticaria, rash, pruritus (I.V.)

Endocrine & metabolic: Hyperlipidemia with rapid infusion (I.V.)

Gastrointestinal: Nausea (I.V.), vomiting (I.V.), diarrhea (I.V.)

Genitourinary: Pelvic cramps

Hematologic: Transient anemia (I.V.), thrombocytopenia

Local: Irritation, burning, itching, phlebitis

Miscellaneous: Anaphylactoid reactions (I.V.)

Overdosage Symptoms of overdose include nausea, vomiting, drowsiness

Drug Interactions Warfarin (increased anticoagulant effect), amphotericin B (decreased antifungal effect of both agents), phenytoin (levels may be increased); potential for increased serum concentrations and cardiotoxic effects of terfenadine, astemizole, and cisapride (I.V. only)

Stability Protect from heat; darkening of solution indicates deterioration

Stability of parenteral admixture at room temperature (25°C): 2 days

Mechanism of Action Inhibits biosynthesis of ergosterol, damaging the fungal cell wall membrane, which increases permeability causing leaking of nutrients

Pharmacokinetics Multiphasic degradation

Protein binding: 91% to 93%

Metabolism: In the liver; substrate and inhibitor CYP3A4

Half-life:

Initial: 40 minutes

Secondary: 126 minutes

Terminal: 24 hours

Elimination: ~50% in feces and <1% in urine as unchanged drug

Usual Dosage Geriatrics and Adults:

Topical: Apply twice daily

(Continued)

Miconazole *(Continued)*

Vaginal: Insert contents of one applicator of vaginal cream (100 mg) or 100 mg suppository at bedtime for 7 days, or 200 mg suppository at bedtime for 3 days

Bladder candidal infections: 200 mg diluted solution instilled in the bladder

I.V.: Initial: 200 mg, then 1.2-3.6 g/day divided every 8 hours for 1-20 weeks depending upon organism

I.T.: 20 mg every 1-2 days

Not dialyzable (0% to 5%)

Administration Administer I.V. dose over 2 hours; administer around-the-clock rather than 4 times/day, 3 times/day, etc (ie, 12-6-12-6, not 9-1-5-9) to promote less variation in peak and trough serum concentration

Monitoring Parameters Signs and symptoms of infection

Test Interactions Increased protein

Patient Information Avoid contact with the eyes; if no response after several weeks of therapy, contact physician

Nursing Implications See Administration

Additional Information

Miconazole: Monistat i.v.™

Miconazole nitrate: Micatin®, Monistat™, Monistat-Derm™

Special Geriatric Considerations No specific data for elderly; use does not require alteration in dose or dose intervals; assess patient's ability to self administer, may be difficult in patients with arthritis or limited range of motion

Dosage Forms

Miconazole nitrate:

Cream:

Topical: 2% (15 g, 30 g, 56.7 g, 85 g)

Vaginal: 2% (45 g is equivalent to 7 doses)

Injection: 1% [10 mg/mL] (20 mL)

Lotion: 2% (30 mL, 60 mL)

Powder, topical: 2% (45 g, 90 g, 113 g)

Spray, topical: 2% (105 mL)

Suppository, vaginal: 100 mg (7s); 200 mg (3s)

Tincture: 2% with alcohol (7.39 mL, 29.57 mL)

Micro-K® 10 *see* Potassium Chloride *on page 763*

Micro-K® Extencaps® *see* Potassium Chloride *on page 763*

Micro-K® LS® *see* Potassium Chloride *on page 763*

Micronase® *see* Glyburide *on page 428*

microNefrin® *see* Epinephrine *on page 336*

Midamor® *see* Amiloride *on page 53*

Midazolam *(MID aye zoe lam)*

Related Information

Antacid Drug Interactions *on page 1096*

Brand Names Versed®

Generic Available No

Therapeutic Category Benzodiazepine; Hypnotic; Sedative

Use Preoperative sedation and provide conscious sedation prior to diagnostic or radiographic procedures

Restrictions C-IV

Contraindications Hypersensitivity to midazolam or any component, cross-sensitivity with other benzodiazepines may occur; uncontrolled pain; existing CNS depression; shock; narrow-angle glaucoma

Warnings Midazolam may cause respiratory depression/arrest; deaths and hypoxic encephalopathy have resulted when these were not promptly recognized and treated appropriately. The danger of apnea or underventilation is greater in the elderly; the peak effect may take longer; reduce dosage increments and slow the rate of injection.

Precautions Use with caution in patients with congestive heart failure, renal impairment, pulmonary disease, hepatic dysfunction

Adverse Reactions

Cardiovascular: Cardiac arrest, hypotension, bradycardia

Central nervous system: Drowsiness, ataxia, amnesia, dizziness, paradoxical excitement, sedation, headache

Gastrointestinal: Nausea, vomiting

Local: Pain and local reactions at injection site (severity less than diazepam)

Ocular: Blurred vision, diplopia

Respiratory: Respiratory depression, apnea, laryngospasm, bronchospasm

Miscellaneous: Physical and psychological dependence with prolonged use, hiccups

Overdosage Symptoms of overdose include sedation, confusion, impaired coordination, diminished reflexes, and coma

Toxicology Treatment for benzodiazepine overdose is supportive; rarely is mechanical ventilation required; flumazenil has been shown to selectively block the binding of benzodiazepines to CNS receptors, resulting in a reversal of benzodiazepine-induced sedation; however, its use may not alter the course of overdose

Drug Interactions

Decreased effect: Theophylline may antagonize the sedative effects of midazolam; rifampin may decrease midazolam concentrations

Increased toxicity: CNS depressants, may increase sedation and respiratory depression; doses of anesthetic agents should be reduced when used in conjunction with midazolam

Increased midazolam serum concentration: cimetidine, ketoconazole, SSRIs, itraconazole, erythromycin

Stability Admixtures do not require protection from light for short-term storage

Mechanism of Action Benzodiazepines appear to potentiate the effects of GABA and other inhibitory neurotransmitters by binding to specific benzodiazepine-receptor sites in various areas of the CNS

Pharmacodynamics

Sedation onset:
I.M.: Within 15 minutes
I.V. within 1-5 minutes
Peak effects: I.M.: 30-60 minutes
Duration: I.M.: Mean: 2 hours, up to 6 hours

Pharmacokinetics

Distribution: V_d: 0.8-2.5 L/kg; increased V_d with congestive heart failure and chronic renal failure; slightly increased V_d in the elderly

Protein binding: 95%

Metabolism: Extensive in the liver (microsomally); substrate CYP3A4

Half-life: Elimination: 1-4 hours; increased half-life with cirrhosis, congestive heart failure, obesity, elderly (5.6 ± 4.8 hours); some elderly males had a marked increase in elimination half-life

Elimination: Excreted as glucuronide conjugated metabolites in urine, ~2% to 10% is excreted in feces

Pharmacokinetics in elderly males were less predictable than in elderly females

Usual Dosage

Geriatrics: Conscious sedation: Initial: 1 mg slow I.V.; administer no more than 1.5 mg in a 2-minute period; if additional titration is needed, administer no more than 1 mg over 2 minutes, waiting another 2 or more minutes to evaluate sedative effect; total dose >3.5 mg is rarely necessary

Adults:

Preoperative sedation: I.M.: 0.07-0.08 mg/kg 30-60 minutes presurgery; usual dose: 5 mg; lower doses may suffice in the elderly

Conscious sedation: I.V.: Initial: 0.5-2 mg slow I.V. over at least 2 minutes; slowly titrate to effect by repeating doses every 2-3 minutes if needed; usual total dose: 2.5-5 mg

Administration See Usual Dosage

Monitoring Parameters Respiratory, cardiovascular and mental status

Patient Information May cause drowsiness; do not drive or operate hazardous machinery until the effects of the drug are gone or until the day after administration

Additional Information Healthy adults <60 years of age: Some patients respond to doses as low as 1 mg; no more than 2.5 mg should be administered over a period of 2 minutes. Additional doses of midazolam may be administered after a 2-minute waiting period and evaluation of sedation after each dose increment. A total dose >5 mg is generally not needed. If narcotics or other CNS depressants are administered concomitantly, the midazolam dose should be reduced by 30%.

Special Geriatric Considerations In the elderly if concomitant CNS depressant medications are used, the midazolam dose will be at least 50% less than doses used in healthy, young, unpremedicated patients (see Warnings and Pharmacokinetics)

Dosage Forms Injection, as hydrochloride: 1 mg/mL (2 mL, 5 mL, 10 mL); 5 mg/mL (1 mL, 2 mL, 5 mL, 10 mL)

(Continued)

Midazolam *(Continued)*

References
Kanto J, Aaltonen L, Himberg JJ, et al, "Midazolam as an Intravenous Induction Agent in the Elderly: A Clinical and Pharmacokinetic Study," *Anesth Analg*, 1986, 65(1):15-20.

Servin F, Enriquez I, Fournet M, et al, "Pharmacokinetics of Midazolam Used as an Intravenous Induction Agent for Patients Over 80 Years of Age," *Eur J Anaesthesiol*, 1987, 4(1):1-7.

Midol® 200 [OTC] *see* Ibuprofen *on page 475*

Migranal® *see* Dihydroergotamine *on page 295*

Miles Nervine® Caplets [OTC] *see* Diphenhydramine *on page 302*

Milkinol® [OTC] *see* Mineral Oil *on this page*

Milk of Magnesia *see* Magnesium Hydroxide *on page 564*

Miltown® *see* Meprobamate *on page 588*

Mineral Oil *(MIN er al oyl)*

Brand Names Agoral® Plain [OTC]; Fleet® Mineral Oil Enema [OTC]; Kondremul® [OTC]; Milkinol® [OTC]; Neo-Cultol® [OTC]; Zymenol® [OTC]

Synonyms Heavy Mineral Oil; Liquid Paraffin; White Mineral Oil

Generic Available Yes

Therapeutic Category Laxative, Lubricant

Use Temporary relief of constipation, relief of fecal impaction, preparation for bowel studies or surgery

Contraindications Patients with colostomy or an ileostomy, appendicitis, ulcerative colitis, diverticulitis

Warnings Lipid pneumonitis results from aspiration of mineral oil which usually occurs in patients who are in a supine (debilitated) position. Elderly patients are particularly at risk, especially if they have any condition which interferes with swallowing or epiglottal function (eg, strokes, Parkinson's disease, Alzheimer's disease, esophageal dysmotility).

Precautions Lipid pneumonitis

Adverse Reactions
Gastrointestinal: Nausea, vomiting, diarrhea, abdominal cramps
Respiratory: Lipid pneumonitis with aspiration
Miscellaneous: Large doses may cause anal leakage causing anal itching, irritation, hemorrhoids, perianal discomfort, soiling of clothes

Drug Interactions May impair absorption of fat-soluble vitamins (A, D, K, E), oral contraceptives, coumarin, sulfonamides; administration of surfactants (docusate) with mineral oil may increase mineral oil absorption and therefore enhance toxic potential of mineral oil resulting in a foreign body reaction in lymphoid tissue

Mechanism of Action Eases passage of stool by decreasing water absorption and lubricating the intestine; retards colonic absorption of water

Pharmacodynamics Onset of action: ~6-8 hours; effect on bowel function is generally seen after 2-3 days of use

Pharmacokinetics
Distribution: Site of action is the colon
Elimination: In feces

Usual Dosage Geriatrics and Adults:
Oral: 15-45 mL/day once daily or in divided doses
Rectal: Retention enema, contents of one enema (range 60-150 mL)/day as a single dose

Monitoring Parameters Monitor for response: Stool frequency, consistency. Avoid use in patients who may aspirate.

Patient Information Do not take with food or meals; do not use if experiencing abdominal pain, nausea, or vomiting; do not take while reclining in bed, sit up; do **not** administer just before bedtime; wear protective undergarments

Nursing Implications Administer on an empty stomach; avoid administration in a reclining position, sit patient up

Additional Information Do not administer with food or meals because of the risk of aspiration; prolonged administration of mineral oil may decrease absorption of lipid-soluble vitamins A, D, E, and K. Light sterile mineral oils are not for injection.

Special Geriatric Considerations Other therapies should be attempted before using mineral oil to relieve constipation to avoid complications with mineral oil; doses, if used, should begin low and should be used as infrequently as possible (see Warnings)

Dosage Forms
Emulsion: 1.4 g/5 mL (480 mL); 2.5 mL/5 mL (420 mL); 2.75 mL/5 mL (480 mL); 4.75 mL/5 mL (240 mL)

Jelly: 2.75 mL/5 mL (180 mL)
Liquid: 500 mL, 1000 mL, 4000 mL
Liquid, rectal: 133 mL

Minipress® *see* Prazosin *on page 772*
Minitran® Patch *see* Nitroglycerin *on page 677*
Minocin® IV Injection *see* Minocycline *on this page*
Minocin® Oral *see* Minocycline *on this page*

Minocycline (mi noe SYE kleen)
Brand Names Dynacin® Oral; Minocin® IV Injection; Minocin® Oral
Therapeutic Category Antibiotic, Tetracycline Derivative
Use Treatment of susceptible bacterial infections of both gram-negative and gram-positive organisms; acne
   Unlabeled use: Rheumatoid arthritis
Contraindications Hypersensitivity to minocycline or any component or tetracycline
Precautions Should be avoided in renal insufficiency; photosensitivity reactions can occur with minocycline, superinfection
Adverse Reactions
   Central nervous system: Lightheadedness, vertigo, dizziness
   Dermatologic: Skin rashes, photosensitivity, pigmentation of nails, exfoliative dermatitis
   Endocrine & metabolic: Diabetes insipidus
   Gastrointestinal: Nausea, vomiting, esophagitis, anorexia, abdominal cramps, diarrhea
   Genitourinary: Azotemia
   Renal: Acute renal failure
Overdosage Symptoms of overdose include photosensitivity, diabetes insipidus, nausea, anorexia, diarrhea
Drug Interactions
   Decreased effect with antacids (aluminum, calcium, zinc, or magnesium), bismuth salts, sodium bicarbonate, barbiturates, carbamazepine, hydantoins; decreased effect of oral contraceptives
   Increased effect of warfarin
Mechanism of Action Inhibits bacterial protein synthesis by binding with the 30S and possibly the 50S ribosomal subunit(s) of susceptible bacteria, cell wall synthesis is not affected
Pharmacokinetics
   Absorption: Well absorbed
   Protein binding: 70% to 75%
   Half-life: 15 hours
   Elimination: Majority of dose deposits for extended periods in fat and eventually is cleared renally
Usual Dosage Geriatrics and Adults:
   Infection: Oral, I.V.: 200 mg stat, 100 mg every 12 hours
   Acne: Oral: 50 mg 1-3 times/day
   Not dialyzable (0% to 5%)
Monitoring Parameters Signs and symptoms of infection; monitor for CNS adverse effects
Test Interactions Increased catecholamines (U), increased uric acid (S); decreased urea nitrogen (B)
Patient Information Complete full course of therapy; use caution if vertigo, dizziness, and driving or operation of machinery; may be taken with food or milk; avoid prolonged exposure to sunlight or tanning equipment
Nursing Implications May be administered with food or milk; unlike other tetracyclines, monitor for signs of vertigo and dizziness
Special Geriatric Considerations Minocycline has not been studied in the elderly but its CNS effects may limit its use (see Adverse Reactions); dose reduction for renal function not necessary
Dosage Forms
   Minocycline hydrochloride:
      Capsule: 50 mg, 100 mg
      Capsule (Dynacin®): 50 mg, 100 mg
      Capsule, pellet-filled (Minocin®): 50 mg, 100 mg
      Injection (Minocin® IV): 100 mg
      Suspension, oral (Minocin®): 50 mg/5 mL (60 mL)

Minodyl® *see* Minoxidil *on next page*

Minoxidil (mi NOKS i dil)

Brand Names Loniten®; Minodyl®; Rogaine® Extra Strength for Men [OTC]; Rogaine® for Men [OTC]; Rogaine® for Women [OTC]

Generic Available Yes: Tablet

Therapeutic Category Vasodilator

Use Management of severe hypertension; treatment of male pattern baldness (alopecia androgenetica)

Contraindications Pheochromocytoma, hypersensitivity to minoxidil or any component

Precautions Use with caution in patients with coronary artery disease or with recent myocardial infarction, pulmonary hypertension, significant renal dysfunction, congestive heart failure

Adverse Reactions
Cardiovascular: Edema, congestive heart failure, tachycardia, angina, pericardial effusion, tamponade, EKG changes
Central nervous system: Dizziness, fatigue, headache
Dermatologic: Hypertrichosis (commonly occurs within 1-2 months of therapy), coarsening facial features, dermatologic reactions, rash, Stevens-Johnson syndrome, sunburn
Endocrine & metabolic: Sodium and water retention
Gastrointestinal: Weight gain
Local: Topical burning, itching
Respiratory: Pulmonary hypertension/edema

Overdosage Symptoms of overdose include hypotension, tachycardia

Toxicology Hypotension usually responds to I.V. fluids or Trendelenburg positioning. If unresponsive to these measures the use of a parenteral vasoconstrictor may be required (eg, norepinephrine 0.1-0.2 mcg/kg/minute titrated to response). Treatment is primarily supportive and symptomatic.

Drug Interactions Increased effect: Other hypotensive agents, hypotensive diuretics; concurrent administration with guanethidine may cause profound orthostatic hypotensive effects

Mechanism of Action Produces vasodilation by directly relaxing arteriolar smooth muscle, with little effect on veins, effects may be mediated by cyclic AMP; stimulation of hair growth is secondary to vasodilation, increased cutaneous blood flow and stimulation of resting hair follicles

Pharmacodynamics
Onset of action: Oral: Hypotensive effects occur within 30 minutes
Peak effects: Within 2-8 hours
Duration: Up to 2-5 days

Pharmacokinetics
Protein binding: None
Metabolism: 88% primarily via glucuronidation
Bioavailability: Oral: 90%
Half-life: 3.5-4.2 hours
Elimination: 12% unchanged in urine

Usual Dosage
Geriatrics: Oral: Initial: 2.5 mg once daily, increase gradually
Adults:
Hypertension: Oral: Initial: 5 mg once daily, increase gradually every 3 days; usual dose: 10-40 mg/day in 1-2 divided doses; maximum: 100 mg/day
Alopecia: Apply twice daily
Dialyzable (50% to 100%)

Monitoring Parameters Blood pressure, standing and sitting/supine, fluid and electrolyte status, signs and symptoms of congestive heart failure, weight

Patient Information Topical product must be used every day. Minoxidil is usually taken with at least two other antihypertensive medications. Take all medications as prescribed; do not discontinue except on advice of physician. Notify the physician if any of the following occur: heart rate ≥20 beats/minute over normal; rapid weight gain >5 pounds (2 kg); unusual swelling of extremities, face, or abdomen; breathing difficulty, especially when lying down; new or aggravated angina symptoms (chest, arm or shoulder pain); severe indigestion; dizziness, lightheadedness, or fainting; nausea or vomiting may occur.

Nursing Implications May cause hirsutism or hypertrichosis (see Monitoring Parameters)

Additional Information Usually given in combination with a diuretic and beta-blocker

Special Geriatric Considerations See Precautions and Adverse Reactions

Dosage Forms
Solution, topical [OTC]: 2% = 20 mg/metered dose (60 mL); 5% = 50 mg/metered dose (60 mL)
Tablet: 2.5 mg, 10 mg

Minute-Gel® see Fluoride on page 392

Miochol-E® see Acetylcholine on page 25

Miostat® Intraocular see Carbachol on page 159

Mirapex® see Pramipexole on page 768

Mirtazapine (mir TAZ a peen)

Related Information
Antidepressant Medication Guidelines on page 1075

Brand Names Remeron™

Generic Available No

Therapeutic Category Antidepressant

Use Treatment of depression

Contraindications Previous hypersensitivity to mirtazapine or mianserin

Precautions Use with caution in patients with cardiovascular or gastrointestinal disorders, prostatic hypertrophy or urinary retention, narrow-angle glaucoma, renal or hepatic impairment

Adverse Reactions
Cardiovascular: Hypotension, tachycardia, palpitations
Central nervous system: Drowsiness, headache, dizziness, excessive sedation, fatigue, insomnia, agitation, restlessness, vertigo, hypomanic or manic switch
Gastrointestinal: Appetite (increased), constipation, nausea, xerostomia, bitter taste, weight gain or loss
Genitourinary: Impotence, decreased libido, erectile dysfunction
Hematologic: Neutropenia (rare), agranulocytosis (rare)
Hepatic: Increased transaminase and transferase levels
Neuromuscular & skeletal: Tremor, myalgia, weakness
Ocular: Blurred vision, abnormal accommodations
Respiratory: Dyspnea

Overdosage Symptoms of overdose include transient somnolence, tachycardia, disorientation; no cases of cardiovascular or respiratory compromise nor seizures have been reported with overdose

Toxicology Supportive therapy

Drug Interactions Substrate and **weak** inhibitor of CYP2D6, 1AZ, and 3A4; increased sedative effects occur with alcohol and benzodiazepines; although no data are available, avoid concurrent use with monoamine oxidase (MAO) inhibitors, or until at least 14 days after stopping an MAO inhibitors, and not starting an MAO inhibitors until at least 14 days after stopping mirtazapine

Mechanism of Action Potent alpha$_2$-adrenergic antagonist, increasing both noradrenergic and serotonergic neurotransmission; antagonist of presynaptic alpha$_2$-adrenergic autoreceptors increasing release of norepinephrine and serotonin; potent blocker of 5-HT$_2$, 5-HT$_3$, and H$_1$ receptors; weak antagonist of alpha$_1$-adrenergic and muscarinic receptors

Pharmacokinetics
Absorption: Food has minimal effect
Distribution: V$_d$: 4.5 L/kg
Protein binding: 85%
Metabolism: By CYP3A4 to N-demethylmirtazapine (active); CYP2D6 to 8-hydroxymirtazapine which is metabolized by CYP1A2
Bioavailability: ~50%
Half-life:
Elderly: 31-39 hours
Adults: 21 hours (13-34 hours)

Usual Dosage Oral: Initial:
Geriatrics: 7.5 mg/day as a single bedtime dose; increase by 7.5-15 mg/day every 1-2 weeks; usual dose: 15-30 mg/day; maximum dose: 45 mg/day
Adults: 15 mg/day as a single bedtime dose; increase by 15 mg/day every 1-2 weeks; usual dose: 30 mg/day; maximum dose: 45 mg/day
Dosage adjustment in moderate-to-severe renal or hepatic impairment: Dosage reductions may be necessary

Monitoring Parameters Signs and symptoms of depression; sleep; appetite and weight

Patient Information Take as a single bedtime dose; avoid alcohol and other sedating medications; impaired driving performance or delayed reaction times
(Continued)

Mirtazapine *(Continued)*

are possible; expect a delay in the onset of therapeutic effects; report side effects

Nursing Implications See Usual Dosage and Adverse Reactions

Special Geriatric Considerations Limited published data specifically in the elderly or addressing *in vivo* drug interactions (see Pharmacokinetics and Usual Dosage)

Dosage Forms Tablet: 15 mg, 30 mg

References

"Mirtazapine - A New Antidepressant," *Med Lett Drugs Ther*, 1996, 38(990):113-4.

Stimmel GL, Dopheide JA, and Stahl SM, "Mirtazapine: An Antidepressant With Noradrenergic and Specific Serotonergic Effects," *Pharmacotherapy*, 1997, 17(1):10-21.

Misoprostol *(mye soe PROST ole)*

Brand Names Cytotec®

Generic Available No

Therapeutic Category Prostaglandin

Use Prevention of NSAID-induced gastric ulcers

Unlabeled use: Treatment of duodenal and gastric ulcers

Contraindications Hypersensitivity to misoprostol, prostaglandins, or any component

Warnings Renal function impairment may increase half-life; does not prevent NSAID-induced duodenal ulcers; elderly have an increased AUC in studies

Precautions Diarrhea (13% to 40%) is dose related; diarrhea usually occurs in first 2 weeks; diarrhea is usually self-limited but may require dose reduction or discontinuation (see Additional Information)

Adverse Reactions

Cardiovascular: Headache

Endocrine & metabolic: Postmenopausal vaginal bleeding

Gastrointestinal: Diarrhea (transient), abdominal pain, nausea, dyspepsia, vomiting, constipation, flatulence

Overdosage Symptoms of overdose include sedation, tremor, convulsions, dyspnea, abdominal pain, diarrhea, hypotension, bradycardia

Toxicology General supportive care; not dialyzable

Drug Interactions Antacids and food diminish absorption; antacids may enhance diarrhea

Mechanism of Action Misoprostol is a synthetic prostaglandin E_1 analog that replaces the protective prostaglandins consumed with prostaglandin-inhibiting therapies (eg, nonsteroidal anti-inflammatory drugs)

Pharmacokinetics

Absorption: Oral: Rapid

Half-life (parent and metabolite combined): 1.5 hours

Time to peak serum concentration (active metabolite): Within 15-30 minutes

Rapidly de-esterified to misoprostol acid

Elimination: In urine (64% to 73% in 24 hours) and feces (15% in 24 hours)

Since elderly have decreased clearance (increased AUC), it may be necessary to reduce dose to 100 mcg 4 times/day

Usual Dosage Oral:

Geriatrics: 100-200 mcg 4 times/day with food; if 200 mcg 4 times/day not tolerated, reduce to 100 mcg 4 times/day or 200 mcg twice daily with food. **Note:** To avoid the diarrhea potential, doses can be initiated at 100 mcg/day and increased 100 mcg/day at 3-day intervals until desired dose is achieved; also, recommend administering with food to decrease diarrhea incidence (see Special Geriatric Considerations).

Adults: 200 mcg 4 times/day with food or 100 mcg 4 times/day or 200 mcg twice daily with food if not tolerated

Monitoring Parameters Monitor for diarrhea, stool occult blood; gastroscopy may be preferred

Patient Information May cause diarrhea when first being used (within 2 weeks); diarrhea incidence and severity may be decreased by taking with food and at bedtime

Nursing Implications Incidence of diarrhea may be lessened by having patient take dose right after meals and at bedtime (see Monitoring Parameters)

Additional Information Although food may decrease absorption, the clinical significance is unknown; administration with food may decrease diarrhea; diarrhea is normally a transient problem

Special Geriatric Considerations Elderly, due to extensive use of NSAIDs and the high percentage of asymptomatic hemorrhage and perforation from

NSAIDs, are at risk for NSAID-induced ulcers and may be candidates for misoprostol use. However, routine use for prophylaxis is not justified. Patients must be selected upon demonstration that they are at risk for NSAID-induced lesions. Misoprostol should not be used as a first-line therapy for gastric or duodenal ulcers.

Dosage Forms Tablet: 100 mcg, 200 mcg

References

Walt RP, "Misoprostol for the Treatment of Peptic Ulcer and Anti-inflammatory Drug-Induced Gastroduodenal Ulceration," *N Engl J Med*, 1992, 327(22):1575-80.

Mitran® Oral *see* Chlordiazepoxide *on page 205*

Mitrolan® Chewable Tablet [OTC] *see* Calcium Polycarbophil *on page 151*

MK594 *see* Losartan *on page 553*

MMR *see* Measles, Mumps, and Rubella Vaccines, Combined *on page 572*

M-M-R® II *see* Measles, Mumps, and Rubella Vaccines, Combined *on page 572*

Moban® *see* Molindone *on page 635*

Mobidin® *see* Salicylates (Various Salts) *on page 842*

Modane® Bulk [OTC] *see* Psyllium *on page 804*

Modane® Soft [OTC] *see* Docusate *on page 312*

Modified Shohl's Solution *see* Sodium Citrate and Citric Acid *on page 861*

Moduretic® *see* Amiloride and Hydrochlorothiazide *on page 54*

Moexipril (mo EKS i pril)

Related Information
ACE Inhibitors Comparison *on page 1019*

Brand Names Univasc®

Generic Available No

Therapeutic Category Angiotensin-Converting Enzyme (ACE) Inhibitors

Use Treatment of hypertension, alone or in combination with thiazide diuretics
Unlabeled use: Since ACE inhibitors as a class are indicated in systolic congestive heart failure, this agent may be added to treatment regimen

Contraindications Hypersensitivity to moexipril; history of angioedema related to treatment with an ACE inhibitor

Warnings Neutropenia, agranulocytosis, angioedema, decreased renal function (hypertension, renal artery stenosis, congestive heart failure), hepatic dysfunction (elimination, activation), proteinuria, first-dose hypotension (hypovolemia, congestive heart failure, dehydrated patients at risk, eg, diuretic use, elderly), elderly (due to renal function changes)

Precautions Use with caution and modify dosage in patients with renal impairment (especially renal artery stenosis), hyponatremia, hypovolemia, severe congestive heart failure or with coadministered diuretic therapy; valvular stenosis, hyperkalemia (>5.7 mEq/L), anesthesia

Adverse Reactions
Cardiovascular: Hypotension, syncope, orthostatic hypotension, arrhythmias, tachycardia, CVA, myocardial infarction, chest pain, palpitations, angina
Central nervous system: Fatigue, vertigo, insomnia, dizziness, headache, somnolence, ataxia, confusion, depression, nervousness
Dermatologic: Rash, urticaria, pemphigus, erythema multiforme, exfoliative dermatitis, flushing, photosensitivity, angioedema
Endocrine & metabolic: Hypoglycemia, hyperkalemia
Gastrointestinal: Nausea, diarrhea, xerostomia, dyspepsia, glossitis, abdominal pain, vomiting, dysgeusia, anorexia, constipation, pancreatitis, ageusia
Genitourinary: Polyuria
Hematologic: Agranulocytosis, neutropenia, anemia, eosinophilia, thrombocytopenia
Hepatic: Hepatitis
Neuromuscular & skeletal: Muscle cramps, myalgia, arthralgia, arthritis, weakness
Otic: Tinnitus
Renal: Deterioration in renal function, especially with renal artery stenosis, oliguria
Respiratory: Chronic cough (nonproductive, persistent); asthma, bronchitis, bronchospasm, dyspnea, pulmonary embolism, sinusitis, rhinitis
Miscellaneous: Diaphoresis

Overdosage Signs and symptoms of overdose include severe hypotension

Toxicology Following initiation of essential overdose management, toxic symptom treatment and supportive treatment should be initiated. Hypotension usually responds to I.V. fluids or Trendelenburg positioning. If unresponsive
(Continued)

Moexipril (Continued)

to these measures, the use of a parenteral inotrope may be required (eg, norepinephrine 0.1-0.2 mcg/kg/minute titrated to response).

Drug Interactions Hypotensive agents or diuretics may increase hypotensive effect; moexipril and potassium or potassium-sparing diuretics may have additive hyperkalemic effect; lithium and ACE inhibitors may cause increased lithium levels; NSAIDs and ACE inhibitors may decrease hypotensive effects

Mechanism of Action Moexipril is a prodrug of moexiprilat which acts as a competitive inhibitor of angiotensin-converting enzyme (ACE); prevents conversion of angiotensin I to angiotensin II, a potent vasoconstrictor; results in lower levels of angiotensin II which causes an increase in plasma renin activity and a reduction in aldosterone secretion

Pharmacodynamics

Onset of action: 2 hours after administration

Peak effect: 3-6 hours

Duration: 24 hours (see Additional Information)

Pharmacokinetics Moexipril is a prodrug and is converted to moexiprilat in the liver

Protein binding: 50% (moexiprilat)

Bioavailability: 13% (reduced with food)

Half-life:

Moexipril: 1 hour

Moexiprilat: 2-10 hours

Elimination: With oral administration, 52% of the dose is recovered in the feces as moexiprilat and 1% as moexipril; only 7% appears in the urine as moexiprilat and 1% as moexipril

In elderly male subjects, the AUC and peak serum concentrations were 30% greater than those of younger subjects; no difference in clinical effect was seen

Usual Dosage

Geriatrics: Same as adults or tablet may be cut in half (3.75 mg) (see Dosing Adjustment in Renal Failure and Additional Information)

Adults: Oral: Initial: 7.5 mg once daily (in patients **not** receiving diuretics) 1 hour prior to a meal; maintenance dose: 7.5-30 mg daily in 1 or 2 divided doses 1 hour before meals

Unlabeled use: Since ACE inhibitors are indicated as a class for treatment of congestive heart failure, patients receiving moexipril may benefit at proper dose; titrate to maintenance dose of 7.5-30 mg/day; no data available to date

Note: If patient is currently on diuretic therapy, the diuretic should be discontinued 2-3 days prior to initiating therapy with moexipril; if this is not possible, cautiously start with 3.75 mg and monitor for hypotension

Dosing adjustment in renal impairment:

Cl_{cr} ≤40 mL/minute: Patients may be cautiously placed on 3.75 mg once daily, then upwardly titrated to a maximum of 15 mg/day

Administration Administer on an empty stomach at least 1 hour before meals

Monitoring Parameters Blood pressure, serum potassium concentration, BUN, serum creatinine, renal function, WBCs

Test Interactions Increases BUN, creatinine, potassium, positive Coombs' [direct]; decreases cholesterol (S); may cause false-positive results in urine acetone determinations using sodium nitroprusside reagent

Patient Information Do not stop therapy except under prescriber advice; notify physician if you develop sore throat, fever, swelling of hands, feet, face, eyes, lips, and tongue; difficult breathing, irregular heartbeats, chest pains, or cough. May cause dizziness, fainting, and lightheadedness, especially in first week of therapy, sit and stand up slowly; may cause changes in taste or rash; do not add a salt substitute (potassium) without advice of physician.

Nursing Implications May cause depression in some patients; discontinue if angioedema of the face, extremities, lips, tongue, or glottis occurs; watch for hypotensive effect within 1-3 hours of first dose or new higher dose (see Precautions, Warnings, Monitoring Parameters, and Special Geriatric Considerations)

Additional Information The antihypertensive effect of moexipril may decrease towards the end of the dosing interval; blood pressure should be monitored prior to dosing. If blood pressure control is not adequate, an increased dose or divided dose may be attempted. Moexipril offers no therapeutic advantage over other ACE inhibitors. To reduce the risk of hypotension, discontinue therapy 2-3 days prior to starting moexipril if possible. If diuretics cannot be stopped for a short period, initiate dose at 3.75 mg/day.

Special Geriatric Considerations Due to frequent decreases in glomerular filtration (also creatinine clearance) with aging, elderly patients may have exaggerated responses to ACE inhibitors; differences in clinical response due to hepatic changes are not observed. ACE inhibitors may be preferred agents in elderly patients with congestive heart failure and diabetes mellitus. Diabetic proteinuria is reduced and insulin sensitivity is enhanced. In general, the side effect profile is favorable in elderly and causes little or no CNS confusion; use lowest dose recommendations initially; adjust dose for renal function in elderly (see Pharmacokinetics).

Dosage Forms Tablet, as hydrochloride: 7.5 mg, 15 mg

References

Konstam MA, Drakup K, Baker DW, et al, "Heart Failure: Evaluation and Care of Patients With Left Ventricular Systolic Dysfunction," *Clinical Practice Guideline No. 11*, Rockville, MD: Agency for Health Care Policy and Research, Public Health Service, U.S. Department of Health and Human Services, 1994.

Lewis EJ, Hunsicker LG, Bain RP, et al, "The Effect of Angiotensin-Converting Enzyme Inhibition on Diabetic Nephropathy," *N Engl J Med*, 1993, 329(20):1456-62.

McAreavey D and Robertson JIS, "Angiotensin Converting Enzyme Inhibitors and Moderate Hypertension," *Drugs*, 1990, 40(3):326-45.

Williams JF, Bristow MR, Fowler MB, et al, "Guidelines for the Evaluation and Management of Heart Failure: Report of the American College of Cardiology/American Heart Association Task Force on Practice Guidelines (Committee on Evaluation and Management of Heart Failure)," *J Am Coll Cardiol*, 1995, 26:1376-8.

Moi-Stir® [OTC] *see* Saliva Substitute on page 846

Moisture® Ophthalmic Drops [OTC] *see* Artificial Tears on page 82

Molindone (moe LIN done)

Related Information

Antipsychotic Agents Comparison on page 1023
Antipsychotic Medication Guidelines on page 1076
Federal OBRA Regulations Recommended Maximum Doses - Antipsychotics on page 1056

Brand Names Moban®

Generic Available No

Therapeutic Category Antipsychotic Agent; Neuroleptic Agent

Use Management of psychotic disorders; nonpsychotic symptoms associated with dementia in elderly, Tourette's syndrome, Huntington's chorea (see Special Geriatric Considerations)

Contraindications Narrow-angle glaucoma, bone marrow suppression, CNS depression, liver or cardiac disease, subcortical brain damage; circulatory collapse, severe hypotension or hypertension, hypersensitivity to molindone or any component

Warnings

Tardive dyskinesia: Prevalence rate may be 40% in elderly; elderly women especially at risk; embarrassment from dyskinesias may lead to greater social isolation; development of the syndrome and the irreversible nature are proportional to duration and total cumulative dose over time. May be reversible if diagnosed early in therapy; intermittent use of antipsychotics (not proven use) helps decrease total cumulative dose.

EPS: Extrapyramidal reactions are more common in elderly with up to 50% developing these reactions after age 60. These reactions may be more common in dementia patients. Drug-induced **Parkinson's syndrome** occurs often. Discontinuation usually resolves symptoms but may take weeks to months (12+) to clear. **Akathisia** is the most common EPS reaction in elderly. The symptoms of motor restlessness are difficult to diagnose in demented elderly; increased nervousness, assertiveness, restlessness with constant movement may indicate this adverse event. Consider decreasing dose if antipsychotic to treat as well as diagnose problem; usually see this reaction within 2-3 months of initiating antipsychotic drug.

Anticholinergic effects: These side effects most common with low potency antipsychotics (eg, thioridazine, chlorpromazine). CNS toxicity occurs more frequently and severely in elderly; increased confusion, memory loss, psychotic behavior, and agitation frequently occur as a consequence of anticholinergic effects to antipsychotic agents. Peripheral anticholinergic action troublesome to elderly; most peripheral anticholinergic effects last only 2-3 weeks (see Adverse Reactions).

Orthostatic hypotension: More common with low potency agents (eg, thioridazine, chlorpromazine, and clozapine) but of concern with all antipsychotic agents; orthostasis due to alpha-receptor blockade by antipsychotic agents. Elderly present many risk factors for orthostatic hypotension: blunted baroreceptor reflexes, decreased vascular tone, decreased vascular volume, (Continued)

Molindone *(Continued)*

and possible presence of cardiac diseases which result in decreased cardiac output.

Sedation: Common side effect with antipsychotic therapy; should not be used as a hypnotic unless insomnia is associated with target behavior symptoms treated with antipsychotic medications (see Special Geriatric Considerations). Anecdotal reports suggesting antipsychotic sedation in nonpsychotic patients is extremely unpleasant due to feelings of depersonalization, derealization, and dysphoria. Due to the long duration of action with antipsychotic drugs, these reactions may last up to 24 hours and result in decreased daytime function.

Cardiac toxicity: Life-threatening arrhythmias have occurred at therapeutic doses of antipsychotics. Thioridazine more commonly demonstrates EKG changes than other antipsychotics; suggested to use high potency antipsychotic agents (ie, haloperidol) in patients with cardiac conduction defects.

Precautions Use with caution in patients with severe cardiovascular disease, seizures, and Parkinson's disease; benefits of therapy must be weighed against risks

Adverse Reactions

Cardiovascular: Hypotension, tachycardia, arrhythmias

Central nervous system: Sedation, drowsiness, restlessness, anxiety, extrapyramidal reactions, pseudoparkinsonian signs and symptoms, seizures, altered central temperature regulation, neuroleptic malignant syndrome (NMS)

Dermatologic: Hyperpigmentation, pruritus, rash, photosensitivity

Endocrine & metabolic: Amenorrhea, galactorrhea, gynecomastia

Gastrointestinal: Xerostomia, constipation, GI upset, weight gain

Genitourinary: Urinary retention

Hematologic: Agranulocytosis (more often in women between fourth and tenth weeks of therapy), leukopenia (usually in patients with large doses for prolonged periods)

Ocular: Blurred vision, retinal pigmentation

Overdosage Symptoms of overdose include deep sleep, coma, extrapyramidal symptoms, abnormal involuntary muscle movements, hypotension or hypertension; agitation, restlessness, fever, hypothermia or hyperthermia, seizures, cardiac arrhythmias, EKG changes

Toxicology Following initiation of essential overdose management, toxic symptom treatment and supportive treatment should be initiated. Hypotension usually responds to I.V. fluids or Trendelenburg positioning. If unresponsive to these measures the use of a parenteral inotrope may be required (eg, norepinephrine 0.1-0.2 mcg/kg/minute titrated to response). Do not use epinephrine. Seizures commonly respond to diazepam (I.V. 5-10 mg bolus in adults every 15 minutes if needed up to a total of 30 mg) or to phenytoin or phenobarbital. Also critical cardiac arrhythmias often respond to I.V. phenytoin (15 mg/kg up to 1 g), while other antiarrhythmics can be used. Neuroleptics often cause extrapyramidal symptoms (eg, dystonic reactions) requiring management with diphenhydramine 1-2 mg/kg up to a maximum of 50 mg I.M. or I.V. slow push followed by a maintenance dose for 48-72 hours. When these reactions are unresponsive to diphenhydramine, benztropine mesylate I.V. 1-2 mg may be effective. These agents are generally effective within 2-5 minutes.

Drug Interactions Administration with CNS depressants will increase CNS depression; may block (weak) antihypertensive effects of guanethidine; anticonvulsants (phenytoin, carbamazepine, and phenobarbital) may decrease serum concentrations of molindone

Stability Protect from light; dispense in amber or opaque vials

Mechanism of Action Mechanism of action is similar to that of chlorpromazine; however, it produces more extrapyramidal effects and less sedation than chlorpromazine; blocks postsynaptic mesolimbic dopaminergic D_1 and D_2 receptors in the brain; exhibits a strong alpha-adrenergic blocking and anticholinergic effect, depresses the release of hypothalamic and hypophyseal hormones; believed to depress the reticular activating system thus affecting basal metabolism, body temperature, wakefulness, vasomotor tone, and emesis

Pharmacodynamics Duration of action: 24-36 hours

Pharmacokinetics

Absorption: Oral: May be affected by the inherent anticholinergic action on the gastrointestinal tissue causing variable absorption. Absorption from tablets is erratic with less variation seen with solutions. These agents are widely distributed in tissues with CNS concentrations exceeding that of plasma due to their lipophilic characteristics.

Protein binding: Antipsychotic agents are bound 90% to 99% to plasma proteins; highly bound to brain and lung tissue and other tissues with a high blood perfusion.

Metabolism: Metabolized in the liver

Time to peak: Following oral administration peak serum concentrations occur within 90 minutes; peak concentrations between 2-4 hours

Elimination: Principally excreted in the urine and feces (90% within 24 hours); <2% to 3% excreted unmetabolized; eliminated through hepatic metabolism (oxidation) where numerous active metabolites are produced; active metabolites excreted in urine; elimination half-lives of antipsychotics ranges from 20-40 hours which may be extended in elderly due to decline in oxidative hepatic reactions (phase I) with age.

The biologic effect of a single dose persists for 24 hours. When the patient has accommodated to initial side effects (sedation), once daily dosing is possible due to the long half-life of antipsychotics.

Steady-state plasma concentrations are achieved in 4-7 days; therefore, if possible, do not make dose adjustments more than once in a 7-day period. Due to the long half-lives of antipsychotics, as needed (prn) use is ineffective since repeated doses are necessary to achieve therapeutic tissue concentrations in the CNS.

Usual Dosage Oral:

Geriatrics (nonpsychotic patients, dementia behavior): Initial: 5-10 mg 1-2 times/day; increase at 4- to 7-day intervals by 5-10 mg/day; increase dosing intervals (bid, tid, etc) as necessary to control response or side effects; maximum daily dose: 112 mg; gradual increases (titration) may prevent some side effects or decrease their severity

Adults: 50-75 mg/day; up to 225 mg/day

Monitoring Parameters Orthostatic blood pressures; tremors; gait changes, abnormal movement in trunk, neck, buccal area, or extremities; monitor target behaviors for which the agent is given

Patient Information May cause drowsiness; avoid alcoholic beverages; do not take within 1 hour of taking antacids; rise slowly from recumbent position; use of supportive stockings may prevent orthostatic hypotension

Nursing Implications Monitor orthostatic blood pressures 3-5 days after initiation of therapy or after a dose increase; observe for tremor and abnormal movement or posturing (extrapyramidal symptoms)

Special Geriatric Considerations See Warnings.

Many elderly patients receive antipsychotic medications for inappropriate nonpsychotic behavior. Before initiating antipsychotic medication, the clinician should investigate any possible reversible cause; any stress or stress from any disease can cause acute "confusion" or worsening of baseline nonpsychotic behavior. Most commonly acute changes in behavior are due to increases in drug dose or addition of new drug to regimen, fluid electrolyte loss, infections, and changes in environment.

Any changes in disease status in any organ system can result in behavior changes.

In the treatment of agitated, demented, elderly patients, authors of meta-analysis of controlled trials of the response to the traditional antipsychotics (phenothiazines, butyrophenones) in controlling agitation have concluded that the use of neuroleptics results in a response rate of 18%. Clearly neuroleptic therapy for behavior control should be limited with frequent attempts to withdraw the agent given for behavior control.

Dosage Forms

Molindone hydrochloride:

Concentrate, oral: 20 mg/mL (120 mL)

Tablet: 5 mg, 10 mg, 25 mg, 50 mg, 100 mg

References

Peabody CA, Warner MD, Whiteford HA, et al, "Neuroleptics and the Elderly," *J Am Geriatr Soc,* 1987, 35(3):233-8.

Risse SC and Barnes R, "Pharmacologic Treatment of Agitation Associated With Dementia," *J Am Geriatr Soc,* 1986, 34(5):368-76.

Saltz BL, Woerner MG, Kane JM, et al, "Prospective Study of Tardive Dyskinesia Incidence in the Elderly," *JAMA,* 1991, 266(17):2402-6.

Seifert RD, "Therapeutic Drug Monitoring: Psychotropic Drugs," *J Pharm Pract,* 1984, 6:403-16.

Mol-Iron® [OTC] see Ferrous Sulfate *on page 379*

Mollifene® Ear Wax Removing Formula [OTC] see Carbamide Peroxide *on page 162*

MOM see Magnesium Hydroxide *on page 564*

Mometasone Furoate (moe MET a sone FYOOR oh ate)

Related Information
Corticosteroids Comparison, Topical *on page 1030*

Brand Names Elocon®

Generic Available No

Therapeutic Category Corticosteroid, Topical (Medium Potency)

Use Relief of the inflammatory and pruritic manifestations of corticosteroid-responsive dermatoses

Contraindications Hypersensitivity to mometasone or any component; fungal, viral, or tubercular skin lesions, herpes simplex or zoster

Precautions Systemic absorption of topical corticosteroids has produced reversible HPA axis suppression. This is more likely to occur when the preparation is used on large surfaces or denuded areas for prolonged periods of time or with an occlusive dressing.

Adverse Reactions
Dermatologic: Acne, hypopigmentation, allergic dermatitis, maceration of the skin, skin atrophy, striae, miliaria, telangiectasia
Endocrine & metabolic: HPA suppression, Cushing's syndrome, growth retardation
Local: Burning, itching, irritation, dryness, folliculitis, hypertrichosis
Miscellaneous: Secondary infection

Mechanism of Action Topical corticosteroids have anti-inflammatory, antipruritic, vasoconstrictive, and antiproliferative actions

Usual Dosage Geriatrics and Adults: Topical: Apply sparingly to area once daily, do not use occlusive dressings

Monitoring Parameters Relief of symptoms

Patient Information Use only as prescribed and for no longer than the period prescribed; apply sparingly in a thin film and rub in lightly; avoid contact with eyes; notify physician if condition persists or worsens

Nursing Implications Use sparingly

Additional Information Considered a moderate-potency steroid; may be used for a limited time on the face; prolonged use may cause atrophic changes

Special Geriatric Considerations Due to age-related changes in skin, limit use of topical glucocorticosteroids (see Precautions)

Dosage Forms
Cream: 0.1% (15 g, 45 g)
Lotion: 0.1% (30 mL, 60 mL)
Ointment, topical: 0.1% (15 g, 45 g)

MOM/Mineral Oil Emulsion *see* Magnesium Hydroxide and Mineral Oil Emulsion *on page 565*

Monacolin K *see* Lovastatin *on page 555*

Monafed® *see* Guaifenesin *on page 437*

Monafed® DM *see* Guaifenesin and Dextromethorphan *on page 439*

Monistat-Derm™ Topical *see* Miconazole *on page 625*

Monistat i.v.™ Injection *see* Miconazole *on page 625*

Monistat™ Vaginal *see* Miconazole *on page 625*

Monocid® *see* Cefonicid *on page 180*

Monodox® Oral *see* Doxycycline *on page 322*

Mono-Gesic® *see* Salsalate *on page 847*

Monoket® *see* Isosorbide Mononitrate *on page 505*

Monopril® *see* Fosinopril *on page 411*

More Attenuated Enders Strain *see* Measles Virus Vaccine, Live *on page 574*

More-Dophilus® [OTC] *see* Lactobacillus acidophilus and Lactobacillus bulgaricus *on page 522*

Moricizine (mor I siz een)

Brand Names Ethmozine®

Generic Available No

Therapeutic Category Antiarrhythmic Agent, Class I-A

Use Treatment of ventricular tachycardia and life-threatening ventricular arrhythmias
Unlabeled use: Moricizine 600-900 mg/day may be effective in treatment of PVCs, complete and nonsustained ventricular tachycardia

Contraindications Pre-existing second or third degree A-V block and in patients with right bundle-branch block when associated with left hemiblock, unless pacemaker is present; cardiogenic shock; known hypersensitivity to the drug

Warnings Considering the known proarrhythmic properties and lack of evidence of improved survival for any antiarrhythmic drug in patients without life-threatening arrhythmias, it is prudent to reserve the use for patients with life-threatening ventricular arrhythmias; CAST II trial demonstrated a trend towards decreased survival for patients treated with moricizine; proarrhythmic effects occur as with other antiarrhythmic agents; hypokalemia, hyperkalemia, hypomagnesemia may effect response to class I agents; use with caution in patients with sick sinus syndrome, hepatic, and renal impairment

Precautions Use with caution in patients with hepatic or renal insufficiency since increases in half-life may occur; EKG changes may occur due to conduction abnormalities from changes in A-V node conduction; congestive heart failure may be aggravated; may alter pacemaker threshold sensitivity; drug fever

Adverse Reactions

Cardiovascular: Proarrhythmia, syncope, cardiac arrest, myocardial infarction, chest pain, CHF, cardiac death, hypotension, bradycardia, thromboembolism

Central nervous system: Dizziness, headache, fatigue, anxiety, depression, agitation, seizure, coma, euphoria, dyskinesia, hallucinations, speech difficulties, confusion, loss of memory, vertigo, somnolence, gait disturbances, akathisia, fever

Dermatologic: Rash, pruritus, dry skin, urticaria

Gastrointestinal: Anorexia, bitter taste, abdominal pain, ileus, vomiting, diarrhea, flatulence, xerostomia

Genitourinary: Urinary incontinence, impotence

Neuromuscular & skeletal: Tremors, myalgia, skeletal pain, paresthesia

Ocular: Nystagmus, periorbital edema, blurred vision, eye pain, diplopia

Otic: Tinnitus

Respiratory: Dyspnea, hyperventilation, cough, pharyngitis, apnea, pulmonary embolism, asthma

Miscellaneous: Temperature intolerance, edema of lips and tongue, diaphoresis, hypothermia

Overdosage Symptoms of overdose include emesis, lethargy, hypotension, conduction disturbances, sinus arrest, arrhythmias

Toxicology General supportive care; gastric lavage may be helpful

Drug Interactions

Theophylline levels decreased

Cimetidine increases moricizine levels

Digoxin and propranolol have increased cardiac effects

Mechanism of Action Reduces the fast inward current carried by sodium ions, shortens Phase I and Phase II repolarization, resulting in decreased action potential duration and effective refractory period

Pharmacokinetics

Protein binding, plasma: 95%

Metabolism: Undergoes significant first-pass metabolism (38%)

Half-life:

Normal patients: 3-4 hours

Cardiac disease patients: 6-13 hours

Elimination: 56% excreted in feces and 39% in urine, some enterohepatic recycling occurs

Usual Dosage Geriatrics and Adults: Hospitalization required to start therapy. Oral: 200-300 mg every 8 hours, adjust dosage at 150 mg/day at 3-day intervals; to switch from another antiarrhythmic agent to moricizine, start moricizine 6-12 hours after last dose of former agent; may need 24-hour postdose with flecainide (see Additional Information)

Dosing adjustment in renal and hepatic impairment: Initial dose: 600 mg or less/day

Monitoring Parameters Holter monitoring may be considered; monitor pulse, EKG, and blood pressure

Patient Information Take as directed; do not change dose except from advice of your physician; report any chest pain and irregular heartbeats

Nursing Implications Giving 30 minutes after a meal delays the rate of absorption, resulting in lower peak plasma concentrations

Additional Information For transferring a patient from another antiarrhythmic agent, discontinue previous antiarrhythmic for 1-2 half-lives before starting moricizine; if this cannot be done, hospitalize patient to make transfer (Continued)

Moricizine *(Continued)*

Special Geriatric Considerations Due to moricizine binding to plasma albumin and alpha-glycoprotein, other highly bound drugs may displace moricizine; since elderly may require multiple drugs, caution with highly bound drugs is necessary; consider changes in renal and hepatic function with age and monitor closely since half-life may be prolonged

Dosage Forms Tablet, as hydrochloride: 200 mg, 250 mg, 300 mg

References

Fenster PE and Nolan PE, "Antiarrhythmic Drugs," *Geriatric Pharmacology*, Bressler R and Katz MD, eds, New York, NY: McGraw-Hill, 1993, 6:105-49.

Morphine Sulfate (MOR feen SUL fate)

Related Information

I.V. Push Recommended Guidelines *on page 1083*
Narcotic Agonist Comparative Pharmacology *on page 1036*
Pharmacokinetics of Narcotic Agonist Analgesics *on page 1037*

Brand Names Astramorph™ PF Injection; Duramorph® Injection; Infumorph™ Injection; Kadian® Capsule; MS Contin® Oral; MSIR® Oral; MS/L®; MS/S®; OMS® Oral; Oramorph SR™ Oral; RMS® Rectal; Roxanol™ Oral; Roxanol Rescudose®; Roxanol SR™ Oral

Synonyms MS

Generic Available Yes

Therapeutic Category Analgesic, Narcotic

Use Relief of moderate to severe acute and chronic pain; pain of myocardial infarction; relieves dyspnea of acute left ventricular failure and pulmonary edema; preanesthetic medication

Restrictions C-II

Contraindications Known hypersensitivity to morphine sulfate; increased intracranial pressure; severe respiratory depression; severe liver or renal insufficiency

Warnings Some preparations contain sulfites which may cause allergic reactions

Precautions Use with caution in patients with hypersensitivity reactions to other phenanthrene derivative opioid agonists (codeine, hydrocodone, hydromorphone, levorphanol, oxycodone, oxymorphone)

Adverse Reactions

Cardiovascular: Palpitations, hypotension, bradycardia, peripheral vasodilation

Central nervous system: CNS depression, increased intracranial pressure

Dermatologic: Pruritus

Endocrine & metabolic: Antidiuretic hormone release

Gastrointestinal: Nausea, vomiting, constipation

Ocular: Miosis

Respiratory: Respiratory depression

Miscellaneous: Physical and psychological dependence, biliary or urinary tract spasm, histamine release

Overdosage Symptoms of overdose include respiratory depression, miosis, hypotension, bradycardia, apnea, pulmonary edema

Toxicology Treatment of an overdose includes support of the patient's airway, establishment of an I.V. line and administration of naloxone 2 mg I.V. with repeat administration as necessary up to a total of 10 mg.

Drug Interactions Increased toxicity: CNS depressants, phenothiazines, tricyclic antidepressants

Stability Refrigerate suppositories; do not freeze; degradation depends on pH and presence of oxygen; relatively stable in pH ≤4; darkening of solutions indicate degradation; usual concentration for continuous I.V. infusion = 0.1-1 mg/mL in D_5W

Mechanism of Action Binds to opiate receptors in the CNS, causing inhibition of ascending pain pathways, altering the perception of and response to pain; produces generalized CNS depression

Pharmacodynamics Enhanced analgesia has been seen in elderly patients on therapeutic doses of narcotics; duration of action may be prolonged in the elderly; see table.

Pharmacokinetics

Absorption: Oral: Variable

Distribution: V_d: Decreased in elderly

Metabolism: In the liver via glucuronide conjugation; susbstrate CYP2D6

Half-life: 2-4 hours

Elimination: 6% to 10% excreted unchanged in urine; total body clearance decreased in elderly

Dosage Form/Route	Analgesia	
	Peak	Duration
Tablets	1 h	4-5 h
Oral solution	1 h	4-5 h
Extended release tablets	1 h	8-12 h
Suppository	20-60 min	3-7 h
Subcutaneous injection	50-90 min	4-5 h
I.M. injection	30-60 min	4-5 h
I.V. injection	20 min	4-5 h

Usual Dosage Doses should be titrated to appropriate effect; when changing routes of administration in chronically treated patients, note that oral doses are ~1/3 to 1/6 as effective as parenteral dose

Geriatrics and Adults:
Oral: Prompt release: 10-30 mg every 4 hours as needed; controlled release: 15-30 mg every 8-12 hours
I.M., I.V., S.C.: 2.5-20 mg/dose every 2-6 hours as needed; usual: 10 mg/dose every 4 hours as needed. Initial I.M. dose for geriatric patients: 2.5-5 mg every 4-6 hours
I.V., S.C. continuous infusion: 0.8-10 mg/hour; may increase depending on pain relief/adverse effects; usual range up to 80 mg/hour
Rectal: 10-20 mg every 4 hours
Epidural: Initial: 5 mg in lumbar region; if inadequate pain relief within 1 hour, administer 1-2 mg, maximum: 10 mg/24 hours; geriatric patients: <5 mg may provide satisfactory pain relief
Intrathecal (1/10 of epidural dose): 0.2-1 mg/dose; repeat doses **not** recommended; use extreme caution in geriatric patients

Monitoring Parameters Pain relief, respiratory and mental status, blood pressure

Reference Range Therapeutic: Surgical anesthesia: 65-80 ng/mL (SI: 227-280 nmol/L); Toxic: 200-5000 ng/mL (SI: 700-17,500 nmol/L)

Test Interactions Increased aminotransferase [ALT (SGPT)/AST (SGOT)] (S)

Patient Information May cause drowsiness; avoid alcoholic beverages; do not crush controlled release tablet

Nursing Implications Do not crush controlled release tablet; observe patient for excessive sedation, respiratory depression

Additional Information Because of its variety of dosage forms, morphine is particularly useful in the treatment of terminal pain. Serum concentrations >20 ng/dL may cause seizures; when converting from immediate release to controlled release morphine, the conversion is on a mg for mg basis. Immediate release morphine (oral, I.M., or S.C.) may be used for breakthrough pain until the dosage is adjusted.

Special Geriatric Considerations The elderly may be particularly susceptible to the CNS depressant and constipating effects of narcotics; for chronic administration of narcotic analgesics, morphine is preferable in the elderly due to its pharmacokinetics and side effect profile as compared to meperidine and methadone (see Pharmacodynamics and Pharmacokinetics)

Dosage Forms
Injection: 0.5 mg/mL (10 mL); 1 mg/mL (10 mL, 30 mL, 60 mL); 2 mg/mL (1 mL, 2 mL, 60 mL); 3 mg/mL (50 mL); 4 mg/mL (1 mL, 2 mL); 5 mg/mL (1 mL, 30 mL); 8 mg/mL (1 mL, 2 mL); 10 mg/mL (1 mL, 2 mL, 10 mL); 15 mg, mL (1 mL, 2 mL, 20 mL)
Injection, preservative free: 0.5 mg/mL (2 mL, 10 mL); 1 mg/mL (2 mL, 10 mL)
Injection, I.V. via PCA pump: 1 mg/mL (10 mL, 30 mL, 60 mL); 5 mg/mL (30 mL)
Injection, for I.V. infusion preparation: 25 mg/mL (4 mL, 10 mL, 20 mL)
Solution, oral: 10 mg/5 mL (5 mL, 10 mL, 100 mL, 120 mL, 500 mL); 20 mg/5 mL (5 mL, 100 mL, 120 mL, 500 mL)
Suppositories, rectal: 5 mg, 10 mg, 20 mg, 30 mg
Tablet: 15 mg, 30 mg
Tablet:
Controlled release: 15 mg, 30 mg, 60 mg, 100 mg
Soluble: 10 mg, 15 mg, 30 mg

References
Ferrell BA, "Pain Management in Elderly People," *J Am Geriatr Soc*, 1991, 39(1):64-73.
(Continued)

Morphine Sulfate *(Continued)*

Kaiko RF, "Age and Morphine Analgesia in Cancer Patients With Postoperative Pain," *Clin Pharmacol Ther*, 1980, 28(6):823-6.

Kaiko RF, Wallenstein SL, Rogers AG, et al, "Narcotics in the Elderly," *Med Clin North Am*, 1982, 66(5):1079-89.

Mosco® Liquid [OTC] *see* Salicylic Acid *on page 845*

Motrin® *see* Ibuprofen *on page 475*

Motrin® IB [OTC] *see* Ibuprofen *on page 475*

6-MP *see* Mercaptopurine *on page 589*

M-Prednisol® Injection *see* Methylprednisolone *on page 611*

M-R-VAX® II *see* Measles and Rubella Vaccines, Combined *on page 571*

MS *see* Morphine Sulfate *on page 640*

MS Contin® Oral *see* Morphine Sulfate *on page 640*

MSIR® Oral *see* Morphine Sulfate *on page 640*

MS/L® *see* Morphine Sulfate *on page 640*

MS/S® *see* Morphine Sulfate *on page 640*

MTX *see* Methotrexate *on page 605*

Muco-Fen-DM® *see* Guaifenesin and Dextromethorphan *on page 439*

Muco-Fen-LA® *see* Guaifenesin *on page 437*

Mumps, Measles and Rubella Vaccines, Combined *see* Measles, Mumps, and Rubella Vaccines, Combined *on page 572*

Mumpsvax® *see* Mumps Virus Vaccine, Live, Attenuated *on this page*

Mumps Virus Vaccine, Live, Attenuated

(mumpz VYE rus vak SEEN, live, a ten YOO ate ed)

Related Information

Immunization Guidelines *on page 1058*

Brand Names Mumpsvax®

Generic Available No

Therapeutic Category Vaccine, Live Virus

Use Selective mumps prophylaxis by promoting active immunity; trivalent MMR preferred

Warnings Do not vaccinate immunocompromised persons, those with a history of anaphylactic reaction following egg ingestion or receipt of neomycin, or patients with cellular or humoral immune deficiencies; persons born prior to 1957 are considered immune and need not be vaccinated; do not use for delayed hypersensitivity skin testing; have epinephrine 1:1000 available when vaccinating for mumps

Adverse Reactions

Central nervous system: Fever ≤100°F, fever >103°F, convulsions, confusion, severe or continuing headache

Dermatologic: Rash

Endocrine & metabolic: Parotitis

Gastrointestinal: Diarrhea

Genitourinary: Orchitis in postpubescent and adult males

Hematologic: Thrombocytopenic purpura

Local: Burning or stinging at injection site

Ocular: Optic neuritis

Miscellaneous: Anaphylactic reactions, lymphoadenopathy

Drug Interactions Decreased effect with concurrent infection, immunoglobulin with in 1 month, other live vaccines with the exception of attenuated measles, rubella, or polio

Stability Refrigerate (2°C to 8°C); protect from light; discard within 8 hours after reconstitution; the powder can be left at room temperature for up to 5 days

Usual Dosage Geriatrics and Adults: 0.5 mL S.C. in outer aspect of the upper arm, no booster (see Additional Information and Administration)

Administration Reconstitute only with diluent provided; administer only S.C. on outer aspect of upper arm

Monitoring Parameters Monitor for anaphylaxis after vaccination, having person remain in office for a period of 15-30 minutes would be more than adequate

Test Interactions Temporary suppression of tuberculosis skin test

Patient Information A little swelling of the glands in the cheeks and under the jaw may occur that lasts for a few days; this could appear from 1-2 weeks after receiving the mumps vaccine

Additional Information MMR is the preferred vaccine for immunizing adults who have no evidence of mumps protection. Federal law requires that the date of administration, the vaccine manufacturer, lot number of vaccine, and the administering person's name, title and address be entered into the patient's permanent medical record; all adults without documentation of live vaccine on or after the first birthday or physician-diagnosed mumps, or laboratory evidence or immunity (particularly males and young adults who work in or congregate in hospitals, colleges, and on military bases) should be vaccinated. It is reasonable to consider persons born before 1957 immune, but there is no contraindication to vaccination of older persons. Susceptible travelers should be vaccinated.

Special Geriatric Considerations Most adults are immune to mumps and vaccination is not necessary for those born prior to 1957; elderly who have lived in isolated communities may have no immunity; for those who fail to demonstrate immunity by testing, vaccination would be desired if exposure is likely (travel to endemic area, etc); the trivalent MMR is preferred, however

Dosage Forms Injection: Single dose

Mupirocin (myoo PEER oh sin)

Brand Names Bactroban®; Bactroban® Nasal

Synonyms Pseudomonic Acid A

Therapeutic Category Antibacterial, Topical; Antibiotic, Topical

Use Topical treatment of impetigo due to *Staphylococcus aureus*, beta-hemolytic *Streptococcus* and *S. pyogenes*; intranasally for the eradication of nasal colonization with methicillin-resistant *Streptococcus aureus* in adult patients and healthcare workers during institutional outbreaks

Contraindications Known hypersensitivity to mupirocin or polyethylene glycol

Warnings Potentially toxic amounts of polyethylene glycol contained in the vehicle may be absorbed percutaneously in patients with extensive burns or open wounds; prolonged use may result in overgrowth of nonsusceptible organisms

Precautions Use with caution in patients with impaired renal function

Adverse Reactions
Cardiovascular: Edema
Dermatologic: Pruritus, rash, erythema, dry skin
Local: Burning, stinging, pain, tenderness

Stability Do not mix with Aquaphor®, coal tar solution, or salicylic acid

Mechanism of Action Binds to bacterial isoleucyl transfer-RNA synthetase resulting in the inhibition of protein and RNA synthesis

Pharmacokinetics
Absorption: Topical: Penetrates outer layers of skin; systemic absorption is minimal through intact skin
Protein binding: 95%
Metabolism: Extensive, principally in the liver and skin to monic acid
Half-life: 17-36 minutes
Elimination: In urine

Usual Dosage Geriatrics and Adults: Topical: Apply small amount 3 times/day for 5-14 days

Monitoring Parameters If no clinical response in 3-5 days, re-evaluate use

Patient Information For topical use only; do not apply into the eye

Nursing Implications See Warnings and Special Geriatric Considerations

Additional Information Contains polyethylene glycol vehicle

Special Geriatric Considerations Not for treatment of pressure sores (see Warnings)

Dosage Forms
Mupirocin calcium:
Ointment:
Intranasal: 2% (1 g single use tube)
Topical: 2% (15 g)

References
Goldfarb J, Crenshaw D, O'Horo J, et al, "Randomized Clinical Trial of Topical Mupirocin Versus Oral Erythromycin for Impetigo," *Antimicrob Agents Chemother*, 1988, 32(12):1780-3.

Murine® Ear Drops [OTC] see Carbamide Peroxide *on page 162*

Murine® Plus Ophthalmic [OTC] see Tetrahydrozoline *on page 901*

Murine® Solution [OTC] see Artificial Tears *on page 82*

Muro 128® Ophthalmic [OTC] see Sodium Chloride *on page 860*

Murocel® Ophthalmic Solution [OTC] see Artificial Tears *on page 82*

Muroptic-5® [OTC] see Sodium Chloride *on page 860*

Muse® Pellet see Alprostadil *on page 38*

Mus-Lax® see Chlorzoxazone *on page 218*

Myambutol® see Ethambutol on page 355

Mycelex® see Clotrimazole on page 242

Mycelex®-7 see Clotrimazole on page 242

Mycelex®-G see Clotrimazole on page 242

Mycobutin® see Rifabutin on page 829

Mycogen II Topical see Nystatin and Triamcinolone on page 687

Mycolog®-II Topical see Nystatin and Triamcinolone on page 687

Myconel® Topical see Nystatin and Triamcinolone on page 687

Mycostatin® see Nystatin on page 686

Myco-Triacet® II see Nystatin and Triamcinolone on page 687

Mydfrin® Ophthalmic Solution see Phenylephrine on page 740

Mykrox® see Metolazone on page 617

Mylanta® [OTC] see Aluminum Hydroxide, Magnesium Hydroxide, and Simethicone on page 44

Mylanta Gas® [OTC] see Simethicone on page 856

Mylanta®-II [OTC] see Aluminum Hydroxide, Magnesium Hydroxide, and Simethicone on page 44

Mylanta® Soothing Antacids [OTC] see Calcium Salts (Oral) on page 152

Myleran® see Busulfan on page 137

Mylicon® [OTC] see Simethicone on page 856

Myochrysine® see Gold Sodium Thiomalate on page 432

Myotonachol™ see Bethanechol on page 117

Myphetapp® [OTC] see Brompheniramine and Phenylpropanolamine on page 130

Mysoline® see Primidone on page 778

Mytrex® F Topical see Nystatin and Triamcinolone on page 687

Mytussin® [OTC] see Guaifenesin on page 437

Mytussin® AC see Guaifenesin and Codeine on page 438

Mytussin® DM [OTC] see Guaifenesin and Dextromethorphan on page 439

Nabumetone (na BYOO me tone)

Brand Names Relafen®

Generic Available No

Therapeutic Category Antipyretic; Nonsteroidal Anti-inflammatory Agent (NSAID), Oral

Use Management of osteoarthritis and rheumatoid arthritis

Unlabeled use: Sunburn, mild to moderate pain

Contraindications Hypersensitivity to nabumetone, any component, aspirin or other nonsteroidal anti-inflammatory drugs (NSAIDs); salicylate allergy

Warnings GI toxicity (bleeding, ulceration, perforation); CNS effects may occur (headaches, confusion, depression); hypersensitivity, anaphylactoid reactions (intermittent tolmetin use more often); renal function decline, acute renal insufficiency, interstitial nephritis, dysuria, cystitis, hematuria, nephrotic syndrome, hyperkalemia in acute renal insufficiency, hyponatremia, papillary necrosis, hepatic function impairment; elderly have increased risk for adverse reactions to NSAIDs (see Special Geriatric Considerations)

Precautions Use with caution in patients with congestive heart failure, hypertension, decreased renal or hepatic function, history of GI disease (bleeding or ulcers), or those receiving anticoagulants; perform ophthalmologic evaluation for those who develop eye complaints during therapy (blurred vision, diminished vision, changes in color vision, retinal changes); NSAIDs may mask signs/symptoms of infections; photosensitivity reported

Adverse Reactions

Cardiovascular: Congestive heart failure, angina, hypertension, hypotension, arrhythmias, edema

Central nervous system: Headache, drowsiness, vertigo, dizziness, fatigue, hallucinations, confusion, depression, emotional lability, psychotic behavior, pyrexia

Dermatologic: Rash, urticaria, angioedema, Stevens-Johnson syndrome, exfoliative dermatitis, bruising, petechiae, purpura

Endocrine & metabolic: Hyperglycemia, hypoglycemia, hyperkalemia, gynecomastia, hyponatremia, fluid retention

Gastrointestinal: Dyspepsia, heartburn, nausea, diarrhea, constipation, flatulence, stomatitis, vomiting, abdominal pain, peptic ulcer, GI bleeding, GI perforation, gingival ulcers, pancreatitis, proctitis, paralytic ulcers, colitis, anorexia, weight loss, dry mucous membranes

Genitourinary: Impotence, azotemia

Hematologic: Neutropenia, anemia, agranulocytosis, bone marrow suppression, hemolytic anemia, hemorrhage, inhibition of platelet aggregation

Hepatic: Hepatitis, elevated LFTs, cholestatic jaundice

Neuromuscular & skeletal: Involuntary muscle movements, muscle weakness, tremors, weakness

Ocular: Vision changes

Otic: Tinnitus

Renal: Dysuria, polyuria, pyuria, oliguria, anuria, acute renal failure

Respiratory: Exacerbation of asthma, dyspnea

Miscellaneous: Thirst, diaphoresis

Toxicology Management of a nonsteroidal anti-inflammatory agent (NSAID) intoxication is primarily supportive and symptomatic. Fluid therapy is commonly effective in managing the hypotension that may occur following an acute NSAID overdose, except when this is due to an acute blood loss. Seizures tend to be very short-lived and often do not require drug treatment although recurrent seizures should be treated with I.V. diazepam. Since many of the NSAIDs undergo enterohepatic cycling, multiple doses of charcoal may be needed to reduce the potential for delayed toxicities. NSAIDs are highly bound to plasma proteins, therefore hemodialysis and peritoneal dialysis are not useful.

Drug Interactions

May increase digoxin, methotrexate, and lithium serum concentrations

Aspirin or other salicylates may decrease NSAID serum concentrations

Other NSAIDs may increase adverse GI effects

Increased prothrombin time with anticoagulants

Decreased antihypertensive effects of ACE inhibitors, beta-blockers, and thiazide diuretics

Effects of loop diuretics may decrease

Increased response to sympathomimetics

Probenecid may increase toxicity of NSAIDs by increase in serum concentrations

Diuretics may increase risk for acute renal insufficiency

Azotemia may be enhanced in elderly receiving loop diuretics

Mechanism of Action Inhibits prostaglandin synthesis, acts on the hypothalamus heat-regulating center to reduce fever, blocks prostaglandin synthetase action which prevents formation of the platelet-aggregating substance thromboxane A_2; decreases pain receptor sensitivity. Other proposed mechanisms of action are lysosomal stabilization, inhibition of kinin and leukotriene production, alteration of chemotactic factors, and inhibition of neutrophil activation. This latter mechanism may be the most significant pharmacologic action to reduce inflammation. Nabumetone is a weak inhibitor of cyclo-oxygenase, however, its acetic acid active metabolite, 6-methoxy-2-naphthylacetic, is a potent inhibitor of cyclo-oxygenase.

Pharmacokinetics

Absorption: Rapidly and completely

Distribution: Readily distributes into body fluids and tissues

Metabolism: Nabumetone is essentially a prodrug which is activated to its active metabolite (acetic acid metabolites) in the liver; these are subsequently eliminated by liver metabolism

Half-life: 22-30 hours for active metabolite

Time to peak: 2-4 hours

Usual Dosage Geriatrics and Adults: Initial: 1000 mg as a single dose daily; dose can be increased to 1500-2000 mg/day; total dose may be divided into 2 doses daily; do not exceed 2000 mg/day

Monitoring Parameters Monitor response (pain, range of motion, grip strength, mobility, ADL function), inflammation; observe for weight gain, edema; monitor renal function; observe for bleeding, bruising; evaluate gastrointestinal effects (abdominal pain, bleeding, dyspepsia); mental confusion, disorientation, CBC, serum, creatinine, BUN, liver function tests

Patient Information Serious gastrointestinal bleeding can occur as well as ulceration and perforation. Pain may or may not be present. Avoid aspirin and aspirin-containing products while taking this medication. If gastric upset occurs, take with food, milk, or antacid. If gastric adverse effects persist, contact physician. May cause drowsiness, dizziness, blurred vision, and confusion. Use caution when performing tasks which require alertness (eg, driving). Do not take for more than 3 days for fever or 10 days for pain without physician advice.

Nursing Implications See Monitoring Parameters, Overdosage, Patient Information, and Special Geriatric Considerations

(Continued)

Nabumetone (Continued)

Additional Information There are no clinical guidelines to predict which NSAID will give response in a particular patient. Trials with each must be initiated until response determined. Consider dose, patient convenience, and cost.

Special Geriatric Considerations In trials with nabumetone, no significant differences were noted between young and elderly in regards to efficacy and safety. However, elderly are a high-risk population for adverse effects from nonsteroidal anti-inflammatory agents. As much as 60% of elderly can develop peptic ulceration and/or hemorrhage asymptomatically. The concomitant use of H_2 blockers, omeprazole, and sucralfate is not effective as prophylaxis with the exception of NSAID-induced duodenal ulcers which may be prevented by the use of ranitidine. Misoprostol and proton pump inhibitors are the only agents proven to help prevent the development of NSAID-induced ulcers. Also, concomitant disease and drug use contribute to the risk for GI adverse effects. Use lowest effective dose for shortest period possible. Consider renal function decline with age. Use of NSAIDs can compromise existing renal function especially when Cl_{cr} is ≤30 mL/minute. Tinnitus may be a difficult and unreliable indication of toxicity due to age-related hearing loss or eighth cranial nerve damage. CNS adverse effects such as confusion, agitation, and hallucination are generally seen in overdose or high dose situations, but elderly may demonstrate these adverse effects at lower doses than younger adults.

Dosage Forms Tablet: 500 mg, 750 mg

References

Brooks PM, Day RO, "Nonsteroidal Anti-inflammatory Drugs - Differences and Similarities," N Engl J Med, 1991, 324(24):1716-25.

Clinch D, Banerjee AK, Ostick G, "Absence of Abdominal Pain in Elderly Patients With Peptic Ulcer," Age Ageing, 1984, 13:120-3.

Clive DM, Stoff JS, "Renal Syndromes Associated With Nonsteroidal Anti-inflammatory Drugs," N Engl J Med, 1984, 310(9):563-72.

Graham DY, "Prevention of Gastroduodenal Injury Induced by Chronic Nonsteroidal Anti-inflammatory Drug Therapy," Gastroenterology, 1989, 96(2 Pt 2 Suppl):675-81.

Gurwitz JH, Avorn J, Ross-Degnan D, et al, "Nonsteroidal Anti-Inflammatory Drug-Associated Azotemia in the Very Old," JAMA, 1990, 264(4):471-5.

Hawkey CJ, Karrasch JA, Szczepaski L, et al, "Omeprazole Compared With Misoprostrol for Ulcers Associated With Nonsteroidal Anti-inflammatory Drugs," N Engl J Med, 1998, 338(11):727-34.

Knodel LC, "Preventing NSAID-Induced Ulcers: The Role of Misoprostol," Consult Pharm, 1989, 4:37-41.

Pounder R, "Silent Peptic Ulceration: Deadly Silence or Golden Silence?" Gastroenterology, 1989, 96:(2 Pt 2 Suppl)626-31.

Yeomans ND, Tulassay Z, Juhasz L, et al, "A Comparison of Omeprazole With Ranitidine for Ulcers Associated With Nonsteroidal Anti-inflammatory Drugs," N Engl J Med, 1998, 338(11):719-26.

N-Acetyl-P-Aminophenol see Acetaminophen on page 16

NaCl see Sodium Chloride on page 860

Nadolol (nay DOE lole)

Related Information
Beta-Blockers Comparison on page 1026

Brand Names Corgard®

Therapeutic Category Antianginal Agent; Beta-Adrenergic Blocker

Use Treatment of hypertension and angina pectoris

Unlabeled use: Prevention of myocardial infarction, prophylaxis of migraine headaches, ventricular arrhythmia treatment, essential tremor, lithium-induced tremor, Parkinson's tremor, aggressive behavior, antipsychotic-induced tremor, anxiety, esophageal varices bleeding, and increased intra-ocular pressure; diastolic congestive heart failure

Contraindications Uncompensated congestive heart failure, cardiogenic shock, bradycardia or heart block, bronchial asthma, bronchospasms, hypersensitivity to beta-blocking agents, diabetes mellitus

Warnings Abrupt withdrawal of beta-blockers may result in an exaggerated cardiac beta-adrenergic responsiveness. Symptomatology has included reports of tachycardia, hypertension, ischemia, angina, myocardial infarction, and sudden death. It is recommended that patients be tapered gradually off of beta-blockers over a 2-week period rather than via abrupt discontinuation.

Precautions Increase dosing interval in patients with renal dysfunction; administer with caution to patients with bronchospastic disease, diabetes mellitus, hyperthyroidism, myasthenia gravis, and renal function decline and severe peripheral vascular disease; abrupt withdrawal of the drug should be avoided, drug should be discontinued over 2 weeks

Adverse Reactions Other adverse effects similar to other beta-blockers

Cardiovascular: Persistent bradycardia, hypotension, chest pain, edema, heart failure, Raynaud's phenomena

Central nervous system: Depression, confusion, dizziness, fatigue, insomnia, lethargy, nightmares, headache

Gastrointestinal: Constipation, diarrhea, nausea

Genitourinary: Impotence

Miscellaneous: Cold extremities

Overdosage Symptoms of overdose include bronchospasm, bradycardia, heart failure, hypotension (see Toxicology)

Toxicology Sympathomimetics (eg, epinephrine or dopamine), glucagon, or a pacemaker can be used to treat the toxic bradycardia, asystole, and/or hypotension; initially fluids may be the best treatment for toxic hypotension; patients should remain supine; serum glucose and potassium should be measured; use supportive measures: lavage, syrup of ipecac. Nadolol may be removed by hemodialysis. I.V. glucose should be administered for hypoglycemia; seizures may be treated with phenytoin or diazepam intravenously; continuous monitoring of blood pressure and EKG is necessary. If PVCs occur, treat with lidocaine or phenytoin; avoid quinidine, procainamide, and disopyramide since these agents further depress myocardial function; bronchospasm can be treated with theophylline or beta$_2$ agonists (epinephrine).

Drug Interactions

Pharmacologic action of beta antagonists may be decreased by aluminum compounds, calcium salts, barbiturates, cholestyramine, colestipol, NSAIDs, penicillins (ampicillin), rifampin, salicylates, sulfinpyrazone, thyroid hormones; hypoglycemic effect of sulfonylureas may be blunted

Pharmacologic effect of beta antagonists may be enhanced with concomitant use of calcium channel blockers, oral contraceptives, flecainide (bioavailability and effect of flecainide also enhanced), haloperidol (hypotensive effects of both drugs), H$_2$ antagonists (decreased metabolism), hydralazine (both drugs hypotensive effects increased), loop diuretics (increased serum concentrations of beta-blockers except atenolol), MAO inhibitors, phenothiazines, propafenone, quinidine, quinolones, thioamines; beta-blockers may decrease clearance of acetaminophen; beta-blockers may increase anticoagulant effects of warfarin (propranolol); benzodiazepine effects enhanced by the lipophilic beta-blockers (atenolol does not interact); significant and fatal increases in blood pressure have occurred after decrease in dose or discontinuation of clonidine in patients receiving both clonidine and beta-blockers together (reduce doses of each cautiously with small decreases); peripheral ischemia of ergot alkaloids enhanced by beta-blockers; beta-blockers increase serum concentration of lidocaine; beta-blockers increase hypotensive effect of prazosin

Mechanism of Action Competitively blocks response to beta$_1$- and beta$_2$-adrenergic stimulation; does not exhibit any membrane stabilizing or intrinsic sympathomimetic activity; low lipid solubility, therefore, little penetration through blood-brain barrier

Pharmacodynamics Duration of effect: 24 hours

Pharmacokinetics

Absorption: Oral: 30% to 50%

Protein binding: 28%

Half-life: Adults: 20-24 hours; increased half-life with decreased renal function

Time to peak serum concentration: Oral: Within 2-4 hours and persist for 17-24 hours

Elimination: Renally eliminated unchanged. Since geriatric patients will have reduced renal function, correct for Cl$_{cr}$

Usual Dosage Oral:

Geriatrics: Initial: 20 mg/day; increase doses 20 mg/increase; usual dose range: 20-240 mg

Adults: Initial: 40 mg once daily; increase gradually; usual dosage: 40-80 mg/day; may need up to 240-320 mg/day; doses as high as 640 mg/day have been used

Dosing interval in renal impairment:

Cl$_{cr}$ >50 mL/minute: Administer every 24 hours

Cl$_{cr}$ 31-50 mL/minute: Administer every 24-36 hours

Cl$_{cr}$ 10-30 mL/minute: Administer every 24-48 hours

Cl$_{cr}$ <10 mL/minute: Administer every 40-60 hours

Moderately dialyzable (20% to 50%)

Monitoring Parameters Blood pressure, orthostatic hypotension, heart rate, CNS effects

(Continued)

Nadolol *(Continued)*

Test Interactions Increased cholesterol (S), glucose, triglycerides, potassium, uric acid; decreased HDL

Patient Information Do not discontinue medication abruptly, sudden stopping of medication may precipitate or cause angina; consult pharmacist or physician before taking with other adrenergic drugs (eg, cold medications); notify physician if any of the following symptoms occur: difficult breathing, night cough, swelling of extremities, slow pulse, dizziness, lightheadedness, confusion, depression, skin rash, fever, sore throat, unusual bleeding or bruising; may produce drowsiness, blurred vision; use with caution while driving or performing tasks requiring alertness; may mask signs of hypoglycemia in diabetics; may be taken without regard to meals

Nursing Implications Advise against abrupt withdrawal; monitor orthostatic blood pressures, apical and peripheral pulse and mental status changes (ie, confusion, depression)

Special Geriatric Considerations Due to alterations in the beta-adrenergic autonomic nervous system, beta-adrenergic blockade may result in less hemodynamic response than seen in younger adults. Studies indicate that despite decreased sensitivity to the chronotropic effects of beta blockade with age, there appears to be an increased myocardial sensitivity to the negative inotropic effect during stress (ie, exercise). Controlled trials have shown the overall response rate for propranolol to be only 20% to 50% in elderly populations. Therefore, all beta-adrenergic blocking drugs may result in a decreased response as compared to younger adults. Must adjust dose for renal function (see Precautions and Usual Dosage).

Dosage Forms Tablet: 20 mg, 40 mg, 80 mg, 120 mg, 160 mg

References

Aagaard GN, "Treatment of Hypertension in The Elderly," *Drug Treatment in the Elderly*, Vestal RE, ed, Boston, MA: ADIS Health Science Press, 1984, 77.

Nafazair® Ophthalmic *see Naphazoline on page 653*

Nafcil™ Injection *see Nafcillin on this page*

Nafcillin *(naf SIL in)*

Related Information

I.V. Medication Recommendations *on page 1080*
Penicillins, Penicillin-Related Antibiotics, & Other Antibiotics *on page 1010*

Brand Names Nafcil™ Injection; Nallpen® Injection; Unipen® Injection; Unipen® Oral

Synonyms Ethoxynaphthamido Penicillin Sodium; Sodium Nafcillin

Generic Available Yes

Therapeutic Category Antibiotic, Penicillin

Use Treatment of susceptible bacterial infections such as osteomyelitis, cellulitis, septicemia, endocarditis, and CNS infections due to penicillinase-producing strains of *Staphylococcus*

Contraindications Hypersensitivity to nafcillin or any component or penicillins

Precautions Extravasation of I.V. infusions should be avoided; modification of dosage is necessary in patients with both severe renal and hepatic impairment; patients with a cephalosporin allergy (anaphylaxis)

Adverse Reactions

Central nervous system: Fever
Dermatologic: Skin rash
Gastrointestinal: Nausea, diarrhea
Hematologic: Neutropenia
Local: Pain, thrombophlebitis
Renal: Rare acute interstitial nephritis
Miscellaneous: Hypersensitivity reactions

Overdosage Symptoms of overdose include neuromuscular hypersensitivity, seizure

Toxicology Many beta-lactam-containing antibiotics have the potential to cause neuromuscular hyperirritability or convulsive seizures. Hemodialysis may be helpful to aid in the removal of the drug from the blood, otherwise most treatment is supportive or symptom directed.

Drug Interactions

Decreased effect of warfarin possible
Increased risk of bleeding with heparin, increased effect with probenecid

Stability Refrigerate oral suspension after reconstitution; discard after 7 days; reconstituted parenteral solution is stable for 3 days at room temperature and 7 days when refrigerated or 12 weeks when frozen; for I.V. infusion in NS or

D$_5$W, solution is stable for 24 hours at room temperature and 96 hours when refrigerated

Mechanism of Action Interferes with bacterial cell wall synthesis during active multiplication causing cell death and resultant bactericidal activity against susceptible bacteria

Pharmacokinetics
Absorption: Oral: Poor and erratic
Protein binding: 90%
Half-life: Adults with normal renal and hepatic function: 0.5-1.5 hours
Time to peak serum concentration:
   Oral: Within 2 hours
   I.M.: 30-60 minutes
Elimination: Primarily in bile, and 10% to 30% in urine as unchanged drug; undergoes enterohepatic recycling

Usual Dosage Geriatrics and Adults:
Oral: 250-500 mg every 4-6 hours, up to 1 g every 4-6 hours for more severe infections
I.M.: 500 mg every 4-6 hours
I.V.: 500 mg to 2 g every 4-6 hours
Dosing interval in renal impairment: No change necessary
Not dialyzable (0% to 5%)

Administration Administer around-the-clock rather than 4 times/day, 3 times/day, etc (ie, 12-6-12-6, not 9-1-5-9) to promote less variation in peak and trough serum concentrations; burning on I.V. administration may be decreased by further diluting the preparation to 250 mL NS or D$_5$W

Monitoring Parameters Watch for signs or symptoms of fluid overload or retention in patients with congestive heart failure; pain/burning with administration

Test Interactions False-positive urinary and serum proteins

Patient Information Report any diarrhea that develops within 2 weeks of completion of therapy to your physician or pharmacist; complete full course of therapy

Nursing Implications See Administration

Additional Information Due to its poor oral absorption, patients switched from I.V. to oral treatment should be given a more suitable oral alternative such as dicloxacillin or cloxacillin

Sodium content of 1 g: 66.7 mg (2.9 mEq)

Special Geriatric Considerations Nafcillin has not been studied exclusively in the elderly, however, given its route of elimination, dosage adjustments based upon age and renal function is not necessary

Dosage Forms
Nafcillin sodium:
   Capsule: 250 mg
   Powder for injection: 500 mg, 1 g, 2 g, 4 g, 10 g
   Solution: 250 mg/5 mL (100 mL)
   Tablet: 500 mg

Naftifine (NAF ti feen)

Brand Names Naftin®
Synonyms Naftifine Hydrochloride
Generic Available No
Therapeutic Category Antifungal Agent, Topical
Use Topical treatment of tinea cruris (jock itch), tinea corporis (ring worm), and tinea pedis (athlete's foot)
Contraindications Hypersensitivity to any component
Warnings For external use only
Adverse Reactions
Dermatologic: Dryness, erythema, itching
Local: Irritation, burning, stinging
Mechanism of Action Synthetic, broad-spectrum antifungal agent in the allylamine class; topical antifungals totally unrelated to the imidazole compounds. As with all allylamine derivatives, most active when the allylamine double bond has the transorientation; the corresponding cis-isomer is much less active. The drug appears to have both fungistatic and fungicidal activity with no systemic adverse effects. Exhibits antifungal activity by selectively inhibiting the enzyme squalene epoxidase in a dose-dependent manner. As a result of this inhibitor, the primary sterol, ergosterol, within the fungal membrane is not synthesized.
(Continued)

Naftifine (Continued)

Pharmacokinetics
Absorption: Systemic, 6% for cream, ≤4% for gel
Half-life: 2-3 days
Elimination: Metabolites excreted in urine and feces

Usual Dosage Geriatrics and Adults: Topical: Apply twice daily

Patient Information External use only; avoid eyes, mouth, and other mucous membranes; do not use occlusive dressings unless directed to do so; discontinue if irritation or sensitivity develops; wash hands after application

Nursing Implications See Patient Information

Special Geriatric Considerations No specific recommendations for use in the elderly

Dosage Forms
Cream, as hydrochloride: 1% (15 g, 30 g, 60 g)
Gel, topical, as hydrochloride: 1% (20 g, 40 g, 60 g)

Naftifine Hydrochloride see Naftifine on previous page

Naftin® see Naftifine on previous page

NaHCO₃ see Sodium Bicarbonate on page 858

Nalbuphine (NAL byoo feen)

Related Information
I.V. Push Recommended Guidelines on page 1083
Pharmacokinetics of Narcotic Agonist Analgesics on page 1037

Brand Names Nubain®

Generic Available Yes

Therapeutic Category Analgesic, Narcotic

Use Relief of moderate to severe pain

Contraindications Hypersensitivity to nalbuphine or any component

Precautions Use with caution in patients with drug dependence (may experience withdrawal symptoms), head trauma or increased intracranial pressure, decreased hepatic or renal function; use with caution in patients with recent myocardial infarction, biliary tract surgery, or sulfite sensitivity; may produce respiratory depression

Adverse Reactions
Cardiovascular: Hypotension, flushing
Central nervous system: CNS depression, dizziness, hallucinations
Dermatologic: Urticaria
Gastrointestinal: Nausea, vomiting, anorexia, xerostomia
Respiratory: Pulmonary edema, respiratory depression

Overdosage Symptoms of overdose include CNS depression, respiratory depression, miosis, hypotension, bradycardia

Toxicology Treatment of an overdose includes support of the patient's airway, establishment of an I.V. line and administration of naloxone 2 mg I.V. with repeat administration as necessary up to a total of 10 mg

Drug Interactions Increased toxicity: Barbiturates, anesthetics

Mechanism of Action Binds to opiate receptors in the CNS, causing inhibition of ascending pain pathways, altering the perception of and response to pain; produces generalized CNS depression

Pharmacodynamics
Peak effect and serum concentrations:
I.M.: Within 30 minutes
I.V.: Within 1-3 minutes

Pharmacokinetics
Metabolism: In the liver
Half-life: 3.5-5 hours
Elimination: Metabolites excreted primarily in feces (via bile) and in urine (~7%)

Usual Dosage Geriatrics and Adults: I.M., I.V., S.C.: 10 mg/70 kg every 3-6 hours

Monitoring Parameters Relief of pain, respiratory and mental status, blood pressure

Patient Information May cause drowsiness; avoid CNS depressants and alcohol

Nursing Implications Observe patient for excessive sedation, respiratory depression, signs of narcotic withdrawal

Special Geriatric Considerations The elderly may be particularly susceptible to CNS effects; monitor closely (see Precautions)

Dosage Forms Injection, as hydrochloride: 10 mg/mL (1 mL, 10 mL); 20 mg/mL (1 mL, 10 mL)

Naldecon® Senior DX [OTC] *see* Guaifenesin and Dextromethorphan *on page 439*

Naldecon® Senior EX [OTC] *see* Guaifenesin *on page 437*

Nalfon® *see* Fenoprofen *on page 372*

Nalidixic Acid (nal i DIKS ik AS id)
Related Information
   Antacid Drug Interactions *on page 1096*
Brand Names NegGram®
Synonyms Nalidixinic Acid
Generic Available Yes
Therapeutic Category Antibiotic, Quinolone
Use Urinary tract infections
Contraindications History of convulsive disorders, hypersensitivity to nalidixic acid or any component
Warnings Has been shown to cause cartilage degeneration in immature animals
Precautions Usefulness may be limited by the emergence of bacterial resistance; use with caution in patients with impaired hepatic or renal function
Adverse Reactions
   Central nervous system: Malaise, drowsiness, vertigo, confusion, toxic psychosis, convulsions, fever, headache, increased intracranial pressure, dizziness, chills
   Dermatologic: Rash, urticaria, photosensitivity
   Endocrine & metabolic: Metabolic acidosis
   Gastrointestinal: Nausea, vomiting
   Hematologic: Leukopenia, thrombocytopenia
   Hepatic: Hepatotoxicity
   Ocular: Visual disturbances
Overdosage Symptoms of overdose include nausea, vomiting, toxic psychosis, convulsions, increased intracranial pressure, metabolic acidosis
Drug Interactions Warfarin (increased anticoagulant effect due to displacement from albumin binding sites), antacids (decreased nalidixic acid absorption)
Mechanism of Action Inhibits DNA polymerization in late stages of chromosomal replication
Pharmacokinetics Achieves significant antibacterial concentrations only in the urinary tract
   Protein binding: 90%.
   Metabolism: Partially in the liver
   Half-life: 6-7 hours (increases significantly with renal impairment)
   Time to peak serum concentration: Oral: Within 1-2 hours
   Elimination: In urine as unchanged drug and 80% as metabolites; small amounts appear in feces
   In one study, nalidixic acid's half-life (11.5 hours) and V_d (.55 L/kg) were significantly greater and its total body clearance significantly decreased (2.9 L/hour) in older volunteers compared to younger volunteers, 2.7 hours, 0.47 L/kg, and 8.3 L/hour, respectively
Usual Dosage Geriatrics and Adults: Oral: 1 g 4 times/day for 2 weeks; then suppressive therapy of 500 mg 4 times/day

   Dosing comments in renal impairment: Cl_{cr} <50 mL/minute: Avoid use
Administration Administer around-the-clock rather than 4 times/day, 3 times/day, etc (ie, 12-6-12-6, not 9-1-5-9) to promote less variation in peak and trough serum concentrations
Monitoring Parameters Signs and symptoms of infection
Test Interactions False-positive urine glucose with Clinitest®, false increase in urinary VMA
Patient Information Avoid undue exposure to direct sunlight; take 1 hour before meals; complete full course of therapy
Nursing Implications See Administration
Special Geriatric Considerations Calculate an estimated creatinine clearance to determine if use is appropriate (see Pharmacokinetics, Precautions, and Usual Dosage)
Dosage Forms
   Suspension, oral: 250 mg/5 mL (473 mL)
   Tablet: 250 mg, 500 mg, 1 g
   (Continued)

Nalidixic Acid *(Continued)*

References
Barbeau G, Belanger PM, "Pharmacokinetics of Nalidixic Acid in Old and Young Volunteers," *J Clin Pharmacol*, 1982, 22(10):490-6.

Nalidixinic Acid *see Nalidixic Acid on previous page*

Nallpen® Injection *see Nafcillin on page 648*

N-allylnoroxymorphine Hydrochloride *see Naloxone on this page*

Naloxone (nal OKS one)

Related Information
Antidotes *on page 1097*
I.V. Push Recommended Guidelines *on page 1083*

Brand Names Narcan® Injection

Synonyms N-allylnoroxymorphine Hydrochloride

Generic Available Yes

Therapeutic Category Antidote for Narcotic Agonists

Use Reverses CNS and respiratory depression in suspected narcotic overdose; coma of unknown etiology; used investigationally for shock, PCP and alcohol ingestion, and Alzheimer's disease

Contraindications Hypersensitivity to naloxone or any component

Warnings May precipitate withdrawal symptoms in patients addicted to opiates, including hypertension, sweating, agitation, irritability

Precautions Use with caution in patients with cardiovascular disease; excessive dosages should be avoided after use of opiates in surgery, because naloxone may cause an increase in blood pressure and reversal of anesthesia

Adverse Reactions
Cardiovascular: Hypertension, hypotension, tachycardia, ventricular arrhythmias, cardiac arrest
Central nervous system: Insomnia, irritability, anxiety
Dermatologic: Rash
Gastrointestinal: Nausea, vomiting
Miscellaneous: Diaphoresis

Overdosage Symptoms of overdose include excitation, hypotension, hypertension, pulmonary edema, arrhythmias

Toxicology Naloxone is the drug of choice for respiratory depression that is known or suspected to be caused by an overdose of an opiate or opioid. **Caution:** Naloxone's effects are due to its action on narcotic reversal, not due to any direct effect upon opiate receptors. Therefore, adverse events occur secondarily to reversal (withdrawal) of narcotic analgesia and sedation, which can cause severe reactions.

Drug Interactions Decreased effect of narcotic analgesics

Stability Protect from light; stable in 0.9% NaCl and D_5W at 4 mcg/mL for 24 hours; do not mix with alkaline solutions

Mechanism of Action Competes and displaces narcotics at narcotic receptor sites

Pharmacodynamics
Onset of action:
I.V.: Within 2 minutes
S.C., I.M., E.T.: Within 2-5 minutes
Duration of effect: 20-60 minutes; shorter than that of most opioids, therefore, repeated doses are usually needed

Pharmacokinetics
Metabolism: Primarily by glucuronidation in the liver
Half-life: 1-1.5 hours
Elimination: In urine as metabolites

Usual Dosage Continuous infusion: I.V.: If continuous infusion is required, calculate dosage/hour based on effective intermittent dose used and duration of adequate response seen, titrate dose

Geriatrics and Adults: Postoperative narcotic depression (partial reversal): I.V.: 0.1-0.2 mg at 2- to 3-minute intervals to desired degree of reversal; may require repeat doses within 1 or 2 hours

Monitoring Parameters Blood pressure, pulse, mental status

Nursing Implications Monitor patients for signs of narcotic reversal; too rapid a reversal of narcotic depression may result in nausea, vomiting, sweating, tachycardia, increased blood pressure, and tremulousness

Additional Information In Talwin® Nx to prevent abuse of tablets via parenteral administration

Special Geriatric Considerations In small trials, naloxone has shown temporary improvement in Alzheimer's disease; however, is not recommended for treatment

Dosage Forms

Naloxone hydrochloride:
Injection: 0.4 mg/mL (1 mL, 2 mL, 10 mL); 1 mg/mL (2 mL, 10 mL)
Injection, neonatal: 0.02 mg/mL (2 mL)

References

Waters C, "Cognitive Enhancing Agents: Current Status in the Treatment of Alzheimer's Disease," *Can J Neurol Sci*, 1988, 15(3):249-56.

Naphazoline (naf AZ oh leen)

Brand Names AK-Con® Ophthalmic; Albalon® Liquifilm® Ophthalmic; Allerest® Eye Drops [OTC]; Clear Eyes® [OTC]; Comfort® Ophthalmic [OTC]; Degest® 2 Ophthalmic [OTC]; Estivin® II Ophthalmic [OTC]; I-Naphline® Ophthalmic; Nafazair® Ophthalmic; Naphcon Forte® Ophthalmic; Naphcon® Ophthalmic [OTC]; Opcon® Ophthalmic; Privine® Nasal [OTC]; VasoClear® Ophthalmic [OTC]; Vasocon Regular® Ophthalmic

Generic Available Yes

Therapeutic Category Adrenergic Agonist Agent, Ophthalmic; Decongestant, Nasal; Nasal Agent, Vasoconstrictor; Ophthalmic Agent, Vasoconstrictor; Vasoconstrictor, Nasal; Vasoconstrictor, Ophthalmic

Use Topical ocular vasoconstrictor; will temporarily relieve congestion, itching, and minor irritation, and to control hyperemia in patients with superficial corneal vascularity

Contraindications Hypersensitivity to naphazoline or any component, narrow-angle glaucoma, prior to peripheral iridectomy (in patients susceptible to angle block)

Precautions Rebound congestion may occur with extended use; use with caution in the presence of hypertension, diabetes, hyperthyroidism, heart disease, coronary artery disease, cerebral arteriosclerosis, or long-standing bronchial asthma

Adverse Reactions

Cardiovascular: Systemic cardiovascular stimulation, hypertension
Central nervous system: Nervousness, dizziness, headache
Gastrointestinal: Nausea
Neuromuscular & skeletal: Weakness
Ocular: Pupillary dilation, increase in intraocular pressure, mydriasis, blurring of vision, transient stinging
Respiratory: Nasal mucosa irritation, dryness, sneezing, rebound congestion
Miscellaneous: Diaphoresis

Overdosage Symptoms of overdose include CNS depression, hypothermia, bradycardia, cardiovascular collapse, coma

Toxicology Following initiation of essential overdose management, toxic symptoms should be treated. The patient should be kept warm and monitored for alterations in vital functions. Seizures commonly respond to diazepam (5-10 mg I.V. bolus every 15 minutes if needed up to a total of 30 mg) or to phenytoin or phenobarbital.

Drug Interactions Anesthetics (discontinue mydriatic prior to use of anesthetics that sensitize the myocardium to sympathomimetics, ie, cyclopropane, halothane), MAO inhibitors, tricyclic antidepressants may cause hypertensive reactions

Stability Store in tight, light-resistant containers

Mechanism of Action Stimulates alpha-adrenergic receptors in the arterioles of the conjunctiva and the nasal mucosa to produce vasoconstriction

Pharmacodynamics

Onset of action: Following topical administration, decongestion occurs within 10 minutes
Duration: 2-6 hours

Pharmacokinetics Elimination is not well defined

Usual Dosage Geriatrics and Adults:

Nasal: 2 drops or sprays in each nostril no more than every 3 hours (drops) or 4-6 hours (spray) as needed
Ophthalmic (0.01% to 0.1%): Instill 1-2 drops into conjunctival sac of affected eye(s) every 3-4 hours; therapy generally should not exceed 3-4 days

Monitoring Parameters Blood pressure in hypertensives

Patient Information Do not use discolored solutions; discontinue eye drops if visual changes or ocular pain occur; do not use nasal products for >3 days without physician's consent

(Continued)

Naphazoline *(Continued)*

Nursing Implications Rebound congestion can result with continued use beyond 3 days

Special Geriatric Considerations Evaluate patient's ability to self-administer; use cautiously in patients with cardiovascular disease

Dosage Forms

Naphazoline hydrochloride: Solution:
Nasal:
Drops: 0.05% (20 mL)
Spray: 0.05% (15 mL)
Ophthalmic: 0.012% (7.5 mL, 30 mL); 0.02% (15 mL); 0.03% (15 mL); 0.1% (15 mL)

Naphazoline and Antazoline (naf AZ oh leen & an TAZ oh leen)

Related Information

Naphazoline *on previous page*

Brand Names Albalon-A® Ophthalmic; Antazoline-V® Ophthalmic; Vasocon-A® [OTC] Ophthalmic

Therapeutic Category Ophthalmic Agent, Vasoconstrictor

Use Topical ocular congestion, irritation and itching

Contraindications Narrow-angle glaucoma, known hypersensitivity to naphazoline or antazoline

Precautions Use with caution in patients with hypothyroidism, heart disease, hypertension or diabetes mellitus

Adverse Reactions

Cardiovascular: Systemic cardiovascular stimulation, hypertension
Central nervous system: Nervousness, dizziness, headache
Gastrointestinal: Nausea
Neuromuscular & skeletal: Weakness
Ocular: Pupillary dilation, increase in intraocular pressure, mydriasis, blurring of vision, transient stinging
Respiratory: nasal mucosa irritation, dryness, sneezing, rebound congestion
Miscellaneous: Diaphoresis

Overdosage Symptoms of overdose include drowsiness, decreased body temperature, bradycardia, short-life hypotension, coma

Toxicology Following initiation of essential overdose management, toxic symptoms should be treated. The patient should be kept warm and monitored for alterations in vital functions. Seizures commonly respond to diazepam (5-10 mg I.V. bolus) every 15 minutes if needed up to a total of 30 mg or to phenytoin or phenobarbital.

Drug Interactions MAO inhibitors

Stability Store in tight, light-resistant containers

Usual Dosage Geriatrics and Adults: Ophthalmic: Instill 1-2 drops every 3-4 hours

Patient Information Discontinue drug and consult physician if ocular pain or visual changes occur, ocular redness or irritation, or condition worsens or persists for more than 72 hours

Nursing Implications Do not use discolored solutions

Special Geriatric Considerations Evaluate patient's ability to self-administer; use with caution in patients with cardiovascular disease

Dosage Forms Solution, ophthalmic: Naphazoline hydrochloride 0.05% and antazoline phosphate 0.5% (15 mL)

Naphazoline and Pheniramine

(naf AZ oh leen & fen NIR a meen)

Related Information

Naphazoline *on previous page*

Brand Names Naphcon-A® Ophthalmic [OTC]

Synonyms Pheniramine and Naphazoline

Therapeutic Category Ophthalmic Agent, Vasoconstrictor

Use Topical ocular vasoconstrictor

Contraindications Hypersensitivity to naphazoline, pheniramine or any component

Warnings Topical antihistamines are potential sensitizers and may produce local sensitivity reactions; because they may produce angle closure, use with caution in persons with a narrow angle or history of glaucoma; use with caution in patients with hypothyroidism, heart disease, hypertension or diabetes mellitus; rebound congestion may occur with extended use

Adverse Reactions

Cardiovascular: Systemic cardiovascular stimulation, hypertension

Central nervous system: Nervousness, dizziness, headache

Gastrointestinal: Nausea

Neuromuscular & skeletal: Weakness

Ocular: Pupillary dilation, increase in intraocular pressure, mydriasis, blurring of vision, transient stinging

Respiratory: Nasal mucosa irritation, dryness, sneezing, rebound congestion

Miscellaneous: Diaphoresis

Drug Interactions MAO inhibitors

Usual Dosage Geriatrics and Adults: Ophthalmic: Instill 1-2 drops every 3-4 hours

Patient Information Discontinue drug and consult physician if ocular pain or visual changes occur, ocular redness or irritation, or condition worsens or persists more than 72 hours

Special Geriatric Considerations Evaluate patient's ability to self-administer; use cautiously in patients with cardiovascular disease

Dosage Forms Solution, ophthalmic: Naphazoline hydrochloride 0.025% and pheniramine 0.3% (15 mL)

Naphcon-A® Ophthalmic [OTC] *see* Naphazoline and Pheniramine *on previous page*

Naphcon Forte® Ophthalmic *see* Naphazoline *on page 653*

Naphcon® Ophthalmic [OTC] *see* Naphazoline *on page 653*

Naprelan® *see* Naproxen *on this page*

Naprosyn® *see* Naproxen *on this page*

Naproxen (na PROKS en)

Related Information

Antacid Drug Interactions *on page 1096*

Brand Names Aleve® [OTC]; Anaprox®; Naprelan®; Naprosyn®

Generic Available No

Therapeutic Category Analgesic, Non-narcotic; Anti-inflammatory Agent; Antipyretic; Nonsteroidal Anti-inflammatory Agent (NSAID), Oral

Use Management of inflammatory disease and rheumatoid disorders, osteoarthritis; ankylosing spondylitis, tendonitis, bursitis, acute gout; mild to moderate pain; dysmenorrhea; fever, sunburn, migraine headache (acute, prophylaxis)

Contraindications Hypersensitivity to naproxen, aspirin, or other nonsteroidal anti-inflammatory drugs (NSAIDs)

Warnings GI toxicity (bleeding, ulceration, perforation); CNS effects may occur (headaches, confusion, depression); hypersensitivity, anaphylactoid reactions (intermittent tolmetin use more often); renal function decline, acute renal insufficiency, interstitial nephritis, dysuria, cystitis, hematuria, nephrotic syndrome, hyperkalemia in acute renal insufficiency, hyponatremia, papillary necrosis, hepatic function impairment; elderly have increased risk for adverse reactions to NSAIDs (see Special Geriatric Considerations)

Precautions Use with caution in patients with congestive heart failure, hypertension, decreased renal or hepatic function, history of GI disease (bleeding or ulcers), or those receiving anticoagulants; perform ophthalmologic evaluation for those who develop eye complaints during therapy (blurred vision, diminished vision, changes in color vision, retinal changes); NSAIDs may mask signs/symptoms of infections; photosensitivity reported

Adverse Reactions

Cardiovascular: Congestive heart failure, angina, hypertension, hypotension, arrhythmias, edema

Central nervous system: Headache, drowsiness, vertigo, dizziness, fatigue, hallucinations, confusion, depression, emotional lability, psychotic behavior, pyrexia

Dermatologic: Rash, urticaria, angioedema, Stevens-Johnson syndrome, exfoliative dermatitis, bruising, petechiae, purpura

Endocrine & metabolic: Hyperglycemia, hypoglycemia, hyperkalemia, gynecomastia, hyponatremia, fluid retention

Gastrointestinal: Dyspepsia, heartburn, nausea, diarrhea, constipation, flatulence, stomatitis, vomiting, abdominal pain, peptic ulcer, GI bleeding, GI perforation, gingival ulcers, pancreatitis, proctitis, paralytic ulcers, colitis, anorexia, weight loss, dry mucous membranes

Genitourinary: Impotence, azotemia

Hematologic: Neutropenia, anemia, agranulocytosis, bone marrow suppression, hemolytic anemia, hemorrhage, inhibition of platelet aggregation

Hepatic: Hepatitis, elevated LFTs, cholestatic jaundice

(Continued)

Naproxen *(Continued)*

Neuromuscular & skeletal: Involuntary muscle movements, muscle weakness, tremors, weakness
Ocular: Vision changes
Otic: Tinnitus
Renal: Dysuria, polyuria, pyuria, oliguria, anuria, acute renal failure
Respiratory: Exacerbation of asthma, dyspnea
Miscellaneous: Thirst, diaphoresis

Overdosage Symptoms include drowsiness, lethargy, disorientation, confusion, dizziness, numbness, paresthesia, nausea, vomiting, gastric irritation, abdominal pain, headache, tinnitus, sweating, blurred vision, muscle twitching, seizures, coma, acute renal failure, increased BUN and serum creatinine, hypotension, tachycardia, and metabolic acidosis

Toxicology Management of a nonsteroidal anti-inflammatory agent (NSAID) intoxication is primarily supportive and symptomatic. Fluid therapy is commonly effective in managing the hypotension that may occur following an acute NSAID overdose, except when this is due to an acute blood loss. Seizures tend to be very short-lived and often do not require drug treatment although recurrent seizures should be treated with I.V. diazepam. Since many of the NSAIDs undergo enterohepatic cycling, multiple doses of charcoal may be needed to reduce the potential for delayed toxicities.

Drug Interactions
May increase digoxin, methotrexate, and lithium serum concentrations
Aspirin or other salicylates may decrease NSAID serum concentrations
Other NSAIDs may increase adverse GI effects
Increased prothrombin time with anticoagulants
Decreased antihypertensive effects of ACE inhibitors, beta-blockers, and thiazide diuretics
Effects of loop diuretics may decrease
Increased response to sympathomimetics
Probenecid may increase toxicity of NSAIDs by increase in serum concentrations
Diuretics may increase risk of acute renal insufficiency
May enhance azotemia in elderly receiving loop diuretics

Mechanism of Action Inhibits prostaglandin synthesis, acts on the hypothalamus heat-regulating center to reduce fever, blocks prostaglandin synthetase action which prevents formation of the platelet-aggregating substance thromboxane A_2; decreases pain receptor sensitivity. Other proposed mechanisms of action for salicylate anti-inflammatory action are lysosomal stabilization, inhibition of kinin and leukotriene production, alteration of chemotactic factors, and inhibition of neutrophil activation. This latter mechanism may be the most significant pharmacologic action to reduce inflammation.

Pharmacodynamics
Analgesia:
Onset of action: 1 hour
Duration: Up to 7 hours
Anti-inflammatory:
Onset of action: Within 2 weeks
Peak: 2-4 weeks

Pharmacokinetics
Absorption: Oral: Almost 100%
Metabolism: Substrate CYP2C9, 2C18
Protein binding: High (>90%); increased free fraction in the elderly
Half-life: 12-15 hours
Time to peak serum concentration: Within 1-2 hours for sodium salt and 2-4 hours for plain naproxen

Usual Dosage Geriatrics and Adults: Oral (as naproxen):
Rheumatoid arthritis, osteoarthritis, and ankylosing spondylitis: 500-1000 mg/day in 2 divided doses; maximum, plain: 1500 mg; maximum, sodium salt: 1375 mg
Mild to moderate pain: Initial: 500 mg, then 250 mg every 6-8 hours; maximum: 1250 mg/day; Aleve®: 220 mg every 8 hours

Monitoring Parameters Monitor response (pain, range of motion, grip strength, mobility, ADL function), inflammation; observe for weight gain, edema; monitor renal function (serum creatinine, BUN); observe for bleeding, bruising; evaluate gastrointestinal effects (abdominal pain, bleeding, dyspepsia); mental confusion, disorientation, CBC, liver function tests

Test Interactions Increased chloride (S), increased sodium (S)

Patient Information Serious gastrointestinal bleeding can occur as well as ulceration and perforation. Pain may or may not be present. Avoid aspirin and aspirin-containing products while taking this medication. If gastric upset occurs, take with food, milk, or antacid. If gastric adverse effects persist, contact physician. May cause drowsiness, dizziness, blurred vision, and confusion. Use caution when performing tasks which require alertness (eg, driving). Do not take for more than 3 days for fever or 10 days for pain without physician's advice.

Nursing Implications Administer with food, milk, or antacids to decrease GI adverse effects; monitor for occult blood loss, periodic ophthalmologic exams

Additional Information There are no clinical guidelines to predict which NSAID will give response in a particular patient. Trials with each must be initiated until response determined. Consider dose, patient convenience, and cost.

Special Geriatric Considerations Elderly are a high-risk population for adverse effects from nonsteroidal anti-inflammatory agents. As much as 60% of elderly can develop peptic ulceration and/or hemorrhage asymptomatically. The concomitant use of H_2 blockers, omeprazole, and sucralfate is not effective as prophylaxis with the exception of NSAID-induced duodenal ulcers which may be prevented by the use of ranitidine. Misoprostol and proton pump inhibitors are the only agents proven to help prevent the development of NSAID-induced ulcers. Also, concomitant disease and drug use contribute to the risk for GI adverse effects. Use lowest effective dose for shortest period possible. Consider renal function decline with age. Use of NSAIDs can compromise existing renal function especially when Cl_{cr} is ≤30 mL/minute. Tinnitus may be a difficult and unreliable indication of toxicity due to age-related hearing loss or eighth cranial nerve damage. CNS adverse effects such as confusion, agitation, and hallucination are generally seen in overdose or high-dose situations, but elderly may demonstrate these adverse effects at lower doses than younger adults.

Dosage Forms
Suspension, oral: 125 mg/5 mL (15 mL, 30 mL, 480 mL)
Tablet (Naprosyn®): 250 mg, 375 mg, 500 mg
Tablet, controlled release (Naprelan®): 375 mg, 500 mg
Tablet, as sodium:
Anaprox®: 220 mg (200 mg base); 275 mg (250 mg base); 550 mg (500 mg base)
Aleve®: 200 mg

References

Brooks PM, Day RO, "Nonsteroidal Anti-inflammatory Drugs - Differences and Similarities," *N Engl J Med*, 1991, 324(24):1716-25.

Clinch D, Banerjee AK, Ostick G, "Absence of Abdominal Pain in Elderly Patients With Peptic Ulcer," *Age Ageing*, 1984, 13:120-3.

Clive DM, Stoff JS, "Renal Syndromes Associated With Nonsteroidal Anti-inflammatory Drugs," *N Engl J Med*, 1984, 310(9):563-72.

Graham DY, "Prevention of Gastroduodenal Injury Induced by Chronic Nonsteroidal Anti-inflammatory Drug Therapy," *Gastroenterology*, 1989, 96(2 Pt 2 Suppl):675-81.

Gurwitz JH, Avorn J, Ross-Degnan D, et al, "Nonsteroidal Anti-Inflammatory Drug-Associated Azotemia in the Very Old," *JAMA*, 1990, 264(4):471-5.

Hawkey CJ, Karrasch JA, Szczepaski L, et al, "Omeprazole Compared With Misoprostrol for Ulcers Associated With Nonsteroidal Anti-inflammatory Drugs," *N Engl J Med*, 1998, 338(11):727-34.

Knodel LC, "Preventing NSAID-Induced Ulcers: The Role of Misoprostol," *Consult Pharm*, 1989, 4:37-41.

Pounder R, "Silent Peptic Ulceration: Deadly Silence or Golden Silence?" *Gastroenterology*, 1989, 96:(2 Pt 2 Suppl)626-31.

Yeomans ND, Tulassay Z, Juhasz L, et al, "A Comparison of Omeprazole With Ranitidine for Ulcers Associated With Nonsteroidal Anti-inflammatory Drugs," *N Engl J Med*, 1998, 338(11):719-26.

Narcan® Injection *see Naloxone on page 652*

Narcotic Agonist Comparative Pharmacology *see page 1036*

Nardil® *see Phenelzine on page 735*

Nasacort® *see Triamcinolone on page 949*

Nasacort® AQ *see Triamcinolone on page 949*

Nasahist B® *see Brompheniramine on page 129*

NāSal™ [OTC] *see Sodium Chloride on page 860*

Nasalcrom® Nasal Solution [OTC] *see Cromolyn Sodium on page 255*

Nasalide® Nasal Aerosol *see Flunisolide on page 390*

Nasal Moist® [OTC] *see Sodium Chloride on page 860*

Nasarel® Nasal Spray *see Flunisolide on page 390*

Natacyn® *see Natamycin on next page*

Natamycin (na ta MYE sin)
Brand Names Natacyn®
Synonyms Pimaricin
Therapeutic Category Antifungal Agent, Ophthalmic
Use Treatment of blepharitis, conjunctivitis, and keratitis caused by susceptible fungi (*Aspergillus, Candida*), *Cephalosporium, Curvularia, Fusarium, Penicillium, Microsporum, Epidermophyton, Blastomyces dermatitidis, Coccidioides immitis, Cryptococcus neoformans, Histoplasma capsulatum, Sporothrix schenckii,* and *Trichomonas vaginalis*
Contraindications Known hypersensitivity to natamycin or any component
Warnings Failure to improve (keratitis) after 7-10 days of administration suggests infection caused by a microorganism not susceptible to natamycin; inadequate as a single agent in fungal endophthalmitis
Precautions If toxicity to natamycin is suspected, discontinue the drug
Adverse Reactions
Ocular: Blurred vision, photophobia, eye pain, eye irritation not present before therapy
Drug Interactions Increased toxicity: Topical corticosteroids (concomitant use contraindicated)
Stability Store at room temperature (8°C to 24°C/46°F to 75°F); protect from excessive heat and light; do not freeze
Mechanism of Action Increases cell membrane permeability in susceptible fungi
Pharmacokinetics
Absorption: Ophthalmic: <2% systemically absorbed
Distribution: Adheres to cornea and is retained in the conjunctival fornices
Usual Dosage Geriatrics and Adults: Ophthalmic: Instill 1 drop in conjunctival sac every 1-2 hours, after 3-4 days reduce to one drop 6-8 times/day; usual course of therapy is 2-3 weeks.
Monitoring Parameters Monitor tolerance to the drug at least twice weekly
Patient Information Shake well before using, do not touch dropper to eye; notify physician if condition worsens or does not improve after 3-4 days
Special Geriatric Considerations Assess patient's ability to self-administer ophthalmic drops
Dosage Forms Suspension, ophthalmic: 5% (15 mL)

Nature's Tears® Solution [OTC] *see* Artificial Tears *on page 82*
Navane® *see* Thiothixene *on page 913*
ND-Stat® *see* Brompheniramine *on page 129*
Nebcin® Injection *see* Tobramycin *on page 929*
NebuPent™ Inhalation *see* Pentamidine *on page 726*

Nedocromil Sodium (ne doe KROE mil SOW dee um)
Related Information
Asthma Guidelines *on page 1040*
Inhaled Medications Comparison *on page 1034*
Brand Names Tilade® Inhalation Aerosol
Generic Available No
Therapeutic Category Antihistamine, Inhalation; Inhalation, Miscellaneous
Use Maintenance therapy in patients with mild to moderate bronchial asthma
Contraindications Hypersensitivity to nedocromil or other ingredients in the preparation
Warnings If systemic or inhaled steroid therapy is at all reduced, monitor patients carefully; nedocromil is **not** a bronchodilator and, therefore, should not be used for reversal of acute bronchospasm
Precautions Coughing and bronchospasm may occur when nedocromil is used; if this is uncontrollable, discontinue use
Adverse Reactions 1% to 10%:
Cardiovascular: Chest pain
Central nervous system: Dizziness, dysphonia, headache, fatigue
Dermatologic: Rash
Gastrointestinal: Nausea, vomiting, dyspepsia, diarrhea, abdominal pain, xerostomia, unpleasant taste
Hepatic: Increased ALT
Neuromuscular & skeletal: Arthritis, tremor
Respiratory: Cough, pharyngitis, rhinitis, bronchitis, upper respiratory infection, bronchospasm, increased sputum production
Overdosage Symptoms include bronchospasm, laryngeal edema
Stability Store at 2°C to 30°C/36°F to 86°F; do not freeze

Mechanism of Action Inhibits the activation of and mediator release from a variety of inflammatory cell types associated with asthma including eosinophils, neutrophils, macrophages, mast cells, monocytes, and platelets; it inhibits the release of histamine, leukotrienes, and slow-reacting substance of anaphylaxis; it inhibits the development of early and late bronchoconstriction responses to inhaled antigen; has no intrinsic bronchodilator activity

Pharmacodynamics Duration of therapeutic effect: 2 hours

Pharmacokinetics
Protein binding, plasma: 89%
Bioavailability: Systemic: 7% to 9% absorption
Half-life: 1.5-2 hours
Elimination: Excreted unchanged in urine

Usual Dosage Geriatrics and Adults: Inhalation: 2 inhalations 4 times/day; may reduce dosage to 2-3 times/day once desired clinical response to initial dose is observed

Administration If patient has aerosol (MDI) bronchodilators in their regimen, these should be used first, 5-10 minutes prior to use of nedocromil

Monitoring Parameters Pulmonary function, spirometry

Patient Information An illustrated patient instruction packet is included with inhaler; must be used regularly to obtain benefit, even though symptoms may be absent; be aware of proper use

Nursing Implications Patients must be clear of mucus before inhalation (as much as possible); see Patient Information, Warnings, and Special Geriatric Considerations

Additional Information Has no known therapeutic systemic activity when delivered by inhalation

Special Geriatric Considerations Elderly may have difficulty using inhaler delivery system, especially if they have physical or medical impairment (ie, Parkinson's disease, stroke, etc); if this prophylactic modality is desired but patient cannot tolerate nedocromil inhalations, consider cromolyn sodium solution for nebulizer use

Dosage Forms Aerosol: 1.75 mg/activation (16.2 g) [112 inhalations]

Nefazodone (nef AY zoe done)

Related Information
Antidepressant Agents Comparison *on page 1021*
Antidepressant Medication Guidelines *on page 1075*

Brand Names Serzone®

Therapeutic Category Antidepressant

Use Treatment of depression

Contraindications Hypersensitivity to nefazodone, trazodone, or any component; concomitant use of any MAO inhibitors, astemizole, terfenadine, or cisapride

Warnings Monitor closely and use with extreme caution in patients with cardiac disease, cerebrovascular disease or seizures; very sedating and can be dehydrating; therapeutic effects may take up to 4 weeks to occur; therapy is normally maintained for several months and optimum response is reached to prevent recurrence of depression, discontinue therapy and re-evaluate if priapism occurs

Adverse Reactions
Cardiovascular: Postural hypotension, bradycardia
Central nervous system: Headache, drowsiness, insomnia, somnolence, agitation, dizziness, confusion (see Additional Information)
Endocrine & metabolic: Decreased libido
Gastrointestinal: Xerostomia, nausea, constipation, vomiting, diarrhea, dyspepsia
Genitourinary: Prolonged priapism, abnormal ejaculation
Neuromuscular & skeletal: Tremor, weakness
Ocular: Blurred vision, amblyopia

Overdosage Symptoms of overdose include drowsiness, nausea, vomiting, hypotension, tachycardia, incontinence, coma, priapism, somnolence

Toxicology Following initiation of essential overdose management, toxic symptoms should be treated. Ventricular arrhythmias often respond to lidocaine 1.5 mg/kg bolus followed by 2 mg/minute infusion with concurrent systemic alkalinization (sodium bicarbonate 0.5-2 mEq/kg I.V.). Seizures usually respond to diazepam I.V. boluses (5-10 mg for adults up to 30 mg). If seizures are unresponsive or recur, phenytoin or phenobarbital may be required. Hypotension is best treated by I.V. fluids and by placing the patient in the Trendelenburg position.

(Continued)

Nefazodone *(Continued)*

Drug Interactions

Decreased effect: Clonidine, methyldopa, diuretics, oral hypoglycemics, anticoagulants, propranolol

Increased toxicity: Inhibits CYP3A4 isoenzyme terfenadine, astemizole, and cisapride (increased concentrations have been associated with serious ventricular arrhythmias and death), fluoxetine, triazolam (reduce triazolam dose by 75%), alprazolam (reduce alprazolam dose by 50%), midazolam, phenytoin, CNS depressants (including alcohol), MAO inhibitors (allow 14 days after MAO inhibitors are stopped or 7 days after nefazodone is stopped); digoxin serum concentrations may increase; protease inhibitors may inhibit nefazodone's metabolism

Mechanism of Action

Inhibits serotonin (5-HT) reuptake and a potent antagonist at type 2 serotonin (5-HT) receptors; down regulates $5-HT_2$ receptors with chronic administration; blocks norepinephrine reuptake presynaptically; has been shown to antagonize alpha$_1$-adrenergic receptors; minimal affinity for cholinergic or histaminic receptors

Pharmacokinetics

Absorption: Nearly complete with oral dosing, however, first-pass effect results in 20% systemic bioavailability

Protein binding: >99%

Metabolism: In the liver to 3 active metabolites; triazoledione, hydroxynefazodone and m-chlorophenylpiperazine (mCPP); hydroxynefazodone is equipotent $5-HT_2$ antagonist and 5-HT reuptake inhibitor as nefazodone; substrate and inhibitor CYP3A4

Half-life: 2-4 hours (parent compound), active metabolites persist longer

Time to peak serum concentration: 30 minutes, prolonged in presence of food

Elimination: Primarily as metabolites in urine and secondarily in feces

Usual Dosage

Oral:

Geriatrics: Initial: 50 mg twice daily; increase dose to 100 mg twice daily in 2 weeks; usual maintenance dose: 200-400 mg/day

Adults: 200 mg/day, administered in two divided doses initially, with a range of 300-600 mg/day in two divided doses thereafter

Monitoring Parameters

Sitting and standing blood pressure and pulse; signs and symptoms of depression including appetite, sleep

Reference Range

Therapeutic plasma concentrations have not yet been defined

Patient Information

Take shortly after a meal or light snack; can be given at bedtime dose if drowsiness occurs; optimum effect may take 2-4 weeks to be achieved; avoid alcohol; may cause painful erections (contact physician if this should occur); avoid sudden changes in position; may cause dizziness

Nursing Implications

Dosing after meals may decrease lightheadedness and postural hypotension, use safety precautions if administered to the elderly; observe patient's activity and compare with admission level; assist with ambulation (see Monitoring Parameters)

Additional Information

Experience with this drug has led some clinicians to realize that it may cause less insomnia, anxiety, and sexual dysfunction than the SSRIs; should consider this agent for patients who cannot tolerate the sexual dysfunction that may result from other antidepressants

Special Geriatric Considerations

Data on nefazodone in the elderly are limited, specifically regarding efficacy; clinical trials in adult patients have found it superior to placebo and similar to imipramine; nefazodone's C_{max} and AUC have been reported to be increased two-fold in the elderly and women after a single dose compared to younger patients, however, these differences were markedly reduced with multiple dosing (see Usual Dosage)

Dosage Forms

Tablet, as hydrochloride: 100 mg, 150 mg, 200 mg, 250 mg

References

Fontaine R, Ontiveros A, Elie R, et al, "A Double-Blind Comparison of Nefazodone, Imipramine, and Placebo in Major Depression," *J Clin Psychiatry*, 1994, 55(6):234-41.

Rickels K, Schweizer E, Clary C, et al, "Nefazodone and Imipramine in Major Depression: A Placebo-Controlled Trial," *Br J Psychiatry*, 1994, 164(6):802-5.

Shea JP, Shulka UA, Rittman KA, "Single Dose Pharmacokinetics of Nefazodone in Elderly Subjects, Renally Impaired Patients, and Patients With Hepatic Cirrhosis in Comparison to Healthy Volunteers," *Clin Pharmacol Ther*, 1988, 43:146.

Neomycin, Polymyxin B, and Dexamethasone
(nee oh MYE sin, pol i MIKS in bee, & deks a METH a sone)

Brand Names AK-Trol®; Dexacidin®; Dexasporin®; Maxitrol®

Generic Available Yes

Therapeutic Category Antibacterial, Topical; Antibiotic, Ophthalmic

Use Steroid-responsive inflammatory ocular conditions in which a corticosteroid is indicated and where bacterial infection or a risk of bacterial infection exists

Contraindications Hypersensitivity to dexamethasone, polymyxin B, neomycin or any component; herpes simplex, vaccinia, and varicella

Warnings Prolonged use may result in glaucoma, defects in visual acuity, posterior subcapsular cataract formation, and secondary ocular infections

Adverse Reactions
Dermatologic: Contact dermatitis, cutaneous sensitization (sensitivity to topical neomycin has been reported to occur in 5% to 15% of patients)
Local: Pain, stinging
Ocular: Development of glaucoma, cataract, increased intraocular pressure, optic nerve damage, visual defects, blurred vision
Miscellaneous: Delayed wound healing, increased incidence to secondary infections

Mechanism of Action Interferes with bacterial protein synthesis by binding to 30S ribosomal subunits; binds to phospholipids, alters permeability, and damages the bacterial cytoplasmic membrane permitting leakage of intracellular constituents; decreases inflammation by suppression of migration of polymorphonuclear leukocytes and reversal of increased capillary permeability; suppresses normal immune response

Usual Dosage Geriatrics and Adults: Ophthalmic:
Ointment: Place a small amount (~½") in the affected eye 3-4 times/day or apply at bedtime as an adjunct with drops
Solution: Instill 1-2 drops into affected eye(s) every 3-4 hours; in severe disease, drops may be used hourly and tapered to discontinuation

Administration Shake well before using; tilt head back, place medication in conjunctival sac, and close eyes; apply finger pressure on lacrimal sac for 1 minute following instillation

Monitoring Parameters Intraocular pressure with use >10 days

Patient Information For the eye; shake well before using; do not touch dropper to eye; notify physician if condition worsens or does not improve in 3-4 days

Nursing Implications See Administration

Special Geriatric Considerations Assess patients ability to self-administer (see Monitoring Parameters)

Dosage Forms
Ophthalmic:
Ointment: Neomycin sulfate 3.5 mg, polymyxin b sulfate 10,000 units, and dexamethasone 0.1% per g (3.5 g)
Suspension: Neomycin sulfate 3.5 mg, polymyxin b sulfate 10,000 units, and dexamethasone 0.1% per mL (5 mL)

Neoral® Oral *see* Cyclosporine *on page 263*

Neosar® Injection *see* Cyclophosphamide *on page 260*

Neostigmine (nee oh STIG meen)
Brand Names Prostigmin®

Generic Available No

Therapeutic Category Antidote, Neuromuscular Blocking Agent; Cholinergic Agent; Diagnostic Agent, Myasthenia Gravis

Use Diagnosis and treatment of myasthenia gravis and prevent and treat postoperative bladder distention and urinary retention; reversal of the effects of nondepolarizing neuromuscular blocking agents after surgery

Contraindications Hypersensitivity to neostigmine, bromides or any component; GI or GU obstruction, peritonitis

Warnings Does **not** antagonize and may prolong the phase I block of depolarizing muscle relaxants (eg, succinylcholine); use with caution in patients with epilepsy, asthma, bradycardia, hyperthyroidism, cardiac arrhythmias, or peptic ulcer; adequate facilities should be available for cardiopulmonary resuscitation when testing and adjusting dose for myasthenia gravis; have atropine and epinephrine ready to treat hypersensitivity reactions; overdosage may result in cholinergic crisis, this must be distinguished from myasthenic crisis; anticholinesterase insensitivity can develop for brief or prolonged periods
(Continued)

Neostigmine *(Continued)*

Precautions Patients may become insensitive to pharmacologic action; this may be brief or prolonged; reduce dose or withhold dose until patient regains sensitivity; monitor respiratory rate

Adverse Reactions

Cardiovascular: A-V block, bradycardia, hypotension, bradyarrhythmias, asystole

Central nervous system: Dysphoria, restlessness, agitation, seizures, headache, drowsiness

Gastrointestinal: Hyperperistalsis, nausea, vomiting, salivation, diarrhea, stomach cramps

Genitourinary: Urge to urinate

Local: Thrombophlebitis

Neuromuscular & skeletal: Muscle spasms, tremor, weakness, fasciculations

Ocular: Miosis, lacrimation, diplopia

Respiratory: Increased bronchial secretions, bronchoconstriction, laryngospasm, respiratory paralysis

Miscellaneous: Diaphoresis (increased), hypersensitivity, hyper-reactive cholinergic responses

Overdosage Symptoms of overdose include muscle weakness, blurred vision, excessive sweating, tearing and salivation, nausea, vomiting, diarrhea, hypertension, bradycardia, muscle weakness, paralysis

Toxicology Atropine sulfate injection should be readily available as an antagonist for the effects of neostigmine

Drug Interactions

Decreased effect: Antagonizes effects of nondepolarizing muscle relaxants (eg, pancuronium, tubocurarine); atropine antagonizes the muscarinic effects of neostigmine; magnesium has skeletal muscle depressant action

Increased effect: Neuromuscular blocking agents effects are increased; aminoglycoside antibiotics have mild nondepolarizing blocking effect which enhances neostigmine effect

Mechanism of Action Inhibits destruction of acetylcholine by acetylcholinesterase which facilitates transmission of impulses across myoneural junction

Pharmacodynamics

Onset of effect:

I.M.: Within 20-30 minutes

I.V.: Within 1-20 minutes

Oral: 45-75 minutes

Duration:

I.M.: 2.5-4 hours

I.V.: 1-2 hours

Oral: 2-4 hours

Pharmacokinetics

Absorption: Oral: Poor, <2%

Metabolism: In the liver

Half-life:

Normal renal function: 0.5-2.1 hours

End stage renal disease: Prolonged

Elimination: 50% excreted renally as unchanged drug

Usual Dosage

Myasthenia gravis: Diagnosis: Geriatrics and Adults: I.M.: 0.02 mg/kg as a single dose

Myasthenia gravis: Treatment: Geriatrics and Adults:

Oral: 15 mg/dose every 3-4 hours up to 375 mg/day maximum; interval between doses must be individualized for maximal response

I.M., I.V., S.C.: 0.5-2.5 mg every 1-3 hours up to 10 mg/24 hours maximum

Reversal of nondepolarizing neuromuscular blockade after surgery in conjunction with atropine: Geriatrics and Adults: I.V.: 0.5-2.5 mg; total dose not to exceed 5 mg; must administer atropine several minutes prior to neostigmine

Bladder atony: Geriatrics and Adults: I.M., S.C.:

Prevention: 0.25 mg every 4-6 hours for 2-3 days

Treatment: 0.5-1 mg every 3 hours for 5 doses after bladder has emptied

Dosing adjustment in renal impairment:

Cl_{cr} 10-50 mL/minute: Administer 50% of normal dose

Cl_{cr} <10 mL/minute: Administer 25% of normal dose

Administration When giving for reversal of neuromuscular blockade, keep patient well ventilated until recovered

Monitoring Parameters Respiratory rate, pulse, blood pressure, signs of cholinergic crisis (see Overdosage)

Test Interactions ↑ aminotransferase [ALT (SGPT)/AST (SGOT)] (S), ↑ amylase (S)

Patient Information Side effects are generally due to exaggerated pharmacologic effects; most common are salivation and muscle fasciculations; notify physician if nausea, vomiting, muscle weakness, severe abdominal pain, or difficulty breathing occurs

Nursing Implications In the diagnosis of myasthenia gravis, all anticholinesterase medications should be discontinued for at least 8 hours before administering neostigmine; monitor for signs of cholinergic crisis (see Overdosage)

Additional Information
Neostigmine bromide: Prostigmin® tablet
Neostigmine methylsulfate: Prostigmin® injection

Special Geriatric Considerations Many elderly will have diseases which may influence the use of neostigmine (see Warnings). Also, many elderly will need doses reduced 50% due to creatinine clearances in the 10-50 mL/minute range (common in the aged); side effects or concomitant disease may warrant use of pyridostigmine.

Dosage Forms
Injection, as methylsulfate: 0.25 mg/mL (1 mL); 0.5 mg/mL (1 mL, 10 mL); 1 mg/mL (10 mL)
Tablet, as bromide: 15 mg

References
Payne JP, Hughes R, and Al Azawi S, "Neuromuscular Blockade by Neostigmine in Anaesthetized Man," *Br J Anaesth*, 1980, 52(1):69-76.

Neo-Synephrine® 12 Hour Nasal Solution [OTC] *see* Oxymetazoline *on page 706*

Neo-Synephrine® Nasal Solution [OTC] *see* Phenylephrine *on page 740*

Neo-Synephrine® Ophthalmic Solution *see* Phenylephrine *on page 740*

Nephro-Calci® [OTC] *see* Calcium Salts (Oral) *on page 152*

Nephro-Fer™ [OTC] *see* Ferrous Fumarate *on page 376*

Nephrox Suspension [OTC] *see* Aluminum Hydroxide *on page 41*

Neptazane® *see* Methazolamide *on page 600*

Nervocaine® *see* Lidocaine *on page 537*

Nestrex® *see* Pyridoxine *on page 807*

1-N-Ethyl Sisomicin *see* Netilmicin *on this page*

Netilmicin (ne til MYE sin)

Related Information
Cephalosporins, Aminoglycosides, Macrolides, & Quinolones *on page 1014*

Brand Names Netromycin®

Synonyms 1-N-Ethyl Sisomicin

Therapeutic Category Antibiotic, Aminoglycoside

Use Short-term treatment of serious or life-threatening infections including septicemia, peritonitis, intra-abdominal abscess, lower respiratory tract infections, urinary tract infections, skin, bone and joint infections caused by sensitive *Pseudomonas aeruginosa*, *Escherichia coli*, *Proteus*, *Klebsiella*, *Serratia*, *Enterobacter*, *Citrobacter*, and *Staphylococcus*

Contraindications Known hypersensitivity to netilmicin (aminoglycosides, bisulfites)

Warnings
Use with caution in patients with pre-existing renal insufficiency, vestibular or cochlear impairment, myasthenia gravis, hypocalcemia, conditions which depress neuromuscular transmission

Parenteral aminoglycosides are associated with nephrotoxicity or ototoxicity; the ototoxicity may be proportional to the amount of drug given and the duration of treatment; tinnitus or vertigo are indications of vestibular injury and impending hearing loss; renal damage is usually reversible

Adverse Reactions
Dermatologic: Rash
Gastrointestinal: Pseudomembranous colitis
Neuromuscular & skeletal: Neuromuscular blockade
Otic: Ototoxicity
Renal: Nephrotoxicity
Respiratory: Respiratory depression
(Continued)

Netilmicin *(Continued)*

Overdosage Symptoms of overdose include ototoxicity, nephrotoxicity, and neuromuscular toxicity

Toxicology Serum concentration monitoring is recommended. Treatment of choice following a single acute overdose appears to be the maintenance of good urine output of at least 3 mL/kg/hour. Dialysis is of questionable value in the enhancement of aminoglycoside elimination. If required, hemodialysis is preferred over peritoneal dialysis in patients with normal renal function. Careful hydration may be all that is required to promote diuresis and, therefore, the enhancement of the drug's elimination. Chelation with penicillins is experimental.

Drug Interactions
Increased/prolonged effect of depolarizing and nondepolarizing neuromuscular blocking agents

Increased toxicity: Concurrent use of amphotericin, vancomycin, ethacrynic acid, or furosemide may increase nephrotoxicity

Mechanism of Action Interferes with protein synthesis in bacterial cell by binding to ribosomal subunit

Pharmacokinetics
Absorption: I.M.: Well absorbed

Distribution: V_d: 0.16-0.34 L/kg

Half-life: 2-3 hours (age and renal function dependent)

Time to peak serum concentration: Within 30-60 minutes

Elimination: By glomerular filtration; since clearance is dependent upon renal function, the clearance has been found to decrease with age and the half-life increase

Usual Dosage Dosage should be based on an estimate of ideal body weight.

Geriatrics:
Intrathecal: 4-8 mg/day
I.M., I.V.: 1.5-5 mg/kg/day in 1-2 divided doses

Adults:
Intrathecal: 4-8 mg/day
I.M., I.V.: 3-5 mg/kg/day in 3 divided doses or as indicated by adjustment for renal function
Once daily or extended interval: I.V.: 5-7 mg/kg/dose given every 24, 36, or 48 hours depending on Cl_{cr} (see Dosing Adjustment in Renal Impairment) (see Special Geriatric Considerations)

Dosing adjustment in renal impairment: 2 mg/kg (2-3 serum concentration measurements should be obtained after the initial dose to measure the half-life in order to determine the frequency of subsequent doses)
Cl_{cr} ≥60 mL/minute: Administer every 24 hours
Cl_{cr} 40-59 mL/minute: Administer every 36 hours
Cl_{cr} 20-39 mL/minute: Administer every 48 hours
Cl_{cr} <20 mL/minute: Individualize dose

Dialyzable (50% to 100%)

Some patients may require larger or more frequent doses (eg, every 6 hours) if serum concentrations document the need (ie, cystic fibrosis or febrile granulocytopenic patients)

Dosing adjustment/comments in hepatic disease: Monitor plasma concentrations

Monitoring Parameters Urinalysis, urine output, BUN, serum creatinine; hearing should be tested before, during, and after treatment; particularly in those at risk for ototoxicity or who will be receiving prolonged therapy (>2 weeks). Obtain peak concentrations 30 minutes after the end of a 30-minute infusion trough concentrations are drawn within 30 minutes before the next dose.

Reference Range
Therapeutic:
Peak: 4-8 µg/mL (SI: 8-17 µmol/L)
Trough: <2 µg/mL (SI: 4 µmol/L) (depends in part on the minimal inhibitory concentration of drug against organism being treated)
Once daily or extended interval: Trough: <0.5 µg/mL
Toxic:
Peak: >12 µg/mL (SI: >21 µmol/L)
Trough: >2 µg/mL (SI: >8.4 µmol/L)

Test Interactions Increased protein; decreased magnesium

Nursing Implications Aminoglycoside serum concentrations are measured in blood taken from Silastic® central catheters can sometimes give falsely high readings

Special Geriatric Considerations The aminoglycosides are important therapeutic interventions for infections due to susceptible organisms and as empiric therapy in seriously ill patients. Their use is not without risk of toxicity, however, these risks can be minimized if initial dosing is adjusted for estimated renal function and appropriate monitoring performed. High dose, once daily aminoglycosides have been advocated as an alternative to traditional dosing regimens. Once daily or extended interval dosing is as effective and may be safer than traditional dosing. The interval must be adjusted for renal function. See Pharmacokinetics and Usual Dosage.

Dosage Forms Injection, as sulfate: 100 mg/mL

References
Welling PG, Baumueller A, Lau CC, et al, "Netilmicin Pharmacokinetics After Single Intravenous Doses to Elderly Male Patients," *Antimicrob Agents Chemother*, 1977, 12:328-34.

Netromycin® *see* Netilmicin *on page 663*

Neucalm® *see* Hydroxyzine *on page 470*

Neupogen® *see* Filgrastim *on page 381*

Neuramate® *see* Meprobamate *on page 588*

Neurontin® *see* Gabapentin *on page 418*

Neut® Injection *see* Sodium Bicarbonate *on page 858*

Neutra-Phos® *see* Potassium Phosphate and Sodium Phosphate *on page 767*

Neutra-Phos®-K *see* Potassium Phosphate *on page 766*

Neutrexin™ Injection *see* Trimetrexate Glucuronate *on page 963*

N.G.T.® Topical *see* Nystatin and Triamcinolone *on page 687*

Niacin (NYE a sin)

Brand Names Nicobid® [OTC]; Nicolar® [OTC]; Nicotinex [OTC]; Slo-Niacin® [OTC]

Synonyms Nicotinic Acid; Vitamin B_3

Generic Available Yes

Therapeutic Category Antilipemic Agent; Vitamin, Water Soluble

Use Adjunctive treatment of hyperlipidemias; peripheral vascular disease and circulatory disorders; treatment of pellagra; dietary supplement

Unlabeled use: Hypercholesterolemia

Contraindications Liver disease, peptic ulcer, severe hypotension, known hypersensitivity to niacin, hemorrhaging

Precautions Monitor liver function tests and blood glucose; may elevate uric acid levels; use with caution in patients predisposed to gout, tartrazine sensitivity

Adverse Reactions

Cardiovascular: Hypotension, tachycardia, syncope, vasovagal attacks, flushing

Central nervous system: Dizziness, headache

Dermatologic: Pruritus, burning, tingling skin, increased sebaceous gland activity; starting low doses and slowly increasing the nicotinic acid dose greatly reduces the potential for severe flushing or itching reactions; the table lists a titration approach that is useful in reducing these reactions

First week	50 mg twice daily
Second week	100 mg twice daily
Third week	200 mg twice daily
Fourth week	250 mg twice daily
Fifth week	500 mg twice daily
Sixth week	1 g twice daily
Seventh week	1.5 g twice daily

Gastrointestinal: GI upset, nausea, vomiting, heartburn, diarrhea

Hepatic: Abnormal liver function tests, jaundice, chronic liver damage

Ocular: Blurred vision

Overdosage Symptoms of overdose include flushing, GI distress, pruritus

Drug Interactions

Adrenergic-blocking agents may have additive vasodilating effect and may produce postural hypotension

Sulfinpyrazone's uricosuric effect may be inhibited

Probenecid's uricosuric effect may be inhibited

Decreased effect of oral hypoglycemics

Decreased toxicity (flush) with aspirin; increased toxicity with lovastatin (myopathy) and possibly with other HMG-CoA reductase inhibitors

(Continued)

Niacin *(Continued)*

Mechanism of Action A component of two coenzymes which is necessary for tissue respiration, lipid metabolism, and glycogenolysis; inhibits the synthesis of very low density lipoproteins

Pharmacodynamics
Onset of action: Vasodilation occurs within 20 minutes
Duration: 20-60 minutes (extended release preparations persist for 8-10 hours)

Pharmacokinetics
Metabolism: Depending upon the dose, niacin converts to niacinamide; following this conversion, niacinamide is metabolized in the liver
Half-life: 45 minutes
Elimination: In urine

Usual Dosage Geriatrics and Adults: Oral (see Additional Information):
Hyperlipidemia: 3-6 g/day in 3 divided doses with or after meals; maximum: 8 g/day
Pellagra: 50 mg 3-10 times/day, maximum: 500 mg/day
Niacin deficiency: 10-20 mg/day, maximum: 100 mg/day

Monitoring Parameters Fractionated serum cholesterol

Test Interactions False elevations in some fluorometric determinations of urinary catecholamines; false-positive urine glucose (Benedict's reagent)

Patient Information May experience transient cutaneous flushing and sensation of warmth, especially of face and upper body; itching or tingling, and headache may occur; may cause GI upset, take with food; if dizziness occurs, avoid sudden changes in posture

Nursing Implications Can cause muscle damage leading to muscle aches and cramps; monitor blood glucose concentration, liver function tests in patients on large doses and long-term therapy

Additional Information If flushing is bothersome or persistent, 325 mg of aspirin 30 minutes before each dose or increasing the dose slowly with weekly increase may minimize this reaction; for explicit guidelines on the risk factors for CHD and when to treat high blood cholesterol (see References); due to liver function test abnormalities induced by sustained release niacin, these dosage forms are not currently recommended

Special Geriatric Considerations The definition of and, therefore, when to treat hyperlipidemia in the elderly is a controversial issue. The National Cholesterol Education Program recommends that all adults 20 years of age and older maintain a plasma cholesterol of <200 mg/dL. By this definition, 60% of all elderly would be considered to have a borderline high (200-230 mg/dL) or high (≥240 mg/dL) plasma cholesterol. However, plasma cholesterol has been shown to be a less reliable predictor of coronary heart disease in the elderly. Therefore, it is the authors' belief that pharmacologic treatment be reserved for those who are unable to obtain a desirable plasma cholesterol concentration by diet alone and for whom the benefits of treatment are believed to outweigh the potential adverse effects, drug interactions, and cost of treatment (see Additional Information).

Dosage Forms
Capsule: 125 mg, 250 mg, 500 mg
Capsule, timed release: 125 mg, 250 mg, 300 mg, 400 mg, 500 mg
Elixir: 50 mg/5 mL (473 mL, 4000 mL)
Injection: 100 mg/mL (30 mL)
Tablet: 25 mg, 50 mg, 100 mg, 250 mg, 500 mg
Tablet, timed release: 250 mg, 500 mg, 750 mg

References
"Summary of the Second Report of the National Cholesterol Education Program (NCEP) Expert Panel on Detection, Evaluation, and Treatment of High Blood Cholesterol in Adults (Adult Treatment Panel II)," *JAMA*, 1993, 269(23):3015-23.

Niacinamide *(nye a SIN a mide)*

Synonyms Nicotinamide; Vitamin B₃

Generic Available Yes

Therapeutic Category Vitamin, Water Soluble

Use Prophylaxis and treatment of pellagra

Contraindications Liver disease, peptic ulcer, severe hypotension, known hypersensitivity to niacin

Warnings Large doses should be administered with caution to patients with gallbladder disease, jaundice; liver disease, or diabetes; use with caution in patients predisposed to gout; some products may contain tartrazine

Adverse Reactions
Cardiovascular: Flushing, tachycardia

Central nervous system: Headache
Dermatologic: Pruritus, increased sebaceous gland activity, skin rash
Gastrointestinal: Vomiting, flatulence
Neuromuscular & skeletal: Paresthesia
Ocular: Blurred vision
Respiratory: Wheezing

Overdosage Symptoms of overdose include flushing, GI distress, pruritus

Mechanism of Action A component of two coenzymes which is necessary for tissue respiration, lipid metabolism, and glycogenolysis

Pharmacokinetics
Absorption: Rapid from GI tract
Metabolism: In the liver
Half-life: 45 minutes
Time to peak serum concentration: 20-70 minutes
Elimination: In urine

Usual Dosage Geriatrics and Adults: Oral: 50 mg 3-10 times/day
Pellagra: 300-500 mg/day

Test Interactions False elevations of urinary catecholamines

Special Geriatric Considerations Should not be confused with niacin (see Usual Dosage)

Dosage Forms Tablet: 50 mg, 100 mg, 125 mg, 250 mg, 500 mg

Nicardipine (nye KAR de peen)

Related Information
Calcium Channel Blocking Agents Comparison *on page 1027*

Brand Names Cardene®; Cardene® SR

Generic Available No

Therapeutic Category Antianginal Agent; Calcium Channel Blocker

Use Chronic stable angina; management of essential hypertension; sustained release and I.V.: Hypertension
Unlabeled use: CHF

Contraindications Severe hypotension or second and third degree heart block; sinus bradycardia; advanced heart block; ventricular tachycardia; cardiogenic shock, hypotension, CHF; hypersensitivity to nicardipine or any component, calcium channel blockers, and adenosine; atrial fibrillation or flutter associated with accessory conduction pathways; not to be given within a few hours of I.V. beta-blocking agents

Warnings Hypotension, CHF; cardiac conduction defects, PVCs, idiopathic hypertrophic subaortic stenosis; may cause platelet inhibition; do not abruptly withdraw (chest pain); hepatic dysfunction, increased angina, increased intracranial pressure with cranial tumors; elderly may have greater hypotensive effect
The FDA's Cardiovascular and Renal Drug Advisory Committee reviewed current data regarding the risk of heart attacks in patients treated with calcium channel blockers and determined that as a class, the calcium channel antagonists are safe; however, they warned that short-acting nifedipine could increase the risk of myocardial infarction in some patients. The committee was in agreement with a statement issued September, 1995 by the National Heart Lung, and Blood Institute of the National Institute of Health, that warned that short-acting nifedipine should be used with great caution especially at higher doses.

Precautions Sick sinus syndrome, severe left ventricular dysfunction, CHF, hepatic or renal impairment, hypertrophic cardiomyopathy (especially obstructive), concomitant therapy with beta-blockers or digoxin, edema

Adverse Reactions
Cardiovascular: Sustained tachycardia, myocardial infarction, increased angina, palpitations, peripheral vascular disease, atypical chest pain, chest pain, flushing, syncope, bradycardia, ventricular extrasystoles, peripheral edema
Central nervous system: Dizziness, lightheadedness, nervousness, psychotic symptoms, malaise, anxiety, equilibrium difficulty, headache, somnolence, insomnia, disturbed dreams, confusion
Dermatologic: Rash
Gastrointestinal: Nausea, constipation, abdominal discomfort and pain, vomiting, xerostomia
Genitourinary: Polyuria, nocturia, urinary incontinence
Neuromuscular & skeletal: Arthralgia, hyperkinesia, weakness, paresthesia
Ocular: Blurred vision
Otic: Tinnitus
Respiratory: Shortness of breath, sore throat, nasal congestion
(Continued)

Nicardipine *(Continued)*

Miscellaneous: Infection, allergic reactions, gingival swelling and inflammation

Overdosage Symptoms of overdose include hypotension, bradycardia, A-V block, hepatic necrosis

Toxicology Ipecac-induced emesis can hypothetically worsen calcium antagonist toxicity, since it can produce vagal stimulation. The potential for seizures precipitously following acute ingestion of large doses of a calcium antagonist may also contraindicate the use of ipecac. Supportive and symptomatic treatment, including I.V. fluids and Trendelenburg positioning, should be initiated as intoxication may cause hypotension. Although calcium (calcium chloride I.V. 1-2 g in adults over 5-10 minutes with repeats as needed) has been used as an "antidote" for acute intoxications, there is limited experience to support its routine use and should be reserved for those cases where definite signs of myocardial depression are evident. Heart block may respond to isoproterenol, glucagon, atropine and/or calcium although a temporary pacemaker may be required.

Drug Interactions

Beta-blockers increased cardiac and A-V conduction depression

Fentanyl increased volume requirements and hypotension; although this drug is new, other drug interactions not reported to the same degree as older agents; however, should be suspect of any drug interaction reported with other calcium channel blockers

Nicardipine metabolism may be inhibited by erythromycin, ketoconazole, itraconazole, protease inhibitors; induced by rifampin, rifabutin

Stability I.V. ampuls must be diluted; dilute each ampul in 240 mL to result in 250 mL of 0.1 mg/mL nicardipine; compatible with D_5W, $D_5\frac{1}{2}NS$, D_5NS, and D_5W with 40 mEq potassium chloride; 0.45% and 0.9% NS; **do not** mix with 5% sodium bicarbonate and lactated Ringer's solution; store at room temperature; protect from light; stable for 24 hours at room temperature

Mechanism of Action Inhibits calcium ion from entering the "slow channels" or select voltage-sensitive areas of vascular smooth muscle and myocardium during depolarization, producing a relaxation of coronary vascular smooth muscle and coronary vasodilation; increases myocardial oxygen delivery in patients with vasospastic angina

Pharmacokinetics

Absorption: Oral: Well absorbed, ~100%

Protein binding: 95%

Metabolism: Extensive first-pass metabolism; only metabolized in the liver; substrate CYP3A4

Bioavailability: Absolute, 35%

Half-life: 2-4 hours

Time to peak serum concentrations: Within 20-120 minutes and an onset of hypotension occurs within 20 minutes

Elimination: As metabolites in urine

Usual Dosage Geriatrics and Adults:

Angina (immediate release): 20 mg 3 times/day; usual range: 60-120 mg/day; increase dose at 3-day intervals

Hypertension: 20 mg 3 times/day; usual range: 60-120 mg/day; maximum blood pressure effect seen in 1-2 hours of administration

Sustained release: 30 mg twice daily

I.V.: Individualize dose

I.V. to oral equivalence:

20 mg every 8 hours orally = 0.5 mg/hour I.V.

30 mg every 8 hours orally = 1.2 mg/hour I.V.

40 mg every 8 hours orally = 2.2 mg/hour I.V.

Monitoring Parameters Heart rate, signs and symptoms of CHF; monitor blood pressure 1, 2, and 8 hours after dosing; measure sustained release blood pressure at 2, 4, and 6 hours after dosing

Reference Range Therapeutic: 28-50 ng/mL

Patient Information Sustained release products should be taken with food and not crushed; limit caffeine intake; avoid alcohol; notify physician if angina pain is not reduced when taking this drug, irregular heartbeat, shortness of breath, swelling, dizziness, constipation, nausea, or hypotension occur; do not stop therapy without advice of physician

Nursing Implications Do not crush sustained release capsules (see Warnings, Precautions, Monitoring Parameters, and Special Geriatric Considerations)

Special Geriatric Considerations Elderly may experience a greater hypotensive response; constipation may be more of a problem in elderly; calcium channel blockers are no more effective in elderly than other therapies; however, they do not cause significant CNS effects which is an advantage over some antihypertensive agents.

Dosage Forms
Nicardipine hydrochloride:
Capsule: 20 mg, 30 mg
Capsule, sustained release: 30 mg, 45 mg, 60 mg
Injection: 2.5 mg/mL (10 mL)

N'ice® Vitamin C Drops [OTC] *see* Ascorbic Acid *on page 82*

Nicobid® [OTC] *see* Niacin *on page 665*

Nicoderm® Patch *see* Nicotine *on this page*

Nicolar® [OTC] *see* Niacin *on page 665*

Nicorette® DS Gum *see* Nicotine *on this page*

Nicorette® Gum *see* Nicotine *on this page*

Nicotinamide *see* Niacinamide *on page 666*

Nicotine (nik oh TEEN)

Brand Names Habitrol™ Patch; Nicoderm® Patch; Nicorette® DS Gum; Nicorette® Gum; Nicotrol® NS Nasal Spray; Nicotrol® Patch [OTC]; ProStep® Patch

Generic Available No

Therapeutic Category Smoking Deterrent

Use Treatment aid to smoking cessation while participating in a behavioral modification program under medical supervision

Contraindications Nonsmokers, patients with a history of hypersensitivity or allergy to nicotine or any components used in the transdermal system, post-myocardial infarction period, patients with life-threatening arrhythmias, or severe or worsening angina pectoris, active temporomandibular joint disease (gum)

Warnings Use with caution in oropharyngeal inflammation and in patients with history of esophagitis, peptic ulcer, coronary artery disease, vasospastic disease, angina, hypertension, hyperthyroidism, pheochromocytoma, diabetes, and hepatic dysfunction; nicotine is known to be one of the most toxic of all poisons; while the gum is being used to help the patient overcome a health hazard, it also must be considered a hazardous drug vehicle.
Nicotine nasal spray: Fatal dose: 40 mg

Precautions Use with caution in patients with peptic ulcer history or active disease, or esophagitis; allergic reactions are frequently encountered; patients must stop smoking when using nicotine therapy since the use of nicotine with cigarettes may result in high concentrations of nicotine in the blood, thus giving serious adverse effects. The possibility of nicotine dependence must be considered; the use of the transdermal systems or gum beyond three months has not been shown to be effective in smoking cessation.

Adverse Reactions
Chewing gum:
Cardiovascular: Tachycardia, flushing, edema, syncope, atrial fibrillation, chest pain
Central nervous system: Headache (mild), insomnia, dizziness, nervousness, irritability, confusion, seizures, depression, euphoria
Dermatologic: Erythema, itching
Endocrine & metabolic: Dysmenorrhea
Gastrointestinal: Nausea, vomiting, indigestion, excessive salivation, belching, increased appetite, mouth or throat soreness, GI distress, eructation, glossitis, stomatitis, gingivitis, aphthous ulcer, anorexia
Neuromuscular & skeletal: Jaw muscle ache, paresthesias, weakness, numbness, myalgia, asthenia, back pain
Respiratory: Hoarseness, coughing, wheezing, sneezing
Miscellaneous: Hiccups, hypersensitivity reactions
Transdermal systems:
Cardiovascular: Tachycardia, atrial fibrillation
Central nervous system: Headache (mild), insomnia, nervousness, dizziness, impaired concentration
Dermatologic: Pruritus, erythema, burning sensation, rash, itching
Endocrine & metabolic: Dysmenorrhea
Gastrointestinal: Increased appetite, dyspepsia, diarrhea, nausea, constipation, dry mouth, abdominal pain
(Continued)

Nicotine *(Continued)*

Neuromuscular & skeletal: Myalgia, paresthesia, arthralgia

Respiratory: Cough, pharyngitis

Miscellaneous: Hypersensitivity reactions

Overdosage Symptoms of overdose include nausea, vomiting, abdominal pain, mental confusion, diarrhea, salivation, tachycardia, respiratory and cardiovascular collapse

Toxicology Treatment after decontamination is symptomatic and supportive; remove patch, rinse area with water and dry, do not use soap as this may increase absorption.

Mechanism of Action Nicotine is one of two naturally-occurring alkaloids which exhibit their primary effects via autonomic ganglia stimulation. The other alkaloid is lobeline which has many actions similar to those of nicotine but is less potent. Nicotine is a potent ganglionic and central nervous system stimulant, the actions of which are mediated via nicotine-specific receptors. Biphasic actions are observed depending upon the dose administered. The main effect of nicotine in small doses is stimulation of all autonomic ganglia; with larger doses, initial stimulation is followed by blockade of transmission. Biphasic effects are also evident in the adrenal medulla; discharge of catecholamines occurs with small doses, whereas prevention of catecholamines release is seen with higher doses as a response to splanchnic nerve stimulation. Stimulation of the central nervous system (CNS) is characterized by tremors and respiratory excitation. However, convulsions may occur with higher doses, along with respiratory failure secondary to both central paralysis and peripheral blockade to respiratory muscles.

Pharmacokinetics

Intranasal nicotine may more closely approximate the time course of plasma nicotine levels observed after cigarette smoking than other dosage forms

Duration of action: Transdermal: 24 hours

Absorption: Transdermal: Slow

Metabolism: In the liver, primarily to cotinine, which is $1/5$ as active; inducer of CYP1A2

Half-life, elimination: 4 hours

Time to peak serum concentration: Transdermal: 8-9 hours

Elimination: Via the kidneys; renal clearance is pH-dependent

Oral:

Absorption: Dependent upon the vigor and duration of chewing

Half-life: ~4 hours

Usual Dosage Geriatrics and Adults:

Gum: Chew 1 piece of gum when urge to smoke, up to 30 pieces/day; most patients require 10-12 pieces of gum/day

Transdermal patch (patients should be advised to completely stop smoking upon initiation of therapy): Apply new patch every 24 hours to nonhairy, clean, dry skin on the upper body or upper outer arm; each patch should be applied to a different site

Initial starting dose: 21 mg/day for 4-8 weeks for most patients

First weaning dose: 14 mg/day for 2-4 weeks

Second weaning dose: 7 mg/day for 2-4 weeks

Initial starting dose for patients <100 pounds, smoke <10 cigarettes/day, have a history of cardiovascular disease: 14 mg/day for 4-8 weeks followed by 7 mg/day for 2-4 weeks

In patients who are receiving >600 mg/day of cimetidine: Decrease to the next lower patch size

Benefits of use of nicotine transdermal patches beyond 3 months have not been demonstrated

Spray: 1-2 sprays/hour; do not exceed more than 5 doses (10 sprays) per hour; each dose (2 sprays) contains 1 mg of nicotine. **Warning:** A dose of 40 mg can cause fatalities

Administration Patients must desire smoking cessation; therapy is initiated for 4-12 weeks at which time the patient should be able to completely stop smoking by the end of treatment; use beyond 3 months is of no increased benefit

Monitoring Parameters Smoking habit, blood pressure, pulse, sleeping, and mood; monitor skin for side effects if transdermal system used

Patient Information Instructions for the proper use of the patch should be given to the patient; notify physician if persistent rash, itching, or burning may occur with the patch; do not smoke while wearing patches

Nursing Implications Patients should be instructed to chew slowly to avoid jaw ache and to maximize benefit; patches cannot be cut; use of an aerosol corticosteroid may diminish local irritation under patches

Special Geriatric Considerations Must evaluate benefit in elderly who may have chronic diseases mentioned in Warning and Contraindications. The transdermal systems are as effective in elderly as they are in younger adults; however, complaints of body aches, dizziness, and asthenia were reported more often in elderly.

Dosage Forms
Patch, transdermal:
Habitrol™: 21 mg/day; 14 mg/day; 7 mg/day (30 systems/box)
Nicoderm®: 21 mg/day; 14 mg/day; 7 mg/day (14 systems/box)
Nicotrol® [OTC]: 15 mg/day (gradually released over 16 hours)
ProStep®: 22 mg/day; 11 mg/day (7 systems/box)
Pieces, chewing gum, as polacrilex: 2 mg/square [OTC] (96 pieces/box); 4 mg/square (96 pieces/box)
Spray, nasal: 0.5 mg/actuation [10 mg/mL - 200 actuations] (10 mL)

References
Benowitz NL, Jacob P 3rd, and Sachs DP, "Deficient C-oxidation of Nicotine," *Clin Pharmacol Ther*, 1995, 57(5):590-4.
Benowitz NL, "Pharmacologic Aspects of Cigarette Smoking and Nicotine Addiction," *N Engl J Med*, 1988, 319(20):1318-30.
Blanchard J, "Nicotine," *Clin Toxicol Rev*, 1993, 15:11-2.
Harchelroad F, Potts K, Burdick J, et al, "Oral Absorption of Nicotine From Transdermal Therapeutic Systems," *Vet Hum Toxicol*, 1992, 34:332.
Ottervanger JP, Festen JM, de Vries AG, et al, "Acute Myocardial Infarction While Using The Nicotine," *Chest*, 1995, 107(6):1765-6.
Ross MP, Revolinski D, and Taurman L, "Green Tobacco Sickness Among Adults in Kentucky," *Vet Hum Toxicol*, 1994, 36:360.
Svensson CK, "Clinical Pharmacokinetics of Nicotine," *Clin Pharmacokinet*, 1987, 12(1):30-40.
Thomas GA, Rhodes J, Mani V, et al, "Transdermal Nicotine as Maintenance Therapy for Ulcerative Colitis," *N Engl J Med*, 1995, 332(15):988-92.

Nicotinex [OTC] *see Niacin on page 665*

Nicotinic Acid *see Niacin on page 665*

Nicotrol® NS Nasal Spray *see Nicotine on page 669*

Nicotrol® Patch [OTC] *see Nicotine on page 669*

Nico-Vert® [OTC] *see Meclizine on page 574*

Nidryl® Oral [OTC] *see Diphenhydramine on page 302*

Nifedipine (nye FED i peen)
Related Information
Calcium Channel Blocking Agents Comparison *on page 1027*
Brand Names Adalat®; Adalat® CC; Procardia®; Procardia XL®
Generic Available Yes: Capsule
Therapeutic Category Antianginal Agent; Calcium Channel Blocker
Use Angina (vasospastic, chronic stable), hypertrophic cardiomyopathy, hypertension (sustained release only), pulmonary hypertension
Unlabeled use: Migraine headache, Raynaud's syndrome, CHF
Contraindications Known hypersensitivity to nifedipine or any other calcium channel blocker and adenosine; sick sinus syndrome, second or third degree A-V block, hypotension (<90 mm Hg systolic)
Warnings Monitor EKG and blood pressure closely in patients receiving I.V. therapy; hypotension, CHF; cardiac conduction defects, PVCs, idiopathic hypertrophic subaortic stenosis; may cause platelet inhibition; do not abruptly withdraw (chest pain); hepatic dysfunction, renal function impairment, increased angina, increased intracranial pressure with cranial tumors; elderly may have greater hypotensive effect
The FDA's Cardiovascular and Renal Drug Advisory Committee reviewed current data regarding the risk of heart attacks in patients treated with calcium channel blockers and determined that as a class, the calcium channel antagonists are safe; however, they warned that short-acting nifedipine could increase the risk of myocardial infarction in some patients. The committee was in agreement with a statement issued September, 1995 by the National Heart Lung, and Blood Institute of the National Institute of Health, that warned that short-acting nifedipine should be used with great caution especially at higher doses.
Precautions May increase frequency, duration, and severity of angina during initiation of therapy; use with caution in patients with congestive heart failure or aortic stenosis (especially with concomitant beta-adrenergic blocker); sick sinus syndrome, severe left ventricular dysfunction, hepatic impairment, hypertrophic cardiomyopathy (especially obstructive), concomitant therapy with beta-blockers or digoxin, edema
(Continued)

Nifedipine *(Continued)*

Adverse Reactions

Cardiovascular: Flushing, hypotension, tachycardia, palpitations, syncope, headache, facial edema, CHF, increased angina, peripheral edema

Central nervous system: Dizziness, fever, giddiness, ataxia, migraine, chills

Dermatologic: Dermatitis, urticaria, petechiae, bruising, Stevens-Johnson syndrome, alopecia, pruritus, rash, urticaria, erythema multiforme, purpura

Endocrine & metabolic: Gynecomastia, hyperglycemia, gout, breast pain, hypokalemia

Gastrointestinal: Nausea, diarrhea, constipation (especially elderly), gingival hyperplasia, weight gain, gastroesophageal reflux, melena, eructation

Genitourinary: Polyuria, nocturia, dysuria, hematuria, urinary incontinence

Hematologic: Thrombocytopenia, leukopenia, anemia, hematomas

Neuromuscular & skeletal: Joint stiffness, arthritis with increased ANA, muscle cramps, arthralgia

Ocular: Blurred vision, transient blindness, periorbital edema

Respiratory: Shortness of breath, rhinitis, sinusitis, nasal congestion, epistaxis

Miscellaneous: Diaphoresis, gingival swelling and inflammation

Overdosage
Symptoms of overdose include peripheral vasodilation, heart-block, hypotension, asystole, nausea, weakness, dizziness, drowsiness, confusion and slurred speech; profound bradycardia and occasionally hyperglycemia

Toxicology
Ipecac-induced emesis can hypothetically worsen calcium antagonist toxicity, since it can produce vagal stimulation. The potential for seizures precipitously following acute ingestion of large doses of a calcium antagonist may also contraindicate the use of ipecac. Supportive and symptomatic treatment, including I.V. fluids and Trendelenburg positioning, should be initiated as intoxication may cause hypotension. Although calcium (calcium chloride I.V. 1-2 g in adults over 5-10 minutes with repeats as needed) has been used as an "antidote" for acute intoxications, there is limited experience to support its routine use and should be reserved for those cases where definite signs of myocardial depression are evident. Heart block may respond to isoproterenol, glucagon, atropine and/or calcium although a temporary pacemaker may be required.

Drug Interactions

Beta-blockers increased cardiac and A-V conduction depression

Fentanyl increased volume requirements and hypotension; although this drug is new, other drug interactions not reported to the same degree as older agents; however, should be suspect of any drug interaction reported with other calcium channel blockers

Nifedipine metabolism may be inhibited by erythromycin, ketoconazole, itraconazole, protease inhibitors; induced by rifampin, rifabutin

Mechanism of Action
Inhibits calcium ion from entering the "slow channels" or select voltage-sensitive areas of vascular smooth muscle and myocardium during depolarization, producing a relaxation of coronary vascular smooth muscle and coronary vasodilation; increases myocardial oxygen delivery in patients with vasospastic angina

Pharmacodynamics

Onset of action:

Oral: Within 20 minutes

S.L.: Within 1-5 minutes

Pharmacokinetics

Protein binding: 92% to 98% (concentration-dependent)

Metabolism: In the liver to inactive metabolites

Bioavailability:

Capsules: 45% to 75%

Sustained release: 65% to 86%

Half-life:

Normal adults: 2-5 hours

Cirrhosis: 7 hours

Elimination: In urine

Usual Dosage
Geriatrics and Adults: Initial: 10 mg 3 times/day as capsules or 30-60 mg once daily as sustained release tablet; maintenance: 10-30 mg 3-4 times/day (capsules); titrate over a 7- to 14-day period; maximum: 180 mg/24 hours (capsules) or 120 mg/day (sustained release), increase sustained release at 7- to 14-day intervals

Monitoring Parameters
Heart rate, blood pressure, signs and symptoms of CHF, peripheral edema

Reference Range Therapeutic: 25-100 ng/mL

Patient Information Sustained release products should not be crushed or chewed; Adalat® CC should be taken on an empty stomach; limit caffeine intake; avoid alcohol; notify physician if angina pain is not reduced when taking this drug, irregular heartbeat, shortness of breath, swelling, dizziness, constipation, nausea, or hypotension occurs; do not stop therapy without advice of physician; the shell of the sustained-release tablet may appear intact in the stool, this is no cause for concern

Nursing Implications May cause some patients to urinate frequently at night; may cause inflamed gums; capsule may be punctured and drug solution administered sublingually or orally to reduce blood pressure in recumbent patient (see Warnings, Precautions, Adverse Reactions, and Special Geriatric Considerations)

Additional Information Capsule may be punctured and drug solution administered sublingually to reduce blood pressure

Special Geriatric Considerations Elderly may experience a greater hypotensive response; constipation may be more of a problem in elderly; calcium channel blockers are no more effective in elderly than other therapies; however, they do not cause significant CNS effects which is an advantage over some antihypertensive agents.

Dosage Forms
Capsule, liquid-filled (Adalat®, Procardia®): 10 mg, 20 mg
Tablet, extended release (Adalat® CC): 30 mg, 60 mg, 90 mg
Tablet, sustained release (Procardia XL®): 30 mg, 60 mg, 90 mg

References
Rosen WJ and Johnson CE, "Evaluation of Five Procedures for Measuring Nonstandard Doses of Nifedipine Liquid," *Am J Hosp Pharm*, 1989, 46(11):2313-7.

Nilstat® see Nystatin *on page 686*

Nimodipine (nye MOE di peen)
Related Information
Calcium Channel Blocking Agents Comparison *on page 1027*

Brand Names Nimotop®

Therapeutic Category Calcium Channel Blocker

Use Improvement of neurological deficits due to spasm following subarachnoid hemorrhage from ruptured congenital intracranial aneurysms who are in good neurological condition postictus

Unlabeled use: Migraine headache

Contraindications Sinus bradycardia; advanced heart block; ventricular tachycardia; cardiogenic shock, hypotension, CHF; hypersensitivity to nimodipine or any component, calcium channel blockers, and adenosine; atrial fibrillation or flutter associated with accessory conduction pathways; not to be given within a few hours of I.V. beta-blocking agents

Warnings Hypotension, CHF; cardiac conduction defects, PVCs, idiopathic hypertrophic subaortic stenosis; may cause platelet inhibition; do not abruptly withdraw (chest pain); hepatic dysfunction, increased angina, decreased neuromuscular transmission with Duchenne's muscular dystrophy; increased intracranial pressure with cranial tumors; elderly may have greater hypotensive effect

The FDA's Cardiovascular and Renal Drug Advisory Committee reviewed current data regarding the risk of heart attacks in patients treated with calcium channel blockers and determined that as a class, the calcium channel antagonists are safe; however, they warned that short-acting nifedipine could increase the risk of myocardial infarction in some patients. The committee was in agreement with a statement issued September, 1995 by the National Heart Lung, and Blood Institute of the National Institute of Health, that warned that short-acting nifedipine should be used with great caution especially at higher doses.

Adverse Reactions
Cardiovascular: Hypotension, bradycardia, first, second, or third degree A-V block, worsening heart failure, palpitations, CHF, myocardial infarction, angina, tachycardia, peripheral edema
Central nervous system: Headache, fatigue, seizures, dizziness, lightheadedness, psychotic symptoms, insomnia
Gastrointestinal: Constipation (more of a problem in elderly), nausea, abdominal discomfort, diarrhea, xerostomia
Genitourinary: Urinary incontinence
Hepatic: Increase in hepatic enzymes
Neuromuscular & skeletal: Paresthesia, weakness
Ocular: Blurred vision
(Continued)

Nimodipine *(Continued)*

Respiratory: May precipitate insufficiency of respiratory muscle function in Duchenne muscular dystrophy

Overdosage Symptoms of overdose include hypotension, peripheral vasodilation

Toxicology Ipecac-induced emesis can hypothetically worsen calcium antagonist toxicity, since it can produce vagal stimulation. The potential for seizures precipitously following acute ingestion of large doses of a calcium antagonist may also contraindicate the use of ipecac. Supportive and symptomatic treatment, including I.V. fluids and Trendelenburg positioning, should be initiated as intoxication may cause hypotension. Although calcium (calcium chloride I.V. 1-2 g in adults over 5-10 minutes with repeats as needed) has been used as an "antidote" for acute intoxications, there is limited experience to support its routine use and should be reserved for those cases where definite signs of myocardial depression are evident. Heart block may respond to isoproterenol, glucagon, atropine, and/or calcium although a temporary pacemaker may be required.

Drug Interactions

Beta-blockers increased cardiac and A-V conduction depression

Fentanyl increased volume requirements and hypotension; although this drug is new, other drug interactions not reported to the same degree as older agents; however, should be suspect of any drug interaction reported with other calcium channel blockers

Nimodipine metabolism may be inhibited by erythromycin, ketoconazole, itraconazole, protease inhibitors; induced by rifampin, rifabutin

Mechanism of Action Nimodipine is a calcium channel blocker; animal studies indicate that nimodipine has a greater effect on cerebral arterials than other arterials; this increased specificity may be due to the drug's increased lipophilicity and cerebral distribution as compared to nifedipine; inhibits calcium ion from entering the "slow channels" or select voltage sensitive areas of vascular smooth muscle and myocardium during depolarization

Pharmacokinetics

Protein binding: >95%

Metabolism: Extensive in the liver; substrate CYP3A4

Bioavailability: 13% absolute

Half-life: 3 hours, increases with reduced renal function

Time to peak serum concentration: Oral: Within 1 hour

Elimination: In feces (32%) and in urine (50% within 4 days)

Usual Dosage Geriatrics and Adults: Oral: 60 mg every 4 hours for 21 days; if capsule cannot be swallowed, extract capsule contents with 18-gauge needle and empty into NG tube; flush with 30 mL normal saline

Monitoring Parameters CNS response, heart rate, blood pressure, signs and symptoms of congestive heart failure

Reference Range No data

Patient Information Do not crush or chew capsule; notify physician if you experience irregular heartbeat, shortness of breath, swelling, constipation, nausea, hypotension, or dizziness; do not stop or interrupt therapy without advice of physician

Nursing Implications If capsules cannot be swallowed, the liquid may be removed by making a hole in each end of the capsule with an 18-gauge needle and extracting the contents into a syringe; if given via NG tube, follow with a flush of 30 mL NS

Special Geriatric Considerations Elderly may experience a greater hypotensive response; constipation may be more of a problem in elderly; studies in the treatment of Alzheimer's disease have not demonstrated clear clinical effect

Dosage Forms Capsule, liquid-filled: 30 mg

Nimotop® *see* Nimodipine *on previous page*

Nisoldipine *(NYE sole di peen)*

Related Information

Calcium Channel Blocking Agents Comparison *on page 1027*

Brand Names Sular®

Generic Available No

Therapeutic Category Calcium Channel Blocker

Use Management of hypertension, may be used alone or in combination with other antihypertensive agents

Contraindications Hypersensitivity to nisoldipine or any component or other dihydropyridine calcium channel blocker; 2nd or 3rd degree AV block (unless has pacemaker), sick sinus syndrome, hypotension

Warnings Increased angina and/or myocardial infarction in patients with coronary artery disease; hypotension, CHF; cardiac conduction defects, PVCs, idiopathic hypertrophic subaortic stenosis; may cause platelet inhibition; do not abruptly withdraw (chest pain); hepatic dysfunction, increased angina, increased intracranial pressure with cranial tumors; elderly may have greater hypotensive effect

The FDA's Cardiovascular and Renal Drug Advisory Committee reviewed current data regarding the risk of heart attacks in patients treated with calcium channel blockers and determined that as a class, the calcium channel antagonists are safe.

Precautions May increase frequency, duration, and severity of angina during initiation of therapy; use with caution in patients with congestive heart failure or aortic stenosis (especially with concomitant beta-adrenergic blocker); sick sinus syndrome, severe left ventricular dysfunction, hepatic impairment, hypertrophic cardiomyopathy (especially obstructive), concomitant therapy with beta-blockers or digoxin, edema

Adverse Reactions

Cardiovascular: Flushing, hypotension, tachycardia, palpitations, syncope, headache, facial edema, CHF, increased angina, peripheral edema

Central nervous system: Dizziness, fever, giddiness, ataxia, migraine, chills

Dermatologic: Dermatitis, urticaria, petechiae, bruising, Stevens-Johnson syndrome, alopecia, pruritus, rash, urticaria, erythema multiforme, purpura

Endocrine & metabolic: Gynecomastia, hyperglycemia, gout, breast pain, hypokalemia

Gastrointestinal: Nausea, diarrhea, constipation (especially elderly), gingival hyperplasia, weight gain, gastroesophageal reflux, melena, eructation, gingival swelling and inflammation

Genitourinary: Polyuria, nocturia, dysuria, hematuria, urinary incontinence

Hematologic: Thrombocytopenia, leukopenia, anemia, hematomas

Neuromuscular & skeletal: Joint stiffness, arthritis with increased ANA, muscle cramps, arthralgia

Ocular: Blurred vision, transient blindness, periorbital edema

Respiratory: Shortness of breath, rhinitis, sinusitis, nasal congestion, epistaxis

Miscellaneous: Diaphoresis

Overdosage The primary cardiac symptoms of calcium blocker overdose includes hypotension and bradycardia. The hypotension is caused by peripheral vasodilation, myocardial depression, and bradycardia. Bradycardia results from sinus bradycardia, second- or third-degree atrioventricular block, or sinus arrest with junctional rhythm. Intraventricular conduction is usually not affected so QRS duration is normal.

The noncardiac symptoms include confusion, stupor, nausea, vomiting, metabolic acidosis and hyperglycemia

Toxicology Following initial gastric decontamination, if possible, repeated calcium administration may promptly reverse the depressed cardiac contractility (but not sinus node depression or peripheral vasodilation); glucagon, epinephrine, and amrinone may treat refractory hypotension; glucagon and epinephrine also increase the heart rate (outside the U.S., 4-aminopyridine may be available as an antidote); dialysis and hemoperfusion are not effective in enhancing elimination although repeat-dose activated charcoal may serve as an adjunct with sustained release preparations.

Drug Interactions

Beta-blockers increased cardiac and A-V conduction depression

Fentanyl increased volume requirements and hypotension; although this drug is new, other drug interactions not reported to the same degree as older agents; however, should be suspect of any drug interaction reported with other calcium channel blockers

Nisoldipine metabolism may be inhibited by erythromycin, ketoconazole, itraconazole, protease inhibitors; induced by rifampin, rifabutin

Drug/Food Interactions High fat meals may result in excessive peak serum concentrations and, therefore, should be avoided

Mechanism of Action As a dihydropyridine calcium channel blocker, structurally similar to nifedipine, nisoldipine impedes the movement of calcium ions into vascular smooth muscle and cardiac muscle. Dihydropyridines are potent vasodilators and are not as likely to suppress cardiac contractility and slow
(Continued)

Nisoldipine *(Continued)*

cardiac conduction as other calcium antagonists such as verapamil and dilti-azem; nisoldipine is 5-10 times as potent a vasodilator as nifedipine.

Pharmacokinetics

Absorption: Well absorbed

Metabolism: Extensive presystemic metabolism in the intestinal wall and the liver; hepatically metabolized to inactive metabolites; substrate CYP3A4

Bioavailability: 5%; T_{max}: 6-12 hours

Half-life: 7-12 hours

Elimination: Hepatic metabolism with metabolites excreted in the urine; only a trace of unchanged drug excreted in urine

Usual Dosage Oral:

Geriatrics: 10 mg/day, increase by 10 mg/week (or longer intervals) to attain adequate blood pressure control; also, those with hepatic disease should be started with 10 mg/day

Adults: Initial: 20 mg once daily, then increase by 10 mg/week (or longer intervals) to attain adequate control of blood pressure; doses >60 mg once daily are not recommended

Administration Avoid taking with high fat meals; avoid grapefruit products before and after dosing

Monitoring Parameters Heart rate, blood pressure, signs and symptoms of CHF, peripheral edema

Patient Information Avoid grapefruit products before and after dosing; administration with a high fat meal can lead to excessive peak drug concentrations and should be avoided; do not crush tablets

Nursing Implications Administer at the same time each day to ensure minimal fluctuation of serum concentrations; do not crush tablets

Additional Information Initial data indicate that once daily doses of 10-40 mg are about as effective as hydrochlorothiazide, lisinopril, or amlodipine; doses of 20-60 mg are about as effective as twice daily verapamil in lowering blood pressure in patients with mild to moderate hypertension; although there are some initial data which may show increased risk of myocardial infarction following treatment of hypertension with calcium channel blockers, controlled trials (eg, ALL-HAT) are ongoing to examine the long-term effects of not only the calcium channel blockers, but also other antihypertensives in preventing heart disease. Until done, patients taking these agents should be encouraged to continue with prescribed antihypertension regimens although a switch from high-dose, short-acting agents to sustained release products may be warranted. Many practitioners agree to avoid calcium channel blockers as primary treatment for hypertension unless diuretics or beta-blockers are contraindicated.

Special Geriatric Considerations Elderly may experience a greater hypotensive response; constipation may be more of a problem in elderly; calcium channel blockers are no more effective in elderly than other therapies; however, they do not cause significant CNS effects which is an advantage over some antihypertensive agents.

Dosage Forms Tablet, extended release: 10 mg, 20 mg, 30 mg, 40 mg

Nitro-Bid® I.V. Injection *see* Nitroglycerin *on next page*

Nitro-Bid® Ointment *see* Nitroglycerin *on next page*

Nitrodisc® Patch *see* Nitroglycerin *on next page*

Nitro-Dur® Patch *see* Nitroglycerin *on next page*

Nitrofurantoin *(nye troe fyoor AN toyn)*

Related Information

Antacid Drug Interactions *on page 1096*

Penicillins, Penicillin-Related Antibiotics, & Other Antibiotics *on page 1010*

Brand Names Furadantin®; Furalan®; Furan®; Furanite®; Macrobid®; Macrodantin®

Generic Available Yes: Tablet and suspension

Therapeutic Category Antibiotic, Miscellaneous

Use Prevention and treatment of urinary tract infections caused by susceptible gram-negative and some gram-positive organisms; *Pseudomonas*, *Serratia*, and most species of *Proteus* are generally resistant to nitrofurantoin

Contraindications Hypersensitivity to nitrofurantoin or any component; renal impairment

Warnings Therapeutic concentrations of nitrofurantoin are not attained in the urine of patients with Cl_{cr} <40 mL/minute

Precautions Use with caution in patients with G-6-PD deficiency, patients with anemia, vitamin B deficiency, diabetes mellitus or electrolyte abnormalities; superinfection

Adverse Reactions
Cardiovascular: Chest pains
Central nervous system: Dizziness, headache, fever, chills, drowsiness
Dermatologic: Rash, exfoliative dermatitis, urticaria
Gastrointestinal: Nausea, vomiting, anorexia, pancreatitis, sore throat
Hematologic: Hemolytic anemia
Hepatic: Hepatotoxicity
Neuromuscular & skeletal: Peripheral neuropathy, arthralgia
Respiratory: Interstitial pneumonitis and/or fibrosis, asthma, cough

Overdosage Symptoms of overdose include vomiting

Drug Interactions
Probenecid decreased renal excretion of nitrofurantoin, antacids decreased absorption of nitrofurantoin
Anticholinergic drugs and food increased absorption of nitrofurantoin
Magnesium trisilicate delays or decreases absorption

Mechanism of Action Inhibits several bacterial enzyme systems including acetyl coenzyme A

Pharmacokinetics
Absorption: Well from the GI tract; the macrocrystalline form is absorbed more slowly due to slower dissolution, but causes less GI distress
Distribution: V_d: 0.8 L/kg
Protein binding: ~40%
Metabolism: 60% of the drug is metabolized by body tissues throughout the body, with the exception of plasma, to inactive metabolites
Bioavailability: Presence of food increases bioavailability
Half-life: 20-60 minutes and is prolonged with renal impairment
Elimination: As metabolites and unchanged drug (40%) in urine and small amounts in bile; renal excretion is via glomerular filtration and tubular secretion

Usual Dosage Geriatrics and Adults: Oral: 50-100 mg every 6 hours
Prophylaxis: 50-100 mg/dose at bedtime (see Special Geriatric Considerations)

Administration Higher peak serum concentrations may cause increased GI upset; administer with meals to slow the rate of absorption and thus decrease adverse effects; administer around-the-clock rather than 4 times/day, 3 times/day, etc (ie, 12-6-12-6, not 9-1-5-9) to promote less variation in peak and trough serum concentration

Monitoring Parameters Signs of pulmonary reaction, signs of numbness or tingling of the extremities; periodic liver function tests; signs and symptoms of infection

Test Interactions Causes false-positive urine glucose with Clinitest®

Patient Information Take with food or milk; may discolor urine to a dark yellow or brown color; complete full course of therapy; notify physician or pharmacist if diarrhea, tingling in extremities, skin rash, or difficulty breathing occurs

Nursing Implications See Administration

Special Geriatric Considerations Because of nitrofurantoin's decreased efficacy in patients with a Cl_{cr} <40 mL/minute and its side effect profile, it is not an antibiotic of choice for acute or prophylactic treatment of urinary tract infections in the elderly.

Dosage Forms
Capsule: 50 mg, 100 mg
Capsule:
Extended release: 100 mg
Macrocrystal: 25 mg, 50 mg, 100 mg
Macrocrystal/monohydrate: 100 mg
Suspension, oral: 25 mg/5 mL (470 mL)

Nitrogard® Buccal see Nitroglycerin *on this page*

Nitroglycerin (nye troe GLI ser in)

Brand Names Deponit® Patch; Minitran® Patch; Nitro-Bid® I.V. Injection; Nitro-Bid® Ointment; Nitrodisc® Patch; Nitro-Dur® Patch; Nitrogard® Buccal; Nitroglyn® Oral; Nitrolingual® Translingual Spray; Nitrol® Ointment; Nitrong® Oral Tablet; Nitrostat® Sublingual; Transdermal-NTG® Patch; Transderm-Nitro® Patch; Tridil® Injection

Synonyms Glyceryl Trinitrate; Nitroglycerol; NTG
(Continued)

Nitroglycerin *(Continued)*

Generic Available Yes

Therapeutic Category Antianginal Agent; Nitrate; Vasodilator, Coronary

Use Angina pectoris; I.V. for congestive heart failure (especially when associated with acute myocardial infarction); pulmonary hypertension; hypertensive emergencies occurring perioperatively (especially during cardiovascular surgery)

Unlabeled use: Oral, sublingual, and topical routes have been used to reduce preload in patients with CHF and myocardial infarction; nitroglycerine ointment has been used as adjunctive treatment of Raynaud's disease. Oral nitrates are used in esophageal spastic disorders.

Contraindications Hypersensitivity to nitroglycerin or any component; closed-angle glaucoma; severe anemia, postural hypotension, early myocardial infarction, head trauma, cerebral hemorrhage, allergy to adhesive (transdermal), uncorrected hypovolemia (I.V.), inadequate cerebral circulation, increased intracranial pressure, constrictive pericarditis, pericardial tamponade; transdermal NTG is not effective for immediate relief of angina

Warnings Do not chew or swallow sublingual dosage form

Precautions Do not use extended release preparations in patients with GI hypermotility or malabsorptive syndrome; use with caution in patients with hypovolemia, constrictive pericarditis, hypertension, and hypotension; use with caution in patients with increased intracranial pressure; do not abruptly withdraw therapy for treatment of angina

Adverse Reactions

Cardiovascular: Flushing, headache, hypotension, reflex tachycardia, severe hypotension and bradycardia have been described; abrupt withdrawal may result in acute coronary vascular insufficiency

Central nervous system: Dizziness, restlessness

Dermatologic: Allergic contact dermatitis may be seen with ointment and patches

Gastrointestinal: Nausea, vomiting

Miscellaneous: Perspiration and collapse, pallor

Overdosage Symptoms of overdose include hypotension, throbbing headache, palpitations, bloody diarrhea, bradycardia, cyanosis, tissue hypoxia, metabolic acidosis, clonic convulsions, circulatory collapse

Toxicology If ingested, perform gastric lavage or induce emesis followed by charcoal administration; keep patient warm and in recumbent position to prevent shock; administer oxygen and artificial ventilation if needed. Monitor methemoglobin levels if indicated; if severely hypotensive, elevate legs; administer I.V. fluids, consider alpha-adrenergics; treat methemoglobinemia if present.

Drug Interactions I.V. nitroglycerin may antagonize the anticoagulant effect of heparin, monitor closely, may need to decrease heparin dosage when nitroglycerin is discontinued; alcohol, beta-blockers, calcium channel blockers may enhance nitroglycerin's hypotensive effect

Stability I.V. infusion solution in NS or D_5W, is stable for 48 hours at room temperature, mixed and stored in glass containers; maximum concentration not to exceed 400 mcg/mL; do not mix with other drugs; store sublingual tablets and ointment in tightly closed container; store at 15°C to 30°C

Mechanism of Action Relax vascular smooth muscle via stimulation of intracellular cyclic GMP production which stimulates a cyclic GMP-dependent protein kinases that alters phosphorylation of the smooth muscle myosin resulting in relaxation of the muscle; venous dilation is predominate action causing peripheral pooling which decreases venous return to heart and, therefore, workload, central venous pressure, and pulmonary capillary wedge pressure; reduction in pulmonary vascular resistance occurs secondary to pulmonary arterial dilation; reduces cardiac oxygen demand by decreasing left ventricular pressure and systemic vascular resistance; dilates coronary arteries and improves collateral flow to ischemic regions

Pharmacodynamics Onset and duration of action is dependent upon dosage form administered; see table.

Pharmacokinetics

Protein binding: 60%

Metabolism: Extensive first-pass

Half-life: 1-4 minutes

Elimination: Excretion of inactive metabolites in urine

Dosage Form	Onset of Effect	Peak Effect	Duration
Sublingual tablet	1-3 min	4-8 min	30-60 min
Lingual spray	2 min	4-10 min	30-60 min
Buccal tablet	2-5 min	4-10 min	2 h
Sustained release	20-45 min	45-120 min	4-8 h
Topical	15-60 min	30-120 min	2-12 h
Transdermal	40-60 min	60-180 min	8-24 h
I.V. drip	Immediate	Immediate	3-5 min

Usual Dosage Geriatrics and Adults:

Buccal: Initial: 1 mg every 5 hours while awake (3 times/day); titrate dosage upward if angina occurs with tablet in place

Oral: 2.5-9 mg every 8-12 hours (see Additional Information)

I.V.: 5 mcg/minute, increase by 5 mcg/minute every 3-5 minutes to 20 mcg/minute, then increase by 10 mcg/minute every 3-5 minutes, up to 200 mcg/minute

Lingual: 1-2 sprays into mouth under tongue every 3-5 minutes for maximum of 3 doses in 15 minutes

Ointment: 1" to 2" every 8 hours (see Additional Information)

Patch, transdermal: 2.5-15 mg/24 hours (recommended to remove patch at bedtime for a drug-free period of 10-12 hours)

Sublingual: 0.2-0.6 mg every 5 minutes for maximum of 3 doses in 15 minutes

Monitoring Parameters Orthostatic blood pressure, blood pressure, heart rate; therapeutic dose may be determined by observing for a decrease in systolic blood pressure by 15 mm Hg, diastolic reduction of 10 mm Hg or an increase in heart rate of 10 bpm

Test Interactions Increased catecholamines (U)

Patient Information Go to hospital or call 911 if no relief after 3 sublingual doses; do not swallow or chew sublingual form; keep in original container and tightly closed; remove and do not reinsert cotton plug; for the sublingual tablets, it is best to get a fresh bottle 3-6 months after opening. Get instructions on proper use of transdermal patches or ointment.

Nitroglycerin

Product	Release Rate		Surface Area (cm²)	Total Content (mg)
	mg/h	mg/24 h		
Deponit®				
5	0.2	5	16	16
10	0.42	10	32	32
Minitran®				
2.5	0.1	2.5	3.3	9
5	0.2	5	6.7	18
10	0.42	10	13.3	36
15	0.625	15	20	54
Nitrocine®				
5	0.2	5	10	62.5
10	0.42	10	20	125
15	0.625	15	30	187.5
Nitrodisc®				
5	0.2	5	8	6
7.5	0.312	7.5	12	24
10	0.42	10	16	32
Nitro-Dur®				
2.5	0.1	2.5	5	20
5	0.2	5	10	40
7.5	0.312	7.5	15	60
10	0.42	10	20	80
15	0.625	15	30	120
Transderm-Nitro®				
2.5	0.1	2.5	5	12.5
5	0.2	5	10	25
10	0.42	10	20	50
15	0.625	15	30	75

(Continued)

Nitroglycerin *(Continued)*

Nursing Implications I.V. must be prepared in glass bottles and use special sets intended for nitroglycerin; transdermal patches labeled as mg/hour; do not crush sublingual drug product

Additional Information I.V. preparations contain alcohol and/or propylene glycol; may need to use nitrate-free internal (10-12 hours/day) to avoid tolerance development; tolerance may possibly be reversed with acetylcysteine; gradually decrease dose in patients receiving NTG for prolonged period to avoid withdrawal reaction

Special Geriatric Considerations Caution should be used when using nitrate therapy in elderly due to hypotension; hypotension is enhanced in elderly due to decreased baroreceptor response, decreased venous tone, and often hypovolemia (dehydration) or other hypotensive drugs

Dosage Forms

Capsule, sustained release: 2.5 mg, 6.5 mg, 9 mg

Injection: 0.5 mg/mL (10 mL); 0.8 mg/mL (10 mL); 5 mg/mL (1 mL, 5 mL, 10 mL, 20 mL); 10 mg/mL (5 mL, 10 mL)

Ointment, topical (Nitrol®): 2% (30 g, 60 g)

Patch, transdermal: Systems designed to deliver 2.5 mg, 5 mg, 7.5 mg, 10 mg, or 15 mg NTG over 24 hours. See table.

Spray, translingual: 0.4 mg/metered spray (13.8 g)

Tablet:

Buccal, controlled release: 1 mg, 2 mg, 3 mg

Sublingual (Nitrostat®): 0.15 mg, 0.3 mg, 0.4 mg, 0.6 mg

Sustained release: 2.6 mg, 6.5 mg, 9 mg

References

Elkayam U, "Tolerance to Organic Nitrates: Evidence, Mechanisms, Clinical Relevance, and Strategies for Prevention," *Ann Intern Med*, 1991, 114(8):667-77.

Nitroglycerol *see* Nitroglycerin *on page 677*

Nitroglyn® Oral *see* Nitroglycerin *on page 677*

Nitrolingual® Translingual Spray *see* Nitroglycerin *on page 677*

Nitrol® Ointment *see* Nitroglycerin *on page 677*

Nitrong® Oral Tablet *see* Nitroglycerin *on page 677*

Nitropress® *see* Nitroprusside *on this page*

Nitroprusside *(nye troe PRUS ide)*

Brand Names Nitropress®

Synonyms Sodium Nitroferricyanide; Sodium Nitroprusside

Generic Available Yes

Therapeutic Category Vasodilator

Use Management of hypertensive crises; congestive heart failure; used for controlled hypotension to reduce bleeding during surgery

Contraindications Hypersensitivity to nitroprusside or components; decreased cerebral perfusion; arteriovenous shunt or coarctation of the aorta (ie, compensatory hypertension)

Warnings Use only as an infusion with 5% dextrose in water; continuously monitor patient's blood pressure; excessive amounts of nitroprusside can cause cyanide toxicity (usually in patients with decreased liver function) or thiocyanate toxicity (usually in patients with decreased renal function, or in patients with normal renal function but prolonged nitroprusside use)

Precautions Use with caution in patients with increased intracranial pressure (head trauma, cerebral hemorrhage); severe renal impairment, hepatic failure, hypothyroidism, hyponatremia

Adverse Reactions

Cardiovascular: Excessive hypotensive response, palpitations

Central nervous system: Restlessness, disorientation, psychosis, headache, increased intracranial pressure

Endocrine & metabolic: Thyroid suppression, thiocyanate toxicity

Gastrointestinal: Nausea, vomiting

Neuromuscular & skeletal: Muscle spasm, weakness

Otic: Tinnitus

Respiratory: Substernal distress, hypoxia

Miscellaneous: Diaphoresis

Overdosage Symptoms of overdose include hypotension, vomiting, hyperventilation, tachycardia, muscular twitching, hypothyroidism, cyanide or thiocyanate toxicity

Toxicology Thiocyanate toxicity includes psychosis, hyper-reflexia, confusion, weakness, tinnitus, seizures, and coma; cyanide toxicity includes acidosis (decreased HCO_3, decreased pH, increased lactate), increase in mixed venous blood oxygen tension, tachycardia, altered consciousness, coma, convulsions, and almond smell on breath. Nitroprusside has been shown to release cyanide *in vivo* with hemoglobin. Cyanide toxicity does not usually occur because of the rapid uptake of cyanide by erythrocytes and its eventual incorporation into cyanocobalamin. However, prolonged administration of nitroprusside or its reduced elimination can lead to cyanide intoxication. In these situations, airway support with oxygen therapy is germane, followed closely with antidotal therapy of amyl nitrate perles, sodium nitrate 300 mg I.V. and sodium thiosulfate 12.5 g I.V.

Stability Discard solution 24 hours after reconstitution and dilution in D_5W; promptly wrap in aluminum foil or other opaque material to protect from light; reconstituted solution should be very faint brown, discard if highly colored (blue, green or red); store powder in carton until ready to use

Mechanism of Action Causes peripheral vasodilation by direct action on venous and arteriolar smooth muscle, thus reducing peripheral resistance; will increase cardiac output by decreasing afterload; reduces aortal and left ventricular impedance

Pharmacodynamics
Onset of action: Hypotensive effects occur in <2 minutes
Duration: Following discontinuation of therapy, effects cease within 1-10 minutes

Pharmacokinetics
Metabolism: Converted to cyanide by erythrocyte and tissue sulfhydryl group interactions; cyanide is converted in the liver by rhodanese to thiocyanate
Half-life: <10 minutes; half-life (thiocyanate): 2.7-7 days
Elimination: In urine

Usual Dosage Geriatrics and Adults: I.V.: Continuous infusion: Start 0.5 mcg/kg/minute, titrate to effect; usual dose: 3 mcg/kg/minute, rarely need >4 mcg/kg/minute; maximum: 10 mcg/kg/minute

Monitoring Parameters Blood pressure, cardiac status, thiocyanate levels

Reference Range Monitor thiocyanate levels if requiring prolonged infusion (>4 days) or ≥4 µg/kg/minute; Therapeutic: 6-29 µg/mL (SI: 103-499 µmol/L)

Nursing Implications I.V. infusion only, not for direct injection; protect from light; brownish solution is usable, discard if bluish in color

Additional Information Nitroprusside is converted to cyanide ions in the bloodstream; decomposes to prussic acid which in the presence of sulfur donor is converted to thiocyanate (liver and kidney rhodanase systems); thiocyanate is then renally eliminated

Special Geriatric Considerations Elderly patients may have an increased sensitivity to nitroprusside possibly due to a decreased baroreceptor reflex, altered sensitivity to vasodilating effects or a resistance of cardiac adrenergic receptors to stimulation by catecholamines

Dosage Forms Injection, as sodium: 10 mg/mL (5 mL); 25 mg/mL (2 mL)

Nitrostat® Sublingual *see Nitroglycerin on page 677*

Nix™ Creme Rinse *see Permethrin on page 730*

Nizatidine (ni ZA ti deen)

Brand Names Axid®; Axid® AR [OTC]
Generic Available No
Therapeutic Category Histamine H_2 Antagonist
Use Treatment and maintenance of duodenal ulcer, benign gastric ulcer, GERD

Contraindications Hypersensitivity to nizatidine or any component; hypersensitivity to other H_2 blockers since a cross-sensitivity has been observed in this class of drugs

Warnings Adjust dosages in renal/hepatic impairment; elderly due to renal decline with age

Precautions Modify dosage in patients with renal and/or hepatic impairment; gastric malignancy may be masked, gynecomastia; cardiac arrhythmias and hypotension; CNS side effects (confusion, depression, psychosis, hallucinations, anxiety)

Adverse Reactions
Cardiovascular: Ventricular (asymptomatic) tachycardia
Central nervous system: Somnolence, headache, fatigue, dizziness, hallucinations, insomnia, fever
Dermatologic: Urticaria, exfoliative dermatitis, rash, pruritus
(Continued)

Nizatidine *(Continued)*

Endocrine & metabolic: Gynecomastia, hyperuricemia
Gastrointestinal: Nausea, vomiting, abdominal pain, diarrhea, constipation
Genitourinary: Impotence, loss of libido
Hematologic: Eosinophilia, thrombocytopenia
Hepatic: Cholestatic and hepatocellular damage
Miscellaneous: Diaphoresis

Overdosage No experience with intentional overdose; reported ingestions of 20 g have had transient side effects seen with recommended doses; animal data have shown respiratory failure, tachycardia, muscle tremors, vomiting, restlessness, hypotension, salivation, emesis, and diarrhea (LD$_{50}$ ~80 mg/kg)

Toxicology Treatment is primarily symptomatic and supportive

Drug Interactions Does not bind to cytochrome P-450 *in vitro*; antacids may decrease absorption (~10%); aspirin (increased levels) with high doses (3.9 g/day), diazepam; food may increase absorption

Mechanism of Action Nizatidine is an H$_2$ receptor antagonist. In healthy volunteers, nizatidine has been effective in suppressing gastric acid secretion induced by pentagastrin infusion or food. Nizatidine reduces gastric acid secretion by 29.4% to 78.4%. This compares with a 60.3% reduction by cimetidine. Nizatidine 100 mg is reported to provide equivalent acid suppression as cimetidine 300 mg.

Pharmacokinetics
Bioavailability: >90% (rapidly absorbed)
Protein binding: ~35%
Time to peak serum concentration: 0.5-3 hours
Elimination:
Renal: Unchanged, 60%
Hepatic: <18%

Usual Dosage Geriatrics and Adults: Oral: 300 mg at bedtime or 150 mg twice daily; maintenance: 150 mg once daily (bedtime); GERD 150 mg twice daily

Dosing interval in renal impairment:
Cl$_{cr}$ 20-50 mL/minute: Administer 150 mg/day for duodenal ulcer; 150 mg every other day for maintenance therapy
Cl$_{cr}$ <20 mL/minute: Administer 150 mg every other day; 150 mg every third day for maintenance therapy

Monitoring Parameters Signs and symptoms of peptic ulcer disease, occult blood with GI bleeding, gastric pH where necessary; monitor renal function to correct dose; monitor for side effects

Test Interactions False-positive tests for urobilinogen

Patient Information May take several days before relief of stomach pain occurs; take with or immediately after meals; inform pharmacist and physician (nurse practitioner) of any concomitant drug therapy; stagger doses with antacids with this medication by taking antacids 30-60 minutes before or after taking nizatidine

Nursing Implications Giving a dose at 6 PM may more effectively suppress nocturnal acid secretion than giving a dose at 10 PM (see Warnings, Precautions, Monitoring Parameters, and Special Geriatric Considerations)

Special Geriatric Considerations H$_2$ blockers are the preferred drugs for treating peptic ulcer disorder (PUD) in elderly due to cost and ease of administration. These agents are no less or more effective than any other therapy. The preferred agents (due to side effects and drug interaction profile and pharmacokinetics) are ranitidine, famotidine, and nizatidine. Treatment for PUD in elderly is recommended for 12 weeks since their lesions are larger, and therefore, take longer to heal; always adjust dose based upon creatinine clearance.

Dosage Forms
Capsule: 150 mg, 300 mg
Tablet [OTC]: 75 mg

References
Fennerty MD and Higbee M, "Drug Therapy of Gastrointestinal Disease," *Geriatric Pharmacology*, Bressler R and Katz MD, eds, New York, NY: McGraw-Hill, 1993, 585-608.

Nizoral® *see* Ketoconazole *on page 513*

Nolvadex® *see* Tamoxifen *on page 887*

No Pain-HP® **[OTC]** *see* Capsaicin *on page 155*

Norcet® *see* Hydrocodone and Acetaminophen *on page 461*

Nordeoxyguanosine *see* Ganciclovir *on page 419*

Nordryl® **Injection** *see* Diphenhydramine *on page 302*

Nordryl® **Oral** *see* Diphenhydramine *on page 302*

Norflex™ *see* Orphenadrine *on page 697*

Norfloxacin (nor FLOKS a sin)
Related Information
Antacid Drug Interactions *on page 1096*
Cephalosporins, Aminoglycosides, Macrolides, & Quinolones *on page 1014*
Brand Names Chibroxin™ Ophthalmic; Noroxin® Oral
Generic Available No
Therapeutic Category Antibiotic, Ophthalmic; Antibiotic, Quinolone
Use Complicated and uncomplicated urinary tract infections caused by susceptible gram-negative and gram-positive bacteria; ophthalmic solution for conjunctivitis
Contraindications Known hypersensitivity to quinolones including cinoxacin and nalidixic acid
Warnings Convulsion in persons with CNS disorders (seizure disorder, increased intracranial pressure, and toxic psychosis); CNS stimulation, tremor, headache, pseudomembranous colitis
Precautions Superinfection, crystalluria, phototoxicity
Adverse Reactions
Central nervous system: Headache, dizziness, fatigue, hallucinations, confusion
Dermatologic: Erythema multiforme
Gastrointestinal: Nausea, xerostomia, flatulence, abdominal pain, vomiting, heartburn, diarrhea
Hematologic: Leukopenia
Hepatic: Increased liver function tests, hepatitis
Neuromuscular & skeletal: Tremors
Renal: Acute renal failure, increased creatinine and BUN
Drug Interactions
Antacids, iron salts, sucralfate, zinc salts may reduce absorption by up to 98% if given at the same time
Antineoplastic agents may decrease norfloxacin levels
Cimetidine may increase levels
Nitrofurantoin may antagonize norfloxacin's effects
Probenecid may decrease urinary excretion
Norfloxacin may increase the effects of anticoagulants, increase nephrotoxicity of cyclosporine, and decrease clearance (increase levels) of theophylline and caffeine, hence, monitor appropriately
Mechanism of Action Exerts a broad spectrum antimicrobial effect. The primary target of the fluoroquinolones is DNA gyrase (topoisomerase II), an essential bacterial enzyme that maintains the superhelical structure of DNA. DNA gyrase is required for DNA replication and transcription, DNA repair, recombination, and transposition.
Pharmacokinetics
Absorption: Oral: Rapid, up to 40%
Protein binding: 15%
Metabolism: In the liver; inhibitor CYP1A2
Half-life: 4.8 hours (can be higher with reduced glomerular filtration rates)
Time to peak serum concentration: Within 1-2 hours
Elimination: In urine and feces (30%); increased area under the curve (AUC), a 30% to 40% decrease in renal clearance without a significant change in half-life has been reported in elderly
Usual Dosage Geriatrics and Adults:
Oral: 400 mg twice daily for 7-21 days depending on infection; do not administer as single or 3-day course of therapy; treat prostatitis for 28 days
Ophthalmic: Instill 1-2 drops in affected eye(s) 4 times/day for up to 7 days
Dosing interval in renal impairment: Oral: $Cl_{cr} \leq 30$ mL/minute/1.73 m²: Administer 400 mg once daily for appropriate duration
Administration Hold antacids and sucralfate for 2-4 hours before and after giving dose
Monitoring Parameters Signs and symptoms of infection, WBC, mental status, culture, and sensitivity
Patient Information Take 1 hour before or 2 hours after meals; do not take with antacids, dairy products, iron, or zinc products; may cause dizziness, headache, or stimulation; avoid excess natural or artificial sunlight exposure; complete full course of therapy
Nursing Implications See Administration
(Continued)

Norfloxacin (Continued)

Special Geriatric Considerations Assess ability to self-administer eye drops; adjust dose for renal function (see Pharmacokinetics and Usual Dosage)

Dosage Forms
Solution, ophthalmic: 0.3% [3 mg/mL] (5 mL)
Tablet: 400 mg

References
Nilsson-Ehle I and Ljungberg B, "Quinolone Disposition in the Elderly: Practical Implications," *Drugs Aging*, 1991, 1(4):279-88.

Norisodrine® *see* Isoproterenol *on page 501*
Normal Saline *see* Sodium Chloride *on page 860*
Normiflo® *see* Ardeparin *on page 80*
Normodyne® *see* Labetalol *on page 520*
Noroxin® Oral *see* Norfloxacin *on previous page*
Norpace® *see* Disopyramide *on page 309*
Norpramin® *see* Desipramine *on page 271*
Nor-tet® Oral *see* Tetracycline *on page 900*

Nortriptyline (nor TRIP ti leen)

Related Information
Antidepressant Agents Comparison *on page 1021*
Antidepressant Medication Guidelines *on page 1075*
Federal OBRA Regulations Recommended Maximum Doses - Antidepressants *on page 1056*
Serum Drug Concentrations Commonly Monitored: Guidelines *on page 1114*

Brand Names Aventyl® Hydrochloride; Pamelor®
Therapeutic Category Antidepressant, Tricyclic
Use Treatment of various forms of depression, often in conjunction with psychotherapy
    Unlabeled use: Panic disorder, chronic urticaria, angioedema, nocturnal pruritus, and neuropathic pain
Contraindications Narrow-angle glaucoma
Precautions Use with caution in patients with cardiac conduction disturbances, history of hyperthyroidism, bipolar illness; renal or hepatic impairment; nortriptyline should not be abruptly discontinued in patients receiving high doses for prolonged periods; to avoid cholinergic crisis; an EKG prior to initiating therapy is advised
Adverse Reactions
Cardiovascular: Postural hypotension, arrhythmias, tachycardia, sudden death
Central nervous system: Sedation, fatigue, anxiety, impaired cognitive function, seizures have occurred occasionally, delirium, headache
Gastrointestinal: Xerostomia, constipation, increased appetite
Genitourinary: Urinary retention
Hematologic: Rarely agranulocytosis, eosinophilia
Hepatic: Jaundice
Neuromuscular & skeletal: Tremors, weakness
Ocular: Blurred vision, increased intraocular pressure
Miscellaneous: Allergic reactions
Overdosage Symptoms of overdose include agitation, confusion, hallucinations, urinary retention, hypothermia, hypotension, tachycardia
Toxicology Following initiation of essential overdose management, toxic symptoms should be treated. Ventricular arrhythmias often respond to phenytoin 15-20 mg/kg with concurrent systemic alkalinization (sodium bicarbonate 0.5-2 mEq/kg I.V.). Arrhythmias unresponsive to this therapy may respond to lidocaine 1 mg/kg I.V. followed by a titrated infusion. Physostigmine (1-2 mg I.V. slowly) may be indicated in reversing cardiac arrhythmias that are due to vagal blockade or for anticholinergic effects. Seizures usually respond to diazepam I.V. boluses (5-10 mg, up to 30 mg). If seizures are unresponsive or recur, phenytoin or phenobarbital may be required.
Drug Interactions
Nortriptyline blocks the uptake of guanethidine and thus prevents the hypotensive effect of guanethidine; nortriptyline may be additive with or may potentiate the action of other CNS depressants, anticholinergic agents, dicumarol; nortriptyline potentiates the pressor and cardiac effects of sympathomimetic agents such as isoproterenol, epinephrine, etc; cimetidine, fluoxetine, methylphenidate, and haloperidol may decrease the

metabolism and/or elevate TCA levels; phenobarbital may increase TCA metabolism; disulfiram may increase bioavailability

With MAO inhibitors, hyperpyrexia, hypertension, tachycardia, confusion, seizures, and death have been reported

Additive anticholinergic effects seen with other anticholinergic agents

Clonidine used concurrently has been reported to cause hypertensive crisis and increase blood pressure

Stability Protect from light

Mechanism of Action Traditionally believed to increase the synaptic concentration of serotonin and/or norepinephrine in the central nervous system by inhibition of their reuptake by the presynaptic neuronal membrane. However, additional receptor effects have been found including desensitization of adenyl cyclase, down regulation of beta-adrenergic receptors, and down regulation of serotonin receptors.

Pharmacodynamics Onset of therapeutic effects: Takes 1-3 weeks before effects are seen; NE >>5-HT

Pharmacokinetics
Distribution: V_d: 21 L/kg
Protein binding: 93% to 95%
Metabolism: Undergoes significant first-pass metabolism; substrate CYP2D6
Half-life: 28-31 hours
Time to peak serum concentration: Oral: Within 7-8.5 hours
Elimination: Primarily detoxified in the liver and excreted as metabolites and small amounts of unchanged drug in the urine; small amounts of biliary elimination occurs.
Geriatric: Single-dose pharmacokinetic studies have found the mean half-life to range from 37-45 hours in older subjects; the mean metabolic clearance was significantly lower compared to younger subjects, 20 vs 54 L/hour

Usual Dosage Oral:
Geriatrics: Initial: 10-25 mg at bedtime; dosage can be increased by 25 mg every 3 days for inpatients and weekly for outpatients if tolerated; usual maintenance dose: 75 mg as a single bedtime dose, however, lower or higher doses may be required to stay within the therapeutic window
Adults: 25 mg 3-4 times/day up to 150 mg/day

Chronic urticaria, angioedema, nocturnal pruritus: 75 mg/day

Monitoring Parameters Blood pressure and pulse; serum concentration, target symptoms

Reference Range Therapeutic: 50-150 ng/mL (SI: 190-570 nmol/L); Toxic: >500 ng/mL (SI: >1900 nmol/L)

Test Interactions Elevated glucose

Patient Information Do not stop abruptly, rise slowly to avoid dizziness; may cause dry mouth, constipation, blurred vision; use sugarless hard candy for dry mouth

Nursing Implications Offer patient sugarless hard candy for dry mouth, monitor for orthostatic changes, weight gain, decreased appetite

Additional Information Maximum antidepressant effect may not be seen for 2 or more weeks after initiation of therapy

Special Geriatric Considerations Since it is the least likely of the TCAs to cause orthostatic hypotension and one of the least anticholinergic and sedating TCAs, it is a preferred agent when a TCA is indicated. Data from a clinical trial comparing fluoxetine to tricyclics suggest that fluoxetine is significantly less effective than nortriptyline in hospitalized elderly patients with unipolar affective disorder, especially those with melancholia and concurrent cardiovascular disease. Paroxetine has been shown to be an equally effective antidepressant compared to nortriptyline n patients with ischemic heart disease. However, nortriptyline was associated a significantly higher rate of adverse cardiac events (sustained increase in heart rate, sinus tachycardia, and asymptomatic increase in ventricular ectopy) compared to placebo.

Dosage Forms
Nortriptyline hydrochloride:
Capsule: 10 mg, 25 mg, 50 mg, 75 mg
Solution: 10 mg/5 mL (473 mL)

References
Dawling S, Crome P, and Braithwaite R, "Pharmacokinetics of Single Oral Doses of Nortriptyline in Depressed Elderly Hospital Patients and Young Healthy Volunteers," *Clin Pharmacokinet*, 1980, 5(4):394-401.

Roose SP, Glassman AH, Attia E, et al, "Comparative Efficacy of Selective Serotonin Reuptake Inhibitors and Tricyclics in the Treatment of Melancholia," *Am J Psychiatry*, 1994, 151(12):1735-9.

Roose SP, Laghrissi-Thode F, Kennedy JS, et al, "Comparison of Paroxetine and Nortriptyline in Depressed Patients With Ischemic Heart Disease," *JAMA*, 1998, 279(4):287-91.

(Continued)

Nortriptyline *(Continued)*

Schneider LS, Cooper TB, Staples FR, et al, "Prediction of Individual Dosage of Nortriptyline in Depressed Elderly Outpatients," *J Clin Psychopharmacol*, 1987, 7(5):311-4.

Turbott J, Norman TR, Burrows GD, et al, "Pharmacokinetics of Nortriptyline in Elderly Volunteers," *Commun Psychopharmacol*, 1980, 4(3):225-31.

Norvasc® see Amlodipine on page 62

Nōstrilla® [OTC] see Oxymetazoline on page 706

Nostril® Nasal Solution [OTC] see Phenylephrine on page 740

Novolin® 70/30 see Insulin Preparations on page 488

Novolin® L see Insulin Preparations on page 488

Novolin® N see Insulin Preparations on page 488

Novolin® R see Insulin Preparations on page 488

NP-27® [OTC] see Tolnaftate on page 939

NPH see Insulin Preparations on page 488

NPH Iletin® I see Insulin Preparations on page 488

NPH Insulin see Insulin Preparations on page 488

NPH-N see Insulin Preparations on page 488

NSC 26271 see Cyclophosphamide on page 260

NTG see Nitroglycerin on page 677

NTZ® Long Acting Nasal Solution [OTC] see Oxymetazoline on page 706

Nubain® see Nalbuphine on page 650

Numorphan® see Oxymorphone on page 707

Nuprin® [OTC] see Ibuprofen on page 475

Nu-Tears® II Solution [OTC] see Artificial Tears on page 82

Nu-Tears® Solution [OTC] see Artificial Tears on page 82

Nutracort® see Hydrocortisone on page 462

Nydrazid® Injection see Isoniazid on page 500

Nystatin *(nye STAT in)*

Brand Names Mycostatin®; Nilstat®; Nystat-Rx®; Nystex®; O-V Staticin®

Generic Available Yes

Therapeutic Category Antifungal Agent, Oral Nonabsorbed; Antifungal Agent, Topical; Antifungal Agent, Vaginal

Use Treatment of susceptible cutaneous, mucocutaneous, and oral cavity fungal infections normally caused by the *Candida* species

Contraindications Hypersensitivity to nystatin or any component

Adverse Reactions
Dermatologic: Contact dermatitis
Gastrointestinal: Nausea, vomiting, diarrhea, stomach pain
Local: Irritation
Miscellaneous: Hypersensitivity reactions

Overdosage Symptoms of overdose include nausea, vomiting, diarrhea

Stability Keep vaginal inserts in refrigerator; protect from temperature extremes, moisture, and light

Mechanism of Action Binds to sterols in fungal cell membrane, changing the cell wall permeability allowing for leakage of cellular contents

Pharmacokinetics
Absorption: Not absorbed through mucous membranes or intact skin; poorly absorbed from the GI tract
Elimination: In feces as unchanged drug

Usual Dosage Geriatrics and Adults:
Intestinal infections: Oral: 500,000-1,000,000 units every 8 hours
Oral candidiasis: 400,000-600,000 units 4 times/day; pastilles: 200,000-400,000 units 4-5 times/day
Cutaneous and mucocutaneous infections: Topical: Apply 2-3 times/day
Vaginal infections: Vaginal tablets: Insert 1-2 tablets/day at bedtime for 2 weeks

Patient Information The oral suspension should be swished about the mouth and retained in the mouth for as long as possible (several minutes) before swallowing. Troches must be allowed to dissolve slowly and should not be chewed or swallowed whole. *Candida* infections should be treated for 48 hours after symptoms have disappeared. Avoid contact with the eyes.

Nursing Implications Administer around-the-clock rather than 4 times/day, 3 times/day, etc (ie, 12-6-12-6, not 9-1-5-9) to promote less variation in peak and trough serum concentrations

Additional Information Very moist topical lesions are treated best with powder

Special Geriatric Considerations For oral infections, patients who wear dentures must have them removed and cleaned in order to eliminate source of reinfection (see Usual Dosage)

Dosage Forms
Cream: 100,000 units/g (15 g, 30 g)
Ointment, topical: 100,000 units/g (15 g, 30 g)
Powder:
  For preparation of oral suspension: 50 million units, 1 billion units, 2 billion units, 5 billion units
  Topical: 100,000 units/g (15 g)
Suspension, oral: 100,000 units/mL (5 mL 60 mL, 480 mL)
Tablet:
  Oral: 500,000 units
  Vaginal: 100,000 units (15 and 30/box with applicator)
Troches: 200,000 units

References
Dismukes WE, Wade JS, Lee JY, et al, "A Randomized, Double-Blind Trial of Nystatin Therapy for the Candidiasis Hypersensitivity Syndrome," *N Engl J Med*, 1990, 323(25):1717-23.

Nystatin and Triamcinolone (nye STAT in & trye am SIN oh lone)

Related Information
Nystatin *on previous page*
Triamcinolone *on page 949*

Brand Names Mycogen II Topical; Mycolog®-II Topical; Myconel® Topical; Myco-Triacet® II; Mytrex® F Topical; N.G.T.® Topical; Tri-Statin® II Topical

Synonyms Triamcinolone and Nystatin

Generic Available Yes

Therapeutic Category Antifungal Agent, Topical; Corticosteroid, Topical (Medium Potency)

Use Treatment of cutaneous candidiasis

Contraindications Known hypersensitivity to nystatin or triamcinolone

Warnings Avoid use of occlusive dressings; limit therapy to least amount necessary for effective therapy

Adverse Reactions
Dermatologic: Dryness, folliculitis, hypertrichosis, acne, hypopigmentation, allergic dermatitis, maceration of the skin, skin atrophy
Local: Burning, itching, irritation
Miscellaneous: Increased incidence of secondary infection

Mechanism of Action Binds to sterols in fungal cell membrane, changing the cell wall permeability allowing for leakage of cellular contents; decreases inflammation by suppression of migration of polymorphonuclear leukocytes and reversal of increased capillary permeability; suppresses the immune system by reducing activity and volume of the lymphatic system suppresses adrenal function at high doses

Usual Dosage Geriatrics and Adults: Topical: Apply sparingly 2-4 times/day

Administration External use only; do not use on open wounds; apply sparingly to occlusive dressings; should not be used in the presence of open or weeping lesions

Patient Information Before applying, gently wash area to reduce risk of infection; apply a thin film to cleansed area and rub in gently and thoroughly until medication vanishes; avoid exposure to sunlight, severe sunburn may occur

Nursing Implications See Administration

Special Geriatric Considerations No specific dose adjustment or use consideration necessary in the elderly; for oral infections, patients who wear dentures must have them removed and cleaned in order to eliminate source of reinfection (see Usual Dosage)

Dosage Forms
Cream: Nystatin 100,000 units and triamcinolone acetonide 0.1% (15 g, 30 g, 45 g, 60 g, 240 g)
Ointment, topical: Nystatin 100,000 units and triamcinolone acetonide 0.1% (15 g, 30 g, 60 g, 120 g)

Nystat-Rx® *see* Nystatin *on previous page*

Nystex® *see* Nystatin *on previous page*

Nytol® Oral [OTC] *see* Diphenhydramine *on page 302*

Occlusal-HP Liquid *see* Salicylic Acid *on page 845*

Ocean Nasal Mist [OTC] *see* Sodium Chloride *on page 860*

Octamide® *see* Metoclopramide *on page 616*

Octocaine® *see* Lidocaine *on page 537*

Ocu-Carpine® Ophthalmic *see* Pilocarpine *on page 748*

OcuClear® Ophthalmic [OTC] *see* Oxymetazoline *on page 706*

OcuCoat® Ophthalmic Solution [OTC] *see* Artificial Tears *on page 82*

OcuCoat® PF Ophthalmic Solution [OTC] *see* Artificial Tears *on page 82*

Ocufen® Ophthalmic *see* Flurbiprofen *on page 400*

Ocuflox™ *see* Ofloxacin *on this page*

Ocular Lubricant (OK yoo lar LOO bri kant)

Brand Names Akwa Tears® Ophthalmic Ointment [OTC]; Dry Eyes® Ophthalmic Ointment [OTC]; Duratears® Naturale® Ophthalmic Ointment [OTC]; HypoTears® Ophthalmic Ointment [OTC]; Lacri-Lube® NP Ophthalmic Ointment [OTC]; Lacri-Lube® S.O.P. Ophthalmic Ointment [OTC]; LubriTears® Ophthalmic Ointment [OTC]; Puralube® Ophthalmic Ointment [OTC]; Refresh PM® Ophthalmic Ointment [OTC]; Stye® Ophthalmic Ointment [OTC]; Tears Renewed® Ophthalmic Ointment [OTC]

Synonyms Petrolatum White and Mineral Oil Ophthalmic Ointment

Therapeutic Category Ophthalmic Agent, Miscellaneous

Use Ocular lubricant

Contraindications Known hypersensitivity to any of the components

Warnings Discontinue if eye pain, vision change, redness or eye irritation occurs or if condition worsens or persists for more than 72 hours

Precautions Do not use with contact lenses

Adverse Reactions Local: Temporary blurring of vision

Stability Store away from heat

Usual Dosage Geriatrics and Adults:
Liquid: Instill 1-2 drops into eye(s) 3-4 times a day as needed
Ointment: Instill ¼" of ointment to the inside of the lower lid as needed

Patient Information If condition worsens or persists more than 72 hours, discontinue use and consult a physician; do not touch tip of tube or dropper to any surface to avoid contamination; do not use with contact lenses

Additional Information Ointment contains petrolatum and mineral oil

Special Geriatric Considerations Ointment is useful at bedtime; make sure patient is able to apply correctly

Dosage Forms Ointment, ophthalmic: 3.5 g

Ocupress® Ophthalmic *see* Carteolol *on page 166*

Ocusert Pilo-20® Ophthalmic *see* Pilocarpine *on page 748*

Ocusert Pilo-40® Ophthalmic *see* Pilocarpine *on page 748*

Ocusulf-10® Ophthalmic *see* Sulfacetamide Sodium *on page 874*

Ocu-Tropine® *see* Atropine *on page 92*

Off-Ezy® Wart Remover [OTC] *see* Salicylic Acid *on page 845*

Ofloxacin (oh FLOKS a sin)

Related Information
Antacid Drug Interactions *on page 1096*
Cephalosporins, Aminoglycosides, Macrolides, & Quinolones *on page 1014*
I.V. Medication Recommendations *on page 1080*

Brand Names Floxin®; Ocuflox™

Generic Available No

Therapeutic Category Antibiotic, Ophthalmic; Antibiotic, Quinolone

Use Quinolone antibiotic for skin and skin structure, lower respiratory and urinary tract infections and sexually transmitted diseases, bacterial conjunctivitis caused by susceptible organisms

Contraindications Known hypersensitivity to quinolones including cinoxacin and nalidixic acid

Warnings Convulsion in persons with CNS disorders (seizure disorder, increased intracranial pressure, and toxic psychosis); CNS stimulation, tremor, headache, pseudomembranous colitis; use with caution in patients with renal impairment; failure to respond to an ophthalmic antibiotic after 2-3 days may indicate the presence of resistant organisms or another causative agent (ie, viral or allergy)

Precautions Superinfection, crystalluria, phototoxicity

Adverse Reactions
Central nervous system: Headache, dizziness, fatigue, drowsiness, insomnia, seizures, nervousness
Dermatologic: Rash, pruritus
Gastrointestinal: Nausea, diarrhea, flatulence, dysgeusia, xerostomia
Genitourinary: Vaginitis, external genital pruritus in women

Hematologic: Eosinophilia
Neuromuscular & skeletal: Tremors
Ocular: Visual disturbance, photophobia

Drug Interactions
Antacids, iron and zinc salts, sucralfate may reduce absorption by up to 98% if given at the same time
Antineoplastic agents may decrease absorption; cimetidine may increase levels
Probenecid may decrease urinary excretion
Ofloxacin may increase effects of anticoagulant, increased nephrotoxicity of cyclosporine, and decrease clearance (increased serum concentrations) of theophylline, hence, monitor appropriately

Drug/Food Interactions Food causes alteration in absorption; best to avoid concomitant administration

Mechanism of Action Ofloxacin, a fluorinated quinolone, is a pyridone carboxylic acid derivative which exerts a broad spectrum antimicrobial effect. Ofloxacin is related to the older quinolone derivatives, nalidixic acid, and oxolinic acid, and to the newer quinolone derivatives, norfloxacin and cipro-floxacin. The primary target of the fluoroquinolones is DNA gyrase (topoisomerase II), an essential bacterial enzyme that maintains the superhelical structure of DNA. DNA gyrase is required for DNA replication and transcription, DNA repair, recombination, and transposition.

Pharmacokinetics
Absorption: Fraction absorbed increases proportionately with the dose; age does not affect absorption
Half-life:
Young adults: 5 hours
Older adults with normal renal function: 6-8 hours
Sick, older, hospitalized adults: Between 9-13 hours
Time to peak serum concentration: Within 1-2 hours
Elimination: Primarily renal with ~5% excreted in feces

Usual Dosage Oral, I.V.:
Geriatrics: 200-400 mg every 12-24 hours (based on estimated renal function) for 7 days to 6 weeks depending on indication.
Adults: 200-400 mg every 12 hours for 3 days to 6 weeks; single 400 mg dose for acute uncomplicated gonorrhea.
Dosing interval in renal impairment (administer normal initial dose and adjust as follows):
Cl_{cr} 10-50 mL/minute: Administer recommended dose every 24 hours
Cl_{cr} <10 mL/minute: Administer half of recommended dose every 24 hours

Monitoring Parameters Signs and symptoms of infection; WBC, mental status

Patient Information Do not take antacids or multivitamins with minerals within 6 hours before or 2 hours after taking drug; take 1 hour before or 2 hours after meals; do not take with dairy products, iron, or zinc products; may cause dizziness, headache, or stimulation; avoid excess natural or artificial sunlight exposure; complete full course of therapy

Nursing Implications Hold antacids for 2-4 hours before and after giving dose

Special Geriatric Considerations Must adjust dose for renal function (see Pharmacokinetics and Usual Dosage)

Dosage Forms
Injection: 200 mg (50 mL); 400 mg (10 mL, 20 mL, 100 mL)
Solution, ophthalmic: 0.3% (1 mL, 5 mL)
Tablet: 200 mg, 300 mg, 400 mg

References
Nilsson-Ehle I and Ljungberg B, "Quinolone Disposition in the Elderly: Practical Implications," *Drugs Aging*, 1991, 1(4):279-88.

Olanzapine (oh LAN za peen)

Related Information
Antipsychotic Agents Comparison *on page 1023*
Antipsychotic Medication Guidelines *on page 1076*
Brand Names Zyprexa®
Synonyms LY170053
Generic Available No
Therapeutic Category Antipsychotic Agent; Neuroleptic Agent
Use Treatment of the manifestations of psychotic disorders
Contraindications Hypersensitivity to the product
(Continued)

Olanzapine *(Continued)*

Warnings Tardive dyskinesia is an adverse effect that may develop in patients treated with antipsychotics. Although olanzapine is a "novel" antipsychotic and has less potential for this adverse effect, patients need to be monitored closely. The prevalence of tardive dyskinesia is higher in elderly, especially elderly women; embarrassment from dyskinesia may cause greater social isolation; olanzapine should be reserved for those who require long-term antipsychotics for treatment of a psychosis and those who need an antipsychotic agent with less potential for development of tardive dyskinesia. Periodic assessment as to the need to continue olanzapine is recommended. If signs and symptoms of tardive dyskinesia develop, taper olanzapine off.

Neuroleptic malignant syndrome (NMS) occurs with the use of antipsychotics. Should this syndrome be diagnosed, the antipsychotic must be discontinued. If the patient requires an antipsychotic after recovery, cautious consideration of reintroduction must be given with very close monitoring.

Tachycardia has been associated with olanzapine. This may be due to the potential for hypotension/orthostatic reaction. Use with caution in patients with hepatic impairment or patients treated concomitantly with hepatotoxic drugs.

Carcinogenic potential has been demonstrated in mice where hemangiomas and hemanigosarcomas were significantly increased. The incidence of mammary tumors was significantly increased in female mice and measurement of serum prolactin concentrations were increased fourfold in rats.

Elderly did not demonstrate any difference in tolerability to olanzapine than younger adults. Caution should be exercised in patients with hepatic impairment or drugs which interfere with the CYP450 1A2 and 2D6 fraction.

Precautions Orthostatic hypotension may occur due to the alpha adrenergic blockade action of olanzapine especially during initiation of this drug. This reaction can be minimized by starting doses at 5 mg and titrating slowly with 5 mg doses. Use with caution in patients with history of myocardial infarction, ischemia, or conduction abnormalities and patients with cerebrovascular disease or predisposed to hypotension (antihypertensives, hypovolemia, dehydration).

Use with caution in patients with a history of seizure. Olanzapine was associated with seizure in 0.9% of patients studied. Use with caution in patients with increased risk of seizure such as CVA, Alzheimer's disease, or any condition which may lower seizure threshold. Many elderly (>65%) may have medical conditions putting them at risk for seizures.

Hyperprolactinemia is found with the use of olanzapine as it is with other D_2 dopamine antagonists. Research *in vitro* indicates 1/3 of human breast cancers are prolactin-dependent. However, no association with such tumors in humans has been found to date. Limited data available and no conclusions can be made.

Transaminase elevations were reported with olanzapine use in a small percentage of patients (2%). No jaundice was experienced. Periodic liver function tests should be performed in patients with hepatic disease.

Dose related somnolence was reported in 26% of patients taking olanzapine. Impairment of cognitive and motor skills puts patients at risk for operating hazardous machinery or driving. Monitor closely.

Body temperature regulation may be impaired such that the ability to reduce core temperature is decreased. Use with caution in those who will be at risk (exposure to heat, dehydration, vigorous exercise, and concomitant use of anticholinergic medications).

Dysphagia leading to aspiration has been reported with other antipsychotics and olanzapine. Use with caution in patients with suicide potential. Olanzapine exhibits anticholinergic action (muscarinic). Constipation, dry mouth, and tachycardia were seen in studies. Monitor patients at risk for urinary incontinence (BPH) and narrow angle glaucoma. Suicide is an inherent problem in schizophrenic patients. Monitor closely and limit the amount of prescription drug available to patient.

Adverse Reactions
Cardiovascular: Peripheral edema, migraine, palpitations, ventricular extrasystoles, chest pain
Central nervous system: Headache, somnolence, insomnia, agitation, nervousness, hostility, dizziness, dystonic reactions, parkinsonian events, akathisia, anxiety, personality changes, fever, amnesia, stuttering, euphoria, tardive dyskinesia, neuroleptic malignant syndrome, hypotonia, obsessive compulsion, stupor, vertigo

Dermatologic: Rash, dermatitis, dry skin, eczema, seborrhea, urticaria, alopecia

Endocrine & metabolic: Breast pain, decreased libido, diabetes mellitus, goiter, dehydration, hyperkalemia, hyperglycemia, hypoglycemia, hyponatremia

Gastrointestinal: Xerostomia, constipation, abdominal pain, weight gain (increased appetite), weight loss, salivation, fecal incontinence, gastritis, gingivitis, glossitis, esophageal ulcer, altered taste

Genitourinary: Hematuria, incontinence (urine), abnormal ejaculation, impotence

Neuromuscular & skeletal: Arthralgia, tremor, pain in extremities, twitching, back pain, neck rigidity, abnormal gait

Ocular: Amblyopia, blepharitis, diplopia, eye pain, nystagmus, macular hypopigmentation, cataract, glaucoma

Otic: Tinnitus

Respiratory: Rhinitis, cough, pharyngitis, hyperventilation, laryngitis, asthma, apnea

Overdosage Drowsiness and slurred speech were only effects in up to 300 mg ingestion. No change in EKG or laboratory values noted.

Toxicology There is no antidote for olanzapine. Following initiation of essential overdose management, toxic symptom treatment and supportive treatment should be initiated. Hypotension usually responds to I.V. fluids or Trendelenburg positioning. If unresponsive to these measures the use of a parenteral inotrope may be required (eg, norepinephrine 0.1-0.2 mcg/kg/minute titrated to response). Do not use epinephrine. Seizures commonly respond to diazepam (I.V. 5-10 mg bolus in adults every 15 minutes if needed up to a total of 30 mg) or to phenytoin or phenobarbital. Also critical cardiac arrhythmias often respond to I.V. phenytoin (15 mg/kg up to 1 g), while other antiarrhythmics can be used. Neuroleptics often cause extrapyramidal symptoms (eg, dystonic reactions) requiring management with diphenhydramine 1-2 mg/kg up to a maximum of 50 mg I.M. or I.V. slow push followed by a maintenance dose for 48-72 hours. When these reactions are unresponsive to diphenhydramine, benztropine mesylate I.V. 1-2 mg may be effective. These agents are generally effective within 2-5 minutes.

Drug Interactions

Decreased effect: Cigarette smoking, levodopa, pergolide, bromocriptine, charcoal, and reduction of effects may be seen with cytochrome P-450 enzyme inducers such as rifampin, omeprazole, carbamazepine

Increased effect: Effects may be potentiated with cytochrome P-450 $1A_2$ inhibitors such as fluvoxamine

Increased toxicity: Increased sedation with alcohol or other CNS depressants, increased risk of hypotension and orthostatic hypotension with antihypertensives

Stability Store at room temperature (20°C to 25°C); protect from light

Mechanism of Action Olanzapine is a thienobenzodiazepine neuroleptic; thought to work by antagonizing dopamine and serotonin activities. It is a selective monoaminergic antagonist with high affinity binding to serotonin $5HT2_A$ and $5HT2_C$, dopamine D_{1-4}, muscarinic M_{1-5}, histamine H_1 and alpha$_1$-adrenergic receptor sites. The exact mechanism of action is unknown. However, it is speculated that is pharmacologic action is a result of antagonism of the combination of dopamine and $5HT_2$ receptors. other receptors antagonized most likely explain side effects, ie, muscarinic-anticholinergic effects; somnolence-histamine receptors; hypotension-alpha$_1$ receptors.

Pharmacokinetics

Absorption: Well absorbed orally

Distribution: V_d: 1000 L

Metabolism: Substrate CYP1A2, 2D6

Peak serum concentrations: 6 hours

Half-life: 21-54 hours (mean half-life: 30 hours)

Time to steady-state: 1 week

Clearance: 30% lower in females

Elimination: Hepatic metabolism cytochrome P-450 fractions $1A_2$ and 2D6

Usual Dosage Oral:

Geriatrics: Initial dose: 5 mg/day with increases of 5 mg/day with 5-7 days to attain a target dose of 10 mg/day within first weeks of initiation. Thereafter, adjust by 5 mg/day at weekly intervals; maximum dose: 20 mg/day (see Special Geriatric Considerations)

Adults >18 years: Usual starting dose: 5-10 mg once daily; increase to 10 mg once daily within 5-7 days, thereafter adjust by 5 mg/day at 1-week intervals, up to a maximum of 20 mg/day (see Additional Information)

(Continued)

Olanzapine *(Continued)*

Monitoring Parameters Orthostatic blood pressures; tremors, gait changes, abnormal movement in trunk, neck, buccal area, or extremities; monitor target behaviors for which the agent is given

Patient Information Patient should be advised of the risk of hypotension, especially at the start of therapy. Also explain other medications that induce hypotension and augment the orthostatic effects of olanzapine. Warn patient that olanzapine may impair judgment, thinking, or motor skills making driving or operating hazardous equipment a risk. Therefore, patient should be cautious until the effects of their dose is experienced and known. Avoid overheating and dehydration.

Nursing Implications Monitor and observe for extrapyramidal effects, orthostatic blood pressure changes for 3-5 days after starting or increasing dose

Special Geriatric Considerations See Warnings.

Studies revealed that elderly had an elimination half-life that was 1.5 times that of younger adults (<65 years of age)

Extrapyramidal syndrome symptoms occur less often than with traditional antipsychotics from the phenothiazine and butyrophenone classes. Many elderly patients receive antipsychotic medications for inappropriate nonpsychotic behavior. Before initiating antipsychotic medication, the clinician should investigate any possible reversible cause; any stress or stress from any disease can cause acute "confusion" or worsening of baseline nonpsychotic behavior. Most commonly acute changes in behavior are due to increases in drug dose or addition of new drug to regimen; fluid electrolyte loss; infections; and changes in environment.

Any changes in disease status in any organ system can result in behavior changes

In the treatment of agitated, demented, elderly patients, authors of meta-analysis of controlled trials of the response to the traditional antipsychotics (phenothiazines, butyrophenones) in controlling agitation have concluded that the use of neuroleptics results in a response rate of 18%. Clearly neuroleptic therapy for behavior control should be limited with frequent attempts to withdraw the agent given for behavior control.

Dosage Forms Tablet: 5 mg, 7.5 mg, 10 mg

References

Baldwin DS and Montgomery SA, "First Clinical Experience With Olanzapine (LY 170053): Results of an Open-label Safety and Dose-Ranging Study in Patients With Schizophrenia," *Int Clin Psychopharmacol* , 1995, 10(4):239-44.

Goldberg RJ, "Managing Psychosis-Related Behavioral Problems in the Elderly," *Consult Pharm*, 1997, 12(Suppl C):4-10.

Littrell K, Peabody CD, and Littrell SH, "Olanzapine: A New Atypical Antipsychotic," *J Psychosoc Nurs Ment Health Serv*, 1996, 34(8):41-6.

"Olanzapine for Schizophrenia," *Med Lett Drugs Ther*, 1997, 39(992):5-6.

Tollefson GD, Beasley CM Jr, Tran PV, et al, "Olanzapine Versus Haloperidol in the Treatment of Schizophrnia and Schizoaffective and Schizophreniform Disorders: Results of an International Collaborative Trial," *Am J Psychiatry*, 1997, 154(4):457-65.

Oleum Ricini *see* Castor Oil *on page 171*

Olsalazine *(ole SAL a zeen)*

Brand Names Dipentum®

Generic Available No

Therapeutic Category 5-Aminosalicylic Acid Derivative; Anti-inflammatory Agent

Use Maintenance of remission of ulcerative colitis in patients intolerant to sulfasalazine

Contraindications Hypersensitivity to salicylates

Warnings Bladder tumors in rats receiving 10-100 times the equivalent dose for man have been found in studies; liver tumors have also been reported in mice. No evidence exists for such problems in people receiving recommended doses.

Precautions Diarrhea appears to be dose related, but is difficult to distinguish from underlying disease symptoms; diarrhea occurs in up to 33% of patients

Adverse Reactions

Dermatologic: Rash, pruritus

Gastrointestinal: Diarrhea, abdominal pain/cramps, nausea, anorexia, dyspepsia

Miscellaneous: Depression, arthralgia, fever, hepatitis, blood dyscrasias (<1%)

Overdosage Symptoms of overdose include decreased motor activity, diarrhea

Toxicology Supportive care and discontinuation of drug may be initiated at a decreased dose after symptoms clear

Mechanism of Action Olsalazine is converted to two molecules of 5-ASA (mesalamine) by colonic bacteria. Mechanism of action is unknown but appears action is topical rather than systemic and decreases inflammation by inhibiting cyclo-oxygenase production of prostaglandins. Other actions may contribute to the anti-inflammatory action such as inhibition of polymorphonuclear cell migration and inhibition of leukotriene production.

Pharmacokinetics
Absorption: 2% to 4%
Protein binding: 98%
Metabolism: 98% to 99% is converted to 5-aminosalicylic acid
Half-life: 0.9 hours; olsalazine-0-sulfate (olsalazine-S) accounts for 0.1% of the dose and has a half-life of 7 days
Time to peak serum concentration: Within 1 hour
Elimination: Primarily in feces

Usual Dosage Geriatrics and Adults: Oral: 1 g twice daily

Monitoring Parameters Stool frequency

Reference Range Olsalazine: 0-4.3 mmol/L; olsalazine sodium: 3.3-12.4 mmol/L. These are not therapeutic guideline levels. These are reported levels after administration that have been observed on study. No correlation to response is known at this time.

Test Interactions Increases in ALT/AST reported

Patient Information Take with food in evenly divided doses; contact physician if rash or diarrhea occur

Nursing Implications Monitor stool frequency

Special Geriatric Considerations No specific data available on elderly to suggest the drug needs alterations in dose. Since so little is absorbed, dosing should not be changed for reasons of age. Diarrhea may pose a serious problem for elderly in that it may cause dehydration, electrolyte imbalance, hypotension, and confusion.

Dosage Forms Capsule, as sodium: 250 mg

Omeprazole (oh ME pray zol)

Related Information
Regimens Used to Treat *Helicobacter pylori* and Ulcers *on page 1033*

Replaces Losec®

Brand Names Prilosec™

Generic Available No

Therapeutic Category Gastric Acid Secretion Inhibitor

Use Short-term (4-8 weeks) treatment of erosive esophagitis (grade ≥2), diagnosed by endoscopy; maintain healing of erosive esophagitis; short-term treatment of symptomatic gastroesophageal reflux disease (GERD) poorly responsive to customary medical treatment; short-term treatment of active duodenal ulcer; short-term treatment of active benign gastric ulcers; long-term treatment of pathological hypersecretory conditions; may be effective in treating gastric ulcers caused by NSAIDs, more studies may be necessary to clearly establish this use; treatment of *H. pylori* in combination with clarithromycin for the treatment of ulcers; heartburn (initial symptoms associated with GERD)

Contraindications Known hypersensitivity to omeprazole

Warnings Omeprazole should be prescribed only for the conditions, dosage and duration described. Bioavailability may be increased in elderly patients.

Precautions Symptomatic response to omeprazole does not preclude gastric malignancy

Adverse Reactions
Cardiovascular: Headache (most frequent at 7%), angina, tachycardia, bradycardia, edema
Central nervous system: Dizziness, fever, fatigue, malaise, apathy, somnolence, nervousness, anxiety
Dermatologic: Rash, urticaria, pruritus, dry skin
Endocrine & metabolic: Hypoglycemia
Gastrointestinal: Diarrhea, nausea, abdominal pain, vomiting, constipation, abdominal edema, anorexia, irritable colon, fecal discoloration, esophageal candidiasis, xerostomia, dysgeusia
Genitourinary: Polyuria, testicular pain
Hematologic: Thrombocytopenia, pancytopenia, leukocytosis
(Continued)

Omeprazole *(Continued)*

Hepatic: Hepatitis, elevated AST/ALT/GGT/alkaline phosphatase, jaundice

Neuromuscular & skeletal: Back pain, weakness occurred frequently in >1% of patients, muscle cramps, myalgia, arthralgia, leg pain

Otic: Tinnitus

Renal: Pyuria, proteinuria, hematuria, glycosuria, increases in serum creatinine

Respiratory: Cough

Overdosage Symptoms of overdose include hypothermia, sedation, convulsions, decreased respiratory rate (animal data)

Toxicology Symptomatic and general supportive care; not dialyzable

Drug Interactions Diazepam may increase half-life with increased CNS effects (toxicity), phenytoin, ketoconazole (decreased absorption); increased effects of warfarin

Mechanism of Action Suppresses gastric acid secretion by inhibiting the parietal cell H+/K+ ATP pump

Pharmacodynamics

Onset of antisecretory action: Oral: Within 1 hour

Maximum effect: 2 hours

Duration: 72 hours

Pharmacokinetics

Protein binding: 95%

Metabolism: Extensive in the liver; inducer CYP1A2; inhibitor CYP2C8, 2C19, 3A4; substrate 2C8, 2C18, 2C19

Half-life: 30-90 minutes

Usual Dosage Geriatrics and Adults: Oral:

Duodenal ulcer: 20 mg/day for 4-8 weeks

Gastric ulcer: 40 mg daily for 4-8 weeks

GERD or erosive esophagitis: 20 mg/day for 4-8 weeks

Maintenance of healing erosive esophagitis: 20 mg/day

Pathological hypersecretory conditions: 60 mg once daily initially; doses up to 120 mg 3 times/day have been administered; administer daily doses >80 mg in divided doses; patients with Zollinger-Ellison syndrome have been treated continuously for over 5 years

Eradication of *H. pylori*: 40 mg once daily with clarithromycin 500 mg three times/day for 2 weeks, then omeprazole 20 mg daily for 2 weeks

Dosing adjustment in renal impairment: No adjustment for dose is necessary for patients with renal or hepatic impairment or for elderly

Monitoring Parameters Monitor symptoms, occult blood; use of gastroscopy is preferred; INR for patients on warfarin

Test Interactions False increase in gastrin

Patient Information Take before eating; do not chew, crush, or open capsule; if need to open capsule for ease of administration, place contents in acid juice (orange juice, tomato juice, etc); may take with antacids concomitantly

Nursing Implications Capsule should be swallowed whole, not chewed, crushed, or opened

Special Geriatric Considerations The incidence of side effects in elderly is no different than that of younger adults (≤65 years of age) despite slight decrease in elimination and increase in bioavailability. Bioavailability may be increased in elderly (≥65 years of age), however, dosage adjustments are not necessary.

Dosage Forms Capsule, delayed release: 10 mg, 20 mg

Omnipen® *see Ampicillin on page 73*

Omnipen®-N *see Ampicillin on page 73*

OMS® Oral *see Morphine Sulfate on page 640*

Ondansetron *(on DAN se tron)*

Related Information

I.V. Push Recommended Guidelines *on page 1083*

Brand Names Zofran®

Generic Available No

Therapeutic Category Antiemetic; Serotonin Antagonist, Antiemetic

Use May be prescribed for patients who are refractory to or have severe adverse reactions to standard antiemetic therapy. Ondansetron may be prescribed for young patients (ie, <45 years of age who are more likely to develop extrapyramidal reactions to high-dose metoclopramide) who are to receive highly emetogenic chemotherapeutic agents as listed:

Agents with high emetogenic potential (>90%) (dose/m^2):
    Carmustine ≥200 mg
    Cisplatin ≥75 mg
    Cyclophosphamide ≥1000 mg
    Cytarabine ≥1000 mg
    Dacarbazine ≥500 mg
    Ifosfamide ≥1000 mg
    Lomustine ≥60 mg
    Mechlorethamine
    Pentostatin
    Streptozocin

or two agents classified as having high or moderately high emetogenic potential as listed:

Agents with moderately high emetogenic potential (60% to 90%) (dose/m^2):
    Carmustine <200 mg
    Cisplatin <75 mg
    Cyclophosphamide 1000 mg
    Cytarabine 250-1000 mg
    Dacarbazine <500 mg
    Doxorubicin ≥75 mg
    Ifosfamide
    Lomustine <60 mg
    Methotrexate ≥250 mg
    Mitomycin
    Mitoxantrone
    Procarbazine

Ondansetron should not be prescribed for chemotherapeutic agents with a low emetogenic potential (eg, bleomycin, busulfan, cyclophosphamide <1000 mg, etoposide, 5-fluorouracil, vinblastine, vincristine)

Contraindications Hypersensitivity to ondansetron or any component

Warnings Ondansetron should be used on a scheduled basis, not as an "as needed" (prn) basis, since data support the use of this drug in the prevention of nausea and vomiting and not in the rescue of nausea and vomiting. Ondansetron should only be used in the first 24-48 hours of receiving chemotherapy. Data do not support any increased efficacy of ondansetron in delayed nausea and vomiting.

Adverse Reactions
    Cardiovascular: Headache, tachycardia, angina
    Central nervous system: Lightheadedness, seizures
    Dermatologic: Rash
    Endocrine & metabolic: Hypokalemia
    Gastrointestinal: Constipation, diarrhea
    Hepatic: Transient elevations in serum concentrations of aminotransferases and bilirubin
    Respiratory: Rarely bronchospasm
    Miscellaneous: There have been two cases of EPS reaction

Overdosage In a few reported cases, the following symptoms have been noted: sudden blindness for 2-3 minutes, severe constipation, syncope, hypotension, transient vasovagal response

Toxicology No antidote; manage with general supportive care; doses 10 times greater than recommended have not shown significant adverse effects

Drug Interactions Metabolized by the hepatic cytochrome P-450 enzymes; therefore, the drug's clearance and half-life may be changed with concomitant use of cytochrome P-450 inducers (eg, barbiturates, carbamazepine, rifampin, phenytoin, and phenylbutazone) or inhibitors (eg, cimetidine, allopurinol, disulfiram, protease inhibitors). Carmustine, etoposide, and cisplatin do not affect the pharmacokinetics of ondansetron in humans.

Stability The injection may be stored between 36°F and 86°F. Ondansetron is stable when mixed in 5% dextrose or 0.9% sodium chloride for 48 hours at room temperature and does not need protection from light.

Ondansetron is physically compatible with the following drugs for Y-site administration: amikacin, aztreonam, bleomycin, carboplatin, cefazolin, ceftazidime, ceftizoxime, cefuroxime, chlorpromazine, doxorubicin, doxycycline, droperidol, etoposide, floxuridine, fluconazole, gentamicin, haloperidol, hydrocortisone, ifosfamide, imipenem-cilastatin, magnesium sulfate, mannitol, mechlorethamine, mesna, methotrexate, miconazole, mitomycin, mitoxantrone, pentostatin, potassium chloride, streptozocin, tetracycline, ranitidine, ticarcillin/clavulanate, vancomycin, vinblastine, and vincristine.

(Continued)

Ondansetron *(Continued)*

Ondansetron is incompatible with the following drugs: acyclovir, aminophylline, amphotericin B, ampicillin, ampicillin/sulbactam, amsacrine, fluorouracil, furosemide, ganciclovir, lorazepam, methylprednisolone, mezlocillin, and piperacillin.

Mechanism of Action Selective 5-HT$_3$ receptor antagonist, blocking serotonin, both peripherally on vagal nerve terminals and centrally in the chemoreceptor trigger zone

Pharmacokinetics

Protein binding: Plasma 70% to 76%

Metabolism: Extensive by hydroxylation, followed by glucuronide or sulfate conjugation; elderly >75 years of age have a decreased hepatic clearance; substrate CYP1A2, 3A4

Half-life: Geriatric patients <75 years of age and Adults: 4 hours

Elimination: In urine and feces; <10% of the parent drug is recovered unchanged in urine

Usual Dosage Geriatrics and Adults:

Oral: 8 mg 3 times/day; first dose 30 minutes prior to chemotherapy; administer for 1-2 days after completion of each chemotherapy treatment

I.V.: 0.15 mg/kg/dose or a single dose 32 mg over 15 minutes, infused 30 minutes before the start of emetogenic chemotherapy, with subsequent doses administered 4 and 8 hours after the first dose; decreased effectiveness has been reported when administered for prolonged therapy (eg, more than 3 doses); dilute in 50 mL D$_5$W or sodium chloride 0.9% for injection; elderly may need dosage adjustment if >75 years of age; however, no dosage adjustment is recommended

Dosing in hepatic impairment: Oral, I.V.: Do not exceed 8 mg/day dose

Postoperative nausea/vomiting: I.V.: 4 mg undiluted over 2-5 minutes; may administer before anesthesia and after procedure

Administration If injected undiluted, administer over a 2- to 5-minute period (see Stability)

Monitoring Parameters Emetic episodes, diarrhea, headache

Patient Information May cause diarrhea and headache

Nursing Implications First dose should be given 30 minutes prior to starting chemotherapy treatment

Additional Information The I.V. product has been used orally successfully

Special Geriatric Considerations Elderly have a slightly decreased hepatic clearance rate; this does not, however, require a dose adjustment

Dosage Forms

Ondansetron hydrochloride:

Injection: 2 mg/mL (20 mL); 32 mg (single-dose vials)

Tablet: 4 mg, 8 mg

References

Marty M, Pouillart P, Scholl S, et al, "Comparison of the 5-hydroxytryptamine 3 (Serotonin) Antagonist Ondansetron (GR 38032F) With High-Dose Metoclopramide in the Control of Cisplatin-Induced Emesis," *N Engl J Med*, 1990, 322(12):816-21.

Pinkerton CR, Williams D, Wootton C, et al, "5-HT$_3$ Antagonist Ondansetron - An Effective Outpatient Antiemetic in Cancer Treatment," *Arch Dis Child*, 1990, 65(8):822-5.

Ony-Clear® Spray *see* Miconazole *on page 625*

Opcon® Ophthalmic *see* Naphazoline *on page 653*

Ophthalgan® Ophthalmic *see* Glycerin *on page 429*

Optigene® Ophthalmic [OTC] *see* Tetrahydrozoline *on page 901*

Optimine® *see* Azatadine *on page 97*

OptiPranolol® *see* Metipranolol *on page 615*

OPV *see* Poliovirus Vaccine, Live, Trivalent, Oral *on page 761*

Orabase® HCA *see* Hydrocortisone *on page 462*

Oracit® *see* Sodium Citrate and Citric Acid *on page 861*

Orajel® Perioseptic [OTC] *see* Carbamide Peroxide *on page 162*

Oraminic® II *see* Brompheniramine *on page 129*

Oramorph SR™ Oral *see* Morphine Sulfate *on page 640*

Orap™ *see* Pimozide *on page 750*

Orasone® *see* Prednisone *on page 776*

Orazinc® Oral [OTC] *see* Zinc Sulfate *on page 995*

Orciprenaline Sulfate *see* Metaproterenol *on page 596*

Oretic® *see* Hydrochlorothiazide *on page 458*

Oreton® Methyl *see* Methyltestosterone *on page 613*

Orex® [OTC] *see* Saliva Substitute *on page 846*

Organidin® NR *see* Guaifenesin *on page 437*

Orgaran® *see* Danaparoid *on page 267*

Original Doan's® [OTC] *see* Salicylates (Various Salts) *on page 842*

Orimune® *see* Poliovirus Vaccine, Live, Trivalent, Oral *on page 761*

Orinase® Diagnostic Injection *see* Tolbutamide *on page 934*

Orinase® Oral *see* Tolbutamide *on page 934*

Ormazine *see* Chlorpromazine *on page 209*

Orphenadrine (or FEN a dreen)

Brand Names Norflex™

Generic Available Yes

Therapeutic Category Skeletal Muscle Relaxant

Use Treatment of muscle spasm associated with acute painful musculoskeletal conditions

Unlabeled use: Orphenadrine 100 mg at bedtime may be useful in the treatment of quinine-resistant leg cramps

Contraindications Glaucoma, GI obstruction, prostatic hypertrophy or GU obstruction, cardiospasm, myasthenia gravis, hypersensitivity to orphenadrine or any component

Warnings Use with caution in patients with CHF or cardiac arrhythmias; some products contain sulfites

Precautions Safety of continuous long-term therapy has not been established

Adverse Reactions Adverse effects are mainly due to its anticholinergic effects

Cardiovascular: Tachycardia, palpitations

Central nervous system: Dizziness, drowsiness, confusion in the elderly, hallucinations, agitation

Gastrointestinal: Xerostomia, nausea, constipation

Genitourinary: Urinary hesitancy and retention

Neuromuscular & skeletal: Tremors

Ocular: Blurred vision, dilated pupils

Overdosage Symptoms of overdose include blurred vision, tachycardia, confusion, seizures, respiratory arrest, dysrhythmias

Toxicology There is no specific treatment; however, most of its clinical toxicity is due to anticholinergic effects. Cholinesterase inhibitors may be useful by reducing acetylcholinesterase. Cholinesterase inhibitors include physostigmine, neostigmine, pyridostigmine, and edrophonium. For anticholinergic overdose with severe life-threatening symptoms, physostigmine 1-2 mg I.V., slowly may be given to reverse these effects. Lethal dose is 2-3 g.

Drug Interactions

Decreased effect of phenothiazines, haloperidol, tacrine

Increased toxicity with amantadine (anticholinergic effects)

Mechanism of Action Has not been identified, may be related to its analgesic properties; acts centrally at the brain stem

Pharmacodynamics

Peak effect: Oral: Within 2-4 hours

Duration: 4-6 hours

Pharmacokinetics

Protein binding: 20%

Metabolism: Extensive

Half-life: 14-16 hours

Elimination: Urine (8% as unchanged drug)

Usual Dosage

Geriatrics: See Special Geriatric Considerations

Adults:

Oral: 100 mg twice daily

I.M., I.V.: 60 mg every 12 hours

Monitoring Parameters Relief of symptoms, mental status, anticholinergic effects

Patient Information May cause drowsiness, dizziness, blurred vision, or fainting; do not crush or chew sustained release product; avoid alcohol, may impair coordination and judgment

Nursing Implications Do not crush sustained release drug product; raise bed rails and institute safety measures; assist with ambulation

Special Geriatric Considerations Because of its anticholinergic side effects, orphenadrine is not a drug of choice in the elderly (constipation, urinary retention, confusion)

(Continued)

Orphenadrine *(Continued)*

Dosage Forms
Orphenadrine citrate:
Injection: 30 mg/mL (2 mL, 10 mL)
Tablet: 100 mg
Tablet, sustained release: 100 mg

Or-Tyl® Injection *see* Dicyclomine *on page 285*

Orudis® *see* Ketoprofen *on page 515*

Orudis® KT [OTC] *see* Ketoprofen *on page 515*

Oruvail® *see* Ketoprofen *on page 515*

Os-Cal® 500 [OTC] *see* Calcium Salts (Oral) *on page 152*

Osmoglyn® Ophthalmic *see* Glycerin *on page 429*

Osteocalcin® Injection *see* Calcitonin *on page 142*

Otrivin® [OTC] *see* Xylometazoline *on page 991*

O-V Staticin® *see* Nystatin *on page 686*

Oxacillin *(oks a SIL in)*

Related Information
Penicillins, Penicillin-Related Antibiotics, & Other Antibiotics *on page 1010*

Brand Names Bactocill®; Prostaphlin®

Synonyms Methylphenyl Isoxazolyl Penicillin

Generic Available Yes

Therapeutic Category Antibiotic, Penicillin

Use Treatment of susceptible bacterial infections such as osteomyelitis, septicemia, endocarditis, and CNS infections due to penicillinase-producing strains of *Staphylococcus* (except methicillin resistant)

Contraindications Hypersensitivity to oxacillin or other penicillins or any component

Precautions Use with caution in patients with severe renal impairment; use with caution in patients with cephalosporin allergy

Adverse Reactions
Central nervous system: Fever
Dermatologic: Rash
Gastrointestinal: Diarrhea, nausea, vomiting
Hematologic: Mild leukopenia, agranulocytosis, thrombocytopenia
Hepatic: Elevated AST, hepatotoxicity
Local: Thrombophlebitis
Renal: Acute interstitial nephritis, hematuria
Miscellaneous: Allergy, serum sickness-like reactions

Overdosage Symptoms of overdose include neuromuscular hypersensitivity, seizure

Toxicology Many beta-lactam-containing antibiotics have the potential to cause neuromuscular hyperirritability or convulsive seizures. Hemodialysis may be helpful to aid in the removal of the drug from the blood, otherwise most treatment is supportive or symptom directed.

Drug Interactions Increased effect with probenecid

Drug/Food Interactions Food decreases bioavailability

Stability Reconstituted parenteral solution is stable for 3 days at room temperature and 7 days when refrigerated; for I.V. infusion in NS or D₅W, solution is stable for 24 hours at room temperature

Mechanism of Action Interferes with bacterial cell wall synthesis during active multiplication causing cell death and resultant bactericidal activity against susceptible bacteria

Pharmacokinetics
Absorption: Oral: ~35% to 67%
Distribution: Penetrates the blood-brain barrier only when meninges are inflamed
Protein binding: 90% to 95%
Metabolism: In the liver to active metabolites
Half-life: 23-60 minutes (prolonged with reduced renal function)
Time to peak serum concentration:
Oral: Within 120 minutes
I.M.: 30-60 minutes
Elimination: By the kidneys and to small degree the bile as parent drug and metabolites

Usual Dosage Geriatrics and Adults:
Oral: 500-1000 mg every 4-6 hours
I.M., I.V.: 250 mg to 2 g/dose every 4-6 hours

Dosing interval in renal impairment: Cl$_{cr}$ <10 mL/minute: Use lower range of the usual dosage

Not dialyzable (0% to 5%)

Administration Administer around-the-clock rather than 4 times/day, 3 times/day, etc (ie, 12-6-12-6, not 9-1-5-9) to promote less variation in peak and trough serum concentrations; I.M. injections should be given deep into a large muscle mass such as the gluteus maximus

Monitoring Parameters Monitor signs and symptoms of infection, WBC, mental status

Test Interactions False-positive urinary and serum proteins

Patient Information Take on an empty stomach 1 hour before meals or 2 hours after meals; complete full course of therapy; call your physician or pharmacist if diarrhea, cramping, or skin rash occur

Nursing Implications See Administration

Additional Information Sodium content of 1 g: 2.5 mEq

Special Geriatric Considerations Oxacillin has not been studied in the elderly; dosing adjustments are not necessary except in renal failure (ie, Cl$_{cr}$ <10 mL/minute)

Dosage Forms
Oxacillin sodium:
Capsule: 250 mg, 500 mg
Powder for injection: 250 mg, 500 mg, 1 g, 2 g, 4 g, 10 g
Powder for oral solution: 250 mg/5 mL (100 mL)

References
Yoshikawa TT, "Antimicrobial Therapy for the Elderly Patient," *J Am Geriatr Soc*, 1990, 38(12):1353-72.

Oxaprozin (oks a PROE zin)

Brand Names Daypro™

Therapeutic Category Analgesic, Non-narcotic; Anti-inflammatory Agent; Antipyretic; Nonsteroidal Anti-inflammatory Agent (NSAID), Oral

Use Acute and long-term use in the management of signs and symptoms of osteoarthritis and rheumatoid arthritis

Unlabeled use: Mild to moderate pain, acute painful shoulder

Contraindications Hypersensitivity to oxaprozin or other NSAIDs; due to the potential cross-sensitivity, use extreme caution when a history of allergy exists to aspirin, iodides, or other NSAIDs; hypersensitivity has caused symptoms of rhinitis, urticaria, asthma, nasal polyps, bronchospasm, angioedema, and anaphylaxis

Warnings GI toxicity (bleeding, ulceration, perforation); CNS effects may occur (headaches, confusion, depression); hypersensitivity, anaphylactoid reactions (intermittent tolmetin use more often); renal function decline, acute renal insufficiency, interstitial nephritis, dysuria, cystitis, hematuria, nephrotic syndrome, hyperkalemia in acute renal insufficiency, hyponatremia, papillary necrosis, hepatic function impairment; elderly have increased risk for adverse reactions to NSAIDs (see Special Geriatric Considerations)

Precautions Use with caution in patients with congestive heart failure, hypertension, decreased renal or hepatic function, history of GI disease (bleeding or ulcers), or those receiving anticoagulants; perform ophthalmologic evaluation for those who develop eye complaints during therapy (blurred vision, diminished vision, changes in color vision, retinal changes); NSAIDs may mask signs/symptoms of infections; photosensitivity reported

Adverse Reactions
Cardiovascular: Congestive heart failure, angina, hypertension, hypotension, arrhythmias, edema
Central nervous system: Headache, drowsiness, vertigo, dizziness, fatigue, hallucinations, confusion, depression, emotional lability, psychotic behavior, pyrexia
Dermatologic: Rash, urticaria, angioedema, Stevens-Johnson syndrome, exfoliative dermatitis, bruising, petechiae, purpura
Endocrine & metabolic: Hyperglycemia, hypoglycemia, hyperkalemia, gynecomastia, hyponatremia, fluid retention
Gastrointestinal: Dyspepsia, heartburn, nausea, diarrhea, constipation, flatulence, stomatitis, vomiting, abdominal pain, peptic ulcer, GI bleeding, GI perforation, gingival ulcers, pancreatitis, proctitis, paralytic ulcers, colitis, anorexia, weight loss, dry mucous membranes
Genitourinary: Impotence, azotemia
Hematologic: Neutropenia, anemia, agranulocytosis, bone marrow suppression, hemolytic anemia, hemorrhage, inhibition of platelet aggregation
Hepatic: Hepatitis, elevated LFTs, cholestatic jaundice
(Continued)

Oxaprozin *(Continued)*

Neuromuscular & skeletal: Involuntary muscle movements, muscle weakness, tremors, weakness

Ocular: Vision changes

Otic: Tinnitus

Renal: Dysuria, polyuria, pyuria, oliguria, anuria, acute renal failure

Respiratory: Exacerbation of asthma, dyspnea

Miscellaneous: Thirst, diaphoresis

Overdosage Symptoms include drowsiness, lethargy, disorientation, confusion, dizziness, numbness, paresthesia, nausea, vomiting, gastric irritation, abdominal pain, headache, tinnitus, sweating, blurred vision, muscle twitching, seizures, coma, acute renal failure, increased BUN and serum creatinine, hypotension, tachycardia, and metabolic acidosis

Toxicology Management of a nonsteroidal anti-inflammatory agent (NSAID) intoxication is primarily supportive and symptomatic. Fluid therapy is commonly effective in managing the hypotension that may occur following an acute NSAID overdose, except when this is due to an acute blood loss. Seizures tend to be very short-lived and often do not require drug treatment although recurrent seizures should be treated with I.V. diazepam. Since many of the NSAIDs undergo enterohepatic cycling, multiple doses of charcoal may be needed to reduce the potential for delayed toxicities. NSAIDs are highly bound to plasma proteins, therefore hemodialysis and peritoneal dialysis are not useful.

Drug Interactions

May increase digoxin, methotrexate, and lithium serum concentrations

Aspirin may decrease NSAID serum concentrations

Other NSAIDs may increase adverse GI effects

Increased prothrombin time with anticoagulants

Decreased antihypertensive effects of ACE inhibitors, beta-blockers, and thiazide diuretics

Increased response to sympathomimetics

Probenecid may increase toxicity of NSAIDs by increase in serum concentrations

Diuretics may increase risk of acute renal function

Azotemia may be enhanced in elderly receiving loop diuretics

Mechanism of Action Inhibits prostaglandin synthesis, acts on the hypothalamus heat-regulating center to reduce fever, blocks prostaglandin synthetase action which prevents formation of the platelet-aggregating substance thromboxane A_2; decreases pain receptor sensitivity. Other proposed mechanisms of action are lysosomal stabilization, inhibition of kinin and leukotriene production, alteration of chemotactic factors, and inhibition of neutrophil activation. This latter mechanism may be the most significant pharmacologic action to reduce inflammation.

Pharmacodynamics Onset of anti-inflammatory action: Up to 7 days

Pharmacokinetics

Absorption: Almost completely

Protein binding: >99%

Half-life: 40-50 hours; with continued dosing, half-life decreases to ~40 hours

Time to peak: 3-5 hours

Elimination: Has a dual pathway, hepatic and renal; with continued dosing, this dual pathway explains the lower half-life of chronic dosing vs single dose half-life

Usual Dosage Geriatrics and Adults: Oral (individualize dosage to lowest effective dose to minimize adverse effects):

Osteoarthritis: 600-1200 mg once daily

Rheumatoid arthritis: 1200 mg once daily

Maximum dose: 1800 mg/day or 26 mg/kg (whichever is lower) in divided doses

See Additional Information

Monitoring Parameters Monitor response (pain, range of motion, grip strength, mobility, ADL function), inflammation; observe for weight gain, edema; monitor renal function; observe for bleeding, bruising; evaluate gastrointestinal effects (abdominal pain, bleeding, dyspepsia); mental confusion, disorientation, CBC, serum, creatinine, BUN, liver function tests

Test Interactions Increased chloride (S), increased sodium (S)

Patient Information Serious gastrointestinal bleeding can occur as well as ulceration and perforation. Pain may or may not be present. Avoid aspirin and aspirin-containing products while taking this medication. If gastric upset occurs, take with food, milk, or antacid. If gastric adverse effects persist, contact physician. May cause drowsiness, dizziness, blurred vision, and confusion. Use caution when performing tasks which require alertness (eg, driving). Do not take for more than 3 days for fever or 10 days for pain without physician's advice.

Nursing Implications See Patient Information, Overdosage, Monitoring Parameters, and Special Geriatric Considerations

Additional Information There are no clinical guidelines to predict which NSAID will give response in a particular patient; trials with each must be initiated until response determined; consider dose, patient convenience, and cost

Special Geriatric Considerations Elderly are a high-risk population for adverse effects from nonsteroidal anti-inflammatory agents. As much as 60% of elderly can develop peptic ulceration and/or hemorrhage asymptomatically. The concomitant use of H_2 blockers, omeprazole, and sucralfate is not generally effective as prophylaxis with the exception of NSAID-induced duodenal ulcers which may be prevented by the use of ranitidine. Misoprostol and proton pump inhibitors are the only agents proven to help prevent the development of NSAID-induced ulcers. Also, concomitant disease and drug use contribute to the risk for GI adverse effects. Use lowest effective dose for shortest period possible. Consider renal function decline with age. Use of NSAIDs can compromise existing renal function especially when Cl_{cr} is ≤30 mL/minute. Tinnitus may be a difficult and unreliable indication of toxicity due to age-related hearing loss or eighth cranial nerve damage. CNS adverse effects such as confusion, agitation, and hallucination are generally seen in overdose or high dose situations, but elderly may demonstrate these adverse effects at lower doses than younger adults.

Dosage Forms Tablet: 600 mg

References

Brooks PM, Day RO, "Nonsteroidal Anti-inflammatory Drugs - Differences and Similarities," *N Engl J Med*, 1991, 324(24):1716-25.

Clinch D, Banerjee AK, Ostick G, "Absence of Abdominal Pain in Elderly Patients With Peptic Ulcer," *Age Ageing*, 1984, 13(2):120-3.

Clive DM, Stoff JS, "Renal Syndromes Associated With Nonsteroidal Anti-inflammatory Drugs," *N Engl J Med*, 1984, 310(9):563-72.

Graham DY, "Prevention of Gastroduodenal Injury Induced by Chronic Nonsteroidal Anti-inflammatory Drug Therapy," *Gastroenterology*, 1989, 96(2 Pt 2 Suppl):675-81.

Gurwitz JH, Avorn J, Ross-Degnan D, et al, "Nonsteroidal Anti-Inflammatory Drug-Associated Azotemia in the Very Old," *JAMA*, 1990, 264(4):471-5.

Hawkey CJ, Karrasch JA, Szczepaski L, et al, "Omeprazole Compared With Misoprostrol for Ulcers Associated With Nonsteroidal Anti-inflammatory Drugs," *N Engl J Med*, 1998, 338(11):727-34.

Knodel LC, "Preventing NSAID-Induced Ulcers: The Role of Misoprostol," *Consult Pharm*, 1989, 4:37-41.

Pounder R, "Silent Peptic Ulceration: Deadly Silence or Golden Silence?" *Gastroenterology*, 1989, 96:(2 Pt 2 Suppl)626-31.

Yeomans ND, Tulassay Z, Juhasz L, et al, "A Comparison of Omeprazole With Ranitidine for Ulcers Associated With Nonsteroidal Anti-inflammatory Drugs," *N Engl J Med*, 1998, 338(11):719-26.

Oxazepam (oks A ze pam)

Related Information

Antacid Drug Interactions *on page 1096*

Anxiolytic/Hypnotic Use in Long-Term Care Facilities *on page 1099*

Benzodiazepines Comparison *on page 1024*

Federal OBRA Regulations Recommended Maximum Doses - Anxiolytics *on page 1057*

Federal OBRA Regulations Recommended Maximum Doses - Hypnotics *on page 1057*

Brand Names Serax®

Generic Available Yes

Therapeutic Category Antianxiety Agent; Benzodiazepine

Use Treatment of anxiety and management of alcohol withdrawal

Restrictions C-IV

Contraindications Hypersensitivity to oxazepam or any component, cross-sensitivity with other benzodiazepines may exist; avoid using in patients with pre-existing CNS depression, severe uncontrolled pain, or narrow-angle glaucoma

Precautions Use with caution in patients with a history of drug dependence

Adverse Reactions

Central nervous system: Drowsiness, confusion, dizziness, ataxia, amnesia, slurred speech, paradoxical excitement or rage

Gastrointestinal: Constipation, xerostomia, diarrhea, nausea, vomiting

Neuromuscular & skeletal: Impaired coordination

Ocular: Blurred vision, diplopia

(Continued)

Oxazepam *(Continued)*

Respiratory: Decrease in respiratory rate, apnea, laryngospasm
Miscellaneous: Physical and psychological dependence with prolonged use

Overdosage Symptoms of overdose include somnolence, confusion, coma, and diminished reflexes

Toxicology Treatment for benzodiazepine overdose is supportive; rarely is mechanical ventilation required
Flumazenil has been shown to selectively block the binding of benzodiazepines to CNS receptors, resulting in a reversal of benzodiazepine-induced sedation; however, its use may not alter the course of overdose

Drug Interactions Increased toxicity: CNS depressants, alcohol

Mechanism of Action Benzodiazepines appear to potentiate the effects of GABA and other inhibitory neurotransmitters by binding to specific benzodiazepine-receptor sites in various areas of the CNS

Pharmacodynamics Studies have shown that the elderly are more sensitive to the effects of benzodiazepines as compared to younger adults

Pharmacokinetics No significant changes in pharmacokinetics are seen in the elderly

Absorption: Oral: Almost completely
Protein binding: 86% to 99%
Metabolism: In the liver to inactive compounds (primarily as glucuronides)
Half-life: 5-20 hours
Time to peak serum concentration: Within 2-4 hours
Elimination: Urinary excretion of unchanged drug (50%) and metabolites; excreted without need for liver metabolism

Usual Dosage Oral:
Geriatrics: Anxiety: 10 mg 2-3 times/day; increase gradually as needed to a total of 30-45 mg/day
Adults:
Anxiety: 10-15 mg 3-4 times/day
Alcohol withdrawal: 15-30 mg 3-4 times/day
Not dialyzable (0% to 5%)

Monitoring Parameters Respiratory, cardiovascular and mental status, symptoms of anxiety

Reference Range Therapeutic: 0.2-1.4 μg/mL (SI: 0.7-4.9 μmol/L)

Patient Information Avoid alcohol and other CNS depressants; may cause drowsiness; avoid activities needing good psychomotor coordination until CNS effects are known; may cause physical or psychological dependence; avoid abrupt discontinuation after prolonged use

Nursing Implications Assist patient with ambulation, monitor for alertness

Special Geriatric Considerations Because of its relatively short half-life and its lack of active metabolites, oxazepam is recommended for use in the elderly when a benzodiazepine is indicated (see Pharmacodynamics)

Dosage Forms
Capsule: 10 mg, 15 mg, 30 mg
Tablet: 15 mg

References
Hicks R, Dysken MW, Davis JM, et al, "The Pharmacokinetics of Psychotropic Medication in the Elderly: A Review," *J Clin Psychiatry*, 1981, 42(10)374-85.

Oxilapine Succinate *see Loxapine on page 556*
Oxpentifylline *see Pentoxifylline on page 728*

Oxybutynin *(oks i BYOO ti nin)*

Brand Names Ditropan®

Generic Available Yes

Therapeutic Category Antispasmodic Agent, Urinary

Use Antispasmodic for bladder (urgency, frequency, urge incontinence) and uninhibited bladder

Contraindications Glaucoma, myasthenia gravis, partial or complete GI obstruction, GU obstruction, ulcerative colitis; patients hypersensitive to the drug; intestinal atony, megacolon, toxic megacolon

Precautions Use with caution in patients with hepatic or renal disease, heart disease, hyperthyroidism, reflux esophagitis; use with caution in elderly, autonomic neuropathy, ulcerative colitis (may cause ileus and toxic megacolon), hypertension, hiatal hernia, and prostatic hypertrophy; use caution in patients with heat prostration, diarrhea (may be early sign of intestinal obstruction)

Adverse Reactions
Cardiovascular: Tachycardia, palpitations

Central nervous system: Drowsiness, fever, dizziness, insomnia, hallucinations, restlessness

Dermatologic: Rash

Endocrine & metabolic: Hot flashes

Gastrointestinal: Xerostomia, nausea, vomiting, constipation, decreased GI motility

Genitourinary: Urinary hesitancy or retention, impotence

Neuromuscular & skeletal: Weakness

Ocular: Blurred vision, mydriasis, amblyopia

Miscellaneous: Decreased diaphoresis

Overdosage Symptoms of overdose include hypotension, circulatory failure, psychotic behavior, flushing, respiratory failure, paralysis, restlessness, tremor, irritability, seizures, delirium, hallucinations, coma

Toxicology Symptomatic and supportive; induce emesis or perform gastric lavage followed by charcoal and a cathartic; physostigmine may be required; treat hyperpyrexia with cooling techniques (ice bags, cold applications, alcohol sponges)

Drug Interactions

Oxybutynin may increase serum concentrations of digoxin

May decrease serum concentrations of haloperidol

May enhance development of tardive dyskinesia; may enhance anticholinergic effect of drugs exhibiting anticholinergic pharmacologic action

Mechanism of Action Direct antispasmodic effect on smooth muscle, also inhibits the action of acetylcholine on smooth muscle (exhibits $1/5$ the anticholinergic activity of atropine, but is 4-10 times the antispasmodic activity); does not block effects at skeletal muscle or at autonomic ganglia; increases bladder capacity, decreases uninhibited contractions, and delays desire to void; therefore, decreases urgency and frequency

Pharmacodynamics

Onset of action: Oral: 30-60 minutes

Peak effects: 3-6 hours

Duration: 6-10 hours

Pharmacokinetics

Absorption: Oral: Rapid

Metabolism: In the liver

Half-life: 1-2.3 hours

Time to peak serum concentration: Within 60 minutes

Elimination: In urine

Usual Dosage Oral (see Additional Information):

Geriatrics: 2.5-5 mg twice daily; increase by 2.5 mg increments every 1-2 days

Adults: 5 mg 2-3 times/day up to 5 mg 4 times/day maximum

Monitoring Parameters Monitor incontinence episodes, postvoid residual (PVR)

Patient Information May impair ability to perform activities requiring mental alertness or physical coordination; alcohol or other sedating drugs may enhance drowsiness

Nursing Implications See Adverse Reactions, Precautions, Monitoring Parameters, and Special Geriatric Considerations

Additional Information Should be discontinued periodically to determine whether the patient can manage without the drug and to minimize resistance to the drug

Special Geriatric Considerations Caution should be used in elderly due to anticholinergic activity (eg, confusion, constipation, blurred vision, and tachycardia)

Dosage Forms

Oxybutynin chloride:

Syrup: 5 mg/5 mL (473 mL)

Tablet: 5 mg

Oxycodone (oks i KOE done)

Related Information

Narcotic Agonist Comparative Pharmacology *on page 1036*

Pharmacokinetics of Narcotic Agonist Analgesics *on page 1037*

Brand Names OxyContin®; OxyIR®; Roxicodone™

Synonyms Dihydrohydroxycodeinone

Generic Available No

Therapeutic Category Analgesic, Narcotic

(Continued)

Oxycodone *(Continued)*

Use Management of moderate to severe pain, normally used in combination with non-narcotic analgesics; controlled release: management of moderate to severe pain where use of an opioid is appropriate for more than a few days

Restrictions C-II

Contraindications Hypersensitivity to oxycodone or any component

Warnings Use with caution in patients with hypersensitivity reactions to other phenanthrene derivative opioid agonists (morphine, hydrocodone, hydromorphone, levorphanol, oxycodone, oxymorphone); respiratory diseases including asthma, emphysema, COPD, or severe liver or renal insufficiency; some preparations contain sulfites which may cause allergic reactions

Adverse Reactions

Cardiovascular: Palpitations, hypotension, bradycardia, peripheral vasodilation

Central nervous system: CNS depression, increased intracranial pressure

Dermatologic: Pruritus

Endocrine & metabolic: Antidiuretic hormone release

Gastrointestinal: Nausea, vomiting, constipation

Ocular: Miosis

Respiratory: Respiratory depression

Miscellaneous: Physical and psychological dependence, histamine release, biliary or urinary tract spasm

Overdosage Symptoms of overdose include CNS depression, respiratory depression, miosis

Toxicology Treatment of an overdose includes support of the patient's airway, establishment of an I.V. line and administration of naloxone 2 mg I.V. with repeat administration as necessary up to a total of 10 mg.

Drug Interactions

Decreased effect with phenothiazines

Increased effect/toxicity with CNS depressants, TCAs, dextroamphetamine

Mechanism of Action Binds to opiate receptors in the CNS, causing inhibition of ascending pain pathways, altering the perception of and response to pain; produces generalized CNS depression

Pharmacodynamics

Onset of action: Oral: Pain relief occurs within 10-15 minutes

Peak effects: 30-60 minutes

Duration: 4-5 hours (immediate release), 12 hours (sustained release); enhanced analgesia has been seen in elderly patients on therapeutic doses of narcotics; duration of action may be increased in the elderly

Pharmacokinetics

Metabolism: In the liver

Half-life: Plasma concentrations in the elderly were 15% higher as compared to younger adults

Immediate release: 3.2 hours

Controlled release: 4.5 hours

Elimination: In urine

Usual Dosage Oral:

Geriatrics: 2.5-5 mg every 6 hours as needed

Adults: 5 mg every 6 hours as needed

Controlled release:

Opioid naive (not currently on opioid): 10 mg every 12 hours

Currently on opioid/ASA or acetaminophen or NSAID combination:

1-5 tablets: 10-20 mg every 12 hours

6-9 tablets: 20-30 mg every 12 hours

10-12 tablets: 30-40 mg every 12 hours

May continue the nonopioid as a separate drug

Currently on opioids: Use standard conversion chart to convert daily dose to oxycodone equivalent. Divide daily dose in 2 (for every 12-hour dosing) and round down to nearest dosage form.

Monitoring Parameters Pain relief, respiratory and mental status, blood pressure

Patient Information May cause drowsiness, avoid alcoholic beverages; do not exceed recommended dose; controlled release "ghost" tablet may appear in stool; do not chew, break, or crush the controlled release form

Nursing Implications Monitor patient for pain relief, excessive sedation, confusion, and constipation; do not allow patient to chew, break, or crush the controlled release form

Additional Information

Oxycodone: Roxicodone™, OxyContin® (controlled release)

Oxycodone and acetaminophen: Oxycet®, Percocet®, Roxicet®, Tylox®
Oxycodone and aspirin: Percodan®, Percodan®-Demi, Codoxy®, Roxiprin®

Special Geriatric Considerations The elderly may be particularly susceptible to the CNS depressant and constipating effects of narcotics (see Pharmacodynamics)

Dosage Forms
Oxycodone hydrochloride:
Capsule, immediate release (OxyIR®): 5 mg
Liquid, oral: 5 mg/5 mL (500 mL)
Solution, oral concentrate: 20 mg/mL (30 mL)
Tablet: 5 mg
Tablet, controlled release (OxyContin®): 10 mg, 20 mg, 40 mg, 80 mg

Oxycodone and Acetaminophen
(oks i KOE done & a seet a MIN oh fen)

Related Information
Acetaminophen *on page 16*
Oxycodone *on page 703*
Pharmacokinetics of Narcotic Agonist Analgesics *on page 1037*

Brand Names Percocet®; Roxicet® 5/500; Roxilox®; Tylox®

Synonyms Acetaminophen and Oxycodone

Generic Available Yes

Therapeutic Category Analgesic, Narcotic

Use Management of moderate to severe pain

Restrictions C-II

Contraindications Hypersensitivity to oxycodone, acetaminophen or any component; severe respiratory depression, severe liver or renal insufficiency

Warnings Some preparations may contain bisulfites which may cause allergies

Precautions Use with caution in patients with hypersensitivity to other phenanthrene derivative opioid agonists (morphine, codeine, hydrocodone, hydromorphone, oxymorphone, levorphanol)

Adverse Reactions
Cardiovascular: Palpitations, hypotension, bradycardia, peripheral vasodilation
Central nervous system: CNS depression, increased intracranial pressure
Dermatologic: Pruritus
Endocrine & metabolic: Antidiuretic hormone release
Gastrointestinal: Nausea, vomiting, constipation
Ocular: Miosis
Respiratory: Respiratory depression
Miscellaneous: Physical and psychological dependence, biliary or urinary tract spasm, histamine release

Overdosage Symptoms of overdose include hepatic necrosis, transient azotemia, renal tubular necrosis with acute toxicity, anemia, renal damage, and GI disturbances with chronic toxicity

Toxicology Treatment of an overdose includes support of the patient's airway, establishment of an I.V. line and administration of naloxone 2 mg I.V. with repeat administration as necessary. Mucomyst® (acetylcysteine) 140 mg/kg orally (loading) followed by 70 mg/kg (maintenance) every 4 hours for 17 doses. Therapy should be initiated based upon laboratory analysis suggesting high probability of hepatotoxic potential.

Drug Interactions
Decreased effect with phenothiazines
Increased effect/toxicity with CNS depressants, TCAs, dextroamphetamine

Usual Dosage Oral (doses should be titrated to appropriate analgesic effects):
Geriatrics: 1 tablet or capsule every 6 hours as needed; do not exceed 4 g/day of acetaminophen
Adults: 1-2 tablets every 4-6 hours as needed for pain

Monitoring Parameters Pain relief, respiratory and mental status, blood pressure

Patient Information May cause drowsiness, avoid alcoholic beverages; do not exceed recommended dose

Nursing Implications Monitor for pain relief, excessive sedation, confusion, and constipation

Special Geriatric Considerations Enhanced analgesia has been seen in elderly patients on therapeutic doses of narcotics; duration of action may be increased in the elderly; the elderly may be particularly susceptible to the CNS depressant and constipating effects of narcotics; if 1 tablet/dose is used, (Continued)

Oxycodone and Acetaminophen *(Continued)*

it may be useful to add an additional 325 mg of acetaminophen to maximize analgesic effect

Dosage Forms

Caplet: Oxycodone hydrochloride 5 mg and acetaminophen 500 mg

Capsule: Oxycodone hydrochloride 5 mg and acetaminophen 500 mg

Solution, oral: Oxycodone hydrochloride 5 mg and acetaminophen 325 mg per 5 mL (5 mL, 500 mL)

Tablet: Oxycodone hydrochloride 5 mg and acetaminophen 325 mg

Oxycodone and Aspirin (oks i KOE done & AS pir in)

Related Information

Aspirin *on page 84*

Oxycodone *on page 703*

Pharmacokinetics of Narcotic Agonist Analgesics *on page 1037*

Brand Names Codoxy®; Percodan®; Percodan®-Demi; Roxiprin®

Synonyms Aspirin and Oxycodone

Generic Available Yes

Therapeutic Category Analgesic, Narcotic

Use Relief of moderate to moderately severe pain

Restrictions C-II

Contraindications Known hypersensitivity to oxycodone or aspirin; severe respiratory depression, severe liver or renal insufficiency

Precautions Use with caution in patients with hypersensitivity to other phenanthrene derivative opioid agonists (morphine, codeine, hydrocodone, hydromorphone, oxymorphone, levorphanol)

Adverse Reactions

Cardiovascular: Palpitations, hypotension, bradycardia, peripheral vasodilation

Central nervous system: CNS depression, increased intracranial pressure

Dermatologic: Pruritus

Endocrine & metabolic: Antidiuretic hormone release

Gastrointestinal: Nausea, vomiting, constipation

Ocular: Miosis

Respiratory: Respiratory depression

Miscellaneous: Physical and psychological dependence, biliary or urinary tract spasm, histamine release

Overdosage Symptoms of overdose include CNS and respiratory depression, gastrointestinal cramping, constipation, tinnitus, headache, dizziness, confusion, metabolic acidosis, hyperpyrexia

Toxicology Naloxone 2 mg I.V. with repeat administration as necessary up to a total of 10 mg; see also Aspirin toxicology

Drug Interactions

Decreased effect with phenothiazines

Increased effect/toxicity with CNS depressants, TCAs, dextroamphetamine

Usual Dosage Geriatrics and Adults: Oral (based on oxycodone combined salts): Percodan®: 1 tablet every 6 hours as needed for pain or Percodan®-Demi: 1-2 tablets every 6 hours as needed for pain

Monitoring Parameters Pain relief, respiratory and mental status, blood pressure

Patient Information May cause drowsiness, avoid alcoholic beverages; do not exceed recommended dose

Nursing Implications Monitor for pain relief, excessive sedation, confusion, and constipation

Special Geriatric Considerations Enhanced analgesia has been seen in elderly patients on therapeutic doses of narcotics; duration of action may be increased; the elderly may be particularly susceptible to the CNS depressant and constipating effects of narcotics; if 1 tablet/dose is used, it may be useful to add an additional 325 mg of aspirin to maximize analgesic effect

Dosage Forms Tablet: Oxycodone hydrochloride 4.5 mg, oxycodone terephthalate 0.38 mg, and aspirin 325 mg; oxycodone hydrochloride 2.25 mg, oxycodone terephthalate 0.19 mg, and aspirin 325 mg

OxyContin® *see* Oxycodone *on page 703*

OxyIR® *see* Oxycodone *on page 703*

Oxymetazoline (oks i met AZ oh leen)

Brand Names Afrin® Children's Nose Drops [OTC]; Afrin® Sinus [OTC]; Allerest® 12 Hour Nasal Solution [OTC]; Chlorphed®-LA Nasal Solution [OTC];

Dristan® Long Lasting Nasal Solution [OTC]; Duramist Plus® [OTC]; Duration® Nasal Solution [OTC]; Neo-Synephrine® 12 Hour Nasal Solution [OTC]; Nōstrilla® [OTC]; NTZ® Long Acting Nasal Solution [OTC]; OcuClear® Ophthalmic [OTC]; Sinarest® 12 Hour Nasal Solution; Sinex® Long-Acting [OTC]; Twice-A-Day® Nasal [OTC]; Visine® L.R. Ophthalmic [OTC]; 4-Way® Long Acting Nasal Solution [OTC]

Generic Available Yes

Therapeutic Category Adrenergic Agonist Agent; Adrenergic Agonist Agent, Ophthalmic; Decongestant, Nasal; Ophthalmic Agent, Vasoconstrictor; Vasoconstrictor, Nasal; Vasoconstrictor, Ophthalmic

Use Symptomatic relief of nasal mucosal congestion and adjunctive therapy of middle ear infections, associated with acute or chronic rhinitis, the common cold, sinusitis, hay fever, or other allergies

Ophthalmic: Relief of redness of eye due to minor eye irritations

Contraindications Hypersensitivity to oxymetazoline or any component

Warnings Rebound congestion may occur with extended use (>3 days); use with caution in the presence of hypertension, diabetes, hyperthyroidism, heart disease, coronary artery disease, cerebral arteriosclerosis, or long-standing bronchial asthma

Adverse Reactions

Cardiovascular: Hypertension, palpitations, reflex bradycardia

Central nervous system: Nervousness, dizziness, insomnia, headache

Gastrointestinal: Nausea

Respiratory: Sneezing; transient burning, stinging, dryness of nasal mucosa; rebound congestion with prolonged use

Overdosage Symptoms of overdose include CNS depression, hypothermia, bradycardia, cardiovascular collapse, coma, apnea

Toxicology Following initiation of essential overdose management, toxic symptoms should be treated. The patient should be kept warm and monitored for alterations in vital functions. Seizures commonly respond to diazepam (5-10 mg I.V. bolus in adults every 15 minutes if needed up to a total of 30 mg) or to phenytoin or phenobarbital; hypotension should be treated with fluids.

Drug Interactions Increased toxicity: MAO inhibitors

Mechanism of Action Stimulates alpha-adrenergic receptors in the arterioles of the nasal mucosa to produce vasoconstriction

Pharmacodynamics

Onset of effect: Intranasal: Within 5-10 minutes

Duration: 5-6 hours

Pharmacokinetics Metabolism: Metabolic fate is unknown

Usual Dosage Geriatrics and Adults (therapy should not exceed 3-5 days):

Intranasal: 0.05% solution: Instill 2-3 drops or 2-3 sprays into each nostril twice daily

Ophthalmic: Instill 1-2 drops into affected eye(s) every 6 hours

Monitoring Parameters Blood pressure in hypertensives

Patient Information Should not be used for self-medication for longer than 3 days, if symptoms persist, drug should be discontinued and a physician consulted; notify physician of insomnia, tremor, or irregular heartbeat; burning, stinging, or drying of the nasal mucosa may occur

Special Geriatric Considerations Evaluate the patient's ability to self-administer; use with caution in patients with cardiovascular disease

Dosage Forms

Oxymetazoline hydrochloride:

Nasal solution:

Drops:

Afrin® Children's Nose Drops: 0.025% (20 mL)

Afrin®, NTZ® Long Acting Nasal Solution: 0.05% (15 mL, 20 mL)

Spray: Afrin® Sinus, Allerest® 12 Hours, Chlorphed®-LA, Dristan® Long Lasting, Duration®, 4-Way® Long Acting, Genasal®, Nasal Relief®, Neo-Synephrine® 12 Hour, Nōstrilla®, NTZ® Long Acting Nasal Solution, Sinex® Long-Acting, Twice-A-Day®: 0.05% (15 mL, 30 mL)

Ophthalmic solution (OcuClear®, Visine® L.R.): 0.025% (15 mL, 30 mL)

Oxymorphone (oks i MOR fone)

Related Information

Narcotic Agonist Comparative Pharmacology on page 1036

Brand Names Numorphan®

Generic Available No

Therapeutic Category Analgesic, Narcotic

(Continued)

Oxymorphone *(Continued)*

Use Management of moderate to severe pain and preoperatively as a sedative and a supplement to anesthesia

Restrictions C-II

Contraindications Hypersensitivity to oxymorphone or any component, increased intracranial pressure; severe respiratory depression

Warnings Some preparations contain sulfites which may cause allergic reactions; use with caution in patients with impaired respiratory function or severe hepatic dysfunction and in patients with hypersensitivity reactions to other phenanthrene derivative opioid agonists (codeine, hydrocodone, hydromorphone, levorphanol, oxycodone, oxymorphone)

Adverse Reactions
Cardiovascular: Hypotension (>10%)
Central nervous system: Fatigue (>10%), drowsiness (>10%), dizziness (>10%), nervousness, headache, restlessness, malaise, confusion, mental depression, hallucinations, paradoxical CNS stimulation, increased intracranial pressure
Dermatologic: Rash, urticaria
Gastrointestinal: Nausea (>10%), vomiting (>10%), constipation (>10%), anorexia, stomach cramps, xerostomia, biliary spasm, paralytic ileus
Genitourinary: Decreased urination, ureteral spasms
Local: Pain at injection site
Neuromuscular & skeletal: Weakness (>10%)
Respiratory: Dyspnea, shortness of breath
Miscellaneous: Histamine release, physical and psychological dependence

Overdosage Symptoms of overdose include respiratory depression, miosis, hypotension, bradycardia, apnea, pulmonary edema, CNS depression

Toxicology Treatment of an overdose includes support of the patient's airway, establishment of an I.V. line and administration of naloxone 2 mg I.V. with repeat administration as necessary up to a total of 10 mg.

Drug Interactions
Decreased effect with phenothiazines
Increased effect/toxicity with CNS depressants, TCAs, dextroamphetamine

Stability Refrigerate suppository

Mechanism of Action Oxymorphone hydrochloride is a potent narcotic analgesic with uses similar to those of morphine. The drug is a semisynthetic derivative of morphine (phenanthrene derivative) and is closely related to hydromorphone (Dilaudid®).

Pharmacodynamics
Onset of analgesia:
I.V., I.M., S.C.: Within 5-10 minutes
Rectal: Within 15-30 minutes
Duration of analgesia: Parenteral, rectal: 3-4 hours; enhanced analgesia has been seen in elderly patients on therapeutic doses of narcotics; duration of action may be increased in the elderly

Pharmacokinetics
Metabolism: Conjugated with glucuronic acid
Elimination: In urine

Usual Dosage Geriatrics and Adults:
I.M., S.C.: 0.5 mg initially, 1-1.5 mg every 4-6 hours as needed
I.V.: 0.5 mg initially
Rectal: 5 mg every 4-6 hours

Monitoring Parameters Pain relief, respiratory and mental status, blood pressure, pulse

Patient Information Avoid alcohol, may cause drowsiness, impaired judgment or coordination; may cause physical and psychological dependence with prolonged use, do not exceed recommended dose

Nursing Implications Monitor patient for pain relief, excessive sedation, confusion, and constipation

Special Geriatric Considerations The elderly may be particularly susceptible to the CNS depressant and constipating effects of narcotics (see Pharmacodynamics)

Dosage Forms
Oxymorphone hydrochloride:
Injection: 1 mg (1 mL); 1.5 mg/mL (1 mL, 10 mL)
Suppository, rectal: 5 mg

References
Sinatra RS and Harrison DM, "Oxymorphone in Patient-Controlled Analgesia," *Clin Pharm*, 1989, 8(8):541, 544.

Oxytetracycline (oks i tet ra SYE kleen)

Brand Names Terramycin® I.M. Injection; Terramycin® Oral; Uri-Tet® Oral

Therapeutic Category Antibiotic, Tetracycline Derivative

Use Treatment of susceptible bacterial infections; both gram-positive and gram-negative, as well as *Rickettsia* and *Mycoplasma* organisms

Contraindications Hypersensitivity to tetracycline or any component

Precautions Photosensitivity can occur with oxytetracycline

Adverse Reactions
Central nervous system: Pseudotumor cerebri
Dermatologic: Photosensitivity
Gastrointestinal: Nausea, vomiting, diarrhea, antibiotic-associated pseudo-membranous colitis, staphylococcal enterocolitis
Hepatic: Hepatotoxicity
Local: Thrombophlebitis
Neuromuscular & skeletal: Injury to growing bones and teeth
Renal: Renal damage
Miscellaneous: Candidal superinfection, discoloration of teeth and enamel hypoplasia, hypersensitivity reactions

Drug Interactions
Antacids, milk, iron, calcium, methoxyflurane, zinc, penicillins, cimetidine, food (particularly dairy products) may decrease absorption
May increase the effects of anticoagulants, digoxin; may increase or decrease lithium level

Drug/Food Interactions Food, particularly dairy products, may decrease absorption

Mechanism of Action Inhibits bacterial protein synthesis by binding with the 30S and possibly the 50S ribosomal subunit(s) of susceptible bacteria, cell wall synthesis is not affected

Pharmacokinetics
Absorption:
Oral: Adequately, ~75%
I.M.: Poor
Metabolism: Small amounts metabolized in the liver
Half-life: 8.5-9.6 hours (increases with renal impairment)
Time to peak serum concentration: Within 2-4 hours
Elimination: In urine, while much higher amounts can be found in bile

Usual Dosage Geriatrics and Adults:
Oral: 250-500 mg every 6 hours
I.M.: 250-500 mg every 12 hours or 300 mg/day divided every 8-12 hours

Administration Injection for intramuscular use only; do not administer with food or antacids

Monitoring Parameters Signs and symptoms of infection, WBC, mental status

Test Interactions Increased catecholamines (U), increased uric acid (S); decreased urea nitrogen (B)

Patient Information Complete full course of therapy; take on an empty stomach 1 hour before or 2 hours after meals; do not take with antacids or vitamins or iron; avoid excessive exposure to natural or artificial sunlight

Nursing Implications Reduce dose in renal insufficiency (see Administration)

Special Geriatric Considerations Oxytetracycline has not been studied in the elderly, however, dose reduction for renal function is not necessary

Dosage Forms
Oxytetracycline hydrochloride:
Capsule: 250 mg
Injection, with lidocaine 2%: 5% [50 mg/mL] (2 mL, 10 mL); 12.5% [125 mg/mL] (2 mL)

Oyst-Cal 500 [OTC] *see* Calcium Salts (Oral) *on page 152*

Oystercal® 500 *see* Calcium Salts (Oral) *on page 152*

P-071 *see* Cetirizine *on page 199*

Pamelor® *see* Nortriptyline *on page 684*

Pamidronate (pa mi DROE nate)

Brand Names Aredia™

Generic Available No

Therapeutic Category Antidote, Hypercalcemia; Bisphosphonate Derivative

Use Hypercalcemia associated with malignancy with or without bone metastases

(Continued)

Pamidronate *(Continued)*

Unlabeled use: Symptomatic treatment of Paget's disease, postmenopausal osteoporosis; reduce severe bone pain in malignancy; prevent steroid-induced osteoporosis

Contraindications Hypersensitivity to biphosphonates

Warnings Has not been tested in patients with serum creatinine >5 mg/dL; renal dysfunction when used to treat hypercalcemia secondary to malignancy

Precautions Patients should maintain adequate intake of calcium and vitamin D; use with caution in patients with pre-existing fractures, for uninterrupted periods of >6 months, and in patients with renal dysfunction (serum creatinine: >5 mg/dL)

Adverse Reactions

Cardiovascular: Fluid overload, hypertension, syncope, tachycardia, atrial fibrillation

Central nervous system: Fatigue, somnolence, insomnia, self-limiting pyrexia (within the first 72 hours)

Endocrine & metabolic: Hypokalemia, hypomagnesemia, hypophosphatemia, hypothyroidism, hypocalcemia

Gastrointestinal: Abdominal pain, nausea, anorexia, constipation, GI bleeding

Genitourinary: Urinary tract infections

Hematologic: Anemia

Hepatic: Elevated liver function tests

Local: Soft tissue erythema, edema or induration, pain on palpation at site of injection

Neuromuscular & skeletal: Generalized pain, bone pain

Ocular: Uveitis, abnormal vision

Respiratory: Rhinitis

Miscellaneous: Transient elevation of body temperature (1°C) at initiation of therapy, moniliasis

Overdosage Symptoms of overdose include hypocalcemia, EKG changes, seizures, bleeding, paresthesia, carpopedal spasm, fever

Toxicology Treat hypocalcemia with I.V. calcium gluconate; general supportive care; fever and hypotension can be treated with corticosteroids

Drug Interactions Calcium (see Additional Information)

Stability Reconstitute with 10 mL of sterile water for injection, USP; resulting solution has a pH of 6-7.4; infusion is stable for 24 hours at room temperature; solution should be diluted with ½ normal or normal saline USP or 5% dextrose injection, USP. Reconstituted with sterile water for injection may be stored in refrigerator at temperatures of 36°F to 46°F (2°C to 8°C) for 24 hours. Do not use calcium-containing solutions such as Ringer's solution as a diluent.

Mechanism of Action Inhibits normal and abnormal bone resorption; this action is achieved without inhibiting bone formation and mineralization; the exact mechanism is not known, but may be due to inhibition of hydroxyapatite crystal dissolution or its action on osteoclasts; decreased phosphate serum concentrations due to release from bone and increase in parathyroid hormone levels (suppressed during hypercalcemia)

Pharmacokinetics Limited data in humans

Half-life:

Alpha (distribution): 1.6 hours

Urinary (elimination): 2.5 hours

Bone: 300 days

Elimination, biphasic: ~50% excreted unchanged in urine within 72 hours

Usual Dosage Geriatrics and Adults (dose is dependent on the severity and symptoms of hypercalcemia): I.V.:

Moderate hypercalcemia (corrected serum calcium 12-13.5 mg/dL): 60-90 mg given as a slow infusion over 24 hours

Severe hypercalcemia (corrected serum calcium >13.5 mg/dL): 90 mg given as a slow infusion over 24 hours

Consider retreatment if needed; allow at least 7 days before retreatment (see Additional Information)

Monitoring Parameters Serum calcium, electrolytes, phosphate, magnesium, potassium, serum creatinine, CBC with differential

Reference Range Calcium (total): Adults: 9.0-11.0 mg/dL (2.05-2.54 mmol/L), may slightly decrease with aging; phosphorus: 2.5-4.5 mg/dL (0.81-1.45 mmol/L)

Patient Information Maintain adequate intake of calcium and vitamin D; report any fever, sore throat, or unusual bleeding to your physician

Nursing Implications Patient should be adequately hydrated while receiving this medication (see Additional Information and Special Geriatric Considerations)

Additional Information Do not mix with calcium containing solutions (ie, lactated Ringer's solution); reconstitute in 10 mL sterile water for injection USP for each vial (results in 30 mg/10 mL); dilute in 0.45% NS, 0.9% NS, or D_5W to administer

Special Geriatric Considerations Has not been studied exclusively in the elderly; monitor serum electrolytes periodically since elderly are often receiving diuretics which can result in decreases in serum calcium, potassium, and magnesium

Dosage Forms Powder for injection, lyophilized, as disodium: 30 mg, 60 mg, 90 mg

References
Drug Facts and Comparisons, St Louis, MO: JB Lippincott Co, 1992, 134f-134m.
Kellihan MJ and Mangino PD, "Pamidronate," *Ann Pharmacother*, 1992, 26(10):1262-9.

p-Aminoclonidine *see* Apraclonidine *on page 78*

Pamisyl® *see* Aminosalicylic Acid *on page 57*

Pamprin IB® [OTC] *see* Ibuprofen *on page 475*

Panadol® [OTC] *see* Acetaminophen *on page 16*

Pancrease® *see* Pancrelipase *on next page*

Pancrease® MT 4 *see* Pancrelipase *on next page*

Pancrease® MT 10 *see* Pancrelipase *on next page*

Pancrease® MT 16 *see* Pancrelipase *on next page*

Pancrease® MT 20 *see* Pancrelipase *on next page*

Pancreatin (PAN kree a tin)

Brand Names Creon®; Digepepsin®; Donnazyme®; Hi-Vegi-Lip®

Generic Available No

Therapeutic Category Enzyme

Use Replacement therapy in symptomatic treatment of malabsorption syndrome caused by pancreatic insufficiency secondary to disease or surgery; presumptive test for pancreatic function in patients with suspected pancreatic insufficiency

Contraindications Hypersensitivity to pancreatin, pancreatic extract, or any component; pork protein

Warnings Pancreatin is inactivated by acids; use microencapsulated products whenever possible, since these products permit better dissolution of enzymes in the duodenum and protect the enzyme preparations from acid degradation in the stomach; pancreatic enzyme replacement should not be used until diagnosis and treatment of primary disorder is accomplished.

Precautions Excessive doses of pancreatic enzyme replacement may result in gastrointestinal adverse effects, ie, nausea, vomiting, diarrhea, and abdominal cramps/pain. Very high doses have been reported to cause hyperuricosuria and hyperuricemia. Patients with a history of sensitivity to pork products, trypsin, pancrelipase, or pancreatin may develop allergic reactions.

Adverse Reactions
1% to 10%: High doses:
Endocrine & metabolic: Hyperuricemia
Gastrointestinal: Nausea, cramps, constipation, diarrhea, perianal irritation
Genitourinary: Hyperuricosuria
Ocular: Lacrimation
Respiratory: Sneezing, bronchospasm
<1%:
Dermatologic: Rash
Respiratory: Shortness of breath, bronchospasm
Miscellaneous: Irritation of the mouth

Overdosage Symptoms of overdose include diarrhea, other transient intestinal upset, hyperuricosuria, hyperuricemia

Drug Interactions
Decreased effect: Calcium carbonate, magnesium hydroxide; oral iron administration may have decreased serum iron concentration
Increased effect: H_2-antagonists (eg, ranitidine, cimetidine), proton pump inhibitors (omeprazole, lansoprazole), and antacids

Mechanism of Action Replaces endogenous pancreatic enzymes to assist in digestion of protein, starch and fats

Pharmacokinetics
Absorption: Not absorbed, acts locally in GI tract
(Continued)

Pancreatin *(Continued)*

Elimination: In feces

Usual Dosage Enteric coated microspheres: The following dosage recommendations are only an approximation for initial dosages. The actual dosage will depend on the digestive requirements of the individual patient which is achieved by titration and monitoring.

Geriatrics and Adults: Oral: 4000-18,000 units of lipase with meals and with snacks

Administration Do not crush enteric coating or chew the microspheres or microtablets. If swallowing difficulties exist, capsules may be opened and contents sprinkled onto a small quantity of food, which is **not hot** and does not require chewing. Swallow immediately; follow with a glass of water or juice; do not store food-enzyme mixture.

Monitoring Parameters Stool frequency and fat content

Patient Information Do not chew capsules, microspheres, or microtablets; take before or with meals; avoid inhaling powder dosage form

Nursing Implications Monitor stool fat content and frequency (3-4 stools per day acceptable)

Additional Information These products are not bioequivalent and, therefore, cannot be interchanged (substituted) without consulting the physician

Special Geriatric Considerations No special considerations necessary since drug is dosed to response; however, drug-induced diarrhea can result in unwanted side effects (confusion, hypotension, lethargy, fluid electrolyte loss)

Dosage Forms

Capsule, enteric coated microspheres (Creon®): Lipase 8000 units, amylase 30,000 units, protease 13,000 units and pancreatin 300 mg

Tablet:

Digepepsin®: Pancreatin 300 mg, pepsin 250 mg, and bile salts 150 mg

Donnazyme®: Lipase 1000 units, amylase 12,500 units, protease 12,500 units and pancreatin 500 mg

Hi-Vegi-Lip®: Lipase 4800 units, amylase 60,000 units, protease 60,000 units and pancreatin 2400 mg

Pancrelipase *(pan kre LI pase)*

Brand Names Cotazym®; Cotazym-S®; Creon® 10; Creon® 20; Ilozyme®; Ku-Zyme® HP; Pancrease®; Pancrease® MT 4; Pancrease® MT 10; Pancrease® MT 16; Pancrease® MT 20; Protilase®; Ultrase® MT12; Ultrase® MT20; Viokase®; Zymase®

Synonyms Lipancreatin

Generic Available No

Therapeutic Category Enzyme, Pancreatic; Pancreatic Enzyme

Use Replacement therapy in symptomatic treatment of malabsorption syndrome caused by pancreatic insufficiency secondary to disease or surgery; presumptive test for pancreatic function in patients with suspected pancreatic insufficiency

Contraindications Hypersensitivity to pancrelipase, pancreatic extract, or any component; pork protein

Warnings Pancrelipase is inactivated by acids; use microencapsulated products whenever possible, since these products permit better dissolution of enzymes in the duodenum and protect the enzyme preparations from acid degradation in the stomach; pancreatic enzyme replacement should not be used until diagnosis and treatment of primary disorder is accomplished.

Precautions Excessive doses of pancreatic enzyme replacement may result in gastrointestinal adverse effects, ie, nausea, vomiting, diarrhea, and abdominal cramps/pain. Very high doses have been reported to cause hyperuricosuria and hyperuricemia. Patients with a history of sensitivity to pork products, trypsin, pancreatin, or pancrelipase may develop allergic reactions.

Adverse Reactions

1% to 10%: High doses:

Endocrine & metabolic: Hyperuricemia

Gastrointestinal: Nausea, cramps, constipation, diarrhea

Genitourinary: Hyperuricosuria

Ocular: Lacrimation

Respiratory: Sneezing, bronchospasm

<1%:

Dermatologic: Rash

Respiratory: Shortness of breath, bronchospasm

Miscellaneous: Irritation of the mouth

Overdosage Symptoms of overdose include diarrhea, other transient intestinal upset, hyperuricosuria, hyperuricemia

Drug Interactions

Decreased effect: Calcium carbonate, magnesium hydroxide; oral iron administration may have decreased serum iron concentration

Increased effect: H_2-antagonists (eg, ranitidine, cimetidine), proton pump inhibitors (omeprazole, lansoprazole), and antacids

Mechanism of Action Replaces endogenous pancreatic enzymes to assist in digestion of protein, starch and fats

Pharmacokinetics

Absorption: Not absorbed, acts locally in GI tract

Elimination: In feces

Usual Dosage See Additional Information

Geriatrics and Adults: 0.7 g (powder) or 4000-48,000 units lipase; actual dose depends on the digestive requirements of the patient and is achieved by titration and monitoring (tablets/capsules) with meals

Enteric coated microspheres and microtablets: The following dosage recommendations are only an approximation for initial dosages. The actual dosage will depend on the digestive requirements of the individual patient. Geriatrics and Adults: 4000-48,000 units of lipase with meals and with snacks or 1-3 tablets/capsules before or with meals and snacks; in severe deficiencies, dose may be increased to 8 tablets/capsules

Patients with pancreatectomy or pancreatic obstruction: 8000-16,000 units lipase at 2-hour intervals or as directed by physician; severe deficiency may require doses up to 88,000 with meals

Occluded feeding tubes: One tablet of Viokase® crushed with one 325 mg tablet of sodium bicarbonate (to activate the Viokase®) in 5 mL of water can be instilled into the nasogastric tube and clamped for 5 minutes; then, flushed with 50 mL of tap water

Administration Do not crush enteric coating or chew the microspheres or microtablets. If swallowing difficulties exist, capsules may be opened and contents sprinkled onto a small quantity of food, which is **not hot** and does not require chewing. Swallow immediately; follow with a glass of water or juice; do not store food-enzyme mixture.

Monitoring Parameters Stool frequency and fat content

Patient Information Do not chew capsules, microspheres, or microtablets; take before or with meals; avoid inhaling powder dosage form

Nursing Implications Monitor stool fat and frequency (3-4 stools daily is acceptable)

Additional Information These products are not bioequivalent and, therefore, cannot be interchanged (substituted) without consulting the physician

Special Geriatric Considerations No special considerations are necessary since drug is dosed to response; however, drug-induced diarrhea can result in unwanted side effects (confusion, hypotension, lethargy, fluid and electrolyte loss)

Dosage Forms

Capsule:

Cotazym®: Lipase 8000 units, protease 30,000 units, amylase 30,000 units

Ku-Zyme® HP: Lipase 8000 units, protease 30,000 units, amylase 30,000 units

Ultrase® MT12: Lipase 12,000 units, protease 39,000 units, amylase 39,000 units

Ultrase® MT20: Lipase 20,000 units, protease 65,000 units, amylase 65,000 units

Enteric coated microspheres (Pancrease®): Lipase 4000 units, protease 25,000 units, amylase 20,000 units

Enteric coated microtablets:

Pancrease® MT 4: Lipase 4500 units, protease 12,000 units, amylase 12,000 units

Pancrease® MT 10: Lipase 10,000 units, protease 30,000 units, amylase 30,000 units

Pancrease® MT 16: Lipase 16,000 units, protease 48,000 units, amylase 48,000 units

Pancrease® MT 20: Lipase 20,000 units, protease 44,000 units, amylase 56,000 units

Enteric coated spheres:

Cotazym-S®: Lipase 5000 units, protease 20,000 units, amylase 20,000 units

Pancrelipase, Protilase®: Lipase 4000 units, protease 25,000 units, amylase 20,000 units

(Continued)

Pancrelipase *(Continued)*

      Zymase®: Lipase 12,000 units, protease 24,000 units, amylase 24,000 units

    Delayed release:

      Creon® 10: Lipase 10,000 units, protease 37,500 units, amylase 33,200 units

      Creon® 20: Lipase 20,000 units, protease 75,000 units, amylase 66,400 units

   Powder (Viokase®): Lipase 16,800 units, protease 70,000 units, amylase 70,000 units per 0.7 g

   Tablet:

      Ilozyme®: Lipase 11,000 units, protease 30,000 units, amylase 30,000 units

      Viokase®: Lipase 8000 units, protease 30,000 units, amylase 30,000 units

Panex 500® [OTC] *see Acetaminophen on page 16*

Panmycin® Oral *see Tetracycline on page 900*

Panscol® [OTC] *see Salicylic Acid on page 845*

Papaverine *(pa PAV er een)*

Brand Names Genabid®; Pavabid®; Pavatine®

Generic Available Yes

Therapeutic Category Vasodilator

Use Papaverine has been used for many conditions where vasodilatation is felt to be of some benefit; however, to date, insufficient scientific evidence exists for any therapeutic value to its use except in testing for impotence

Oral: Relief of peripheral and cerebral ischemia associated with arterial spasm; smooth muscle relaxant

Parenteral: Various vascular spasms associated with muscle spasms as in myocardial infarction, angina, peripheral and pulmonary embolism, peripheral vascular disease, angiospastic states, and visceral spasm (ureteral, biliary, and GI colic); testing for impotence

Contraindications Complete atrioventricular block; Parkinson's disease

Warnings May, in large doses, depress cardiac conduction (eg, A-V node) leading to arrhythmias; may interfere with levodopa therapy of Parkinson's disease

Precautions Use with caution in patients with glaucoma; administer I.V. cautiously since apnea and arrhythmias may result; hepatic hypersensitivity noted with jaundice, eosinophilia, and abnormal LFTs

Adverse Reactions

Cardiovascular: Flushing of the face, tachycardia, hypotension, arrhythmias with rapid I.V. use

Central nervous system: Depression, dizziness, vertigo, drowsiness, sedation, lethargy, headache

Dermatologic: Pruritus

Gastrointestinal: Xerostomia, nausea, constipation

Hepatic: Hepatic hypersensitivity

Local: Thrombosis at the I.V. administration site

Respiratory: Apnea with rapid I.V. use

Miscellaneous: Diaphoresis

Overdosage Symptoms of overdose include constipation, diplopia, weakness, drowsiness, liver damage, nystagmus, respiratory depression, anxiety, ataxia, gastric upset, urticaria, macular eruptions

Toxicology

Acute overdose: Gastric lavage or emesis, then follow with catharsis; with coma and respiratory depression, administer general supportive care and respiratory support

Chronic overdose: Discontinue medication; administer supportive care

Parenteral overdose: Administer general supportive care, monitor vital signs, blood gases, and blood chemistry

Treat convulsions with diazepam, phenytoin, or phenobarbital; refractory seizures may be treated with general anesthesia (thiopental, halothane) and muscular paralysis with neuromuscular blocking agents; treat hypotension with I.V. fluids, elevation of legs, and vasopressor agents (dopamine/norepinephrine); cardiovascular effects may be treated with calcium gluconate; monitor EKG and serum calcium; dialysis (peritoneal or charcoal hemoperfusion) does not show any benefit

Drug Interactions

Additive effects with CNS depressants or morphine

Papaverine decreases the effects of levodopa

May enhance hypotensive action of drugs causing hypotension; use with caution in elderly

Stability Protect from heat or freezing; refrigerate injection at 2°C to 8°C (35°F to 46°F); solutions should be clear to pale yellow; precipitates with lactated Ringer's

Mechanism of Action Smooth muscle spasmolytic producing a generalized smooth muscle relaxation including: vasodilatation, gastrointestinal sphincter relaxation, bronchiolar muscle relaxation, and potentially a depressed myocardium; muscle relaxation may occur due to inhibition or cyclic nucleotide phosphodiesterase, increasing cyclic AMP; muscle relaxation is unrelated to nerve innervation; papaverine increases cerebral blood flow in normal subjects; oxygen uptake is unaltered; atrioventricular conduction and intraventricular conduction are depressed with large doses

Pharmacodynamics Peak concentrations: 1-2 hours

Pharmacokinetics

Absorption: Sustained preparations erratically absorbed

Protein binding: 90%

Metabolism: Rapidly in the liver

Bioavailability: Oral: ~54%

Half-life: 30-120 minutes

Elimination: Primarily as metabolites in urine

Usual Dosage Geriatrics and Adults:

Oral: 100-300 mg 3-5 times/day (start with lowest dose in elderly due to hypotensive potential)

Oral, sustained release: 150-300 mg every 12 hours; may increase to 150 mg every 8 hours or 300 mg every 12 hours

I.M., I.V.: 30-120 mg every 3 hours as needed

Cardiac extrasystoles: 2 doses 10 minutes apart; I.V. should be given over 1-2 minutes

Treatment of impotence: Self-injection of papaverine 2.5-37.5 mg, but usually titrated up to 30 mg, combined with small doses of phentolamine mesylate 0.08-1.25 mg, usually 0.5-1 mg into corpus cavernosum of the penis

Monitoring Parameters Monitor blood pressure

Patient Information Inform patient about potential for dizziness, hypotension, drowsiness; alcohol may enhance these effects; may cause flushing, sweating, headache, tiredness, jaundice, skin rash, nausea, anorexia, abdominal discomfort, constipation, or diarrhea

Nursing Implications Rapid I.V. administration may result in arrhythmias and fatal apnea

Additional Information Therapeutic value is lacking

Special Geriatric Considerations Vasodilators have been used to treat dementia upon the premise that dementia is secondary to a cerebral blood flow insufficiency. The hypothesis is that if blood flow could be increased, cognitive function would be increased. This hypothesis is no longer valid. The use of vasodilators for cognitive dysfunction is not recommended or proven by appropriate scientific study.

Dosage Forms

Papaverine hydrochloride:

Capsule, sustained release: 150 mg

Injection: 30 mg/mL

Tablet: 30 mg, 60 mg, 100 mg, 150 mg, 200 mg, 300 mg

Tablet, timed release: 200 mg

References

Erwin WG, "Senile Dementia of the Alzheimer Type," *Clin Pharm*, 1984, 3:497-504.

Higbee MD, "Noncholinergic Approaches to Treating Senile Dementia of the Alzheimer's Type," *Consult Pharm*, 1992, 7(6):635-41.

Waters C, "Cognitive Enhancing Agents: Current Status in the Treatment of Alzheimer's Disease," *Can J Neurol Sci*, 1988, 15:249-56.

Yesavage JA, Tinklenberg JR, Hollister LE, et al, "Vasodilators in Senile Dementias: A Review of the Literature," *Arch Gen Psychiatry*, 1979, 36:220-3.

Parabromdylamine *see* Brompheniramine *on page 129*

Paracetamol *see* Acetaminophen *on page 16*

Paraflex® *see* Chlorzoxazone *on page 218*

Parafon Forte™ DSC *see* Chlorzoxazone *on page 218*

Parepectolin® *see* Kaolin and Pectin With Opium *on page 512*

Parlodel® *see* Bromocriptine *on page 128*

Parnate® *see* Tranylcypromine *on page 946*

Paroxetine (pa ROKS e teen)

Related Information
Antidepressant Agents Comparison *on page 1021*
Antidepressant Medication Guidelines *on page 1075*

Brand Names Paxil™

Therapeutic Category Antidepressant; Selective Serotonin Reuptake Inhibitor (SSRI)

Use Treatment of depression; obsessive-compulsive disorder; panic disorders

Contraindications Hypersensitivity to paroxetine or any component; do not use within 14 days of MAO inhibitors

Warnings Use cautiously in patients with a history of seizures, mania, renal disease, cardiac disease, suicidal patients; avoid ECT

Adverse Reactions
Cardiovascular: Bradycardia, hypotension, palpitations, tachycardia, vasodilation, postural hypotension
Central nervous system: Headache, nervousness, anxiety, somnolence, dizziness, insomnia, migraine, seizures, extrapyramidal reactions (rare)
Dermatologic: Alopecia
Endocrine & metabolic: Hyponatremia possibly due to SIADH
Gastrointestinal: Constipation, diarrhea, nausea, xerostomia, anorexia, flatulence, vomiting, gastritis, thirst
Genitourinary: Ejaculatory disturbances, decreased libido
Hematologic: Anemia, leukopenia
Hepatic: Increased LFTs
Neuromuscular & skeletal: Akinesia, arthritis, tremors, paresthesia, weakness
Ocular: Eye pain
Otic: Ear pain
Respiratory: Asthma
Miscellaneous: Bruxism, diaphoresis

Overdosage Symptoms of overdose include nausea, vomiting, drowsiness, sinus tachycardia, and dilated pupils

Toxicology There are no specific antidotes, following attempts at decontamination, treatment is supportive and symptomatic; forced diuresis, dialysis, and hemoperfusion are unlikely to be beneficial

Drug Interactions
Decreased effect with phenobarbital, phenytoin (also decreased phenytoin effects), digoxin (decreased AUC)
Increased effect/toxicity with alcohol, cimetidine, MAO inhibitors (hyperpyrexic crisis), *L*-tryptophan; increased effect/toxicity of TCAs, fluoxetine, sertraline, phenothiazines, procyclidine, class 1C antiarrhythmics, warfarin; increased toxicity with dexfenfluramine (possible)
May inhibit the metabolism of codeine, tramadol, and to active metabolite (decreased analgesic response)

Mechanism of Action Selectively inhibits the CNS neuronal reuptake of serotonin, thereby enhancing serotonergic activity and inhibiting adrenergic activity in the locus ceruleus; minimal or no effect on reuptake of norepinephrine, dopamine, or cholinergic receptors; no effects on the regulation of beta receptors

Pharmacodynamics Maximum antidepressant effect usually seen after 4 weeks

Pharmacokinetics
Metabolism: Substrate and inhibitor CYP2D6
Half-life: 21 hours
Elimination: Metabolites are excreted in bile and urine

Elderly: Half-life and steady-state concentration increase disproportionately to dose with single and multiple dosing; see table.

Paroxetine

	Median Half-life (h)	Css (ng/mL)
Elderly 20 mg	30	46
Elderly 30 mg	38	80

Usual Dosage Oral:
Depression:
Geriatrics: Initial: 10 mg once daily, preferably in the morning; usual dose: 20-30 mg/day; maximum: 40 mg/day
Adults: 20 mg once daily (maximum: 50 mg/day), preferably in the morning

Obsessive compulsive disorder: Geriatrics and Adults: Initial: 20 mg every morning, increase to 40 mg/day

Panic attack: Geriatrics and Adults: Initial: 10 mg every morning; maximum: 60 mg/day

Administration Best given in the morning unless too sedating; then administer as divided dose or at bedtime

Monitoring Parameters Improvement of depression symptoms, anxiety, sleep disturbance, weight and appetite, hepatic and renal function tests, blood pressure, heart rate

Reference Range Not established

Test Interactions Elevated LFTs

Patient Information If currently on another antidepressant, notify physician; refrain from alcohol; if taking warfarin, anticonvulsants, or other drugs with CNS effects, notify physician

Nursing Implications See Administration and Monitoring Parameters

Special Geriatric Considerations Paroxetine's favorable side effect profile make it a useful alternative to the traditional tricyclic antidepressants; paroxetine is the most sedating of the currently available selective serotonin reuptake inhibitors (see Usual Dosage and Pharmacokinetics). Paroxetine has been shown to be an equally effective antidepressant compared to nortriptyline in patients with ischemic heart disease. However, nortriptyline was associated a significantly higher rate of adverse cardiac events (sustained increase in heart rate, sinus tachycardia, and asymptomatic increase in ventricular ectopy) compared to placebo. Data from a clinical trial comparing fluoxetine to tricyclics suggest that fluoxetine is significantly less effective than nortriptyline in hospitalized elderly patients with unipolar major affective disorder, especially those with melancholia and concurrent cardiovascular diseases.

Dosage Forms Tablet: 10 mg, 20 mg, 30 mg, 40 mg

References

Grimsley SR and Jann MW, "Paroxetine, Sertraline, and Fluvoxamine: New Selective Serotonin Reuptake Inhibitors," *Clin Pharm*, 1992, 11(11):930-57.

Hebenstreit GF, Fellerer K, Zochling R, et al, "A Pharmacokinetic Dose Titration Study in Adult and Elderly Depressed Patients," *Acta Psychiatr Scand Suppl*, 1989, 350:81-4.

Lundmark J, Scheel Thomsen I, Fjord-Larsen T, et al, "Paroxetine: Pharmacokinetic and Antidepressant Effect in the Elderly," *Acta Psychiatr Scand Suppl*, 1989, 350:76-80.

Roose SP, Glassman AH, Attia E, et al, "Comparative Efficacy of Selective Serotonin Reuptake Inhibitors and Tricyclics in the Treatment of Melancholia," *Am J Psychiatry*, 1994, 151(12):1735-9.

Roose SP, Laghrissi-Thode F, Kennedy JS, et al, "Comparison of Paroxetine and Nortriptyline in Depressed Patients With Ischemic Heart Disease," *JAMA*, 1998, 279(4):287-91.

Schone W and Ludwig M, "A Double-Blind Study of Paroxetine Compared With Fluoxetine in Geriatric Patients With Major Depression," *J Clin Psychopharmacol*, 1993, 13(6 Suppl 2):34S-9S.

Parsidol® *see* Ethopropazine *on page 360*

PAS *see* Aminosalicylic Acid *on page 57*

Pathocil® *see* Dicloxacillin *on page 284*

Pavabid® *see* Papaverine *on page 714*

Pavatine® *see* Papaverine *on page 714*

Paxil™ *see* Paroxetine *on previous page*

Paxipam® *see* Halazepam *on page 443*

PBZ® *see* Tripelennamine *on page 965*

PBZ-SR® *see* Tripelennamine *on page 965*

PCA *see* Procainamide *on page 780*

PCE® **Oral** *see* Erythromycin *on page 344*

Pectin and Kaolin *see* Kaolin and Pectin *on page 512*

PediaCare® **Oral** *see* Pseudoephedrine *on page 802*

Pediaflor® *see* Fluoride *on page 392*

Pediapred® **Oral** *see* Prednisolone *on page 774*

PediaProfen™ *see* Ibuprofen *on page 475*

Pediatric Triban® *see* Trimethobenzamide *on page 961*

Pediazole® *see* Erythromycin and Sulfisoxazole *on page 346*

Pedi-Boro® **[OTC]** *see* Aluminum Acetate and Calcium Acetate *on page 41*

Penbutolol (pen BYOO toe lole)

Related Information

Beta-Blockers Comparison *on page 1026*

Brand Names Levatol®

Generic Available No

Therapeutic Category Beta-Adrenergic Blocker

(Continued)

Penbutolol *(Continued)*

Use Treatment of mild to moderate arterial hypertension

Contraindications Uncompensated congestive heart failure, cardiogenic shock, bradycardia or heart block, bronchial asthma, bronchospasms, hypersensitivity to beta-blocking agents, diabetes mellitus

Warnings Abrupt withdrawal of beta-blockers may result in an exaggerated cardiac beta-adrenergic responsiveness. Symptomatology has included reports of tachycardia, hypertension, ischemia, angina, myocardial infarction, and sudden death. It is recommended that patients be tapered gradually off of beta-blockers over a 2-week period rather than via abrupt discontinuation.

Precautions Increase dosing interval in patients with renal dysfunction; administer with caution to patients with bronchospastic disease, diabetes mellitus, hyperthyroidism, myasthenia gravis, and renal function decline and severe peripheral vascular disease; abrupt withdrawal of the drug should be avoided, drug should be discontinued over 2 weeks

Adverse Reactions Other adverse effects similar to other beta-blockers
Cardiovascular: Persistent bradycardia, hypotension, chest pain, edema, heart failure, Raynaud's phenomena
Central nervous system: Depression, confusion, dizziness, nightmares, fatigue, insomnia, lethargy, headache
Gastrointestinal: Constipation, diarrhea, nausea
Genitourinary: Impotence
Miscellaneous: Cold extremities

Overdosage Symptoms of overdose include bradycardia, congestive heart failure, hypotension, bronchospasm, hypoglycemia (see Toxicology)

Toxicology Sympathomimetics (eg, epinephrine or dopamine), glucagon, or a pacemaker can be used to treat the toxic bradycardia, asystole, and/or hypotension; initially fluids may be the best treatment for toxic hypotension; patients should remain supine; serum glucose and potassium should be measured; use supportive measures: lavage, syrup of ipecac. I.V. glucose should be administered for hypoglycemia; seizures may be treated with phenytoin or diazepam intravenously; continuous monitoring of blood pressure and EKG is necessary. If PVCs occur, treat with lidocaine or phenytoin; avoid quinidine, procainamide, and disopyramide since these agents further depress myocardial function; bronchospasm can be treated with theophylline or $beta_2$ agonists (epinephrine).

Drug Interactions
Other hypotensive agents, diuretics and phenothiazines may increase hypotensive effects of penbutolol
Penbutolol may enhance neuromuscular blocking agents and will antagonize beta-sympathomimetic drugs; other drug interactions similar to propranolol may occur

Mechanism of Action Blocks both $beta_1$- and $beta_2$-receptors and has mild intrinsic sympathomimetic activity; has negative inotropic and chronotropic effects and can significantly slow A-V nodal conduction; lipid solubility is high which may result in CNS side effects

Pharmacokinetics
Absorption: Well absorbed, ~100%
Protein binding: 80% to 98%
Metabolism: Extensive in the liver (oxidation and conjugation)
Bioavailability: Oral: ~100%
Half-life: 5 hours
Elimination: Hepatic oxidation and conjugation with metabolites; excreted renally

Usual Dosage Oral:
Geriatrics: Initial: 10 mg once daily
Adults: Initial: 20 mg once daily, full effect of a 20 or 40 mg dose is seen by the end of a 2-week period, full effect not seen for 4-6 weeks; doses of 40-80 mg have been tolerated but have shown little additional antihypertensive effects

Monitoring Parameters Blood pressure, orthostatic hypotension, heart rate, CNS effects

Patient Information Do not discontinue medication abruptly, sudden stopping of medication may precipitate or cause angina; consult pharmacist or physician before taking with other adrenergic drugs (eg, cold medications); notify physician if any of the following symptoms occur: difficult breathing, night cough, swelling of extremities, slow pulse, dizziness, lightheadedness, confusion, depression, skin rash, fever, sore throat, unusual bleeding or bruising;

may produce drowsiness, dizziness, lightheadedness, blurred vision, confusion; use with caution while driving or performing tasks requiring alertness; may mask signs of hypoglycemia in diabetics; may be taken without regard to meals

Nursing Implications Advise against abrupt withdrawal; monitor orthostatic blood pressures, apical and peripheral pulse and mental status changes (ie, confusion, depression)

Special Geriatric Considerations Due to alterations in the beta-adrenergic autonomic nervous system, beta-adrenergic blockade may result in less hemodynamic response than seen in younger adults. Studies indicate that despite decreased sensitivity to the chronotropic effects of beta blockade with age, there appears to be an increased myocardial sensitivity to the negative inotropic effect during stress (ie, exercise). Controlled trials have shown the overall response rate for propranolol to be only 20% to 50% in elderly populations. Therefore, all beta-adrenergic blocking drugs may result in a decreased response as compared to younger adults.

Dosage Forms Tablet, as sulfate: 20 mg

Penecort® see Hydrocortisone on page 462

Penetrex™ Oral see Enoxacin on page 332

Penicillamine (pen i SIL a meen)

Related Information
Antacid Drug Interactions on page 1096

Brand Names Cuprimine®; Depen®

Synonyms D-3-Mercaptovaline; β,β-Dimethylcysteine; D-Penicillamine

Generic Available No

Therapeutic Category Antidote, Copper Toxicity; Antidote, Lead Toxicity; Chelating Agent, Oral

Use Treatment of Wilson's disease, cystinuria, adjunct in the treatment of rheumatoid arthritis; lead poisoning, primary biliary cirrhosis

Contraindications Hypersensitivity to penicillamine and possibly penicillin; rheumatoid arthritis patients with renal insufficiency; patients with previous penicillamine-related aplastic anemia or agranulocytosis

Warnings Leukopenia, thrombocytopenia, proteinuria, hematuria, nephrotic syndrome, autoimmune syndrome, polymyositis, diffuse alveolitis, dermatomyositis, Goodpasture's syndrome, obliterative bronchiolitis, myasthenia gravis, and pemphigoid-like reaction; lupus erythematosus reaction

Precautions Patients on penicillamine should receive pyridoxine supplementation 25 mg/day; drug fever, skin rash, pemphigoid rash, oral ulcerations, hypogeusia, hypoglycemia, cross-sensitivity with penicillin may exist; delayed wound healing

Adverse Reactions High evidence of adverse effects (>50%), medical supervision essential

Central nervous system: Fever, hyperpyrexia
Dermatologic: Rash, pruritus, pemphigus, increased friability of the skin, alopecia, lichen planus, TEN, increased skin irritability, excessive wrinkling in skin
Endocrine & metabolic: Iron deficiency, mammary hyperplasia
Gastrointestinal: Oral lesions, nausea, vomiting, ageusia, epigastric pain, diarrhea, reactivate peptic ulcers, pancreatitis, cholestasis
Hematologic: Leukopenia, thrombocytopenia, eosinophilia, aplastic anemia, bone marrow suppression
Hepatic: Hepatic dysfunction, increased alkaline phosphatase, and LDH
Neuromuscular & skeletal: Arthralgia
Ocular: Optic neuritis
Otic: Tinnitus
Renal: Nephrotic syndrome, proteinuria, membranous glomerulopathy
Miscellaneous: Allergic reactions, lymphadenopathy, SLE-like syndrome

Overdosage Symptoms of overdose include proteinuria, leukopenia, thrombocytopenia, skin rashes, bruising, nausea, vomiting, dysgeusia, diarrhea

Toxicology Toxic effects will reverse upon discontinuation of drug therapy; general supportive care; renal effects may take 1 year to reverse

Drug Interactions
Concomitant use of gold therapy, antimalarials, or cytotoxic agents should not be used due to similar toxic/adverse effects
Penicillamine has decreased absorption when taken with food (50% to 60%), antacids (65%), and iron compounds (35%)
Digoxin blood concentrations decreased by penicillamine

Stability Store in tight, well-closed containers
(Continued)

Penicillamine *(Continued)*

Mechanism of Action Chelates with lead, copper, mercury, iron, and other heavy metals to form stable, soluble complexes that are excreted in the urine; depresses circulating IgM rheumatoid factor, depresses T-cell but not B-cell activity; combines with cystine to form a compound which is more soluble, thus cystine calculi is prevented

Pharmacokinetics
  Absorption: Oral: 40% to 70%
  Protein binding: 80% bound to albumin
  Half-life: 1.7-3.2 hours
  Time to peak serum concentration: Within 1 hour
  Elimination: Primarily (30% to 60%) in urine as unchanged drug with small amounts of hepatic metabolism

Usual Dosage Geriatrics and Adults: Oral:
  Rheumatoid arthritis: 125-250 mg/day, may increase dose at 1- to 3-month intervals up to 1-1.5 g/day (750 mg maximum daily dose for elderly)
  Wilson's disease: 1 g/day in 4 divided doses, doses titrated to maintain urinary copper excretion >1 mg/day (750 mg maximum daily dose for elderly)
  Cystinuria: 1-4 g/day divided every 6 hours
  Lead poisoning: 250 mg/dose divided every 8-12 hours
  Primary biliary cirrhosis: 250 mg/day to start, increase by 250 mg every 2 weeks up to a maintenance dose of 1 g/day, usually given 250 mg 4 times/day (750 mg maximum daily dose for elderly)

Monitoring Parameters CBC: WBC <3500/mm^2, neutrophils <2000/mm^2 or monocytes >500/mm^2 indicate need to stop therapy immediately; quantitative 24-hour urine protein at 1- to 2-week intervals initially (first 2-3 months); urinalysis, LFTs occasionally; platelet counts <100,000/mm^3 indicate need to stop therapy until numbers of platelets increase

Patient Information Take at least 1 hour before a meal; loss of taste may occur; probable severe allergic reaction if patient allergic to penicillin; report any signs of toxicity to physician; patients with cystinuria should drink copious amounts of water; report any unusual bleeding, bruising, persistent fever, fatigue, sore throat, shortness of breath

Nursing Implications For patients who cannot swallow, content of capsules may be administered in 15-30 mL of chilled puréed fruit or fruit juice; patients should be warned to report promptly any symptoms suggesting toxicity (see Monitoring Parameters)

Additional Information Approximately 33% of patients will experience an allergic reaction

Special Geriatric Considerations Close monitoring of elderly is necessary; since steady-state serum/tissue concentrations rise slowly, "go slow" with dose increase intervals; steady-state concentrations decline slowly after discontinuation suggesting extensive tissue distribution. Skin rashes and taste abnormalities occur more frequently in elderly than in young adults; leukopenia, thrombocytopenia, and proteinuria occur with equal frequency in both younger adults and elderly. Since toxicity may be dose related, it is recommended not to exceed 750 mg/day in elderly.

Dosage Forms
  Capsule: 125 mg, 250 mg
  Tablet: 250 mg

References
Stein HB, Patterson AC, Offer RC, et al, "Adverse Effects of D-Penicillamine in Rheumatoid Arthritis," *Ann Intern Med*, 1980, 92:24-9.

Penicillin G Benzathine *(pen i SIL in jee BENZ a theen)*

Related Information
  I.V. Medication Recommendations *on page 1080*
  Penicillins, Penicillin-Related Antibiotics, & Other Antibiotics *on page 1010*

Brand Names Bicillin® L-A; Permapen®

Synonyms Benzathine Benzylpenicillin; Benzathine Penicillin G; Benzylpenicillin Benzathine

Therapeutic Category Antibiotic, Penicillin

Use Active against most gram-positive organisms; some gram-negative organisms such as *Neisseria gonorrhoeae* and some anaerobes and spirochetes; used only for the treatment of mild to moderately severe infections caused by organisms susceptible to low concentrations of penicillin G, or for prophylaxis of infections caused by these organisms

Contraindications Known hypersensitivity to penicillin or any component

Precautions Use with caution in patients with impaired renal function, impaired cardiac function, or seizure disorder; history of cephalosporin allergy

Adverse Reactions

Central nervous system: Convulsions, confusion, drowsiness, fever

Dermatologic: Rash

Endocrine & metabolic: Electrolyte imbalance

Hematologic: Hemolytic anemia, positive Coombs' reaction

Local: Pain at injection site, thrombophlebitis

Neuromuscular & skeletal: Myoclonus

Renal: Acute interstitial nephritis

Miscellaneous: Jarisch-Herxheimer reaction, hypersensitivity reactions, anaphylaxis

Overdosage Symptoms of overdose include neuromuscular hypersensitivity, seizure

Toxicology Many beta-lactam-containing antibiotics have the potential to cause neuromuscular hyperirritability or convulsive seizures. Hemodialysis may be helpful to aid in the removal of the drug from the blood, otherwise most treatment is supportive or symptom directed

Drug Interactions Probenecid, tetracyclines, aminoglycosides, anticoagulants (I.M. administration only)

Stability Store in refrigerator

Mechanism of Action Interferes with bacterial cell wall synthesis during active multiplication causing cell death and resultant bactericidal activity against susceptible bacteria

Pharmacokinetics

Absorption: I.M.: Slow

Time to peak serum concentration: Within 12-24 hours; serum concentrations are usually detectable for 1-4 weeks depending on the dose; larger doses result in more sustained concentrations rather than higher concentrations; following equal, simple I.M. injections, the elderly have serum penicillin concentrations approximately twice that of younger adults 48, 96, and 144 hours postadministration

Usual Dosage Geriatrics and Adults: I.M.: Dosage frequency depends on infection being treated

Group A streptococcal upper respiratory infection: 1.2 million units as a single dose

Prophylaxis of recurrent rheumatic fever: 1.2 million units every 3-4 weeks or 600,000 units twice monthly

Early syphilis: 2.4 million units as a single dose

Syphilis >1 year duration: 2.4 million units once weekly for 3 doses

Administration Administer by deep I.M. injection in the upper outer quadrant of the buttock do **not** administer I.V., intra-arterially, or S.C.

Monitoring Parameters Signs and symptoms of infection

Test Interactions Positive Coombs' [direct], false-positive urinary and/or serum proteins

Nursing Implications See Administration

Additional Information A single dose of 600,000 to 1,200,000 units is effective in the prevention of rheumatic fever secondary to streptococcal pharyngitis; used when patient cannot be kept in a hospital environment and neurosyphilis has been ruled out

Special Geriatric Considerations Not indicated as single drug therapy for neurosyphilis, but may be given 1 time/week for 3 weeks following I.V. treatment (see Penicillin G for dosing); no adjustment for renal function or age is necessary (see Pharmacokinetics)

Dosage Forms Injection: 300,000 units/mL (10 mL); 600,000 units/mL (1 mL, 2 mL, 4 mL)

References

Collart P, Poitevin M, Milovanovic A, et al, "Kinetic Study of Serum Penicillin Concentrations After Single Doses of Benzathine and Benethamine Penicillins in Young and Old People," *Br J Vener Dis*, 1980, 56(6):355-62.

WHO Study Group, "Rheumatic Fever and Rheumatic Heart Disease," *WHO Tech Rep Ser*, 1988, 764:1-58.

Penicillin G Benzathine and Procaine Combined

(pen i SIL in jee BENZ a theen & PROE kane KOM bined)

Related Information

Penicillins, Penicillin-Related Antibiotics, & Other Antibiotics *on page 1010*

Brand Names Bicillin® C-R 900/300 Injection; Bicillin® C-R Injection

Synonyms Penicillin G Procaine and Benzathine Combined

Therapeutic Category Antibiotic, Penicillin

(Continued)

Penicillin G Benzathine and Procaine Combined
(Continued)

Use Active against most gram-positive organisms; some gram-negative such as *Neisseria gonorrhoeae* and some anaerobes and spirochetes

Contraindications Known hypersensitivity to penicillin or any component

Precautions Use with caution in patients with impaired renal function, impaired cardiac function, seizure disorder, or history of cephalosporin allergy

Adverse Reactions

Central nervous system: Convulsions, confusion, drowsiness, fever

Dermatologic: Rash

Endocrine & metabolic: Electrolyte imbalance

Hematologic: Hemolytic anemia, positive Coombs' reaction

Local: Thrombophlebitis

Neuromuscular & skeletal: Myoclonus

Renal: Acute interstitial nephritis

Miscellaneous: Jarisch-Herxheimer reaction, hypersensitivity reactions, anaphylaxis

Overdosage Symptoms of overdose include neuromuscular hypersensitivity, seizure

Drug Interactions Probenecid, tetracyclines, aminoglycosides

Stability Store in the refrigerator

Mechanism of Action Interferes with bacterial cell wall synthesis during active multiplication causing cell death and resultant bactericidal activity against susceptible bacteria

Usual Dosage Geriatrics and Adults: I.M.: 2.4 million units in a single dose

Administration Administer by deep I.M. injection in the upper outer quadrant of the buttock do **not** administer I.V., intravascularly, or intra-arterially

Test Interactions Positive Coombs' [direct], increased protein

Nursing Implications See Administration

Special Geriatric Considerations No adjustment for renal function or age is necessary (see Usual Dosage)

Dosage Forms

Injection: 300,000 units = 150,000 units each of penicillin G benzathine and penicillin G procaine (10 mL); 600,000 units = 300,000 units each penicillin G benzathine and penicillin G procaine (1 mL); 1,200,000 units = 600,000 units each penicillin G benzathine and penicillin G procaine (2 mL); 2,400,000 units = 1,200,000 units each penicillin G benzathine and penicillin G procaine (4 mL)

Injection: Penicillin G benzathine 900,000 units and penicillin G procaine/dose 300,000 units (2 mL)

Penicillin G, Parenteral, Aqueous
(pen i SIL in jee, pa REN ter al, AYE kwee us)

Related Information

Penicillins, Penicillin-Related Antibiotics, & Other Antibiotics *on page 1010*

Brand Names Pfizerpen®

Synonyms Benzylpenicillin Potassium; Benzylpenicillin Sodium; Crystalline Penicillin

Generic Available Yes

Therapeutic Category Antibiotic, Penicillin

Use Active against most gram-positive organisms except *Staphylococcus aureus*; some gram-negative such as *Neisseria gonorrhoeae* and some anaerobes and spirochetes; although ceftriaxone is now the drug of choice for lyme disease and gonorrhea

Contraindications Known hypersensitivity to penicillin or any component

Warnings Contains ~2 mEq sodium/1 million units

Precautions Avoid I.V., intravascular or intra-arterial administration or injection into or near major peripheral nerves or blood vessels since such injections may cause severe and/or permanent neurovascular damage; use with caution in patients with severe renal impairment; use with caution in patients with cephalosporin allergy

Adverse Reactions

Central nervous system: Convulsions, confusion, drowsiness, fever

Dermatologic: Rash

Endocrine & metabolic: Electrolyte imbalance

Hematologic: Hemolytic anemia, positive Coombs' reaction

Local: Thrombophlebitis

Neuromuscular & skeletal: Myoclonus

Renal: Acute interstitial nephritis

Miscellaneous: Jarisch-Herxheimer reaction, hypersensitivity reactions, anaphylaxis

Overdosage Symptoms of overdose include neuromuscular hypersensitivity, seizure

Toxicology Many beta-lactam-containing antibiotics have the potential to cause neuromuscular hyperirritability or convulsive seizures. Hemodialysis may be helpful to aid in the removal of the drug from the blood, otherwise most treatment is supportive or symptom directed.

Drug Interactions Probenecid (increased levels), tetracyclines, aminoglycosides, anticoagulants (I.M. administration only)

Stability Reconstituted parenteral solution is stable for 7 days when refrigerated; for I.V. infusion in NS or D_5W, solution is stable for 24 hours at room temperature

Mechanism of Action Interferes with bacterial cell wall synthesis during active multiplication causing cell death and resultant bactericidal activity against susceptible bacteria

Pharmacokinetics

Distribution: Penetration across the blood-brain barrier is poor, despite inflamed meninges

Protein binding: 65%

Metabolism: In the liver (30%) to penicilloic acid

Half-life: 20-50 minutes; prolonged half-life reported in some elderly (~1 hour) compared to younger subjects presumably due to decreased renal function

Time to peak serum concentration: I.V.: Within 1 hour

Elimination: In urine

Usual Dosage Geriatrics and Adults:

I.V.: 3-5 million units every 4-6 hours; higher doses and/or more frequent administration may be necessary for some infections such as meningitis

Neurosyphilis: 3-4 million units every 4 hours for 10-14 days

Dosing interval in renal impairment:

Cl_{cr} 10-30 mL/minute: Administer every 8-12 hours

Cl_{cr} <10 mL/minute: Administer every 12-18 hours

Moderately dialyzable (20% to 50%)

Monitoring Parameters Fever, mental status, WBC count, appetite

Test Interactions Positive Coombs' [direct], increased protein

Patient Information Complete full course of treatment; notify physician if rash, itching, hives, diarrhea, or any other unusual finding

Nursing Implications Dosage modification required in patients with renal insufficiency; administer around-the-clock rather than 4 times/day to avoid variations in peak and trough concentrations

Special Geriatric Considerations Despite a reported prolonged half-life, it is usually not necessary to adjust the dose of penicillin G or VK in the elderly to account for renal function changes with age, however, it is advised to calculate an estimated creatinine clearance and adjust dose accordingly (see Usual Dosage)

Dosage Forms

Penicillin G potassium:

Injection: 200,000 units, 500,000 units, 1 million units, 5 million units, 10 million units, 20 million units

Injection:

Frozen, premixed: 1 million units, 2 million units, 3 million units

Powder 1 million units, 5 million units, 10 million units, 20 million units

Injection, as sodium: 5 million units

References

Hansen JM, Kampmann J, and Laursen H, "Renal Excretion of Drugs in the Elderly," *Lancet*, 1970, 1(657):1170.

Leikola E and Vartia KO, "On Penicillin Levels in Young and Geriatric Subjects," *J Gerontol*, 1957, 12:48-52.

Yoshikawa TT, "Antimicrobial Therapy for the Elderly Patient," *J Am Geriatr Soc*, 1990, 38(12):1353-72.

Penicillin G Procaine (pen i SIL in jee PROE kane)

Related Information

Penicillins, Penicillin-Related Antibiotics, & Other Antibiotics *on page 1010*

Brand Names Crysticillin® A.S.; Pfizerpen®-AS; Wycillin®

Synonyms APPG; Aqueous Procaine Penicillin G; Procaine Benzylpenicillin; Procaine Penicillin G

Generic Available Yes

Therapeutic Category Antibiotic, Penicillin

(Continued)

Penicillin G Procaine *(Continued)*

Use Moderately severe infections due to *Neisseria gonorrhoeae*, *Treponema pallidum* and other penicillin G-sensitive microorganisms that are susceptible to low but prolonged serum penicillin concentrations

Contraindications Known hypersensitivity to penicillin or any component; also contraindicated in patients hypersensitive to procaine

Precautions Modify dosage in patients with severe renal impairment; use with caution in patients with cephalosporin allergy

Adverse Reactions
Cardiovascular: Myocardial depression, vasodilation, conduction disturbances
Central nervous system: Confusion, drowsiness, CNS stimulation, seizures
Hematologic: Hemolytic anemia, positive Coombs' reaction
Local: Sterile abscess at injection site, pain at injection site
Neuromuscular & skeletal: Myoclonus
Renal: Interstitial nephritis
Miscellaneous: Pseudoanaphylactic reactions, Jarisch-Herxheimer reaction, hypersensitivity reactions

Overdosage Symptoms of overdose include neuromuscular hypersensitivity, seizure

Toxicology Many beta-lactam-containing antibiotics have the potential to cause neuromuscular hyperirritability or convulsive seizures. Hemodialysis may be helpful to aid in the removal of the drug from the blood, otherwise most treatment is supportive or symptom directed.

Drug Interactions Probenecid, tetracycline, aminoglycosides, anticoagulants (I.M. administration)

Stability Store in refrigerator

Mechanism of Action Interferes with bacterial cell wall synthesis during active multiplication causing cell death and resultant bactericidal activity against susceptible bacteria

Pharmacokinetics
Absorption: I.M.: Slow
Distribution: Penetration across the blood-brain barrier is poor, despite inflamed meninges
Protein binding: 65%
Half-life: 20-50 minutes
Time to peak serum concentration: Within 1-4 hours and can persist within the therapeutic range for 15-24 hours
Elimination: 60% to 90% of drug is excreted unchanged via renal tubular excretion; ~30% of dose inactivated in the liver
Renal clearance is delayed in patients with impaired renal function

Usual Dosage Geriatrics and Adults: I.M.: 0.6-2.4 million units every 6-12 hours

Uncomplicated gonorrhea: 1 g probenecid orally, then 4.8 million units procaine penicillin divided into 2 injection sites 30 minutes later. When used in conjunction with an aminoglycoside for the treatment of endocarditis caused by susceptible *S. viridans*: 1.2 million units every 6 hours for 2-4 weeks.
Neurosyphilis: I.M.: 2-4 million units/day with 500 mg probenecid by mouth 4 times/day for 10-14 days; penicillin G aqueous I.V. is the preferred agent
Dosing interval in renal impairment:
Cl_{cr} 10-30 mL/minute: Administer every 8-12 hours
Cl_{cr} <10 mL/minute: Administer every 12-18 hours
Moderately dialyzable (20% to 50%)

Administration Procaine suspension for deep I.M. injection only; administer around-the-clock rather than 4 times/day, 3 times/day, etc (ie, 12-6-12-6, not 9-1-5-9) to promote less variation in peak and trough serum concentrations; when doses are repeated, rotate the injection site; avoid I.V., intravascular, or intra-arterial administration of penicillin G procaine since severe and/or permanent neurovascular damage may occur; renal and hematologic systems should be evaluated periodically during prolonged therapy

Monitoring Parameters Fever, mental status, WBC count, appetite

Test Interactions Positive Coombs' [direct], false-positive urinary and/or serum proteins

Patient Information Notify physician if skin rash, itching, hives or severe diarrhea occurs; complete full course of therapy

Nursing Implications See Administration

Special Geriatric Considerations Dosage does not usually need to be adjusted in the elderly, however, if multiple doses are to be given, adjust dose for renal function (see Usual Dosage)

Dosage Forms Injection, suspension: 300,000 units/mL (10 mL); 500,000 units/mL (1.2 mL); 600,000 units/mL (1 mL, 2 mL, 4 mL)

References

Yoshikawa TT, "Antimicrobial Therapy for the Elderly Patient," *J Am Geriatr Soc*, 1990, 38(12):1353-72.

Penicillin G Procaine and Benzathine Combined *see* Penicillin G Benzathine and Procaine Combined *on page 721*

Penicillins, Penicillin-Related Antibiotics, & Other Antibiotics *see page 1010*

Penicillin V Potassium (pen i SIL in vee poe TASS ee um)

Related Information

Penicillins, Penicillin-Related Antibiotics, & Other Antibiotics *on page 1010*

Brand Names Beepen-VK®; Betapen®-VK; Ledercillin® VK; Pen.Vee® K; Robicillin® VK; V-Cillin K®; Veetids®

Synonyms Pen VK; Phenoxymethyl Penicillin

Generic Available Yes

Therapeutic Category Antibiotic, Penicillin

Use Treatment of moderate to severe susceptible bacterial infections; no longer recommended for dental procedure prophylaxis; prophylaxis in rheumatic fever; infections caused by susceptible organisms involving the respiratory tract, otitis media, sinusitis, skin, and urinary tract

Contraindications Known hypersensitivity to penicillin or any component

Precautions Use with caution in patients with renal impairment, dosage adjustment may be necessary; use with caution in patients with cephalosporin allergy

Adverse Reactions

Central nervous system: Convulsions, fever

Dermatologic: Rash

Gastrointestinal: nausea, diarrhea, vomiting, oral candidiasis

Hematologic: Hemolytic anemia, positive Coombs' reaction

Renal: Acute interstitial nephritis

Miscellaneous: Hypersensitivity reactions, anaphylaxis

Overdosage Symptoms of overdose include neuromuscular hypersensitivity, seizure

Toxicology Many beta-lactam-containing antibiotics have the potential to cause neuromuscular hyperirritability or convulsive seizures. Hemodialysis may be helpful to aid in the removal of the drug from the blood, otherwise most treatment is supportive or symptom directed.

Drug Interactions Probenecid, tetracycline, aminoglycosides (synergism)

Stability Refrigerate suspension after reconstitution; discard after 14 days

Mechanism of Action Interferes with bacterial cell wall synthesis during active multiplication causing cell death and resultant bactericidal activity against susceptible bacteria

Pharmacokinetics

Absorption: Oral: 60% to 73% from GI tract

Protein binding: 80%

Half-life: 30 minutes, prolonged in patients with renal impairment

Time to peak serum concentration: Oral: Within 30-60 minutes

Elimination: Penicillin V and its metabolites are excreted in urine mainly by tubular secretion

Usual Dosage Geriatrics and Adults: 125-500 mg every 6 hours

Dosing adjustment in renal impairment: Do not exceed 250 mg every 6 hours

Administration Administer on an empty stomach (ie, 1 hour prior to, or 2 hours after meals) to increase total absorption; administer around-the-clock rather than 4 times/day, 3 times/day, etc (ie, 12-6-12-6, not 9-1-5-9) to promote less variation in peak and trough serum concentrations

Monitoring Parameters Fever, WBC count, mental status, appetite

Test Interactions False-positive or negative urinary glucose determination using Clinitest®; positive Coombs' [direct]; false-positive urinary and/or serum proteins

Patient Information Take on an empty stomach 1 hour before or 2 hours after meals; complete full course of therapy, do not skip doses

Nursing Implications See Administration

(Continued)

Penicillin V Potassium *(Continued)*

Additional Information 0.7 mEq of potassium per 250 mg penicillin V; 250 mg equals 400,000 units of penicillin; each gram contains 2.6 mEq of potassium

Special Geriatric Considerations Dosage adjustment in the elderly is usually not necessary (see Usual Dosage)

Dosage Forms
Powder for oral solution: 125 mg/5 mL (3 mL, 100 mL, 150 mL, 200 mL); 250 mg/5 mL (100 mL, 150 mL, 200 mL)
Tablet: 125 mg, 250 mg, 500 mg

Pentacarinat® Injection *see* Pentamidine *on this page*

Pentam-300® Injection *see* Pentamidine *on this page*

Pentamidine *(pen TAM i deen)*

Brand Names NebuPent™ Inhalation; Pentacarinat® Injection; Pentam-300® Injection

Generic Available No

Therapeutic Category Antibiotic, Miscellaneous

Use Treatment and prevention of pneumonia caused by *Pneumocystis carinii*
Unlabeled use: Treatment of trypanosomiasis

Contraindications Hypersensitivity to pentamidine isethionate or any component (inhalation and injection)

Precautions Use with caution in patients with diabetes mellitus, renal or hepatic dysfunction; hypertension or hypotension

Adverse Reactions
Cardiovascular: Hypotension, tachycardia
Central nervous system: Dizziness, fever, fatigue
Dermatologic: Rash
Endocrine & metabolic: Hypoglycemia, hyperglycemia, hypocalcemia, hyperkalemia
Gastrointestinal: Vomiting, metallic taste, pancreatitis
Hematologic: Megaloblastic anemia, granulocytopenia, leukopenia, thrombocytopenia
Local: Pain at injection site
Renal/Hepatic: Mild renal or hepatic injury
Respiratory: Irritation of the airway, cough, bronchospasm, dyspnea, chest pain/congestion, pharyngitis
Miscellaneous: Jarisch-Herxheimer-like reaction

Stability Reconstituted solution is stable for 24 hours at room temperature; do not refrigerate due to the possibility of crystallization; do not use NS as a diluent, NS is **incompatible** with pentamidine

Mechanism of Action It is proposed to interfere with RNA/DNA, phospholipids, and protein synthesis through inhibition of oxidative phosphorylation and/or interference with incorporation of nucleotides and nucleic acids into RNA and DNA, in protozoa

Pharmacokinetics
Absorption: I.M.: Well absorbed; systemic accumulation of pentamidine does not appear to occur following inhalation therapy
Half-life, terminal: 6.4-9.4 hours; may be prolonged in patients with severe renal impairment
Elimination: 33% to 66% excreted in urine as unchanged drug

Usual Dosage Geriatrics and Adults:
Treatment: I.M., I.V. (I.V. preferred): 4 mg/kg/day once daily for 14 days
Prevention: Inhalation: 300 mg every 4 weeks via Respirgard® II nebulizer
Dosing interval in renal impairment:
Cl_{cr} 10-50 mL/minute: Administer every 24-36 hours
Cl_{cr} <10 mL/minute: Administer every 48 hours

Administration Infuse I.V. slowly over a period of at least 60 minutes or administer deep I.M.; patients receiving I.V. or I.M. pentamidine should be lying down and blood pressure should be monitored closely during administration of drug and several times thereafter until it is stable (see Stability)

Monitoring Parameters Inhaler technique, BUN, serum creatinine, blood glucose, CBC, platelet count, LFTs, serum calcium should be monitored before, during, and after acute treatment, EKG

Test Interactions Decreased glucose

Patient Information Get instructions on how to use inhaler

Nursing Implications See Administration and Stability

Special Geriatric Considerations 10% of acquired immunodeficiency syndrome (AIDS) cases are in the elderly and this figure is expected to increase; pentamidine has not as yet been studied exclusively in this population; adjust dose for renal function

Dosage Forms
Pentamidine isethionate:
Inhalation: 300 mg
Injection: 300 mg

Pentasa® Oral *see Mesalamine on page 591*

Pentazocine (pen TAZ oh seen)

Related Information
Pharmacokinetics of Narcotic Agonist Analgesics *on page 1037*
Brand Names Talwin®; Talwin® NX
Generic Available No
Therapeutic Category Analgesic, Narcotic
Use Relief of moderate to severe pain; has also been used as a sedative prior to surgery and as a supplement to surgical anesthesia
Restrictions C-IV
Contraindications Hypersensitivity to pentazocine or any component, increased intracranial pressure (unless the patient is mechanically ventilated)
Warnings Pentazocine may precipitate opiate withdrawal symptoms in patients who have been receiving opiates regularly; injection contains sulfites which may cause allergic reaction
Precautions Use with caution in seizure-prone patients, acute MI, patients undergoing biliary tract surgery, patients with renal and hepatic dysfunction, and patients with a history of prior opioid dependence or abuse
Adverse Reactions
Cardiovascular: Palpitations, hypotension, bradycardia, peripheral vasodilation
Central nervous system: CNS depression, sedation, dizziness, euphoria, lightheadedness, hallucinations, confusion, disorientation, increased intracranial pressure, seizures may occur in seizure-prone patients
Dermatologic: Pruritus, rash
Endocrine & metabolic: Antidiuretic hormone release
Gastrointestinal: Nausea, vomiting, constipation, biliary spasm
Genitourinary: Urinary tract spasm
Local: Tissue damage and irritation with I.M./S.C. use
Ocular: Miosis
Respiratory: Respiratory depression
Miscellaneous: Physical and psychological dependence, histamine release
Overdosage Symptoms of overdose include drowsiness, sedation, respiratory depression, coma
Toxicology Treatment of an overdose includes support of the patient's airway, establishment of an I.V. line and administration of naloxone 2 mg I.V. with repeat administration as necessary up to a total of 10 mg.
Drug Interactions
May potentiate or reduce analgesic effect of opiate agonist (eg, morphine) depending on patients tolerance to opiates can precipitate withdrawal in narcotic addicts
Increased effect/toxicity with tripelennamine (can be lethal), CNS depressants (phenothiazines, tranquilizers, anxiolytics, sedatives, hypnotics, or alcohol)
Stability Store at room temperature, protect from heat and from freezing
Mechanism of Action Binds to opiate receptors in the CNS, causing inhibition of ascending pain pathways, altering the perception of and response to pain; produces generalized CNS depression; partial agonist-antagonist
Pharmacodynamics
Onset of action:
Oral, I.M., S.C.: Within 15-30 minutes
I.V.: Within 2-3 minutes
Duration:
Parenteral: 2-3 hours
Oral: 4-5 hours
Pharmacokinetics
Protein binding: 60%
Bioavailability: Oral: ~20% due to large first-pass effect; increased oral bioavailability to 60% to 70% in patients with cirrhosis
Metabolism: In liver via oxidative and glucuronide conjugation pathways
Half-life: 2-3 hours, increased half-life with decreased hepatic function
(Continued)

Pentazocine (Continued)

Elimination: Excreted unchanged in urine

Usual Dosage

Geriatrics:
  Oral: 50 mg every 4 hours
  I.M.: 30 mg every 4 hours

Adults:
  Oral: 50-100 mg every 3-4 hours
  I.M., S.C.: 30-60 mg every 3-4 hours
  I.V.: 30 mg every 3-4 hours

Dosing adjustment in renal impairment:
  Cl_{cr} 10-50 mL/minute: Administer 75% of normal dose
  Cl_{cr} <10 mL/minute: Administer 50% of normal dose

Dosing adjustment in hepatic impairment: Reduce dose or avoid use in patients with liver disease

Monitoring Parameters Relief of pain, respiratory and mental status, blood pressure

Patient Information May cause drowsiness; avoid alcohol and CNS depressants; may be addicting if used for prolonged periods; will cause withdrawal in patients currently dependent on narcotics

Nursing Implications Rotate injection site for I.M., S.C. use; avoid intra-arterial injection; observe patient for excessive sedation, respiratory depression, implement safety measures, assist with ambulation; observe for narcotic withdrawal

Additional Information

Pentazocine hydrochloride: Talwin® NX tablet (with naloxone); naloxone is used to prevent abuse by dissolving tablets in water and using as injection
Pentazocine lactate: Talwin® injection

Special Geriatric Considerations Pentazocine is not recommended for use in the elderly because of its propensity to cause delirium and agitation; adjust dose for renal function (see Warnings and Precautions)

Dosage Forms

Injection, as lactate: 30 mg/mL (1 mL, 1.5 mL, 2 mL, 10 mL)
Tablet: Pentazocine hydrochloride 50 mg and naloxone hydrochloride 0.5 mg

Pentobarbital (pen toe BAR bi tal)

Related Information

Anxiolytic/Hypnotic Use in Long-Term Care Facilities on page 1099
Federal OBRA Regulations Recommended Maximum Doses - Hypnotics on page 1057

Brand Names Nembutal®

Synonyms Pentobarbital Sodium

Generic Available Yes: 100 mg capsule, 2 mL Tubex®

Therapeutic Category Barbiturate; Sedative

Special Geriatric Considerations Use of this agent as a hypnotic in the elderly is not recommended due to its long half-life and addiction potential

Pentobarbital Sodium see Pentobarbital on this page

Pentoxifylline (pen toks I fi leen)

Brand Names Trental®

Synonyms Oxpentifylline

Generic Available No

Therapeutic Category Blood Viscosity Reducer Agent

Use Symptomatic management of peripheral vascular disease, mainly intermittent claudication

Unlabeled uses: Psychopathologic symptoms secondary to cerebrovascular insufficiency, diabetic angiopathy/neuropathy, TIAs, strokes, high altitude sickness, Raynaud's disease, sickle cell thalassemias, leg ulcers, hearing disorders; more studies are needed for these uses

Contraindications Hypersensitivity to pentoxifylline or any component and other xanthine derivatives (caffeine, theophylline)

Precautions Dose may need adjustment in patients with impaired renal function and in the elderly

Adverse Reactions

Cardiovascular: Mild hypotension, angina, arrhythmias
Central nervous system: Agitation, dizziness, headache
Gastrointestinal: Nausea, dyspepsia, vomiting
Ocular: Blurred vision
Otic: Earache

Overdosage Symptoms of overdose include hypotension, flushing, convulsions, deep sleep, agitation, tremors, bradycardia with first or second degree A-V block

Toxicology Gastric lavage and activated charcoal; symptomatic treatment for cardiovascular, respiratory, and neurologic events

Drug Interactions Warfarin's effects may be enhanced

Mechanism of Action Mechanism of action remains unclear; is thought to reduce blood viscosity and improve blood flow by altering the rheology of red blood cells

Pharmacokinetics
Absorption: Oral: Well absorbed
Half-life: 24-48 minutes (metabolites half-life: 60-96 minutes)
Time to peak serum concentration: Within 1 hour
Metabolism: Undergoes first-pass metabolism; metabolized in the liver and
Elimination: Mainly in urine

Usual Dosage Geriatrics and Adults: Oral: 400 mg 3 times/day with meals; may reduce to 400 mg twice daily if GI or CNS side effects occur

Monitoring Parameters PT, PTT if used in conjunction with other agents that may affect coagulation or platelet aggregation

Test Interactions Decrease calcium (S), decreased magnesium (S), false-positive theophylline levels

Patient Information Take with food or meals; if GI or CNS side effects continue, contact physician; while effects may be seen in 2-4 weeks, continue treatment for at least 8 weeks

Special Geriatric Considerations Pentoxiphylline's value in the treatment of intermittent claudication is controversial; walking distance improved statistically in some clinical trials, but the actual distance was minimal when applied to improving physical activity (see Usual Dosage and Monitoring Parameters).

Dosage Forms Tablet, controlled release: 400 mg

Pen.Vee® K see Penicillin V Potassium on page 725

Pen VK see Penicillin V Potassium on page 725

Pepcid® see Famotidine on page 367

Pepcid® AC Acid Controller [OTC] see Famotidine on page 367

Pepto-Bismol® [OTC] see Bismuth on page 122

Pepto® Diarrhea Control [OTC] see Loperamide on page 548

Percocet® see Oxycodone and Acetaminophen on page 705

Percodan® see Oxycodone and Aspirin on page 706

Percodan®-Demi see Oxycodone and Aspirin on page 706

Perdiem® Plain [OTC] see Psyllium on page 804

Pergolide (PER go lide)

Brand Names Permax®

Generic Available No

Therapeutic Category Anti-Parkinson's Agent; Ergot Alkaloid

Use Adjunctive treatment to levodopa/carbidopa in the management of Parkinson's Disease

Contraindications Known hypersensitivity to pergolide mesylate or other ergot derivatives

Precautions High incidence of syncope and orthostatic hypotension upon initiation of therapy; use with caution in patients prone to cardiac dysrhythmias and in patients with a history of confusion or hallucinations

Adverse Reactions
Cardiovascular: Myocardial infarction, postural hypotension, syncope, arrhythmias, peripheral edema
Central nervous system: Dizziness, somnolence, insomnia, confusion, hallucinations, anxiety
Gastrointestinal: Nausea, constipation
Neuromuscular & skeletal: Dyskinesias
Respiratory: Rhinitis

Overdosage Symptoms of overdose include vomiting, hypotension, agitation, hallucinations, ventricular extrasystoles, possible seizures; limited data on overdose

Toxicology Treatment is supportive and may require antiarrhythmias and/or neuroleptics for agitation; hypotension, when unresponsive to I.V. fluids or Trendelenburg positioning, often responds to norepinephrine infusions started at 0.1-0.2 mcg/kg/minute followed by a titrated infusion. If signs of CNS stimulation are present, a neuroleptic may be indicated; antiarrhythmics may
(Continued)

Pergolide (Continued)

be indicated, monitor EKG; activated charcoal is useful to prevent further absorption and to hasten elimination.

Drug Interactions
Decreased effect: Dopamine antagonists, metoclopramide
Increased toxicity: Highly plasma protein bound drugs

Mechanism of Action Pergolide is a semisynthetic ergot alkaloid similar to bromocriptine but stated to be more potent and longer-acting; it is a centrally-active dopamine agonist stimulating both D_1 and D_2 receptors

Pharmacokinetics
Absorption: Oral: Well absorbed
Metabolism: Extensive in the liver (on first-pass)
Elimination: ~50% in urine and 50% in feces

Usual Dosage Geriatrics and Adults: Oral: Start with 0.05 mg/day for 2 days, then increase dosage by 0.1 or 0.15 mg/day every 3 days over next 12 days, increase dose by 0.25 mg/day every 3 days until optimal therapeutic dose is achieved; usual dosage range: 2-3 mg/day in 3 divided doses

Monitoring Parameters Blood pressure, both standing and sitting/supine, symptoms of parkinsonism, dyskinesias, mental status

Patient Information Take with food or milk; rise slowly from sitting or lying down; report any confusion or change in mental status

Nursing Implications Raise bed rails and institute safety measures; aid patient with ambulation; may cause postural hypotension and drowsiness

Additional Information When adding pergolide to levodopa/carbidopa, the dose of the latter can usually and should be decreased. Patients no longer responsive to bromocriptine may benefit by being switched to pergolide.

Special Geriatric Considerations See Precautions and Adverse Reactions

Dosage Forms Tablet, as mesylate: 0.05 mg, 0.25 mg, 1 mg

References
Collier DS, Berg MJ, and Fincham RW, "Parkinsonism Treatment: Part III - Update," Ann Pharmacother, 1992, 26(2):227-33.
Koller WC, Silver DE, and Lieberman A, "An Algorithm for the Management of Parkinson's Disease," Neurology, 1994, 44(12 Suppl 10):S1-52.
Staedt J, Wassmuth F, Ziemann U, et al, "Pergolide: Treatment of Choice in Restless Legs Syndrome (RLS) and Nocturnal Myoclonus Syndrome (NMS): A Double-Blind Randomized Crossover Trial of Pergolide Versus L-Dopa," J Neural Transm, 1997, 104(4-5):961-8.
Stern MB, "Contemporary Approaches to the Pharmacotherapeutic Management of Parkinson's Disease: An Overview," Neurology, 1997, 49(1 Suppl 1):S2-9.
Watts RL, "The Role of Dopamine Agonists in Early Parkinson's Disease," Neurology, 1997, 49(1 Suppl 1):S34-48.

Periactin® see Cyproheptadine on page 265

Peri-Colace® [OTC] see Docusate and Casanthranol on page 313

Peridex® Oral Rinse see Chlorhexidine Gluconate on page 206

PerioGard® see Chlorhexidine Gluconate on page 206

Permapen® see Penicillin G Benzathine on page 720

Permax® see Pergolide on previous page

Permethrin (per METH rin)

Brand Names Elimite™ Cream; Nix™ Creme Rinse

Therapeutic Category Antiparasitic Agent, Topical; Pediculocide; Scabicidal Agent

Use Single application treatment of infestation with Pediculus humanus capitis (head louse) and its nits, or Sarcoptes scabiei (scabies)

Contraindications Known hypersensitivity to pyrethyroid, pyrethrin or to chrysanthemums

Precautions Treatment with Nix™ may temporarily exacerbate the symptoms of itching, redness, swelling; for external use only

Adverse Reactions
Cardiovascular: Edema
Dermatologic: Pruritus, numbness or scalp discomfort, erythema, rash of the scalp
Local: Burning, stinging, tingling

Mechanism of Action Inhibits sodium ion influx through nerve cell membrane channels in parasites resulting in delayed repolarization and thus paralysis of the pest

Pharmacokinetics
Absorption: Topical: Minimal, <2%
Metabolism: In the liver
Elimination: In urine

Usual Dosage Geriatrics and Adults: Topical:

Head lice: After hair has been washed with shampoo, rinsed with water and towel dried, apply a sufficient volume to saturate the hair and scalp. Leave on hair for 10 minutes before rinsing off with water; remove remaining nits; may repeat in 1 week if lice or nits still present

Scabies: Apply cream from head to toe; leave on for 8-14 hours before washing off with water, a single application is usually adequate; may repeat in 1 week

Administration Because scabies and lice are so contagious, use caution to avoid spreading or infecting oneself; wear gloves when applying (see Usual Dosage)

Patient Information Avoid contact with eyes during application; shake well before using; notify physician if irritation persists; clothing and bedding should be washed in hot water or dry cleaned to kill the scabies mite

Nursing Implications See Administration

Special Geriatric Considerations Because of its minimal absorption, permethrin is a drug of choice and is preferred over lindane

Dosage Forms
Cream: 5% (60 g)
Creme rinse: 1% (60 mL with comb)

Permitil® Oral *see* Fluphenazine *on page 395*

Perphenazine (per FEN a zeen)
Related Information
Antacid Drug Interactions *on page 1096*
Antipsychotic Agents Comparison *on page 1023*
Antipsychotic Medication Guidelines *on page 1076*
Federal OBRA Regulations Recommended Maximum Doses - Antipsychotics *on page 1056*

Brand Names Trilafon®

Generic Available Yes

Therapeutic Category Antiemetic; Antipsychotic Agent; Neuroleptic Agent; Phenothiazine Derivative

Use Management of manifestations of psychotic disorders; depressive neurosis; alcohol withdrawal; nausea and vomiting; nonpsychotic symptoms associated with dementia in elderly, Tourette's syndrome; Huntington's chorea; spasmodic torticollis and Reye's syndrome (see Special Geriatric Considerations)

Contraindications Hypersensitivity to perphenazine or any component, cross-sensitivity with other phenothiazines may exist; avoid use in patients with narrow-angle glaucoma, bone marrow suppression, severe liver or cardiac disease; subcortical brain damage; circulatory collapse; severe hypotension or hypertension

Warnings

Tardive dyskinesia: Prevalence rate may be 40% in elderly; elderly women especially at risk; embarrassment from dyskinesias may lead to greater social isolation; development of the syndrome and the irreversible nature are proportional to duration and total cumulative dose over time. May be reversible if diagnosed early in therapy; intermittent use of antipsychotics (not proven use) helps decrease total cumulative dose.

EPS: Extrapyramidal reactions are more common in elderly with up to 50% developing these reactions after age 60. These reactions may be more common in dementia patients. Drug-induced **Parkinson's syndrome** occurs often. Discontinuation usually resolves symptoms but may take weeks to months (12+) to clear. **Akathisia** is the most common EPS reaction in elderly. The symptoms of motor restlessness are difficult to diagnose in demented elderly; increased nervousness, assertiveness, restlessness with constant movement may indicate this adverse event. Consider decreasing dose if antipsychotic to treat as well as diagnose problem; usually see this reaction within 2-3 months of initiating antipsychotic drug.

Anticholinergic effects: These side effects most common with low potency antipsychotics (eg, thioridazine, chlorpromazine). CNS toxicity occurs more frequently and severely in elderly; increased confusion, memory loss, psychotic behavior, and agitation frequently occur as a consequence of anticholinergic effects to antipsychotic agents. Peripheral anticholinergic action troublesome to elderly; most peripheral anticholinergic effects last only 2-3 weeks (see Adverse Reactions).

Orthostatic hypotension: More common with low potency agents (eg, thioridazine, chlorpromazine, and clozapine) but of concern with all antipsychotic agents; orthostasis due to alpha-receptor blockade by antipsychotic agents.

(Continued)

Perphenazine (Continued)

Elderly present many risk factors for orthostatic hypotension: blunted baroreceptor reflexes, decreased vascular tone, decreased vascular volume, and possible presence of cardiac diseases which result in decreased cardiac output.

Sedation: Common side effect with antipsychotic therapy; should not be used as a hypnotic unless insomnia is associated with target behavior symptoms treated with antipsychotic medications (see Special Geriatric Considerations). Anecdotal reports suggesting antipsychotic sedation in nonpsychotic patients is extremely unpleasant due to feelings of depersonalization, derealization, and dysphoria. Due to the long duration of action with antipsychotic drugs, these reactions may last up to 24 hours and result in decreased daytime function.

Cardiac toxicity: Life-threatening arrhythmias have occurred at therapeutic doses of antipsychotics. Thioridazine more commonly demonstrates EKG changes than other antipsychotics; suggested to use high potency antipsychotic agents (ie, haloperidol) in patients with cardiac conduction defects.

Precautions Use with caution in patients with cardiovascular disease, seizures, and Parkinson's disease; benefits of therapy must be weighed against risks

Adverse Reactions Sedation and anticholinergic effects are more pronounced than extrapyramidal effects

Cardiovascular: EKG changes, hypotension (especially orthostatic), tachycardia, arrhythmias, abnormal T waves with prolonged ventricular repolarization

Central nervous system: Drowsiness, restlessness, anxiety, extrapyramidal reactions, dystonic reactions, pseudoparkinsonian signs and symptoms, tardive dyskinesia, neuroleptic malignant syndrome, seizures, altered central temperature regulation

Dermatologic: Hyperpigmentation, pruritus, rash, contact dermatitis, photosensitivity (rare)

Endocrine & metabolic: Amenorrhea, galactorrhea, gynecomastia

Gastrointestinal: Xerostomia (problem for denture user), constipation, adynamic ileus, GI upset, weight gain

Genitourinary: Overflow incontinence, urinary retention, priapism, sexual dysfunction (up to 60%)

Hematologic: Agranulocytosis, leukopenia

Hepatic: Cholestatic jaundice

Ocular: Retinal pigmentation (more common than with chlorpromazine), blurred vision, decreased visual acuity (may be irreversible)

Overdosage Symptoms of overdose include deep sleep, coma, extrapyramidal symptoms, abnormal involuntary muscle movements, hypotension or hypertension; agitation, restlessness, fever, hypothermia or hyperthermia, seizures, cardiac arrhythmias, EKG changes

Toxicology Following initiation of essential overdose management, toxic symptom treatment and supportive treatment should be initiated. Hypotension usually responds to I.V. fluids or Trendelenburg positioning. If unresponsive to these measures the use of a parenteral inotrope may be required (eg, norepinephrine 0.1-0.2 mcg/kg/minute titrated to response). Seizures commonly respond to diazepam (I.V. 5-10 mg bolus every 15 minutes if needed up to a total of 30 mg) or to phenytoin or phenobarbital. Also critical cardiac arrhythmias often respond to I.V. phenytoin (15 mg/kg up to 1 g), while other antiarrhythmics can be used. Neuroleptics often cause extrapyramidal symptoms (eg, dystonic reactions) requiring management with diphenhydramine 1-2 mg/kg up to a maximum of 50 mg I.M. or I.V. slow push followed by a maintenance dose for 48-72 hours. When these reactions are unresponsive to diphenhydramine, benztropine mesylate I.V. 1-2 mg may be effective. These agents are generally effective within 2-5 minutes.

Drug Interactions

Alcohol may increase CNS sedation

Anticholinergic agents may decrease pharmacologic effects; increase anticholinergic side effects; may enhance tardive dyskinesia

Aluminum salts may decrease absorption of phenothiazines

Barbiturates may decrease phenothiazine serum concentrations

Bromocriptine may have decreased efficacy when administered with phenothiazines

Guanethidine's hypotensive effect is decreased by phenothiazines

Lithium administration with phenothiazines may increase disorientation

Meperidine and phenothiazine coadministration increases sedation and hypotension

Methyldopa administration with phenothiazine (trifluoperazine) may significantly increase blood pressure

Norepinephrine, epinephrine have decreased pressor effect when administered with chlorpromazine; therefore, be aware of possible decreased effectiveness or when any phenothiazine is used

Phenytoin serum concentrations may increase or decrease with phenothiazines; tricyclic antidepressants may have increased serum concentrations with concomitant administration with phenothiazines

Propranolol administered with phenothiazines may increase serum concentrations of both drugs

Valproic acid may have increased half-life when administered with phenothiazines (chlorpromazine)

Stability Do not mix with beverages containing caffeine (coffee, cola), tannins (tea), or pectinates (apple juice) since physical incompatibility exists; use ~60 mL diluent for each 5 mL of concentrate; protect all dosage forms from light, clear or slightly yellow solutions may be used; should be dispensed in amber or opaque vials/bottles. Solutions may be diluted or mixed with fruit juices or other liquids but must be administered immediately after mixing; do not prepare bulk dilutions or store bulk dilutions.

Mechanism of Action Blocks postsynaptic mesolimbic dopaminergic D_1 and D_2 receptors in the brain; exhibits a strong alpha-adrenergic blocking and anticholinergic effect, depresses the release of hypothalamic and hypophyseal hormones; believed to depress the reticular activating system thus affecting basal metabolism, body temperature, wakefulness, vasomotor tone, and emesis

Pharmacokinetics

Absorption: Oral: Well absorbed; absorption may be affected by the inherent anticholinergic action on the gastrointestinal tissue causing variable absorption. Absorption from tablets is erratic with less variation seen with solutions. These agents are widely distributed in tissues with CNS concentrations exceeding that of plasma due to their lipophilic characteristics.

Protein binding: Antipsychotic agents are bound 90% to 99% to plasma or proteins; highly bound to brain and lung tissue and other tissues with a high blood perfusion

Metabolism: Metabolized in the liver; substrate and inhibitor CYP2D6

Time to peak: Peak serum concentrations occur within 4-8 hours; peak concentrations between 2-4 hours

Elimination: Excreted in urine and bile; excretion occurs through hepatic metabolism (oxidation) where numerous active metabolites are produced; active metabolites excreted in urine; elimination half-lives of antipsychotics ranges from 20-40 hours which may be extended in elderly due to decline in oxidative hepatic reactions (phase I) with age.

The biologic effect of a single dose persists for 24 hours. When the patient has accommodated to initial side effects (sedation), once daily dosing is possible due to the long half-life of antipsychotics.

Steady-state plasma concentrations are achieved in 4-7 days; therefore, if possible, do not make dose adjustments more than once in a 7-day period. Due to the long half-lives of antipsychotics, as needed (prn) use is ineffective since repeated doses are necessary to achieve therapeutic tissue concentrations in the CNS.

Usual Dosage

Geriatrics (nonpsychotic patient; dementia behavior): Oral: Initial: 2-4 mg 1-2 times/day; increase at 4- to 7-day intervals by 2-4 mg/day. Increase dose intervals (bid, tid, etc) as necessary to control behavior response or side effects. Maximum daily dose: 32 mg; gradual increase (titration) may prevent some side effects or decrease their severity.

Adults:

Psychoses: 4-16 mg 2-4 times/day; I.M.: 5 mg every 6 hours

Nausea/vomiting: 8-16 mg/day in divided doses

I.M.: 5-10 mg

I.V. (severe): 1 mg at 1- to 2-minute intervals up to a total of 5 mg

Not dialyzable (0% to 5%)

Monitoring Parameters Orthostatic blood pressures; tremors, gait changes, abnormal movement in trunk, neck, buccal area, or extremities; monitor target behaviors for which the agent is given

Reference Range 0.8-1.2 ng/mL; serum concentrations are controversial and dosing to response is recommended

(Continued)

Perphenazine (Continued)

Test Interactions Increased cholesterol (S), increased glucose; decreased uric acid (S)

Patient Information Oral concentrate must be diluted in 2-4 oz of liquid (water, fruit juice, carbonated drinks, milk, or pudding); do not take antacid within 1 hour of taking drug; avoid alcohol; avoid excess sun exposure (use sun block); may cause drowsiness, rise slowly from recumbent position; use of supportive stockings may help prevent orthostatic hypotension

Nursing Implications Monitor for hypotension when administering I.M. or I.V.; dilute oral concentration to at least 2 oz with water, juice, or milk; for I.V. use, injection should be diluted to at least 0.5 mg/mL with NS and given at a rate of 1 mg/minute. Monitor for orthostatic hypotension 3-5 days after initiation of therapy or a dose increase; observe for tremor and abnormal movement or posturing.

Special Geriatric Considerations See Warnings.

Many elderly patients receive antipsychotic medications for inappropriate nonpsychotic behavior. Before initiating antipsychotic medication, the clinician should investigate any possible reversible cause; any stress or stress from any disease can cause acute "confusion" or worsening of baseline nonpsychotic behavior. Most commonly acute changes in behavior are due to increases in drug dose or addition of new drug to regimen; fluid electrolyte loss; infections; and changes in environment.

Any changes in disease status in any organ system can result in behavior changes.

In the treatment of agitated, demented, elderly patients, authors of meta-analysis of controlled trials of the response to the traditional antipsychotics (phenothiazines, butyrophenones) in controlling agitation have concluded that the use of neuroleptics results in a response rate of 18%. Clearly neuroleptic therapy for behavior control should be limited with frequent attempts to withdraw the agent given for behavior control.

Dosage Forms

Concentrate, oral: 16 mg/5 mL (118 mL)

Injection: 5 mg/mL (1 mL)

Tablet: 2 mg, 4 mg, 8 mg, 16 mg

References

Peabody CA, Warner MD, Whiteford HA, et al, "Neuroleptics and the Elderly," *J Am Geriatr Soc*, 1987, 35(3):233-8.

Risse SC and Barnes R, "Pharmacologic Treatment of Agitation Associated With Dementia," *J Am Geriatr Soc*, 1986, 34(5):368-76.

Saltz BL, Woerner MG, Kane JM, et al, "Prospective Study of Tardive Dyskinesia Incidence in the Elderly," *JAMA*, 1991, 266(17):2402-6.

Seifert RD, "Therapeutic Drug Monitoring: Psychotropic Drugs," *J Pharm Pract*, 1984, 6:403-16.

Perphenazine and Amitriptyline see Amitriptyline and Perphenazine on page 62

Persantine® see Dipyridamole on page 307

Pertussin® CS [OTC] see Dextromethorphan on page 278

Pertussin® ES [OTC] see Dextromethorphan on page 278

Pethidine Hydrochloride see Meperidine on page 584

Petrolatum White and Mineral Oil Ophthalmic Ointment see Ocular Lubricant on page 688

PFA see Foscarnet on page 409

Pfizerpen® see Penicillin G, Parenteral, Aqueous on page 722

Pfizerpen®-AS see Penicillin G Procaine on page 723

PGE₁ see Alprostadil on page 38

Phanatuss® Cough Syrup [OTC] see Guaifenesin and Dextromethorphan on page 439

Pharmacokinetics of Narcotic Agonist Analgesics see page 1037

Pharmaflur® see Fluoride on page 392

Phazyme® [OTC] see Simethicone on page 856

Phenadex® Senior [OTC] see Guaifenesin and Dextromethorphan on page 439

Phenantoin see Mephenytoin on page 585

Phenaphen® With Codeine see Acetaminophen and Codeine on page 18

Phenazine® see Promethazine on page 791

Phenazopyridine (fen az oh PEER i deen)

Brand Names Azo-Standard® [OTC]; Baridium® [OTC]; Prodium® [OTC]; Pyridiate®; Pyridium®; Urodine®; Urogesic®

Synonyms Phenylazo Diamino Pyridine Hydrochloride

Generic Available Yes

Therapeutic Category Analgesic, Urinary; Local Anesthetic, Urinary

Use Symptomatic relief of urinary burning, itching, frequency and urgency in association with urinary tract infection or following urologic procedures

Contraindications Hypersensitivity to phenazopyridine or any component; kidney or liver disease

Warnings Long-term administration has induced neoplasia in rats and mice

Precautions Yellowish tinge of the skin or sclera may indicate accumulation due to impaired renal function. If this occurs, discontinue therapy; phenazopyridine should only be given for 2 days when used with an antibiotic for the treatment of a urinary tract infection. Do not use in patients with Cl_{cr} <50 mL/minute.

Adverse Reactions

Central nervous system: Vertigo, headache

Dermatologic: Skin pigmentation, rash

Hematologic: Methemoglobinemia, hemolytic anemia

Hepatic: Hepatitis

Renal: Acute renal failure

Overdosage Symptoms of overdose include methemoglobinemia, hemolytic anemia, skin pigmentation, renal and hepatic impairment

Toxicology Antidote: Methylene blue 1-2 mg/kg I.V. or 100-200 g ascorbic acid orally

Mechanism of Action Exerts local anesthetic or analgesic action on urinary tract mucosa through an unknown mechanism

Pharmacokinetics

Metabolism: In the liver and other tissues

Elimination: In urine (where it exerts its action); renal excretion (as unchanged drug) is rapid and accounts for 65% of the drug's elimination

Usual Dosage Geriatrics and Adults: Oral: 100-200 mg 3-4 times/day after meals for 2 days

Monitoring Parameters Relief of urinary discomfort

Test Interactions Phenazopyridine may cause delayed reactions with glucose oxidase reagents (Clinistix®, Tes-Tape®); occasional false-positive tests occur with Tes-Tape®; cupric sulfate tests (Clinitest®) are not affected; interference may also occur with urine ketone tests (Acetest®, Ketostix®) and urinary protein tests; tests for urinary steroids and porphyrins may also occur

Patient Information Take by mouth after meals; tablets may color the urine orange or red and may stain clothing. This medication treats the painful symptoms of a urinary tract infection but does not cure the infection.

Nursing Implications Colors urine orange or red; stains clothing and is difficult to remove; administer after meals

Special Geriatric Considerations Use of this agent in the elderly is limited since accumulation of phenazopyridine can occur in patients with renal insufficiency; it should not be used in patients with a Cl_{cr} <50 mL/minute

Dosage Forms Tablet, as hydrochloride: 100 mg, 200 mg

Phendry® Oral [OTC] *see* Diphenhydramine *on page 302*

Phenelzine (FEN el zeen)

Related Information

Antidepressant Medication Guidelines *on page 1075*

Brand Names Nardil®

Therapeutic Category Antidepressant, Monoamine Oxidase Inhibitor

Use Symptomatic treatment of depressed patients refractory to or intolerant to other antidepressants or electroconvulsive therapy

Contraindications Pheochromocytoma, hepatic or renal disease, cerebrovascular defect, cardiovascular disease, hypersensitivity to phenelzine or any component

Warnings Hypertensive crisis within several hours of ingestion of a contraindicated substance (such as tyramine-containing foods)

Adverse Reactions

Cardiovascular: Hypotension, edema, tachycardia

Central nervous system: Drowsiness, nervousness

Dermatologic: Skin rash

Gastrointestinal: Xerostomia, constipation, anorexia

Genitourinary: Urinary retention, impotence

Hematologic: Leukopenia

Hepatic: Hepatocellular (hepatitis-like) damage

Neuromuscular & skeletal: Peripheral neuropathy, trembling, paresthesia

(Continued)

Phenelzine *(Continued)*

Ocular: Blurred vision

Overdosage Symptoms of overdose include tachycardia, palpitations, muscle twitching, seizures

Toxicology Competent supportive care is the most important treatment for an overdose with a monoamine oxidase (MAO) inhibitor. Both hypertension or hypotension can occur with intoxication. Hypotension may respond to I.V. fluids or vasopressors and hypertension usually responds to an alpha-adrenergic blocker. While treating the hypertension, care is warranted to avoid sudden drops in blood pressure, since this may worsen the MAO inhibitor toxicity. Muscle irritability and seizures often respond to diazepam, while hyperthermia is best treated antipyretics and cooling blankets. Cardiac arrhythmias are best treated with phenytoin or procainamide.

Drug Interactions

Increased effect/toxicity of barbiturates, psychotropics, rauwolfia alkaloids, CNS depressants

Increased toxicity with dexfenfluramine (possible), disulfiram (seizures), fluoxetine and other serotonin active agents (increased cardiac effect), tricyclic antidepressants (increased cardiovascular instability), meperidine (increased cardiovascular instability), phenothiazine (hypertensive crisis), sympathomimetics (hypertensive crisis), levodopa (hypertensive crisis), dextroamphetamine

Note: Many of these interactions can occur weeks after the MAO inhibitor has been stopped; in patients undergoing general anesthesia, discontinue the MAO inhibitors several weeks before to avoid cardiovascular effects

Drug/Food Interactions Avoid tyramine-containing foods (may increase blood pressure) (see Warnings)

Stability Protect from light

Mechanism of Action Inhibits the enzymes monoamine oxidase A and B which is responsible for the intraneuronal metabolism of norepinephrine and serotonin, and dopamine and phenylethylamine, respectively. Also involved in the down regulation of $beta_2$- and $alpha_2$-nonadrenergic receptors and serotonin alpha-receptors

Pharmacodynamics

Onset of action: Expect to see some clinical response in 2-4 weeks, provided that the dosing is adequate

Duration of action: May continue to have a therapeutic effect and interactions 2 weeks after discontinuing therapy

Geriatric patients receiving an average of 55 mg/day developed a mean platelet MAO activity inhibition of about 85%

Pharmacokinetics

Absorption: Oral: Well absorbed; undergoes acetylation in the liver

Older patients have been reported to have higher blood concentrations than younger adults after 2 weeks of continuous treatment

Elimination: In urine primarily as metabolites and unchanged drug

Usual Dosage Oral:

Geriatrics: Initial: 7.5 mg/day, increase by 7.5-15 mg/day every 3-4 days as tolerated; usual therapeutic dose: 15-60 mg/day in 3-4 divided doses

Adults: 15 mg 3 times/day; may increase to 60-90 mg/day

Monitoring Parameters Blood pressure, heart rate; diet; weight; mood if depressive symptoms

Reference Range Inhibition of platelet monoamine oxidase (≥80%) correlates with clinical response

Test Interactions Decreased glucose

Patient Information Avoid tyramine-containing foods: red wine, aged cheese (except cottage, ricotta, and cream), smoked or pickled fish, beef or chicken liver, dried sausage, fava or broad bean pods, yeast, vitamin supplements. Report severe headaches, irregular heartbeats, skin rash, insomnia, sedation, changes in strength, sensations of pain, burning, touch, or vibration, or any other unusual symptoms to your physician; avoid alcohol; get up slowly from chair or bed.

Nursing Implications Watch for postural hypotension; monitor blood pressure carefully, especially at therapy onset or if other CNS drugs or cardiovascular drugs are added; check for dietary and drug restriction

Special Geriatric Considerations The MAO inhibitors are effective and generally well tolerated by older patients. It is their potential interactions with tyramine or tryptophan-containing foods (see Warnings) and other drugs (see Drug Interactions), and their effects on blood pressure that have limited their use. The MAO inhibitors are usually reserved for patients who do not tolerate or respond to the traditional "cyclic" or "second generation" antidepressants. The brain activity of monoamine oxidase increases with age and even more so in patients with Alzheimer's disease. Therefore, the MAO inhibitors may have an increased role in patients with Alzheimer's disease who are depressed. Phenelzine is less stimulating than tranylcypromine (see Pharmacokinetics and Pharmacodynamics).

Dosage Forms Tablet, as sulfate: 15 mg

References

Alexopoulos GS, "Treatment of Depression," *Clinical Geriatric Psychopharmacology*, 2nd ed, 137-74, Salzman C, ed, Baltimore, MD: Williams & Wilkins, 1992.

Georgotas A, Friedman E, McCarthy M, et al, "Resistant Geriatric Depression and Therapeutic Response to Monoamine-Oxidase Inhibitors," *Biol Psychiatry*, 1983, 18:195-205.

Goff DC and Jenike MA, "Treatment-Resistant Depression in the Elderly," *J Am Geriatr Soc*, 1986, 34(1):63-70.

Jenike MA, "MAO Inhibitors as Treatment for Depressed Patients With Primary Degenerative Dementia (Alzheimer's Disease)," *Am J Psychiatry*, 1985, 142:763.

Phenerbel-S® see Ergotamine *on page 343*

Phenergan® see Promethazine *on page 791*

Phenetron® see Chlorpheniramine *on page 208*

Pheniramine and Naphazoline see Naphazoline and Pheniramine *on page 654*

Phenobarbital (fee noe BAR bi tal)

Related Information

Antiepileptic Drug Interactions Comparison *on page 1022*
I.V. Push Recommended Guidelines *on page 1083*
Serum Drug Concentrations Commonly Monitored: Guidelines *on page 1114*

Brand Names Barbita®; Luminal®; Solfoton®

Synonyms Phenobarbitone; Phenylethylmalonylurea

Generic Available Yes

Therapeutic Category Anticonvulsant, Barbiturate; Barbiturate; Hypnotic; Sedative

Use Management of generalized tonic-clonic (grand mal) and partial seizures; sedation, hypnosis; lowering of bilirubin in chronic cholestasis

Restrictions C-IV

Contraindications Hypersensitivity to phenobarbital or any component; pre-existing CNS depression, severe uncontrolled pain, porphyria, severe respiratory disease with dyspnea or obstruction

Warnings Abrupt withdrawal may precipitate status epilepticus; use with caution in patients with a history of depression, suicidal threats, or a history of drug abuse; pain may have signs masked; vitamin D requirements may be increased (induced metabolism); rise cautiously in elderly (see Special Geriatric Considerations)

Precautions Use with caution in patients with renal or hepatic impairment; abrupt withdrawal in patients with epilepsy may precipitate status epilepticus; use with caution in patients with myxedema or myasthenia gravis; barbiturates may be habit forming

Adverse Reactions

Cardiovascular: Hypotension, cardiac arrhythmias, bradycardia, syncope, circulatory collapse, arterial spasm, and gangrene with inadvertent intra-arterial injection

Central nervous system: Drowsiness, lethargy, CNS depression, impaired judgment, paradoxical excitement, cognitive impairment, defects in general comprehension, short-term memory deficits, decreased attention span, ataxia, hypothermia, hallucinations, lethargy

Dermatologic: Rash, skin eruptions, exfoliative dermatitis

Gastrointestinal: Nausea, vomiting

Hematologic: Megaloblastic anemia

Hepatic: Hepatitis

Local: Thrombophlebitis with I.V. use

Neuromuscular & skeletal: Osteomalacia, hyperkinetic activity

Renal: Oliguria

Respiratory: Respiratory depression, apnea (especially with rapid I.V. use)

Overdosage Symptoms of overdose include CNS depression, respiratory depression, hypotension, tachycardia, areflexia

Toxicology Treatment is mainly supportive; emesis may be induced if the patient is conscious and has not lost his/her gag reflex; activated charcoal may be administered; if renal function is normal, forced diuresis is helpful.

(Continued)

Phenobarbital *(Continued)*

Alkalinization of the urine with I.V. sodium bicarbonate helps enhance elimination; hemodialysis and hemoperfusion may be used in severe barbiturate intoxications.

Drug Interactions

Decreased effect of phenothiazines, haloperidol, quinidine, cyclosporine, TCAs, corticosteroids, theophylline, ethosuximide, lamotrigine, warfarin, oral contraceptives, chloramphenicol, griseofulvin, doxycycline, beta-blockers

Increased effect/toxicity of phenobarbital with propoxyphene, benzodiazepines, CNS depressants, valproic acid, methylphenidate, chloramphenicol

Stability Protect elixir from light; not stable in aqueous solutions; use only clear solutions; do not add to acidic solutions, precipitation may occur

Mechanism of Action Interferes with transmission of impulses from the thalamus to the cortex of the brain resulting in an imbalance in central inhibitory and facilitatory mechanisms

Pharmacodynamics

Hypnosis after oral dose:

Onset of action: Within 20-60 minutes

Duration: 6-10 hours

I.V.:

Onset: Within 5 minutes with peak effect within 30 minutes

Duration: 4-10 hours; the elderly may be more sensitive to the sedative effects of phenobarbital

Pharmacokinetics

Absorption: Oral: 70% to 90%

Protein binding: 20% to 45%

Metabolism: In liver via hydroxylation and glucuronide conjugation; inducer CYP1A2, 2B6, 2C8, 3A4

Half-life: 53-140 hours; half-life may be increased in elderly; clearance can be increased with alkalinization of urine or with oral multiple dose activated charcoal

Time to peak serum concentration: Oral: Within 1-6 hours

Elimination: 20% to 50% excreted unchanged in urine

Usual Dosage Geriatric patients should be started at the lowest recommended dose

Geriatrics and Adults:

Anticonvulsant: 2-4 mg/kg/day at bedtime or in divided doses; adjust dose until serum concentration is therapeutic; in status epilepticus, load with 15 mg/kg I.V. given over 10-15 minutes

Status epilepticus: I.V.: 15-20 mg/kg; may possibly be increased to up to 25 mg/kg at a rate not to exceed 100 mg/minute

Geriatrics and Adults:

Sedation: Oral, I.M.: 30-120 mg/day in 2-3 divided doses

Hypnotic: Oral, I.M., I.V., S.C.: 100-320 mg at bedtime

Hyperbilirubinemia: Oral: 90-180 mg/day in 2-3 divided doses

Preoperative sedation: I.M.: 100-200 mg 1-1.5 hours before procedure

Moderately dialyzable (20% to 50%)

Monitoring Parameters Phenobarbital serum concentrations, mental status, CBC, LFTs, seizure activity

Reference Range Adults: Therapeutic: 15-40 µg/mL (SI: 65-172 µmol/L); Toxic: >40 µg/mL (SI: >172 µmol/L)

Test Interactions Increased alkaline phosphatase (S), increased ammonia (B); decreased bilirubin (S), decreased calcium (S)

Patient Information May cause drowsiness, avoid alcohol and other CNS depressants

Nursing Implications Observe patient for excessive sedation, respiratory depression

Additional Information Sodium content of injection (65 mg, 1 mL): 6 mg (0.3 mEq)

Phenobarbital: Barbita®, Solfoton®

Phenobarbital sodium: Luminal®

Special Geriatric Considerations Using barbiturates in the elderly may induce paradoxical stimulation, cause or aggravate depression and confusion. Due to its long half-life and risk of dependence, phenobarbital is not recommended as a sedative or hypnotic in the elderly; interpretive guidelines from the Health Care Financing Administration discourage the use of this agent as a sedative/hypnotic in long-term care residents

Dosage Forms
Capsule: 16 mg
Elixir: 15 mg/5 mL (5 mL, 10 mL, 20 mL); 20 mg/5 mL (3.75 mL, 5 mL, 7.5 mL, 120 mL, 473 mL, 946 mL, 4000 mL)
Injection, as sodium: 30 mg/mL (1 mL); 60 mg/mL (1 mL); 65 mg/mL (1 mL); 130 mg/mL (1 mL)
Powder for injection: 120 mg
Tablet: 8 mg, 15 mg, 16 mg, 30 mg, 32 mg, 60 mg, 65 mg, 100 mg

Phenobarbitone *see* Phenobarbital *on page 737*

Phenoxybenzamine (fen oks ee BEN za meen)
Brand Names Dibenzyline®
Generic Available No
Therapeutic Category Alpha-Adrenergic Blocking Agent, Oral; Vasodilator, Coronary
Use Symptomatic management of pheochromocytoma; treatment of hypertensive crisis caused by sympathomimetic amines
  Unlabeled use: Micturition problems associated with neurogenic bladder, functional outlet obstruction, and partial prostatic obstruction
Contraindications Shock and other conditions where a fall in blood pressure would be undesirable
Warnings Do not administer with drugs that stimulate beta-adrenergic receptors as this may cause hypotension and tachycardia
Precautions Use with caution in patients with renal damage, congestive heart failure, or cerebral or coronary arteriosclerosis; can exacerbate symptoms of respiratory tract infections
Adverse Reactions
Cardiovascular: Postural hypotension, tachycardia, syncope, shock
Central nervous system: Lethargy, headache
Gastrointestinal: Vomiting, nausea, diarrhea, xerostomia
Genitourinary: Inhibition of ejaculation
Neuromuscular & skeletal: Weakness
Respiratory: Nasal congestion
Overdosage Symptoms of overdose include hypotension, tachycardia, lethargy, dizziness, shock
Toxicology Place patient in Trendelenburg's position; norepinephrine may be used in severe hypotension; do not use epinephrine; keep patient flat for 24 hours or more as phenoxybenzamine's effect is prolonged
Drug Interactions
Decreased effect with alpha agonists
Increased toxicity with beta-blockers, epinephrine (hypotension, tachycardia)
Mechanism of Action Irreversible noncompetitive alpha-adrenergic blockade of postganglionic synapses in exocrine glands and smooth muscle; relaxes the urethra and increases the opening of the bladder
Pharmacodynamics
Onset of action: Oral: Within 2 hours
Peak effects: Within 4-6 hours
Duration: 4 or more days
Pharmacokinetics
Half-life: 24 hours
Elimination: Primarily in urine and feces
Usual Dosage Geriatrics and Adults: Oral:
Initial: 10 mg twice daily, increase by 10 mg every other day until optimum dose is achieved. Usual range: 20-40 mg 2-3 times/day
Urinary incontinence: 10 mg 1-3 times/day
Monitoring Parameters Blood pressure, pulse, urine output
Patient Information Avoid alcoholic beverages; if dizziness occurs, avoid sudden changes in posture; may cause nasal congestion and constricted pupils; may inhibit ejaculation; avoid cough, cold or allergy medications containing sympathomimetics
Nursing Implications Monitor vital signs
Special Geriatric Considerations Because of the risk of adverse effects, avoid the use of this medication in the elderly if possible
Dosage Forms Capsule, as hydrochloride: 10 mg

Phenoxymethyl Penicillin *see* Penicillin V Potassium *on page 725*
Phenylalanine Mustard *see* Melphalan *on page 582*
Phenylazo Diamino Pyridine Hydrochloride *see* Phenazopyridine *on page 734*

Phenylephrine (fen il EF rin)

Brand Names AK-Dilate® Ophthalmic Solution; AK-Nefrin® Ophthalmic Solution; Alconefrin® Nasal Solution [OTC]; Doktors® Nasal Solution [OTC]; I-Phrine® Ophthalmic Solution; Isopto® Frin Ophthalmic Solution; Mydfrin® Ophthalmic Solution; Neo-Synephrine® Nasal Solution [OTC]; Neo-Synephrine® Ophthalmic Solution; Nostril® Nasal Solution [OTC]; Prefrin™ Ophthalmic Solution; Relief® Ophthalmic Solution; Rhinall® Nasal Solution [OTC]; Sinarest® Nasal Solution [OTC]; St. Joseph® Measured Dose Nasal Solution [OTC]; Vicks Sinex® Nasal Solution [OTC]

Generic Available Yes

Therapeutic Category Adrenergic Agonist Agent; Adrenergic Agonist Agent, Ophthalmic; Alpha-Adrenergic Blocking Agent, Ophthalmic; Decongestant, Nasal; Nasal Agent, Vasoconstrictor; Ophthalmic Agent, Mydriatic

Use Treatment of hypotension, vascular failure in shock; as a vasoconstrictor in regional analgesia; symptomatic relief of nasal and nasopharyngeal mucosal congestion; as a mydriatic in ophthalmic procedures and treatment of wide-angle glaucoma

Contraindications Pheochromocytoma, severe hypertension, tachyarrhythmias; hypersensitivity to phenylephrine or any component

Warnings Injection may contain sulfites which may cause allergic reactions in some patients; do not use if solution turns brown or contains a precipitate. Administer all dosage forms with caution to patients with hypertension, hyperthyroidism, diabetes mellitus, cardiovascular disease, ischemic heart disease, increased intraocular pressure, or prostatic hypertrophy. Elderly patients are more likely to experience adverse reactions to sympathomimetics. Overdosage may cause hallucinations, seizures, CNS depression, and death.

Precautions Topical phenylephrine should only be used for 3-5 days. Rebound congestion may occur after the effects of the topical application subside.

Adverse Reactions

Cardiovascular: Hypertension, angina, reflex bradycardia, arrhythmias, palpitations

Central nervous system: Headache, restlessness, anxiety, excitability

Genitourinary: Dysuria

Neuromuscular & skeletal: Tremors (with systemic use)

Respiratory: Rebound nasal congestion

Overdosage Symptoms of overdose include vomiting, hypertension, palpitations, paresthesia, ventricular extrasystoles

Toxicology Treatment is supportive; in extreme cases, I.V. phentolamine may be used

Drug Interactions

Decreased effect with alpha-blockers, beta-blockers

Increased effect/toxicity with oxytocic drugs, sympathomimetics (tachycardia, arrhythmias), MAO inhibitors

Stability Stable for 48 hours in 5% dextrose in water at pH 3.5-7.5; do not use brown colored solutions

Mechanism of Action Potent, direct-acting, alpha-adrenergic stimulator with weak beta-adrenergic activity; causes vasoconstriction of the arterioles of the nasal mucosa and conjunctiva; activates the dilator muscle of the pupil to cause contraction; produces vasoconstriction of arterioles in the body

Pharmacodynamics

Onset of action: Parenteral injection: Effects occur immediately

Duration:

I.M., S.C.: 45-60 minutes

I.V.: 20-30 minutes

Pharmacokinetics

Half-life: 2.5 hours

Metabolism: To phenolic conjugates

Elimination: Urine (90%)

Usual Dosage

Ophthalmic preparations for pupil dilation:

Geriatrics: Instill 1 drop of 2.5% solution, may repeat in 1 hour if necessary

Adults: Instill 1 drop of 2.5% or 10% solution, may repeat in 10-60 minutes as needed

Nasal decongestant:

Geriatrics: Administer 2-3 drops or 1-2 sprays every 4 hours of 0.125% to 0.25% solution as needed; do not use more than 3 days

Adults: Administer 2-3 drops or 1-2 sprays every 4 hours of 0.25% solution as needed; the 0.5% or 1% solution may be used in cases of extreme nasal congestion; do not use nasal solutions more than 3 days

Ophthalmic decongestant: Instill 1-2 drops of 0.12% solution 2-4 times/day

Hypotension/shock: Geriatrics and Adults:

I.M., S.C.: 2-5 mg/dose every 1-2 hours as needed (initial dose should not exceed 5 mg)

I.V. bolus: 0.1-0.5 mg/dose every 10-15 minutes as needed (initial dose should not exceed 0.5 mg)

I.V. infusion: 10 mg in 250 mL D_5W or NS (1:25,000 dilution) (40 mcg/mL); start at 100-180 mcg/minute (2-5 mL/minute; 50-90 drops/minute) initially. When blood pressure is stabilized, maintenance rate: 40-60 mcg/minute (20-30 drops/minute).

Paroxysmal supraventricular tachycardia: Geriatrics and Adults: I.V.: 0.25-0.5 mg/dose over 20-30 seconds

Monitoring Parameters Blood pressure, pulse, EKG (systemic), relief of symptoms (topical)

Patient Information Nasal decongestant should not be used for >3 days in a row, hereby reducing problems of rebound congestion. Consult physician or pharmacist before using. Notify physician of insomnia, weakness, dizziness, tremor, or irregular heartbeat.

Nursing Implications May cause necrosis or sloughing tissue if extravasation occurs during I.V. administration or S.C. administration; monitor elderly patients closely while on phenylephrine

Special Geriatric Considerations Phenylephrine I.V. should be used with extreme caution in the elderly. The 10% ophthalmic solution has caused increased blood pressure in elderly patients and its use should, therefore, be avoided. Since topical decongestants can be obtained over-the-counter, elderly patients should be counseled about their proper use and in what disease states they should be avoided (see Warnings).

Dosage Forms

Phenylephrine hydrochloride:

Injection (Neo-Synephrine®): 1% [10 mg/mL] (1 mL)

Nasal solution:

Drops:

Neo-Synephrine®: 0.125% (15 mL)

Alconefrin® 12: 0.16% (30 mL)

Alconefrin® 25, Neo-Synephrine®, Children's Nostril®, Rhinall®: 0.25% (15 mL, 30 mL, 40 mL)

Alconefrin®, Neo-Synephrine®: 0.5% (15 mL, 30 mL)

Spray:

Alconefrin® 25, Neo-Synephrine®, Rhinall®: 0.25% (15 mL, 30 mL, 40 mL)

Neo-Synephrine®, Nostril®, Sinex®: 0.5% (15 mL, 30 mL)

Neo-Synephrine®: 1% (15 mL)

Ophthalmic solution:

AK-Nefrin®, Isopto® Frin, Prefrin™ Liquifilm®, Relief®: 0.12% (0.3 mL, 15 mL, 20 mL)

AK-Dilate®, Mydfrin®, Neo-Synephrine®, Phenoptic®: 2.5% (2 mL, 3 mL, 5 mL, 15 mL)

AK-Dilate®, Neo-Synephrine®, Neo-Synephrine® Viscous: 10% (1 mL, 2 mL, 5 mL, 15 mL)

Phenylethylmalonylurea see Phenobarbital *on page 737*

Phenylpropanolamine (fen il proe pa NOLE a meen)

Brand Names Acutrim® Precision Release® [OTC]; Control® [OTC]; Dex-A-Diet® [OTC]; Dexatrim® [OTC]; Maigret-50; Prolamine® [OTC]; Propadrine; Propagest® [OTC]; Stay Trim® Diet Gum [OTC]; Westrim® LA [OTC]

Synonyms *dl*-Norephedrine Hydrochloride; PPA

Generic Available Yes

Therapeutic Category Adrenergic Agonist Agent; Anorexiant; Decongestant; Nasal Agent, Vasoconstrictor

Use Anorexiant and nasal decongestant

Unlabeled use: Urinary incontinence, stress type

Contraindications Known hypersensitivity to phenylpropanolamine

Warnings Elderly patients are more likely to experience adverse reactions to sympathomimetics; overdosage may cause hallucinations, seizures, CNS depression, and death

(Continued)

Phenylpropanolamine *(Continued)*

Precautions Administer with caution to patients with hypertension, hyperthyroidism, diabetes mellitus, cardiovascular disease, ischemic heart disease, increased intraocular pressure, or prostatic hypertrophy

Adverse Reactions

Cardiovascular: Palpitations, reflex bradycardia, arrhythmias, hypertension, angina, stimulating sympathomimetic agents

Central nervous system: Anxiety, nervousness, restlessness, headache

Gastrointestinal: Xerostomia, nausea

Genitourinary: Dysuria

Overdosage Symptoms of overdose include vomiting, hypertension, palpitations, paresthesias, excitation, seizures

Toxicology Treatment is supportive; in extreme cases, I.V. phentolamine may be used

Drug Interactions

Decreased effect of antihypertensives

Increased effect/toxicity with tricyclic antidepressants, MAO inhibitors, increased effect of caffeine

Mechanism of Action Releases tissue stores of epinephrine and thereby produces an alpha- and beta-adrenergic stimulation; this causes vasoconstriction and nasal mucosa blanching; also appears to depress central appetite centers; increases urethral resistance to prevent urine leakage during times of increased intra-abdominal pressure

Pharmacokinetics

Absorption: Oral: Well absorbed

Bioavailability: Close to 100%

Metabolism: In the liver to norephedrine

Half-life: 4.6-6.6 hours

Elimination: In urine primarily as unchanged drug (80% to 90%)

Usual Dosage Oral:

Geriatrics:

Decongestant: 25 mg every 4-6 hours as needed

Urinary incontinence: 75 mg twice daily (use sustained release capsules)

Adults: Decongestant: 25 mg every 4 hours or 50 mg every 8 hours as needed, not to exceed 150 mg/day; sustained release: 75 mg every 12 hours

Monitoring Parameters Blood pressure, pulse, relief of symptoms, episodes of urinary incontinence

Patient Information Do not exceed recommended doses; consult physician or pharmacist before using; notify physician of insomnia, weakness, dizziness, tremor, or irregular heartbeat

Additional Information Phenylpropanolamine is found in many combination cough and cold products

Special Geriatric Considerations Not recommended for use an as anorexiant in the elderly. Phenylpropanolamine is ~75% effective in controlling mild to moderate stress incontinence. Elderly patients should be counseled about the proper use of over-the-counter cough and cold preparations (see Warnings).

Dosage Forms

Phenylpropanolamine hydrochloride:

Capsule: 37.5 mg

Capsule: timed release: 25 mg, 75 mg

Tablet: 25 mg

Tablet:

Precision release: 75 mg

Timed release: 75 mg

References

Romanowski GL, Shimp LA, Balson AB, et al, "Urinary Incontinence in the Elderly: Etiology and Treatment," *Drug Intell Clin Pharm*, 1988, 22(7-8):525-33.

Phenylpropanolamine and Brompheniramine *see* Brompheniramine and Phenylpropanolamine *on page 130*

Phenytoin *(FEN i toyn)*

Related Information

Antacid Drug Interactions *on page 1096*

Antiepileptic Drug Interactions Comparison *on page 1022*

Serum Drug Concentrations Commonly Monitored: Guidelines *on page 1114*

Brand Names Dilantin®; Diphenylan Sodium®

Synonyms Diphenylhydantoin; DPH

Generic Available Yes

Therapeutic Category Antiarrhythmic Agent, Class I-B; Anticonvulsant, Hydantoin

Use Management of generalized tonic-clonic (grand mal), simple partial and complex partial seizures; prevention of seizures following head trauma/neurosurgery; ventricular arrhythmias, including those associated with digitalis intoxication, also used for epidermolysis bullosa; trigeminal neuralgia

Contraindications Hypersensitivity to phenytoin or any component; heart block, sinus bradycardia

Warnings Do not withdraw abruptly in seizure patients; elderly and patients with hepatic disease may accumulate and cause toxicity; discontinue in hepatic failure; patients with a low serum albumin or Cl_{cr} <10 mL/minute, may have an increase unbound (free) concentration; use with caution in patients with hypotension and myocardial insufficiency; do not use phenytoin in sinus bradycardia, second or third degree A-V block, sinoatrial block, or in patients with Adams-Stokes syndrome

Precautions May increase frequency of petit mal seizures; I.V. form may cause hypotension, skin necrosis at I.V. site; avoid I.V. administration in small veins; use with caution in patients with porphyria; discontinue if rash or lymphadenopathy occurs

Adverse Reactions

Dose-related:

Central nervous system: Ataxia, slurred speech, dizziness, drowsiness, lethargy, confusion, fever, mood changes, coma

Dermatologic: Rash, hirsutism, coarsening of facial features

Endocrine & metabolic: Folic acid depletion, hyperglycemia

Gastrointestinal: Nausea, vomiting, gingival hyperplasia

Neuromuscular & skeletal: Peripheral neuropathy, tenderness, osteomalacia

Ocular: Nystagmus, blurred vision, diplopia, amblyopia

I.V.:

Cardiovascular: Hypotension, bradycardia, and other cardiac arrhythmias

Local: Venous irritation and pain, thrombophlebitis

Rarely:

Dermatologic: Stevens-Johnson syndrome

Endocrine & metabolic: Gynecomastia

Gastrointestinal: Loss of taste

Genitourinary: Urinary retention, urinary incontinence, polyuria, oliguria, vaginitis, vaginal candidiasis, dysuria, Peyronies disease, urethral pain

Hematologic: Blood dyscrasias, pseudolymphoma, lymphoma, leukopenia, agranulocytosis, pancytopenia, folic acid, induced macrocytic anemia, thrombocytopenia

Hepatic: Hepatitis

Neuromuscular & skeletal: Dyskinesias

Ocular: Photophobia, eye pain

Otic: Tinnitus

Miscellaneous: SLE-like syndrome, lymphadenopathy

Overdosage Symptoms of overdose include unsteady gait, slurred speech, confusion, nausea, hypothermia, fever, hypotension, respiratory depression, coma

Drug Interactions

Phenytoin may decrease the serum concentration or effectiveness of lamotrigine, valproic acid, ethosuximide, primidone, warfarin, corticosteroids, cyclosporin, theophylline, chloramphenicol, rifampin, doxycycline, quinidine, mexiletine, disopyramide, dopamine, or nondepolarizing skeletal muscle relaxants

Protein binding of phenytoin can be affected by valproic acid or salicylates

Serum phenytoin concentrations may be increased by cimetidine, chloramphenicol, INH, trimethoprim, or sulfonamides and decreased by rifampin, cisplatin, vinblastine, bleomycin, folic acid, or continuous NG feeds; do not use extended release capsules for enteral feeding (NG)

Stability Parenteral solution may be used as long as there is no precipitate and it is not hazy; slightly yellowed solution may be used; refrigeration may cause precipitate, sometimes the precipitate is resolved by allowing the solution to reach room temperature again; drug may precipitate with pH ≤11.5; do not mix with other medications; may dilute with normal saline for I.V. infusion, but must be diluted to concentration <6 mg/mL

Mechanism of Action Stabilizes neuronal membranes and decreases seizure activity by increasing efflux or decreasing influx of sodium ions across (Continued)

Phenytoin *(Continued)*

cell membranes in the motor cortex during generation of nerve impulses; prolongs effective refractory period and suppresses ventricular pacemaker automaticity, shortens action potential in the heart

Pharmacokinetics

Absorption: Oral: Slow

Distribution: V_d: 0.6-0.7 L/kg

Protein binding: 90% to 95%

Metabolism: Inducer CYP2B6, 3A4; substrate CYP2C9

Bioavailability and peak serum concentrations are dependent upon formulation administered

Time to peak: Oral:

Extended release capsule: Within 4-12 hours

Immediate release preparation: Within 2-3 hours

Elimination: <5% excreted unchanged in urine

Highly variable clearance, dependent upon intrinsic hepatic function and dose administered; major metabolite (via oxidation) HPPA undergoes enterohepatic recycling and elimination in urine as glucuronides

Increased clearance and decreased serum concentrations with febrile illness

Usual Dosage Geriatrics and Adults:

Status epilepticus: I.V.:

Loading dose: 15-18 mg/kg in a single or divided dose at a rate of 25 mg/minute; maintenance, anticonvulsant: usual: 300 mg/day or 5-6 mg/kg/day in 3 divided doses or 1-2 divided doses using extended release; do not exceed 25-50 mg/minute infusion rate with I.V. use; recommended to initiate status epilepticus loading with 25 mg/minute, especially if elderly have any cardiovascular disease, to avoid adverse effects

Anticonvulsant: Oral:

Loading dose: 15-20 mg/kg; based on phenytoin serum concentrations and recent dosing history; administer oral loading dose in 3 divided doses given every 2-4 hours to decrease GI adverse effects and to ensure complete oral absorption; maintenance dose: same as I.V.; doses >400 mg should be divided to avoid possible gastric irritation and reduced absorption

Arrhythmias:

Loading dose: I.V.: 1.25 mg/kg IVP every 5 minutes may repeat up to total loading dose: 15 mg/kg; do not exceed 25-50 mg/minute infusion rate with I.V. use

Maintenance dose: Oral: 250 mg 4 times/day for 1 day, 250 mg twice daily for 2 days, then maintenance at 300-400 mg/day in divided doses 1-4 times/day

See tables.

Adjustment of Serum Concentration in Patients With Low Serum Albumin

Measured Total Phenytoin Concentration (mcg/mL)	Patient's Serum Albumin (g/dL)			
	3.5	3	2.5	2
	Adjusted Total Phenytoin Concentration (mcg/mL)*			
5	6	7	8	10
10	13	14	17	20
15	19	21	25	30

*Adjusted concentration = measured total concentration / [(0.2 x albumin) + 0.1].

Adjustment of Serum Concentration in Patients With Renal Failure (Cl$_{cr}$ ≤10 mL/min) (Product Information From Parke-Davis)

Measured Total Phenytoin Concentration (mcg/mL)	Patient's Serum Albumin (g/dL)				
	4	3.5	3	2.5	2
	Adjusted Total Phenytoin Concentration (mcg/mL)*				
5	10	11	13	14	17
10	20	22	25	29	33
15	30	33	38	43	50

*Adjusted concentration = measured total concentration / [(0.1 x albumin) + 0.1].

Monitoring Parameters Monitor serum concentration (see Reference Range) and note time for serum assays; gait, CNS effects, speech; free concentrations for patients with low serum albumin

Reference Range

Therapeutic: 10-20 µg/mL (SI: 40-79 µmol/L); for status epilepticus, initial serum concentrations should be between 20-25 µg/mL with later serum concentrations (24 hours) in the 10-20 µg/mL range; some recommend the therapeutic range be extended to 5-20 µg/mL; free serum concentration: 0.5-2 µg/mL

Toxicity is measured clinically, and some patients require levels outside the suggested therapeutic range; Toxic: 30-50 µg/mL (SI: 120-200 µmol/L)

Lethal: >100 µg/mL (SI: >400 µmol/L)

Do not obtain serum for analysis 8-12 hours after administration; spurious elevations will be seen due to slow distribution of phenytoin

Test Interactions Increased glucose, alkaline phosphatase (S); decreased thyroxine (S), calcium (S)

Patient Information Shake oral suspension well prior to each dose; do not change brand or dosage form without consulting physician; may cause drowsiness; report any incoordination, blurred vision; good oral hygiene may help prevent gingival tissue hyperplasia

Nursing Implications I.V. injections should be followed by normal saline flushes through the same needle or I.V. catheter to avoid local irritation of the vein; must be diluted to concentrations <6 mg/mL, in normal saline, for I.V. infusion; patients with enteral feeding tubes should have feeding stopped 2 hours before and after dosing with suspension

Additional Information Not recommended to be given I.M. unless no other route exists due to erratic absorption; best to not switch brands once stabilized

Special Geriatric Considerations Elderly may have reduced hepatic clearance due to age decline in phase I metabolism; elderly may have low albumin which will increase free fraction and, therefore, pharmacologic response; monitor closely in those who are hypoalbuminemic; free fraction measurements advised, also elderly may display a higher incidence of adverse effects (cardiovascular) when using the I.V. loading regimen; therefore, recommended to decrease loading I.V. dose to 25 mg/minute (see Warnings)

Dosage Forms

Phenytoin sodium:

Capsule, extended: 30 mg, 100 mg

Capsule, prompt: 30 mg, 100 mg

Injection: 50 mg/mL (2 mL, 5 mL)

Suspension, oral: 30 mg/5 mL (5 mL, 240 mL); 125 mg/5 mL (5 mL, 240 mL)

Tablet, chewable: 50 mg

Phillips® Milk of Magnesia [OTC] *see* Magnesium Hydroxide *on page 564*

Phos-Ex® *see* Calcium Acetate *on page 145*

Phos-Flur® *see* Fluoride *on page 392*

PhosLo® *see* Calcium Acetate *on page 145*

Phosphate, Potassium *see* Potassium Phosphate *on page 766*

Phospholine Iodide® Ophthalmic *see* Echothiophate Iodide *on page 327*

Phosphonoformate *see* Foscarnet *on page 409*

Phosphonoformic Acid *see* Foscarnet *on page 409*

3-Phosphoryloxymethyl Phenytoin Disodium *see* Fosphenytoin *on page 412*

p-Hydroxyampicillin *see* Amoxicillin *on page 67*

Phyllocontin® *see* Aminophylline *on page 55*

Phylloquinone *see* Phytonadione *on page 747*

Physostigmine (fye zoe STIG meen)

Related Information

Antidotes *on page 1097*

Glaucoma Drug Therapy Comparison *on page 1032*

Brand Names Antilirium®

Synonyms Eserine Salicylate

Generic Available No

Therapeutic Category Antidote, Anticholinergic Agent; Cholinergic Agent; Cholinergic Agent, Ophthalmic

Use Reverse toxic CNS effects caused by anticholinergic drugs; used as miotic in treatment of glaucoma

(Continued)

Physostigmine *(Continued)*

Unlabeled use: Alzheimer's disease

Contraindications Hypersensitivity to physostigmine or any component; GI or GU obstruction, asthma, diabetes, gangrene, cardiovascular disease

Precautions Use with caution in patients with epilepsy, bradycardia. Discontinue if excessive salivation or emesis, frequent urination or diarrhea occur. Reduce dosage if excessive sweating or nausea occur. Administer I.V. slowly or at a controlled rate not faster than 1 mg/minute. Due to the possibility of hypersensitivity or overdose/cholinergic crisis, atropine should be readily available.

Adverse Reactions

Cardiovascular: Palpitations, bradycardia

Central nervous system: Restlessness, hallucinations, seizures

Gastrointestinal: Nausea, vomiting, salivation

Genitourinary: Frequent urge to urinate

Local: Topical stinging, burning, lacrimation

Neuromuscular & skeletal: Muscle twitching, weakness

Ocular: Miosis, blurred vision, eye pain

Respiratory: Dyspnea, bronchospasm, respiratory paralysis, pulmonary edema

Miscellaneous: Diaphoresis

Overdosage Symptoms of overdose include muscle weakness, blurred vision, excessive sweating, tearing and salivation, nausea, vomiting, bronchospasm, seizures

Toxicology Physostigmine has proven useful in the treatment of central nervous system effects caused by anticholinergic agents. However, physostigmine has been associated with intoxications as well. If physostigmine is used in excess or in the absence of an anticholinergic overdose, patients may manifest signs of cholinergic toxicity. At this point an anticholinergic agent (eg, atropine 0.015-0.05 mg/kg) may be necessary.

Drug Interactions Increased toxicity with bethanechol, methacholine, succinylcholine

Mechanism of Action Inhibits destruction of acetylcholine by acetylcholinesterase which facilitates transmission of impulses across myoneural junction

Pharmacodynamics

Onset of action:

Ophthalmic: Within 2 minutes

Parenteral: Within 5 minutes

Pharmacokinetics

Absorption: I.M., S.C., ophthalmic: Readily absorbed

Distribution: Crosses the blood-brain barrier readily and reverses both central and peripheral anticholinergic effects

Metabolism: In the liver

Half-life: 1-2 hours

Usual Dosage Geriatrics and Adults:

I.M., I.V., S.C.: 0.5-2 mg to start, repeat every 20 minutes until response occurs or adverse effect occurs; maximum I.V. rate: 1 mg/minute

I.M., I.V. to reverse the anticholinergic effects of atropine or scopolamine given as preanesthetic medications: Administer twice the dose, on a weight basis of the anticholinergic drug

Ointment, ophthalmic: Administer 1/4" up to 3 times/day

Solution, ophthalmic: Instill 1-2 drops up to 4 times/day

Monitoring Parameters Blood pressure, pulse, intraocular pressure

Test Interactions Increased aminotransferase [ALT (SGPT)/AST (SGOT)] (S), increased amylase (S)

Nursing Implications Too rapid administration (I.V. rate not to exceed 1 mg/minute) can cause bradycardia, hypersalivation leading to respiratory difficulties and seizures

Special Geriatric Considerations Studies on the use of physostigmine in Alzheimer's disease have reported variable results. Doses generally were in the range of 2-4 mg 4 times/day. Limitations to the use of physostigmine include a short half-life requiring frequent dosing, variable absorption from the GI tract, and no commercially available oral product; therefore, not recommended for treatment of Alzheimer's disease.

Dosage Forms

Injection, as salicylate: 1 mg/mL (2 mL)

Ointment, ophthalmic, as sulfate: 0.25% (3.5 g, 3.7 g)

References

Jenike MA, Albert MS, Heller H, et al, "Oral Physostigmine Treatment for Patients With Presenile and Senile Dementia of the Alzheimer's Type: A Double-Blind Placebo-Controlled Trial," *J Clin Psychiatry*, 1990, 51(1):3-7.

Theesen KA, Boyd JA, "Dementia of the Alzheimer's Type: An Update," *Consult Pharm*, 1990, 5:535-40.

Phytomenadione *see* Phytonadione *on this page*

Phytonadione (fye toe na DYE one)

Related Information

Anticoagulant Therapy Guidelines *on page 1069*

Brand Names AquaMEPHYTON®; Konakion®; Mephyton®

Synonyms Methylphytyl Napthoquinone; Phylloquinone; Phytomenadione; Vitamin K_1

Generic Available No

Therapeutic Category Vitamin, Fat Soluble

Use Prevention and treatment of hypoprothrombinemia caused by drug-induced or anticoagulant-induced vitamin K deficiency; phytonadione is more effective and is preferred to other vitamin K preparations in the presence of impending hemorrhage; oral absorption depends on the presence of bile salts

Contraindications Hypersensitivity to phytonadione or any component

Warnings Severe reactions resembling anaphylaxis or hypersensitivity have occurred rarely during or immediately after I.V. administration (even with proper dilution and rate of administration); restrict I.V. administration for emergency use only; ineffective in hereditary hypoprothrombinemia and hypoprothrombinemia caused by severe liver disease

Adverse Reactions

Cardiovascular: Transient flushing reaction, rarely hypotension, cyanosis

Central nervous system: Dizziness (rarely), pain

Gastrointestinal: Abnormal taste, GI upset (oral)

Hematologic: Hemolysis in patients with G-6-PD deficiency

Local: Tenderness at injection site

Respiratory: Dyspnea

Miscellaneous: Diaphoresis, anaphylaxis, hypersensitivity reactions

Drug Interactions Decreased effect: Warfarin sodium, dicumarol, anisindione effects antagonized by phytonadione; mineral oil decreases the absorption of oral vitamin K

Stability Protect injection from light at all times; may be autoclaved

Mechanism of Action Promotes liver synthesis of clotting factors (II, VII, IX, X); however, the exact mechanism as to this stimulation is unknown. Phytonadione (vitamin K_1) is a lipid soluble synthetic analog of vitamin K. it possesses the same type and degree of activity as the naturally occurring vitamin K.

Pharmacodynamics

Onset of increased coagulation factors:

Oral: Within 6-12 hours

Parenteral: Within 1-2 hours; patient may become normal after 12-14 hours

Pharmacokinetics

Absorption: Oral: Absorbed from the intestines in the presence of bile

Metabolism: In the liver rapidly

Elimination: In bile and urine

Usual Dosage Geriatrics and Adults: I.V. route should be restricted for emergency use only

Minimum daily requirement (not well established): 0.03 mcg/kg/day

Oral anticoagulant overdose: Oral, I.M., I.V., S.C.: 0.5-10 mg/dose; rarely up to 25-50 mg has been used; may repeat in 6-8 hours if given by I.M., I.V., S.C. route; may repeat 12-48 hours after oral route

Vitamin K deficiency (due to drugs, malabsorption or decreased synthesis of vitamin K):

Oral: 5-25 mg/24 hours

I.M., I.V.: 10 mg

Administration I.V. administration: Dilute in normal saline, D_5W or D_5NS and infuse slowly; rate of infusion should not exceed 1 mg/minute. **This route should be used only if administration by another route is not feasible.** I.V. administration should not exceed 1 mg/minute; for I.V. infusion, dilute in PF (preservative free) D_5W or normal saline.

Monitoring Parameters PT, INR

Nursing Implications See Administration

Additional Information Injection contains benzyl alcohol 0.9% as preservative

(Continued)

747

Phytonadione *(Continued)*

Special Geriatric Considerations See Usual Dosage; see Anticoagulation Guidelines in the Appendix, reversal of oral anticoagulant effect

Dosage Forms
Injection:
Aqueous colloidal: 2 mg/mL (0.5 mL); 10 mg/mL (1 mL, 2.5 mL, 5 mL)
Aqueous (I.M. only): 2 mg/mL (0.5 mL); 10 mg/mL (1 mL)
Tablet: 5 mg

References
Barash P, Kitahata LM, and Mandel S, "Acute Cardiovascular Collapse After Intravenous Phytonadione," *Anesth Analg*, 1976, 55(2):304-6.
Hopkins CS, "Adverse Reaction to a Cremophor-Containing Preparation of Intravenous Vitamin K," *Intensive Therapy Clin Monit*, 1988, 9:254-5.
Martinez-Abad M, Delgado F, Palop V, et al, "Vitamin K₁ and Anaphylactic Shock," *DICP*, 1991, 25(7-8):871-2.

Pilagan® Ophthalmic *see* Pilocarpine *on this page*

Pilocar® Ophthalmic *see* Pilocarpine *on this page*

Pilocarpine *(pye loe KAR peen)*

Related Information
Glaucoma Drug Therapy Comparison *on page 1032*

Brand Names Adsorbocarpine® Ophthalmic; Akarpine® Ophthalmic; Isopto® Carpine Ophthalmic; Ocu-Carpine® Ophthalmic; Ocusert Pilo-20® Ophthalmic; Ocusert Pilo-40® Ophthalmic; Pilagan® Ophthalmic; Pilocar® Ophthalmic; Pilopine HS® Ophthalmic; Piloptic® Ophthalmic; Pilostat® Ophthalmic; Salagen® Oral

Generic Available Yes: Solution

Therapeutic Category Cholinergic Agent, Ophthalmic; Ophthalmic Agent, Miotic

Use Management of chronic simple glaucoma, chronic and acute angle-closure glaucoma; counter effects of cycloplegics; treatment of xerostomia

Contraindications Hypersensitivity to pilocarpine or any component; acute inflammatory disease of anterior chamber

Precautions Use with caution in patients with corneal abrasion; narrow-angle glaucoma (may promote acute-angle closure)

Adverse Reactions
Cardiovascular: Hypertension, tachycardia
Central nervous system: Headache, browache
Gastrointestinal: Salivation, nausea, vomiting, diarrhea
Genitourinary: Urination
Local: Stinging, burning, lacrimation
Ocular: Miosis, ciliary spasm, blurred vision, retinal detachment, photophobia, acute iritis, conjunctival and ciliary congestion early in therapy, decreased night vision
Miscellaneous: Diaphoresis, hypersensitivity reactions

Overdosage Symptoms of overdose include bronchospasm, bradycardia, involuntary urination, vomiting, hypotension, tremors

Toxicology Atropine is the treatment of choice for intoxications manifesting with significant muscarinic symptoms. Atropine I.V. 2-4 mg every 3-60 minutes should be repeated to control symptoms and then continued as needed for 1-2 days following the acute ingestion. Epinephrine 0.1-1 mg S.C. may be useful in reversing severe cardiovascular or pulmonary sequel.

Stability Refrigerate gel

Mechanism of Action Directly stimulates cholinergic receptors in the eye causing miosis (by contraction of the iris sphincter), loss of accommodation (by constriction of ciliary muscle), and lowering of intraocular pressure (with decreased resistance to aqueous humor outflow)

Pharmacodynamics
Ophthalmic:
Onset of action: Miosis occurs within 10-30 minutes
Duration: 4-8 hours
Intraocular pressure reduction requires an hour to begin and persists for 4-12 hours
Ocusert® Pilo application:
Onset of action: 90-120 minutes; miosis occurs within 10-30 minutes
Peak effect: Within 30-40 minutes
Duration: 4-8 hours; reduced intraocular pressure is detectable within 60 minutes and lasts 4-14 hours, depending on concentration

Usual Dosage Geriatrics and Adults: Ophthalmic:
Nitrate solution: Shake well before using; instill 1-2 drops 2-4 times/day

Hydrochloride solution:
    Instill 1-2 drops up to 6 times/day; adjust the concentration and frequency
        as required to control elevated intraocular pressure
    To counteract the mydriatic effects of sympathomimetic agents: Instill 1
        drop of a 1% solution in the affected eye
Gel: Instill ½" ribbon into lower conjunctival sac once daily at bedtime
Ocular systems: Systems are labeled in terms of mean rate of release of
    pilocarpine over 7 days; begin with 20 mcg/hour at night and adjust based
    on response

Monitoring Parameters Intraocular pressure, fundoscopic exam, visual field testing

Patient Information May sting on instillation, do not touch dropper to eye; visual acuity may be decreased after administration; night vision may be decreased; distance vision may be altered. Do not leave damaged Ocusert® system in the eye; read package instructions for insertion; after topical instillation, finger pressure should be applied to lacrimal sac to decrease drainage into the nose and throat and minimize possible systemic absorption.

Nursing Implications Usually causes difficulty in dark adaptation; advise patients to use caution while night driving or performing hazardous tasks in poor illumination; after topical instillation, finger pressure should be applied to lacrimal sac to decrease drainage into the nose and throat and minimize possible systemic absorption

Special Geriatric Considerations Assure the patient or a caregiver can adequately administer ophthalmic medication dosage form

Dosage Forms See table.

Pilocarpine

Dosage Form	Strength %	1 mL	2 mL	15 mL	30 mL	3.5 g
Gel	4					x
Solution as hydrochloride	0.25			x		
	0.5			x	x	
	1	x	x	x	x	
	2	x	x	x	x	
	3			x	x	
	4	x	x	x	x	
	6			x	x	
	8		x			
	10			x		
Solution as nitrate	1			x		
	2			x		
	4			x		
Ocusert® Pilo-20: Releases 20 mcg/hour for 1 week						
Ocusert® Pilo-40: Releases 40 mcg/hour for 1 week						

Pilocarpine and Epinephrine (pye loe KAR peen & ep i NEF rin)

Related Information
    Epinephrine *on page 336*
    Pilocarpine *on previous page*

Brand Names E-Pilo-x® Ophthalmic; P$_x$E$_x$® Ophthalmic

Therapeutic Category Ophthalmic Agent, Miotic

Use Treatment of glaucoma; counter effect of cycloplegics

Contraindications Hypersensitivity to pilocarpine, epinephrine or any component; acute inflammatory disease of anterior chamber

Precautions Use with caution in patients with corneal abrasion and narrow-angle glaucoma

Adverse Reactions
    Cardiovascular: Tachycardia, hypertension
    Central nervous system: Headache, brow ache
    Gastrointestinal: Salivation
    Local: Stinging, itching
    Ocular: Miosis, ciliary spasm, blurred vision, retinal detachment vitreous hemorrhages, photophobia, acute iritis, lacrimation
    Miscellaneous: Hypersensitivity reactions

Pharmacodynamics
    Onset of action: Miosis occurs within 10-30 minutes
    (Continued)

Pilocarpine and Epinephrine *(Continued)*

Peak effect: Within 30-40 minutes

Duration: 4-8 hours; reduced intraocular pressure is detectable within 60 minutes and lasts 4-14 hours, depending on concentration

Usual Dosage Geriatrics and Adults: Instill 1-2 drops up to 6 times/day

Monitoring Parameters Intraocular pressure, funduscopic exam, visual field testing

Patient Information May sting on instillation, do not touch dropper to eye

Nursing Implications Usually causes difficulty in dark adaptation; advise patients to use caution while night driving or performing hazardous tasks in poor illumination

Special Geriatric Considerations Assess patient's ability to self-administer ophthalmic drops; use with caution in patients with cardiovascular disease

Dosage Forms Solution, ophthalmic: Epinephrine bitartrate 1% and pilocarpine hydrochloride 1%, 2%, 4%, 6% (15 mL)

Pilopine HS® Ophthalmic *see* Pilocarpine *on page 748*

Piloptic® Ophthalmic *see* Pilocarpine *on page 748*

Pilostat® Ophthalmic *see* Pilocarpine *on page 748*

Pimaricin *see* Natamycin *on page 658*

Pimozide *(PI moe zide)*

Related Information

Antipsychotic Agents Comparison *on page 1023*

Antipsychotic Medication Guidelines *on page 1076*

Brand Names Orap™

Generic Available No

Therapeutic Category Antipsychotic Agent; Neuroleptic Agent

Use Suppression of severe motor and phonic tics in patients with Tourette's disorder who have failed to respond to other standard treatment

Contraindications Simple tics other than Tourette's, phonic tics and drug-induced motor tics (eg, amphetamines, methylphenidate, pemoline), history of cardiac dysrhythmias, administration with other medications is known to prolong Q-T interval, known hypersensitivity to pimozide, use with caution in patients with hypersensitivity to other neuroleptics; do not use in patients with severe CNS depression or comatose patients; use in patients receiving macrolide antibiotics such as clarithromycin, erythromycin, azithromycin, and dirithromycin

Warnings Tardive dyskinesia may develop, especially in elderly females taking high doses; prolongation of Q-T intervals with sudden death has occurred in patients receiving doses of approximately 1 mg/kg; sudden death and grand mal seizures have occurred at doses >20 mg/kg; prolongation of Q-T interval may be responsible for sudden deaths since this may predispose patient to ventricular arrhythmias; recommend baseline EKG and EKG with dosage increases to observe for serious adverse effects; carcinogenic potential suggested in mice studies, however, no clinical significance known in man; neuroleptic malignant syndrome can occur with the use of neuroleptics

Precautions Hypokalemia is associated with ventricular arrhythmias, therefore correct any existing deficiency before starting pimozide; use with caution in elderly as anticholinergic side effects are caused by pimozide; use with caution in patients with renal/hepatic impairment; may caused decreased alertness

Adverse Reactions

Cardiovascular: Ventricular dysrhythmias, sudden death, Q-T interval increase, hypertension, hypotension, postural hypotension, chest pain, palpitations, tachycardia, syncope

Central nervous system: Extrapyramidal effects (usually in first few days of treatment), tardive dyskinesia, motor restlessness, akathisia, dystonias, opisthotonos, oculogyric crisis, neuroleptic malignant syndrome, seizures, headache, sedation, drowsiness, insomnia, speech difficulties, akinesia, dizziness, nervousness, anxiety, Parkinson's syndrome, depression, hyperpyrexia

Dermatologic: Rash

Gastrointestinal: Diarrhea, constipation, thirst, xerostomia, belching, salivation, anorexia, nausea, vomiting, GI distress, dysgeusia

Genitourinary: Nocturia, polyuria, impotence

Neuromuscular & skeletal: Tremors, hyper-reflexia

Ocular: Visual disturbances, light sensitivity, spots before eyes

Respiratory: Respiratory failure

Miscellaneous: Diaphoresis

Overdosage Symptoms of overdose include hypotension, coma, respiratory depression, EKG abnormalities, extrapyramidal symptoms

Toxicology Following attempts at decontamination, treatment is supportive and symptomatic. Seizures can be treated with diazepam, phenytoin, or phenobarbital; monitor EKG until normal EKG is achieved; use I.V. fluids for hypotension/circulating collapse, plasma, vasopressors (norepinephrine) **do not use epinephrine**; observe patient for 4 days

Drug Interactions Pimozide lowers seizures threshold, therefore may interfere with anticonvulsant therapy; Q-T interval may be increased when pimozide is used with tricyclic antidepressants, phenothiazines, or other antiarrhythmias; pimozide will increase sedation associated with CNS depressant drugs

Mechanism of Action A potent centrally-acting dopamine receptor antagonist resulting in its characteristic neuroleptic effects

Pharmacokinetics
Absorption: Oral: 50%
Protein binding: 99%
Metabolism: In the liver with significant first-pass decay
Half-life: 50 hours
Time to peak serum concentration: Within 6-8 hours
Elimination: Metabolites excreted in urine

Usual Dosage
Geriatrics: Recommend initial dose of 1 mg/day; periodically attempt gradual reduction of dose to determine if tic persists; follow up for 1-2 weeks before concluding the tic is a persistent disease phenomenon and not a manifestation of drug withdrawal; see EKG note under adult dosing
Adults: **Note:** Recommend obtaining a baseline EKG and done periodically, especially with dose increases or addition of drugs which may interact. Oral: Initial: 1-2 mg/day, increase dosage as needed every other day; maximum dose: 10 mg.
Dosing adjustment in hepatic impairment: Reduction of dose is necessary in patients with liver disease

Monitoring Parameters Monitor EKG, blood pressure, and CNS side effects

Test Interactions Increased prolactin (S)

Patient Information May cause drowsiness; use caution when driving or performing tasks which require alertness; do not stop medication without physician advice

Nursing Implications Must obtain baseline EKG and an EKG with dose increases (see Adverse Reactions and Monitoring Parameters)

Additional Information Treatment with pimozide exposes the patient to serious risks; a decision to use pimozide chronically in Tourette's disorder is one that deserves full consideration by the patient (or patient's family) as well as by the treating physician. Because the goal of treatment is symptomatic improvement, the patient's view of the need for treatment and assessment of response are critical in evaluating the impact of therapy and weighing its benefits against the risks.

Special Geriatric Considerations No specific clinical studies in the use of this drug in elderly; use with extreme caution in elderly due to cardiovascular effects; consider cardiovascular effects of drugs the elderly patient may be receiving

In the treatment of agitated, demented, elderly patients, authors of meta-analysis of controlled trials of the response to the traditional antipsychotics (phenothiazines, butyrophenones) in controlling agitation have concluded that the use of neuroleptics results in a response rate of 18%. Clearly neuroleptic therapy for behavior control should be limited with frequent attempts to withdraw the agent given for behavior control.

Dosage Forms Tablet: 2 mg

References
Peabody CA, Warner MD, Whiteford HA, et al, "Neuroleptics and the Elderly," *J Am Geriatr Soc*, 1987, 35(3):233-8.
Risse SC and Barnes R, "Pharmacologic Treatment of Agitation Associated With Dementia," *J Am Geriatr Soc*, 1986, 34(5):368-76.
Saltz BL, Woerner MG, Kane JM, et al, "Prospective Study of Tardive Dyskinesia Incidence in the Elderly," *JAMA*, 1991, 266(17):2402-6.
Seifert RD, "Therapeutic Drug Monitoring: Psychotropic Drugs," *J Pharm Pract*, 1984, 6:403-16.

Pindolol (PIN doe lole)

Related Information
Beta-Blockers Comparison on page 1026

Brand Names Visken®

(Continued)

Pindolol *(Continued)*

Generic Available Yes

Therapeutic Category Beta-Adrenergic Blocker

Use Management of hypertension

Unlabeled use: Ventricular arrhythmias/tachycardia, antipsychotic-induced akathisia, situational anxiety; aggressive behavior associated with dementia

Contraindications Uncompensated congestive heart failure, cardiogenic shock, bradycardia or heart block, asthma, bronchospasm, COPD

Warnings Use with caution in patients with inadequate myocardial function; acute withdrawal may exacerbate symptoms; use with caution in patients undergoing anesthesia, bronchospastic disease, hyperthyroidism, impaired hepatic function, diabetes mellitus, hyperthyroidism. Abrupt withdrawal of the drug should be avoided, drug should be discontinued over 1-2 weeks; may potentiate hypoglycemia in a diabetic patient and mask signs and symptoms; sweating will continue.

Adverse Reactions

Cardiovascular: A-V block, edema, hypotension, impaired myocardial contractility

Central nervous system: Dizziness, fatigue, insomnia, depression

Gastrointestinal: Ischemic colitis, nausea, vomiting, diarrhea, GI distress

Genitourinary: Sexual dysfunction

Neuromuscular & skeletal: Myalgia

Respiratory: Bronchospasm

Miscellaneous: Cold extremities

Overdosage Symptoms of overdose include severe hypotension, bradycardia, heart failure, and bronchospasm

Toxicology Sympathomimetics (eg, epinephrine or dopamine), glucagon or a pacemaker can be used to treat the toxic bradycardia, asystole, and/or hypotension; initially fluids may be the best treatment for toxic hypotension.

Drug Interactions

Decreased effect with NSAIDs, sympathomimetics

Increased effect with diuretics, other antihypertensives

Mechanism of Action Blocks both beta$_1$- and beta$_2$-receptors and has mild intrinsic sympathomimetic activity; pindolol has negative inotropic and chronotropic effects and can significantly slow A-V nodal conduction

Pharmacodynamics One study found that beta blockade lasted longer in elderly patients as compared to younger patients

Pharmacokinetics

Absorption: Oral: Rapid, 50% to 95%

Protein binding: 50%

Metabolism: In the liver (60% to 65%) to conjugates

Half-life: 2.5-4 hours (increased with renal insufficiency, and cirrhosis); half-life is not significantly prolonged in the elderly, though some accumulation of drug may occur (related to renal function)

Time to peak: Within 1-2 hours

Elimination: In urine (35% to 50% unchanged drug)

Usual Dosage

Geriatrics: Initial: 5 mg once daily, increase as necessary by 5 mg/day every 3-4 weeks (see Pharmacokinetics)

Adults: Initial: 5 mg twice daily, increase as necessary by 10 mg/day every 3-4 weeks; maximum daily dose: 60 mg

Monitoring Parameters Blood pressure, standing and sitting/supine, pulse, respiratory function, signs of congestive heart failure

Test Interactions Increased cholesterol (S), decreased glucose; decreased bilirubin (S)

Patient Information Do not discontinue medication abruptly; consult pharmacist or physician before taking over-the-counter cold preparations

Nursing Implications Do not discontinue abruptly (see Monitoring Parameters)

Special Geriatric Considerations Due to alterations in the beta-adrenergic autonomic nervous system, beta-adrenergic blockade may result in less hemodynamic response than seen in younger adults. Studies indicate that despite decreased sensitivity to the chronotropic effects of beta blockade with age, there appears to be an increased myocardial sensitivity to the negative inotropic effect during stress (ie, exercise). Controlled trials have shown the overall response rate for propranolol to be only 20% to 50% in elderly populations. Therefore, all beta-adrenergic blocking drugs may result in a decreased response as compared to younger adults (see Pharmacodynamics and Pharmacokinetics).

Dosage Forms Tablet: 5 mg, 10 mg

References

Gretzer I, Alvan G, Duner H, et al, "Beta-Blocking Effect and Pharmacokinetics of Pindolol in Young and Elderly Hypertensive Patients," *Eur J Clin Pharmacol*, 1986, 31(4):415-8.

Pink Bismuth® [OTC] *see* Bismuth *on page 122*

Piperacillin (pi PER a sil in)

Related Information

I.V. Medication Recommendations *on page 1080*

Penicillins, Penicillin-Related Antibiotics, & Other Antibiotics *on page 1010*

Brand Names Pipracil®

Generic Available No

Therapeutic Category Antibiotic, Penicillin

Use Treatment of *Pseudomonas aeruginosa* infections in combination with an aminoglycoside which are susceptible to piperacillin; also effective against other gram-negative microorganisms and nonpenicillinase-producing anaerobes (including *B. fragilis*) and gram-positive organisms; normally used with other antibiotics (ie, aminoglycosides)

Contraindications Hypersensitivity to piperacillin or any component or penicillins

Precautions Dosage modification required in patients with impaired renal function; use with caution in patients with cephalosporin allergy

Adverse Reactions

Central nervous system: Convulsions, confusion, drowsiness, seizures, fever

Dermatologic: Rash, exfoliative dermatitis

Endocrine & metabolic: Electrolyte imbalance, hypokalemia

Gastrointestinal: Diarrhea

Hematologic: Hemolytic anemia, eosinophilia, neutropenia, prolonged bleeding time

Hepatic: Positive Coombs' reaction, elevated liver enzymes

Local: Thrombophlebitis

Neuromuscular & skeletal: Myoclonus

Renal: Acute interstitial nephritis

Miscellaneous: Hypersensitivity reactions, anaphylaxis, serum sickness-like reaction

Overdosage Symptoms of overdose include neuromuscular hypersensitivity, seizure

Toxicology Many beta-lactam-containing antibiotics have the potential to cause neuromuscular hyperirritability or convulsive seizures. Hemodialysis may be helpful to aid in the removal of the drug from the blood, otherwise most treatment is supportive or symptom directed.

Drug Interactions

Decreased effect if administration is within 1 hour prior to or 4 hours after aminoglycosides in patients with renal impairment

Increased serum concentrations with probenecid

Stability Reconstituted solution is stable (I.V. infusion) in NS or D_5W for 24 hours at room temperature, 7 days when refrigerated or 4 weeks when frozen; after freezing, thawed solution is stable for 24 hours at room temperature or 48 hours when refrigerated; 40 g bulk vial should **not** be frozen after reconstitution; incompatible with aminoglycosides

Mechanism of Action Interferes with bacterial cell wall synthesis during active multiplication causing cell death and resultant bactericidal activity against susceptible bacteria

Pharmacodynamics Bactericidal

Pharmacokinetics

Absorption: I.M.: 70% to 80%

Protein binding: 22%

Half-life: Adults: 36-80 minutes (dose-dependent), prolonged with moderately severe renal or hepatic impairment

Time to peak serum concentration: Within 30-50 minutes

Elimination: Principally in urine and partially in feces (via bile)

Usual Dosage

Geriatrics:

I.M.: 1-2 g every 8-12 hours

I.V.: 2-4 g every 6-8 hours

Adults: I.M., I.V.: 2-4 g/dose every 4-8 hours

Dosing interval in renal impairment:

Cl_{cr} 20-40 mL/minute: Administer every 8 hours

Cl_{cr} <20 mL/minute: Administer every 12 hours

Moderately dialyzable (20% to 50%)

(Continued)

Piperacillin *(Continued)*

Monitoring Parameters Temperature, WBC count, mental status, appetite; bleeding time, especially in patients with renal impairment

Test Interactions False-positive urinary and serum proteins, positive Coombs' test [direct]

Nursing Implications Administer 1 hour apart from aminoglycosides; extended spectrum includes *Pseudomonas aeruginosa*; dosage modification required in patients with impaired renal function

Additional Information Sodium content of 1 g: 1.85 mEq

Special Geriatric Considerations Antipseudomonal penicillins should not be used alone and are often combined with an aminoglycoside as empiric therapy for lower respiratory infections and sepsis in which gram-negative (including *Pseudomonas*) and/or anaerobes are of a high probability; because of piperacillin's lower sodium content, it is preferred over ticarcillin in patients with a history of heart failure and/or renal or hepatic disease; adjust dose for renal function

Dosage Forms Powder for injection, as sodium: 2 g, 3 g, 4 g, 40 g

References

Donowitz GR and Mandell GL, "Beta-Lactam Antibiotics," *N Engl J Med*, 1988, 318(7):419-26 and 318(8):490-500.

Yoshikawa TT, "Antimicrobial Therapy for the Elderly Patient," *J Am Geriatr Soc*, 1990, 38(12):1353-72.

Piperacillin and Tazobactam (pi PER a sil in & ta zoe BAK tam)

Related Information

I.V. Medication Recommendations *on page 1080*

Penicillins, Penicillin-Related Antibiotics, & Other Antibiotics *on page 1010*

Piperacillin *on previous page*

Brand Names Zosyn™

Synonyms Tazobactam and Piperacillin

Therapeutic Category Antibiotic, Penicillin

Use Treatment of infections of lower respiratory tract, urinary tract, skin and skin structures, gynecologic, bone and joint infections, and septicemia caused by susceptible organisms. Tazobactam expands activity of piperacillin to include beta-lactamase producing strains of *S. aureus*, *H. influenzae*, *Enterobacteriaceae*, *Pseudomonas*, *Klebsiella*, *Citrobacter*, *Serratia*, *Bacteroides*, and other gram-negative anaerobes.

Contraindications Hypersensitivity to piperacillin, tazobactam, other penicillins, or any component

Warnings Use with caution in patients with known hypersensitivity to cephalosporins or other beta-lactamase inhibitors; use with caution in patients with a history of seizures and in patients with renal function impairment

Adverse Reactions

Cardiovascular: Hypertension, hypotension, edema

Central nervous system: Insomnia, headache, dizziness, agitation, confusion

Dermatologic: Rash

Gastrointestinal: Diarrhea, constipation, nausea, vomiting, dyspepsia, pseudomembranous colitis

Hematologic: Leukopenia

Respiratory: Bronchospasm

Overdosage Symptoms of overdose include neuromuscular hypersensitivity, seizures

Toxicology Many beta-lactam-containing antibiotics have the potential to cause neuromuscular hyperirritability or convulsive seizures. Hemodialysis may be helpful to aid in the removal of the drug from the blood, otherwise most treatment is supportive or symptom directed.

Drug Interactions

Increased duration of neuromuscular blockers

Increased/prolonged levels with probenecid

Stability Store at controlled room temperature; after reconstitution, stable for 24 hours at room temperature and 1 week when refrigerated; unused portions should be discarded after 24 hours at room temperature and 48 hours when refrigerated; not compatible with lactated Ringer's solution

Mechanism of Action Piperacillin interferes with bacterial cell wall synthesis during active multiplication, causing cell wall death and resultant bactericidal activity against susceptible bacteria; tazobactam prevents degradation of piperacillin by binding to the active side on beta-lactamase

Pharmacokinetics Both AUC and peak serum concentrations are dose proportional

Distribution: Distributes well into lungs, intestinal mucosa, skin, muscle, uterus, ovary, prostate, gallbladder, and bile; penetration into CSF is low in subject with noninflamed meninges

Metabolism:
Piperacillin: 6% to 9%
Tazobactam: ~26%

Protein binding:
Piperacillin: ~26% to 33%
Tazobactam: 31% to 32%

Half-life:
Piperacillin: 1 hour
Metabolite: 1-1.5 hours
Tazobactam: 0.7-0.9 hour

Elimination: Both piperacillin and tazobactam are directly proportional to renal function
Piperacillin: 50% to 70% eliminated unchanged in urine, 10% to 20% excreted in bile
Tazobactam: Found in urine at 24 hours, with 26% as the inactive metabolite

Hemodialysis removes 30% to 40% of piperacillin and tazobactam; peritoneal dialysis removes 11% to 21% of tazobactam and 6% of piperacillin; hepatic impairment does not affect the kinetics of piperacillin or tazobactam significantly

Usual Dosage Geriatrics and Adults: I.V.: 3.375 g (3 g piperacillin/0.375 g tazobactam) every 6 hours

Dosing interval in renal impairment:
Cl_{cr} >40 mL/minute: No change
Cl_{cr} 20-40 mL/minute: Administer 2.25 g every 6 hours
Cl_{cr} <20 mL/minute: Administer 2.25 g every 8 hours
Hemodialysis: Administer 2.25 g every 8 hours with an additional dose of 0.75 g after each dialysis

Administration See Stability

Monitoring Parameters Signs and symptoms of infection, mental status, WBC; bleeding time, especially in patients with renal impairment

Test Interactions Positive Coombs' [direct] test 3.8%, increased ALT, increased AST

Nursing Implications Administer 1 hour apart from aminoglycosides; administer around-the-clock (ie, 6-12-6-12) (see Stability)

Special Geriatric Considerations Has not been studied exclusively in the elderly (see Usual Dosage); adjust dose for renal function

Dosage Forms Injection: Piperacillin sodium 2 g and tazobactam sodium 0.25 g; piperacillin sodium 3 g and tazobactam sodium 0.375 g; piperacillin sodium 4 g and tazobactam sodium 0.5 g (vials at an 8:1 ratio of piperacillin sodium to tazobactam sodium)

Piperazine (PI per a zeen)

Brand Names Vermizine®

Generic Available Yes

Therapeutic Category Anthelmintic

Use Treatment of pinworm and roundworm infections (used as an alternative to first-line agents, mebendazole, or pyrantel pamoate)

Contraindications Seizure disorders, liver or kidney impairment, hypersensitivity to piperazine or any component

Precautions Use with caution in patients with anemia or malnutrition

Adverse Reactions
Central nervous system: Dizziness, vertigo, seizures, EEG changes, headache
Gastrointestinal: Nausea, vomiting, diarrhea
Hematologic: Hemolytic anemia
Neuromuscular & skeletal: Weakness
Ocular: Visual impairment
Respiratory: Bronchospasm
Miscellaneous: Hypersensitivity reactions

Drug Interactions Pyrantel pamoate (antagonistic mode of action)

Mechanism of Action Causes muscle paralysis of the roundworm by blocking the effects of acetylcholine at the neuromuscular junction

Pharmacokinetics
Absorption: Well absorbed from GI tract
Time to peak plasma concentration: 1 hour
(Continued)

Piperazine *(Continued)*

Elimination: In urine as metabolites and unchanged drug

Usual Dosage Geriatrics and Adults: Oral:

Pinworms: 65 mg/kg/day as a single daily dose for 7 days, in severe infections, repeat course after a 1-week interval; not to exceed 2.5 g/day

Roundworms: 3.5 g/day for 2 days (in severe infections, repeat course, after a 1-week interval)

Monitoring Parameters Stool exam for worms and ova

Patient Information Take on an empty stomach; contact physician if headache, dizziness, poor coordination, muscle weakness, seizures, nausea, vomiting, diarrhea, or rash occur; wash bed clothes, towels, night clothes, and maintain good hygiene to prevent spread or reinfection

Nursing Implications Cure rates may be decreased with massive infections or in patients with hypermotility of the GI tract; administer on an empty stomach

Special Geriatric Considerations Not a drug of choice (see Adverse Reactions); monitor closely in the elderly

Dosage Forms

Piperazine citrate:

Syrup: 500 mg/5 mL (473 mL, 4000 mL)

Tablet: 250 mg

Pipracil® *see* Piperacillin *on page 753*

Pirbuterol *(peer BYOO ter ole)*

Related Information

Inhaled Medications Comparison *on page 1034*

Brand Names Maxair™ Autohaler™; Maxair™ Inhaler

Generic Available No

Therapeutic Category Adrenergic Agonist Agent; Beta$_2$-Adrenergic Agonist Agent; Bronchodilator

Use Prevention and treatment of reversible bronchospasm including asthma

Contraindications Hypersensitivity to pirbuterol, adrenergic amines, or any ingredient

Warnings Administer with caution to individuals with unstable vasomotor systems, diabetes, hyperthyroidism, prostatic hypertrophy, or a history of seizures; also administer with caution to elderly patients, psychoneurotic individuals, and to patients with long-standing bronchial asthma and emphysema who have developed degenerative heart disease

Precautions Excessive use may result in tolerance; deaths have been reported after excessive use; though the exact cause is unknown, cardiac arrest after a severe asthmatic crisis is suspected

Adverse Reactions

Cardiovascular: Tachycardia, palpitations, elevation or depression of blood pressure

Central nervous system: Nervousness, CNS stimulation, hyperactivity, insomnia

Gastrointestinal: GI upset

Neuromuscular: Tremors (may be more common in the elderly)

Overdosage Symptoms of overdose include hypertension, tachycardia, seizures, angina, hypokalemia, and tachyarrhythmias

Toxicology In cases of overdose, supportive therapy should be instituted, and prudent use of a cardioselective beta-adrenergic blocker (eg, atenolol or metoprolol) should be considered, keeping in mind the potential for induction of bronchoconstriction in an asthmatic individual. Dialysis has not been shown to be of value in the treatment of an overdose with this agent.

Drug Interactions

Decreased therapeutic effect: Beta-adrenergic blockers (eg, propranolol)

Increased therapeutic effect: Inhaled ipratropium may increase duration of bronchodilation, nifedipine may increase FEV-1

Increased toxicity (cardiovascular): MAO inhibitors, tricyclic antidepressants, sympathomimetic agents (eg, amphetamine, dopamine, dobutamine), inhaled anesthetics (eg, enflurane)

Mechanism of Action Relaxes bronchial smooth muscle by action on beta$_2$-receptors with little effect on heart rate (minor beta$_1$ activity)

Pharmacodynamics

Onset of action: Within 5 minutes

Peak effect: 30-60 minutes

Duration of action: 3-5 hours

Pharmacokinetics
  Metabolism: In the liver
  Elimination: Urine as unchanged drug and metabolites
Usual Dosage Geriatrics and Adults: 2 inhalations (puffs) every 4-6 hours; some patients may be controlled on 1 puff every 4 hours; do not exceed 12 puffs/day
Monitoring Parameters Pulmonary function, blood pressure, pulse
Patient Information Patient instructions are available with product. Do not exceed recommended dosage; rinse mouth with water following each inhalation to help with dry throat and mouth. May cause nervousness, restlessness, insomnia - if these effects continue after dosage reduction, notify physician. Also notify physician if palpitations, tachycardia, chest pain, muscle tremors, dizziness, headache, flushing, or if breathing difficulty persists. Autohaler™ is breath-activated; follow instructions with product.
Nursing Implications Before using, the inhaler must be shaken well; assess lung sounds, pulse, and blood pressure before administration and during peak of medication; observe patient for wheezing after administration, if this occurs, call physician
Special Geriatric Considerations Elderly patients may find it useful to utilize a spacer device when using a metered dose inhaler; difficulty in using the inhaler often limits its effectiveness. The Autohaler™ may be easier for the elderly to use.
Dosage Forms
  Pirbuterol acetate: Aerosol for oral inhalation:
    Maxair™ Inhaler: 0.2 mg per actuation (25.6 g)
    Maxair™ Autohaler™: 0.2 mg per actuation (2.8 g, 14 g)

Piroxicam (peer OKS i kam)

Brand Names Feldene®
Generic Available No
Therapeutic Category Analgesic, Non-narcotic; Anti-inflammatory Agent; Antipyretic; Nonsteroidal Anti-inflammatory Agent (NSAID), Oral
Use Management of inflammatory disorders; symptomatic treatment of acute and chronic rheumatoid arthritis, osteoarthritis, and sunburn
Contraindications Hypersensitivity to piroxicam, any component, aspirin or other nonsteroidal anti-inflammatory drugs (NSAIDs); active GI bleeding
Warnings GI toxicity (bleeding, ulceration, perforation); CNS effects may occur (headaches, confusion, depression); hypersensitivity, anaphylactoid reactions (intermittent tolmetin use more often); renal function decline, acute renal insufficiency, interstitial nephritis, dysuria, cystitis, hematuria, nephrotic syndrome, hyperkalemia in acute renal insufficiency, hyponatremia, papillary necrosis, hepatic function impairment; elderly have increased risk for adverse reactions to NSAIDs (see Special Geriatric Considerations)
Precautions Use with caution in patients with congestive heart failure, hypertension, decreased renal or hepatic function, history of GI disease (bleeding or ulcers), or those receiving anticoagulants; perform ophthalmologic evaluation for those who develop eye complaints during therapy (blurred vision, diminished vision, changes in color vision, retinal changes); NSAIDs may mask signs/symptoms of infections; photosensitivity reported
Adverse Reactions
  Cardiovascular: Congestive heart failure, angina, hypertension, hypotension, arrhythmias, edema
  Central nervous system: Headache, drowsiness, vertigo, dizziness, fatigue, hallucinations, confusion, depression, emotional lability, psychotic behavior, pyrexia
  Dermatologic: Rash, urticaria, angioedema, Stevens-Johnson syndrome, exfoliative dermatitis, bruising, petechiae, purpura
  Endocrine & metabolic: Hyperglycemia, hypoglycemia, hyperkalemia, gynecomastia, hyponatremia, fluid retention
  Gastrointestinal: Dyspepsia, heartburn, nausea, diarrhea, constipation, flatulence, stomatitis, vomiting, abdominal pain, peptic ulcer, GI bleeding, GI perforation, gingival ulcers, pancreatitis, proctitis, paralytic ulcers, colitis, anorexia, weight loss, dry mucous membranes
  Genitourinary: Impotence, azotemia
  Hematologic: Neutropenia, anemia, agranulocytosis, bone marrow suppression, hemolytic anemia, hemorrhage, inhibition of platelet aggregation
  Hepatic: Hepatitis, elevated LFTs, cholestatic jaundice
  Neuromuscular & skeletal: Involuntary muscle movements, muscle weakness, tremors, weakness
  Ocular: Vision changes
  (Continued)

Piroxicam *(Continued)*

Otic: Tinnitus
Renal: Dysuria, polyuria, pyuria, oliguria, anuria, acute renal failure
Respiratory: Exacerbation of asthma, dyspnea
Miscellaneous: Thirst, diaphoresis

Overdosage Symptoms include drowsiness, lethargy, disorientation, confusion, dizziness, numbness, paresthesia, nausea, vomiting, gastric irritation, abdominal pain, headache, tinnitus, sweating, blurred vision, muscle twitching, seizures, coma, acute renal failure, increased BUN and serum creatinine, hypotension, tachycardia, and metabolic acidosis

Toxicology Management of a nonsteroidal anti-inflammatory agent (NSAID) intoxication is primarily supportive and symptomatic. Fluid therapy is commonly effective in managing the hypotension that may occur following an acute NSAID overdose, except when this is due to an acute blood loss. Seizures tend to be very short-lived and often do not require drug treatment although recurrent seizures should be treated with I.V. diazepam. Since many of the NSAIDs undergo enterohepatic cycling, multiple doses of charcoal may be needed to reduce the potential for delayed toxicities.

Drug Interactions

May increase digoxin, methotrexate, and lithium serum concentrations
Aspirin or other salicylates may decrease NSAID serum concentrations
Other NSAIDs may increase adverse GI effects
Increased prothrombin time with anticoagulants
Decreased antihypertensive effects of ACE inhibitors, beta-blockers, and thiazide diuretics
Effects of loop diuretics may decrease
Increased response to sympathomimetics
Probenecid may increase toxicity of NSAIDs by increase in serum concentrations
Diuretics may increase risk of acute renal insufficiency
Azotemia may be enhanced in elderly receiving loop diuretics

Mechanism of Action Inhibits prostaglandin synthesis, acts on the hypothalamus heat-regulating center to reduce fever, blocks prostaglandin synthetase action which prevents formation of the platelet-aggregating substance thromboxane A_2; decreases pain receptor sensitivity. Other proposed mechanisms of action are lysosomal stabilization, inhibition of kinin and leukotriene production, alteration of chemotactic factors, and inhibition of neutrophil activation. This latter mechanism may be the most significant pharmacologic action to reduce inflammation.

Pharmacodynamics

Onset of analgesia: Oral: Within 1 hour
Duration: 2-3 days
Onset of anti-inflammatory effect: 7-12 days
Peak effect: 2-3 weeks

Pharmacokinetics

Protein binding: 99%
Metabolism: In the liver; substrate CYP2C9, 2C18
Half-life: 45-50 hours
Time to peak serum concentration: 3-5 hours after ingestion
Elimination: Excreted as unchanged drug (5%) and metabolites primarily in urine and to a small degree in feces

Usual Dosage Geriatrics and Adults: Oral: 10-20 mg/day once daily; although associated with increase in GI adverse effects, doses >20 mg/day have been used (ie, 30-40 mg/day); maximum recommended dose: 20 mg/day; assess therapeutic effect after 2 weeks of therapy before increasing doses

Note: Some clinicians have used 10 mg every other day to initiate therapy in elderly to help avoid side effects and produce effect at minimal dose

Monitoring Parameters Monitor response (pain, range of motion, grip strength, mobility, ADL function), inflammation; observe for weight gain, edema; monitor renal function; observe for bleeding, bruising; evaluate gastrointestinal effects (abdominal pain, bleeding, dyspepsia); mental confusion, disorientation, CBC, serum, creatinine, BUN, liver function tests

Test Interactions Increased chloride (S), increased sodium (S)

Patient Information Serious gastrointestinal bleeding can occur as well as ulceration and perforation. Pain may or may not be present. Avoid aspirin and aspirin-containing products while taking this medication. If gastric upset occurs, take with food, milk, or antacid. If gastric adverse effects persist, contact physician. May cause drowsiness, dizziness, blurred vision, and confusion. Use caution when performing tasks which require alertness (eg, driving). Do not take for more than 3 days for fever or 10 days for pain without physician's advice.

Nursing Implications Administer with food to decrease GI adverse effect; monitor CBC, BUN, serum creatinine, liver enzymes; periodic ophthalmologic exams with chronic use

Additional Information Because of its long half-life, may be dosed once daily. There are no clinical guidelines to predict which NSAID will give response in a particular patient. Trials with each must be initiated until response determined. Consider dose, patient convenience, and cost.

Special Geriatric Considerations Elderly are a high-risk population for adverse effects from nonsteroidal anti-inflammatory agents. As much as 60% of elderly can develop peptic ulceration and/or hemorrhage asymptomatically. The concomitant use of H_2 blockers, omeprazole, and sucralfate is not generally effective as prophylaxis with the exception of NSAID-induced duodenal ulcers which may be prevented by the use of ranitidine. Misoprostol and proton pump inhibitors are the only agents proven to help prevent the development of NSAID-induced ulcers. Also, concomitant disease and drug use contribute to the risk for GI adverse effects. Use lowest effective dose for shortest period possible. Consider renal function decline with age. Use of NSAIDs can compromise existing renal function especially when Cl_{cr} is ≤30 mL/minute. Tinnitus may be a difficult and unreliable indication of toxicity due to age-related hearing loss or eighth cranial nerve damage. CNS adverse effects such as confusion, agitation, and hallucination are generally seen in overdose or high dose situations, but elderly may demonstrate these adverse effects at lower doses than younger adults.

Dosage Forms Capsule: 10 mg, 20 mg

References

Brooks PM, Day RO, "Nonsteroidal Anti-inflammatory Drugs - Differences and Similarities," *N Engl J Med*, 1991, 324(24):1716-25.

Clinch D, Banerjee AK, Ostick G, "Absence of Abdominal Pain in Elderly Patients With Peptic Ulcer," *Age Ageing*, 1984, 13:120-3.

Clive DM, Stoff JS, "Renal Syndromes Associated With Nonsteroidal Anti-inflammatory Drugs," *N Engl J Med*, 1984, 310(9):563-72.

Graham DY, "Prevention of Gastroduodenal Injury Induced by Chronic Nonsteroidal Anti-inflammatory Drug Therapy," *Gastroenterology*, 1989, 96(2 Pt 2 Suppl):675-81.

Gurwitz JH, Avorn J, Ross-Degnan D, et al, "Nonsteroidal Anti-Inflammatory Drug-Associated Azotemia in the Very Old," *JAMA*, 1990, 264(4):471-5.

Hawkey CJ, Karrasch JA, Szczepaski L, et al, "Omeprazole Compared With Misoprostrol for Ulcers Associated With Nonsteroidal Anti-inflammatory Drugs," *N Engl J Med*, 1998, 338(11):727-34.

Knodel LC, "Preventing NSAID-Induced Ulcers: The Role of Misoprostol," *Consult Pharm*, 1989, 4:37-41.

Pounder R, "Silent Peptic Ulceration: Deadly Silence or Golden Silence?" *Gastroenterology*, 1989, 96(2 Pt 2 Suppl):626-31.

Yeomans ND, Tulassay Z, Juhasz L, et al, "A Comparison of Omeprazole With Ranitidine for Ulcers Associated With Nonsteroidal Anti-inflammatory Drugs," *N Engl J Med*, 1998, 338(11):719-26.

p-Isobutylhydratropic Acid *see* Ibuprofen *on page 475*

Pitressin® Injection *see* Vasopressin *on page 983*

Placidyl® *see* Ethchlorvynol *on page 356*

Plantago Seed *see* Psyllium *on page 804*

Plantain Seed *see* Psyllium *on page 804*

Plaquenil® *see* Hydroxychloroquine *on page 467*

Plavix® *see* Clopidogrel *on page 240*

Plendil® *see* Felodipine *on page 370*

Pneumococcal Polysaccharide Vaccine *see* Pneumococcal Vaccine *on this page*

Pneumococcal Vaccine (noo moe KOK al vak SEEN)

Related Information

Immunization Guidelines *on page 1058*

Brand Names Pneumovax® 23; Pnu-Imune® 23

Synonyms Pneumococcal Polysaccharide Vaccine

Therapeutic Category Vaccine, Inactivated Bacteria

Use Immunity to pneumococcal lobar pneumonia and bacteremia in individuals ≥2 years of age who are at high risk of morbidity and mortality from pneumococcal infection; patients with a chronic disease which predisposes them to pneumococcal pneumonia (pulmonary, cardiovascular disease, diabetes, alcoholism, liver disease); patients with immunodeficiency due to drugs and/or disease; persons whose living environments place them at risk (nursing homes, hospitals, community epidemics)

(Continued)

Pneumococcal Vaccine (Continued)

Contraindications Active infections, immunosuppressive therapy, Hodgkin's disease patients, hypersensitivity to pneumococcal vaccine or any component

Warnings Hypersensitivity reactions (have epinephrine 1:1000 available); limited effectiveness in preventing infections in patients with skull fractures, external communication with CSF, immune deficiency diseases, certain myeloproliferative diseases, immunosuppressive drugs, splenectomy (vaccination should still be administered)

Precautions Should be administered with caution in individuals who have had episodes of pneumococcal infection within the preceding 3 years - pre-existing pneumococcal antibodies may result in increased reactions to the vaccine; may cause relapse in patients with stable idiopathic thrombocytopenia purpura; patients with cardiac and/or pulmonary disease whom adverse effects to vaccine may be undesirable; revaccination may result in an Arthus reaction or other systemic reactions which may be more frequent and severe; those who received the 14 valent vaccine may benefit from 23 valent vaccine only if at high risk for pneumococcal pneumonia; those at less risk do not have significant benefit

Adverse Reactions Booster doses are associated with an increase in adverse reactions and are currently not recommended

Central nervous system: Fever, Guillain-Barré syndrome
Dermatologic: Rash
Local: Erythema, induration, and soreness at the injection site (2-3 days)
Neuromuscular & skeletal: Myalgia, arthralgia, paresthesia
Miscellaneous: Anaphylaxis (rare)

Drug Interactions Immunosuppressive agents

Stability Refrigerate at 2°C to 8°C (36°F to 46°F); at room temperature (25°C) Pnu-Imune® 23 is stable for several days; Pneumovax® 23 is stable for 1 month at temperatures 15°C to 30°C (59°F to 86°F)

Usual Dosage Geriatrics and Adults: I.M., S.C.: 0.5 mL as a one time only dose; recent studies indicate that high-risk patients (ie, severe COPD, immunosuppressed patients) should have this vaccine administered every 6 years

Patient Information Be aware of adverse effects

Nursing Implications Do not inject I.V., avoid intradermal, administer S.C. or I.M. (deltoid muscle or lateral midthigh); no dilution or reconstitution necessary

Additional Information Federal law requires that the date of administration, the vaccine manufacturer, lot number of vaccine, and the administering person's name, title and address be entered into the patient's permanent medical record; inactivated bacteria vaccine

Special Geriatric Considerations Elderly have ~3 times the incidence of pneumococcal pneumonia than younger adults and 30% of all pneumococcal meningitis occurs in persons >50 years of age with a 20% mortality. Limited data on elderly; however, the elderly, compared to young adults, develop slightly lower antibody titers; provides 60% to 70% protection for bacterial pneumonia. 90% protection for pneumococcal pneumonia strains; 20% of elderly with pneumococcal pneumonia have an associated bacteremia with a 17% to 40% fatality. All persons ≥65 years of age should receive the pneumococcal vaccine including previously unvaccinated persons and persons who have not been vaccinated within 5 years. All persons of unknown vaccination status should receive once dose of vaccine.

Dosage Forms Injection: 25 mcg each of 23 polysaccharide isolates/0.5 mL dose (1 mL, 5 mL)

References

Davidson M, Bulkow LR, Grabman J, et al, "Immunogenicity of Pneumococcal Revaccination in Patients With Chronic Disease," Arch Intern Med, 1994, 154(19):2209-14.

Gardner P and Schaffner W, "Immunization of Adults," N Engl J Med, 1993, 328(17):1252-8.

U.S. Department of Health and Human Services, "Prevention of Pneumococcal Disease. Recommendations of the Advisory Committee on Immunization Practices (ACIP)," MMWR Morb Mortal Wkly Rep, 1997, 46(RR-8):1-24.

Pneumomist® see Guaifenesin on page 437

Pneumovax® 23 see Pneumococcal Vaccine on previous page

Pnu-Imune® 23 see Pneumococcal Vaccine on previous page

Point-Two® see Fluoride on page 392

Poladex® see Dexchlorpheniramine on page 276

Polaramine® see Dexchlorpheniramine on page 276

Poliovirus Vaccine, Inactivated

(POE lee oh VYE rus vak SEEN, in ak ti VAY ted)

Related Information

Immunization Guidelines *on page 1058*

Brand Names IPOL™

Synonyms Enhanced-potency Inactivated Poliovirus Vaccine; IPV; Salk Vaccine

Therapeutic Category Vaccine, Live Virus and Inactivated Virus

Use Active immunization for prevention of poliomyelitis from types 1, 2, and 3; routine primary polio vaccination of adults who reside in the U.S. is not recommended unless patient is at increased risk due to contact or travel

Contraindications Acute febrile illness, including respiratory infections; allergy to streptomycin, polymyxin B, or neomycin; immunodeficiency conditions

Warnings Hypersensitivity reactions, have epinephrine 1:1000 available

Precautions Review patient history and allergy status; HIV infection

Adverse Reactions

Cardiovascular: Fever

Central nervous system: Drowsiness, Guillain-Barré syndrome

Gastrointestinal: Decreased appetite

Local: Erythema, induration, pain at injection site

Drug Interactions Immunosuppressive drugs and therapy may blunt response to vaccine

Stability Refrigerate at 2°C to 8°C (36°F to 46°F); do not freeze

Usual Dosage Geriatrics and Adults: S.C.: 3 doses of 0.5 mL; the first 2 doses should be administered at an interval of 1-2 months; the third dose should be given at least 6 months and preferably 12 months after the second dose (see Additional Information)

Reference Range >1:8 titer

Patient Information Be aware of adverse reactions

Nursing Implications Do not administer I.V.

Additional Information If <3 months exist for series, administer 3 doses at 1-month intervals; if <1 month is available, it is recommended to give OPV single dose or IPV single dose; for adults incompletely vaccinated, administer remainder of doses needed to complete series

Special Geriatric Considerations For elderly who cannot document a primary immunization series or at risk due to contact or travel, administer the initial series; boosters may be necessary for travel since antibody titers may diminish with age

Dosage Forms Injection: Suspension of three types of poliovirus (types 1, 2 and 3) grown in human diploid cell cultures (0.5 mL)

References

Gardner P and Schaffner W, "Immunization of Adults," *N Engl J Med*, 1993, 328(17):1252-8.

Poliovirus Vaccine, Live, Trivalent, Oral

(POE lee oh VYE rus vak SEEN, live, try VAY lent, OR al)

Related Information

Immunization Guidelines *on page 1058*

Brand Names Orimune®

Synonyms OPV; Sabin Vaccine; TOPV

Therapeutic Category Vaccine, Live Virus

Use Poliovirus immunization to prevent poliomyelitis types 1, 2, and 3

Contraindications Persistent vomiting or diarrhea, patients allergic to sorbitol, streptomycin, or neomycin, known hypersensitivity to poliovirus vaccine; defer administration in presence of any acute illness; patients with any immunodeficiency condition (drug induced or disease)

Precautions The vaccine will not modify or prevent cases of existing or incubating poliomyelitis; do not administer TOPV after ISG administration; if given a short time after ISG, repeat dose of TOPV in 3 months

Adverse Reactions Central nervous system: Paralytic poliomyelitis

Drug Interactions May temporarily suppress tuberculin skin test sensitivity (4-6 weeks), immunosuppressive agents, immune globulin

Stability Keep in freezer; vaccine must remain frozen to retain potency; thawed dose must be refrigerated at 2°C to 8°C (36°F to 46°F) and used within 30 days

Usual Dosage Geriatrics and Adults: Oral: Two 0.5 mL doses 8 weeks apart; third dose of 0.5 mL 6-12 months after second dose

(Continued)

Poliovirus Vaccine, Live, Trivalent, Oral *(Continued)*

Booster dose: If an individual is at increased risk due to contact, travel, or occupation and has completed a primary series of immunization, a single booster dose (0.5 mL) orally is suggested

Reference Range >1:8 titer

Nursing Implications Do not administer parenterally; administer directly or dilute with distilled water, simple syrup USP, or milk; may be administered on bread or sugar cubes

Additional Information Federal law requires that the date of administration, the vaccine manufacturer, lot number of vaccine, and the administering person's name, title and address be entered into the patient's permanent medical record

Special Geriatric Considerations For elderly who cannot document a primary immunization series or at risk due to contact or travel, administer the initial series; boosters may be necessary for travel since antibody titers may diminish with age

Dosage Forms Oral: Mixture of type 1, 2, and 3 viruses in monkey kidney tissue (0.5 mL)

References

Gardner P and Schaffner W, "Immunization of Adults," *N Engl J Med*, 1993, 328(17):1252-8.

Polycillin® *see* Ampicillin *on page 73*

Polycillin-N® *see* Ampicillin *on page 73*

Polycitra® *see* Sodium Citrate and Potassium Citrate Mixture *on page 862*

Polymox® *see* Amoxicillin *on page 67*

Polyvinyl Alcohol *see* Artificial Tears *on page 82*

Ponstel® *see* Mefenamic Acid *on page 579*

Pork NPH Iletin® II *see* Insulin Preparations *on page 488*

Pork Regular Iletin® II *see* Insulin Preparations *on page 488*

Posture® [OTC] *see* Calcium Salts (Oral) *on page 152*

Potasalan® *see* Potassium Chloride *on next page*

Potassium Acid Phosphate *(poe TASS ee um AS id FOS fate)*

Brand Names K-Phos® Original

Generic Available No

Therapeutic Category Electrolyte Supplement, Oral; Potassium Salt; Urinary Acidifying Agent

Use Acidifies urine and lowers urinary calcium concentration; reduces odor and rash caused by ammoniacal urine; to increase the antibacterial activity of methenamine

Contraindications Severe renal impairment, hyperkalemia, hyperphosphatemia, and infected magnesium ammonium phosphate stones

Warnings Use with caution in patients receiving other potassium supplementation and in patients with renal insufficiency, or severe tissue breakdown as seen in chemotherapy or hemodialysis

Precautions Use cautiously, serum potassium needs regulation; use caution in patients receiving digitalis products, Addison's disease, dehydrated patients, renal insufficiency, hepatic disease, peripheral or pulmonary edema, hypertension, hypernatremia, hypoparathyroidism, acute pancreatitis, osteomalacia

Adverse Reactions

Cardiovascular: Arrhythmia

Central nervous system: Tetany, dizziness, fatigue, tingling or numbness of lips

Endocrine & metabolic: Hyperphosphatemia, hyperkalemia, hypocalcemia

Gastrointestinal: Nausea; vomiting; diarrhea; abdominal discomfort; a mild laxative effect may occur, but resolves with dose reduction; weight gain

Genitourinary: Decreased urine output

Neuromuscular & skeletal: Pain/weakness of extremities, bone pain, arthralgia

Respiratory: Shortness of breath

Miscellaneous: Thirst, edema

Overdosage Symptoms of overdose include muscle weakness, paralysis, peaked T waves, flattened P waves, prolongation of QRS complex, ventricular arrhythmias

Toxicology Removal of potassium can be accomplished by various means; removal through the GI tract with Kayexalate® administration; by way of the kidney through diuresis, mineralocorticoid administration or increased sodium intake; by hemodialysis or peritoneal dialysis; or by shifting potassium back into the cells by insulin and glucose infusion or sodium bicarbonate; calcium chloride will reverse cardiac effects.

Drug Interactions

Antacids containing magnesium, calcium or aluminum binds phosphate and decreased absorption

Potassium or potassium-sparing diuretics may increase chance of hyperkalemia

Salicylates have increased serum concentrations

Angiotensin-converting enzyme inhibitors may increase serum potassium

Mechanism of Action The principal intracellular cation; involved in transmission of nerve impulses, muscle contractions, enzyme activity, and glucose utilization

Pharmacokinetics

Absorption: Absorbed well from upper GI tract

Distribution: Enters cells via active transport from extracellular fluid

Elimination: Largely by the kidneys, but also small amount via the skin and feces, with most intestinal potassium being reabsorbed

Usual Dosage Geriatrics and Adults: Oral: 1000 mg dissolved in 6-8 oz of water 4 times/day with meals and at bedtime; for best results, soak tablets in water for 2-5 minutes, then stir and swallow

Monitoring Parameters Serum potassium, sodium, phosphate, calcium; serum salicylates (if taking salicylates); signs of muscle weakness, cramps

Test Interactions Decreased ammonia (B)

Patient Information Dissolve tablets completely before drinking; avoid taking magnesium, calcium, or aluminum antacids at the same time; patients may pass old kidney stones when starting therapy; notify physician if experiencing nausea, vomiting, or abdominal pain, muscle weakness, or cramps

Special Geriatric Considerations A complete drug history should be taken to rule out potential drug interactions since elderly frequently may be taking potassium and potassium-sparing diuretics, salicylates, or antacids; use with caution in renal impairment (low Cl_{cr})

Dosage Forms Tablet, sodium free: 500 mg [potassium 3.67 mEq]

Potassium Chloride (poe TASS ee um KLOR ide)

Related Information

I.V. Medication Recommendations *on page 1080*

Brand Names Cena-K®; Gen-K®; K+ 10®; Kaochlor®; Kaochlor® SF; Kaon-Cl®; Kaon Cl-10®; Kato®; Kay Ciel®; K+ Care®; K-Dur® 10; K-Dur® 20; K-Lease®; K-Lor™; Klor-Con®; Klor-Con® 8; Klor-Con® 10; Klor-Con/25®; Klorvess®; Klotrix®; K-Lyte/Cl®; K-Norm®; K-Tab®; Micro-K® 10; Micro-K® Extencaps®; Micro-K® LS®; Potasalan®; Rum-K®; Slow-K®; Ten-K®

Synonyms KCl

Generic Available Yes

Therapeutic Category Electrolyte Supplement, Oral; Electrolyte Supplement, Parenteral; Potassium Salt

Use Treatment or prevention of hypokalemia

Unlabeled use: Treatment of hypertension

Contraindications Severe renal impairment, untreated Addison's disease, acute dehydration, heat cramps, hyperkalemia, severe tissue trauma; liquid potassium preparation should be used in patients with esophageal compression or delayed gastric emptying time

Warnings Potassium injections should be administered only in patients with adequate urine flow; patients with impaired potassium excretion (renal failure) can develop hyperkalemia and cardiac arrhythmias or arrest; potassium tablets have been reported to produce stenotic or ulcerative lesions in gastrointestinal tract

Precautions Use with caution in patients with cardiac disease, patients receiving potassium-sparing drugs; patients must be on a cardiac monitor during intermittent infusions

Adverse Reactions

Cardiovascular: Cardiac arrhythmias, heart block, hypotension

Central nervous system: Parethesias, mental confusion

Endocrine & metabolic: Hyperkalemia

Gastrointestinal: Nausea, vomiting, diarrhea, abdominal pain, GI lesions

Local: Pain at the site of injection, phlebitis

Neuromuscular & skeletal: Muscle weakness

Overdosage See Adverse Reactions

Toxicology Removal of potassium can be accomplished by various means; removal through the GI tract with Kayexalate® administration; by way of the (Continued)

Potassium Chloride *(Continued)*

kidney through diuresis, mineralocorticoid administration or increased sodium intake; by hemodialysis or peritoneal dialysis; or by shifting potassium back into the cells by insulin and glucose infusion.

Drug Interactions Potassium-sparing diuretics, salt substitutes, digitalis, angiotensin-converting enzyme inhibitors

Stability Store at room temperature, protect from freezing; use only clear solutions; use admixtures within 24 hours

Mechanism of Action Needed for the conduction of nerve impulses in heart, brain, and skeletal muscle; contraction of cardiac, skeletal and smooth muscles; maintenance of normal renal function

Pharmacokinetics

Absorption: Well from upper GI tract; enters cells via active transport from extracellular fluid

Elimination: Largely by the kidneys, but also small amount via skin and feces, with most intestinal potassium being reabsorbed

Usual Dosage I.V. doses should be incorporated into the patient's maintenance I.V. fluids, intermittent I.V. potassium administration should be reserved for severe depletion situations in patients undergoing EKG monitoring.

Geriatrics and Adults:

Normal daily requirement: Oral, I.V.: 30-80 mEq/day

Prevention during diuretic therapy: Oral: 10-40 mEq/day in 1-2 divided doses

Treatment: Oral, I.V.: 20-100 mEq/day

I.V. intermittent infusion: 10-20 mEq/hour, not to exceed 40 mEq/hour and 150 mEq/day. See table.

Potassium Dosage/Rate of Infusion Guidelines

Serum Potassium+	Maximum Infusion Rate	Maximum Concentration	Maximum 24-Hour Dose
>2.5 mEq/L	10 mEq/h	40 mEq/L	200 mEq
<2.5 mEq/L	40 mEq/h	80 mEq/L	400 mEq

Monitoring Parameters Serum potassium, blood pressure, pulse, EKG (as needed), signs of muscle weakness, cramps

Reference Range 3.5-5.0 mEq/L (3.5-5.0 mmol/L)

Test Interactions Decreased ammonia (B)

Patient Information Swallow tablets whole, do not crush or chew; take with food, water, or juice

Nursing Implications Maximum concentration (peripheral line): 80 mEq/L; usual rate: 10 mEq/hour; maximum concentration (central line): 30 mEq/100 mL; may not be given I.V. push or I.V. retrograde; oral liquid potassium supplements should be diluted (2-6 parts diluent) with water or fruit juice during administration; wax matrix tablets must be swallowed and not allowed to dissolve in mouth

Special Geriatric Considerations Elderly may require less potassium than younger adults due to decreased renal function; for elderly who do not respond to replacement therapy, check serum magnesium; due to long-term diuretic use, elderly may be hypomagnesemic

Dosage Forms

Capsule, controlled release, micro encapsulated (Micro-K®): 600 mg [8 mEq]; 750 mg [10 mEq]

Injection: 1.5 mEq/mL, 2 mEq/mL, 3 mEq/mL

Liquid, oral: 10 mEq/15 mL, 15 mEq/15 mL, 20 mEq/15 mL, 30 mEq/15 mL, 40 mEq/15 mL, 45 mEq/15 mL

Powder, oral: 15 mEq, 20 mEq, 25 mEq packet

Tablet:

Effervescent, as potassium chloride: 25 mEq

Effervescent, as potassium bicarbonate: 20 mEq, 25 mEq, 50 mEq

Extended release (K+8®): 8 mEq

Sustained release, microcrystalloids (K-Dur®): 750 mg [10 mEq]; 1500 mg [20 mEq]

Wax matrix:

Kaon-Cl®: 500 mg [6.7 mEq]

Slow-K®: 600 mg [8 mEq]; 750 mg [10 mEq]

Potassium Gluconate (poe TASS ee um GLOO coe nate)

Brand Names Kaon®; Kaylixir®; K-G®

Generic Available Yes

Therapeutic Category Electrolyte Supplement, Oral; Potassium Salt

Use Treatment of potassium deficiency (hypokalemia) or prevention of hypokalemia

Unlabeled use: Treatment of hypertension

Contraindications Severe renal impairment, untreated Addison's disease, acute dehydration, heat cramps, hyperkalemia, severe tissue trauma; liquid potassium preparation should be used in patients with esophageal compression or delayed gastric emptying time

Warnings Patients with impaired potassium excretion (renal failure) can develop hyperkalemia and cardiac arrhythmias or arrest; potassium tablets have been reported to produce stenotic or ulcerative lesions in gastrointestinal tract

Precautions Use with caution in patients with cardiac disease, patients receiving potassium-sparing drugs; patients must be on a cardiac monitor during intermittent infusions

Adverse Reactions
Cardiovascular: Cardiac arrhythmias, heart block, hypotension
Central nervous system: Parethesias, mental confusion
Endocrine & metabolic: Hyperkalemia
Gastrointestinal: Nausea, vomiting, diarrhea, abdominal pain, GI lesions
Local: Phlebitis
Neuromuscular & skeletal: Muscle weakness

Overdosage See Adverse Reactions

Toxicology Removal of potassium can be accomplished by various means; removal through the GI tract with Kayexalate® administration; by way of the kidney through diuresis, mineralocorticoid administration or increased sodium intake; by hemodialysis or peritoneal dialysis; or by shifting potassium back into cells by insulin and glucose infusion

Drug Interactions Potassium-sparing diuretics, salt substitutes
Digitalis: Low serum concentrations of potassium may result in arrhythmias
Angiotensin-converting enzyme inhibitors may increase serum concentrations of potassium

Stability Store at room temperature, protect from freezing; use only clear solutions; use admixtures within 24 hours

Mechanism of Action Needed for the conduction of nerve impulses in heart, brain, and skeletal muscle; contraction of cardiac, skeletal and smooth muscles; maintenance of normal renal function

Pharmacokinetics
Absorption: Well from upper GI tract
Distribution: Enters cells via active transport from extracellular fluid
Elimination: Largely by the kidneys, but also small amount via skin and feces, with most intestinal potassium being reabsorbed

Usual Dosage Geriatrics and Adults: Oral:
Normal daily requirement: 40-80 mEq/day
Prevention during diuretic therapy: 10-40 mEq/day in 1-2 divided doses
Treatment of hypokalemia: 20-100 mEq/day in 2-4 divided doses

Monitoring Parameters Serum potassium, blood pressure, pulse, EKG (as needed), signs of muscle weakness, cramps; serum magnesium for failure to respond to replacement

Reference Range 3.5-5 mEq/L (3.5-5 mmol/L)

Test Interactions Decreased ammonia (B)

Patient Information Take with food, water, or fruit juice; swallow tablets whole; do not crush or chew

Nursing Implications Maximum concentration (peripheral line): 80 mEq/L; maximum concentration (central line): 30 mEq/100 mL; oral liquid potassium supplements should be diluted (2-6 parts diluent) with water or fruit juice during administration; wax matrix tablets must be swallowed and not chewed

Additional Information 9.4 g potassium gluconate is approximately equal to 40 mEq potassium (4.3 mEq potassium/g salt)

Special Geriatric Considerations Elderly may require less potassium than younger adults due to decreased renal function; for elderly who do not respond to replacement therapy, check serum magnesium; long-term use of diuretics may result in hypomagnesemia

Dosage Forms
Elixir: 20 mEq/15 mL (5 mL, 15 mL, 118 mL, 473 mL, 946 mL, 4000 mL)
Tablet: 500 mg, 595 mg

Potassium Phosphate (poe TASS ee um FOS fate)

Brand Names Neutra-Phos®-K

Synonyms Phosphate, Potassium

Generic Available Yes

Therapeutic Category Electrolyte Supplement, Oral; Electrolyte Supplement, Parenteral; Phosphate Salt; Potassium Salt

Use Source of potassium and phosphorus in parenteral nutrition and large volume I.V. fluids; treatment of conditions associated with excessive renal phosphate and potassium loss, inadequate GI absorption of these electrolytes, or inadequate phosphate and potassium in the diet

Contraindications Hyperphosphatemia, hyperkalemia, low calcium levels, severe renal impairment

Warnings Use with caution in patients with renal insufficiency, cardiac disease, metabolic alkalosis; admixture of phosphate and calcium in I.V. fluids can result in calcium phosphate precipitation; cases where severe tissue breakdown occurs (eg, hemolysis, chemotherapy)

Precautions Use cautiously, serum potassium needs regulation; use caution in patients receiving digitalis products, Addison's disease, dehydrated patients, renal insufficiency, hepatic disease, peripheral or pulmonary edema, hypertension, hypernatremia, hypoparathyroidism, acute pancreatitis, osteomalacia

Adverse Reactions

Cardiovascular: Arrhythmia

Central nervous system: Tetany, dizziness, fatigue, tingling or numbness of lips

Endocrine & metabolic: Hyperphosphatemia, hyperkalemia, hypocalcemia

Gastrointestinal: Nausea; vomiting; diarrhea; abdominal discomfort; a mild laxative effect may occur, but resolves with dose reduction; weight gain

Genitourinary: Decreased urine output

Neuromuscular & skeletal: Pain/weakness of extremities, bone pain, arthralgia

Respiratory: Shortness of breath

Miscellaneous: Thirst, edema

Overdosage Symptoms of overdose include muscle weakness, paralysis, peaked T waves, flattened P waves, prolongation of QRS complex, ventricular arrhythmias, tetany, calcium-phosphate precipitation

Toxicology Removal of potassium can be accomplished by various means; removal through the GI tract with Kayexalate® administration; by way of the kidney through diuresis, mineralocorticoid administration or increased sodium intake; by hemodialysis or peritoneal dialysis; or by shifting potassium back into the cells by insulin, glucose infusion, or sodium bicarbonate; calcium chloride reverses cardiac effects.

Drug Interactions

Decreased effect/serum concentrations with aluminum- and magnesium-containing antacids or sucralfate which can act as phosphate binders

Increased effect/serum concentrations with potassium-sparing diuretics, ACE inhibitors, or salt substitutes

Digitalis: Low serum concentrations of potassium predispose patient to arrhythmias

Stability Store at room temperature, protect from freezing; use only clear solutions; up to 10-15 mEq of calcium may be added per liter before precipitate may occur

Stability of parenteral admixture at room temperature (25°C): 24 hours

Usual Dosage I.V. doses should be incorporated into the patient's maintenance I.V. fluids; intermittent I.V. infusion should be reserved for severe depletion situations in patients undergoing continuous EKG monitoring. It is difficult to determine total body phosphorus deficit; the following dosages are empiric guidelines:

Geriatrics and Adults: Normal requirements elemental phosphorus: Oral: 1200 mg/day

Treatment: It is difficult to provide concrete guidelines for the treatment of severe hypophosphatemia because the extent of total body deficits and response to therapy are difficult to predict. Aggressive doses of phosphate may result in a transient serum elevation followed by redistribution into intracellular compartments or bone tissue. It is recommended that repletion of severe hypophosphatemia (<1 mg/dL) be done I.V. because large doses of oral phosphate may cause diarrhea and intestinal absorption may be unreliable

Geriatrics and Adults: I.V. phosphate repletion:
Initial dose: 0.08 mmol/kg if recent uncomplicated hypophosphatemia
Initial dose: 0.16 mmol/kg if prolonged hypophosphatemia with presumed total body deficits; increase dose by 25% to 50% if patient symptomatic with severe hypophosphatemia
Do not exceed 0.24 mmol/kg/day; administer over 6 hours by I.V. infusion

With orders for I.V. phosphate, there is considerable confusion associated with the use of millimoles (mmol) versus milliequivalents (mEq) to express the phosphate requirement. Because inorganic phosphate exists as monobasic and dibasic anions, with the mixture of valences dependent on pH, ordering by mEq amounts is unreliable and may lead to large dosing errors. In addition, I.V. phosphate is available in the sodium and potassium salt; therefore, the content of these cations must be considered when ordering phosphate. The most reliable method of ordering I.V. phosphate is by millimoles, then specifying the potassium or sodium salt. For example, an order for 15 mmol of phosphate as potassium phosphate in 1 liter of normal saline would also provide 22 mEq of potassium.

Phosphate maintenance electrolyte requirement in parenteral nutrition: Geriatrics and Adults: 2 mmol/kg/24 hours or 35 mmol/kcal/24 hours; maximum: 15-30 mmol/24 hours

Maintenance: Geriatrics and Adults:
I.V. solutions: 15-30 mmol/24 hours I.V. or 50-150 mmol/24 hours in divided doses
Fleet® Phospho®-Soda: Laxative: Oral: Single dose: 20-30 mL mixed with 120 mL cold water

Administration For intermittent infusion, if peripheral line, dilute to a maximum concentration of 0.05 mmol/mL; if central line, dilute to a maximum concentration of 0.12 mmol/mL; maximum rate of infusion: 0.06 mmol/kg/hour; do **not** infuse with calcium containing IV. fluids (ie, TPN)

Monitoring Parameters Serum potassium, phosphate, magnesium (failure to respond), calcium, EKG, salicylate serum concentrations if patient is taking salicylates; signs of muscle weakness, cramps

Reference Range Geriatrics and Adults: 2.5-5 mg/dL

Test Interactions Decreased ammonia (B)

Nursing Implications Injection must be diluted in appropriate I.V. solution and volume prior to administration and administered over a minimum of 4 hours

Special Geriatric Considerations A complete drug history should be taken to rule out potential drug interactions since elderly frequently may be taking potassium and potassium-sparing diuretics or salicylates as antacids; elderly may require less potassium than younger adults due to decreased renal function; for elderly who do not respond to replacement therapy, check serum magnesium; long-term use of diuretics may result in hypomagnesemia

Dosage Forms
Injection: Potassium 4.4 mEq and phosphate 3 mmol per mL (15 mL)
Powder packet (Neutra-Phos®-K): Potassium 556 mg [14.25 mEq] and phosphorus 250 mg [8 mmol] per packet

Potassium Phosphate and Sodium Phosphate
(poe TASS ee um FOS fate & SOW dee um FOS fate)

Brand Names K-Phos® Neutral; Neutra-Phos®; Uro-KP-Neutral®

Synonyms Sodium Phosphate and Potassium Phosphate

Generic Available Yes

Therapeutic Category Electrolyte Supplement, Oral; Phosphate Salt; Potassium Salt

Use Treatment of conditions associated with excessive renal phosphate loss or inadequate GI absorption of phosphate; to acidify the urine to lower calcium concentrations; to increase the antibacterial activity of methenamine; reduce odor and rash caused by ammonia in urine

Contraindications Severe renal impairment, hyperkalemia, hyperphosphatemia, and infected magnesium ammonium phosphate stones

Warnings Use with caution in patients with renal disease, hyperkalemia, cardiac disease, Addison's disease, hyperkalemia, infected urolithiasis or struvite stone formation, patients with severely impaired renal function

Precautions Use cautiously in sodium-restricted patients; serum potassium needs regulation; use caution in patients receiving digitalis products, Addison's disease, dehydrated patients, renal insufficiency, hepatic disease, peripheral or pulmonary edema, hypertension, hypernatremia, hypoparathyroidism, acute pancreatitis, osteomalacia
(Continued)

Potassium Phosphate and Sodium Phosphate
(Continued)

Adverse Reactions
Cardiovascular: Arrhythmia

Central nervous system: Tetany, dizziness, fatigue, tingling or numbness of lips

Endocrine & metabolic: Hyperphosphatemia, hyperkalemia, hypocalcemia

Gastrointestinal: Nausea; vomiting; diarrhea; abdominal discomfort; a mild laxative effect may occur, but resolves with dose reduction; weight gain

Genitourinary: Decreased urine output

Neuromuscular & skeletal: Pain/weakness of extremities, bone pain, arthralgia

Respiratory: Shortness of breath

Miscellaneous: Thirst, edema

Overdosage Symptoms of overdose include muscle weakness, paralysis, peaked T waves, flattened P waves, prolongation of QRS complex, ventricular arrhythmias, tetany, calcium phosphate precipitation

Toxicology Removal of potassium can be accomplished by various means; removal through the GI tract with Kayexalate® administration; by way of the kidney through diuresis, mineralocorticoid administration or increased sodium intake; by hemodialysis or peritoneal dialysis; or by shifting potassium back into the cells by insulin and glucose infusion; calcium chloride reverses cardiac effects.

Drug Interactions
Decreased effect/serum concentrations with aluminum- and magnesium-containing antacids or sucralfate which can act as phosphate binders

Increased effect/serum concentrations with potassium-sparing diuretics or ACE inhibitors

Salicylates may have increased serum concentrations

Digitalis: Low serum concentrations of potassium are predisposed to arrhythmias

Usual Dosage All dosage forms to be mixed in 6-8 oz of water prior to administration

Geriatrics and Adults: 1-2 capsules (250-500 mg phosphorus/8-16 mmol) 4 times/day after meals and at bedtime; do not exceed 8 doses in 24 hours; if urine is difficult to acidify, administer 1 dose (tablet/capsule/powder) every 2 hours, not to exceed 8 doses in 24 hours

Monitoring Parameters Serum potassium, sodium, magnesium (failure to respond to replacement), calcium, phosphate, EKG; signs of muscle weakness, cramps

Patient Information Do not swallow, open capsule and dissolve in 6-8 oz of water; powder packets are to be mixed in 6-8 oz of water; tablets should be crushed and mixed in 6-8 oz of water

Nursing Implications Tablets may be crushed and stirred vigorously to speed dissolution

Special Geriatric Considerations A complete drug history should be taken to rule out potential drug interactions since elderly frequently may be taking potassium and potassium-sparing diuretics or salicylates as antacids; elderly may require less potassium than younger adults due to decreased renal function; for elderly who do not respond to replacement therapy, check serum magnesium; long-term use of diuretics may result in hypomagnesemia

Dosage Forms
Powder, concentrate: Phosphate 8 mmol, sodium 7.125 mEq, and potassium 7.125 mEq per 75 mL when reconstituted

Tablet: Phosphate 8 mmol, sodium 13 mEq, and potassium 1.1 mEq (114 mg of phosphorus)

PPA see Phenylpropanolamine on page 741

PPD see Tuberculin Purified Protein Derivative on page 971

Pramipexole (pra mi PEX ole)
Brand Names Mirapex®

Generic Available No

Therapeutic Category Anti-Parkinson's Agent; Dopaminergic Agent (Antiparkinson's)

Use Treatment of the signs and symptoms of idiopathic Parkinson's disease; has been studied without levodopa in early disease and in combination with levodopa in advanced disease

Contraindications Hypersensitivity to pramipexole or any other component

Warnings The use of dopamine agonists may cause orthostatic hypotension, particularly during dose escalation; patients should be carefully monitored for the signs and symptoms of orthostatic hypotension; during clinical trials of pramipexole, clinically significant orthostatic hypotension did not occur more frequently with pramipexole as compared to placebo; this may be due to the nature of the population enrolled; pramipexole is associated with an increased risk of hallucinations, especially in older patients.

Precautions Use with caution in patients with renal insufficiency; may cause or exacerbate dyskinesias when given with levodopa

Adverse Reactions

Early Parkinson's disease:

Central nervous system: Dizziness, somnolence, insomnia, hallucinations, confusion, amnesia

Gastrointestinal: Nausea, constipation

Neuromuscular & skeletal: Asthenia

Ocular: Vision abnormalities

Late Parkinson's disease (with levodopa):

Cardiovascular: Postural hypotension

Central nervous system: Insomnia, dizziness, hallucinations, dream abnormalities, confusion, somnolence, amnesia, dyskinesias, EPS, dystonia

Gastrointestinal: Constipation, dry mouth

Genitourinary: Urinary frequency

Neuromuscular & skeletal: Asthenia, gait abnormalities

Ocular: Vision abnormalities

Overdosage No clinical experience with massive overdosage

Toxicology Management of overdose may require general supportive measures, along with gastric lavage, intravenous fluids, and electrocardiogram monitoring

Drug Interactions

Increased effect: Cimetidine increased the AUC and half-life of pramipexole by 50% and 40% respectively

Decreased clearance: Drugs secreted by the cationic transport system may decrease the clearance of pramipexole by 20% (this includes cimetidine, ranitidine, diltiazem, triamterene, verapamil, quinidine, and quinine)

Decreased effect: Dopamine antagonists such as phenothiazines, haloperidol, metoclopramide

Mechanism of Action Nonergot dopamine agonist with high relative *in vitro* specificity and full intrinsic activity at the D_2 subfamily of dopamine receptors in the striatum; binds with higher affinity to D_3 than to D_2 or D_4 receptor subtypes

Pharmacokinetics

Absorption: Rapid, T_{max}: 2 hours; food delays T_{max} by 1 hour

Metabolism: Minimal

Bioavailability: >90%

Half-life: Adults: 8 hours; elderly: 12 hours

Elimination: 90% eliminated unchanged in the urine

Clearance is decreased in the elderly, likely due to decreased renal function. Clearance in Parkinson's patients was 30% less than healthy elderly volunteers. Clearance is decreased 60% when creatinine clearance is 40 mL/minute; 75% when clearance is 20 mL/minute.

Usual Dosage

Geriatrics: See dosage in renal impairment

Adults: Suggested dosing schedule:

Week 1: 0.125 mg 3 times/day

Week 2: 0.25 mg 3 times/day

Week 3: 0.5 mg 3 times/day

Week 4: 0.75 mg 3 times/day

Week 5: 1 mg 3 times/day

Week 6: 1.25 mg 3 times/day

Week 7: 1.5 mg 3 times/day

Usual dosage range: 1.5-4.5 mg/day

Dosing adjustment in renal impairment:

Cl_{cr} >60 mL/minute:

Starting dose: 0.125 mg 3 times/day

Maximum dose: 1.5 mg 3 times/day

Cl_{cr} 35-59 mL/minute:

Starting dose: 0.125 mg twice daily

Maximum dose: 1.5 mg twice daily

Cl_{cr} 15-34 mL/minute:

Starting dose: 0.125 mg/day

(Continued)

Pramipexole *(Continued)*

Maximum dose: 1.5 mg/day

Cl_{cr} <15 mL/minute: Not studied in this group

Monitoring Parameters Blood pressure, standing and sitting/lying down; mental status

Patient Information If pramipexole causes nausea, may take with food; rise slowly from sitting/lying down position; drowsiness may occur, use caution when driving until used to the effects of pramipexole; avoid alcohol and other CNS depressants

Nursing Implications Monitor for signs and symptoms of orthostatic hypotension, change in mental status

Special Geriatric Considerations See Warnings, Pharmacokinetics, and Usual Dosage

Dosage Forms Tablet: 0.125 mg, 0.25 mg, 1 mg, 1.5 mg

References

Lieberman A, Ranhosky A, and Korts D, "Clinical Evaluation of Pramipexole in Advanced Parkinson's Disease: Results of a Double-Blind, Placebo-Controlled, Parallel-Group Study," *Neurology,* 1997, 49(1):162-8.

"Safety and Efficacy of Pramipexole in Early Parkinson Disease. Parkinson Study Group," *JAMA,* 1997, 278(2):125-30.

Stern MB, "Contemporary Approaches to the Pharmacotherapeutic Management of Parkinson's Disease: An Overview," *Neurology,* 1997, 49(1 Suppl 1):S2-9.

Watts RL, "The Role of Dopamine Agonists in Early Parkinson's Disease," *Neurology,* 1997, 49(1 Suppl 1):S34-48.

Pravachol® *see* Pravastatin *on this page*

Pravastatin *(PRA va stat in)*

Brand Names Pravachol®

Therapeutic Category Antilipemic Agent; HMG-CoA Reductase Inhibitor

Use Adjunct to diet for the reduction of elevated total and LDL-cholesterol levels in patients with hypercholesterolemia (type IIa, IIb, and IIc)

Contraindications Previous hypersensitivity, active liver disease, or persistent, unexplained liver function enzyme elevations

Warnings May elevate aminotransferases (see Monitoring Parameters); may also cause myalgia and rhabdomyolysis or muscle weakness/myopathy

Precautions Use with caution in patients who consume large quantities of alcohol or patients having a history of liver disease

Adverse Reactions

Central nervous system: Headache, dizziness

Dermatologic: Rash

Gastrointestinal: Flatulence, abdominal cramps, diarrhea, constipation, nausea, dyspepsia, heartburn, dysgeusia

Neuromuscular & skeletal: Myalgia

Ocular: Lenticular opacities, blurred vision

Miscellaneous: Elevated creatinine phosphokinase (CPK)

Overdosage Treatment is symptomatic

Drug Interactions

Increased effect with cholestyramine

Increased effect/toxicity of oral anticoagulants

Concurrent use with cyclosporine, gemfibrozil, clofibrate, erythromycin, clarithromycin, troleandomycin, itraconazole, or protease inhibitors may increase risk of rhabdomyolysis or myopathy

Mechanism of Action Pravastatin is a competitive inhibitor of 3-hydroxy-3-methylglutaryl coenzyme A (HMG-CoA) reductase, which is the rate-limiting enzyme involved in *de novo* cholesterol synthesis

Pharmacokinetics

Absorption: Poor

Metabolism: In the liver to at least two metabolites; substrate CYP3A4

Bioavailability: 17%

Half-life: 2-3 hours

Elimination: Up to 20% excreted in urine (8% unchanged)

Usual Dosage Geriatrics and Adults: Oral: 10-20 mg once daily at bedtime, may increase to 40 mg/day at bedtime; recommended to start with 10 mg in the elderly with most responding to 10-20 mg/day

Monitoring Parameters Serum cholesterol (total and fractionated), CPK serum concentrations; LFTs before and every 4-6 weeks during the first 12-15 months of therapy and periodically thereafter or LFTs before and every 4-6 weeks during the first 3 months of therapy and then every 6-12 weeks during the next 12 months and periodically thereafter

Patient Information Promptly report any unexplained muscle pain, tenderness or weakness, especially if accompanied by malaise or fever; follow prescribed diet

Nursing Implications The best effect is seen when administered at night; monitor for symptoms of adverse effects (see Adverse Reactions and Special Geriatric Considerations)

Special Geriatric Considerations Effective and well tolerated in the elderly. The definition of and, therefore, when to treat hyperlipidemia in the elderly is a controversial issue. The National Cholesterol Education Program recommends that all adults 20 years of age and older maintain a plasma cholesterol <200 mg/dL. By this definition, 60% of all elderly would be considered to have a borderline high (200-239 mg/dL) or high (≥240 mg/dL) plasma cholesterol. However, plasma cholesterol has been shown to be a less reliable predictor of coronary heart disease in the elderly. Therefore, it is the authors' belief that pharmacologic treatment be reserved for those who are unable to obtain a desirable plasma cholesterol concentration by diet alone and for whom the benefits of treatment are believed to outweigh the potential adverse effects, drug interactions, and cost of treatment.

Dosage Forms Tablet, as sodium: 10 mg, 20 mg, 40 mg

References

Lintott CJ and Scott RS, "HMG-CoA Reductase Inhibitor Use in the Aged: A Review of Clinical Experience," *Drugs Aging*, 1992, 2(6):518-29.

"Summary of the Second Report of the National Cholesterol Education Program (NCEP) Expert Panel on Detection, Evaluation, and Treatment of High Blood Cholesterol in Adults," *JAMA*, 1993, 269(23):3015-23.

Prazepam (PRA ze pam)

Related Information

Antacid Drug Interactions *on page 1096*

Benzodiazepines Comparison *on page 1024*

Federal OBRA Regulations Recommended Maximum Doses - Anxiolytics *on page 1057*

Brand Names Centrax®

Generic Available No

Therapeutic Category Antianxiety Agent; Anticonvulsant, Benzodiazepine; Benzodiazepine

Use Treatment of anxiety and management of alcohol withdrawal

Restrictions C-IV

Contraindications Hypersensitivity to prazepam or any component, cross-sensitivity with other benzodiazepines may exist; avoid using in patients with pre-existing CNS depression, severe uncontrolled pain, or narrow-angle glaucoma

Warnings May cause drug dependency; avoid abrupt discontinuance in patients with prolonged therapy or seizure disorders

Precautions Use with caution in patients with a history of drug dependence

Adverse Reactions

Central nervous system: Drowsiness, dizziness, confusion, sedation, ataxia, headache

Gastrointestinal: Xerostomia, constipation, diarrhea, nausea, vomiting

Neuromuscular & skeletal: Impaired coordination

Ocular: Blurred vision

Respiratory: Decreased respiratory rate, apnea, laryngospasm

Miscellaneous: Physical and psychological dependence with prolonged use

Overdosage Symptoms of overdose include somnolence, confusion, coma, and diminished reflexes

Toxicology Treatment for benzodiazepine overdose is supportive; rarely is mechanical ventilation required

Flumazenil has been shown to selectively block the binding of benzodiazepines to CNS receptors, resulting in a reversal of benzodiazepine-induced sedation; however, its use may not alter the course of overdose

Drug Interactions Benzodiazepines may decrease the effect of levodopa

Decreased metabolism: Cimetidine, fluoxetine

Increased metabolism: Rifampin

Increased toxicity: CNS depressants, alcohol

Mechanism of Action Benzodiazepines appear to potentiate the effects of GABA and other inhibitory neurotransmitters by binding to specific benzodiazepine-receptor sites in various areas of the CNS

Pharmacodynamics

Peak effects: Within 6 hours

Duration: 48 hours; studies have shown that the elderly are more sensitive to the effects of benzodiazepines as compared to younger adults

(Continued)

Prazepam (Continued)

Pharmacokinetics

Distribution: V_d is increased in elderly

Half-life:

Parent: 78 minutes

Desmethyldiazepam: 30-100 hours; significantly prolonged in elderly men (127.8 hours) as compared to young men (61.8 hours) and older women (75.4 hours)

Metabolism: Prazepam, itself, is pharmacologically inactive; first-pass hepatic metabolism

Elimination: Renal excretion of unchanged drug and primarily N-desmethyldiazepam (active)

Usual Dosage Oral:

Geriatrics: Initial: 5 mg 2-3 times/day

Adults: 30 mg/day in divided doses; may increase gradually to 60 mg/day

Monitoring Parameters Respiratory, cardiovascular and mental status, symptoms of anxiety

Patient Information Avoid alcohol and other CNS depressants; may cause drowsiness; avoid activities needing good psychomotor coordination until CNS effects are known; may cause physical or psychological dependence; avoid abrupt discontinuation after prolonged use

Nursing Implications Assist patient with ambulation, monitor for alertness

Additional Information Prazepam offers no significant advantage over other benzodiazepines

Special Geriatric Considerations Because of its long-acting metabolite, prazepam is not considered a drug of choice in the elderly (see Pharmacokinetics and Pharmacodynamics); long-acting benzodiazepines have been associated with falls in the elderly; interpretive guidelines from the Health Care Financing Administration (HCFA) discourage the use of this agent in residents of long-term care facilities

Dosage Forms

Capsule: 5 mg, 10 mg, 20 mg

Tablet: 10 mg

References

Allen MD, Greenblatt DJ, Harmatz JS, et al, "Desmethyldiazepam Kinetics in the Elderly After Oral Prazepam," *Clin Pharmacol Ther,* 1986, 28:196-202.

Prazosin (PRA zoe sin)

Brand Names Minipress®

Synonyms Furazosin

Generic Available Yes

Therapeutic Category Alpha-Adrenergic Blocking Agent, Oral; Vasodilator, Coronary

Use Hypertension

Unlabeled use: Severe congestive heart failure (in conjunction with diuretics and cardiac glycosides), overflow incontinence secondary to prostatic obstruction; Raynaud's vasospasm

Contraindications Hypersensitivity to prazosin or any component

Warnings Can cause marked hypotension and syncope with sudden loss of consciousness with the first few doses. Anticipate a similar effect if therapy is interrupted for a few days, if dosage is increased rapidly, or if another antihypertensive drug is introduced.

Precautions Marked orthostatic hypotension, syncope, and loss of consciousness may occur with first dose ("first-dose phenomenon"). This reaction is more likely to occur in patients receiving beta-blockers, diuretics, low sodium diets or larger first doses (ie, >1 mg/dose in adults); avoid rapid increase in dose; use with caution in patients with renal impairment.

Adverse Reactions

Cardiovascular: Orthostatic hypotension, syncope, palpitations, tachycardia, edema

Central nervous system: Dizziness, lightheadedness, nightmares, drowsiness, headache

Dermatologic: Rash

Endocrine & metabolic: Fluid retention

Gastrointestinal: Nausea, xerostomia

Genitourinary: Polyuria, priapism, sexual dysfunction

Neuromuscular & skeletal: Weakness

Respiratory: Nasal congestion

Miscellaneous: Hypothermia

Overdosage Symptoms of overdose include hypotension and drowsiness

Toxicology Hypotension usually responds to I.V. fluids or Trendelenburg positioning. If unresponsive to these measures the use of a parenteral vasoconstrictor may be required (eg, norepinephrine 0.1-0.2 mcg/kg/minute titrated to response). Treatment is primarily supportive and symptomatic.

Drug Interactions Increased effect (hypotensive) with diuretics and antihypertensive medications (especially beta-blockers)

Mechanism of Action Competitively inhibits postsynaptic alpha$_1$-adrenergic receptors which results in vasodilation of veins and arterioles and a decrease in total peripheral resistance and blood pressure; in the treatment of BPH, improvement in symptoms and urine flow is due to the relaxation of smooth muscle produced by the alpha$_1$ blockade in the bladder neck and prostate; since the bladder body does not have many alpha receptors, contractility is not affected

Pharmacodynamics
Onset of hypotensive effect: Within 2 hours; maximum decrease: 2-4 hours
Duration: 10-24 hours

Pharmacokinetics
Distribution: V_d: 0.5 L/kg (hypertensive adults)
Protein binding: 92% to 97%
Metabolism: Extensive in the liver; metabolites may be active
Bioavailability: Oral: 43% to 82%
Half-life: 2-4 hours; increased half-life with congestive heart failure
Elimination: 6% to 10% excreted renally as unchanged drug
In the elderly, half-life and volume of distribution may be increased and the oral absorption decreased, though the clinical significance is unknown

Usual Dosage Oral (first dose given at bedtime):
Geriatrics: Initial: 1 mg 1-2 times/day
Adults: Initial: 1 mg/dose 2-3 times/day; usual maintenance dose: 3-15 mg/day in divided doses 2-4 times/day; maximum daily dose: 20 mg

Monitoring Parameters Blood pressure, standing and sitting/supine

Patient Information Rise from sitting/lying carefully, may cause dizziness; take first dose at bedtime

Nursing Implications Syncope may occur usually within 90 minutes of the initial dose; administer initial dose at bedtime (see Monitoring Parameters)

Special Geriatric Considerations Adverse effects such as dry mouth and urinary problems can be particularly bothersome in the elderly (see Warnings and Pharmacokinetics)

Dosage Forms Capsule, as hydrochloride: 1 mg, 2 mg, 5 mg

References
Rubin PC, Scott PJ, and Reid JL, "Prazosin Disposition in Young and Elderly Subjects," *Br J Clin Pharmacol*, 1981, 12(3):401-4.

Precose® see Acarbose on page 14

Predaject® **Injection** see Prednisolone on next page

Predalone Injection see Prednisolone on next page

Predcor-TBA® **Injection** see Prednisolone on next page

Pred Forte® **Ophthalmic** see Prednisolone on next page

Pred-G® **Ophthalmic** see Prednisolone and Gentamicin on page 776

Pred Mild® **Ophthalmic** see Prednisolone on next page

Prednicarbate (PRED ni kar bate)

Brand Names Dermatop®

Generic Available No

Therapeutic Category Corticosteroid, Topical (Medium Potency)

Use Relief of the inflammatory and pruritic manifestations of corticosteroid-responsive dermatoses

Contraindications Hypersensitivity to prednicarbate or any component; fungal, viral, or tubercular skin lesions, herpes simplex or zoster

Precautions Systemic absorption of topical corticosteroids has produced reversible HPA axis suppression. This is more likely to occur when the preparation is used on large surface or denuded areas for prolonged periods of time or with an occlusive dressing.

Adverse Reactions
Dermatologic: Acne, hypopigmentation, allergic dermatitis, maceration of the skin, skin atrophy, striae, miliaria, telangiectasia
Endocrine & metabolic: HPA suppression, Cushing's syndrome, growth retardation
Local: Burning, itching, irritation, dryness, folliculitis, hypertrichosis
Miscellaneous: Secondary infection
(Continued)

Prednicarbate *(Continued)*

Mechanism of Action Topical corticosteroids have anti-inflammatory, anti-pruritic, vasoconstrictive, and antiproliferative actions

Usual Dosage Geriatrics and Adults: Topical: Apply a thin film to affected area twice daily

Monitoring Parameters Relief of symptoms

Patient Information Use only as prescribed and for no longer than the period prescribed; apply sparingly in a thin film and rub in lightly; avoid contact with eyes; notify physician if condition persists or worsens

Nursing Implications Use sparingly

Additional Information Considered a moderate-potency steroid; has been shown that the atrophic activity of prednicarbate is many times less than agents with similar clinical potency, nevertheless, avoid prolonged use on the face

Special Geriatric Considerations Due to age-related changes in skin, limit use of topical corticosteroids (see Precautions)

Dosage Forms Cream: 0.1% (15 g, 60 g)

References
Rumbaugh MM, "High Potency Topical Corticosteroids," *US Pharmacist*, 1993, 18(6):30-41.

Prednicen-M® *see* Prednisone *on page 776*

Prednisolone *(pred NIS oh lone)*

Related Information
Antacid Drug Interactions *on page 1096*
Asthma Guidelines *on page 1040*
Corticosteroids Comparison, Systemic *on page 1029*

Brand Names AK-Pred® Ophthalmic; Articulose-50® Injection; Delta-Cortef® Oral; Econopred® Ophthalmic; Econopred® Plus Ophthalmic; Inflamase® Forte Ophthalmic; Inflamase® Mild Ophthalmic; Key-Pred® Injection; Key-Pred-SP® Injection; Metreton® Ophthalmic; Pediapred® Oral; Predaject® Injection; Predalone Injection; Predcor-TBA® Injection; Pred Forte® Ophthalmic; Pred Mild® Ophthalmic; Prednisol® TBA Injection; Prelone® Oral

Synonyms Deltahydrocortisone; Metacortandralone

Generic Available Yes

Therapeutic Category Adrenal Corticosteroid; Anti-inflammatory Agent; Anti-inflammatory Agent, Ophthalmic; Corticosteroid, Ophthalmic; Corticosteroid, Systemic

Use Treatment of palpebral and bulbar conjunctivitis; corneal injury from chemical, radiation, thermal burns, or foreign body penetration; endocrine disorders, rheumatic disorders, collagen diseases, dermatologic diseases, allergic states, ophthalmic diseases, respiratory diseases, hematologic disorders, neoplastic diseases, edematous states, and gastrointestinal diseases; useful in patients unable to activate prednisone (ie, liver disease)

Contraindications Acute superficial herpes simplex keratitis; systemic fungal infections; varicella; hypersensitivity to prednisolone or any component

Precautions Use with caution in patients with hypothyroidism, cirrhosis, hypertension, congestive heart failure, nonspecific ulcerative colitis, thromboembolic disorders and in patients at increased risk for peptic ulcer disease; gradually taper dose to withdraw therapy

Adverse Reactions
Cardiovascular: Hypertension, edema, accelerated atherogenesis
Central nervous system: Euphoria, mental changes, headache, vertigo, seizures, psychoses, pseudotumor cerebri
Dermatologic: Folliculitis, hypertrichosis, acneiform eruption dermatitis, maceration, skin atrophy, acne, impaired wound healing, hirsutism, striae, miliaria, telangiectasia
Endocrine & metabolic: Growth suppression, Cushing's syndrome, pituitary-adrenal axis suppression, alkalosis, glucose intolerance, hypokalemia, postmenopausal bleeding, hot flashes
Gastrointestinal: Peptic ulcer, nausea, vomiting, pancreatitis
Local: Burning, irritation
Neuromuscular & skeletal: Muscle weakness, osteoporosis, fractures, aseptic necrosis of femoral and humeral heads, steroid myopathy
Ocular: Cataracts, glaucoma
Miscellaneous: Increased susceptibility to infection

Toxicology When consumed in excessive quantities for prolonged periods, systemic hypercorticism and adrenal suppression may occur; in those cases, discontinuation and withdrawal of the corticosteroid should be done judiciously

Drug Interactions

Steroids decrease the effect of anticholinesterases, isoniazid, salicylates, insulin, oral hypoglycemics

Decreased effect: Barbiturates, phenytoin, rifampin

Increased effect (hypokalemia) of potassium-depleting diuretics

Increased risk of digoxin toxicity (due to hypokalemia)

Increased effect: Estrogens, ketoconazole

Mechanism of Action Decreases inflammation by suppression of migration of polymorphonuclear leukocytes and reversal of increased capillary permeability; suppresses the immune system by reducing activity and volume of the lymphatic system

Pharmacokinetics

Half-life: 3.6 hours; biologic: 18-36 hours

Protein binding: 65% to 91% (concentration dependent)

Metabolism: Primarily in the liver, but also metabolized in most tissues, to inactive compounds

Elimination: In urine principally as glucuronides, sulfates, and unconjugated metabolites

Usual Dosage Dose depends upon condition being treated and response of patient; alternate day dosing may be attempted in some disease states

Geriatrics: Use the lowest effective dose

Adults:

Oral, I.M.: 5-60 mg/day

Rheumatoid arthritis: Oral: Initial: 5-7.5 mg/day; adjust dose as necessary

Ophthalmic suspension: Instill 1-2 drops into conjunctival sac every hour during day, every 2 hours at night until favorable response is obtained, then use 1 drop every 4 hours

Monitoring Parameters Blood pressure, blood glucose, electrolytes, symptoms of fluid retention; if ophthalmic product is used more than 10 days, monitor intraocular pressure

Test Interactions Increased amylase (S), chloride (S), increased cholesterol (S), increased glucose, increased protein, increased sodium (S); decreased calcium (S), decreased chloride (S), decreased potassium (S), decreased thyroxine (S)

Patient Information Take oral form after meals or with food or milk; do not abruptly discontinue if on long-term therapy; carry an identification card or bracelet advising that you are on steroids; notify physician of any signs of infection

Nursing Implications Administer with food or milk; parenteral product is not for I.V. use - only administer I.M., intralesional, intra-articular, or soft tissue injections

Additional Information

Prednisolone: Cortalone®, Delta-Cortef®, Prelone®

Prednisolone acetate: Key-Pred®, Predaject®, Predate®, Predcor®

Prednisolone acetate, ophthalmic: AK-Tate®, Econopred®, Econopred® Plus, Ocu-Pred®, Pred Forte®, Pred Mild®

Prednisolone sodium phosphate: Hydeltrasol®, Key-Pred-SP®, Nor-Pred S®, Predate® S

Prednisolone sodium phosphate, ophthalmic: AK-Pred®, Inflamase®, Inflamase® Mild, I-Pred®, Predair®

Prednisolone tebutate: Hydeltra-T.B.A.®, Nor-Pred T.B.A.®, Predalone T.B.A.®, Predate® TBA, Predcor-TBA®

Special Geriatric Considerations Useful in patients with inability to activate prednisone (liver disease). Because of the risk of adverse effects, systemic corticosteroids should be used cautiously in the elderly, in the smallest possible dose, and for the shortest possible time.

Dosage Forms

Prednisolone acetate:

Injection: 25 mg/mL (10 mL, 30 mL); 50 mg/mL (10 mL, 30 mL); 100 mg/mL (10 mL)

Suspension, ophthalmic: 0.12% (5 mL, 10 mL); 0.125% (5 mL, 10 mL); 1% (1 mL, 5 mL, 10 mL, 15 mL)

Prednisolone sodium phosphate:

Injection: 20 mg/mL (2 mL, 5 mL, 10 mL)

Liquid, oral: 5 mg/5 mL (120 mL)

Solution, ophthalmic: 0.125% (5 mL, 10 mL, 15 mL); 0.5% (5 mL)

Injection, as tebutate: 20 mg/mL (1 mL, 5 mL, 10 mL)

Syrup: 15 mg/5 mL (240 mL)

Tablet: 5 mg

Prednisolone Acetate and Sodium Sulfacetamide *see* Sulfacetamide Sodium and Prednisolone *on page 875*

Prednisolone and Gentamicin
(pred NIS oh lone & jen ta MYE sin)

Related Information
Gentamicin *on page 422*
Prednisolone *on page 774*

Brand Names Pred-G® Ophthalmic

Synonyms Gentamicin and Prednisolone

Therapeutic Category Antibiotic, Ophthalmic; Corticosteroid, Ophthalmic

Use Treatment of steroid responsive inflammatory conditions and superficial ocular infections due to strains of microorganisms susceptible to gentamicin

Contraindications Known hypersensitivity to a drug component, dendritic keratitis, fungal diseases, vaccinia, varicella and most other viral infections, mycobacterial infection of the eye. The product's use is contraindicated after uncomplicated removal of a corneal foreign body.

Warnings Prolonged use may result in glaucoma, damage to the optic nerve, defects in visual acuity, posterior subcapsular cataract formation, and secondary ocular infections

Adverse Reactions
Local: Burning, stinging
Ocular: Elevation of intraocular pressure, glaucoma, infrequent optic nerve damage, posterior subcapsular cataract formation, superficial punctate keratitis
Miscellaneous: Delayed wound healing, development of secondary infection, allergic sensitization

Usual Dosage Geriatrics and Adults: Ophthalmic: Instill 1 drop 2-4 times/day; during the initial 24-48 hours, the dosing frequency may be increased if necessary

Monitoring Parameters With use >10 days, monitor intraocular pressure

Nursing Implications Shake well before using

Special Geriatric Considerations No specific recommendations for use in elderly necessary

Dosage Forms
Ointment, ophthalmic: Prednisolone acetate 0.6% and gentamicin sulfate 0.3% (3.5 g)
Suspension, ophthalmic: Prednisolone acetate 1% and gentamicin sulfate 0.3% (2 mL, 5 mL, 10 mL)

Prednisol® TBA Injection *see* Prednisolone *on page 774*

Prednisone (PRED ni sone)

Related Information
Antacid Drug Interactions *on page 1096*
Asthma Guidelines *on page 1040*
Corticosteroids Comparison, Systemic *on page 1029*

Brand Names Deltasone®; Liquid Pred®; Meticorten®; Orasone®; Prednicen-M®; Sterapred®

Synonyms Deltacortisone; Deltadehydrocortisone

Generic Available Yes

Therapeutic Category Adrenal Corticosteroid; Anti-inflammatory Agent; Corticosteroid, Systemic

Use Treatment of a variety of diseases including adrenocortical insufficiency, hypercalcemia, rheumatic and collagen disorders, dermatologic, ocular, respiratory, gastrointestinal and neoplastic diseases, organ transplantation and a variety of diseases including those of hematologic, allergic, inflammatory, and autoimmune in origin

Contraindications Serious infections, except septic shock or tuberculous meningitis; systemic fungal infections; hypersensitivity to prednisone or any component; varicella

Precautions Use with caution in patients with hypothyroidism, cirrhosis, hypertension, congestive heart failure, nonspecific ulcerative colitis, thromboembolic disorders, and patients at increased risk for peptic ulcer disease; gradually taper dose to withdraw therapy

Adverse Reactions
Cardiovascular: Hypertension, edema, accelerated atherogenesis
Central nervous system: Euphoria, mental changes, headache, vertigo, seizures, psychoses, pseudotumor cerebri

Dermatologic: Folliculitis, hypertrichosis, acneiform eruption dermatitis, maceration, skin atrophy, acne, impaired wound healing, hirsutism

Endocrine & metabolic: Growth suppression, Cushing's syndrome, pituitary-adrenal axis suppression, alkalosis, glucose intolerance, hypokalemia, postmenopausal bleeding, hot flashes

Gastrointestinal: Peptic ulcer, nausea, vomiting, pancreatitis

Neuromuscular & skeletal: Muscle weakness, osteoporosis, fractures, aseptic necrosis of femoral and humeral heads, steroid myopathy

Ocular: Cataracts, glaucoma

Miscellaneous: Increased susceptibility to infection

Toxicology When consumed in excessive quantities for prolonged periods, systemic hypercorticism and adrenal suppression may occur; in those cases, discontinuation and withdrawal of the corticosteroid should be done judiciously

Drug Interactions

Steroids decrease the effect of anticholinesterases, isoniazid, salicylates, insulin, oral hypoglycemics

Decreased effect: Barbiturates, phenytoin, rifampin

Increased effect (hypokalemia) of potassium-depleting diuretics

Increased risk of digoxin toxicity (due to hypokalemia)

Increased effect: Estrogens, ketoconazole

Mechanism of Action Decreases inflammation by suppression of migration of polymorphonuclear leukocytes and reversal of increased capillary permeability; suppresses the immune system by reducing activity and volume of the lymphatic system; suppresses adrenal function at high doses

Pharmacokinetics Converted rapidly to prednisolone in the liver (active); see Prednisolone for full kinetic information

Usual Dosage Oral (dose depends upon condition being treated and response of patient; alternate day dosing may be attempted):

Geriatrics: Use the lowest effective dose

Adults: 5-60 mg/day in divided doses 1-4 times/day

Monitoring Parameters Blood pressure, blood glucose, electrolytes, symptoms of fluid retention

Test Interactions Increased amylase (S), chloride (S), increased cholesterol (S), increased glucose, increased protein, increased sodium (S); decreased calcium (S), decreased chloride (S), decreased potassium (S), decreased thyroxine (S)

Patient Information Take with food or milk or after meals; do not discontinue or decrease the drug without contacting your physician; carry an identification card or bracelet advising that you are on steroids; notify physician if signs of infection occur

Nursing Implications Administer with meals to decrease GI upset; withdraw therapy with gradual tapering of dose

Additional Information Not available in injectable form, prednisolone must be used

Special Geriatric Considerations Because of the risk of adverse effects, systemic corticosteroids should be used cautiously in the elderly, in the smallest possible dose, and for the shortest possible time

Dosage Forms

Solution:

Concentrate: 5 mg/mL (5 mL, 30 mL)

Oral: 5 mg/5 mL (10 mL, 20 mL, 500 mL)

Syrup: 5 mg/5 mL (120 mL, 240 mL)

Tablet: 1 mg, 2.5 mg, 5 mg, 10 mg, 20 mg, 50 mg

Primaclone see Primidone on this page
Primatene® Mist [OTC] see Epinephrine on page 336
Primaxin® see Imipenem and Cilastatin on page 478

Primidone (PRI mi done)

Related Information
Serum Drug Concentrations Commonly Monitored: Guidelines on page 1114

Brand Names Mysoline®

Synonyms Desoxyphenobarbital; Primaclone

Generic Available Yes: Tablet

Therapeutic Category Anticonvulsant, Barbiturate

Use Management of grand mal, complex partial, and psychomotor or focal seizures

Unlabeled use: Benign familial tremor (essential tremor)

Contraindications Hypersensitivity to primidone, phenobarbital, or any component; porphyria

Warnings Do not abruptly withdraw therapy

Precautions Use with caution in patients with renal or hepatic impairment, pulmonary insufficiency; monitor for hematologic effects every 6 months; drowsiness may occur, therefore, patients should exercise caution when performing hazardous tasks

Adverse Reactions
Central nervous system: Drowsiness, vertigo, ataxia, lethargy, behavior change (mood changes with paranoia)
Dermatologic: Rash
Gastrointestinal: Nausea, vomiting
Genitourinary: Impotence
Hematologic: Leukopenia, malignant lymphoma-like syndrome, megaloblastic anemia
Ocular: Diplopia, nystagmus
Miscellaneous: Systemic lupus-like syndrome

Overdosage Symptoms of overdose include unsteady gait, slurred speech, confusion, jaundice, hypothermia, fever, hypotension

Toxicology Repeated oral doses of activated charcoal significantly reduces the half-life of primidone resulting from an enhancement of nonrenal elimination. The usual dose is 30-60 g every 4-6 hours for 3-4 days unless the patient has no bowel movement causing the charcoal to remain in the GI tract. Assure adequate hydration and renal function. Urinary alkalinization with I.V. sodium bicarbonate also helps to enhance elimination. Hemodialysis or hemoperfusion is of uncertain value. Patients in stage IV coma due to high serum drug concentrations may require charcoal hemoperfusion.

Drug Interactions
Primidone may decrease serum concentrations of ethosuximide, lamotrigine, valproic acid, griseofulvin
Succinimides may also decrease primidone and phenobarbital serum concentrations
Methylphenidate, nicotinamide, and isoniazid may increase primidone serum concentrations
Phenytoin (hydantoins) may increase primidone serum concentrations
Valproic acid may increase phenobarbital concentrations derived from primidone
Acetazolamide decrease primidone concentrations
Primidone and carbamazepine concomitantly given together may influence each others serum concentration (decrease or increased)

Stability Protect from light

Mechanism of Action Decreases neuron excitability, raises seizure threshold similar to phenobarbital; primidone has two active metabolites, phenobarbital and phenylethylmalonamide (PEMA); PEMA may enhance the activity of phenobarbital

Pharmacokinetics
Distribution: V_d: 2-3L/kg (adults)
Protein binding: 99%
Metabolism: In the liver to phenobarbital (active) and phenylethylmalonamide (PEMA); inducer of CYP1A2, 2B6, 2C8, 3A4
Bioavailability: 60% to 80%
Half-life:
Primidone: 10-12 hours
PEMA: 16 hours

Phenobarbital: 52-118 hours (age-dependent with elderly generally having the longer half-life)

Time to peak serum concentration: Oral: Within 4 hours

Elimination: Urinary excretion of both active metabolites and unchanged primidone (15% to 25%)

Usual Dosage Geriatrics and Adults: Oral:

Initial: 125-250 mg/day at bedtime; increase by 125-250 mg/day every 3-7 days

Usual dose: 750-1500 mg/day in divided doses 3-4 times/day with maximum dosage of 2 g/day

Essential tremor: 750 mg early in divided doses (see Additional Information)

Dosing interval in renal impairment:

Cl_{cr} 50-80 mL/minute: Administer every 8 hours

Cl_{cr} 10-50 mL/minute: Administer every 8-12 hours

Cl_{cr} <10 mL/minute: Administer every 12-24 hours

Moderately dialyzable (20% to 50%)

Monitoring Parameters Monitor CBC, serum concentrations of primidone, and if applicable, other anticonvulsants when given concomitantly

Reference Range

Therapeutic: Adults: 5-12 µg/mL (SI: 23-55 µmol/L); Toxic effects rarely present with serum concentrations <10 µg/mL (SI: 46 µmol/L) if phenobarbital concentrations are low

Dosage of primidone is adjusted with reference mostly to the phenobarbital serum concentration

Toxic: >15 µg/mL (SI: >69 µmol/L)

Test Interactions Increased alkaline phosphatase (S); decreased calcium (S)

Patient Information May cause drowsiness; if stomach upset occurs, take with food; do not stop therapy without consulting physician

Nursing Implications Observe patient for excessive sedation (see Monitoring Parameters and Reference Range)

Additional Information Bioequivalence problems have been noted with primidone from one manufacturer to another, therefore, brand interchange is not recommended

Special Geriatric Considerations Due to CNS effects, monitor closely when initiating drug in elderly (see Adverse Reactions). Monitor CBC at 6-month intervals to compare with baseline obtained at start of therapy. Since elderly metabolize phenobarbital at a slower rate than younger adults, it is suggested to measure both primidone and phenobarbital serum concentrations together. Adjust dose for renal function in elderly when initiating or changing dose.

Dosage Forms

Suspension, oral: 250 mg/5 mL (240 mL)

Tablet: 50 mg, 250 mg

Principen® *see* Ampicillin *on page 73*

Prinivil® *see* Lisinopril *on page 543*

Privine® Nasal [OTC] *see* Naphazoline *on page 653*

Probalan® *see* Probenecid *on this page*

Pro-Banthine® *see* Propantheline *on page 794*

Proben-C® *see* Colchicine and Probenecid *on page 249*

Probenecid (proe BEN e sid)

Brand Names Benemid®; Probalan®

Generic Available Yes

Therapeutic Category Adjuvant Therapy, Penicillin Level Prolongation; Uric Acid Lowering Agent

Use Prevention of gouty arthritis; hyperuricemia; prolong serum concentration of penicillin/cephalosporin

Contraindications Hypersensitivity to probenecid or any component; high dose aspirin therapy; moderate to severe renal impairment

Precautions Rapid lowering of uric acid may precipitate acute gout; use with caution in patients with peptic ulcer; use extreme caution in the use of probenecid with penicillin in patients with renal insufficiency; probenecid may not be effective in patients with a Cl_{cr} <30 mL/minute

Adverse Reactions

Cardiovascular: Flushing

Central nervous system: Dizziness, headache

Dermatologic: Rash

Gastrointestinal: Anorexia, nausea, vomiting

Genitourinary: Polyuria, uric acid stones

(Continued)

Probenecid *(Continued)*

Hematologic: Anemia, leukopenia
Hepatic: Hepatic necrosis
Renal: Nephrotic syndrome

Overdosage Symptoms of overdose include nausea, vomiting, tonic-clonic seizures, coma

Toxicology Activated charcoal is especially effective at binding probenecid

Drug Interactions
Decreased effect with high-dose salicylates
Increased effect/toxicity of acyclovir, thiopental, benzodiazepines, dapsone, methotrexate, sulfonylureas, zidovudine, penicillins, and cephalosporins

Mechanism of Action Competitively inhibits the reabsorption of uric acid at the proximal convoluted tubule, thereby promoting its excretion and reducing serum uric acid levels; increases plasma levels of weak organic acids (penicillins, cephalosporins or other beta-lactam antibiotics) by competitively inhibiting their renal tubular secretion

Pharmacodynamics Onset of action: Effect on penicillin levels is reached in about 2 hours

Pharmacokinetics
Absorption: Rapid and complete from GI tract
Metabolism: In the liver
Half-life: 6-12 hours (dose dependent)
Time to peak: Within 2-4 hours
Elimination: In urine

Usual Dosage Geriatrics and Adults: Oral:
Hyperuricemia: 250 mg twice daily for one week; increase by 250-500 mg/day until uric acid normalizes; maximum: 2-3 g/day
Prolongation of penicillin serum levels: 500 mg 4 times/day
Dosing adjustment in renal impairment: Cl_{cr} <30 mL/minute: Avoid use

Monitoring Parameters Uric acid, renal function, CBC

Test Interactions False-positive glucosuria with Clinitest®

Patient Information Take with food or antacids; drink plenty of fluids to reduce the risk of uric acid stones; the frequency of acute gouty attacks may increase during the first 6-12 months of therapy; avoid taking large doses of aspirin or other salicylates

Nursing Implications Administer with food or antacids

Special Geriatric Considerations Since probenecid loses its effectiveness when the Cl_{cr} is <30 mL/minute, its usefulness in the elderly is limited

Dosage Forms Tablet: 500 mg

Probenecid and Colchicine *see* Colchicine and Probenecid *on page 249*

Procainamide *(proe kane A mide)*

Related Information
I.V. Push Recommended Guidelines *on page 1083*
Serum Drug Concentrations Commonly Monitored: Guidelines *on page 1114*

Brand Names Procanbid®; Promine®; Pronestyl®; Rhythmin®

Synonyms PCA; Procaine Amide Hydrochloride

Generic Available Yes

Therapeutic Category Antiarrhythmic Agent, Class I-A

Use Ventricular tachycardia, premature ventricular contractions considered life-threatening, paroxysmal atrial tachycardia, and atrial fibrillation; to prevent recurrence of ventricular tachycardia, paroxysmal supraventricular tachycardia, atrial fibrillation or flutter

Contraindications Complete heart block; second or third degree heart block without pacemaker; torsade de pointes (twisting of the points) an unusual ventricular tachycardia; prolonged Q-T syndrome; hypokalemia; hypersensitivity to the drug or procaine, or related drugs; myasthenia gravis; SLE

Warnings Long-term administration leads to the development of a positive antinuclear antibody test in 50% of patients which may lead to a lupus erythematosus-like syndrome (in 20% to 30% of patients); assess relative benefits and risks if ANA titer becomes positive and consider alternative agent; discontinue PCA with SLE symptoms and change to alternative agent; serious blood dyscrasias have been reported; neutropenia and granulocytosis induced on rare occasions and associated more commonly with sustained release products; proarrhythmic potential is low

Precautions Marked A-V conduction disturbances, bundle-branch block or severe cardiac glycoside intoxication, ventricular arrhythmias in patients with organic heart disease or coronary occlusion, supraventricular tachyarrhythmias unless digitalis levels adequate to prevent marked increases in ventricular rates; drug may accumulate in patients with renal or hepatic dysfunction; some tablets contain tartrazine; injection may contain bisulfite

Adverse Reactions

Cardiovascular: Pericarditis, flushing, hypotension, tachycardia, arrhythmias, A-V block, Q-T prolongation, widening QRS complex

Central nervous system: Lightheadedness, fever, clouded sensorium, inability to concentrate, confusion, disorientation, depression, psychosis, hallucination, fatigue

Dermatologic: Rash, urticaria, pruritus

Gastrointestinal: Nausea, vomiting, GI complaints, anorexia, diarrhea, abdominal pain, bitter taste

Hematologic: Agranulocytosis, neutropenia, thrombocytopenia, positive ANA titer in 70% or more of patients

Hepatic: Positive Coombs' test

Neuromuscular & skeletal: Arthralgia, myalgia

Respiratory: Pleural effusion

Miscellaneous: Drug fever, systemic lupus erythematosus

Overdosage Symptoms of overdose include hypotension, widening of QRS complex, junctional tachycardia, intraventricular conduction delay, oliguria, lethargy, confusion

Toxicology Hypotension usually responds to I.V. fluids or Trendelenburg positioning. If unresponsive to these measures the use of a parenteral inotrope may be required (eg, norepinephrine 0.1-0.2 mcg/kg/minute titrated to response). Concurrent sodium bicarbonate and sodium lactate infusions have been effective in reversing the drug-induced cardiac toxicity.

Drug Interactions

Cimetidine, ranitidine, trimethoprim, and amiodarone may increase plasma PCA and NAPA concentrations, PCA dosage adjustment may be required

PCA may potentiate skeletal muscle relaxants and anticholinergic drugs may have enhanced effects

Propranolol may increase PCA levels

PCA may enhance neuromuscular blockade of succinylcholine

May enhance quinidine and lidocaine cardiac response (depression)

Stability Use only clear or slightly yellow solutions; stability of parenteral admixture at room temperature (25°C) and refrigeration (4°C): 24 hours

Mechanism of Action Decreases myocardial excitability and conduction velocity and depresses myocardial contractility, by increasing the electrical stimulation threshold of ventricle, HIS-Purkinje system and through direct cardiac effects

Pharmacodynamics Onset of action: I.M.: 10-30 minutes

Pharmacokinetics

Protein binding: 15% to 20%

Distribution: V_d: 2 L/kg, decreased V_d with congestive heart failure or shock

Metabolism: By acetylation in the liver to produce N-acetyl procainamide (NAPA) (active metabolite)

Bioavailability: 75% to 95% orally

Half-life (PCA):

Adults with normal renal function: 2.5-4.7 hours; half-life dependent upon hepatic acetylator phenotype, cardiac function, and renal function

NAPA (adults with normal renal function): 6-8 hours

Anephric half-life (procainamide): 11 hours

NAPA: 42 hours; half-life for procainamide and NAPA increases with age; clearance is 4.3 L/minute/kg for patients >60 years, whereas those younger have a clearance of procainamide of 7.7 L/minute/kg

Time to peak:

Capsule: Within 45 minutes to 2.5 hours

I.M.: 15-60 minutes

Elimination: Urinary excretion (25% as NAPA)

Usual Dosage Geriatrics and Adults: Must be titrated to patient's response

Oral: 250-500 mg/dose every 3-6 hours or 500 mg to 1 g every 6 hours sustained release; usual dose: 50 mg/kg/24 hours or 2-4 g/24 hours; must individualize dose; if possible, start with lowest doses in elderly

I.V.: Load: 50-100 mg/dose, repeated every 5-10 minutes until patient controlled; or load with 15-18 mg/kg, maximum loading dose: 1-1.5 g; maintenance: 2-6 mg/minute continuous I.V. infusion, usual maintenance: 3-4 mg/minute; use lowest recommended doses for elderly

Patients with chronic hepatic disease have a reduced urinary clearance of PCA, therefore, reduce dose 50%

(Continued)

Procainamide (Continued)

Dosing interval in renal impairment:
Cl$_{cr}$ 10-50 mL/minute: Administer every 6-12 hours
Cl$_{cr}$ <10 mL/minute: Administer every 8-24 hours
Moderately dialyzable (20% to 50%)

Monitoring Parameters Blood pressure, apical pulse, pulse, EKG; monitor for SLE, obtain CBC to monitor WBC every 2 weeks for first 3 months of treatment

Reference Range
Therapeutic: 4.9-12 µg/mL (SI: 15-37 µmol/L) for procainamide, <30 µg/mL (SI: <127 µmol/L) for sum of procainamide and NAPA. Optimal ranges must be ascertained for individual patients, with EKG monitoring; Toxic: >10-12 µg/mL (SI: >42-51 µmol/L).

Patient Information Do not discontinue therapy unless instructed by physician; notify physician or pharmacist if soreness of mouth, throat or gums, unexplained fever, symptoms of upper respiratory tract infection. Do not break or chew sustained release tablets. Sustained release tablets contain a wax core that slowly releases the drug. When this process is complete, the empty, nonabsorbable wax core is eliminated.

Nursing Implications Dilute I.V. with D$_5$W; maximum rate: 25-50 mg/minute

Special Geriatric Considerations Monitor closely since clearance is reduced in those >60 years of age; if clinically possible, start doses at lowest recommended dose; also, elderly frequently have drug therapy which may interfere with the use of procainamide; adjust dose for renal function in elderly (see Drug Interactions, Pharmacokinetics, and Usual Dosage)

Dosage Forms
Procainamide hydrochloride:
Capsule: 250 mg, 375 mg, 500 mg
Injection: 100 mg/mL (10 mL); 500 mg/mL (2 mL)
Tablet: 250 mg, 375 mg, 500 mg
Tablet, sustained release: 250 mg, 500 mg, 750 mg, 1000 mg
Tablet, sustained release (Procanbid®): 500 mg, 1000 mg

References
Fenster PE and Nolan PE, "Antiarrhythmic Drugs," *Geriatric Pharmacology*, Bressler R and Katz MD, eds, New York, NY: McGraw-Hill, 1993, 6:105-49.

Procaine Amide Hydrochloride *see* Procainamide *on page 780*

Procaine Benzylpenicillin *see* Penicillin G Procaine *on page 723*

Procaine Penicillin G *see* Penicillin G Procaine *on page 723*

Pro-Cal-Sof® [OTC] *see* Docusate *on page 312*

Procanbid® *see* Procainamide *on page 780*

Procardia® *see* Nifedipine *on page 671*

Procardia XL® *see* Nifedipine *on page 671*

Prochlorperazine (proe klor PER a zeen)

Related Information
Antacid Drug Interactions *on page 1096*
Antipsychotic Medication Guidelines *on page 1076*
I.V. Push Recommended Guidelines *on page 1083*

Brand Names Compazine®

Generic Available Yes: Injection and tablet

Therapeutic Category Antiemetic; Antipsychotic Agent; Neuroleptic Agent; Phenothiazine Derivative

Use Management of nausea and vomiting; acute and chronic psychosis; nonpsychotic symptoms associated with dementia (not commonly used) (see Special Geriatric Considerations)

Contraindications Hypersensitivity to prochlorperazine or any component; cross-sensitivity with other phenothiazines may exist; avoid use in patients with narrow-angle glaucoma; bone marrow suppression; severe liver or cardiac disease; subcortical brain damage; severe hypotension or hypertension

Warnings High incidence of extrapyramidal reactions occurs; injection contains sulfites which may cause allergic reactions; hypotension with parenteral use

Tardive dyskinesia: Prevalence rate may be 40% in elderly; elderly women especially at risk; embarrassment from dyskinesias may lead to greater social isolation; development of the syndrome and the irreversible nature are proportional to duration and total cumulative dose over time. May be reversible if diagnosed early in therapy; intermittent use of antipsychotics (not proven use) helps decrease total cumulative dose.

EPS: Extrapyramidal reactions are more common in elderly with up to 50% developing these reactions after age 60. These reactions may be more common in dementia patients. Drug-induced **Parkinson's syndrome** occurs often. Discontinuation usually resolves symptoms but may take weeks to months (12+) to clear. **Akathisia** is the most common EPS reaction in elderly. The symptoms of motor restlessness are difficult to diagnose in demented elderly; increased nervousness, assertiveness, restlessness with constant movement may indicate this adverse event. Consider decreasing dose if antipsychotic to treat as well as diagnose problem; usually see this reaction within 2-3 months of initiating antipsychotic drug.

Anticholinergic effects: These side effects most common with low potency antipsychotics (eg, thioridazine, chlorpromazine). CNS toxicity occurs more frequently and severely in elderly; increased confusion, memory loss, psychotic behavior, and agitation frequently occur as a consequence of anticholinergic effects to antipsychotic agents. Peripheral anticholinergic action troublesome to elderly; most peripheral anticholinergic effects last only 2-3 weeks (see Adverse Reactions).

Orthostatic hypotension: More common with low potency agents (eg, thioridazine, chlorpromazine, and clozapine) but of concern with all antipsychotic agents; orthostasis due to alpha-receptor blockade by antipsychotic agents. Elderly present many risk factors for orthostatic hypotension: blunted baroreceptor reflexes, decreased vascular tone, decreased vascular volume, and possible presence of cardiac diseases which result in decreased cardiac output.

Sedation: Common side effect with antipsychotic therapy; should not be used as a hypnotic unless insomnia is associated with target behavior symptoms treated with antipsychotic medications (see Special Geriatric Considerations). Anecdotal reports suggesting antipsychotic sedation in nonpsychotic patients is extremely unpleasant due to feelings of depersonalization, derealization, and dysphoria. Due to the long duration of action with antipsychotic drugs, these reactions may last up to 24 hours and result in decreased daytime function.

Cardiac toxicity: Life-threatening arrhythmias have occurred at therapeutic doses of antipsychotics. Thioridazine more commonly demonstrates EKG changes than other antipsychotics; suggested to use high potency antipsychotic agents (ie, haloperidol) in patients with cardiac conduction defects.

Precautions Extrapyramidal reactions associated with prochlorperazine are relatively high; use with caution in patients with severe cardiovascular disorder, seizures, and Parkinson's disease; benefits of therapy must be weighed against risks

Adverse Reactions

Cardiovascular: Hypotension (especially with I.V. use), orthostatic hypotension, tachycardia, arrhythmias, abnormal T waves with prolonged ventricular repolarization

Central nervous system: Sedation, drowsiness, restlessness, anxiety, extrapyramidal reactions, pseudoparkinsonian signs and symptoms, tardive dyskinesia, neuroleptic malignant syndrome, seizures, altered central temperature regulation

Dermatologic: Hyperpigmentation, pruritus, rash, photosensitivity

Endocrine & metabolic: Amenorrhea, galactorrhea, gynecomastia

Gastrointestinal: GI upset, xerostomia (problem for denture users), constipation, adynamic ileus, weight gain

Genitourinary: Urinary retention, overflow incontinence, priapism, sexual dysfunction (up to 60%), impotence

Hematologic: Agranulocytosis, leukopenia (usually in patients with large doses for prolonged periods), thrombocytopenia, hemolytic anemia, eosinophilia

Hepatic: Cholestatic jaundice (rare)

Ocular: Retinal pigmentation, blurred vision

Miscellaneous: Anaphylactoid reactions

Incidence of extrapyramidal reactions are higher with prochlorperazine than chlorpromazine

Overdosage Symptoms of overdose include deep sleep, coma, extrapyramidal symptoms, abnormal involuntary muscle movements, hypotension or hypertension; agitation, restlessness, fever, hypothermia or hyperthermia, seizures, cardiac arrhythmias, EKG changes

(Continued)

Prochlorperazine *(Continued)*

Toxicology Following initiation of essential overdose management, toxic symptom treatment and supportive treatment should be initiated. Hypotension usually responds to I.V. fluids or Trendelenburg positioning. If unresponsive to these measures the use of a parenteral inotrope may be required (eg, norepinephrine 0.1-0.2 mcg/kg/minute titrated to response). Do not use epinephrine. Seizures commonly respond to diazepam (I.V. 5-10 mg bolus in adults every 15 minutes if needed up to a total of 30 mg) or to phenytoin or phenobarbital. Also critical cardiac arrhythmias often respond to I.V. phenytoin (15 mg/kg up to 1 g), while other antiarrhythmics can be used. Neuroleptics often cause extrapyramidal symptoms (eg, dystonic reactions) requiring management with diphenhydramine 1-2 mg/kg up to a maximum of 50 mg I.M. or I.V. slow push followed by a maintenance dose for 48-72 hours. When these reactions are unresponsive to diphenhydramine, benztropine mesylate I.V. 1-2 mg may be effective. These agents are generally effective within 2-5 minutes.

Drug Interactions

Alcohol may increase CNS sedation

Anticholinergic agents may decrease pharmacologic effects; increase anticholinergic side effects; may enhance tardive dyskinesia

Aluminum salts may decrease absorption of phenothiazines

Barbiturates may decrease phenothiazine serum concentrations

Bromocriptine may have decreased efficacy when administered with phenothiazines

Guanethidine's hypotensive effect is decreased by phenothiazines

Lithium administration with phenothiazines may increase disorientation

Meperidine and phenothiazine coadministration increases sedation and hypotension

Methyldopa administration with phenothiazine (trifluoperazine) may significantly increase blood pressure

Norepinephrine, epinephrine have decreased pressor effect when administered with chlorpromazine; therefore, be aware of possible decreased effectiveness or when any phenothiazine is used

Phenytoin serum concentrations may increase or decrease with phenothiazines; tricyclic antidepressants may have increased serum concentrations with concomitant administration with phenothiazines

Propranolol administered with phenothiazines may increase serum concentrations of both drugs

Valproic acid may have increased half-life when administered with phenothiazines (chlorpromazine)

Stability Protect all dosage forms from light, clear or slightly yellow solutions may be used; should be dispensed in amber or opaque vials/bottles. Solutions may be diluted or mixed with fruit juices or other liquids but must be administered immediately after mixing; do not prepare bulk dilutions or store bulk dilutions.

Mechanism of Action Blocks postsynaptic mesolimbic dopaminergic D_1 and D_2 receptors in the brain, including the medullary chemoreceptor trigger zone; exhibits a strong alpha-adrenergic and anticholinergic blocking effect and depresses the release of hypothalamic and hypophyseal hormones; believed to depress the reticular activating system, thus affecting basal metabolism, body temperature, wakefulness, vasomotor tone and emesis

Pharmacodynamics

Onset of action:

Oral: Within 30-40 minutes

I.M.: Within 10-20 minutes

Rectal: Within 60 minutes

Duration: Effect persists longest with I.M. and oral extended release doses (12 hours) and shortest following rectal and immediate release oral administration (3-4 hours)

Pharmacokinetics

Half-life: 23 hours

Elimination: Primarily by hepatic metabolism

Usual Dosage

Geriatrics (nonpsychotic patient; dementia behavior): Initial: 2.5-5 mg 1-2 times/day; increase dose at 4- to 7-day intervals by 2.5-5 mg/day; increase dosing intervals (bid, tid, etc) as necessary to control response or side effects; maximum daily dose should probably not exceed 75 mg in elderly; gradual increases (titration) may prevent some side effects or decrease their severity

Adults, antiemetic:
Oral: 5-10 mg 3-4 times/day; usual maximum: 40 mg/day; doses up to 150 mg/day may be required in some patients
I.M.: 5-10 mg every 3-4 hours; usual maximum: 40 mg/day; doses up to 10-20 mg every 4-6 hours may be required in some patients; do not dilute with any diluent containing parabens (see Nursing Implications)
I.V.: 2.5-10 mg; maximum 10 mg/dose or 40 mg/day; may repeat dose every 3-4 hours as needed; do not dilute with any diluent containing parabens
Rectal: 25 mg twice daily
Not dialyzable (0% to 5%)

Monitoring Parameters Orthostatic blood pressures; tremors, gait changes, abnormal movement in trunk, neck, buccal area, or extremities; monitor target behaviors for which the agent is given

Test Interactions False-positives for phenylketonuria, urinary amylase, uroporphyrins, urobilinogen

Patient Information Do not take antacid within 1 hour of taking drug; avoid alcohol; avoid excess sun exposure (use sun block); may cause drowsiness, rise slowly from recumbent position; use of supportive stockings may help prevent orthostatic hypotension

Nursing Implications Avoid skin contact with oral suspension or solution; may cause contact dermatitis; monitor orthostatic blood pressures 3-5 days after initiation of therapy or a dose increase; observe for tremor and abnormal movement or posturing (extrapyramidal symptoms)

Special Geriatric Considerations Due to side effect profile (dystonias, EPS) this is not a preferred drug in elderly for antiemetic therapy (see Warnings)

Many elderly patients receive antipsychotic medications for inappropriate nonpsychotic behavior. Before initiating antipsychotic medication, the clinician should investigate any possible reversible cause; any stress or stress from any disease can cause acute "confusion" or worsening of baseline nonpsychotic behavior. Most commonly acute changes in behavior are due to increases in drug dose or addition of new drug to regimen, fluid electrolyte loss, infections, and changes in environment.

Any changes in disease status in any organ system can result in behavior changes.

In the treatment of agitated, demented, elderly patients, authors of meta-analysis of controlled trials of the response to the traditional antipsychotics (phenothiazines, butyrophenones) in controlling agitation have concluded that the use of neuroleptics results in a response rate of 18%. Clearly neuroleptic therapy for behavior control should be limited with frequent attempts to withdraw the agent given for behavior control.

Dosage Forms
Prochlorperazine edisylate:
Injection: 5 mg/mL (2 mL, 10 mL)
Syrup: 5 mg/5 mL (120 mL)
Prochlorperazine maleate:
Capsule, sustained action: 10 mg, 15 mg, 30 mg
Tablet: 5 mg, 10 mg, 25 mg
Suppository, rectal: 2.5 mg, 5 mg, 25 mg

References
Peabody CA, Warner MD, Whiteford HA, et al, "Neuroleptics and the Elderly," *J Am Geriatr Soc*, 1987, 35(3):233-8.
Risse SC and Barnes R, "Pharmacologic Treatment of Agitation Associated With Dementia," *J Am Geriatr Soc*, 1986, 34(5):368-76.
Saltz BL, Woerner MG, Kane JM, et al, "Prospective Study of Tardive Dyskinesia Incidence in the Elderly," *JAMA*, 1991, 266(17):2402-6.
Seifert RD, "Therapeutic Drug Monitoring: Psychotropic Drugs," *J Pharm Pract*, 1984, 6:403-16.

Procort® [OTC] see Hydrocortisone on page 462

Procrit® see Epoetin Alfa on page 338

Proctocort™ see Hydrocortisone on page 462

Procyclidine (proe SYE kli deen)
Brand Names Kemadrin®
Generic Available No
Therapeutic Category Anticholinergic Agent; Anti-Parkinson's Agent
Use Relieve symptoms of parkinsonian syndrome and drug-induced extrapyramidal symptoms
(Continued)

Procyclidine *(Continued)*

Contraindications Patients with narrow-angle glaucoma; hypersensitivity to any component; pyloric or duodenal obstruction, stenosing peptic ulcers; bladder neck obstructions; achalasia; myasthenia gravis

Precautions Use with caution in hot weather or during exercise. Elderly patients frequently develop increased sensitivity and require strict dosage regulation; side effects may be more severe in elderly patients with atherosclerotic changes. Use with caution in patients with tachycardia, cardiac arrhythmias, hypertension, hypotension, prostatic hypertrophy (especially in the elderly) or any tendency toward urinary retention, liver or kidney disorders and obstructive disease of the GI or GU tract. May exacerbate mental symptoms and precipitate a toxic psychosis when used to treat extrapyramidal reactions resulting from phenothiazines. When given in large doses or to susceptible patients, may cause weakness and inability to move particular muscle groups. Anticholinergic agents can aggravate tardive dyskinesia caused by neuroleptic agents.

Adverse Reactions

Cardiovascular: Tachycardia, hypotension

Central nervous system: Lightheadedness, hallucinations, memory loss, drowsiness, nervousness, coma **(elderly may be at increased risk for confusion and hallucinations)**

Gastrointestinal: Xerostomia, nausea, vomiting, constipation

Genitourinary: Urinary hesitancy or retention

Neuromuscular & skeletal: Muscle weakness

Ocular: Blurred vision, mydriasis

Miscellaneous: Heat intolerance

Overdosage Symptoms of overdose include CNS depression, confusion, nervousness, hallucinations, dizziness, blurred vision, nausea, vomiting, hyperthermia

Toxicology Anticholinergic toxicity is caused by strong binding of the drug to cholinergic receptors. Cholinesterase inhibitors reduce acetylcholinesterase, the enzyme that breaks down acetylcholine and thereby allows acetylcholine to accumulate and compete for receptor binding with the offending anticholinergic. For anticholinergic overdose with severe life-threatening symptoms, physostigmine 1-2 mg S.C. or I.V., slowly may be given to reverse these effects.

Drug Interactions

Decreased effect of levodopa (decreased absorption), metoclopramide, cisapride

Increased toxicity (central anticholinergic syndrome): Narcotic analgesics, phenothiazines, and other antipsychotics, tricyclic antidepressants, some antihistamines, quinidine, disopyramide

Antagonistic effect: Tacrine, donepezil

Mechanism of Action Thought to act by blocking excess acetylcholine at cerebral synapses; many of its effects are due to its pharmacologic similarities with atropine

Pharmacodynamics

Onset of action: Oral: Within 30-40 minutes

Duration: 4-6 hours; effects may still be seen at 12 hours after the dose

Pharmacokinetics

Half-life: 12 hours

Metabolism: In the liver

Elimination: In urine

Usual Dosage Oral:

Geriatrics: Initial: 2.5 mg once or twice daily, gradually increasing as necessary

Adults:

Parkinsonism: 2.5 mg 3 times/day; gradually increase to 5 mg 3-4 times/day

Drug-induced extrapyramidal symptoms: 2.5 mg 3 times/day; increase as necessary by 2.5 mg/day; most patients require 10-20 mg/day

Monitoring Parameters Symptoms of EPS or Parkinson's, pulse, anticholinergic effects (ie, CNS < bowel and bladder function)

Patient Information Take after meals or with food if GI upset occurs; do not discontinue drug abruptly; notify physician if adverse GI effects, rapid or pounding heartbeat, confusion, eye pain, rash, fever, or heat intolerance occurs. Observe caution when performing hazardous tasks or those that require alertness such as driving, as may cause drowsiness. Avoid alcohol and other CNS depressants. May cause dry mouth which adequate fluid intake or hard sugar-free candy may relieve. Difficult urination or constipation may occur, notify physician if effects persist; may increase susceptibility to heat stroke.

Nursing Implications Do not discontinue drug abruptly

Special Geriatric Considerations Anticholinergic agents are generally not well tolerated in the elderly (constipation, urine retention, confusion) and their use should be avoided when possible (see Precautions, Adverse Reactions). In the elderly, anticholinergic agents should not be used as prophylaxis against extrapyramidal symptoms.

Dosage Forms Tablet, as hydrochloride: 5 mg

References

Feinberg M, "The Problems of Anticholinergic Adverse Effects in Older Patients," *Drugs Aging*, 1993, 3(4):335-48.

Prodium® [OTC] *see* Phenazopyridine *on page 734*

Progestasert® *see* Progesterone *on this page*

Progesterone (proe JES ter one)

Brand Names Progestasert®

Synonyms Pregnenedione; Progestin

Generic Available Yes

Therapeutic Category Progestin

Use Endometrial carcinoma or renal carcinoma as well as secondary amenorrhea or abnormal uterine bleeding due to hormonal imbalance

Contraindications Thrombophlebitis, cerebral apoplexy, undiagnosed vaginal bleeding, hypersensitivity to progesterone or any component; carcinoma of the breast

Precautions Use with caution in patients with impaired liver function

Adverse Reactions

Cardiovascular: Edema, central thrombosis and embolism

Dermatologic: Allergic rash or pruritus

Endocrine & metabolic: Breakthrough bleeding or spotting, breast tenderness

Gastrointestinal: Secretions, weight gain or loss, anorexia

Hepatic: Cholestatic jaundice

Local: Pain at injection site, thrombophlebitis

Respiratory: Pulmonary embolism

Toxicology Toxicity is unlikely following single exposures of excessive doses, and supportive treatment is adequate in most cases

Stability Refrigerate suppositories

Mechanism of Action Natural steroid hormone that induces secretory changes in the endometrium, promotes mammary gland development, relaxes uterine smooth muscle, blocks follicular maturation and ovulation and maintains pregnancy

Pharmacodynamics Duration of action: 24 hours

Pharmacokinetics

Absorption: Inactivated by liver when taken orally, absorbed rapidly after injection

Metabolism: Substrate CYP3A4

Half-life: 5 minutes

Elimination: In urine

Usual Dosage Geriatrics and Adults: I.M.: 5-10 mg/day for 6-8 days

Monitoring Parameters Before starting therapy, a physical exam including the breasts and pelvis are recommended, also a Pap smear; signs or symptoms of depression, glucose in diabetics

Test Interactions Liver function tests, coagulation tests, thyroid, metyrapone test, and endocrine function tests

Patient Information Diabetics should monitor their blood glucose closely

Nursing Implications Patients should receive a copy of the patient labeling for the drug; administer deep I.M. only

Additional Information May be used to prepare suppositories

Special Geriatric Considerations Not a progestin of choice in the elderly for hormonal cycling (see Adverse Reactions)

Dosage Forms

Injection: 50 mg/mL in oil (10 mL vials)

Powder for prescription compounding

Progestin *see* Progesterone *on this page*

Prolamine® [OTC] *see* Phenylpropanolamine *on page 741*

Prolixin Decanoate® Injection *see* Fluphenazine *on page 395*

Prolixin Enanthate® Injection *see* Fluphenazine *on page 395*

Prolixin® Injection *see* Fluphenazine *on page 395*

Prolixin®️ Oral *see* Fluphenazine *on page 395*

Proloprim®️ *see* Trimethoprim *on page 962*

Promazine (PROE ma zeen)

Related Information
Antacid Drug Interactions *on page 1096*
Antipsychotic Agents Comparison *on page 1023*
Antipsychotic Medication Guidelines *on page 1076*
Federal OBRA Regulations Recommended Maximum Doses - Antipsychotics *on page 1056*

Brand Names Sparine®️

Generic Available Yes: Injection only

Therapeutic Category Antipsychotic Agent; Neuroleptic Agent; Phenothiazine Derivative

Use Management of manifestations of psychotic disorders; depressive neurosis; alcohol withdrawal; nausea and vomiting; nonpsychotic symptoms associated with dementia in elderly, Tourette's syndrome; Huntington's chorea; spasmodic torticollis and Reye's syndrome (see Special Geriatric Considerations)

Contraindications Hypersensitivity to promazine or any component; severe CNS depression, cross-sensitivity to other phenothiazines may exist; avoid use in patients with narrow-angle glaucoma, blood dyscrasias, severe liver or cardiac disease; subcortical brain damage; circulatory collapse; severe hypotension or hypertension

Warnings
Tardive dyskinesia: Prevalence rate may be 40% in elderly; elderly women especially at risk; embarrassment from dyskinesias may lead to greater social isolation; development of the syndrome and the irreversible nature are proportional to duration and total cumulative dose over time. May be reversible if diagnosed early in therapy; intermittent use of antipsychotics (not proven use) helps decrease total cumulative dose.

EPS: Extrapyramidal reactions are more common in elderly with up to 50% developing these reactions after age 60. These reactions may be more common in dementia patients. Drug-induced **Parkinson's syndrome** occurs often. Discontinuation usually resolves symptoms but may take weeks to months (12+) to clear. **Akathisia** is the most common EPS reaction in elderly. The symptoms of motor restlessness are difficult to diagnose in demented elderly; increased nervousness, assertiveness, restlessness with constant movement may indicate this adverse event. Consider decreasing dose if antipsychotic to treat as well as diagnose problem; usually see this reaction within 2-3 months of initiating antipsychotic drug.

Anticholinergic effects: These side effects most common with low potency antipsychotics (eg, thioridazine, chlorpromazine). CNS toxicity occurs more frequently and severely in elderly; increased confusion, memory loss, psychotic behavior, and agitation frequently occur as a consequence of anticholinergic effects to antipsychotic agents. Peripheral anticholinergic action troublesome to elderly; most peripheral anticholinergic effects last only 2-3 weeks (see Adverse Reactions).

Orthostatic hypotension: More common with low potency agents (eg, thioridazine, chlorpromazine, and clozapine) but of concern with all antipsychotic agents; orthostasis due to alpha-receptor blockade by antipsychotic agents. Elderly present many risk factors for orthostatic hypotension: blunted baroreceptor reflexes, decreased vascular tone, decreased vascular volume, and possible presence of cardiac diseases which result in decreased cardiac output.

Sedation: Common side effect with antipsychotic therapy; should not be used as a hypnotic unless insomnia is associated with target behavior symptoms treated with antipsychotic medications (see Special Geriatric Considerations). Anecdotal reports suggesting antipsychotic sedation in nonpsychotic patients is extremely unpleasant due to feelings of depersonalization, derealization, and dysphoria. Due to the long duration of action with antipsychotic drugs, these reactions may last up to 24 hours and result in decreased daytime function.

Cardiac toxicity: Life-threatening arrhythmias have occurred at therapeutic doses of antipsychotics. Thioridazine more commonly demonstrates EKG changes than other antipsychotics; suggested to use high potency antipsychotic agents (ie, haloperidol) in patients with cardiac conduction defects.

Precautions Use with caution in patients with severe cardiovascular disorder, seizures, and Parkinson's disease; benefits of therapy must be weighed against risks

Adverse Reactions Anticholinergic effects are more pronounced than extrapyramidal effects

Cardiovascular: Hypotension (especially with I.V. use), orthostatic hypotension, tachycardia, arrhythmias, abnormal T waves with prolonged ventricular repolarization

Central nervous system: Sedation, drowsiness, restlessness, anxiety, extrapyramidal reactions, pseudoparkinsonian signs and symptoms, tardive dyskinesia, neuroleptic malignant syndrome, seizures, altered central temperature regulation

Dermatologic: Hyperpigmentation, pruritus, rash, photosensitivity

Endocrine & metabolic: Amenorrhea, galactorrhea, gynecomastia

Gastrointestinal: GI upset, xerostomia (problem for denture users), constipation, adynamic ileus, weight gain

Genitourinary: Urinary retention, overflow incontinence, priapism, sexual dysfunction (up to 60%), impotence

Hematologic: Agranulocytosis, leukopenia (usually in patients with large doses for prolonged periods), thrombocytopenia, hemolytic anemia, eosinophilia

Hepatic: Cholestatic jaundice (rare)

Ocular: Retinal pigmentation, blurred vision

Miscellaneous: Anaphylactoid reactions

Toxicology Following initiation of essential overdose management, toxic symptom treatment and supportive treatment should be initiated. Hypotension usually responds to I.V. fluids or Trendelenburg positioning. If unresponsive to these measures the use of a parenteral inotrope may be required (eg, norepinephrine 0.1-0.2 mcg/kg/minute titrated to response). Do not use epinephrine. Seizures commonly respond to diazepam (I.V. 5-10 mg bolus in adults every 15 minutes if needed up to a total of 30 mg) or to phenytoin or phenobarbital. Also critical cardiac arrhythmias often respond to I.V. phenytoin (15 mg/kg up to 1 g), while other antiarrhythmics can be used. Neuroleptics often cause extrapyramidal symptoms (eg, dystonic reactions) requiring management with diphenhydramine 1-2 mg/kg up to a maximum of 50 mg I.M. or I.V. slow push followed by a maintenance dose for 48-72 hours. When these reactions are unresponsive to diphenhydramine, benztropine mesylate I.V. 1-2 mg may be effective. These agents are generally effective within 2-5 minutes.

Drug Interactions

Alcohol may increase CNS sedation

Anticholinergic agents may decrease pharmacologic effects; increase anticholinergic side effects; may enhance tardive dyskinesia

Aluminum salts may decrease absorption of phenothiazines

Barbiturates may decrease phenothiazine serum concentrations

Bromocriptine may have decreased efficacy when administered with phenothiazines

Guanethidine's hypotensive effect is decreased by phenothiazines

Lithium administration with phenothiazines may increase disorientation

Meperidine and phenothiazine coadministration increases sedation and hypotension

Methyldopa administration with phenothiazine (trifluoperazine) may significantly increase blood pressure

Norepinephrine, epinephrine have decreased pressor effect when administered with chlorpromazine; therefore, be aware of possible decreased effectiveness or when any phenothiazine is used

Phenytoin serum concentrations may increase or decrease with phenothiazines; tricyclic antidepressants may have increased serum concentrations with concomitant administration with phenothiazines

Propranolol administered with phenothiazines may increase serum concentrations of both drugs

Valproic acid may have increased half-life when administered with phenothiazines (chlorpromazine)

Stability Protect all dosage forms from light, clear or slightly yellow solutions may be used; should be dispensed in amber or opaque vials/bottles. Solutions may be diluted or mixed with fruit juices or other liquids but must be administered immediately after mixing; do not prepare bulk dilutions or store bulk dilutions.

Mechanism of Action Blocks postsynaptic mesolimbic dopaminergic D_1 and D_2 receptors in the brain; exhibits a strong alpha-adrenergic blocking and (Continued)

Promazine *(Continued)*

anticholinergic effect; depresses the release of hypothalamic and hypophyseal hormones; believed to depress the reticular activating system thus affecting basal metabolism, body temperature, wakefulness, vasomotor tone, and emesis

Pharmacokinetics

Absorption: May be affected by the inherent anticholinergic action on the gastrointestinal tissue causing variable absorption. Absorption from tablets is erratic with less variation seen with solutions. These agents are widely distributed in tissues with CNS concentrations exceeding that of plasma due to their lipophilic characteristics.

Protein binding: Antipsychotic agents are bound 90% to 99% to plasma proteins; highly bound to brain and lung tissue and other tissues with a high blood perfusion

Time to peak concentration: Oral: 2-4 hours

Elimination: Excretion occurs through hepatic metabolism (oxidation) where numerous active metabolites are produced; active metabolites excreted in urine; elimination half-lives of antipsychotics ranges from 20-40 hours which may be extended in elderly due to decline in oxidative hepatic reactions (phase I) with age

The biologic effect of a single dose persists for 24 hours. When the patient has accommodated to initial side effects (sedation), once daily dosing is possible due to the long half-life of antipsychotics.

Steady-state plasma concentrations are achieved in 4-7 days; therefore, if possible, do not make dose adjustments more than once in a 7-day period. Due to the long half-lives of antipsychotics, as needed (prn) use is ineffective since repeated doses are necessary to achieve therapeutic tissue concentrations in the CNS.

Usual Dosage

Geriatrics (nonpsychotic patients; dementia behavior): Initial: 25 mg 1-2 times/day; increase dose at 4- to 7-day intervals by 25 mg/day; increase dose intervals (bid, tid, etc) as necessary to control response or side effects; maximum daily dose: 500 mg; gradual increases (titration) may prevent some side effects or decrease their severity

Adults: Oral, I.M.: 10-200 mg every 4-6 hours; I.M. injection preferred, I.V. not recommended

Not dialyzable (0% to 5%)

Test Interactions Increased cholesterol (S), increased glucose; decreased uric acid (S)

Patient Information Do not take antacid within 1 hour of taking drug; avoid alcohol; avoid excess sun exposure (use sun block); may cause drowsiness, rise slowly from recumbent position; use of supportive stockings may help prevent orthostatic hypotension

Nursing Implications I.M. injections should be deep injections; if giving I.V., dilute to at least 25 mg/mL and administer slowly; watch for hypotension; protect injection from light; monitor orthostatic blood pressures 3-5 days after initiation of therapy or a dose increase; observe for tremor and abnormal movement or posturing (extrapyramidal symptoms)

Special Geriatric Considerations See Warnings.

Many elderly patients receive antipsychotic medications for inappropriate nonpsychotic behavior. Before initiating antipsychotic medication, the clinician should investigate any possible reversible cause; any stress or stress from any disease can cause acute "confusion" or worsening of baseline nonpsychotic behavior. Most commonly acute changes in behavior are due to increases in drug dose or addition of new drug to regimen; fluid electrolyte loss; infections; and changes in environment.

Any changes in disease status in any organ system can result in behavior changes

In the treatment of agitated, demented, elderly patients, authors of meta-analysis of controlled trials of the response to the traditional antipsychotics (phenothiazines, butyrophenones) in controlling agitation have concluded that the use of neuroleptics results in a response rate of 18%. Clearly neuroleptic therapy for behavior control should be limited with frequent attempts to withdraw the agent given for behavior control.

Dosage Forms

Promazine hydrochloride:

Injection: 25 mg/mL (10 mL); 50 mg/mL (1 mL, 2 mL, 10 mL)

Tablet: 25 mg, 50 mg, 100 mg

References

Peabody CA, Warner MD, Whiteford HA, et al, "Neuroleptics and the Elderly," *J Am Geriatr Soc*, 1987, 35(3):233-8.

Risse SC and Barnes R, "Pharmacologic Treatment of Agitation Associated With Dementia," *J Am Geriatr Soc*, 1986, 34(5):368-76.

Saltz BL, Woerner MG, Kane JM, et al, "Prospective Study of Tardive Dyskinesia Incidence in the Elderly," *JAMA*, 1991, 266(17):2402-6.

Seifert RD, "Therapeutic Drug Monitoring: Psychotropic Drugs," *J Pharm Pract*, 1984, 6:403-16.

Prometa® *see* Metaproterenol *on page 596*

Prometh® *see* Promethazine *on this page*

Promethazine (proe METH a zeen)

Related Information

Antacid Drug Interactions *on page 1096*
I.V. Push Recommended Guidelines *on page 1083*

Brand Names Anergan®; Phenazine®; Phenergan®; Prometh®; Prorex®

Generic Available Yes

Therapeutic Category Antiemetic; Antihistamine; Phenothiazine Derivative; Sedative

Use Symptomatic treatment of various allergic conditions, antiemetic, motion sickness, and as a sedative

Contraindications Hypersensitivity to promethazine or any component; narrow-angle glaucoma

Warnings Do not administer S.C. or intra-arterially, necrotic lesions may occur; injection may contain sulfites which may cause allergic reactions in some patients. Antihistamines are more likely to cause dizziness, excessive sedation, syncope, toxic confusion states, and hypotension in the elderly. Phenothiazine-type side effects (especially EPS) are more prone to develop in the elderly.

Precautions Use with caution in patients with cardiovascular disease, impaired liver function, asthma, sleep apnea, seizures, hypertensive crisis; avoid in patients with Reye's syndrome

Adverse Reactions

Cardiovascular: Tachycardia, bradycardia with I.V. administration
Central nervous system: Sedation (pronounced), confusion, fatigue, excitation, extrapyramidal reactions with high doses, dystonia, faintness with I.V. administration
Dermatologic: Photosensitivity
Gastrointestinal: Xerostomia, abdominal pain, nausea, diarrhea
Genitourinary: Urinary retention
Hematologic: Thrombocytopenia
Hepatic: Jaundice
Ocular: Blurred vision
Respiratory: Irregular respiration, bronchospasm
Miscellaneous: Allergic reactions

Overdosage Symptoms of overdose include CNS depression, respiratory depression, possible CNS stimulation, dry mouth, fixed and dilated pupils, hypotension

Toxicology Following initiation of essential overdose management, toxic symptom treatment and supportive treatment should be initiated. Hypotension usually responds to I.V. fluids or Trendelenburg positioning. If unresponsive to these measures the use of a parenteral vasopressor may be required (eg, norepinephrine 0.1-0.2 mcg/kg/minute titrated to response). Seizures commonly respond to diazepam (I.V. 5-10 mg bolus every 15 minutes if needed up to a total of 30 mg); or to phenytoin or phenobarbital. Also critical cardiac arrhythmias often respond to I.V. phenytoin (15 mg/kg up to 1 g), while other antiarrhythmics can be used. Neuroleptics often cause extrapyramidal symptoms (eg, dystonic reactions) requiring management with diphenhydramine 1-2 mg/kg up to a maximum of 50 mg I.M. or I.V. slow push followed by a maintenance dose for 48-72 hours. When these reactions are unresponsive to diphenhydramine, benztropine mesylate I.V. 1-2 mg may be effective. These agents are generally effective within 2-5 minutes. Cholinesterase inhibitors including physostigmine, neostigmine, pyridostigmine, and edrophonium may be useful in treating life-threatening anticholinergic symptoms. Physostigmine 1-2 mg I.V., slowly may be given to reverse these effects.

Drug Interactions Increased toxicity with epinephrine (increased blood pressure), CNS depressants, alcohol

Stability Protect from light and from freezing

Mechanism of Action Blocks postsynaptic mesolimbic dopaminergic receptors in the brain; exhibits a strong alpha-adrenergic blocking effect and (Continued)

Promethazine *(Continued)*

depresses the release of hypothalamic and hypophyseal hormones; competes with histamine for the H_1-receptor; reduces stimuli to the brainstem reticular system

Pharmacodynamics
Onset of action: Within 20 minutes (3-5 minutes with I.V. injection)
Duration: 4-6 hours

Pharmacokinetics
Metabolism: In the liver
Elimination: Principally as inactive metabolites in urine and feces

Usual Dosage Geriatrics and Adults:
Antihistamine:
Oral: 25 mg at bedtime or 12.5 mg 3 times/day
I.M., I.V., rectal: 25 mg, may repeat in 2 hours
Antiemetic: Oral, I.M., I.V., rectal: 12.5-25 mg every 4 hours as needed
Motion sickness: Oral: 25 mg 30 minutes to 1 hour before departure, then every 12 hours as needed
Sedation: Oral, I.M., I.V., rectal: 25-50 mg/dose
Not dialyzable (0% to 5%)

Administration When administering IVP, do not give any faster than 25 mg/minute

Monitoring Parameters Relief of symptoms, mental status

Test Interactions Alters the flare response in intradermal allergen tests

Patient Information May cause drowsiness; avoid the use of alcohol and other CNS depressants; may cause photosensitivity

Nursing Implications Rapid I.V. administration may produce a transient fall in blood pressure, rate of administration should not exceed 25 mg/minute; slow I.V. administration may produce a slightly elevated blood pressure; avoid extravasation since tissue necrosis has occurred with extravasation; monitor patient's mental status, monitor for EPS

Additional Information Promethazine is available in various combinations; these include codeine, phenylephrine, phenylephrine and codeine

Special Geriatric Considerations Because promethazine is a phenothiazine (and can, therefore, cause side effects such as extrapyramidal symptoms), it is not considered an antihistamine of choice in the elderly (see Warnings)

Dosage Forms
Promethazine hydrochloride:
Injection: 25 mg/mL (1 mL, 10 mL); 50 mg/mL (1 mL, 10 mL)
Suppository, rectal: 12.5 mg, 25 mg, 50 mg
Syrup: 6.25 mg/5 mL (5 mL, 120 mL, 240 mL, 480 mL, 4000 mL); 25 mg/5 mL (120 mL, 480 mL, 4000 mL)
Tablet: 12.5 mg, 25 mg, 50 mg

Promine® *see Procainamide on page 780*
Pronestyl® *see Procainamide on page 780*
Propacet® *see Propoxyphene and Acetaminophen on page 796*
Propadrine *see Phenylpropanolamine on page 741*

Propafenone *(proe pa FEEN one)*

Brand Names Rythmol®

Therapeutic Category Antiarrhythmic Agent, Class I-C

Use Life-threatening ventricular arrhythmias
Unlabeled use: Supraventricular tachycardias, including those patients with Wolff-Parkinson-White syndrome

Contraindications Hypersensitivity to propafenone or any component; patients with uncontrolled congestive heart failure or bronchospastic disorders; cardiogenic shock, conduction disorders (A-V block, sick sinus syndrome), bradycardia

Warnings The CAST study issued warnings for increased mortality for any class IC antiarrhythmic agent; may be proarrhythmia, nonallergic bronchospasm, worsening or induction of CHF, decreased A-V conduction including A-V block; alterations of pacemaker thresholds; use cautiously in patients with hepatic and renal impairment; elderly may be at risk for toxicity due to decreased renal and hepatic function with age

Precautions Propafenone may cause elevation of ANA titers; both renal and hepatic tissue changes (interstitial nephritis, fatty degeneration respectively) reported in animal studies at doses above those recommended in humans; agranulocytosis has been reported

Adverse Reactions The majority of adverse reactions are noncardiac; for other less frequent (rare) side effects, refer to product information circular

Cardiovascular: New or worsened arrhythmias (proarrhythmic effect); prolonged A-V conduction; aggravated existing A-V block; first degree A-V block; CHF; ventricular tachycardia, palpitations, and proarrhythmia in high doses

Central nervous system: Dizziness, headache, loss of balance, fatigue, numbness, abnormal speech, bad dreams; occasionally: depression, confusion, memory loss, psychosis, vertigo

Gastrointestinal: Bitter or metallic taste sensation, dyspepsia, nausea, vomiting, flatulence, anorexia, abdominal pain, and constipation

Hematologic: Leukopenia, thrombocytopenia, agranulocytosis

Neuromuscular & skeletal: Weakness, paresthesia

Ocular: Blurred vision

Otic: Tinnitus

Overdosage Symptoms of overdose include hypotension, somnolence, bradycardia, conduction disturbances, convulsions, ventricular arrhythmias most severe 3 hours after ingestion

Toxicology Treatment is supportive; I.V. fluids and the Trendelenburg position are employed for hypotension; bradycardia can be treated with atropine but may require a pacemaker; ventricular arrhythmias are often resistant to conventional therapy; however, lidocaine 1.5 mg/kg bolus followed by 1-2 mg/minute may be effective; magnesium may be helpful in wide complex tachycardia; however, defibrillation, or isoproterenol may be needed; not dialyzable

Drug Interactions Increases effect of levels of local anesthetics, cimetidine, quinidine, anticoagulants, beta-blockers, cyclosporine, digoxin (reduce dose of digoxin 25%); rifampin increases propafenone clearance (decreases serum concentration); phenytoin, phenobarbital may do the same

Mechanism of Action Direct myocardial membrane stabilization; decreased velocity of phase O (upstroke), decreased velocity in Purkinje fibers; increased diastolic excitability threshold; prolonged effective refractory period; reduced spontaneous automaticity; exhibits beta-blockade activity

Pharmacokinetics

Absorption: Well absorbed

Metabolism: Two genetically determined metabolism groups exist: fast or slow metabolizers; 10% of Caucasians are slow metabolizers; substrate CYP1A2, 2D6, 3A4; inhibitor CYP2D6

Half-life after a single dose (100-300 mg): 2-8 hours; half-life after chronic dosing ranges from 10-32 hours

Time to peak serum concentration: 2 hours with a 150 mg dose and 3 hours after a 300 mg dose; this agent exhibits nonlinear pharmacokinetics; when dose is increased from 300-900 mg/day, serum concentrations increase tenfold; this nonlinearity is thought to be due to saturable first-pass hepatic enzyme metabolism

Usual Dosage Geriatrics and Adults: Oral: 150 mg every 8 hours, increase dose at 3- to 4-day intervals; increase to 225 mg every 8 hours; increase up to 300 mg every 8 hours (maximum dose); patients who exhibit significant widening of QRS complex or second or third degree A-V block may need dose reduction

Dosing adjustment in hepatic impairment: Dose reduction is necessary

Monitoring Parameters EKG, blood pressure, pulse (particularly at initiation of therapy), signs and symptoms of CHF; titrate dose according to response and tolerance

Patient Information Take dose the same way each day, either with or without food; very important to take drug correctly, do not double the next dose if present dose is missed; report any palpitations, chest pain, difficult breathing, blurred vision, fever, sore throat, bleeding, bruising, or drowsiness; may impair coordination and judgment

Nursing Implications Watch for signs of infection; monitor heart sounds and pulses for rate, rhythm and quality

Additional Information An oral sodium channel blocker similar to flecainide; in clinical trials was used effectively to treat atrial flutter, atrial fibrillation, and other arrhythmias, but are not labeled indications; can worsen or even cause new ventricular arrhythmias (proarrhythmic effect)

Special Geriatric Considerations Elderly may have age-related decreases in hepatic phase I metabolism; propafenone is dependent upon liver metabolism, therefore, monitor closely in elderly and dose more gradually during initial treatment (see Warnings). No differences in clearance noted with (Continued)

Propafenone *(Continued)*

impaired renal function and, therefore, no adjustment for renal function in elderly is necessary.

Dosage Forms Tablet, as hydrochloride: 150 mg, 225 mg, 300 mg

References

Fenster PE and Nolan PE, "Antiarrhythmic Drugs," *Geriatric Pharmacology*, Bressler R and Katz MD, eds, New York, NY: McGraw-Hill, 1993, 6:105-49.

Propagest® [OTC] *see* Phenylpropanolamine *on page 741*

Propantheline (proe PAN the leen)

Brand Names Pro-Banthine®

Generic Available Yes: 15 mg tablet

Therapeutic Category Antispasmodic Agent, Gastrointestinal

Use Adjunctive treatment of peptic ulcer, irritable bowel syndrome, pancreatitis, ureteral and urinary bladder spasm; to reduce duodenal motility during diagnostic radiologic procedures

Contraindications Narrow-angle glaucoma, known hypersensitivity to propantheline; ulcerative colitis; toxic megacolon; obstructive disease of the GI or urinary tract

Precautions Use with caution in febrile patients, patients with hyperthyroidism, hepatic, cardiac, or renal disease, hypertension, GI infections

Adverse Reactions

Cardiovascular: Tachycardia, palpitations, flushing, orthostatic hypotension
Central nervous system: Insomnia, drowsiness, dizziness, nervousness
Dermatologic: Rash
Gastrointestinal: Xerostomia, nausea, vomiting, constipation
Genitourinary: Urinary retention, impotence
Ocular: Mydriasis, blurred vision
Miscellaneous: Diaphoresis

Overdosage Symptoms of overdose include CNS disturbances, flushing, respiratory failure, paralysis, coma, urinary retention, hyperthermia

Toxicology Anticholinergic toxicity is caused by strong binding of the drug to cholinergic receptors; for anticholinergic overdose with severe life-threatening symptoms, physostigmine 1-2 mg S.C. or I.V., slowly may be given to reverse these effects

Drug Interactions

Decreased effect with antacids (decreased absorption); decreased effect of sustained release dosage forms (decreased absorption), metoclopramide, cisapride

Increased effect/toxicity with anticholinergics, disopyramide, narcotic analgesics, bretylium, type I antiarrhythmics, antihistamines, phenothiazines, TCAs, corticosteroids (increased IOP), CNS depressants (sedation), adenosine, amiodarone, beta-blockers, amoxapine

Antagonistic effect: Tacrine, donepezil

Mechanism of Action Competitively blocks the action of acetylcholine at postganglionic parasympathetic receptor sites

Pharmacodynamics

Onset of action: Oral: Within 30-45 minutes
Duration: 4-6 hours

Pharmacokinetics

Metabolism: In the liver and GI tract
Elimination: In urine, bile, and other body fluids

Usual Dosage Oral:

Geriatrics: 7.5 mg 2-3 times/day increasing as necessary to a maximum of 30 mg 3 times/day

Adults: 15 mg 3 times/day before meals or food and 30 mg at bedtime

Monitoring Parameters Anticholinergic effects, blood pressure, pulse, urinary output, postvoid residual, GI symptoms

Patient Information Take 30 minutes before meals and at bedtime. Maintain good oral hygiene habits, because lack of saliva may increase chance of cavities. Observe caution while driving or performing other tasks requiring alertness, as may cause drowsiness, dizziness, or blurred vision. Notify physician if skin rash, flushing or eye pain occurs; or if difficulty in urinating, constipation or sensitivity to light becomes severe or persists.

Nursing Implications Administer 30 minutes before meals so that the drug's peak effect occurs at the proper time; monitor for anticholinergic effects, orthostatic changes

Additional Information Because propantheline is a quaternary ammonium compound, it does not cross the blood-brain barrier and is less likely to cause CNS effects as compared to atropine

Special Geriatric Considerations The primary use of propantheline in the geriatric population is for treatment of urinary incontinence due to detrusor instability. Even though it does not cross the blood-brain barrier, CNS effects have been reported. Orthostatic hypotension may also occur, therefore, avoid long-term use in the elderly.

Dosage Forms Tablet, as bromide: 7.5 mg, 15 mg

Propecia® see Finasteride on page 383

Propine® Ophthalmic see Dipivefrin on page 306

Propoxyphene (proe POKS i feen)

Related Information
Narcotic Agonist Comparative Pharmacology on page 1036
Pharmacokinetics of Narcotic Agonist Analgesics on page 1037

Brand Names Darvon®; Darvon-N®; Dolene®

Synonyms Dextropropoxyphene

Generic Available Yes: Capsule

Therapeutic Category Analgesic, Narcotic

Use Management of mild to moderate pain

Restrictions C-IV

Contraindications Hypersensitivity to propoxyphene or any component

Warnings Give with caution in patients dependent on opiates, substitution may result in acute opiate withdrawal symptoms, use with caution in patients with severe renal or hepatic dysfunction; when given in excessive doses, either alone or in combination with other CNS depressants, propoxyphene is a major cause of drug-related deaths; do not exceed recommended dosage

Adverse Reactions
Central nervous system: Dizziness, lightheadedness, delirium, dysphoria, hallucinations, disorientation, mental clouding, toxic psychosis, depression, sedation, paradoxical excitement and insomnia, headache, psychic dependence

Dermatologic: Rashes

Gastrointestinal: GI upset, nausea, vomiting, constipation, dry mouth, anorexia

Hepatic: Increased liver enzymes, reversible jaundice

Neuromuscular & skeletal: Weakness

Miscellaneous: Psychologic and physical dependence with prolonged use

Overdosage Symptoms of overdose include CNS, respiratory, depression, hypotension, pulmonary edema, seizures

Toxicology Treatment of an overdose includes support of the patient's airway, establishment of an I.V. line and administration of naloxone 2 mg I.V. with repeat administration as necessary up to a total of 10 mg.

Drug Interactions
Decreased effect with charcoal, cigarette smoking
Increased effect/toxicity of carbamazepine, warfarin, tricyclic antidepressants, propranolol, metoprolol, ritonavir
Increased toxicity with CNS depressants

Mechanism of Action Binds to opiate receptors in the CNS, causing inhibition of ascending pain pathways, altering the perception of and response to pain; produces generalized CNS depression

Pharmacodynamics
Onset of effect: Oral: Within 30-60 minutes
Duration: 4-6 hours

Pharmacokinetics
Bioavailability: Oral: 30% to 70% due to first-pass effect
Metabolism: In the liver to an active metabolite (norpropoxyphene) and inactive metabolites; metabolism is decreased in the elderly and hepatic dysfunction; inhibitor CYP3A4; propoxyphene and norpropoxyphene accumulate in renal failure
Half-life: 8-24 hours (mean: ~15 hours)
Half-life: Norpropoxyphene: 34 hours

Usual Dosage Oral:
Geriatrics:
Hydrochloride: 65 mg every 4-6 hours as needed for pain
Napsylate: 100 mg every 4-6 hours as needed for pain
(Continued)

Propoxyphene *(Continued)*

Adults:

Hydrochloride: 65 mg every 3-4 hours as needed for pain; maximum: 390 mg/day

Napsylate: 100 mg every 4 hours as needed for pain; maximum: 600 mg/day

Monitoring Parameters Pain relief, respiratory and mental status, blood pressure

Reference Range Therapeutic: 0.1-0.4 µg/mL (SI: 0.3-1.2 µmol/L) (therapeutic ranges published vary between laboratories and may not correlate with clinical effect); Toxic: >0.5 µg/mL (SI: >1.5 µmol/L)

Test Interactions Abnormal LFTs

Patient Information May cause drowsiness, dizziness, or blurring of vision; avoid alcohol and other sedatives; may take with food

Nursing Implications Monitor for excessive sedation

Additional Information Some studies have found no significant difference in pain relief between propoxyphene and aspirin or acetaminophen

Propoxyphene hydrochloride: Darvon®
Propoxyphene napsylate: Darvon-N®

Special Geriatric Considerations The elderly may be particularly susceptible to the CNS depressant and constipating effects of narcotics (see Pharmacokinetics, Usual Dosage, and Additional Information); propoxyphene is not considered the analgesic of choice in elderly when mild to moderate pain requires a narcotic analgesic. This is due to the higher incidence of adverse CNS effects seen in the elderly population. Also a concern is the addiction potential in elderly; avoid use, if possible.

Dosage Forms

Capsule, as hydrochloride: 65 mg
Tablet, as napsylate: 100 mg

References

Ferrell BA, "Pain Management in Elderly People," *J Am Geriatr Soc*, 1991, 39(1):64-73.

Propoxyphene and Acetaminophen

(proe POKS i feen & a seet a MIN oh fen)

Related Information

Acetaminophen *on page 16*
Pharmacokinetics of Narcotic Agonist Analgesics *on page 1037*
Propoxyphene *on previous page*

Brand Names Darvocet-N®; Darvocet-N® 100; Genagesic®; Propacet®; Wygesic®

Generic Available Yes

Therapeutic Category Analgesic, Narcotic

Use Management of mild to moderate pain

Restrictions C-IV

Contraindications Hypersensitivity to propoxyphene, acetaminophen or any component

Warnings Give with caution in patients dependent on opiates, substitution may result in acute opiate withdrawal symptoms, use with caution in patients with severe renal or hepatic dysfunction; when given in excessive doses, either alone or in combination with other CNS depressants, propoxyphene is a major cause of drug-related deaths; do not exceed recommended dosage

Adverse Reactions

Central nervous system: Dizziness, lightheadedness, delirium, dysphoria, hallucinations, disorientation, mental clouding, toxic psychosis, depression, sedation, paradoxical excitement and insomnia, headache, psychic dependence

Dermatologic: Rashes

Gastrointestinal: GI upset, nausea, vomiting, constipation, dry mouth, anorexia

Hepatic: Increased liver enzymes, reversible jaundice

Neuromuscular & skeletal: Weakness

Miscellaneous: Psychological and physical dependence with prolonged use

Toxicology Treatment of an overdose includes support of the patient's airway, establishment of an I.V. line and administration of naloxone 2 mg I.V. with repeat administration as necessary up to a total of 10 mg. Mucomyst® (acetylcysteine) 140 mg/kg orally (loading) followed by 70 mg/kg (maintenance) every 4 hours for 17 doses. Therapy should be initiated based upon laboratory analysis suggesting high probability of acetaminophen hepatotoxic potential.

Drug Interactions
 Decreased effect with charcoal, cigarette smoking
 Increased effect/toxicity of carbamazepine, warfarin, tricyclic antidepressants, propranolol, metoprolol, ritonavir
 Increased toxicity with CNS depressants

Usual Dosage Geriatrics and Adults:
 Darvocet-N® 50: 1-2 tablets every 4 hours as needed; maximum: 600 mg propoxyphene napsylate/day
 Darvocet-N® 100: 1 tablet every 4 hours as needed; maximum: 600 mg propoxyphene napsylate/day
 Dolene® AP-65: 1 tablet every 4 hours as needed

Monitoring Parameters Pain relief, respiratory and mental status, blood pressure

Test Interactions Abnormal LFTs

Patient Information Do not exceed recommended dose; may cause drowsiness, avoid alcoholic beverages

Nursing Implications Monitor for excessive sedation

Additional Information Some studies have found no significant difference in pain relief between propoxyphene and aspirin or acetaminophen

 Propoxyphene hydrochloride and acetaminophen: Dolene® AP-65, Wygesic®, Genagesic®
 Propoxyphene napsylate and acetaminophen: Darvocet-N®, Darvocet-N® 100; Propacet®
 Propoxyphene napsylate 100 mg and propoxyphene hydrochloride contain same amount of propoxyphene

Special Geriatric Considerations Elderly may be particularly susceptible to the CNS depressant and constipating effects of narcotics; do not exceed 4 g/day of acetaminophen (see Warnings, Usual Dosage, and Additional Information); propoxyphene is not considered the analgesic of choice in elderly when mild to moderate pain requires a narcotic analgesic. This is due to the higher incidence of adverse CNS effects seen in the elderly population. Also a concern is the addiction potential in elderly; avoid use, if possible.

Dosage Forms Tablet: Propoxyphene napsylate 50 mg and acetaminophen 325 mg; propoxyphene napsylate 100 mg and acetaminophen 650 mg; propoxyphene hydrochloride 65 mg and acetaminophen 650 mg

Propranolol (proe PRAN oh lole)

Related Information
 Beta-Blockers Comparison *on page 1026*
 I.V. Push Recommended Guidelines *on page 1083*

Brand Names Betachron E-R® Capsule; Inderal®; Inderal® LA

Generic Available Yes

Therapeutic Category Antianginal Agent; Antiarrhythmic Agent, Class II; Beta-Adrenergic Blocker

Use Management of hypertension, angina pectoris, pheochromocytoma, essential tremor, and arrhythmias (such as atrial fibrillation, PVCs, and flutter, A-V nodal re-entrant tachycardias, and catecholamine-induced arrhythmias); prevention of myocardial infarction, migraine headache; symptomatic treatment of hypertrophic subaortic stenosis, digitalis-induced arrhythmias, resistant tachyarrhythmias, migraine prophylaxis

 Unlabeled use: Tremor due to Parkinson's disease, alcohol withdrawal, aggressive behavior, antipsychotic-induced akathisia, esophageal varices bleeding, anxiety, schizophrenia, acute panic, and gastric bleeding in portal hypertension

Contraindications Uncompensated congestive heart failure, cardiogenic shock, bradycardia or heart block, asthma, hyperactive airway disease, chronic obstructive lung disease, Raynaud's syndrome, diabetes mellitus, and those with hypersensitivity to beta-blocking agents

Warnings In patients with angina pectoris, exacerbation of angina and, in some cases, myocardial infarction, occurred following abrupt discontinuance of therapy abrupt withdrawal of the drug should be avoided; drug should be discontinued over 2 weeks

Precautions Use with caution in patients with renal or hepatic impairment administer to CHF patients with caution; administer with caution to patients with bronchospastic disease, diabetes mellitus, hyperthyroidism, myasthenia gravis, renal function decline, and severe peripheral vascular disease; abrupt withdrawal of the drug should be avoided, drug should be discontinued over 2 weeks.

(Continued)

Propranolol *(Continued)*

Adverse Reactions
Cardiovascular: Hypotension, impaired myocardial contractility, congestive heart failure, bradycardia, worsening of A-V conduction disturbances

Central nervous system: Lightheadedness, insomnia, vivid dreams, lethargy, depression

Endocrine & metabolic: Hypoglycemia, hyperglycemia

Gastrointestinal: Nausea, vomiting, diarrhea, GI distress, constipation

Hematologic: Agranulocytosis

Neuromuscular & skeletal: Weakness

Respiratory: Bronchospasm

Miscellaneous: Cold extremities

Overdosage
Symptoms of overdose include severe hypotension, bradycardia, heart failure and bronchospasm; isoproterenol may be used to counteract (see Toxicology)

Toxicology
Sympathomimetics (eg, epinephrine or dopamine), glucagon or a pacemaker can be used to treat the toxic bradycardia, asystole, and/or hypotension. Initially, fluids may be the best treatment for toxic hypotension. Patients should remain supine; serum glucose and potassium should be measured; use supportive measures: lavage, syrup of ipecac; propranolol not significantly removed by hemodialysis; I.V. glucose should be administered for hypoglycemia. Seizures may be treated with phenytoin or diazepam intravenously; continuous monitoring of blood pressure and EKG is necessary. If PVCs occur, treat with lidocaine or phenytoin; avoid quinidine, procainamide, and disopyramide since these agents further depress myocardial function; bronchospasm can be treated with theophylline or beta$_2$ agonists (epinephrine).

Drug Interactions
Phenobarbital, rifampin may increase propranolol clearance and may decrease its activity

Cimetidine, SSRIs, mibefradil, ritonavir may reduce propranolol clearance and may increase its effects

Aluminum-containing antacid may reduce GI absorption of propranolol; nonsteroidal anti-inflammatory agents, salicylates, sympathomimetics, thyroid hormones, insulins, lidocaine, calcium channel blockers, nifedipine, catecholamine depleting drugs, clonidine, disopyramide, prazosin, theophylline

Stability
Compatible in saline, incompatible with HCO_3^-; protect injection from light

Mechanism of Action
Competitively blocks response to beta$_1$- and beta$_2$-adrenergic stimulation; demonstrates high membrane stabilization activity but has no intrinsic sympathomimetic activity; highly lipid soluble, therefore, penetrates the blood-brain barrier

Pharmacodynamics
Onset of action: Oral: Beta blockade occurs within 1-2 hours

Duration: ~6 hours

Pharmacokinetics
Extensive first-pass effect

Distribution: V_d: 3.9 L/kg

Protein binding: 93%

Metabolism: In the liver to active and inactive compounds; substrate CYP1A2, 2C18, 2D6

Bioavailability: 30% to 40%

Half-life: 4-6 hours

Elimination: Primarily in urine (96% to 99%)

Usual Dosage
Arrhythmias:

Adults:

Oral: 10-80 mg/dose every 6-8 hours

I.V.: 1 mg/dose slow IVP; repeat every 5 minutes up to a total of 5 mg

Geriatrics: Initial: 10 mg twice daily or 60 mg once daily as sustained release capsules; increase dosage every 3-7 days; usual dose range: 10-320 mg given 1-2 times/day

Hypertension: Geriatrics and Adults: Oral: Initial: 40 mg twice daily or 60-80 mg once daily as sustained release capsules; increase dosage every 3-7 days; usual dose: ≤320 mg divided in 2-3 doses/day or once daily as sustained release; maximum daily dose: 640 mg

Migraine headache prophylaxis: Geriatrics and Adults: Oral: Initial: 80 mg/day divided every 6-8 hours; increase by 20-40 mg/dose every 3-4 weeks to a maximum of 160-240 mg/day given in divided doses every 6-8 hours

Thyrotoxicosis: Geriatrics and Adults:
  Oral: 10-40 mg/dose every 6 hours
  I.V.: 1-3 mg/dose slow IVP as a single dose
Not dialyzable (0% to 5%)

Monitoring Parameters Blood pressure, orthostatic hypotension, heart rate, CNS effects

Reference Range Therapeutic: 50-100 ng/mL (SI: 190-390 nmol/L) at end of dose interval

Test Interactions Increased thyroxine (S), cholesterol (S), glucose, triglycerides, potassium, uric acid; decreased HDL

Patient Information Do not discontinue abruptly, sudden stopping of medication may precipitate or cause angina; consult pharmacist or physician before taking with other adrenergic drugs (eg, cold medications); notify physician if any of the following symptoms occur: difficult breathing, night cough, swelling of extremities, slow pulse, dizziness, lightheadedness, confusion, depression, skin rash, fever, sore throat, unusual bleeding, or bruising; may produce drowsiness, dizziness, lightheadedness, blurred vision, confusion; use with caution while driving or performing tasks requiring alertness; take at the same time each day, may be taken without regard to meals; may mask signs of hypoglycemia in diabetes

Nursing Implications I.V. dose much smaller than oral dose; I.V. administration should not exceed 1 mg/minute; monitor EKG and CVP; patient's therapeutic response may be evaluated by looking at blood pressure, apical and radial pulses, fluid I & O, daily weight, respirations, and circulation in extremities before and during therapy; modify dosage in patients with renal insufficiency

Special Geriatric Considerations Since bioavailability increased in elderly about twofold, geriatric patients may require lower maintenance doses, therefore, as serum and tissue concentrations increase beta$_1$ selectivity diminishes; due to alterations in the beta-adrenergic autonomic nervous system, beta-adrenergic blockade may result in less hemodynamic response than seen in younger adults. Studies indicate that despite decreased sensitivity to the chronotropic effects of beta blockade with age, there appears to be an increased myocardial sensitivity to the negative inotropic effect during stress (ie, exercise). Controlled trials have shown the overall response rate for propranolol to be only 20% to 50% in elderly populations. Therefore, all beta-adrenergic blocking drugs may result in a decreased response as compared to younger adults. Due to propranolol's CNS penetration and nonselective action, it may not be the beta-blocker of choice for use in elderly.

Dosage Forms
Propranolol hydrochloride:
  Capsule, sustained action: 60 mg, 80 mg, 120 mg, 160 mg
  Injection: 1 mg/mL (1 mL)
  Solution, oral (strawberry-mint flavor): 4 mg/mL (5 mL, 500 mL); 8 mg/mL (5 mL, 500 mL)
  Solution, oral, concentrate: 80 mg/mL (30 mL)
  Tablet: 10 mg, 20 mg, 40 mg, 60 mg, 80 mg, 90 mg

References
Aagaard GN, "Treatment of Hypertension in The Elderly," *Drug Treatment in the Elderly*, Vestal RE, ed, Boston, MA: ADIS Health Science Press, 1984, 77.

Propranolol and Hydrochlorothiazide
(proe PRAN oh lole & hye droe klor oh THYE a zide)

Related Information
Hydrochlorothiazide *on page 458*
Propranolol *on page 797*

Brand Names Inderide®

Generic Available Yes: Immediate release

Therapeutic Category Antihypertensive, Combination

Use Management of hypertension

Special Geriatric Considerations Combination products are not recommended for first-line therapy and divided doses of diuretics may increase the incidence of nocturia in the elderly

Dosage Forms
Capsule, long-acting (Inderide® LA):
  80/50 Propranolol hydrochloride 80 mg and hydrochlorothiazide 50 mg
  120/50 Propranolol hydrochloride 120 mg and hydrochlorothiazide 50 mg
  160/50 Propranolol hydrochloride 160 mg and hydrochlorothiazide 50 mg
Tablet (Inderide®):
  40/25 Propranolol hydrochloride 40 mg and hydrochlorothiazide 25 mg
(Continued)

Propranolol and Hydrochlorothiazide *(Continued)*

80/25 Propranolol hydrochloride 80 mg and hydrochlorothiazide 25 mg

Propulsid® *see* Cisapride *on page 228*

2-Propylpentanoic Acid *see* Valproic Acid and Derivatives *on page 977*

Propylthiouracil (proe pil thye oh YOOR a sil)

Synonyms PTU

Generic Available Yes

Therapeutic Category Antithyroid Agent

Use Palliative treatment of hyperthyroidism as an adjunct to ameliorate hyperthyroidism in preparation for surgical treatment or radioactive iodine therapy and in the management of thyrotoxic crisis

Contraindications Hypersensitivity to propylthiouracil or any component

Warnings Use of antithyroid drugs may cause agranulocytosis, thyroid, hyperplasia, thyroid carcinoma (PTU for longer than 1 year)

Precautions Use with caution in patients >40 years of age because PTU may cause hypoprothrombinemia and bleeding, monitor prothrombin time during therapy; use with extreme caution in patients receiving other drugs known to cause agranulocytosis; monitor thyroid function tests periodically (T_4, TSH)

Adverse Reactions

Cardiovascular: Edema, cutaneous vasculitis, periarteritis

Central nervous system: Headache, drowsiness, CNS stimulation, depression, neuritis, vertigo, drug fever

Dermatologic: Rash, urticaria, pruritus, exfoliative dermatitis

Gastrointestinal: Nausea, vomiting, ageusia

Hematologic: Aplastic anemia, agranulocytosis, thrombocytopenia, bleeding

Hepatic: Jaundice, hepatitis

Neuromuscular & skeletal: Arthralgia, paresthesia

Renal: Nephritis

Respiratory: Pneumonitis

Miscellaneous: Lupus-like syndrome

Overdosage Symptoms of overdose include nausea, vomiting, arthralgia, pancytopenia, epigastric distress, and signs of hypothyroidism

Toxicology General supportive care; monitor bone marrow response, forced diuresis, peritoneal and hemodialysis as well as charcoal hemoperfusion **have not** been helpful in overdose situation

Drug Interactions Activity of oral anticoagulants may be increased by the antivitamin K activity of PTU

Mechanism of Action Inhibits the synthesis of thyroid hormones by blocking the oxidation of iodine in the thyroid gland; blocks synthesis of thyroxine and triiodothyronine; does not inactivate circulatory T_4 and T_3

Pharmacodynamics For significant therapeutic effects, 24-36 hours are required and remissions of hyperthyroidism do not usually occur before 4 months of continued therapy

Pharmacokinetics

Protein binding: 75% to 80%

Metabolism: Hepatic

Half-life: 1-2 hours

Time to peak serum concentration: Oral: Within 1 hour and persist for 2-3 hours

Elimination: 35% in urine

Usual Dosage Oral:

Geriatrics: Initial: 150-300 mg/day in divided doses every 8 hours

Adults: Initial: 300-450 mg/day in divided doses every 8 hours

Geriatrics and Adults: Maintenance: 100-150 mg/day in divided doses every 8-12 hours

Monitoring Parameters Monitor signs of hypo- and hyperthyroidism, T_4, T_3, TSH, CBC, prothrombin time (see Precautions)

Test Interactions Increased prothrombin time

Patient Information Do not exceed prescribed dosage; take at regular intervals around-the-clock; notify physician or pharmacist if fever, sore throat, unusual bleeding or bruising, headache, or general malaise occurs

Nursing Implications See Warnings, Precautions, Monitoring Parameters, and Special Geriatric Considerations

Additional Information Periodic blood counts are recommended with chronic therapy (see Warnings)

Special Geriatric Considerations The use of antithyroid thioamides is as effective in elderly as they are in younger adults; however, the expense, potential adverse effects, and inconvenience (compliance, monitoring) make them undesirable. The use of radioiodine, due to ease of administration and less concern for long-term side effects and reproduction problems, makes it a more appropriate therapy (see Warnings and Precautions)

Dosage Forms Tablet: 50 mg

References

Johnson DG and Campbell S, "Hormonal and Metabolic Agents," *Geriatric Pharmacology*, Bressler R and Katz MD, eds, New York, NY: McGraw-Hill, 1993, 427-50.

Raby C, Lagorce JF, Jambut-Absil AC, et al, "The Mechanism of Action of Synthetic Antithyroid Drugs: Iodine Complexation During Oxidation of Iodide," *Endocrinology*, 1990, 126(3):1683-91.

2-Propylvaleric Acid *see* Valproic Acid and Derivatives *on page 977*

Prorex® *see* Promethazine *on page 791*

Proscar® *see* Finasteride *on page 383*

Pro-Sof® Plus [OTC] *see* Docusate and Casanthranol *on page 313*

ProSom™ *see* Estazolam *on page 349*

Prostaglandin E₁ *see* Alprostadil *on page 38*

Prostaphlin® *see* Oxacillin *on page 698*

ProStep® Patch *see* Nicotine *on page 669*

Prostigmin® *see* Neostigmine *on page 661*

Prostin VR Pediatric® Injection *see* Alprostadil *on page 38*

Protilase® *see* Pancrelipase *on page 712*

Protostat® Oral *see* Metronidazole *on page 620*

Protriptyline (proe TRIP ti leen)

Related Information

Antidepressant Agents Comparison *on page 1021*
Antidepressant Medication Guidelines *on page 1075*
Federal OBRA Regulations Recommended Maximum Doses - Antidepressants *on page 1056*

Brand Names Vivactil®

Therapeutic Category Antidepressant, Tricyclic

Use Treatment of various forms of depression, often in conjunction with psychotherapy

Unlabeled use: Obstructive sleep apnea

Contraindications Narrow-angle glaucoma, hypersensitivity to protriptyline or any component

Precautions Use with caution in patients with cardiac conduction disturbances, history of hyperthyroid; protriptyline should not be abruptly discontinued in patients receiving high doses for prolonged periods to avoid cholinergic crisis; an EKG prior to initiation of therapy is advised

Adverse Reactions

Cardiovascular: Postural hypotension, arrhythmias, tachycardia, sudden death

Central nervous system: Sedation, dizziness, fatigue, anxiety, confusion, insomnia, impaired cognitive function, delirium, seizures; extrapyramidal symptoms are possible

Dermatologic: Photosensitivity

Endocrine & metabolic: SIADH

Gastrointestinal: Xerostomia, increased appetite, weight gain, constipation, decreased lower esophageal sphincter tone may cause GE reflux, dysgeusia

Genitourinary: Urinary retention, sexual dysfunction

Hematologic: Rarely agranulocytosis, leukopenia, eosinophilia

Hepatic: Jaundice, cholestatic jaundice

Neuromuscular & skeletal: Tremors, weakness

Ocular: Blurred vision, increased intraocular pressure

Miscellaneous: Allergic reactions

Overdosage Symptoms of overdose include agitation, confusion, hallucinations, urinary retention, hypothermia, hypotension, tachycardia

Toxicology Following initiation of essential overdose management, toxic symptoms should be treated. Ventricular arrhythmias often respond to phenytoin 15-20 mg/kg with concurrent systemic alkalinization (sodium bicarbonate 0.5-2 mEq/kg I.V.). Arrhythmias unresponsive to this therapy may respond to lidocaine 1 mg/kg I.V. followed by a titrated infusion. Physostigmine (1-2 mg I.V. slowly) may be indicated in reversing cardiac arrhythmias that are due to vagal blockade or for anticholinergic effects. Seizures usually respond to diazepam I.V. boluses (5-10 mg, up to 30 mg). If seizures are unresponsive or recur, phenytoin or phenobarbital may be required.

(Continued)

Protriptyline *(Continued)*

Drug Interactions
May decrease effects of guanethidine and clonidine

May increase effects of CNS depressants, adrenergic agents, dicumarol, anticholinergic agents

With MAO inhibitors, hyperpyrexia, tachycardia, hypertension, seizures, and death may occur; interactions similar to other tricyclics may occur

Cimetidine, fluoxetine, methylphenidate, and haloperidol may decrease the metabolism and/or increase TCA levels

Phenobarbital may increase TCA metabolism; use with clonidine may result in hypertensive crisis

Mechanism of Action Traditionally believed to increase the synaptic concentration of serotonin and/or norepinephrine in the central nervous system by inhibition of their reuptake by the presynaptic neuronal membrane. However, additional receptor effects have been found including desensitization of adenyl cyclase, down regulation of beta-adrenergic receptors, and down regulation of serotonin receptors.

Pharmacodynamics Onset of therapeutic effects: Takes 1-3 weeks before effects are seen; NE >>5-HT

Pharmacokinetics
Protein binding: 92%

Metabolism: Undergoes first-pass metabolism (10% to 25%); extensively metabolized in the liver by N-oxidation, hydroxylation and glucuronidation

Half-life: 54-92 hours, averaging 74 hours

Time to peak serum concentration: Oral: Within 24-30 hours

Elimination: In urine

Usual Dosage Oral:
Geriatrics: Initial dose: 5-10 mg/day; increase every 3-7 days by 5-10 mg; usual dose: 15-20 mg/day

Adults: 15-60 mg in 3-4 divided doses

Monitoring Parameters Blood pressure, pulse, target symptoms, mental status; occasional use of serum concentrations may be necessary in cases where response or toxicity are in question

Reference Range Therapeutic: 70-250 ng/mL (SI: 266-950 nmol/L); Toxic: >500 ng/mL (SI: >1900 nmol/L)

Test Interactions Elevated glucose

Patient Information Do not drink alcoholic beverages, may cause dry mouth, constipation, blurred vision, dizziness, avoid sudden changes in position

Nursing Implications Offer patient sugarless hard candy for dry mouth; monitor sitting and standing blood pressure and pulse

Special Geriatric Considerations Little data on its use in the elderly; strong anticholinergic properties which may limit its use; more often stimulating rather than sedating. Data from a clinical trial comparing fluoxetine to tricyclics suggest that fluoxetine is significantly less effective than nortriptyline in hospitalized elderly patients with unipolar major affective disorder, especially those with melancholia and concurrent cardiovascular diseases.

Dosage Forms Tablet, as hydrochloride: 5 mg, 10 mg

References
Roose SP, Glassman AH, Attia E, et al, "Comparative Efficacy of Selective Serotonin Reuptake Inhibitors and Tricyclics in the Treatment of Melancholia," *Am J Psychiatry*, 1994, 151(12):1735-9.

Proventil® *see* Albuterol *on page 29*

Proventil® HFA *see* Albuterol *on page 29*

Provera® Oral *see* Medroxyprogesterone Acetate *on page 578*

Proxigel® Oral [OTC] *see* Carbamide Peroxide *on page 162*

Prozac® *see* Fluoxetine *on page 394*

Pseudoephedrine *(soo doe e FED rin)*
Brand Names Actifed® Allergy Tablet (Day) [OTC]; Afrin® Tablet [OTC]; Cenafed® [OTC]; Children's Silfedrine® [OTC]; Decofed® Syrup [OTC]; Drixoral® Non-Drowsy [OTC]; Efidac/24® [OTC]; Neofed® [OTC]; PediaCare® Oral; Sudafed® [OTC]; Sudafed® 12 Hour [OTC]; Sufedrin® [OTC]; Triaminic® AM Decongestant Formula [OTC]

Synonyms d-Isoephedrine Hydrochloride

Generic Available Yes

Therapeutic Category Adrenergic Agonist Agent; Decongestant

Use Temporary symptomatic relief of nasal congestion due to common cold, upper respiratory allergies, and sinusitis; also promotes nasal or sinus drainage

Unlabeled use: Urinary incontinence (stress type) due to urethral sphincter weakness

Contraindications Hypersensitivity to pseudoephedrine or any component; MAO inhibitor therapy

Warnings Administer with caution to patients with hypertension, hyperthyroidism, diabetes mellitus, cardiovascular disease, ischemic heart disease, increased intraocular pressure, or prostatic hypertrophy. Elderly patients are more likely to experience adverse reactions to sympathomimetics. Overdosage may cause hallucinations, seizures, CNS depression, and death.

Adverse Reactions

Cardiovascular: Tachycardia, palpitations, arrhythmias

Central nervous system: Nervousness, excitability, dizziness, insomnia, drowsiness, headache

Gastrointestinal: Nausea, vomiting

Genitourinary: Dysuria

Neuromuscular & skeletal: Tremors

Overdosage Symptoms of overdose include seizures, nausea, vomiting, cardiac arrhythmias, hypertension, agitation

Toxicology There is no specific antidote for pseudoephedrine intoxication and the bulk of the treatment is supportive. Hyperactivity and agitation usually respond to reduced sensory input, however with extreme agitation haloperidol may be required. Hyperthermia is best treated with external cooling measures, or when severe or unresponsive, muscle paralysis with pancuronium may be needed. Hypertension is usually transient and generally does not require treatment unless severe. For diastolic blood pressures >110 mm Hg, a nitroprusside infusion should be initiated. Seizures usually respond to diazepam I.V. and/or phenytoin maintenance regimens.

Drug Interactions

Decreased effect: Beta-blockers, methyldopa

Increased toxicity/effect: Tricyclic antidepressants, MAO inhibitors (increased blood pressure), sympathomimetics

Mechanism of Action Stimulates alpha-adrenergic receptors of the vascular smooth muscle, thus constricting dilated arterioles within the nasal mucosa and reducing blood flow to the engaged area; increases urethral sphincter tone due to alpha-adrenergic actions; pseudoephedrine exerts beta-adrenergic effects as well as it alpha-adrenergic effect

Pharmacodynamics

Onset of action: Oral: Decongestant effects occur within 15-30 minutes

Duration: 4-6 hours (up to 12 hours with extended release formulation administration)

Pharmacokinetics

Metabolism: Partially in liver

Half-life: 9-16 hours

Elimination: 70% to 90% of dose excreted in urine as unchanged drug and 1% to 6% as norpseudoephedrine (active); renal elimination is dependent on urine pH and flow rate; alkaline urine decreases renal elimination of pseudoephedrine

Usual Dosage

Nasal congestion:

Geriatrics: 30-60 mg every 6 hours as needed

Adults: 60 mg every 4-6 hours; maximum: 240 mg/24 hours; sustained release: 120 mg every 12 hours

Urinary incontinence: Geriatrics and Adults: 15-30 mg 3 times/day

Monitoring Parameters Blood pressure, pulse, relief of symptoms, urinary output, episodes of incontinence

Patient Information Do not crush sustained release products; consult pharmacist or physician before using; do not exceed recommended dose; notify physician of insomnia, weakness, dizziness, tremor, or irregular heartbeat

Additional Information Pseudoephedrine is found in many combination cough and cold products

Pseudoephedrine hydrochloride: Cenafed® syrup [OTC], Decofed® syrup [OTC], Neofed® [OTC], Novafed®, Sudafed® [OTC], Sudafed® 12 Hour [OTC], Sudafed® tablet [OTC], Sufedrin® [OTC]

Pseudoephedrine sulfate: Afrinol® [OTC]

Special Geriatric Considerations Elderly patients should be counseled about the proper use of over-the-counter cough and cold preparations (see Warnings). Elderly are more predisposed to adverse effects of sympathomimetics since they frequently have cardiovascular diseases and diabetes mellitus as well as multiple drug therapies. It may be advisable to treat with a (Continued)

Pseudoephedrine *(Continued)*

short-acting/immediate-release formulation before initiating sustained-release/long-acting formulations.

Dosage Forms
Pseudoephedrine hydrochloride:
Capsule: 60 mg
Capsule, timed release: 120 mg
Drops, oral: 7.5 mg/0.8 mL (15 mL)
Liquid: 15 mg/5 mL (120 mL); 30 mg/5 mL (120 mL, 240 mL, 473 mL)
Syrup: 15 mg/5 mL (118 mL)
Tablet: 30 mg, 60 mg
Tablet, timed release: 120 mg
Tablet, extended release, as sulfate: 120 mg, 240 mg

Pseudoephedrine and Triprolidine *see* Triprolidine and Pseudoephedrine *on page 966*

Pseudomonic Acid A *see* Mupirocin *on page 643*

Psor-a-set® Soap [OTC] *see* Salicylic Acid *on page 845*

Psorion® Cream *see* Betamethasone *on page 114*

P&S® Shampoo [OTC] *see* Salicylic Acid *on page 845*

Psyllium *(SIL i yum)*

Brand Names Effer-Syllium® [OTC]; Fiberall® Powder [OTC]; Fiberall® Wafer [OTC]; Hydrocil® [OTC]; Konsyl-D® [OTC]; Konsyl® [OTC]; Metamucil® [OTC]; Metamucil® Instant Mix [OTC]; Modane® Bulk [OTC]; Perdiem® Plain [OTC]; Reguloid® [OTC]; Serutan® [OTC]; Siblin® [OTC]; Syllact® [OTC]; V-Lax® [OTC]

Synonyms Plantago Seed; Plantain Seed; Psyllium Hydrophilic Mucilloid

Generic Available Yes

Therapeutic Category Laxative, Bulk-Producing

Use Treatment of chronic atonic or spastic constipation and in constipation associated with rectal disorders; treatment of diverticulosis and diverticulitis; management of irritable bowel syndrome; nonspecific acute diarrhea

Contraindications Fecal impaction, GI obstruction; hypersensitivity to psyllium

Warnings May contribute to fecal impaction if insufficient fluid intake exists or other predisposing causes

Precautions Some products contain aspartame which is metabolized in the GI tract to phenylalanine; rectal bleeding may indicate a more serious medical condition which may require further evaluation; impaction and obstruction may occur in diseases which inhibit passage through the gastrointestinal tract (eg, strictures, ileus); use caution in patients with intestinal ulceration, bowel adhesions, or stenosis; not to be used for acute constipation

Adverse Reactions
Gastrointestinal: Esophageal or bowel obstruction, bloating, flatulence, abdominal cramps
Ocular: Rhinoconjunctivitis
Respiratory: Bronchospasm
Miscellaneous: Anaphylaxis upon inhalation in susceptible (hypersensitive) individuals

Overdosage Symptoms of overdose include abdominal pain, diarrhea, flatulence, possible impaction

Drug Interactions Digitalis, nitrofurantoin, salicylates may have their absorption decreased by psyllium

Mechanism of Action Absorbs water in the intestine to form a viscous liquid which promotes peristalsis and reduces transit time through mechanical distention; fiber decreases intraluminal pressures in the colon and rectum which is beneficial in treatment of diverticular disease and irritable bowel syndrome

Pharmacodynamics Onset of action: 12-24 hours, but full effect may take 2-3 days; considered the safest and most physiologic laxative agent

Pharmacokinetics Absorption: Oral: Generally not absorbed, small amounts of grain extracts present in the preparation have been reportedly absorbed following colonic hydrolysis

Usual Dosage Geriatrics and Adults: Oral: 1-2 rounded teaspoonfuls (5-11 g) or 1-2 packets 1-3 times/day in water or fruit juice (see Additional Information)

Monitoring Parameters Monitor for diarrhea, abdominal pain, bowel obstruction, or impaction

Patient Information Must be mixed in a glass of water or juice; drink a full glass of liquid with each dose; must drink fluids throughout the day to be effective and avoid impaction; report bleeding or failure to respond to physician, pharmacist, or nurse; do not use for acute constipation

Nursing Implications Inhalation of psyllium dust may cause sensitivity to psyllium (runny nose, watery eyes, wheezing); fiber therapy increases stool frequency; do not use for acute constipation (see Monitoring Parameters)

Additional Information 3.4 g psyllium hydrophilic mucilloid per 7 g powder is equivalent to a rounded teaspoonful or one packet; fiber therapy results in increased frequency of defecation. Diabetic patients may need or prefer sugar-free products; psyllium using aspartame is available for diabetic patients. Bloating and flatulence are mostly a problem in first 4 weeks of therapy.

Special Geriatric Considerations Elderly may have insufficient fluid intake which may predispose them to fecal impaction and bowel obstruction. Patients should have a 1 month trial, with at least 14 g/day, before effects in bowel function are determined.

Dosage Forms
Chewable pieces: 3.4 g
Granules: 4.03 g per rounded teaspoon (100 g, 250 g); 2.5 g per rounded teaspoon
Powder, effervescent: 3 g per dose (270 g, 480 g); 3.4 g per dose (single dose packets)
Powder: Psyllium 50% and dextrose 50% (6.5 g, 325 g, 420 g, 480 g, 500 g); psyllium hydrophilic: 3.4 g per rounded teaspoon (210 g, 300 g, 420 g, 630 g)
Wafer: 3.4 g

Psyllium Hydrophilic Mucilloid *see Psyllium on previous page*
Pteroylglutamic Acid *see Folic Acid on page 407*
PTU *see Propylthiouracil on page 800*
Puralube® Ophthalmic Ointment [OTC] *see Ocular Lubricant on page 688*
Puralube® Tears Solution [OTC] *see Artificial Tears on page 82*
Purge® [OTC] *see Castor Oil on page 171*
Purinethol® *see Mercaptopurine on page 589*
PₓEₓ® Ophthalmic *see Pilocarpine and Epinephrine on page 749*

Pyrazinamide (peer a ZIN a mide)
Synonyms Pyrazinoic Acid Amide
Therapeutic Category Antitubercular Agent
Use Adjunctive treatment of tuberculosis when primary and secondary agents cannot be used or have failed
Contraindications Severe hepatic damage; hypersensitivity to pyrazinamide or any component, acute gout
Precautions Use with caution in patients with renal failure, gout, or diabetes mellitus
Adverse Reactions
Central nervous system: Malaise, fever
Dermatologic: Urticaria, rash, photosensitivity
Endocrine & metabolic: Gout, hyperuricemia
Gastrointestinal: Nausea, vomiting, anorexia
Hepatic: Hepatotoxicity, jaundice
Neuromuscular & skeletal: Arthralgia
Overdosage Symptoms of overdose include gout, gastric upset, hepatic damage
Drug Interactions Isoniazid (decreased INH serum concentrations)
Mechanism of Action Converted to pyrazinoic acid in susceptible strains of *Mycobacterium* which lowers the pH of the environment
Pharmacodynamics Bacteriostatic or bactericidal depending on the drug's concentration at the site of infection
Pharmacokinetics
Absorption: Oral: Well absorbed
Distribution: Widely distributed into body tissues and fluids including the liver, lung, and CSF
Protein binding: 50%
Metabolism: In the liver
Half-life: 9-10 hours, increased with reduced renal or hepatic function
Time to peak serum concentration: Within 2 hours
Elimination: In urine (4% as unchanged drug)
(Continued)

Pyrazinamide *(Continued)*

Usual Dosage Oral:

Geriatrics: Start with a lower daily dose (15 mg/kg) and increase as tolerated

Adults: 15-30 mg/kg/day in 3-4 divided doses; maximum daily dose: 2 g/day

Alternative dose: A dosing regimen of 50-70 mg/kg twice weekly (based upon lean body weight) has been recommended to improve patient compliance

Monitoring Parameters Periodic liver function tests, serum uric acid, sputum culture, chest x-ray 2-3 months into treatment and at completion

Test Interactions May interfere with Acetest® and Ketostix® urine tests to produce a pink-brown color

Patient Information Compliance must be stressed; inform physician if fever, malaise, weakness, nausea or vomiting, darkened urine, skin or eye discoloration (yellow), or swollen or painful joints develop

Special Geriatric Considerations Pyrazinamide is used in the 2-month intensive treatment phase of a 6-month treatment plan. Most elderly acquired their *Mycobacterium tuberculosis* infection before effective chemotherapy was available; however, older persons with new infections (not reactivation), or who are from areas where drug-resistant *M. tuberculosis* is endemic, or who are HIV-infected should receive 3-4 drug therapies including pyrazinamide.

Dosage Forms Tablet: 500 mg

References

Bass JB Jr, Farer LS, Hopewell PC, et al, "Treatment of Tuberculosis and Tuberculosis Infection in Adults and Children," *Am J Respir Crit Care Med*, 1994, 149(5):1359-74.

Van Scoy RE and Wilkowske CJ, "Antituberculous Agents: Isoniazid, Rifampin, Streptomycin, Ethambutol, and Pyrazinamide," *Mayo Clin Proc*, 1983, 58(4):233-40.

Yoshikawa TT, "Tuberculosis in Aging Adults," *J Am Geriatr Soc*, 1992, 40(2):178-87.

Pyrazinoic Acid Amide *see Pyrazinamide on previous page*

Pyridiate® *see Phenazopyridine on page 734*

Pyridium® *see Phenazopyridine on page 734*

Pyridostigmine *(peer id oh STIG meen)*

Brand Names Mestinon® Injection; Mestinon® Oral; Regonol® Injection

Generic Available No

Therapeutic Category Antidote, Neuromuscular Blocking Agent; Cholinergic Agent

Use Symptomatic treatment of myasthenia gravis; also used as an antidote for nondepolarizing neuromuscular blockers, prevent and treat postoperative bladder distention

Contraindications Hypersensitivity to pyridostigmine, bromides, or any component; GI or GU obstruction

Warnings Does **not** antagonize and may prolong the phase I block of depolarizing muscle relaxants (eg, succinylcholine); use with caution in patients with epilepsy, asthma, bradycardia, hyperthyroidism, cardiac arrhythmias, or peptic ulcer; adequate facilities should be available for cardiopulmonary resuscitation when testing and adjusting dose for myasthenia gravis; have atropine and epinephrine ready to treat hypersensitivity reactions; overdosage may result in cholinergic crisis, this must be distinguished from myasthenic crisis; anticholinesterase insensitivity can develop for brief or prolonged periods

Precautions Patients may become insensitive to pharmacologic action; this may be brief or prolonged; reduce dose or withhold dose until patient regains sensitivity; monitor respiratory rate

Adverse Reactions

Cardiovascular: Bradycardia, A-V block, hypotension, asystole

Central nervous system: Headache, seizures, drowsiness, dysphoria, restlessness, agitation

Dermatologic: Rash

Gastrointestinal: Nausea, vomiting, diarrhea, salivation, stomach cramps, hyperperistalsis

Genitourinary: Urge to urinate

Neuromuscular & skeletal: Muscle cramps, weakness, tremor, fasciculations

Ocular: Miosis, lacrimation

Respiratory: Increased bronchial secretions, bronchospasm

Miscellaneous: Diaphoresis

Overdosage Symptoms of overdose include muscle weakness, blurred vision, excessive sweating, tearing and salivation, nausea, vomiting, diarrhea, hypertension, bradycardia, paralysis

Toxicology Atropine is the treatment of choice for intoxications manifesting with significant muscarinic symptoms. Atropine I.V. 2-4 mg every 3-60 minutes should be repeated to control symptoms and then continued as needed for 1-2 days following the acute ingestion.

Drug Interactions
Decreased effect with corticosteroids, magnesium, antiarrhythmics
Increased effect of depolarizing neuromuscular relaxants (succinylcholine) effect
Increased effect/toxicity with edrophonium, aminoglycosides

Stability Protect from light

Mechanism of Action Inhibits destruction of acetylcholine by acetylcholinesterase which facilitates transmission of impulses across myoneural junction

Pharmacodynamics
Onset of action:
Oral, I.M.: Within 15-30
I.V.: Within 2-5 minutes
Duration:
Oral: 3-6 hours
I.M., I.V.: 2-4 hours

Pharmacokinetics
Absorption: Oral: Very poor (10% to 20%) from GI tract
Metabolism: In the liver

Usual Dosage Geriatrics and Adults:
Myasthenia gravis:
Oral: Initial: 60 mg 3 times/day with maintenance dose ranging from 60 mg to 1.5 g/day; sustained release: 180-540 mg once or twice daily
I.M., I.V.: 2 mg every 2-3 hours or 1/30th of oral dose
Reversal of nondepolarizing neuromuscular blocker: I.V.: 10-20 mg preceded by atropine (I.V. 0.6-1.2 mg)

Administration When giving for reversal of neuromuscular blockade, keep patient well ventilated until recovered

Monitoring Parameters Symptoms of myasthenia gravis, blood pressure, pulse, respiratory rate, signs of cholinergic crisis (see Overdosage)

Test Interactions Increased aminotransferase [ALT (SGPT)/AST (SGOT)] (S), increased amylase (S)

Patient Information Side effects are generally due to exaggerated pharmacologic effects; most common are salivation and muscle fasciculations; notify physician if nausea, vomiting, muscle weakness, severe abdominal pain, or difficulty breathing occurs; take drug as ordered; take with food; report adverse reactions to physician promptly; do not chew or crush sustained release tablets

Nursing Implications Do not crush sustained release drug product; observe patient closely for cholinergic symptoms especially if I.V. dose is used

Additional Information Not a cure; patient may develop resistance to the drug; normally, sustained release dosage form is used at bedtime for patients who complain of morning weakness

Special Geriatric Considerations Many elderly may have pulmonary or cardiovascular diseases which will require cautious use of pyridostigmine; see Precautions, Warnings, and Adverse Reactions

Dosage Forms
Pyridostigmine bromide:
Injection: 5 mg/mL (2 mL, 5 mL)
Syrup (raspberry flavor): 60 mg/5 mL (480 mL)
Tablet: 60 mg
Tablet, sustained release: 180 mg

Pyridoxine (peer i DOKS een)

Related Information
Antidotes on page 1097

Brand Names Nestrex®

Synonyms Vitamin B_6

Generic Available Yes

Therapeutic Category Antidote, Cycloserine Toxicity; Antidote, Hydralazine Toxicity; Antidote, Isoniazid Toxicity; Vitamin, Water Soluble

Use Prevents and treats vitamin B_6 deficiency, adjunct to treatment of acute toxicity from isoniazid, cycloserine, or hydralazine overdose

Contraindications Hypersensitivity to pyridoxine or any component

Warnings Dependence and withdrawal may occur with doses >200 mg/day
(Continued)

807

Pyridoxine *(Continued)*

Adverse Reactions
Central nervous system: Sensory neuropathy, seizures

Neuromuscular & skeletal: Paresthesia

Miscellaneous: Following I.V. administration of very large doses, headache, nausea, decreased serum folic acid secretions (especially in patients with homocystinuria), increased AST, allergic reactions

Overdosage Signs and symptoms of overdose include ataxia, sensory neuropathy with doses of 50 mg to 2 g daily over prolonged periods

Drug Interactions Decreased serum concentrations of levodopa, phenobarbital, and phenytoin (patients taking levodopa without carbidopa should avoid supplemental vitamin B_6 >5 mg/day; includes many multivitamin preparations)

Stability Protect from light

Mechanism of Action Precursor to pyridoxal, which functions in the metabolism of proteins, carbohydrates, and fats; pyridoxal also aids in the release of liver and muscle stored glycogen

Pharmacokinetics
Absorption: Enteral, parenteral: Well absorbed

Metabolism: In 4-pyridoxic acid, and other metabolites

Half-life: 2-3 weeks

Elimination: Urinary excretion

Usual Dosage Geriatrics and Adults:

Dietary deficiency: Oral: 10-20 mg/day for 3 weeks

Drug-induced neuritis (eg, isoniazid, hydralazine, penicillamine, cycloserine): Oral treatment: 100-200 mg/24 hours; prophylaxis: 10-100 mg/24 hours

For the treatment of seizures and/or coma from acute isoniazid toxicity, a dose of pyridoxine hydrochloride equal to the amount of INH ingested can be given I.M./I.V. in divided doses together with other anticonvulsants

For the treatment of acute hydralazine toxicity, a pyridoxine dose of 25 mg/kg in divided doses I.M./I.V. has been used

Administration Administer slow I.V.

Monitoring Parameters When administering large I.V. doses, monitor respiratory rate, heart rate, and blood pressure

Reference Range >50 ng/mL (SI: 243 nmol/L) (varies considerably with method). A broad range is ~25-80 ng/mL (SI: 122-389 nmol/L). HPLC method for pyridoxal phosphate has normal range of 3.5-18 ng/mL (SI: 17-88 nmol/L).

Test Interactions Urobilinogen

Patient Information Dietary sources of pyridoxine include red meats, bananas, potatoes, yeast, lima beans, whole grain cereals; do not exceed recommended doses

Nursing Implications Burning may occur at the injection site after I.M. or S.C. administration; seizures have occurred following I.V. administration of very large doses

Additional Information
For the treatment of seizures and/or coma from acute isoniazid toxicity, a dose of pyridoxine hydrochloride equal to the amount of INH ingested can be given I.M./I.V. in divided doses together with other anticonvulsants

For the treatment of acute hydrazine toxicity, pyridoxine 25 mg/kg/dose I.M./I.V. has been used

Special Geriatric Considerations Use with caution in patients with Parkinson's disease treated with levodopa

Dosage Forms
Pyridoxine hydrochloride:

Injection: 100 mg/mL (10 mL, 30 mL)

Tablet: 25 mg, 50 mg, 100 mg

Tablet, extended release: 100 mg

Quazepam *(KWAY ze pam)*

Related Information
Antacid Drug Interactions *on page 1096*

Anxiolytic/Hypnotic Use in Long-Term Care Facilities *on page 1099*

Benzodiazepines Comparison *on page 1024*

Brand Names Doral®

Generic Available No

Therapeutic Category Benzodiazepine; Hypnotic; Sedative

Use Short-term treatment of insomnia

Restrictions C-IV

Contraindications Narrow-angle glaucoma, known hypersensitivity to quazepam, cross-sensitivity with other benzodiazepines may occur; severe uncontrolled pain, sleep apnea

Warnings Abrupt discontinuance may precipitate withdrawal or rebound insomnia

Precautions Has potential for drug dependence and abuse, use with caution in patients with a history of drug dependence

Adverse Reactions
Central nervous system: Daytime sedation, ataxia, amnesia, confusion, dizziness, hallucinations, headache
Gastrointestinal: Xerostomia, nausea, vomiting
Hepatic: Cholestatic jaundice
Miscellaneous: Physical and psychological dependence may occur with prolonged use

Overdosage Symptoms of overdose include somnolence, confusion, coma, and diminished reflexes

Toxicology Treatment for benzodiazepine overdose is supportive; rarely is mechanical ventilation required
Flumazenil has been shown to selectively block the binding of benzodiazepines to CNS receptors, resulting in a reversal of benzodiazepine-induced sedation; however, its use may not alter the course of overdose

Drug Interactions Benzodiazepines may decrease the effect of levodopa
Decreased metabolism: Cimetidine, fluoxetine
Increased metabolism: Rifampin
Increased toxicity: CNS depressants, alcohol

Mechanism of Action Benzodiazepines appear to potentiate the effects of GABA and other inhibitory neurotransmitters by binding to specific benzodiazepine-receptor sites in various areas of the CNS

Pharmacodynamics Studies have shown that the elderly are more sensitive to the effects of benzodiazepines as compared to younger adults

Pharmacokinetics
Absorption: Oral: Rapidly absorbed
Protein binding: 95%.
Metabolism: In the liver to at least one active compound
Half-life:
Geriatrics:
Parent: 53 hours
Active metabolite: 190 hours
Adults:
Parent: 25-41 hours
Active metabolite: 40-114 hours

Usual Dosage Oral:
Geriatrics: Initial: 7.5-15 mg at bedtime, if giving 15 mg initially, decrease to 7.5 mg on the second or third night
Adults: Initial: 15 mg at bedtime, in some patients the dose may be reduced to 7.5 mg after a few nights

Monitoring Parameters Respiratory, cardiovascular and mental status

Patient Information Avoid alcohol and other CNS depressants; may cause drowsiness; avoid activities needing good psychomotor coordination until CNS effects are known; may cause physical or psychological dependence; avoid abrupt discontinuation after prolonged use; may cause "hangover" effect

Nursing Implications Provide safety measures (ie, side rails, night light, call button); remove smoking materials from area; supervise ambulation

Additional Information More likely than short-acting benzodiazepine to cause daytime sedation and fatigue; is classified as a long-acting benzodiazepine hypnotic (like flurazepam - Dalmane®), this long duration of action may prevent withdrawal symptoms when therapy is discontinued.

Special Geriatric Considerations Two short-term placebo controlled studies found minimal daytime drowsiness or other side effects with quazepam in elderly patients; there is little clinical experience with this drug in the elderly, but because of its long duration of action, it is probably not a drug of choice (see Pharmacodynamics); long-acting benzodiazepines have been associated with falls in the elderly; interpretive guidelines from the Health Care Financing Administration (HCFA) discourage the use of this agent in residents of long-term care facilities

Dosage Forms Tablet: 7.5 mg, 15 mg

References
Martinez HT and Serna CT, "Short-Term Treatment With Quazepam of Insomnia in Geriatric Patients," *Clin Ther*, 1982, 5(2):174-8.
(Continued)

Quazepam *(Continued)*

Winsauer HJ and O'Hair DE, "Quazepam: Short-Term Treatment of Insomnia in Geriatric Outpatients," *Curr Ther Res*, 1984, 35(2):228-34.

Questran® *see* Cholestyramine Resin *on page 220*
Questran® Light *see* Cholestyramine Resin *on page 220*

Quetiapine (kwe TYE a peen)

Related Information
Antipsychotic Agents Comparison *on page 1023*
Brand Names Seroquel®
Synonyms Quetiapine Fumarate
Generic Available No
Therapeutic Category Antipsychotic Agent
Use Management of psychotic disorders; this antipsychotic drug belongs to a new chemical class, the dibenzothiazepine derivatives
Contraindications Known hypersensitivity to this drug or any of its ingredients
Warnings
Neuroleptic malignant syndrome (NMS): A potentially fatal symptom complex has been reported in association with administration of antipsychotic drugs. Clinical manifestations of NMS are hyperpyrexia, muscle rigidity, altered mental status, and evidence of autonomic instability (irregular pulse or blood pressure, tachycardia, diaphoresis, and cardiac dysrhythmia). Management of NMS should include immediate discontinuation of antipsychotic drugs and other drugs not essential to concurrent therapy, intensive symptomatic treatment and medication monitoring, and treatment of any concomitant serious medical problems for which specific treatment are available.
Tardive dyskinesia (TD): No cases of tardive dyskinesia have been reported. However, it cannot be concluded that quetiapine does not cause this symptom complex until more clinical use of this agent has been evaluated.
Use with caution in hepatic impairment since quetiapine is extensively metabolized in the liver. Expect higher serum/tissue concentrations which may require dosage adjustments. Carcinogenicity at $1\frac{1}{2}$ to $4\frac{1}{2}$ times human doses caused thyroid gland follicular adenomas in male mice and rats; mammary adenocarcinomas were increased in female rats at all doses. The relevance to humans is unknown.
Elderly in studies did not demonstrate any difference in tolerability compared to younger adults. The studies did demonstrate a decreased rate of clearance by 30% to 50%. Concomitant diseases and/or medications could result in changes of clearance or pharmacodynamics and, therefore, may require dosage adjustments.
Precautions
Quetiapine may induce orthostatic hypotension and syncope which may be prevented by initiating doses at 25 mg twice daily; cataracts and lens changes may occur, and therefore, ophthalmologic examination (slit lamp) should be done at the start of therapy and at 6-month intervals
Seizures occurred in studies; use with caution in patients with seizure history or in patients with concomitant diseases lowering seizure threshold such as Alzheimer's disease, stroke, or CNS infections
Thyroid function tests in clinical studies demonstrated that some patients had TSH elevations requiring thyroid replacement
Lipid changes: During clinical trials, quetiapine increased cholesterol (11% increase) and triglycerides (17% increase) from baseline
Transaminase (ALT) elevations which were transient and reversible have occurred during clinical trials; 6% of patients had elevations greater than 3 times upper normal. These elevations occurred within 3 weeks of initiating quetiapine and returned to normal while continuing therapy.
Priapism was reported in one patient
Dysphagia in the form of esophageal dysmotility and aspiration are associated with antipsychotic drugs. Elderly may be at risk due to concomitant drug therapy or disease (eg, Alzheimer's disease, stroke, etc).
Cognitive and motor impairment due to somnolence is a common (18%) adverse effect, especially at the start of therapy. Also concomitant drug therapy may potentiate cognitive and motor impairment.
Body temperature regulation disruption has not been reported with quetiapine, however, this is a common problem with antipsychotic therapy. Patients should be cautioned who participate in strenuous activities, receive anticholinergic drugs, or are likely to be dehydrated.

Suicide is an inherent threat with those suffering from schizophrenia. Close monitoring is required. Prescription amounts should be limited for outpatients.

Adverse Reactions

Cardiovascular: Postural hypotension (7%), tachycardia (7%), bradycardia, palpitations, vasodilation, prolonged P-T interval, irregular pulse, bundle branch block, T-wave inversion, A-V block, atrial fibrillation, elevated S-T segment, T-wave flattening, increased QRS interval, angina pectoris, congestive heart failure, peripheral edema, cyanosis (up to 1%)

Central nervous system: Headache (19%), somnolence (18%), dizziness (10%), ataxia, vertigo, incoordination, catatonic reactions, disturbing dreams, confusion, amnesia, psychosis, hallucinations, paranoia, delusions, mania, apathy, depersonalization, stupor, aphasia, emotional lability, fever

Dermatologic: Pruritus, eczema, acne, seborrhea, maculopapular rash, skin ulcers, exfoliative dermatitis, skin discoloration (rare), psoriasis, ecchymosis

Endocrine & metabolic: Hyperlipidemia, dehydration, hyperglycemia, hypoglycemia, hypokalemia, increased libido, gynecomastia, hypothyroidism, hyperthyroid, diabetes mellitus

Gastrointestinal: Constipation (5%), dry mouth (7%), increased salivation, anorexia, increased appetite, dysphagia, glossitis, gingivitis, gastritis, stomatitis, gastroesophageal reflux, mouth ulcers, rectal hemorrhage, melena, hematemesis, hemorrhoids, flatulence, thirst, fecal incontinence, tongue edema, intestinal obstruction, abdominal pain, weight gain, weight loss, taste perversion

Genitourinary: Vaginitis, vaginal moniliasis, abnormal ejaculation, cystitis, leukorrhea, vaginal hemorrhage, vulvovaginitis, orchitis (up to 1%), nocturia, polyuria, urinary incontinence, impotence

Hematologic: Leukopenia (≥1%), leukocytosis, anemia, hypochromic anemia, thrombocytopenia (rare), eosinophilia

Neuromuscular & skeletal: Involuntary movements, gait disturbances, hyperkinesis, myoclonus, hemiplegia, choreoathetosis, neuralgia, asthenia (4%), back pain (2%), myasthenia, arthralgia, arthritis, leg cramps, bone pain, pathological fracture

Ocular: Conjunctivitis, vision changes, dry eyes, blepharitis, eye pain (up to 1%), glaucoma (rare)

Otic: Tinnitus, deafness

Renal: Elevated creatinine, glucosuria

Respiratory: Pharyngitis, rhinitis (3%), cough, dyspnea, epistaxis, asthma

Miscellaneous: Bruxism, alcohol intolerance, diaphoresis, hiccups

Overdosage No fatalities reported with cases where doses have been up to 9600 mg.

Signs and symptoms of overdose are extensions of quetiapine's pharmacologic action including sedation, drowsiness, hypotension, tachycardia, first degree heart block, hypokalemia

Toxicology There is no antidote for quetiapine. With obtundation, seizure, and dystonic reactions, the possibility of aspiration exists. Monitor cardiovascular status and obtain continuous EKG. Treat any arrhythmia with procainamide, quinidine, or disopyramide. Keep in mind disopyramide is very anticholinergic and may pose a problem in elderly. Treat hypotension and circulatory collapse with such measures as I.V. fluids, sympathomimetics. Do **not** use epinephrine or dopamine since beta-adrenergic action may worsen hypotension since quetiapine causes alpha blockade. If extrapyramidal side effects are severe, treat with anticholinergics. Monitor patient closely and administer general supportive care.

Drug Interactions Major interactions occur with drugs that inhibit or induce cytochrome P-450 3A4 fraction (eg, ketoconazole, itraconazole, fluconazole, erythromycin)

Cimetidine: Decreases clearance of quetiapine (20%)

Phenytoin: Increases clearance of quetiapine; may have to adjust dose

Thioridazine: Increases clearance of quetiapine (65%)

Lorazepam: Clearance of lorazepam is reduced by quetiapine (20%)

Dopamine agonists, levodopa: Quetiapine may antagonize dopamine and levodopa

Hepatic enzyme inducers may result in the need to increase quetiapine doses: Rifampin, glucocorticoids, barbiturates, carbamazepine

Drug/Food Interactions Bioavailability is increased when taken with meals

Mechanism of Action An antagonist at multiple neurotransmitter receptors in the brain: serotonin $5HT_{1A}$ and $5HT_2$, dopamine D_1 and D_2, histamine H_1 and (Continued)

Quetiapine *(Continued)*

adrenergic alpha$_1$ and alpha$_2$ receptors; quetiapine fumarate has no appreciable affinity at cholinergic muscarininc and benzodiazepine receptors

Mechanism of action of quetiapine fumarate, as with other antipsychotic drugs, is unknown. However, it has been proposed that this drug's antipsychotic activity is mediated through a combination of dopamine type 2 (D$_2$) and serotonin type 2 (5-HT$_2$) antagonism. Antagonism at receptors other than dopamine and 5HT$_2$ with similar receptor affinities may explain some of the other effects of quetiapine fumarate. The drug's antagonism of histamine H$_1$ receptors may explain the somnolence observed with it. The drug's antagonism of adrenergic alpha$_1$-receptors may explain the orthostatic hypotension observed with it.

Pharmacokinetics

Absorption: Accumulation is predictable upon multiple dosing

Distribution: Widely distributed in body; V$_d$: 10 L/kg

Metabolism: Both metabolites are pharmacologically inactive

Bioavailability: Tablet is 100% bioavailable relative to solution; marginally affected by administration with food, with C$_{max}$ and AUC values increased by 25% and 15% respectively

Half-life, mean terminal: ~6 hours; steady state achieved in 2 days

Time to peak plasma concentrations: 1.5 hours

Elimination: Mainly via hepatic metabolism; reduced clearance seen in elderly when compared to younger adults (40% reduction)

Usual Dosage

Geriatrics and Adults: Oral: Initial: 25 mg twice daily; increase dose in increments of 25-50 mg 2-3 times/day on second and third day as tolerated; elderly may require a slower rate of titration; antipsychotic efficacy is seen in a daily dose range of 150-750 mg/day; do not exceed 800 mg/day.

Dose reductions should be attempted periodically to establish lowest effective dose in patients with psychosis or to establish need to continue treating agitated symptoms in demented elderly. Patients being restarted after 1 week of no drug need to be titrated as above.

Dosing comments in severe renal impairment:

Cl$_{cr}$ 10-30 mL/minute/1.73 m^2: 25% lower mean oral clearance than normal subjects; plasma quetiapine concentrations in subjects with renal insufficiency were within the range of concentrations seen in normal subjects receiving same dose; dosage adjustment is therefore not needed

Dosing comments in hepatic insufficiency: 30% lower mean oral clearance of quetiapine than normal subjects; higher plasma concentrations expected in hepatically impaired subjects; dosage adjustment may be needed

Monitoring Parameters Patients should have eyes checked every 6 months for cataracts while on this medication; monitor for response and behavior control

Test Interactions Asymptomatic increases in AST, cholesterol, triglycerides

Patient Information May cause drowsiness, dizziness, and/or headache; might increase risk of cataracts; care should be exercised when operating machinery/cars

Additional Information Quetiapine has a very low incidence of extrapyramidal symptoms such as restlessness and abnormal movement; is at least as effective as conventional antipsychotics (see Warnings, Precautions, and Monitoring Parameters)

Special Geriatric Considerations See Warnings.

Extrapyramidal syndrome symptoms occur less often than with traditional antipsychotics from the phenothiazine and butyrophenone classes. Many elderly patients receive antipsychotic medications for inappropriate nonpsychotic behavior. Before initiating antipsychotic medication, the clinician should investigate any possible reversible cause; any stress or stress from any disease can cause acute "confusion" or worsening of baseline nonpsychotic behavior. Most commonly acute changes in behavior are due to increases in drug dose or addition of new drug to regimen; fluid electrolyte loss; infections; and changes in environment.

Any changes in disease status in any organ system can result in behavior changes

In the treatment of agitated, demented elderly patients, authors of meta-analyses of controlled trials of the response to the traditional antipsychotics (eg, phenothiazines, butyrophenones) in controlling agitation, have concluded that the use of neuroleptics results in a response rate of 18%.

Clearly neuroleptic therapy for behavior control should be limited with frequent attempts to withdraw the agent given for behavior control.

Dosage Forms Tablet, as fumarate: 25 mg, 100 mg, 200 mg

References

Goldberg RJ, "Managing Psychosis-Related Behavioral Problems in the Elderly," *Consult Pharm*, 1997, 12(Suppl C):4-10.

Quetiapine Fumarate *see* Quetiapine *on page 810*

Quibron®-T *see* Theophylline *on page 902*

Quibron®-T/SR *see* Theophylline *on page 902*

Quiess® *see* Hydroxyzine *on page 470*

Quinaglute® Dura-Tabs® *see* Quinidine *on page 815*

Quinalan® *see* Quinidine *on page 815*

Quinalbarbitone Sodium *see* Secobarbital *on page 851*

Quinapril (KWIN a pril)

Related Information

ACE Inhibitors Comparison *on page 1019*

Brand Names Accupril®

Generic Available No

Therapeutic Category Angiotensin-Converting Enzyme (ACE) Inhibitors

Use Management of hypertension and treatment of systolic congestive heart failure

Contraindications Hypersensitivity to captopril or any component or any ACE inhibitor

Warnings Neutropenia, agranulocytosis, angioedema, decreased renal function (hypertension, renal artery stenosis, CHF), hepatic dysfunction (elimination, activation), proteinuria, first-dose hypotension (hypovolemia, CHF, dehydrated patients at risk, eg, diuretic use, elderly), elderly (due to renal function changes)

Precautions Use with caution and modify dosage in patients with renal impairment; use with caution in patients with collagen vascular disease, CHF, hypovolemia, valvular stenosis, hyperkalemia (>5.7 mEq/L), anesthesia

Adverse Reactions

Cardiovascular: Arrhythmias, orthostatic blood pressure changes, CVA, myocardial infarction, angina, palpitations, chest pain, hypotension, tachycardia, syncope, cardiogenic shock, heart failure

Central nervous system: Nervousness, depression, confusion, somnolence, fatigue, dizziness, headache, insomnia, malaise, vertigo

Dermatologic: Rash, exfoliative dermatitis, photosensitivity, pruritus, dermatopolymyositis, angioedema

Endocrine & metabolic: Hyperkalemia

Gastrointestinal: Ageusia, pancreatitis, xerostomia, constipation, anorexia, nausea, vomiting, abdominal pain, GI hemorrhage

Genitourinary: Impotence

Hematologic: Neutropenia, agranulocytosis, thrombocytopenia (0.5% to 1%)

Hepatic: Hepatitis

Neuromuscular & skeletal: Myalgia, arthralgia, paresthesia

Ocular: Blurred vision

Renal: Increased BUN, serum creatinine, proteinuria, oliguria, worsening of renal failure

Respiratory: Chronic cough (nonproductive, persistent; more often in women and seen in 15% to 30% of patients), asthma, bronchospasm

Miscellaneous: Diaphoresis

Overdosage Symptoms of overdose include hypotension

Toxicology Following initiation of essential overdose management, toxic symptom treatment and supportive treatment should be initiated. Hypotension usually responds to I.V. fluids or Trendelenburg positioning. If unresponsive to these measures, the use of a parenteral inotrope may be required (eg, norepinephrine 0.1-0.2 mcg/kg/minute titrated to response). Seizures commonly respond to diazepam (I.V. 5-10 mg bolus in adults every 15 minutes if needed up to a total of 30 mg) or to phenytoin or phenobarbital.

Drug Interactions

ACE inhibitors (quinapril) and potassium-sparing diuretics may cause additive hyperkalemic effect

ACE inhibitors (quinapril) and indomethacin or nonsteroidal anti-inflammatory agents may cause reduced antihypertensive response to ACE inhibitors (quinapril)

Allopurinol and quinapril may cause neutropenia

Antacids and ACE inhibitors may decrease absorption of ACE inhibitors

(Continued)

Quinapril *(Continued)*

Phenothiazines and ACE inhibitors may increase ACE inhibitor effect

Probenecid and ACE inhibitors (quinapril) may increase ACE inhibitors (quinapril) levels

Rifampin and ACE inhibitors (enalapril) may decrease ACE inhibitor effect

Digoxin and ACE inhibitors may increase serum digoxin concentrations

Lithium and ACE inhibitors may increase lithium serum concentration

Tetracycline and ACE inhibitors (quinapril) may decrease tetracycline absorption (up to 37%)

Food decreases quinapril absorption; rate, but not extent, of ramipril and fosinopril is reduced by concomitant administration with food; food does not reduce absorption of enalapril, lisinopril or benazepril; quinapril has a decreased rate and extent (25% to 30%) of absorption when taken with a high fat meal

Stability Unstable in aqueous solutions; to prepare solution for oral administration, mix prior to administration and use within 10 minutes

Mechanism of Action Competitive inhibitor of angiotensin-converting enzyme (ACE); prevents conversion of angiotensin I to angiotensin II, a potent vasoconstrictor; results in lower levels of angiotensin II which causes an increase in plasma renin activity and a reduction in aldosterone secretion; a CNS mechanism may also be involved in hypotensive effect as angiotensin II increases adrenergic outflow from CNS; vasoactive kallikreins may be decreased in conversion to active hormones by ACE inhibitors, thus reducing blood pressure

Pharmacodynamics

Onset of action: Within 1 hour

Duration: 24 hours; data demonstrate excellent tissue penetration with a long tissue half-life

Pharmacokinetics

Absorption: Oral: 60%

Metabolism: To some degree in liver; active metabolite quinaprilat

Half-life (quinaprilat): 2 hours; prolonged with renal impairment (see Usual Dosage)

Elimination: As metabolites in urine and feces

Usual Dosage Oral:

Geriatrics: Initial: 2.5-5 mg/day; increase dosage at increments of 2.5-5 mg at 1- to 2-week intervals; see following creatinine clearance recommendations (see Additional Information)

Adults: Initial: 10 mg once daily, adjust at 1- to 2-week intervals according to blood pressure response at peak and trough blood concentrations; in general, the normal dosage range is 40-80 mg/day

Congestive heart failure: Initial: 2.5-5 mg twice daily; titrate with daily dose increases of 2.5-5 mg at weekly intervals to a "target dose" of 20 mg twice daily

Dosing adjustment in renal impairment (daily initial dose):

Cl_{cr} >60 mL/minute: Administer 10 mg; elderly: 5 mg

Cl_{cr} 30-60 mL/minute: Administer 5 mg; elderly: 2.5

Cl_{cr} 10-30 mL/minute: Administer 2.5 mg

Monitoring Parameters Serum calcium levels, BUN, serum creatinine, renal function, WBC, and potassium

Test Interactions Increased potassium (S)

Patient Information Do not discontinue medication without advice of physician; notify physician if sore throat, swelling, palpitations, cough, chest pains, difficulty swallowing, swelling of face, eyes, tongue, lips, hoarseness, sweating, vomiting, or diarrhea occurs; may cause dizziness, lightheadedness during first few days; may also cause changes in taste perception; do not use salt substitutes containing potassium without consulting a physician

Nursing Implications May cause depression in some patients; discontinue if angioedema of the face, extremities, lips, tongue, or glottis occurs; watch for hypotensive effects within 1-3 hours of first dose or new higher dose (see Precautions and Special Geriatric Considerations)

Additional Information Patients taking diuretics are at risk for developing hypotension on initial dosing; to prevent this, discontinue diuretics 2-3 days prior to initiating quinapril; may restart diuretics if blood pressure is not controlled by quinapril alone

Special Geriatric Considerations Due to frequent decreases in glomerular filtration (also creatinine clearance) with aging, elderly patients may have exaggerated responses to ACE inhibitors; differences in clinical response due to hepatic changes are not observed. ACE inhibitors may be preferred agents in elderly patients with CHF and diabetes mellitus. Diabetic proteinuria is reduced and insulin sensitivity is enhanced. In general, the side effect profile is favorable in elderly and causes little or no CNS confusion; use lowest dose recommendations initially. Adjust for renal function.

Dosage Forms Tablet, as hydrochloride: 5 mg, 10 mg, 20 mg, 40 mg

References

Konstam MA, Drakup K, Baker DW, et al, "Heart Failure: Evaluation and Care of Patients With Left Ventricular Systolic Dysfunction," *Clinical Practice Guideline No 11*, Rockville, MD: Agency for Health Care Policy and Research, Public Health Service, U.S. Department of Health and Human Services, 1994.

Lewis EJ, Hunsicker LG, Bain RP, et al, "The Effect of Angiotensin-Converting Enzyme Inhibition on Diabetic Nephropathy," *N Engl J Med*, 1993, 329(20):1456-62.

McAreavey D and Robertson JIS, "Angiotensin Converting Enzyme Inhibitors and Moderate Hypertension," *Drugs*, 1990, 40(3):326-45.

Williams JF, Bristow MR, Fowler MB, et al, "Guidelines for the Evaluation and Management of Heart Failure: Report of the American College of Cardiology/American Heart Association Task Force on Practice Guidelines (Committee on Evaluation and Management of Heart Failure)," *J Am Coll Cardiol*, 1995, 26:1376-8.

Quinidex® Extentabs® *see* Quinidine *on this page*

Quinidine (KWIN i deen)

Related Information

Antacid Drug Interactions *on page 1096*

Serum Drug Concentrations Commonly Monitored: Guidelines *on page 1114*

Brand Names Cardioquin®; Quinaglute® Dura-Tabs®; Quinalan®; Quinidex® Extentabs®; Quinora®

Synonyms Quinidine Polygalacturonate

Generic Available Yes

Therapeutic Category Antiarrhythmic Agent, Class I-A

Use Prophylaxis after cardioversion of atrial fibrillation and/or flutter to maintain normal sinus rhythm; also used to prevent recurrence of paroxysmal supraventricular tachycardia, paroxysmal A-V junctional rhythm, paroxysmal ventricular tachycardia, paroxysmal atrial fibrillation, and atrial or ventricular premature contractions; also has activity against *Plasmodium falciparum* malaria

Contraindications Patients with complete A-V block with an A-V junctional or idioventricular pacemaker; patients with intraventricular conduction defects (marked widening of QRS complex); patients with cardiac glycoside-induced A-V conduction disorders; myasthenia gravis; thrombocytopenia associated with quinidine administration; digitalis intoxication, aberrant ectopic rhythms, history of drug-induced torsade de pointes, history of long Q-T syndrome, hypersensitivity to the drug or cinchona derivatives

Warnings May cause syncope, most likely due to ventricular tachycardia or fibrillation; syncope may subside spontaneously, but occasionally may be fatal; discontinue quinidine if syncope occurs; hepatotoxicity, atrial flutter/fibrillation or conversion to sinus rhythm, cardiotoxicity, hypersensitivity; use caution in renal/hepatic impairment or patients with cardiac insufficiency

Precautions Myocardial depression, sick sinus syndrome, incomplete A-V block, cardiac glycoside intoxication, hepatic and/or renal insufficiency, myasthenia gravis; hemolysis may occur in patients with G-6-PD (glucose-6-phosphate dehydrogenase) deficiency; quinidine-induced hepatotoxicity, including granulomatous hepatitis, increased serum AST and alkaline phosphatase concentrations, and jaundice may occur

Adverse Reactions

Cardiovascular: Hypotension, tachycardia, heart block, torsade de pointes, syncope, vascular collapse, ventricular fibrillation, severe hypotension with rapid I.V. administration

Central nervous system: Headache, fever, vertigo, confusion, delirium, dementia

Dermatologic: Angioedema, rash

Gastrointestinal: GI disturbances, nausea, vomiting, abdominal pain, cramps

Hematologic: Blood dyscrasias, thrombotic thrombocytopenic

Hepatic: Purpura

Ocular: Impaired vision

Otic: Tinnitus, impaired hearing

Respiratory: Respiratory depression

Overdosage Symptoms of overdose include ataxia, lethargy, respiratory distress, apnea, severe hypotension, anuria, absence of P waves, broadening QRS complex, PR and Q-T intervals, ventricular arrhythmias, hallucinations, and seizures.

(Continued)

Quinidine *(Continued)*

Toxicology Electrolyte balance should be monitored and treated, especially when refractory arrhythmias develop. Sodium bicarbonate 1-2 mEq/kg I.V. may decrease drug toxicity. Phenytoin or lidocaine are often effective at controlling drug-induced arrhythmias, while phenytoin is preferred due to its beneficial effects on A-V conduction velocity.

Drug Interactions

Quinidine potentiates nondepolarizing and depolarizing muscle relaxants

Verapamil, amiodarone, alkalinizing agents, metronidazole, ketoconazole, fluconazole, miconazole (I.V.), and cimetidine may increase quinidine serum concentrations

Phenobarbital, phenytoin, and rifampin may decrease quinidine serum concentrations

Quinidine may increase plasma concentration of digoxin, closely monitor digoxin concentrations, digoxin dosage may need to be reduced (by one-half) when quinidine is initiated, new steady-state digoxin plasma concentrations occur in 5-7 days; beta-blockers + quinidine may increase bradycardia

Quinidine may enhance coumarin anticoagulants

Quinidine alters pharmacokinetics of flecainide, propafenone, and metoprolol

Stability Do not use discolored parenteral solution

Mechanism of Action Depresses phase O (upstroke) of the action potential; decreases myocardial excitability and conduction velocity, and myocardial contractility by decreasing sodium influx during depolarization and potassium efflux in repolarization; also reduces calcium transport across cell membrane

Pharmacokinetics

Distribution: V_d: 2-3.5 L/kg, decreased V_d with congestive heart failure, malaria; increased V_d with cirrhosis; V_d is not significantly changed with age

Protein binding: 80% to 90% (younger adults); decreased protein binding with cyanotic congenital heart disease, cirrhosis, or acute myocardial infarction

Metabolism: Extensive in the liver (50% to 90%) to inactive compounds; inhibitor CYP2D6, 3A4; substrate CYP3A4

Bioavailability: 80% (sulfate), 70% (gluconate); 87% (elderly)

Half-life, plasma: 6-8 hours (average 5.7 hours) in young adults; increased half-life with elderly (average 9.7 hours), cirrhosis and congestive heart failure

Elimination: In urine (15% to 25% as unchanged drug)

Usual Dosage Note: Dosage expressed in terms of the salt: 267 mg of quinidine gluconate = 275 mg of quinidine polygalacturonate = 200 mg of quinidine sulfate

Geriatrics and Adults: Test dose: 200 mg (sulfate or its equivalent) administered several hours before full dosage (to determine possibility of idiosyncratic reaction)

Oral:

Sulfate: 100-600 mg/dose every 4-6 hours; begin at 200 mg/dose and titrate to desired effect

Gluconate: 324-972 mg every 8-12 hours

Polygalacturonate: 275 mg every 8-12 hours

I.M.: 400 mg/dose every 4-6 hours

I.V.: 200-400 mg/dose diluted and given at a rate ≤10 mg/minute

Slightly dialyzable (5% to 20%)

Monitoring Parameters EKG, apical pulse, heart rate, serum concentrations; monitor for syncope initially, diarrhea, periodic CBC, renal and liver function tests

Reference Range Therapeutic: 2-5 µg/mL (SI: 6.2-15.4 µmol/L). Patient-dependent therapeutic response occurs at levels of 3-6 µg/mL (SI: 9.2-18.5 µmol/L). Optimal therapeutic serum concentration is method dependent: >6 µg/mL (SI: >18 µmol/L).

Test Interactions Increased prothrombin time

Patient Information Patients should notify their physician if rash, fever, diarrhea, unusual bleeding or bruising, ringing in the ears or visual disturbances occur. Complete blood counts, liver and renal function tests should be routinely performed during long-term administration; do not chew or crush sustained release dose forms

Nursing Implications When injecting I.M., aspirate carefully to avoid injection into a vessel; administer around-the-clock rather than 4 times/day, 3 times/day, etc (ie, 12-6-12-6, not 9-1-5-9) to promote less variation in peak and trough serum concentrations; do not crush sustained release drug product

Additional Information Sulfate form is the standard dosage preparation

Special Geriatric Considerations Clearance may be decreased with a resultant increased half-life; must individualize dose; bioavailability and half-life are increased in elderly due to decreases in both renal and hepatic function with age

Dosage Forms
Injection, as gluconate: 80 mg/mL (10 mL)
Tablet, as polygalacturonate: 275 mg
Tablet, as sulfate: 200 mg, 300 mg
Tablet:
Sustained action, as sulfate: 300 mg
Sustained release, as gluconate: 324 mg

References
Fenster PE and Nolan PE, "Antiarrhythmic Drugs," *Geriatric Pharmacology*, Bressler R and Katz MD, eds, New York, NY: McGraw-Hill, 1993, 6:105-49.

Quinidine Polygalacturonate *see* Quinidine *on page 815*

Quinine (KWYE nine)
Brand Names Formula Q®
Generic Available Yes
Therapeutic Category Antimalarial Agent; Skeletal Muscle Relaxant
Use Suppression or treatment of chloroquine-resistant *P. falciparum* malaria; treatment of *Babesia microti* infection
Unlabeled use: Prevention and treatment of nocturnal recumbency leg muscle cramps
Contraindications Tinnitus, optic neuritis, G-6-PD deficiency, hypersensitivity to quinine or any component, history of black water fever, and thrombocytopenia with quinine or quinidine
Precautions Use with caution in patients with cardiac arrhythmias (quinine has quinidine-like activity) and in patients with myasthenia gravis
Adverse Reactions
Cardiovascular: Flushing of the skin, anginal symptoms
Central nervous system: Fever, headache
Dermatologic: Rash, pruritus
Endocrine & metabolic: Hypoglycemia
Gastrointestinal: Nausea, vomiting, epigastric pain, diarrhea
Hematologic: Hemolysis, thrombocytopenia
Hepatic: Hepatitis
Ocular: Nightblindness, diplopia, optic atrophy, blurred vision
Otic: Tinnitus, impaired hearing
Miscellaneous: Hypersensitivity reactions
Overdosage Symptoms of overdose include cinchonism (tinnitus, headache, nausea, abdominal pain, visual disturbance) blood dyscrasias, photosensitivity, cardiac arrhythmias, hypotension, renal injury, hemolysis, hypoprothrombinemia
Drug Interactions
Decreased serum concentrations with phenobarbital, phenytoin, and rifampin
Increased effect of nondepolarizing/depolarizing muscle relaxants and coumarin anticoagulants
Increased serum concentrations with verapamil, amiodarone, alkalinizing agents, and cimetidine
Increased plasma concentration of digoxin, closely monitor digoxin concentrations, digoxin dosage may need to be reduced (by one-half) when quinine is initiated, new steady-state digoxin plasma concentrations occur in 5-7 days
Stability Protect from light
Mechanism of Action Depresses oxygen uptake and carbohydrate metabolism; intercalates into DNA, disrupting the parasite's replication and transcription; affects calcium distribution within muscle fibers and decreases the excitability of the motor end-plate region
Pharmacokinetics
Absorption: Oral: Readily absorbed, mainly from the upper small intestine
Protein binding: 70% to 95%
Metabolism: Primarily in the liver
Half-life (adults): 8-14 hours
Time to peak serum concentration: Within 1-3 hours after dose
Elimination: In bile and saliva with <5% excreted unchanged in urine
Not effectively removed by peritoneal dialysis, removed by hemodialysis
Usual Dosage Geriatrics and Adults: Oral:
Chloroquine-resistant malaria: 650 mg every 8 hours for 5-7 days in conjunction with another agent
(Continued)

Quinine *(Continued)*

   Babesiosis: 650 mg every 6-8 hours for 7 days
   Leg cramps: 250-300 mg at bedtime
Reference Range Toxic: >10 µg/mL
Test Interactions Positive Coombs' [direct], increased prothrombin time
Patient Information Avoid use of aluminum-containing antacids because of drug absorption problems; swallow dose whole to avoid bitter taste; take with food; notify physician if diarrhea, nausea, and other GI complaints or blurred vision, vertigo, confusion or dizziness occurs
Nursing Implications Administer by slow I.V. infusion
Additional Information Parenteral dosage form may be obtained from Centers for Disease Control if needed
Special Geriatric Considerations Efficacy in nocturnal leg cramps is not well supported in the medical and pharmacy literature, however, some patients do respond; nonresponders should be evaluated for other possible etiologies
Dosage Forms
   Quinine sulfate:
      Capsule: 64.8 mg, 65 mg, 200 mg, 300 mg, 325 mg
      Tablet: 162.5 mg, 260 mg

Quinora® *see Quinidine on page 815*

Quinsana Plus® [OTC] *see Tolnaftate on page 939*

Rabies Immune Globulin (Human)
   (RAY beez i MYUN GLOB yoo lin HYU man)
Related Information
   Immunization Guidelines *on page 1058*
Brand Names Hyperab®; Imogam®
Synonyms RIG
Generic Available No
Therapeutic Category Immune Globulin
Use Part of postexposure prophylaxis of persons with rabies exposure who lack a history or pre-exposure or postexposure prophylaxis with rabies vaccine or a recently documented neutralizing antibody response to previous rabies vaccination; although it is preferable to administer RIG with the first dose of vaccine, it can be given up to 8 days after vaccination
Contraindications Inadvertent I.V. administration; allergy to thimerosal or any component; do not administer in repeated doses once vaccine is initiated
Warnings Use with caution in individuals with thrombocytopenia, bleeding disorders, or prior allergic reactions to immune globulins
Precautions Use with caution in patients who are reported to be allergic to human immunoglobulins and thimerosal
Adverse Reactions
   Central nervous system: Fever (mild)
   Dermatologic: Urticaria, angioedema
   Local: Soreness at injection site
   Neuromuscular & skeletal: Stiffness, soreness of muscles
   Miscellaneous: Anaphylactic shock
Drug Interactions
   Decreased effect: Live vaccines, corticosteroids, immunosuppressive agents; should not be administered within 3 months
Stability Refrigerate
Mechanism of Action Rabies immune globulin is a solution of globulins dried from the plasma or serum of selected adult human donors who have been immunized with rabies vaccine and have developed high titers of rabies antibody. It generally contains 10% to 18% of protein of which not less than 80% is monomeric immunoglobulin G.
Usual Dosage Geriatrics and Adults: I.M.: 20 units/kg in a single dose (RIG should always be administered in conjunction with rabies vaccine (HDCV)); infiltrate ½ of the dose locally around the wound; administer the remainder I.M.
Administration Intramuscular injection only; injection should be made into the deltoid muscle or anterolateral aspect of the thigh
Monitoring Parameters Monitor for adverse effects
Nursing Implications Severe adverse reactions can occur if patient receives RIG I.V. (see Administration)
Special Geriatric Considerations No special considerations are needed for initiating therapy; no specific data relevant to elderly to date

Dosage Forms Injection: 150 units/mL (2 mL, 10 mL)

Rabies Virus Vaccine (RAY beez VYE rus vak SEEN)

Related Information
Immunization Guidelines *on page 1058*

Brand Names Imovax® Rabies I.D. Vaccine; Imovax® Rabies Vaccine

Synonyms HDCV; Human Diploid Cell Cultures Rabies Vaccine; Human Diploid Cell Cultures Rabies Vaccine (Intradermal use)

Generic Available No

Therapeutic Category Vaccine, Inactivated Virus

Use Veterinarians, animal handlers, certain laboratory workers, and persons living in or visiting countries for longer than 1 month where rabies is a constant threat.

Complete pre-exposure prophylaxis does not eliminate the need for additional therapy with rabies vaccine after a rabies exposure. The Food and Drug Administration has not approved the I.D. use of rabies vaccine for postexposure prophylaxis. Recommendations for I.D. use of HDCV are currently being discussed. The decision for postexposure rabies vaccination depends on the species of biting animal, the circumstances of biting incident, and the type of exposure (bite, saliva contamination of wound, and so on). The type of and schedule for postexposure prophylaxis depends upon the person's previous rabies vaccination status or the result of a previous or current serologic test for rabies antibody. For postexposure prophylaxis, rabies vaccine should always be administered I.M., **not** I.D.

Contraindications Developing febrile illness (during pre-exposure therapy only); allergy to neomycin, gentamicin, or amphotericin B

Warnings Rabies vaccine is available only in I.M. form; cannot be given intradermally

Precautions
Imovax® rabies vaccine and rabies vaccine adsorbed: Inject I.M. only in deltoid muscle; vaccine failure possible if injected in gluteal muscle. Do **not** inject I.D.

Imovax® rabies I.D. vaccine: Injection I.D> only; do **not** inject I.M.

Adverse Reactions
Cardiovascular: Edema

Central nervous system: Dizziness, malaise, encephalomyelitis, transverse myelitis, fever, pain, headache, neuroparalytic reactions

Dermatologic: Itching, erythema

Gastrointestinal: Nausea, abdominal pain

Local: Local discomfort

Neuromuscular & skeletal: Myalgia

Miscellaneous: Serum sickness reactions occur in 6% of those receiving I.D. booster doses 2-21 days following vaccination

Drug Interactions Decreased effect with immunosuppressive agents, corticosteroids, antimalarial drugs (ie, chloroquine); persons on these drugs should receive RIG (3 doses/1 mL each) by the I.M. route

Stability Refrigerate; reconstituted vaccine should be used immediately

Mechanism of Action Rabies vaccine is an inactivated virus vaccine which promotes immunity by inducing an active immune response. The production of specific antibodies requires about 7-10 days to develop. Rabies immune globulin or antirabies serum, equine (ARS) is given in conjunction with rabies vaccine to provide immune protection until an antibody response can occur.

Pharmacodynamics
Onset of effect: I.M.: Rabies antibody appears in the serum within 7-10 days

Peak effect: Within 30-60 days and persists for at least 1 year

Usual Dosage Geriatrics and Adults:
Pre-exposure prophylaxis: Two 1 mL doses I.M. 1 week apart, third dose 3 weeks after second. If exposure continues, booster doses can be given every 2 years, or an antibody titer determined and a booster dose given if the titer is inadequate.

Postexposure prophylaxis: All postexposure treatment should begin with immediate cleansing of the wound with soap and water

Persons not previously immunized as above: Rabies immune globulin 20 units/kg body weight, half infiltrated at bite site if possible, remainder I.M.; and 5 doses of rabies vaccine, 1 mL I.M., one each on days 0, 3, 7, 14, 28

Persons who have previously received postexposure prophylaxis with rabies vaccine, received a recommended I.M. pre-exposure series of rabies vaccine or have a previously documented rabies antibody titer considered

(Continued)

Rabies Virus Vaccine *(Continued)*

adequate: Two doses of rabies vaccine, 1 mL I.M., one each on days 0 and 3

Administration See Precautions

Monitoring Parameters Monitor for local adverse effects

Reference Range Antibody titers ≥115 as determined by rapid fluorescent-focus inhibition test are indicative of adequate response; collect titers on day 28 postexposure

Additional Information Federal law requires that the date of administration, the vaccine manufacturer, lot number of vaccine, and the administering person's name, title and address be entered into the patient's permanent medical record

Special Geriatric Considerations No specific data for use in elderly; use as recommended in elderly patients for whom this vaccine would be indicated (see Use)

Dosage Forms
Injection:
I.M. (HDCV): Rabies antigen 2.5 units/mL (1 mL)
Intradermal: Rabies antigen 0.25 units/mL (1 mL)

Raloxifene *(ral OX i feen)*

Brand Names Evista®

Synonyms Keoxifene Hydrochloride

Therapeutic Category Selective Estrogen Receptor Modulator (SERM)

Use Prevention of osteoporosis in postmenopausal women

Contraindications Pregnancy or possible pregnancy; active or past history of venous thromboembolic events, including DVT, PE, and retinal vein thrombosis

Warnings Severe hepatic insufficiency; lowered serum total and LDL cholesterol, but not total HDL or triglycerides; raloxifene should be stopped 72 hours prior to or during prolonged immobilization due to risk of thromboembolic events

Adverse Reactions Reported in clinical trials by more than 2% of subjects:
Cardiovascular: Hot flashes, migraine, leg cramps
Central nervous system: Depression, insomnia
Dermatologic: Rash
Endocrine & metabolic: Weight gain, peripheral edema
Gastrointestinal: Nausea, dyspepsia, vomiting, flatulence, gastroenteritis
Genitourinary: Vaginitis, urinary tract infection, cystitis, leukorrhea, endometrial disorder
Neuromuscular & skeletal: Arthralgia, myalgia, arthritis
Respiratory: Sinusitis, pharyngitis, cough, pneumonia, laryngitis
Miscellaneous: Diaphoresis

Drug Interactions Effects on highly protein bound drugs are unclear; use caution with highly protein bound drugs, warfarin, clofibrate, indomethacin, naproxen, ibuprofen, diazepam, phenytoin, or tamoxifen

Mechanism of Action A selective estrogen receptor modulator (ie, it affects some of the same receptors that estrogen does, but not all, and in some instances, it antagonizes or blocks estrogen); it acts like estrogen to prevent bone loss and improve lipid profiles, but it has the potential to block some estrogen effects such as those that lead to breast cancer and uterine cancer

Pharmacokinetics
Absorption: ~60%
Distribution: V_d: 2348 L/kg
Protein binding: >95% to albumin and alpha$_1$-acid glycoprotein
Metabolism: First-pass effect with glucuronide conjugates
Half-life: 28-32.5 hours
Elimination: Feces; <0.2% as unchanged drug in the urine
Note: No age-related differences in raloxifene pharmacokinetics have been identified

Usual Dosage Geriatrics and Adults: Oral: One tablet (60 mg)/day may be administered any time of the day without regard to meals

Dosing comments in hepatic impairment: Safety has not been established

Monitoring Parameters INR if on warfarin, lipid profile, bone mineral density

Patient Information Take without regard to meals; will not reduce hot flashes or flushes associated with estrogen deficiency; supplement calcium and vitamin D if indicated

Nursing Implications raloxifene should be stopped 72 hours prior to or during prolonged immobilization due to risk of thromboembolic events

Additional Information The decrease in estrogen-related adverse effects with the selective estrogen-receptor modulators in general and raloxifene in particular should improve compliance and decrease the incidence of cardiovascular events and fractures while not increasing breast cancer

Special Geriatric Considerations No need to cycle with progesterone (see Pharmacokinetics, Usual Dosage, and Patient Information)

Dosage Forms Tablet, as hydrochloride: 60 mg

References

Delmas PD, Bjarnason NH, Mitlak BH, et al, "Effects of Raloxifene on Bone Mineral Density, Serum Cholesterol Concentrations, and Uterine Endometrium in Postmenopausal Women," *N Engl J Med*, 1997, 337(23):1641-7.

Ramipril (ra MI pril)

Related Information

ACE Inhibitors Comparison *on page 1019*

Brand Names Altace™

Generic Available No

Therapeutic Category Angiotensin-Converting Enzyme (ACE) Inhibitors

Use Treatment of hypertension, alone or in combination with thiazide diuretics; postmyocardial infarction congestive failure

Unlabeled use: Systolic congestive heart failure

Contraindications Hypersensitivity to ramipril or ramiprilat, or any other angiotensin-converting enzyme inhibitors

Warnings Neutropenia, agranulocytosis, angioedema, decreased renal function (hypertension, renal artery stenosis, CHF), hepatic dysfunction (elimination, activation), proteinuria, first-dose hypotension (hypovolemia, CHF, dehydrated patients at risk, eg, diuretic use, elderly), elderly (due to renal function changes)

Precautions Use with caution and modify dosage in patients with renal impairment (decrease dosage) (especially renal artery stenosis), severe congestive heart failure or with coadministered diuretic therapy. Severe hypotension may occur in patients who are sodium and/or volume depleted, initiate lower doses and monitor closely when starting therapy in these patients; may cause hyperkalemia.

Adverse Reactions

Cardiovascular: Arrhythmias, orthostatic blood pressure changes, angina, palpitations, chest pain, hypotension, tachycardia, syncope, myocardial infarction

Central nervous system: Nervousness, depression, confusion, somnolence, fatigue, dizziness, headache, insomnia, malaise, vertigo, anxiety

Dermatologic: Rash, photosensitivity, pruritus, purpura, angioedema

Endocrine & metabolic: Hyperkalemia

Gastrointestinal: Ageusia, pancreatitis, xerostomia, constipation, anorexia, nausea, vomiting, diarrhea, dysphagia, gastroenteritis, increased salivation, abdominal pain, dysgeusia, dyspepsia

Genitourinary: Impotence

Hematologic: Eosinophilia, leukopenia

Hepatic: Hepatitis

Neuromuscular & skeletal: Myalgia, arthralgia, muscle cramps, arthritis, paresthesia, weakness

Ocular: Blurred vision

Otic: Tinnitus

Renal: Proteinuria, increased BUN, serum creatinine, oliguria

Respiratory: Chronic cough (nonproductive, persistent; more often in women and seen in 15% to 30% of patients), asthma, bronchospasm, dyspnea, upper respiratory infections

Miscellaneous: Diaphoresis

Overdosage Severe hypotension

Toxicology Following initiation of essential overdose management, toxic symptom treatment and supportive treatment should be initiated. Hypotension usually responds to I.V. fluids or Trendelenburg positioning. If unresponsive to these measures, the use of a parenteral inotrope may be required (eg, norepinephrine 0.1-0.2 mcg/kg/minute titrated to response). Seizures commonly respond to diazepam (I.V. 5-10 mg bolus in adults every 15 minutes if needed up to a total of 30 mg) or to phenytoin or phenobarbital.

Drug Interactions

ACE inhibitors (ramipril) and potassium-sparing diuretics may cause additive hyperkalemic effect

(Continued)

Ramipril *(Continued)*

ACE inhibitors (ramipril) and indomethacin or nonsteroidal anti-inflammatory agents may cause reduced antihypertensive response to ACE inhibitors (ramipril)

Allopurinol and ACE inhibitors (ramipril) may cause neutropenia

Antacids and ACE inhibitors may decrease absorption of ACE inhibitors

Phenothiazines and ACE inhibitors may increase ACE inhibitor effect

Probenecid and ACE inhibitors (ramipril) may increase ACE inhibitors (ramipril) levels

Rifampin and ACE inhibitors (enalapril) may decrease ACE inhibitor effect

Digoxin and ACE inhibitors may increase serum digoxin concentrations

Lithium and ACE inhibitors may increase lithium serum concentration

Tetracycline and ACE inhibitors (quinapril) may decrease tetracycline absorption (up to 37%)

Food decreases ramipril absorption (see Additional Information); rate, but not extent, of ramipril and fosinopril is reduced by concomitant administration with food; food does not reduce absorption of enalapril, lisinopril, or benazepril

Stability Stable for 24 hours at room temperature or 48 hours under refrigeration.

Mechanism of Action Ramipril is an angiotensin-converting enzyme (ACE) inhibitor which prevents the formation of angiotensin II from angiotensin I and exhibits pharmacologic effects that are similar to captopril. Ramipril must undergo enzymatic saponification by esterases in the liver to its biologically active metabolite, ramiprilat. The pharmacodynamic effects of ramipril result from the high-affinity, competitive, reversible binding of ramiprilat to angiotensin-converting enzyme thus preventing the formation of the potent vasoconstrictor angiotensin II. This isomerized enzyme-inhibitor complex has a slow rate of dissociation, which results in high potency and a long duration of action; a CNS mechanism may also be involved in the hypotensive effect as angiotensin II increases adrenergic outflow from CNS; vasoactive kallikreins may be decreased in conversion to active hormones by ACE inhibitors, thus reducing blood pressure

Pharmacodynamics

Onset of action: Reduction of blood pressure occurs in 2 hours

Duration: 24 hours

Pharmacokinetics

Absorption: Well absorbed from GI tract (50% to 60%)

Distribution: Plasma concentrations decline in a triphasic fashion; rapid decline is a distribution phase to peripheral compartment, plasma protein and tissue ACE (half-life 2-4 hours); 2nd phase is an apparent elimination phase representing the clearance of free ramiprilat (half-life: 9-18 hours); and final phase is the terminal elimination phase representing the equilibrium phase between tissue binding and dissociation (half-life: >50 hours)

Metabolism: Hepatic to the active form, ramiprilat

Half-life: Ramiprilat: >50 hours

Time to peak serum concentration: ~1 hour

Elimination: Ramipril and its metabolites are eliminated primarily through the kidneys (60%) and feces (40%)

Usual Dosage Geriatrics and Adults: Oral: 2.5-5 mg once daily (if a lower initial dose is desired, a 1.25 mg capsule is available), maximum: 20 mg/day (see Special Geriatric Considerations); must adjust dose for renal function for elderly since glomerular filtration rates are decreased; may see exaggerated hypotensive effects if renal clearance is not considered (see Additional Information)

Congestive heart failure: Initial: 1.25-2.5 mg twice daily; titrate over several weeks to a "target dose" of 5 mg twice daily (see renal impairment adjustment below and Additional Information)

Dosing adjustment in renal impairment: Cl_{cr} <40 mL/minute: Initial: 1.25 mg/day, titrate upward to 5 mg/day maximum

Monitoring Parameters Serum calcium levels, BUN, serum creatinine, renal function, WBC, and potassium

Test Interactions Increases BUN, creatinine, potassium, positive Coombs' [direct]; decreases cholesterol (S); may cause false-positive results in urine acetone determinations using sodium nitroprusside reagent

Patient Information Notify physician if vomiting, diarrhea, excessive perspiration, or dehydration should occur; also if swelling of face, lips, tongue, or difficulty in breathing occurs or if persistent cough develops; do not stop therapy or use potassium salt substitutes without physician's advice; may be taken with food

Nursing Implications May cause depression in some patients; discontinue if angioedema of the face, extremities, lips, tongue, or glottis occurs; watch for hypotensive effects within 1-3 hours of first dose or new higher dose (see Warnings, Precautions, Monitoring Parameters, and Special Geriatric Considerations)

Additional Information Some patients may have a decreased hypotensive effect between 12 and 16 hours; consider dividing total daily dose into 2 doses 12 hours apart. If patient is receiving a diuretic, a potential for first-dose hypotension is increased. To decrease this potential, stop diuretic for 2-3 days prior to initiating ramipril. If diuretic cannot be stopped temporarily, then initiate therapy with 1.25 mg daily. Continue diuretic if needed to control blood pressure. Capsules should be swallowed whole; if this cannot be done, capsule contents may be mixed with applesauce; also, contents may be mixed with apple juice or water. Mixtures in juice and water are stable for 24 hours at room temperature or 48 hours with refrigeration.

Special Geriatric Considerations Due to frequent decreases in glomerular filtration (also creatinine clearance) with aging, elderly patients may have exaggerated responses to ACE inhibitors; differences in clinical response due to hepatic changes are not observed. ACE inhibitors may be preferred agents in elderly patients with CHF and diabetes mellitus. Diabetic proteinuria is reduced and insulin sensitivity is enhanced. In general, the side effect profile is favorable in elderly and causes little or no CNS confusion; use lowest dose recommendations initially.

Dosage Forms Capsule: 1.25 mg, 2.5 mg, 5 mg, 10 mg

References

Konstam MA, Drakup K, Baker DW, et al, "Heart Failure: Evaluation and Care of Patients With Left Ventricular Systolic Dysfunction," *Clinical Practice Guideline No 11*, Rockville, MD: Agency for Health Care Policy and Research, Public Health Service, U.S. Department of Health and Human Services, 1994.

McAreavey D and Robertson JIS, "Angiotensin Converting Enzyme Inhibitors and Moderate Hypertension," *Drugs*, 1990, 40(3):326-45.

Williams JF, Bristow MR, Fowler MB, et al, "Guidelines for the Evaluation and Management of Heart Failure: Report of the American College of Cardiology/American Heart Association Task Force on Practice Guidelines (Committee on Evaluation and Management of Heart Failure)," *J Am Coll Cardiol*, 1995, 26:1376-8.

Ranitidine (ra NI ti deen)

Related Information

Antacid Drug Interactions *on page 1096*
I.V. Medication Recommendations *on page 1080*
I.V. Push Recommended Guidelines *on page 1083*

Brand Names Zantac®; Zantac® 75 [OTC]

Generic Available No

Therapeutic Category Histamine H_2 Antagonist

Use Short-term treatment of active duodenal ulcers and benign gastric ulcers; long-term prophylaxis of duodenal ulcer and gastric hypersecretory states, gastroesophageal reflux, erosive esophagitis

Zantac® 75 [OTC]: Relief of symptoms of heartburn, acid indigestion, and sour stomach

Unlabeled use: Upper GI bleeding, prevention of acid-aspiration pneumonitis, prevention of stress-induced ulcers, and prevention of duodenal NSAID ulcers

Contraindications Hypersensitivity to ranitidine or any component

Warnings Use with caution in people (elderly) with reduced renal function, liver disease may impair clearance

Precautions Modify dosage in patients with renal and/or hepatic impairment; gastric malignancy may be masked, gynecomastia; cardiac arrhythmias and hypotension (I.V.); CNS side effects (confusion, depression, psychosis, hallucinations, anxiety)

Adverse Reactions

Cardiovascular: Bradycardia or tachycardia, arrhythmias, edema
Central nervous system: Headache, dizziness, sedation, hallucinations, agitation, anxiety, depression, vertigo, insomnia, malaise, mental confusion
Dermatologic: Alopecia, erythema multiforme, rash
Endocrine & metabolic: Gynecomastia
Gastrointestinal: Constipation, nausea, vomiting, diarrhea, pancreatitis
Genitourinary: Impotence, loss of libido
Hematologic: Agranulocytosis, granulocytopenia, thrombocytopenia, hemolytic anemia, reversible leukopenia, pancytopenia
(Continued)

Ranitidine (Continued)

Hepatic: Hepatitis
Neuromuscular & skeletal: Arthralgias
Ocular: Blurred vision
Renal: Increase in serum creatinine

Overdosage Symptoms of overdose include muscular tremors, vomiting, rapid respiration

Toxicology LD_{50} ~80 mg/kg; treatment is primarily symptomatic and supportive.

Drug Interactions

Binds weakly to cytochrome P-4502D6, and 3A4 and, therefore, does not cause significant inhibition of drug metabolism

Antacids may decrease absorption; decreased absorption of diazepam may occur (ranitidine)

Increased serum concentrations of procainamide (ranitidine)

Increased hypoglycemic effects observed with sulfonylureas

Serum concentrations may be increased (case reports with ranitidine)

May decrease warfarin clearance and increase anticoagulant effect (ranitidine) but conflicting data are available

Stability Solution for I.V. infusion in NS or D_5W is stable for 48 hours at room temperature or 30 days when frozen; is stable for 24 hours in TPN solutions; is stable only for 12 hours in total nutrient admixtures (TPN) when lipids are added

Mechanism of Action Competitive inhibition of histamine at H_2 receptors of the gastric parietal cells, which inhibits gastric acid secretion; gastric volume and hydrogen ion concentration reduced

Pharmacodynamics

Efficacy of healing rate: 63% to 77% at 4 weeks; 82% to 95% at 8 weeks
Duration of effect: Oral: 12 hours; I.V.: 6-8 hours

Pharmacokinetics

Absorption: Oral: ~50% to 60%
Protein binding: 15%
Metabolism: In the liver (<10%)
Half-life: 2-2.5 hours; minimally penetrates the blood-brain barrier
Time to peak serum concentration: Within 1-3 hours and persist for 8 hours, 15 minutes for I.M.
Elimination: Primarily in urine (35% as unchanged drug) and feces

Usual Dosage Geriatrics and Adults:

Short-term treatment of ulceration: 150 mg/dose twice daily or 300 mg at bedtime (100 mg orally twice daily has been found as effective as 150 mg twice daily)

Prophylaxis of recurrent duodenal ulcer: 150 mg at bedtime

Gastric hypersecretory conditions: Oral: 150 mg twice daily, more frequent doses may be necessary up to 6 g/day

GERD: Oral: 150 mg twice daily

Erosive esophagitis: Oral: 150 mg 4 times/day

I.M., I.V.: 50 mg/dose every 6-8 hours (dose not to exceed 400 mg/day)

Zantac® 75 [OTC]: 75 mg as needed up to twice daily; do not take maximum dose for more than 14 days continuously unless directed by physician

Dosing interval in renal impairment:

Oral: Cl_{cr} <50 mL/minute: Administer each dose every 24 hours
I.V.: Cl_{cr} <50 mL/minute: Administer each dose every 18-24 hours
Slightly dialyzable (5% to 20%)

Monitoring Parameters Signs and symptoms of peptic ulcer disease, occult blood with GI bleeding, gastric pH where necessary; monitor renal function to correct dose; monitor for side effects

Test Interactions False-positive urine protein using Multistix® (test with sulfasalicylic acid), gastric acid secretion test, skin tests allergen extracts, serum creatinine and serum transaminase concentrations, urine protein test

Patient Information It may take several days before this medicine begins to relieve stomach pain; antacids may be taken with ranitidine unless your physician has told you not to use them; wait 30-60 minutes between taking the antacid and ranitidine; inform prescribers of any concomitant medications
Zantac® 75 [OTC]: Do not take maximum dose for more than 14 days continuously unless directed by physician

Nursing Implications I.M. solution does not need to be diluted before use; monitor creatinine clearance for renal impairment; giving dose at 6 PM may be better than 10 PM bedtime, the highest acid production usually starts at approximately 7 PM, thus giving at 6 PM controls acid secretion better;

observe caution in patients with renal function impairment and hepatic function impairment

Additional Information Giving dose at 6 PM may be better than 10 PM bedtime, the highest acid production usually starts at approximately 7 PM, thus giving at 6 PM controls acid secretion better; administer I.V. administration over a 30 minute period to avoid bradycardia; causes fewer adverse reactions and interactions than cimetidine; most patient's ulcers have healed within 4 weeks, however, elderly require 12 weeks of therapy; long-term therapy may cause vitamin B_{12} deficiency

Special Geriatric Considerations H_2 blockers are the preferred drugs for treating PUD in elderly due to cost and ease of administration. These agents are no less or more effective than any other therapy. The preferred agents, due to side effects and drug interaction profile and pharmacokinetics are ranitidine, famotidine, and nizatidine. Treatment for PUD in elderly is recommended for 12 weeks since their lesions are larger; therefore, take longer to heal. Always adjust dose based upon creatinine clearance.

Dosage Forms
Ranitidine hydrochloride:
    Capsule (GELdose™): 150 mg, 300 mg
    Granules, effervescent (EFFERdose™): 150 mg
    Infusion, preservative free, in NaCl 0.45%: 1 mg/mL (50 mL)
    Injection: 25 mg/mL (2 mL, 10 mL, 40 mL)
    Syrup (peppermint flavor): 15 mg/mL (473 mL)
    Tablet: 75 mg [OTC]; 150 mg, 300 mg
    Tablet, effervescent (EFFERdose™): 150 mg

References
Fennerty MD and Higbee M, "Drug Therapy of Gastrointestinal Disease," *Geriatric Pharmacology*, Bressler R and Katz MD, eds, New York, NY: McGraw-Hill, 1993, 585-608.

Morris DL, Markham SJ, Beechey A, et al, "Ranitidine—Bolus or Infusion Prophylaxis for Stress Ulcer," *Crit Care Med*, 1988, 16(3):229-32.

Roberts CJ, "Clinical Pharmacokinetics of Ranitidine," *Clin Pharmacokinet*, 1984, 9(3):211-21.

Raxar® *see* Grepafloxacin *on page 435*

Recombinant Plasminogen Activator *see* Reteplase *on page 827*

Recombivax HB® *see* Hepatitis B Vaccine *on page 453*

Redisol® *see* Cyanocobalamin *on page 257*

Redutemp® [OTC] *see* Acetaminophen *on page 16*

Refresh® **Ophthalmic Solution** [OTC] *see* Artificial Tears *on page 82*

Refresh® **Plus Ophthalmic Solution** [OTC] *see* Artificial Tears *on page 82*

Refresh PM® **Ophthalmic Ointment** [OTC] *see* Ocular Lubricant *on page 688*

Regimens Used to Treat *Helicobacter pylori* and Ulcers *see page 1033*

Reglan® *see* Metoclopramide *on page 616*

Regonol® **Injection** *see* Pyridostigmine *on page 806*

Regulace® [OTC] *see* Docusate and Casanthranol *on page 313*

Regular (Concentrated) Iletin® **II U-500** *see* Insulin Preparations *on page 488*

Regular Iletin® **I** *see* Insulin Preparations *on page 488*

Regular Insulin *see* Insulin Preparations *on page 488*

Regular Purified Pork Insulin *see* Insulin Preparations *on page 488*

Regular Strength Bayer® **Enteric 500 Aspirin** [OTC] *see* Aspirin *on page 84*

Regulax SS® [OTC] *see* Docusate *on page 312*

Reguloid® [OTC] *see* Psyllium *on page 804*

Rela® *see* Carisoprodol *on page 165*

Relafen® *see* Nabumetone *on page 644*

Relaxadon® *see* Hyoscyamine, Atropine, Scopolamine, and Phenobarbital *on page 472*

Relief® **Ophthalmic Solution** *see* Phenylephrine *on page 740*

Remeron™ *see* Mirtazapine *on page 631*

Reposans-10® **Oral** *see* Chlordiazepoxide *on page 205*

Requip™ *see* Ropinirole *on page 838*

Reserpine (re SER peen)
Brand Names Serpalan®; Serpasil®
Generic Available Yes
Therapeutic Category Alpha-Adrenergic Blocking Agent, Oral; Rauwolfia Alkaloid
Use Management of mild to moderate hypertension
(Continued)

Reserpine *(Continued)*

Unlabeled use: Management of tardive dyskinesia

Contraindications Any ulcerative condition, gallstones, mental depression, electroshock therapy, hypersensitivity to reserpine or any component

Precautions Electroshock therapy: discontinue reserpine 7 days before electroshock therapy; may increase GI motility and secretions; acute hypersensitivity reactions may occur; some products may contain tartrazine; use cautiously in patients with renal insufficiency

Adverse Reactions

Cardiovascular: Hypotension, bradycardia

Central nervous system: Drowsiness, fatigue, mental depression, parkinsonism

Endocrine & metabolic: Sodium and water retention

Gastrointestinal: Abdominal cramps, nausea, vomiting, increased gastric acid secretion, diarrhea

Genitourinary: Impotence, dysuria

Respiratory: Nasal congestion

Overdosage Symptoms of overdose include hypotension, bradycardia, CNS depression, sedation, coma, hypothermia, vomiting, diarrhea, miosis, tremors

Toxicology Hypotension usually responds to I.V. fluids or Trendelenburg positioning. If unresponsive to these measures the use of a parenteral vasopressor may be required (eg, norepinephrine 0.1-0.2 mcg/kg/minute titrated to response). Anticholinergic agents may be useful in reducing the parkinsonian effects; avoid the use of digoxin in these patients. Since reserpine is long-acting, observe the patient for at least 72 hours.

Drug Interactions

Decreased effect of indirect-acting sympathomimetics, levodopa

Increased effect/toxicity of other antihypertensives, digoxin, quinidine, general anesthesia, MAO inhibitors, direct-acting sympathomimetics

Stability Protect oral dosage forms from light

Mechanism of Action Reduces blood pressure via depletion of sympathetic biogenic amines (norepinephrine and dopamine); this also commonly results in sedative effects

Pharmacodynamics

Onset of action: Within 3-6 days

Duration: 2-6 weeks

Pharmacokinetics

Absorption: Oral: ~40%

Protein binding: 96%

Metabolism: Extensive in the liver (>90%)

Half-life: 50-100 hours

Elimination: Principal excretion in feces (30% to 60%) and small amounts in urine (10%)

Usual Dosage Oral:

Geriatrics: Initial: 0.05 mg once daily increasing by 0.05 mg every week as necessary

Adults: 0.5 mg/day for 1-2 weeks, then decrease to 0.1-0.25 mg once daily

Monitoring Parameters Blood pressure, standing and sitting/supine, symptoms of depression

Test Interactions Decreased catecholamines (U)

Patient Information Take with food or milk; impotency is reversible; notify physician if a weight gain of more than 5 pounds has taken place during therapy; may cause drowsiness

Nursing Implications Observe for mental depression and alert family members to report any symptoms

Additional Information Full antihypertensive effects may take as long as 3 weeks; at high doses, mental depression is possible and might lead to suicide

Special Geriatric Considerations Some studies advocate the use of reserpine because of its low cost, long half-life, and efficacy, but it is generally not considered a first-line drug. If it is to be used, doses should not exceed 0.25 mg and the patient should be monitored for depressed mood.

Dosage Forms

Injection: 2.5 mg/mL (2 mL)

Tablet: 0.1 mg, 0.25 mg, 1 mg

References

Adelman AM, Daly MP, and Michocki RJ, "Alternate Drugs," *Clin Geriatr Med*, 1990, 6(2):423-44.

Reserpine and Hydrochlorothiazide *see* Hydrochlorothiazide and Reserpine *on page 459*

Respa-DM® *see* Guaifenesin and Dextromethorphan *on page 439*

Respa-GF® see Guaifenesin on page 437
Respbid® see Theophylline on page 902
Restoril® see Temazepam on page 889
Retavase® see Reteplase on this page

Reteplase (RE ta plase)

Brand Names Retavase®

Synonyms Recombinant Plasminogen Activator; r-PA

Therapeutic Category Thrombolytic Agent

Use Improvement of ventricular function following acute myocardial infarction, for the reduction of the incidence of CHF and the reduction of mortality associated with acute myocardial infarction

Contraindications Active internal bleeding; history of cerebrovascular accident; recent intracranial or intraspinal surgery or trauma; intracranial neoplasm; arteriovenous malformations or aneurysm; known bleeding diathesis; severe uncontrolled hypertension; history of severe allergic reactions to reteplase, alteplase, anistreplase, or streptokinase

Adverse Reactions

Cardiovascular: Hypotension, arrhythmias, trauma arrhythmias

Central nervous system: Intracranial hemorrhage

Hematologic: Bleeding, anemia, genitourinary bleeding, gastrointestinal bleeding, injection site bleeding

Miscellaneous: Allergic reactions, anaphylaxis

Overdosage Symptoms of overdose include increased incidence of intracranial bleeding

Drug Interactions Increased effect: Anticoagulants, aspirin, ticlopidine, dipyridamole, clopidogrel; abciximab and heparin are at least additive

Stability Dosage kits should be stored at 2°C to 25°C (36°F to 77°F) and remain sealed until use in order to protect from light

Mechanism of Action Reteplase is a nonglycosylated form of tPA produced by recombinant DNA technology using E. coli; it initiates local fibrinolysis by binding to fibrin in a thrombus (clot) and converts entrapped plasminogen to plasmin

Pharmacodynamics Onset: 30-90 minutes

Pharmacokinetics

Half-life: 13-16 minutes

Elimination: Hepatic and renal, cleared from the plasma at a rate of 250-450 mL/minute

Usual Dosage Geriatrics and Adults: 10 units I.V. over 2 minutes, followed by a second dose 30 minutes later of 10 units I.V. over 2 minutes; withhold second dose if serious bleeding or anaphylaxis occurs

Administration Reteplase should be reconstituted using the diluent, syringe, needle, and dispensing pin provided with each kit and the each reconstituted dose should be given I.V. over 2 minutes; no other medication should be added to the injection solution

Monitoring Parameters Monitor for signs of bleeding (hematuria, GI bleeding, gingival bleeding)

Nursing Implications See Administration

Additional Information The dosage of reteplase in clinical trials was expressed in terms of million unit (MU); however, reteplase is being marketed in units (U) with 1 unit equivalent to 1 million units, reteplase units are expressed using a reference standard specific for reteplase and are not comparable with units used for other thrombolytic agents, 10 units is equivalent to 17.4 mg

Special Geriatric Considerations No specific changes in use in elderly are necessary; use as indicated in Usual Dosage

Dosage Forms Injection: Powder in vials, each vial contains reteplase 10.8 units; supplied with 2 mL diluent (preservative free)

Reversol® see Edrophonium on page 328
Rēv-Eyes™ see Dapiprazole on page 269
Rexolate® see Salicylates (Various Salts) on page 842
Rezine® see Hydroxyzine on page 470
Rezulin® see Troglitazone on page 968
R-Gel® [OTC] see Capsaicin on page 155
Rheaban® [OTC] see Attapulgite on page 94
Rheumatrex® see Methotrexate on page 605
Rhinall® Nasal Solution [OTC] see Phenylephrine on page 740
Rhinocort™ see Budesonide on page 131

Rhinosyn-DMX® [OTC] *see* Guaifenesin and Dextromethorphan *on page 439*

rHuEPO-α *see* Epoetin Alfa *on page 338*

Rhythmin® *see* Procainamide *on page 780*

Ribavirin (rye ba VYE rin)

Brand Names Virazole®

Synonyms RTCA; Tribavirin

Generic Available No

Therapeutic Category Antiviral Agent, Inhalation Therapy

Use Treatment of patients with respiratory syncytial virus (RSV) infections; may also be used in other viral infections including influenza A and B and adenovirus; specially indicated for treatment of severe lower respiratory tract RSV infections in patients with an underlying compromising condition (immunodeficiency and immunosuppression)

Warnings Use with caution in patients requiring assisted ventilation because precipitation of the drug in the respiratory equipment may interfere with safe and effective patient ventilation; also monitor carefully in patients with COPD and asthma for deterioration of respiratory function. Ribavirin is potentially mutagenic, tumor-promoting, and gonadotoxic; there is evidence that ribavirin is teratogenic in small animals. Health care workers who are pregnant or may become pregnant should be advised of the potential risks of exposure and counseled about risk reduction strategies including alternate job responsibilities; virus resistance does not appear to develop; incubation period for RSV is 4-8 days.

Adverse Reactions

Cardiovascular: Hypotension, cardiac arrest

Dermatologic: Rash, skin irritation

Hematologic: Anemia

Ocular: Conjunctivitis

Respiratory: Mild bronchospasm, worsening of respiratory function, bacterial pneumonia, pneumothorax, apnea, ventilator dependence

Drug Interactions Decreased effect of zidovudine

Stability Do not use any water containing an antimicrobial agent to reconstitute drug; reconstituted solution is stable for 24 hours at room temperature

Mechanism of Action Inhibits replication of RNA and DNA viruses; inhibits influenza virus RNA polymerase activity and inhibits the initiation and elongation of RNA fragments resulting in inhibition of viral protein synthesis

Pharmacokinetics

Absorption: Systemically from the respiratory tract following nasal and oral inhalation; absorption is dependent upon respiratory factors and method of drug delivery; maximal absorption occurs with the use of the aerosol generator via an endotracheal tube; highest concentrations are found in the respiratory tract and erythrocytes

Metabolism: Occurs intracellularly and may be necessary for drug action

Plasma half-life: Adults: 24 hours, much longer in the erythrocyte (16-40 days), which can be used as a marker for intracellular metabolism

Time to peak serum concentration: Inhalation: Within 60-90 minutes

Elimination: Hepatic metabolism is major route of elimination with 40% of the drug cleared renally as unchanged drug and metabolites

Usual Dosage Geriatrics and Adults:

Aerosol inhalation: Use with Viratek® small particle aerosol generator (SPAG-2) at a concentration of 20 mg/mL (6 g reconstituted with 300 mL of sterile water without preservatives)

Aerosol only: 12-18 hours/day for 3 days, up to 7 days in length

Administration Read the Viratek® Small Particle Aerosol Generator (SPAG) Model SPAG-2 Operator's Manual before use

Monitoring Parameters Respiratory function

Nursing Implications Keep accurate I & O record, discard solutions placed in the SPAG-2 unit at least every 24 hours and before adding additional fluid (see Administration)

Additional Information RSV season is usually December to April; viral shedding period for RSV is usually 3-8 days

Special Geriatric Considerations No specific recommendations are necessary in elderly (see Usual Dosage and Adverse Reactions)

Dosage Forms Powder for aerosol: 6 g (100 mL)

Ridaura® *see* Auranofin *on page 95*

Ridenol® [OTC] *see* Acetaminophen *on page 16*

Rifabutin (rif a BYOO tin)

Brand Names Mycobutin®

Synonyms Ansamycin

Therapeutic Category Antibiotic, Miscellaneous; Antitubercular Agent

Use Prevention of disseminated *Mycobacterium avium* complex (MAC) in patients with advanced HIV infection; also utilized in multiple drug regimens for treatment of MAC

Contraindications Hypersensitivity to rifabutin or any other rifamycins; rifabutin is contraindicated in patients with a WBC <1000/mm^3 or a platelet count <50,000/mm^3

Warnings Rifabutin as a single agent must not be administered to patients with active tuberculosis since its use may lead to the development of tuberculosis that is resistant to both rifabutin and rifampin; rifabutin should be discontinued in patients with AST >500 IU/L or if total bilirubin is >3 mg/dL. Use with caution in patients with liver impairment; modification of dosage should be considered in patients with renal impairment.

Adverse Reactions

Cardiovascular: Chest pain

Central nervous system: Fever, headache, seizures, confusion, insomnia

Dermatologic: Rash

Gastrointestinal: Abdominal pain, diarrhea, dyspepsia, nausea, vomiting, dysgeusia, anorexia, flatulence, eructation

Genitourinary: Urine discoloration

Hematologic: Thrombocytopenia, anemia, leukopenia, neutropenia

Hepatic: Elevated liver enzymes

Neuromuscular & skeletal: Arthralgia, myalgia

Ocular: Uveitis

Overdosage Symptoms of overdose include nausea, vomiting, hepatotoxicity, lethargy, CNS depression

Toxicology Treatment is supportive; lavage with activated charcoal is preferred to ipecac as emesis is frequently present with overdose; hemodialysis will remove rifabutin, its effect on outcome is unknown

Drug Interactions Decreased plasma concentration (because of induced liver enzymes) of verapamil, diltiazem, nifedipine (possibly other calcium channel blockers), methadone, digoxin, cyclosporine, corticosteroids, oral anticoagulants, theophylline, barbiturates, chloramphenicol, ketoconazole, itraconazole, oral contraceptives, quinidine, halothane; rifabutin's metabolism may be inhibited by clarithromycin, fluconazole, protease inhibitors

Mechanism of Action Inhibits DNA-dependent RNA polymerase at the beta subunit which prevents chain initiation

Pharmacokinetics

Absorption: Oral: Readily absorbed 53%

Distribution: V$_d$: 9.32 L/kg; distributes to body tissues including the lungs, liver, spleen, eyes, and kidneys

Protein binding: 85%

Metabolism: To active and inactive metabolites; inducer CYP3A4

Bioavailability: Absolute, 20% in HIV patients

Half-life, terminal: 45 hours (range: 16-69 hours)

Peak serum concentration: Within 2-4 hours

Elimination: Renal and biliary clearance of unchanged drug is 10%; 30% excreted in feces; 53% in urine unchanged

Usual Dosage Geriatrics and Adults: Oral: 300 mg once daily; for patients who experience gastrointestinal upset, rifabutin can be administered 150 mg twice daily with food

Administration May be mixed with food (ie, applesauce)

Monitoring Parameters Periodic liver function tests, CBC with differential, platelet count, hemoglobin, hematocrit

Patient Information May discolor urine, tears, sweat, or other body fluids to a red-orange color; soft contact lenses may be permanently stained; report to physician any severe or persistent flu-like symptoms, nausea, vomiting, dark urine or pale stools, or unusual bleeding or bruising; can be taken with meals or sprinkled on applesauce

Nursing Implications Administer with meals

Special Geriatric Considerations No specific recommendations for elderly

Dosage Forms Capsule: 150 mg

Extemporaneous Preparations Rifabutin is insoluble in water and ethanol; prepare powder packets or compound with a suspending agent and shake well before using

Rifadin® see Rifampin *on next page*

Rifampicin *see* Rifampin *on this page*

Rifampin (RIF am pin)
Related Information
Penicillins, Penicillin-Related Antibiotics, & Other Antibiotics *on page 1010*
Brand Names Rifadin®; Rimactane®
Synonyms Rifampicin
Therapeutic Category Antibiotic, Miscellaneous; Antitubercular Agent
Use Management of active tuberculosis; eliminate meningococci from asymptomatic carriers; prophylaxis of *Haemophilus influenzae* type b infection; used in combination therapy against *Staphylococcus aureus*; used with oral vancomycin for resistant *C. difficile* diarrhea
Contraindications Hypersensitivity to rifampin or any component
Precautions Use with caution in patients with liver impairment; modification of dosage should be considered in patients with severe liver impairment; monitor closely if intermittent therapy is used; hypersensitivity reactions and thrombocytopenia occur more frequently in this setting
Adverse Reactions
Central nervous system: Drowsiness, fatigue, ataxia, confusion, fever, headache

Dermatologic: Rash, pruritus

Gastrointestinal: Nausea, vomiting, diarrhea, stomatitis, abdominal cramps

Hematologic: Eosinophilia, blood dyscrasias (leukopenia, thrombocytopenia)

Hepatic: Hepatitis

Local: Irritation at the I.V. site

Renal: Renal failure

Miscellaneous: Discoloration of urine, feces, saliva, sputum, sweat, and tears (reddish orange); flu-like syndrome
Overdosage Symptoms of overdose include nausea, vomiting, hepatotoxicity
Toxicology Asymptomatic increases in liver enzymes occur in 10% to 20% of patients; most often these increases occur in the first 6 months of treatment and are transient. If AST or ALT increases to 5 times baseline or signs of hepatitis are present, rifampin (and isoniazid) should be stopped; therapy can be reinitiated with close monitoring once symptoms have resolved and/or liver enzymes have returned to normal.
Drug Interactions Rifampin induces liver enzymes which may decrease the plasma concentration of the following drugs: acetaminophen, benzodiazepines (only those that undergo oxidation), beta-blockers, clofibrate, digitoxin, disopyramide, estrogens, phenytoin, and other hydantoins, mexiletine, calcium channel blockers, sulfones, sulfonylureas, enalapril (decreased blood pressure control), verapamil, methadone, digoxin, cyclosporine, corticosteroids, oral anticoagulants, theophylline, barbiturates, chloramphenicol, ketoconazole, itraconazole, oral contraceptives, quinidine, halothane, tocainide
Stability Reconstituted I.V. solution is stable for 24 hours at room temperature; rifampin oral suspension can be compounded with simple syrup or wild cherry syrup at a concentration of 10 mg/mL; the suspension is stable for 4 weeks at room temperature or in a refrigerator when stored in a glass amber prescription bottle
Mechanism of Action Inhibits bacterial RNA synthesis by binding to the beta subunit of DNA-dependent RNA polymerase, blocking RNA transcription
Pharmacodynamics
Peak serum concentrations: Within 2-4 hours

Duration: Up to 24 hours
Pharmacokinetics
Absorption: Oral: Well absorbed

Half-life: 3-4 hours, prolonged with hepatic impairment

Protein binding: 80%

Metabolism: In the liver; inducer CYP1A2, 2C9, 3A4

Highly lipophilic; crosses the blood-brain barrier well, undergoes enterohepatic recycling

Time to peak serum concentration: Within 2-4 hours; food may delay or slightly reduce peak serum concentration

Elimination: Principally in feces (60% to 65%) and urine (~30%)

Plasma rifampin concentrations are not significantly affected by hemodialysis or peritoneal dialysis

In a small (n=6) single-dose study, rifampin's pharmacokinetic parameters in elderly subjects were not significantly different compared to values of younger subjects reported in the literature
Usual Dosage Geriatrics and Adults: I.V. infusion dose is the same as for the oral route

Tuberculosis: Oral: 10 mg/kg/day; maximum: 600 mg/day

American Thoracic Society and CDC currently recommend twice weekly therapy as part of a short-course regimen which follows 1-2 months of daily treatment of uncomplicated pulmonary tuberculosis in the compliant patient. Adults: 10 mg/kg (up to 600 mg) twice weekly

H. influenzae prophylaxis: 600 mg every 24 hours for 4 days

Meningococcal prophylaxis: 600 mg every 12 hours for 2 days

Nasal carriers of *Staphylococcus aureus*: 600 mg/day for 5-10 days in combination with other antibiotics

Administration Administer on an empty stomach (ie, 1 hour prior to, or 2 hours after meals) to increase total absorption

Monitoring Parameters Liver function tests (ALT and AST) at baseline and 1, 3, and 6 months; sputum culture; chest x-ray 2-3 months into treatment and at completion

Test Interactions Increased bilirubin (S), positive Coombs' [direct]; inhibit standard assay's ability to measure serum folate and B_{12}

Patient Information May discolor urine, tears, sweat, or other body fluids to a red-orange color; take 1 hour before or 2 hours after a meal on an empty stomach; soft contact lenses may be permanently stained

Nursing Implications Evaluate hepatic status and mental status (see Administration)

Additional Information Since resistant strains occur rapidly, is normally used with other anti-TB drugs

Special Geriatric Considerations Rifampin, in combination with isoniazid, is the foundation of tuberculosis treatment; since most older patients acquired their *Mycobacterium tuberculosis* infection before effective chemotherapy was available, either a 9-month regimen of isoniazid and rifampin or a 6-month regimen of isoniazid and rifampin with pyrazinamide (the first 2 months) should be effective

Dosage Forms

Capsule: 150 mg, 300 mg

Injection: 600 mg

References

Advenier C, Gobert C, Houin G, et al, "Pharmacokinetic Studies of Rifampicin in the Elderly," *Ther Drug Monit*, 1983, 5(1):61-5.

Bass JB Jr, Farer LS, Hopewell PC, et al, "Treatment of Tuberculosis and Tuberculosis Infection in Adults and Children," *Am J Respir Crit Care Med*, 1994, 149(5):1359-74.

Van Scoy RE and Wilkowske CJ, "Antituberculous Agents: Isoniazid, Rifampin, Streptomycin, Ethambutol, and Pyrazinamide," *Mayo Clin Proc*, 1983, 58(4):233-40.

Yoshikawa TT, "Tuberculosis in Aging Adults," *J Am Geriatr Soc*, 1992, 40(2):178-87.

rIFN-A *see* Interferon Alfa-2a *on page 490*

RIG *see* Rabies Immune Globulin (Human) *on page 818*

Rilutek® *see* Riluzole *on this page*

Riluzole (RIL yoo zole)

Brand Names Rilutek®

Synonyms 2-Amino-6-Trifluoromethoxy-benzothiazole; RP54274

Generic Available No

Therapeutic Category Miscellaneous Product

Use Amyotrophic lateral sclerosis (ALS): Treatment of patients with ALS; riluzole can extend survival or time to tracheostomy

Contraindications Severe hypersensitivity reactions to riluzole or any of the tablet components

Warnings Among 4000 patients given riluzole for ALS, there were 3 cases of marked neutropenia (ANC <500/mm³), all seen within the first 2 months of treatment. Use with caution in patients with concomitant renal insufficiency. Use with caution in patients with current evidence or history of abnormal liver function. Monitor liver chemistries (see Precautions).

Precautions Measure liver function tests, specifically SGPT (ALT) before therapy and **every month** for just 3 months of therapy, then **every 3 months** during the remainder of the first year, then periodically thereafter. If elevations in ALT occur, monitor more often. Usually, maximum increases in ALT occur in the first 3 months of treatment. These are usually transient. There is no experience with ALT >5 ULN. No reported experience rechallenge in the literature and, therefore, no recommendations can be made at this time.

Adverse Reactions Many adverse reactions are dose-related. Most common side effects reported were asthenia, abdominal pain, nausea, vomiting, diarrhea, vertigo, asthma, rhinitis, hypertension, and dizziness.

(Continued)

Riluzole *(Continued)*

Cardiovascular: Hypertension, tachycardia, palpitations, hypertension, syncope, heart failure, angina, myocardial infarction, ventricular extrasystoles, atrial fibrillation, bundle branch block, pericarditis, bradycardia, mesenteric artery occlusion, ventricular fibrillation, ventricular tachycardia, shock, lower extremity embolus, cerebral hemorrhage, edema

Central nervous system: Headache, depression, insomnia, somnolence, vertigo, agitation, hallucination, paranoia, manic episodes, extrapyramidal syndrome, emotional lability, delusions, apathy, confusion, amnesia, delirium, disturbed dreams, euphoria, psychiatric depression, schizophrenic reaction, tetany, malaise

Dermatologic: Pruritus, eczema, exfoliative dermatitis, alopecia, urticaria, psoriasis, seborrhea, erythema multiforme, furunculosis, skin moniliasis, granuloma, angioedema

Endocrine & metabolic: Increased libido, hypokalemia, hyponatremia, hypercalcemia, hypercholesteremia, gout, thyroid neospasm, diabetes mellitus, diabetes insipidus, parathyroid disorder, breast pain

Gastrointestinal: Nausea, vomiting, diarrhea, anorexia, dry mouth, dyspepsia, stomatitis, flatulence, oral moniliasis, intestinal obstruction, fecal impaction, fecal incontinence, tenesmus, gastritis, ulceration (GI), esophageal stenosis (up to 1%), hematemesis, melena, biliary pain, proctitis, pseudomembranous enterocolitis, enlarged salivary glands, pancreatitis, gingival hemorrhage, weight loss, thirst, weight gain, loss of taste

Genitourinary: Urinary urgency, incontinence, dysuria, hematuria, impotence, prostatic carcinoma, priapism (up to 1%), nocturitis, uterine fibroids, vaginal moniliasis, urinary tract infections

Hepatic: Hepatitis, jaundice, cholecystitis

Neuromuscular & skeletal: Hypertonia, paresthesia, tremor, hypokinesis, abnormal gait, myoclonus, peripheral neuritis, myasthenia, bone neoplasm (up to 1%), bone necrosis, osteoporosis

Ocular: Amblyopia, blepharitis, cataracts, diplopia, glaucoma, photophobia

Otic: Ear pain, vestibular dysfunction

Renal: Kidney stones

Respiratory: Decreased lung function, rhinitis, cough, sinusitis, asthma, hypoventilation, laryngitis, pleural effusion, stridor (up to 1%), lung edema, lung carcinoma, epistaxis, hemoptysis, hyperventilation, respiratory acidosis

Miscellaneous: Hiccups, yawning, breast abscess

Toxicology No specific antidote or treatment information available; treatment should be supportive and directed toward alleviating symptoms

Drug Interactions Cytochrome P-450 1A2 (CYP 1A2) substrate

Decreased effect: Drugs that induce CYP 1A2 (eg, cigarette smoke, charbroiled food, rifampin, omeprazole) could increase the rate of riluzole elimination

Increased toxicity: Inhibitors of CYP 1A2 (eg, caffeine, theophylline, amitriptyline, quinolones) could decrease the rate of riluzole elimination

Drug/Food Interactions High fat meals decrease absorption

Stability Protect from bright light

Mechanism of Action Mechanism of action is unknown; its action may be related to inhibitory effect on glutamate release, inactivation of voltage-dependent sodium channels; and ability to interfere with intracellular events that follow transmitter binding at excitatory amino acid receptors

Pharmacokinetics

Absorption: Well absorbed (90%); a high fat meal decreases absorption of riluzole (decreasing AUC by 20% and peak blood concentrations by 45%)

Protein binding: 96% bound to plasma proteins, mainly albumin and lipoproteins

Metabolism: Extensively to 6 major and a number of minor metabolites. Metabolism is mostly hepatic and consists of cytochrome P-450 dependent hydroxylation and glucuronidation; principle isozyme is CYP 1A2

Bioavailability: Oral: Absolute (50%)

Usual Dosage Geriatrics and Adults: Oral: 50 mg every 12 hours; no increased benefit can be expected from higher daily doses, but adverse events are increased

Dosage adjustment in smoking: Cigarette smoking is known to induce CYP 1A2; patients who smoke cigarettes would be expected to eliminate riluzole faster. There is no information, however, on the effect of, or need for, dosage adjustment in these patients.

Dosage adjustment in special populations: Females and Japanese patients may possess a lower metabolic capacity to eliminate riluzole compared with male and Caucasian subjects, respectively

Dosage adjustment in renal impairment: Use with caution in patients with concomitant renal insufficiency

Dosage adjustment in hepatic impairment: Use with caution in patients with current evidence or history of abnormal liver function indicated by significant abnormalities in serum transaminase, bilirubin or GGT levels. Baseline elevations of several LFTs (especially elevated bilirubin) should preclude use of riluzole.

Monitoring Parameters Monitor serum aminotransferases including ALT levels before and during therapy. Evaluate serum ALT levels every month during the first 3 months of therapy, every 3 months during the remainder of the first year and periodically thereafter. Evaluate ALT levels more frequently in patients who develop elevations. Maximum increases in serum ALT usually occurred within 3 months after the start of therapy and were usually transient when <5 x ULN.

In trials, if ALT levels were <5 x ULN, treatment continued and ALT levels usually returned to below 2 x ULN within 2-6 months. Treatment in studies was discontinued, however, if ALT levels exceed 5 x ULN, so that there is no experience with continued treatment of ALS patients once ALT values exceed 5 x ULN.

If a decision is made to continue treatment in patients when the ALT exceeds 5 x ULN, frequent monitoring (at least weekly) of complete liver function is recommended. Discontinue treatment if ALT exceeds 10 x ULN or if clinical jaundice develops.

Test Interactions Increased LFTs, increased alkaline phosphatase, positive direct Coombs' test, increased gamma globulins, increase lactic dehydrogenase

Patient Information Take at least 1 hour before or 2 hours after a meal to avoid decreased bioavailability. Report any febrile illness to your physician. Take riluzole at the same time of the day each day. If a dose is missed, take the next tablet as originally planned.

Nursing Implications Warn patients about the potential for dizziness, vertigo or somnolence and advise them not to drive or operate machinery until they have gained sufficient experience on riluzole to gauge whether or not it affects their mental or motor performance adversely. Whether alcohol increases the risk of serious hepatotoxicity with riluzole is unknown; discourage riluzole-treated patients from drinking alcohol in excess.

Additional Information May be obtained through Rhone-Poulenc Rorer Inc (Collegeville, PA) for compassionate use (through treatment IND process) by calling 800-727-6737 for treatment of amyotrophic lateral sclerosis; may be more effective for amyotrophic lateral sclerosis of bulbar onset; in animal models, riluzole was a potent inhibitor of seizures induced by ouabain

Special Geriatric Considerations In clinical trials, no difference was demonstrated between elderly and younger adults. However, renal changes with age can be expected to result in higher serum concentrations of the parent drug and its metabolites.

Dosage Forms Tablet: 50 mg

References

Bensimon G, Lacomblez L, Meininger V, et al, "A Controlled Trial of Riluzole in Amyotrophic Lateral Sclerosis. ALS/Riluzole Study Group," N Engl J Med, 1994, 330(9):585-91

Rimactane® see Rifampin on page 830

Rimantadine (ri MAN ta deen)

Brand Names Flumadine®

Therapeutic Category Antiviral Agent, Oral

Use Prophylaxis and treatment of influenza A viral infection

Contraindications Hypersensitivity to drugs of the adamantine class (rimantadine or amantadine)

Warnings Use with caution in patients with liver disease, a history of recurrent and eczematoid dermatitis, uncontrolled psychosis or severe psychoneurosis, seizures in those receiving CNS stimulant drugs

Adverse Reactions

Cardiovascular: Hypertension, tachycardia, heart block, orthostatic hypotension, syncope

Central nervous system: Insomnia, dizziness, headache, nervousness, fatigue, impaired concentration, ataxia, confusion, irritability, hallucinations
(Continued)

Rimantadine *(Continued)*

Gastrointestinal: Nausea, vomiting, anorexia, xerostomia, abdominal pain, diarrhea, dyspepsia, constipation, dysgeusia

Genitourinary: Urinary retention

Neuromuscular & skeletal: Tremors

Ocular: Eye pain

Otic: Tinnitus

Respiratory: Dyspnea, bronchospasm, cough

Overdosage Symptoms of overdose include agitation, hallucinations, cardiac arrhythmias, and death

Toxicology I.V. physostigmine, 1-2 mg repeated as needed up to 2 mg/hour may be beneficial; supportive therapy

Drug Interactions Acetaminophen and aspirin decrease rimantadine plasma concentration and AUC 10% to 11%; cimetidine reduced rimantadine clearance

Mechanism of Action Believed to inhibit early viral replication, perhaps by inhibiting viral uncoating

Pharmacokinetics

Absorption: Tablet and syrup essentially completely absorbed

Distribution: 40% bound to plasma protein

Metabolism: 90%

Half-life:

Adults: Mean: 25.4 hours

Elderly (healthy): Mean: 32 hours

At steady-state, AUC, plasma concentration, and half-life are 20% to 30% greater in persons >60 years of age; elderly nursing home residents were found to have steady-state plasma concentrations 2-4 times greater than elderly by community residents

Usual Dosage Oral:

Prophylaxis:

Geriatrics: 100 mg/day

Adults: 100 mg twice daily

Treatment:

Geriatrics: 100 mg/day

Adults: 100 mg twice daily

Dosing adjustment in renal/hepatic impairment: Cl_{cr} ≤10 mL/minute: Dosage should be reduced to 100 mg/day

Monitoring Parameters Signs and symptoms of toxicity, especially CNS

Reference Range No relationship between plasma concentration and antiviral effects has been established

Nursing Implications See Monitoring Parameters

Special Geriatric Considerations Dosing must be individualized (100 mg 1-2 times/day); it is recommended that nursing home patients receive 100 mg/day (see Pharmacokinetics)

Dosage Forms

Rimantadine hydrochloride:

Syrup: 50 mg/5 mL (60 mL, 240 mL, 480 mL)

Tablet: 100 mg

References

Douglas RG Jr, "Prophylaxis and Treatment of Influenza," *N Engl J Med*, 1990, 322(7):443-50.

Guay DR, "Amantadine and Rimantadine Prophylaxis of Influenza A in Nursing Homes," *Drugs Aging*, 1994, 5(1):8-19.

Patriarca PA, Kater NA, Kendal AP, et al, "Safety of Prolonged Administration of Rimantadine Hydrochloride in the Prophylaxis of Influenza A Virus Infections in Nursing Homes," *Antimicrob Agents Chemother*, 1984, 26(1):101-3.

Rimexolone *(ri MEKS oh lone)*

Brand Names Vexol®

Generic Available No

Therapeutic Category Anti-inflammatory Agent, Ophthalmic; Corticosteroid, Ophthalmic

Use Treatment of inflammation after ocular surgery and the treatment of anterior uveitis

Contraindications Fungal, viral, or untreated pus-forming bacterial ocular infections; hypersensitivity to any component

Warnings Prolonged use has been associated with the development of corneal or scleral perforation, optic nerve damage, elevated IOP, defects in visual acuity and posterior subcapsular cataracts; may mask or enhance the establishment of acute purulent untreated infections of the eye; in diseases that cause thinning of the cornea or sclera, perforation with topical steroids has occurred

Adverse Reactions
Cardiovascular: Hyperemia
Dermatologic: Pruritus
Ocular: Temporary mild blurred vision; stinging, burning eyes, corneal thinning, increased intraocular pressure, glaucoma, damage to the optic nerve, defects in visual activity, cataracts, secondary ocular infection, perforation of the globe, ocular pain, discomfort, discharge, foreign body sensation

Toxicology Systemic toxicity is unlikely from the ophthalmic preparation

Mechanism of Action Decreases inflammation by suppression of migration of polymorphonuclear leukocytes and reversal of increased capillary permeability

Pharmacokinetics
Absorption: Through aqueous humor
Metabolism: Any drug absorbed is metabolized in the liver
Elimination: By the kidneys and feces

Usual Dosage Geriatrics and Adults: Ophthalmic: Instill 1 drop in conjunctival sac 2-4 times/day up to every 4 hours; may use every 1-2 hours during first 1-2 days; when favorable response is attained, reduce dosage to 1 drop every 4 hours; later can reduce to 1 drop 3-4 times/day

Postoperative inflammation: Instill 1-2 drops 4 times/day beginning 24 hours following surgery; continue for 2 weeks postoperatively

Monitoring Parameters Intraocular pressure and periodic examination of lens (with prolonged use)

Patient Information Shake well before using, do not touch dropper to the eye

Nursing Implications Monitor the dosing interval closely; IOP must be monitored; watch for ocular adverse effects

Special Geriatric Considerations No special considerations; must limit the time steroids are used to prevent adverse effects

Dosage Forms Suspension, ophthalmic: 1% (5 mL, 10 mL)

Riopan® [OTC] *see* Magaldrate *on page 560*

Riopan Plus® [OTC] *see* Magaldrate and Simethicone *on page 562*

Risperdal® *see* Risperidone *on this page*

Risperidone (ris PER i done)

Related Information
Antipsychotic Agents Comparison *on page 1023*
Antipsychotic Medication Guidelines *on page 1076*
Federal OBRA Regulations Recommended Maximum Doses - Antipsychotics *on page 1056*

Brand Names Risperdal®

Therapeutic Category Antipsychotic Agent; Neuroleptic Agent

Use Management of psychotic disorders (eg, schizophrenia); nonpsychotic symptoms associated with dementia in elderly

Contraindications Known hypersensitivity to risperidone or any component of the product

Warnings Long-term use (>8 weeks) not evaluated; neuroleptic malignant syndrome has been reported with antipsychotics. Risperidone causes less tardive dyskinesia, EPS, anticholinergic effects, and hypotension than phenothiazine and butyrophenone classes of antipsychotics, especially when doses do not exceed 6 mg/day. Nonetheless, the following information needs to be kept in mind even with this "novel antipsychotic:"

Tardive dyskinesia: Prevalence rate may be 40% in elderly; elderly women especially at risk; embarrassment from dyskinesias may lead to greater social isolation; development of the syndrome and the irreversible nature are proportional to duration and total cumulative dose over time. May be reversible if diagnosed early in therapy; intermittent use of antipsychotics (not proven use) helps decrease total cumulative dose.

EPS: Extrapyramidal reactions are more common in elderly with up to 50% developing these reactions for those over 60 years of age. These reactions may be more common in dementia patients. Drug-induced **Parkinson's syndrome** occurs often. Discontinuation usually resolves symptoms but may take weeks to months (12+) to clear. **Akathisia** is the most common EPS reaction in elderly. The symptoms of motor restlessness are difficult to diagnose in demented elderly; increased nervousness, assertiveness, restlessness with constant movement may indicate this adverse event. Consider decreasing dose if antipsychotic to treat as well as diagnose
(Continued)

Risperidone *(Continued)*

problem; usually see this reaction within 2-3 months of initiating antipsychotic drug.

Anticholinergic effects: These side effects most common with low potency antipsychotics (eg, thioridazine, chlorpromazine). CNS toxicity occurs more frequently and severely in elderly; increased confusion, memory loss, psychotic behavior, and agitation frequently occur as a consequence of anticholinergic effects to antipsychotic agents. Peripheral anticholinergic action troublesome to elderly; most peripheral anticholinergic effects last only 2-3 weeks (see Adverse Reactions).

Orthostatic hypotension: More common with low potency agents (eg, thioridazine, chlorpromazine, and clozapine) but of concern with all antipsychotic agents; orthostasis due to alpha-receptor blockade by risperidone and other antipsychotic agents. Elderly present many risk factors for orthostatic hypotension: blunted baroreceptor reflexes, decreased vascular tone, decreased vascular volume, and possible presence of cardiac diseases which result in decreased cardiac output.

Sedation: Common side effect with antipsychotic therapy; should not be used as a hypnotic unless insomnia is associated with target behavior symptoms treated with antipsychotic medications (see Special Geriatric Considerations). Anecdotal reports suggesting antipsychotic sedation in nonpsychotic patients is extremely unpleasant due to feelings of depersonalization, derealization, and dysphoria. Due to the long duration of action with antipsychotic drugs, these reactions may last up to 24 hours and result in decreased daytime function.

Cardiac toxicity: Risperidone or its 9-hydroxyrisperidone metabolite have shown to increase the Q-T interval in some patients. Drugs which lengthen Q-T intervals have been associated with the development of torsade de pointes, a life-threatening event. Use with caution in patients with cardiac disease. Life-threatening arrhythmias have occurred at therapeutic doses of antipsychotics. Thioridazine more commonly demonstrates EKG changes than other antipsychotics; suggested to use high potency antipsychotic agents (ie, haloperidol) in patients with cardiac conduction defects.

Precautions Use with caution in patients with cardiovascular disease, seizures, and Parkinson's disease; benefits of therapy must be weighed against risks of therapy

Adverse Reactions

Anticholinergic: Xerostomia (problem for denture user), urinary retention, constipation, adynamic ileus, overflow incontinence, blurred vision

Cardiovascular: Hypotension (especially orthostatic), tachycardia, arrhythmias, abnormal T waves with prolonged ventricular repolarization, EKG changes

Central nervous system: Sedation, drowsiness, restlessness, anxiety, extrapyramidal reactions, dystonic reactions, pseudoparkinsonian signs and symptoms, tardive dyskinesia, neuroleptic malignant syndrome, seizures, altered central temperature regulation

Dermatologic: Photosensitivity (rare)

Endocrine & metabolic: Amenorrhea, galactorrhea, gynecomastia

Gastrointestinal: Constipation, adynamic ileus, GI upset, xerostomia (problem for denture user), weight gain

Genitourinary: Urinary retention, overflow incontinence, priapism, sexual dysfunction (up to 60%)

Hematologic: Agranulocytosis, leukopenia (usually in patients with large doses for prolonged periods)

Hepatic: Cholestatic jaundice

Ocular: Blurred vision, retinal pigmentation, decreased visual acuity (may be irreversible)

Overdosage In reports of doses ranging from 20-30 mg, no fatalities have occurred; symptoms of overdose include drowsiness, sedation, hypotension, tachycardia, extrapyramidal symptoms, seizures

Toxicology Following initiation of essential overdose management, toxic symptom treatment and supportive treatment should be initiated. Hypotension usually responds to I.V. fluids or Trendelenburg positioning. If unresponsive to these measures the use of a parenteral inotrope may be required (eg, norepinephrine 0.1-0.2 mcg/kg/minute titrated to response). Do not use epinephrine, dopamine, or other sympathomimetics with beta-agonist activity as this may worsen hypotension. Seizures commonly respond to diazepam (I.V. 5-10 mg bolus in adults every 15 minutes if needed up to a total of 30 mg) or to phenytoin or phenobarbital. Also critical cardiac arrhythmias often respond to I.V. phenytoin (15 mg/kg up to 1 g), while other antiarrhythmics can be used. Neuroleptics often cause extrapyramidal symptoms (eg, dystonic reactions) requiring management with diphenhydramine 1-2 mg/kg up to a maximum of 50 mg I.M. or I.V. slow push followed by a maintenance dose for 48-72 hours. When these reactions are unresponsive to diphenhydramine, benztropine mesylate I.V. 1-2 mg may be effective. These agents are generally effective within 2-5 minutes.

Drug Interactions
May antagonize effects of levodopa
Carbamazepine decreased risperidone serum concentrations
Clozapine decreases clearance of risperidone

Mechanism of Action Risperidone is a benzisoxazole derivative, mixed serotonin-dopamine antagonist; binds to $5-HT_2$ receptors in the CNS and in the periphery with a very high affinity; binds to dopamine D_2 receptors with less affinity. The binding affinity to the dopamine D_2 receptor is 20 times lower than the $5-HT_2$ affinity. The addition of serotonin antagonism to dopamine antagonism (classic neuroleptic mechanism) is thought to improve negative symptoms of psychoses and reduce the incidence of extrapyramidal side effects.

Pharmacokinetics
Absorption: Oral: Rapid
Metabolism: Extensively by cytochrome P-4502D6
Protein binding: Plasma: 90%
Half-life: 24 hours (risperidone and its active metabolite)
Time to peak plasma concentration: Within 1 hour

Usual Dosage Oral:
Geriatrics: **Dosing adjustment in renal, hepatic impairment, and elderly:** Starting dose of 0.5 mg once or twice daily is advisable; dosages >6 mg/day increase incidence of extrapyramidal side effects; increase dose at 0.5 mg twice daily at weekly intervals if possible; if rapid escalation in dose is needed, then initial increases at 1 mg twice daily for 3 days may be used to achieve a target dose of 3 mg twice daily
Adults: Recommended starting dose: 1 mg twice daily; slowly increase to the optimum range of 4-8 mg/day; daily dosages >5 mg do not appear to confer any additional benefit, and the incidence of extrapyramidal reactions is higher than with lower doses; maximum dose: 16 mg/day; periodically assess the need to continue maintenance therapy; reinitiating risperidone in patients who have had a respite from therapy need to follow the initial 3-day dosing schedule (see Additional Information)

Monitoring Parameters Orthostatic blood pressures; tremors; gait changes, abnormal movement in trunk, neck, buccal area, or extremities; monitor target behaviors for which the agent is given

Patient Information Explain to patients that orthostatic hypotension may occur at initiation of therapy; may cause impairment of alertness and judgment; enhanced sedation will occur with the ingestion of alcohol; photosensitivity may occur; use sunscreen or avoid exposure to sunlight and ultraviolet light

Nursing Implications Monitor and observe for extrapyramidal effects, orthostatic blood pressure changes for 3-5 days after starting or increasing dose

Additional Information For patients being switched to risperidone when treated with other antipsychotic agents, it is suggested to discontinue the prior therapy immediately and initiate risperidone. For parenteral depot dosage forms, initiate risperidone at the point of the next scheduled injection.

Special Geriatric Considerations See Warnings.

Extrapyramidal syndrome symptoms occur less with this agent when total daily dose remains <6 mg as compared with phenothiazines and butyrophenone classes of antipsychotics

Many elderly patients receive antipsychotic medications for inappropriate nonpsychotic behavior. Before initiating antipsychotic medication, the clinician should investigate any possible reversible cause; any stress or stress from any disease can cause acute "confusion" or worsening of baseline nonpsychotic behavior. Most commonly acute changes in behavior are due to increases in drug dose or addition of new drug to regimen; fluid electrolyte loss; infections; and changes in environment.

Any changes in disease status in any organ system can result in behavior changes

Some clinicians prefer to initiate therapy with 0.25-0.5 mg once daily and titrate upward as necessary
(Continued)

Risperidone *(Continued)*

In the treatment of agitated, demented, elderly patients, authors of meta-analysis of controlled trials of the response to the traditional antipsychotics (phenothiazines, butyrophenones) in controlling agitation have concluded that the use of neuroleptics results in a response rate of 18%. Clearly neuroleptic therapy for behavior control should be limited with frequent attempts to withdraw the agent given for behavior control.

Dosage Forms
Solution, oral: 1 mg/mL
Tablet: 1 mg, 2 mg, 3 mg, 4 mg

References
Cohen LJ, "Risperidone," *Pharmacotherapy*, 1994, 14(3):253-65.

Ritalin® *see* Methylphenidate *on page 609*

Ritalin-SR® *see* Methylphenidate *on page 609*

rIFN-b *see* Interferon Beta-1b *on page 493*

RMS® Rectal *see* Morphine Sulfate *on page 640*

Robafen® AC *see* Guaifenesin and Codeine *on page 438*

Robafen DM® [OTC] *see* Guaifenesin and Dextromethorphan *on page 439*

Robaxin® *see* Methocarbamol *on page 604*

Robicillin® VK *see* Penicillin V Potassium *on page 725*

Robinul® *see* Glycopyrrolate *on page 430*

Robinul® Forte *see* Glycopyrrolate *on page 430*

Robitussin® [OTC] *see* Guaifenesin *on page 437*

Robitussin® A-C *see* Guaifenesin and Codeine *on page 438*

Robitussin® Cough Calmers [OTC] *see* Dextromethorphan *on page 278*

Robitussin®-DM [OTC] *see* Guaifenesin and Dextromethorphan *on page 439*

Robitussin® Pediatric [OTC] *see* Dextromethorphan *on page 278*

Robomol® *see* Methocarbamol *on page 604*

Rocaltrol® *see* Calcitriol *on page 143*

Rocephin® *see* Ceftriaxone *on page 192*

Roferon-A® *see* Interferon Alfa-2a *on page 490*

Rogaine® Extra Strength for Men [OTC] *see* Minoxidil *on page 630*

Rogaine® for Men [OTC] *see* Minoxidil *on page 630*

Rogaine® for Women [OTC] *see* Minoxidil *on page 630*

Rolaids® Calcium Rich [OTC] *see* Calcium Salts (Oral) *on page 152*

Rondec® Drops *see* Carbinoxamine and Pseudoephedrine *on page 164*

Rondec® Filmtab® *see* Carbinoxamine and Pseudoephedrine *on page 164*

Rondec® Syrup *see* Carbinoxamine and Pseudoephedrine *on page 164*

Rondec-TR® *see* Carbinoxamine and Pseudoephedrine *on page 164*

Ropinirole *(roe PIN i role)*

Brand Names Requip™

Therapeutic Category Anti-Parkinson's Agent; Dopaminergic Agent (Antiparkinson's)

Use Treatment of idiopathic Parkinson's disease; in patients with early Parkinson's disease who were not receiving concomitant levodopa therapy as well as in patients with advanced disease on concomitant levodopa

Contraindications Hypersensitivity to ropinirole

Warnings Syncope, sometimes associated with bradycardia, was observed in association with ropinirole in both early Parkinson's disease (without L-dopa) patients and advanced Parkinson's disease (with L-dopa) patients. Dopamine agonists appear to impair the systemic regulation of blood pressure resulting in postural hypotension, especially during dose escalation. Parkinson's disease patients appear to have an impaired capacity to respond to a postural challenge. Parkinson's patients being treated with dopaminergic agonists ordinarily require careful monitoring for signs and symptoms of postural hypotension, especially during dose escalation, and should be informed of this risk. In patients with Parkinson's disease who were not treated with L-dopa, 5.2% of those treated with ropinirole reported hallucinations as compared to 1.4% on a placebo.

Precautions Ropinirole may potentiate dopaminergic side effects of levodopa and may cause and/or exacerbate pre-existing dyskinesia. Cases of retroperitoneal fibrosis, pulmonary infiltrates, pleural effusion, and pleural thickening have been reported in patients treated with ergot-derived dopaminergic agents (ropinirole is a nonergot-derived dopamine agonist).

Adverse Reactions
Early Parkinson's disease:
Cardiovascular: Syncope, dependent/leg edema, orthostatic symptoms
Central nervous system: Dizziness (40%), somnolence (40%), headache, fatigue, pain, confusion, hallucinations
Gastrointestinal: Nausea (60%), dyspepsia, constipation, abdominal pain
Neuromuscular & skeletal: Asthenia
Ocular: Abnormal vision
Respiratory: Pharyngitis
Miscellaneous: Viral infection, diaphoresis (increased)
Advanced Parkinson's disease (with levodopa):
Cardiovascular: Hypotension, syncope
Central nervous system: Dizziness (26%), aggravated parkinsonism, somnolence (20%), headache (17%), insomnia, hallucinations, confusion, pain, paresis, amnesia, anxiety, abnormal dreaming
Gastrointestinal: Nausea (30%), abdominal pain, vomiting, constipation, diarrhea, dysphagia, flatulence, increased salivation, xerostomia, weight loss
Genitourinary: Urinary tract infections
Neuromuscular & skeletal: Dyskinesias (34%), falls (10%), hypokinesia, paresthesia, tremor, arthralgia, arthritis
Miscellaneous: Injury, increased diaphoresis, increased drug level

Overdosage No reports of intentional overdose; symptoms reported with accidental overdosage were agitation, increased dyskinesia, sedation, orthostatic hypotension, chest pain, confusion, nausea and vomiting

Drug Interactions Ropinirole is metabolized by CYP1A2 so there is the potential for interaction when given with inhibitors or inducers of this enzyme
Ciprofloxacin increased C_{max} and AUC of ropinirole
Estrogens decreased clearance of ropinirole
Decreased effect: Dopamine antagonists (phenothiazine, haloperidol, metoclopramide)

Mechanism of Action Ropinirole has a high relative *in vitro* specificity and full intrinsic activity at the D_2 and D_3 dopamine receptor subtypes, binding with higher affinity to D_3 than to D_2 or D_4 receptor subtypes. Although precise mechanism of action of ropinirole is unknown, it is believed to be due to stimulation of postsynaptic dopamine D_2-type receptors within the caudate-putamen in the brain.

Pharmacokinetics
Absorption: Not affected by food; T_{max} increased by 2.5 hours when drug taken with a meal; absolute bioavailability was 55%, indicating first-pass effect
Distribution: V_d: 525 L; removal of drug by hemodialysis is unlikely
Metabolism: Extensively by liver to inactive metabolites; CYP1A2 was the major enzyme responsible for metabolism of ropinirole
Half-life, elimination: ~6 hours
Time to peak concentration: ~1-2 hours
Clearance of ropinirole is reduced by 30% in patients >65 years of age

Usual Dosage Geriatrics and Adults: Oral: The dosage should be increased to achieve a maximum therapeutic effect, balanced against the principal side effects of nausea, dizziness, somnolence and dyskinesia
Recommended starting dose is 0.25 mg three times/day; based on individual patient response, the dosage should be titrated with weekly increments as described below:
•Week 1: 0.25 mg 3 times/day; total daily dose: 0.75 mg
•Week 2: 0.5 mg 3 times/day; total daily dose: 1.5 mg
•Week 3: 0.75 mg 3 times/day; total daily dose: 2.25 mg
•Week 4: 1 mg 3 times/day; total daily dose: 3 mg
After week 4, if necessary, daily dosage may be increased by 1.5 mg per day on a weekly basis up to a dose of 9 mg/day, and then by up to 3 mg/day weekly to a total of 24 mg/day

Patient Information Ropinirole can be taken with or without food. Hallucinations can occur and elderly are at a higher risk than younger patients with Parkinson's disease. Postural hypotension may develop with or without symptoms such as dizziness, nausea, syncope, and sometimes sweating. Hypotension and/or orthostatic symptoms may occur more frequently during initial therapy or with an increase in dose at any time. Use caution when rising rapidly after sitting or lying down, especially after having done so for prolonged periods and especially at the initiation of treatment with ropinirole. Because of additive sedative effects, caution should be used when taking
(Continued)

Ropinirole *(Continued)*

CNS depressants (eg, benzodiazepines, antipsychotics, antidepressants) in combination with ropinirole.

Nursing Implications See Usual Dosage and Patient Information

Additional Information If ropinirole needs to be discontinued, it should be done so gradually over a 7-day period. Decrease dosing to twice daily for 4 days and then once daily for 3 days.

Special Geriatric Considerations Since the dose is titrated to clinical response, no specific dosage adjustment is necessary in the elderly (see Pharmacokinetics)

Dosage Forms Tablet, as hydrochloride: 0.25 mg, 0.5 mg, 1 mg, 2 mg, 5 mg

References

Stern MB, "Contemporary Approaches to the Pharmacotherapeutic Management of Parkinson's Disease: An Overview," *Neurology*, 1997, 49(1 Suppl 1):S2-9.

Watts RL, "The Role of Dopamine Agonists in Early Parkinson's Disease," *Neurology*, 1997, 49(1 Suppl 1):S34-48.

Rowasa® Rectal *see* Mesalamine *on page 591*

Roxanol™ Oral *see* Morphine Sulfate *on page 640*

Roxanol Rescudose® *see* Morphine Sulfate *on page 640*

Roxanol SR™ Oral *see* Morphine Sulfate *on page 640*

Roxicet® 5/500 *see* Oxycodone and Acetaminophen *on page 705*

Roxicodone™ *see* Oxycodone *on page 703*

Roxilox® *see* Oxycodone and Acetaminophen *on page 705*

Roxiprin® *see* Oxycodone and Aspirin *on page 706*

RP54274 *see* Riluzole *on page 831*

r-PA *see* Reteplase *on page 827*

RTCA *see* Ribavirin *on page 828*

Rubella and Measles Vaccines, Combined *see* Measles and Rubella Vaccines, Combined *on page 571*

Rubella and Mumps Vaccines, Combined

(rue BEL a & mumpz vak SEENS, kom BINED)

Related Information

Immunization Guidelines *on page 1058*

Brand Names Biavax®ᵢᵢ

Generic Available No

Therapeutic Category Vaccine

Use Promote active immunity to rubella and mumps by inducing production of antibodies

Contraindications Known hypersensitivity to neomycin, eggs; primary immunodeficient patients; patients receiving immunosuppressant drugs except corticosteroids

Adverse Reactions

Central nervous system: Febrile seizures, fever

Gastrointestinal: Diarrhea

Local: Soreness, burning, stinging, mild lymphoadenopathy

Miscellaneous: Allergic reactions, parotitis

Drug Interactions Immune globulin, whole blood

Stability Refrigerate (36°F to 46°F); discard unused portion within 8 hours; protect from light

Usual Dosage Geriatrics and Adults: 1 vial in outer aspect of the upper arm; children vaccinated before 12 months of age should be revaccinated

Administration Administer S.C. only

Monitoring Parameters Local adverse reactions

Test Interactions Temporary suppression of TB skin test

Patient Information

Mumps vaccine: A little swelling of the glands in the cheeks and under the jaw that lasts for a few days; this could happen from 1-2 weeks after getting the mumps vaccine; this happens rarely

Rubella vaccine: Swelling of the lymph glands in the neck or a rash that lasts 1-2 days; this could happen 1-2 weeks after vaccination

Mild pain or stiffness in the joints that may last up to 3 days; may occur from 1-3 weeks after vaccination

Painful swelling of the joints (arthritis). About 10/100 adults have this adverse effect, usually lasting a few days to a week. Rarely, this swelling has been reported to last longer. Damage to joints is very rare.

Pain or numbness, or "pins and needles" feeling in the hands and feet that lasts for a short time; this happens rarely

Additional Information Federal law requires that the date of administration, the vaccine manufacturer, lot number of vaccine, and the administering person's name, title and address be entered into the patient's permanent medical record

Special Geriatric Considerations Most adults are immune to mumps and vaccination is not necessary for those born prior to 1957. Elderly who lived in isolated communities may have no history of infection and no immunity; testing may be necessary. For those who fail to demonstrate immunity by testing, vaccination may be desirable if exposure is likely (travel to endemic areas etc). The MMR is preferred for adults.

Dosage Forms
Injection (mixture of 2 viruses):
1. Wistar RA 27/3 strain of rubella virus
2. Jeryl Lynn (B level) mumps strain grown cell cultures of chick embryo

References
Gardner P and Schaffner W, "Immunization of Adults," *N Engl J Med*, 1993, 328(17):1252-8.

Rubella, Measles and Mumps Vaccines, Combined *see* Measles, Mumps, and Rubella Vaccines, Combined *on page 572*

Rubella Virus Vaccine, Live (rue BEL a VYE rus vak SEEN, live)
Related Information
Immunization Guidelines *on page 1058*
Brand Names Meruvax® II
Synonyms German Measles Vaccine
Generic Available No
Therapeutic Category Vaccine, Live Virus
Use Provide vaccine-induced immunity to rubella
Contraindications Hypersensitivity to neomycin, patients receiving ACTH, corticosteroids, irradiation; patients with respiratory infections; active tuberculosis; immunosuppressed patients (drug induced or disease)
Precautions Hypersensitivity, allergic reactions to the vaccine; do not administer with other live vaccines; do not vaccinate for at least 3 months following patient receiving blood transfusion and immune serum globulin; may temporarily depress tuberculin skin testing
Adverse Reactions
Central nervous system: Malaise, fever, headache, rarely encephalitis, polyneuritis
Dermatologic: Urticaria, rash
Hematologic: Thrombocytopenia
Local: Local tenderness and erythema
Neuromuscular & skeletal: Arthralgias
Respiratory: Sore throat
Miscellaneous: Lymphadenopathy, hypersensitivity, allergic reactions to the vaccine
Drug Interactions Whole blood, immune globulin
Stability Refrigerate, discard reconstituted vaccine after 8 hours; store at 2°C to 8°C (36°F to 46°F); ship vaccine at 10°C; may use dry ice
Mechanism of Action Antibody titers after immunization last 6 years without significant decline; 90% of those vaccinated have protection for at least 15 years
Usual Dosage S.C.: 1000 $TCID_{50}$ of rubella (entire single-dose vial) into outer aspect of upper arm; do not administer I.V.
Monitoring Parameters See Adverse Reactions
Patient Information Patient may experience burning or stinging at the injection site; joint pain usually occurs 1-10 weeks after vaccination and persists 1-3 days
Nursing Implications Reconstituted vaccine should be used within 8 hours; S.C. injection only; federal law requires that the date of administration, the vaccine manufacturer, lot number of vaccine, and the administering person's name, title, and address be entered into the patient's permanent record
Special Geriatric Considerations Not a vaccine necessary for most adults and elderly adults; however, necessary to protect persons without immunity traveling into endemic or epidemic countries; may need to test for rubella immunity if no record of disease of vaccination is available
Dosage Forms Injection: 1000 $TCID_{50}$ (Wistar RA 27/3 Strain) single dose
References
Gardner P and Schaffner W, "Immunization of Adults," *N Engl J Med*, 1993, 328(17):1252-8.

Rubeola Vaccine *see* Measles Virus Vaccine, Live *on page 574*
Rubramin-PC® *see* Cyanocobalamin *on page 257*

Rufen® *see Ibuprofen on page 475*

Rum-K® *see Potassium Chloride on page 763*

Ru-Vert-M® *see Meclizine on page 574*

Rythmol® *see Propafenone on page 792*

Sabin Vaccine *see Poliovirus Vaccine, Live, Trivalent, Oral on page 761*

Safe Tussin® 30 [OTC] *see Guaifenesin and Dextromethorphan on page 439*

Sal-Acid® Plaster [OTC] *see Salicylic Acid on page 845*

Salactic® Film [OTC] *see Salicylic Acid on page 845*

Salagen® Oral *see Pilocarpine on page 748*

Salbutamol *see Albuterol on page 29*

Saleto-200® [OTC] *see Ibuprofen on page 475*

Saleto-400® *see Ibuprofen on page 475*

Salflex® *see Salsalate on page 847*

Salgesic® *see Salsalate on page 847*

Salicylates (Various Salts) (sa LIS i lates)

Related Information
Antacid Drug Interactions *on page 1096*

Brand Names Arthropan®; Asproject®; Extra Strength Doan's® [OTC]; Magan®; Mobidin®; Original Doan's® [OTC]; Rexolate®; Tusal®

Synonyms Choline Salicylate; Magnesium Salicylate; Sodium Salicylate; Sodium Thiosalicylate

Generic Available Yes

Therapeutic Category Analgesic, Non-narcotic; Anti-inflammatory Agent

Use Treatment of mild to moderate pain, inflammation, and fever; management of rheumatic fever, rheumatoid arthritis, osteoarthritis, and gout (see Mechanism of Action)

Contraindications Bleeding disorders (factor VII or IX deficiencies), hypersensitivity to salicylates or other nonsteroidal anti-inflammatory drugs (NSAIDs); tartrazine dye and asthma

Warnings Tinnitus or impaired hearing may indicate toxicity; discontinue use 1 week prior to surgical procedures

Precautions Use with caution in patients with platelet and bleeding disorders, renal dysfunction, hepatic disease, history of salicylate-induced gastric irritation, peptic ulcer disease, erosive gastritis, bleeding disorders, hypoprothrombinemia, and vitamin K deficiency; use cautiously in asthmatics, especially those with aspirin intolerance and nasal polyps

Adverse Reactions
Central nervous system: Fever, dizziness, mental confusion, CNS depression, headache, lassitude

Dermatologic: Rash, urticaria, angioedema

Gastrointestinal: Nausea, vomiting, GI distress, bleeding, ulcers

Hematologic: Leukopenia, thrombocytopenia

Hepatic: Hepatotoxicity (high dose)

Otic: Tinnitus

Respiratory: Bronchospasm, hyperventilation

Miscellaneous: Thirst, diaphoresis

Overdosage 10-30 g; symptoms of overdose include tinnitus, headache, dizziness, confusion, metabolic acidosis, hyperpyrexia, hyperpnea, tachypnea, nausea, vomiting, irritability, disorientation, hallucinations, lethargy, stupor, dehydration, hyperventilation, hyperthermia, hyperactivity, depression leading to coma, respiratory failure, and collapse; laboratory abnormalities include hypokalemia, hypoglycemia or hyperglycemia with alterations in pH

Aspirin or Other Salicylate Toxicity

Toxic Symptoms	Treatment
Overdose	Induce emesis with ipecac, and/or lavage with saline, followed with activated charcoal
Dehydration	I.V. fluids with KCl (no D_5W only)
Metabolic acidosis (must be treated)	Sodium bicarbonate
Hyperthermia	Cooling blankets or sponge baths
Coagulopathy/hemorrhage	Vitamin K I.V.
Hypoglycemia (with coma, seizures, or change in mental status)	Dextrose 25 g I.V.
Seizures	Diazepam 5-10 mg I.V.

Toxicology The "Done" nomogram is very helpful for estimating the severity of aspirin poisoning and directing treatment using serum salicylate concentrations. Treatment can also be based upon symptomatology; see table.

Drug Interactions

May increase nephrotoxicity of cyclosporin; diclofenac + K$^+$ sparing diuretics may increase serum K$^+$

Concomitant insulin or oral hypoglycemic agents may increase or decrease serum glucose

May increase digoxin, methotrexate, and lithium serum concentrations

Aspirin or other salicylates may decrease NSAID serum concentrations

Other NSAIDs may increase adverse GI effects

Increased prothrombin time with anticoagulants

Decreased antihypertensive effects of ACE inhibitors, beta-blockers, and thiazide diuretics

Increased response to sympathomimetics

Probenecid may increase toxicity of NSAIDs by increase in serum concentrations

Effects of loop diuretics may decrease; concomitant use with loop diuretics may enhance azotemia in elderly

Mechanism of Action Inhibits prostaglandin synthesis; acts on the hypothalamus heat-regulating center to reduce fever through vasodilation of peripheral vessels; decreases pain receptor sensitivity. Other proposed mechanisms of action for salicylate anti-inflammatory action are lysosomal stabilization, inhibition of kinin and leukotriene production, alteration of chemotactic factors, and inhibition of neutrophil activation. This latter mechanism may be the most significant pharmacologic action to reduce inflammation. Nonacetylated salicylates are **not** as potent in prostaglandin synthesis inhibition and, therefore, tend to have less adverse effects on gastrointestinal and renal tissues. They do not inhibit platelet function as aspirin does since they are not acetylated and, therefore, cannot acetylate platelet cyclooxygenase.

Pharmacokinetics

Absorption: From the stomach and small intestine

Distribution: Readily into most body fluids and tissues

Aspirin is hydrolyzed to salicylate (active) by esterases in the GI mucosa, red blood cells, synovial fluid and blood

Metabolism: Metabolism of salicylate occurs primarily by hepatic microsomal enzymes

Half-life, aspirin: 15-20 minutes; metabolic pathways are saturable such that salicylates half-life is dose-dependent ranging from 3 hours at lower doses (300-600 mg), 5-6 hours (after 1 g) and 15-30 hours with higher doses; in therapeutic anti-inflammatory doses, half-lives generally range from 6-12 hours

Time to peak plasma concentration: ~1-2 hours

Usual Dosage Geriatrics and Adults:

Sodium salicylate: Oral: 325-650 mg every 4 hours

Sodium thiosalicylate: I.M.:

Acute gout: 100 mg every 3-4 hours for 2 days, then 100 mg/day until resolved

Rheumatic fever: 100-150 mg every 4-8 hours for 3 days, then 100 mg twice/day until asymptomatic

Musculoskeletal pain: 50-100 mg/day or every other day

Magnesium salicylate: Oral: 650 mg every 4 hours or 1090 mg 3 times/day; may increase dose to 3.6-4.8 g/day in divided dose (3-4 doses); use caution in patients with renal failure and reduced renal function (ie, elderly due to possible magnesium accumulation) with products containing magnesium (see Additional Information)

Monitoring Parameters Serum concentrations, renal function; hearing changes or tinnitus; monitor for response (ie, pain, inflammation, range of motion, grip strength); observe for abnormal bleeding, bruising, weight gain

Reference Range

Sample size: 1.5-2 mL blood (purple top tube)

Timing of serum samples: Peak serum concentrations usually occur 2 hours after ingestion; the half-life increases with the dosage (eg, the half-life after 300 mg is 3 hours, and after 1 g is 5-6 hours, and after 8-10 g is 10-15 hours).

Salicylate serum concentrations correlate with the pharmacological actions and adverse effects observed. Anti-inflammatory therapeutic serum concentrations 150-300 mcg/mL. See table.

(Continued)

Salicylates (Various Salts) *(Continued)*

Serum Salicylate: Clinical Correlations

Serum Salicylate Concentration (mcg/mL)	Desired Effects	Adverse Effects/Intoxication
~100	Antiplatelet Antipyresis Analgesia	GI intolerance and bleeding, hypersensitivity, hemostatic defects
150-300	Anti-inflammatory	Mild salicylism
250-400	Treatment of rheumatic fever	Nausea/vomiting, hyperventilation, salicylism, flushing, sweating, thirst, headache, diarrhea, and tachycardia
>400-500		Respiratory alkalosis, hemorrhage, excitement, confusion, asterixis, pulmonary edema, convulsions, tetany, metabolic acidosis, fever, coma, cardiovascular collapse, renal and respiratory failure

Test Interactions False-negative results for glucose oxidase urinary glucose tests (Clinistix®); false-positives using the cupric sulfate method (Clinitest®); also, interferes with Gerhardt test (urinary ketone analysis), VMA determination; 5-HIAA, xylose tolerance test, and T_3 and T_4; increased PBI; increased uric acid

Patient Information Watch for any signs of bleeding (stool); take with food to minimize GI distress; report ringing in ears, persistent GI pain to physician or pharmacist

Nursing Implications See Monitoring Parameters, Reference Range, and Special Geriatric Considerations

Additional Information Liquid dosage form may be useful for those who have difficulty swallowing tablets or caplets. These agents do not appear to inhibit platelet aggregation. Nonacetylated salicylates have less GI toxicity and renal effects than aspirin and other NSAIDs. They also do not cause reactions in aspirin sensitive patients.

Choline salicylate: Arthropan®

Sodium thiosalicylate: Asproject®; Rexolate®; Tusal®

Magnesium salicylate: Extra Strength Doan's® [OTC]; Magan®; Mobidin®; Original Doan's® [OTC]

Special Geriatric Considerations Elderly are a high-risk population for adverse effects from nonsteroidal anti-inflammatory agents. As much as 60% of elderly can develop peptic ulceration and/or hemorrhage asymptomatically. The concomitant use of H_2 blockers, omeprazole, and sucralfate is not effective as prophylaxis with the exception of NSAID-induced duodenal ulcers which may be prevented by the use of ranitidine. Misoprostol and proton pump inhibitors are the only agents proven to help prevent the development of NSAID-induced ulcers. Also, concomitant disease and drug use contribute to the risk for GI adverse effects. Use lowest effective dose for shortest period possible. Consider renal function decline with age. Use of NSAIDs can compromise existing renal function especially when Cl_{cr} is ≤30 mL/minute. Tinnitus may be a difficult and unreliable indication of toxicity due to age-related hearing loss or eighth cranial nerve damage. CNS adverse effects such as confusion, agitation, and hallucination are generally seen in overdose or high dose situations, but elderly may demonstrate these adverse effects at lower doses than younger adults (see Additional Information).

Dosage Forms

Injection: 50 mg/mL

Liquid: 870 mg/mL (choline salicylate)

Tablet, enteric coated: 325 mg, 545 mg, 600 mg, 650 mg

References

Emmerson BT, "The Management of Gout," *N Engl J Med*, 1996, 334(7):445-51.

Gurwitz JH, Avorn J, Ross-Degnan D, et al, "Nonsteroidal Anti-Inflammatory Drug-Associated Azotemia in the Very Old," *JAMA*, 1990, 264(4):471-5.

Hawkey CJ, Karrasch JA, Szczepaski L, et al, "Omeprazole Compared With Misoprostrol for Ulcers Associated With Nonsteroidal Anti-inflammatory Drugs," *N Engl J Med*, 1998, 338(11):727-34.

Weissmann G, "Aspirin," *Sci Am*, 1991, 264(1):84-90.

Yeomans ND, Tulassay Z, Juhasz L, et al, "A Comparison of Omeprazole With Ranitidine for Ulcers Associated With Nonsteroidal Anti-inflammatory Drugs," *N Engl J Med*, 1998, 338(11):719-26.

Salicylazosulfapyridine *see* Sulfasalazine *on page 877*

Salicylic Acid (sal i SIL ik AS id)

Brand Names Clear Away® Disc [OTC]; Compound W® [OTC]; Dr Scholl's® Disk [OTC]; Dr Scholl's® Wart Remover [OTC]; DuoFilm® [OTC]; DuoPlant® Gel [OTC]; Freezone® Solution [OTC]; Gordofilm® Liquid; Mediplast® Plaster [OTC]; Mosco® Liquid [OTC]; Occlusal-HP Liquid; Off-Ezy® Wart Remover [OTC]; Panscol® [OTC]; Psor-a-set® Soap [OTC]; P&S® Shampoo [OTC]; Sal-Acid® Plaster [OTC]; Salactic® Film [OTC]; Sal-Plant® Gel [OTC]; Trans-Ver-Sal® AdultPatch [OTC]; Trans-Ver-Sal® PediaPatch [OTC]; Trans-Ver-Sal® PlantarPatch [OTC]; Wart-Off® [OTC]

Generic Available Yes

Therapeutic Category Keratolytic Agent; Shampoo, Keratolytic

Use Topically for its keratolytic effect in controlling seborrheic dermatitis or psoriasis of body and scalp, dandruff, and other scaling dermatoses; also used to remove warts, corns, and calluses

Contraindications Hypersensitivity to salicylic acid or any components; prolonged use in diabetics and patients with impaired circulation; use on moles, birth marks, warts with hair growing from them, genital or facial warts, or use on irritated or inflamed skin

Warnings Should not be used systemically, severe irritating effect on GI mucosa; use with caution in areas of ischemia; prolonged use over large areas, may result in salicylate toxicity; do not apply on irritated, reddened, or infected skin; for external use only; avoid contact with eyes, face, and other mucous membranes

Precautions For external use only; avoid exposing eyes, mucous membranes, or normal skin surrounding warts

Adverse Reactions
>10%: Local: Burning and irritation at site of exposure on normal tissue
1% to 10%:
  Central nervous system: Dizziness, mental confusion, headache
  Otic: Tinnitus
  Respiratory: Hyperventilation

Overdosage Signs and symptoms of salicylate toxicity include nausea, vomiting, dizziness, tinnitus, loss of hearing, lethargy, diarrhea, psychic disturbances

Drug Interactions Interactions have been reported from topical use (see Drug Interactions from Salicylates monograph)

Mechanism of Action Produces desquamation of hyperkeratotic epithelium via dissolution of the intercellular cement which causes the cornified tissue to swell, soften, macerate, and desquamate. Salicylic acid is keratolytic at concentrations of 3% to 6%; it becomes destructive to tissue at concentrations >6%. Concentrations of 6% to 60% are used to remove corns and warts and in the treatment of psoriasis and other hyperkeratotic disorders.

Pharmacokinetics
Absorption: Absorbed percutaneously, but systemic toxicity is unlikely with normal use
Time to peak serum concentration: Topical: Within 5 hours of application with occlusion
Elimination: Salicyluric acid (52%), salicylate glucuronides (42%), and salicylic acid (6%) are major metabolites identified in urine after percutaneous absorption

Usual Dosage
Lotion, cream, gel: Apply a thin layer to affected area once or twice daily
Plaster: Cut to size that covers the corn or callus, apply and leave in place for 48 hours; do not exceed 5 applications over a 14-day period
Solution: Apply a thin layer directly to wart using brush applicator once daily as directed for 1 week or until wart is removed

Patient Information When applying in concentrations >10%, protect surrounding tissue with petrolatum; do not use on open skin, avoid contact with eyes, mouth, and other mucous membranes

Nursing Implications For warts: Before applying product, soak area in warm water for 5 minutes; dry area thoroughly, then apply medication

Special Geriatric Considerations No specific considerations are needed if used according to recommended doses and duration of use. Many elderly may have diabetes or impaired circulation and avoidance of topical salicylic acid would be advised (see Contraindications).

(Continued)

Salicylic Acid *(Continued)*
Dosage Forms
Cream: 2% (30 g)

Disk: 40%

Gel: 5% (60 g); 6% (30 g); 17% (7.5 g)

Liquid: 13.6% (9.3 mL); 17% (9.3 mL, 13.5 mL, 15 mL); 16.7% (15 mL)

Lotion: 3% (120 mL)

Ointment: 3% (90 g)

Patch, transdermal: 15% (20 mm); 40% (20 mm)

Plaster: 40%

Soap: 2% (97.5 g)

Strip: 40%

Salicylsalicylic Acid *see Salsalate on next page*

SalineX® [OTC] *see Sodium Chloride on page 860*

Salivart® [OTC] *see Saliva Substitute on this page*

Saliva Substitute (sa LYE va SUB stee tute)
Brand Names Moi-Stir® [OTC]; Orex® [OTC]; Salivart® [OTC]; Xero-Lube® [OTC]

Therapeutic Category Gastrointestinal Agent, Miscellaneous

Use Relief of dry mouth and throat in xerostomia

Usual Dosage Geriatrics and Adults: Use as needed

Special Geriatric Considerations Saliva production has not been shown to change with aging, however, many drugs used by the elderly can cause dry mouth; these patients may benefit from a saliva substitute

Dosage Forms
Solution: 60 mL, 75 mL, 120 mL, 180 mL

Swabstix: 300s

Salk Vaccine *see Poliovirus Vaccine, Inactivated on page 761*

Salmeterol (sal ME te role)
Related Information
Asthma Guidelines *on page 1040*

Inhaled Medications Comparison *on page 1034*

Brand Names Serevent®

Generic Available No

Therapeutic Category Adrenergic Agonist Agent; Beta$_2$-Adrenergic Agonist Agent; Bronchodilator

Use Bronchodilator in reversible airway obstruction due to asthma or COPD; prevention of exercise-induced bronchospasm

Contraindications Hypersensitivity to salmeterol, adrenergic amines or any ingredients

Warnings Not to be used for the treatment of acute symptoms; if patient has an increased need for short-acting, "as needed" beta agonists, medical evaluation should be obtained; patients should be warned not to exceed recommended dose; use with caution in patients with unstable vasomotor symptoms, diabetes, hyperthyroidism, prostatic hypertrophy, or a history of seizures; also use caution in the elderly and those patients with cardiovascular disorders such as coronary artery disease, arrhythmias and hypertension

Precautions Excessive use may result in tolerance; deaths have been reported after excessive use; though the exact cause is unknown, cardiac arrest after a severe asthmatic crisis is suspected

Adverse Reactions
Cardiovascular: Tachycardia, palpitations, elevation or depression of blood pressure

Central nervous system: Nervousness, CNS stimulation, hyperactivity, insomnia

Gastrointestinal: GI upset

Neuromuscular & skeletal: Tremors (may be more common in the elderly)

Overdosage Symptoms of overdose include hypertension, tachycardia, seizures, angina, hypokalemia, and tachyarrhythmias

Toxicology Prudent use of a cardioselective beta-adrenergic blocker (eg, atenolol or metoprolol); keep in mind the potential for induction of bronchoconstriction in an asthmatic. Dialysis has not been shown to be of value in the treatment of an overdose with this agent.

Drug Interactions
Decreased therapeutic effect: Beta-adrenergic blockers (eg, propranolol)

Increased toxicity (cardiovascular): MAO inhibitors, tricyclic antidepressants

Mechanism of Action Relaxes bronchial smooth muscle by action on beta$_2$-receptors with little effect on heart rate

Pharmacodynamics
Onset of effective bronchodilation: 10-20 minutes
Peak effect: Within 3 hours
Duration: 12 hours

Pharmacokinetics
Protein binding: 94% to 98%
Metabolism: Extensive by hydroxylation in the liver; systemic levels are low or undetectable

Usual Dosage Geriatrics and Adults:
Inhalation: 42 mcg (2 puffs) every 12 hours
Prevention of exercise-induced bronchospasm: 2 puffs 30-60 minutes before exercise; do not repeat dose for 12 hours

Monitoring Parameters Pulmonary function tests, blood pressure, pulse

Patient Information Not to be used for the relief of acute attacks; do not exceed recommended dosage; rinse mouth with water following each inhalation to help with dry throat and mouth; follow specific instructions accompanying inhaler; if more than one inhalation is necessary, wait at least 1 full minute between inhalations. May cause nervousness, restlessness, insomnia - if these effects continue after dosage reduction, notify physician; also notify physician if palpitations, tachycardia, chest pain, muscle tremors, dizziness, headache, flushing or if breathing difficulty persists

Nursing Implications Not to be used for the relief of acute attacks; monitor lung sounds, pulse, blood pressure

Special Geriatric Considerations Geriatric patients were included in four clinical studies of salmeterol; no apparent differences in efficacy and safety were noted in geriatric patients compared to younger adults. Because salmeterol is only to be used for prevention of bronchospasm, patients also need a short-acting beta-agonist to treat acute attacks. Elderly patients should be carefully counseled about which inhaler to use and the proper scheduling of doses; a spacer device may be utilized to maximize effectiveness.

Dosage Forms Aerosol, oral, as xinafoate: 21 mcg/spray [60 inhalations] (6.5 g), [120 inhalations] (13 g)

Salmonine® Injection see Calcitonin on page 142

Sal-Plant® Gel [OTC] see Salicylic Acid on page 845

Salsalate (SAL sa late)
Brand Names Argesic®-SA; Artha-G®; Disalcid®; Marthritic®; Mono-Gesic®; Salflex®; Salgesic®; Salsitab®
Synonyms Disalicylic Acid; Salicylsalicylic Acid
Generic Available Yes
Therapeutic Category Analgesic, Non-narcotic; Anti-inflammatory Agent; Antipyretic; Nonsteroidal Anti-inflammatory Agent (NSAID), Oral; Salicylate
Use Treatment of mild to moderate pain, inflammation and fever; management of rheumatic fever, rheumatoid arthritis, osteoarthritis, and gout (see Mechanism of Action)
Contraindications Known hypersensitivity to salsalate; bleeding disorders (factor VII or IX deficiencies), hypersensitivity to salicylates or other nonsteroidal anti-inflammatory drugs (NSAIDs); tartrazine dye and asthma
Warnings Tinnitus or impaired hearing may indicate toxicity; discontinue use 1 week prior to surgical procedures
Precautions Use with caution in patients with platelet and bleeding disorders, renal dysfunction, hepatic disease, history of salicylate-induced gastric irritation, peptic ulcer disease, erosive gastritis, bleeding disorders, hypoprothrombinemia, and vitamin K deficiency; use cautiously in asthmatics, especially those with aspirin intolerance and nasal polyps
Adverse Reactions
Central nervous system: Fever, dizziness, mental confusion, CNS depression, lassitude, headache
Dermatologic: Rash, urticaria, angioedema
Gastrointestinal: Nausea, vomiting, GI distress, bleeding, ulcers, thirst
Hematologic: Leukopenia, thrombocytopenia
Hepatic: Hepatotoxicity (high dose)
Otic: Tinnitus
Respiratory: Hyperventilation, bronchospasm
Miscellaneous: Diaphoresis
(Continued)

Salsalate *(Continued)*

Overdosage 10-30 g; symptoms of overdose include tinnitus, headache, dizziness, confusion, metabolic acidosis, hyperpyrexia, hyperpnea, tachypnea, nausea, vomiting, irritability, disorientation, hallucinations, lethargy, stupor, dehydration, hyperventilation, hyperthermia, hyperactivity, depression leading to coma, respiratory failure, and collapse; laboratory abnormalities include hypokalemia, hypoglycemia or hyperglycemia with alterations in pH

Toxicology The "Done" nomogram is very helpful for estimating the severity of aspirin poisoning and directing treatment using serum salicylate concentrations. Treatment can also be based upon symptomatology; see table.

Aspirin or Other Salicylate Toxicity

Toxic Symptoms	Treatment
Overdose	Induce emesis with ipecac, and/or lavage with saline, followed with activated charcoal
Dehydration	I.V. fluids with KCl (no D_5W only)
Metabolic acidosis (must be treated)	Sodium bicarbonate
Hyperthermia	Cooling blankets or sponge baths
Coagulopathy/hemorrhage	Vitamin K I.V.
Hypoglycemia (with coma, seizures, or change in mental status)	Dextrose 25 g I.V.
Seizures	Diazepam 5-10 mg I.V.

Drug Interactions
May increase nephrotoxicity of cyclosporin
Diclofenac + K^+ sparing diuretics may increase serum K^+
Concomitant insulin or oral hypoglycemic agents may increase or decrease serum glucose
May increase digoxin, methotrexate, and lithium serum concentrations
Aspirin or other salicylates may decrease NSAID serum concentrations
Other NSAIDs may increase adverse GI effects
Increased prothrombin time with anticoagulants
Decreased antihypertensive effects of ACE inhibitors, beta-blockers, and thiazide diuretics
Increased response to sympathomimetics
Probenecid may increase toxicity of NSAIDs by increase in serum concentrations
Effects of loop diuretics may decrease
Concomitant use with loop diuretics may enhance azotemia in elderly

Mechanism of Action Inhibits prostaglandin synthesis; acts on the hypothalamus heat-regulating center to reduce fever through vasodilation of peripheral vessels; decreases pain receptor sensitivity. Other proposed mechanisms of action for salicylate anti-inflammatory action are lysosomal stabilization, inhibition of kinin and leukotriene production, alteration of chemotactic factors, and inhibition of neutrophil activation. This latter mechanism may be the most significant pharmacologic action to reduce inflammation. Nonacetylated salicylates are **not** as potent in prostaglandin synthesis inhibition and, therefore, tend to have less adverse effects on gastrointestinal and renal tissues. They do not inhibit platelet function as aspirin does since they are not acetylated and, therefore, cannot acetylate platelet cyclooxygenase.

Pharmacodynamics Onset of action: Within 3-4 days of continuous dosing

Pharmacokinetics
Absorption: Oral: Completely from the small intestine; insoluble in gastric acid secretions and, therefore, is not absorbed until it reaches the small intestine
Protein binding: 90%
Half-life: 7-8 hours; half-life increases with dose, 15-30 hours with higher doses hydrolyzed in the liver to 2 moles of salicylic acid (active)
Elimination: Almost totally excreted renally

Usual Dosage Geriatrics and Adults: Oral: 500-1000 mg 2-4 times/day

Monitoring Parameters Serum concentrations, renal function; hearing changes or tinnitus; monitor for response (ie, pain, inflammation, range of motion, grip strength); observe for abnormal bleeding, bruising, weight gain

Reference Range
Sample size: 1.5-2 mL blood (purple top tube)

Timing of serum samples: Peak serum concentrations usually occur 2 hours after ingestion; the half-life increases with the dosage (eg, the half-life after

300 mg is 3 hours, and after 1 g is 5-6 hours, and after 8-10 g is 10-15 hours).

Salicylate serum concentrations correlate with the pharmacological actions and adverse effects observed. Anti-inflammatory therapeutic serum concentrations 150-300 mcg/mL. See table.

Serum Salicylate: Clinical Correlations

Serum Salicylate Concentration (mcg/mL)	Desired Effects	Adverse Effects/Intoxication
~100	Antiplatelet Antipyresis Analgesia	GI intolerance and bleeding, hypersensitivity, hemostatic defects
150-300	Anti-inflammatory	Mild salicylism
250-400	Treatment of rheumatic fever	Nausea/vomiting, hyperventilation, salicylism, flushing, sweating, thirst, headache, diarrhea, and tachycardia
>400-500		Respiratory alkalosis, hemorrhage, excitement, confusion, asterixis, pulmonary edema, convulsions, tetany, metabolic acidosis, fever, coma, cardiovascular collapse, renal and respiratory failure

Test Interactions False-negative results for glucose oxidase urinary glucose tests (Clinistix®); false-positives using the cupric sulfate method (Clinitest®); also, interferes with Gerhardt test (urinary ketone analysis), VMA determination; 5-HIAA, xylose tolerance test, and T_3 and T_4; increased PBI; increased uric acid

Patient Information Avoid alcohol; do not self-medicate with other drug products containing aspirin; use antacids to relieve upset stomach; watch for any signs of bleeding (stool); take with food to minimize GI distress; report ringing in ears, persistent GI pain to physician or pharmacist

Nursing Implications See Monitoring Parameters, Reference Range, and Special Geriatric Considerations

Additional Information Does not appear to inhibit platelet aggregation; salsalate causes less GI and renal toxicity than aspirin and other NSAIDs (see Mechanism of Action)

Special Geriatric Considerations Elderly are a high-risk population for adverse effects from nonsteroidal anti-inflammatory agents. As much as 60% of elderly can develop peptic ulceration and/or hemorrhage asymptomatically. The concomitant use of H_2 blockers, omeprazole, and sucralfate is not effective as prophylaxis with the exception of NSAID-induced duodenal ulcers which may be prevented by the use of ranitidine. Misoprostol and proton pump inhibitors are the only agents proven to help prevent the development of NSAID-induced ulcers. Also, concomitant disease and drug use contribute to the risk for GI adverse effects. Use lowest effective dose for shortest period possible. Consider renal function decline with age. Use of NSAIDs can compromise existing renal function especially when Cl_{cr} is ≤30 mL/minute. Tinnitus may be a difficult and unreliable indication of toxicity due to age-related hearing loss or eighth cranial nerve damage. CNS adverse effects such as confusion, agitation, and hallucinations are generally seen in overdose or high dose situations, but elderly may demonstrate these adverse effects at lower doses than younger adults (see Additional Information).

Dosage Forms

Capsule: 500 mg

Tablet: 500 mg, 750 mg

References

Gurwitz JH, Avorn J, Ross-Degnan D, et al, "Nonsteroidal Anti-Inflammatory Drug-Associated Azotemia in the Very Old," *JAMA*, 1990, 264(4):471-5.

Hawkey CJ, Karrasch JA, Szczepaski L, et al, "Omeprazole Compared With Misoprostol for Ulcers Associated With Nonsteroidal Anti-inflammatory Drugs," *N Engl J Med*, 1998, 338(11):727-34.

Weissmann G, "Aspirin," *Sci Am*, 1991, 264(1):84-90.

Yeomans ND, Tulassay Z, Juhasz L, et al, "A Comparison of Omeprazole With Ranitidine for Ulcers Associated With Nonsteroidal Anti-inflammatory Drugs," *N Engl J Med*, 1998, 338(11):719-26.

Salsitab® *see* Salsalate *on page 847*

Salt *see* Sodium Chloride *on page 860*

Sandimmune® Injection *see* Cyclosporine *on page 263*

Sandimmune® Oral *see* Cyclosporine *on page 263*

Sandoglobulin® *see* Immune Globulin *on page 482*

Sani-Supp® Suppository [OTC] *see* Glycerin *on page 429*

Sansert® *see* Methysergide *on page 614*

Santyl® *see* Collagenase *on page 251*

Scabene® *see* Lindane *on page 538*

Scalpicin® *see* Hydrocortisone *on page 462*

Scopolamine (skoe POL a meen)

Brand Names Isopto® Hyoscine Ophthalmic; Transderm Scop® Patch

Synonyms Hyoscine

Generic Available Yes

Therapeutic Category Anticholinergic Agent; Anticholinergic Agent, Ophthalmic; Anticholinergic Agent, Transdermal; Ophthalmic Agent, Mydriatic

Use Preoperative medication to produce amnesia and decrease salivation and respiratory secretions; ophthalmic: to produce cycloplegia and mydriasis prior to refraction; treatment of iridocyclitis; patch: prevention of nausea and vomiting associated with motion, anesthesia or opiate analgesia

Contraindications Hypersensitivity to scopolamine or any component; narrow-angle glaucoma; acute hemorrhage

Precautions Use with caution in the elderly or in individuals with hepatic or renal impairment since adverse CNS effects occur more often in these patients; use with caution in patients with pyloric obstruction, urinary bladder neck obstruction or intestinal obstruction, cardiovascular disease, hypertension

Adverse Reactions

Cardiovascular: Tachycardia, palpitations

Central nervous system: Disorientation, drowsiness, hallucinations, confusion, psychosis, delirium **(the elderly are at increased risk for confusion and hallucinations)**

Gastrointestinal: Xerostomia, constipation

Genitourinary: Urinary retention

Ocular: Blurred vision, cycloplegia, mydriasis, photophobia, increased intraocular pressure, local irritation

Miscellaneous: Anaphylaxis, allergic reactions **Note:** Systemic adverse effects have been reported with both the transdermal and ophthalmic preparations. Drug withdrawal has occurred in patients using the transdermal system for longer than 3 days; symptoms include dizziness, nausea, vomiting, headache, and equilibrium disturbance.

Overdosage Symptoms of overdose include dilated pupils, flushed skin, tachycardia, hypertension, EKG abnormalities, CNS manifestations resembling acute psychosis; CNS depression, circulatory collapse, respiratory failure

Toxicology Pure scopolamine intoxication is extremely rare. However, for a scopolamine overdose with severe life-threatening symptoms, physostigmine 1-2 mg S.C. or I.V. slowly should be given to reverse the toxic effects.

Drug Interactions

Decreased effect due to impaired absorption of acetaminophen, levodopa, ketoconazole, digoxin, riboflavin, potassium chloride in wax matrix preparations

Decreased effect of metoclopramide, cisapride

Increased effect/toxicity with anticholinergic agents

Antagonistic effect: Tacrine, donepezil

Stability Avoid acid solutions, because hydrolysis occurs at pH <3

Mechanism of Action Blocks the action of acetylcholine at parasympathetic sites in smooth muscle, secretory glands and the CNS; increases cardiac output, dries secretions, antagonizes histamine and serotonin

Pharmacodynamics Peak effects: 20-60 minutes; may take 3-7 days for full recovery

Pharmacokinetics Absorption: Well absorbed by all routes of administration

Usual Dosage Geriatrics and Adults:

Preoperatively and Antiemetic: I.M., I.V., S.C.: 0.3-0.65 mg

Motion sickness: Apply 1 patch behind the ear at least 4 hours before the antiemetic effect is required; if therapy is required for longer than 3 days, remove the first patch and apply a new one behind the other ear

Ophthalmic:

Refraction: Instill 1-2 drops of 0.25% to eye(s) 1 hour before procedure

Iridocyclitis: Instill 1-2 drops of 0.25% to eye(s) up to 3 times/day

Monitoring Parameters Blood pressure, pulse, anticholinergic effects

Patient Information Report any changes of vision; wait 5 minutes after instilling ophthalmic preparation before using any other drops; do not blink excessively; after instilling ophthalmic preparation, apply pressure to the side of the nose near the eye to minimize systemic absorption; put patch on at least 4 hours before traveling; once applied, do not remove the patch for 3 full days. May cause dry mouth, drowsiness, blurred vision. If eye pain, blurred vision, dizziness, or rapid pulse occurs, remove patch and consult physician. Wash hands thoroughly after handling the patch.

Nursing Implications Disc (patch) is programmed to deliver *in vivo* 0.5 mg over 3 days; wash hands before and after applying the disc to avoid drug contact with eyes; after instilling ophthalmic preparation, apply pressure to the side of the nose near the eye to minimize systemic absorption

Additional Information Produces more CNS depression, mydriasis, and cycloplegia but less effective in preventing reflex bradycardia and affecting the intestines than atropine

Scopolamine: Transderm Scop®
Scopolamine hydrobromide: Isopto® hyoscine

Special Geriatric Considerations Because of its long duration of action as a mydriatic agent, it should be avoided in elderly patients. Anticholinergic agents are not well tolerated in the elderly and their use should be avoided when possible (see Precautions, Adverse Reactions).

Dosage Forms
Disc, transdermal: 1.5 mg/disc (4's)
Injection, as hydrobromide: 0.3 mg/mL (1 mL); 0.4 mg/mL (0.5 mL, 1 mL); 0.86 mg/mL (0.5 mL); 1 mg/mL (1 mL)
Solution, ophthalmic, as hydrobromide: 0.25% (5 mL, 15 mL)

References
Feinberg M, "The Problems of Anticholinergic Adverse Effects in Older Patients," *Drugs Aging*, 1993, 3(4):335-48.

Scot-Tussin® [OTC] *see* Guaifenesin *on page 437*

Scot-Tussin DM® Cough Chasers [OTC] *see* Dextromethorphan *on page 278*

Scot-Tussin® Senior Clear [OTC] *see* Guaifenesin and Dextromethorphan *on page 439*

SeaMist® [OTC] *see* Sodium Chloride *on page 860*

Sebizon® Topical Lotion *see* Sulfacetamide Sodium *on page 874*

Secobarbital *(see koe BAR bi tal)*
Related Information
Anxiolytic/Hypnotic Use in Long-Term Care Facilities *on page 1099*
Federal OBRA Regulations Recommended Maximum Doses - Hypnotics *on page 1057*
Brand Names Seconal™ Injection
Synonyms Quinalbarbitone Sodium; Secobarbital Sodium
Generic Available Yes
Therapeutic Category Barbiturate; Hypnotic; Sedative
Special Geriatric Considerations Use of this agent in the elderly is not recommended due to its long half-life and addiction potential

Secobarbital and Amobarbital *see* Amobarbital and Secobarbital *on page 65*

Secobarbital Sodium *see* Secobarbital *on this page*

Seconal™ Injection *see* Secobarbital *on this page*

Sectral® *see* Acebutolol *on page 15*

Selegiline *(seh LEDGE ah leen)*
Brand Names Eldepryl®
Synonyms Deprenyl; L-Deprenyl
Generic Available No
Therapeutic Category Anti-Parkinson's Agent
Use Adjunct in the management of parkinsonian patients who are exhibiting a decrease in response to levodopa/carbidopa
Unlabeled use: Early Parkinson's disease
Investigational use: Alzheimer's disease
Contraindications Known hypersensitivity to selegiline
Warnings Do not use at daily doses exceeding 10 mg/day because of the risks associated with nonselective inhibition of MAO
(Continued)

Selegiline (Continued)

Precautions At doses ≤10 mg/day patients can safely consume tyramine-containing foods without the risk of uncontrolled hypertension

Adverse Reactions

Cardiovascular: Orthostatic hypotension, arrhythmias, hypertension

Central nervous system: Hallucinations, confusion, depression, insomnia, agitation, loss of balance

Gastrointestinal: Nausea, vomiting, xerostomia

Neuromuscular & skeletal: Increased involuntary movements, bradykinesia

Overdosage Symptoms of overdose include tachycardia, palpitations, muscle twitching, seizures

Toxicology Competent supportive care is the most important treatment; both hypertension or hypotension can occur with intoxication. Hypotension may respond to I.V. fluids or vasopressors, and hypertension usually responds to an alpha-adrenergic blocker. While treating the hypertension, care is warranted to avoid sudden drops in blood pressure, since this may worsen the MAO inhibitor toxicity. Muscle irritability and seizures often respond to diazepam, while hyperthermia is best treated antipyretics and cooling blankets. Cardiac arrhythmias are best treated with phenytoin or procainamide.

Drug Interactions Increased toxicity: Dexfenfluramine (possible); meperidine in combination with selegiline has caused agitation, delirium, and death; it may be prudent to avoid other opioids as well; fluoxetine increased pressor effects; avoid other SSRIs as well; avoid use with nonselective MAO inhibitors

Mechanism of Action Potent monoamine oxidase (MAO) type-B inhibitor; MAO-B plays a major role in the metabolism of dopamine; selegiline may also increase dopaminergic activity by interfering with dopamine reuptake at the synapse

Pharmacodynamics

Onset of action: Oral: Within 60 minutes

Duration: 24-72 hours

Pharmacokinetics

Metabolism: To amphetamine and methamphetamine in the liver

Half-life: 9 minutes

Usual Dosage Oral:

Geriatrics: Initial: 5 mg in the morning; may increase to a total of 10 mg/day

Adults: 5 mg twice daily with breakfast and lunch or 10 mg in the morning

Monitoring Parameters Blood pressure, symptoms of parkinsonism

Patient Information Do not take more than the prescribed dose; explain the tyramine reaction to patients and tell them to report severe headaches or other unusual symptoms to physician

Nursing Implications Selegiline is a monoamine oxidase inhibitor type "B"; there should **not** be a problem with tyramine-containing products as long as the typical doses are employed

Additional Information When adding selegiline to levodopa/carbidopa the dose of the latter can usually (and should) be decreased. Studies are investigating the use of selegiline in early Parkinson's disease to slow the progression of the disease.

Special Geriatric Considerations Selegiline is also being studied in Alzheimer's disease, but further studies are needed to assess its usefulness (see Warnings and Adverse Reactions). A recent study (Sano, 1997) suggests that selegiline with or without vitamin E may slow the progression of Alzheimer's disease.

Dosage Forms Capsule, as hydrochloride: 5 mg

References

Burke WJ, Roccaforte WH, Wengel SP, et al, "L-deprenyl in the Treatment of Mild Dementia of the Alzheimer Type: Results of a 15-Month Trial," *J Am Geriatr Soc*, 1993, 41(11):1219-25.

Lawlor BA, Aisen PS, and Green C, "Selegiline in the Treatment of Behavioural Disturbances in Alzheimer's Disease," *Int J Geriatr Psychiatry*, 1997, 12(3):319-22.

Sano M, Ernesto C, Thomas RG, et al, "A Controlled Trial of Selegiline, Alpha-Tocopherol, or Both as Treatment for Alzheimer's Disease," *N Engl J Med*, 1997, 336(17):1216-22.

Stern MB, "Contemporary Approaches to the Pharmacotherapeutic Management of Parkinson's Disease: An Overview," *Neurology*, 1997, 49(1 Suppl 1):S2-9.

The Parkinson Study Group, "Effect of Deprenyl on the Progression of Disability in Early Parkinson's Disease," *N Engl J Med*, 1989, 321(20):1364-71.

The Parkinson Study Group, "Effects of Tocopherol and Deprenyl on the Progression of Disability in Early Parkinson's Disease," *N Engl J Med*, 1993, 328(3):176-83.

Selestoject® *see* Betamethasone *on page 114*

Semilente® *see* Insulin Preparations *on page 488*

Senexon® [OTC] *see* Senna *on next page*

Senna (SEN na)

Brand Names Black Draught® [OTC]; Senexon® [OTC]; Senna-Gen® [OTC]; Senokot® [OTC]; Senolax® [OTC]; X-Prep® Liquid [OTC]

Synonyms Sennosides

Therapeutic Category Laxative, Stimulant

Use Short-term treatment of constipation; evacuate the colon for bowel or rectal examinations

Contraindications Hypersensitivity to senna or any component; nausea and vomiting; undiagnosed abdominal pain, appendicitis, intestinal obstruction or perforation

Warnings Laxatives used excessively may lead to fluid/electrolyte imbalance; stimulant cathartics may lead to abuse or dependency with chronic use (laxative abuse syndrome); cathartic colon, which may present as ulcerative colitis, occurs with chronic use of stimulant cathartics; melanosis coli is a dark pigmentation of the colonic mucosa from chronic use of anthraquinone derivatives

Precautions Habit-forming and may result in laxative dependence and loss of normal bowel function with prolonged use; rectal bleeding or failure to respond requires further evaluation for possibly serious medical problems

Adverse Reactions
Cardiovascular: Palpitations
Central nervous system: Dizziness, syncope
Endocrine & metabolic: Fluid and electrolyte loss
Gastrointestinal: Nausea, vomiting, diarrhea, abdominal cramps, bloating, flatulence, perianal irritation
Neuromuscular & skeletal: Weakness
Miscellaneous: Diaphoresis

Overdosage Symptoms of overdose include hypokalemia, hypocalcemia, metabolic acidosis or alkalosis, abdominal pain, diarrhea, malabsorption, weight loss and protein-losing enteropathy

Drug Interactions MAO inhibitors, disulfiram, metronidazole, procarbazine

Mechanism of Action Active metabolite (aglycone) acts as a local irritant on the colon, stimulates Auerbach's plexus to produce peristalsis; alters water and electrolyte secretion

Pharmacodynamics Onset of action: Oral: Within 6-10 hours

Pharmacokinetics
Metabolism: In the liver
Elimination: In feces (via bile) and urine

Usual Dosage Geriatrics and Adults:
Granules: 1 teaspoonful at bedtime, not to exceed 2 teaspoonfuls twice daily
Syrup: 2-3 teaspoonfuls at bedtime, not to exceed 3 teaspoonfuls twice daily
Tablet: 2 tablets at bedtime, not to exceed 4 tablets twice daily (8 tablets total)

Monitoring Parameters Monitor stools daily for consistency, occult or gross blood; also with chronic use, monitor serum electrolytes; monitor for dehydration and hypotension

Test Interactions Decreased calcium (S), decreased potassium (S)

Patient Information May discolor urine or feces (yellow-brown); do not use in presence of nausea, vomiting, or abdominal pain; stimulant laxative use should be limited; notify physician if unrelieved by laxative, rectal bleeding occurs, or signs of electrolyte imbalance develop (dizziness, weakness, muscle cramps); take with a full glass of water

Nursing Implications May discolor urine or feces; liquid syrups contain 7% alcohol; liquids 3.5% to 4.9% alcohol (see Monitoring Parameters and Special Geriatric Considerations)

Additional Information Long-term, chronic use should be avoided; patients should be encouraged to increase fluid intake, fiber intake, and exercise

Special Geriatric Considerations Elderly are often predisposed to constipation due to disease, immobility, drugs, and a decreased "thirst reflex" with age enhancing the possibility of dehydration. Avoid stimulant cathartic use on a chronic basis if possible. Use osmotic, lubricant, stool softeners, and bulk agents as prophylaxis. Patients should be instructed for proper dietary fiber and fluid intake as well as regular exercise. Monitor closely for fluid/electrolyte imbalance, CNS signs of fluid/electrolyte loss, and hypotension.

Dosage Forms
Granules: 326 mg/teaspoonful
Liquid: 33.3 mg/mL (75 mL, 150 mL, 360 mL)
Suppository: 652 mg
Syrup: 218 mg/5 mL (60 mL, 240 mL)
Tablet: 187 mg, 217 mg, 600 mg

Senna-Gen® [OTC] *see Senna on previous page*

Sennosides *see Senna on previous page*

Senokot® [OTC] *see Senna on previous page*

Senolax® [OTC] *see Senna on previous page*

Septra® *see Co-Trimoxazole on page 253*

Septra® DS *see Co-Trimoxazole on page 253*

Serax® *see Oxazepam on page 701*

Serentil® *see Mesoridazine on page 592*

Serevent® *see Salmeterol on page 846*

Seromycin® Pulvules® *see Cycloserine on page 262*

Seroquel® *see Quetiapine on page 810*

Serpalan® *see Reserpine on page 825*

Serpasil® *see Reserpine on page 825*

Sertraline (SER tra leen)

Related Information
Antidepressant Agents Comparison *on page 1021*
Antidepressant Medication Guidelines *on page 1075*

Brand Names Zoloft™

Generic Available No

Therapeutic Category Antidepressant; Selective Serotonin Reuptake Inhibitor (SSRI)

Use Treatment of major depression
Unlabeled use: Obsessive-compulsive disorder

Contraindications Hypersensitivity to sertraline or any component; patients receiving MAO inhibitors currently or in the past 2 weeks

Warnings Do not use in combination with monoamine oxidase inhibitor or within 14 days of discontinuing treatment or initiating treatment with a monoamine oxidase inhibitor due to the risk of serotonin syndrome; use with caution in patients with pre-existing seizure disorders, patients in whom weight loss is undesirable, patients with recent myocardial infarction, unstable heart disease, hepatic or renal impairment, patients taking other psychotropic medications, agitated or hyperactive patients as drug may produce or activate mania or hypomania; because the risk of suicide is inherent in depression, patient should be closely monitored until depressive symptoms remit and prescriptions should be written for minimum quantities to reduce the risk of overdose. A weak uricosuric effect has been noted; its significance is unknown.

Adverse Reactions In clinical trials, dizziness and nausea were two most frequent side effects that led to discontinuation of therapy in the elderly

Cardiovascular: Palpitations
Central nervous system: Insomnia, agitation, dizziness, headache, somnolence, nervousness, fatigue, extrapyramidal reactions (rare)
Dermatologic: Dermatological reactions
Gastrointestinal: Xerostomia, diarrhea or loose stools, nausea, constipation, vomiting
Genitourinary: Sexual dysfunction in men, micturition disorders, hyponatremia
Neuromuscular & skeletal: Pain, tremors
Ocular: Visual difficulty
Otic: Tinnitus
Miscellaneous: Diaphoresis

Toxicology Establish and maintain an airway, ensure adequate oxygenation and ventilation. Activated charcoal with 70% sorbitol may be as or more effective than emesis or lavage. Monitoring of cardiac and vital signs is recommended along with general symptomatic and supportive measures. There is no specific antidote for sertraline. Forced diuresis, dialysis, hemoperfusion and exchange transfusion are unlikely to enhance elimination due to sertraline's large volume of distribution.

Drug Interactions MAO inhibitors (see Warnings); alcohol, benzodiazepines (decreased clearance), tolbutamide (decreased clearance), warfarin (increased PT); desipramine (slight increase in desipramine concentration); increased toxicity with dexfenfluramine (possible); inhibits conversion of codeine and tramadol to active metabolites (decreased analgesic effects)

Mechanism of Action Selectively inhibits the CNS neuronal reuptake of serotonin, thereby enhancing serotonergic activity and inhibiting adrenergic activity in the locus ceruleus. Minimal or no effect on reuptake of norepinephrine or dopamine and does not significantly bind to alpha-adrenergic, histamine, or cholinergic receptors; as a result, it may be useful in patients at risk

for sedation, hypotension, and anticholinergic effects of tricyclic antidepressants.

Pharmacodynamics Maximum antidepressant effects usually seen after 4 weeks

Pharmacokinetics

Protein binding: 87% to 99% bound to plasma proteins

Metabolism: Extensive first-pass metabolism; substrate for CYP3A4 and inhibitor of CYP2D6. Its principle metabolite, N-desmyethylsertraline, is 8 times less active as a serotonin reuptake inhibitor and 4 times less active in its inhibition of norepinephrine and dopamine, and is considered to have little or no clinical activity.

Half-life, elimination: 26 hours

Time to peak plasma concentration: 4.5-8.4 hours after single daily doses of 50-200 mg for 14 days; food appears to increase both the area under the curve and peak plasma concentrations, while decreasing time to peak plasma concentration

Elimination: Both sertraline and N-desmyethylsertraline are further metabolized to ketones and hydroxylates which are eliminated in the urine and feces

Sertraline's clearance has been found to be reduced by 40% in the elderly

Usual Dosage Oral:

Geriatrics: Start treatment with 25 mg/day in the morning and increase by 25 mg/day increments every 2-3 days if tolerated to 75-100 mg/day; additional increases may be necessary; maximum dose: 200 mg/day

Adults: Start with 50 mg/day in the morning and increase by 50 mg/day increments every 2-3 days if tolerated to 100 mg/day; additional increases may be necessary; maximum dose: 200 mg/day. If somnolence is noted, administer at bedtime.

Monitoring Parameters Improvement of depressive symptoms, anxiety, sleep disturbance, weight, and appetite

Patient Information If currently on another antidepressant drug, patients should notify their physician. Although sertraline has not been shown to increase the effects of alcohol, it is recommended to refrain from drinking while on this medication. May experience some weight loss, but it is usually minimal. If on warfarin, digoxin, an oral hypoglycemic drug, or a drug having an effect on the central nervous system, such as a medication for insomnia or anxiety, patients should notify physician. There are no known interactions between sertraline and over-the-counter medications; however, these should be used with caution and the directions for their use should be followed carefully.

Nursing Implications Monitor nutritional intake and weight; if patient becomes anxious or overstimulated, notify physician; if somnolent, administer dose at bedtime (see Monitoring Parameters and Usual Dosage). Offer hard, sugarless candy or ice chips for dry mouth.

Special Geriatric Considerations Sertraline's favorable side effect profile makes it a useful alternative to the traditional tricyclic antidepressants; its potential stimulation effect and anorexia may be bothersome. Has the shortest half-life of the currently marketed serotonin-reuptake inhibitors. Data from a clinical trial comparing fluoxetine to tricyclics suggest that fluoxetine is significantly less effective than nortriptyline in hospitalized elderly patients with unipolar major affective disorder, especially those with melancholia and concurrent cardiovascular diseases.

Dosage Forms Tablet, as hydrochloride: 25 mg, 50 mg, 100 mg

References

Cohn CK, Shrivastava R, Mendels J, et al, "Double-Blind, Multicenter Comparison of Sertraline and Amitriptyline in Elderly Depressed Patients," *J Clin Psychiatry*, 1990, 51(Suppl B):28-33.

Drug Facts and Comparisons, St Louis, MO: JB Lippincott Co, 1992, 263r-4a.

Grimsley SR and Jann MW, "Paroxetine, Sertraline, and Fluvoxamine: New Selective Serotonin Reuptake Inhibitors," *Clin Pharm*, 1992, 11(11):930-57.

Reimherr FW, Chouinard G, Cohn CK, et al, "Antidepressant Efficacy of Sertraline: A Double-Blind Placebo- and Amitriptyline-Controlled, Multicenter Comparison Study in Outpatients With Major Depression," *J Clin Psychiatry*, 1990, 51(Suppl B):18-27.

Roose SP, Glassman AH, Attia E, et al, "Comparative Efficacy of Selective Serotonin Reuptake Inhibitors and Tricyclics in the Treatment of Melancholia," *Am J Psychiatry*, 1994, 151(12):1735-9.

Serum Drug Concentrations Commonly Monitored: Guidelines *see page 1114*

Serutan® [OTC] *see Psyllium on page 804*

Serzone® *see Nefazodone on page 659*

Siblin® [OTC] *see Psyllium on page 804*

Silace-C® [OTC] *see Docusate and Casanthranol on page 313*

Siladryl® Oral [OTC] *see* Diphenhydramine *on page 302*

Silafed® Syrup [OTC] *see* Triprolidine and Pseudoephedrine *on page 966*

Silain® [OTC] *see* Simethicone *on this page*

Silphen® Cough [OTC] *see* Diphenhydramine *on page 302*

Silphen DM® [OTC] *see* Dextromethorphan *on page 278*

Siltussin® [OTC] *see* Guaifenesin *on page 437*

Siltussin DM® [OTC] *see* Guaifenesin and Dextromethorphan *on page 439*

Silvadene® *see* Silver Sulfadiazine *on this page*

Silver Sulfadiazine (SIL ver sul fa DYE a zeen)

Brand Names Silvadene®; SSD® AF; SSD® Cream; Thermazene®

Therapeutic Category Antibacterial, Topical

Use Adjunct in the prevention and treatment of infection in second and third degree burns

Contraindications Hypersensitivity to silver sulfadiazine or any component

Precautions Use with caution in patients with G-6-PD deficiency and renal impairment; sulfadiazine may accumulate in patients with impaired hepatic or renal function; systemic absorption is significant and adverse reactions may be due to the sulfa component

Adverse Reactions

Dermatologic: Itching, rash, erythema multiforme, skin discoloration, photosensitivity

Hematologic: Hemolytic anemia, leukopenia, agranulocytosis, aplastic anemia

Hepatic: Hepatitis

Local: Pain, burning

Renal: Interstitial nephritis

Drug Interactions Silver may inactivate topical proteolytic enzymes

Stability Discard if cream is darkened (reacts with heavy metals resulting in release of silver)

Mechanism of Action Acts upon the bacterial cell wall and cell membrane and is bactericidal

Pharmacokinetics

Absorption: Significant percutaneous absorption of sulfadiazine can occur especially when applied to extensive burns

Half-life: 10 hours, prolonged in patients with renal insufficiency

Time to peak serum concentration: Within 3-11 days of continuous therapy

Elimination: ~50% excreted unchanged in urine

Usual Dosage Geriatrics and Adults: Topical: Apply once or twice daily with a sterile gloved hand; apply to a thickness of $^1/_{16}$"; burned area should be covered with cream at all times

Administration See Patient Information

Patient Information Bathe daily to aid in debridement (if not contraindicated); apply liberally to burned areas; for external use only; notify physician if condition persists or worsens

Nursing Implications Evaluate the development of granulation and cleanliness of wound; monitor for local side effects (see Adverse Reactions)

Additional Information Contains methylparaben and propylene glycol; use of analgesic might be needed before application

Special Geriatric Considerations No specific recommendations for use in the elderly (see Usual Dosage)

Dosage Forms Cream, topical: 1% [10 mg/g] (20 g, 50 g, 100 g, 400 g, 1000 g)

Simethicone (sye METH i kone)

Brand Names Degas® [OTC]; Flatulex [OTC]; Gas-X® [OTC]; Maalox Anti-Gas® [OTC]; Mylanta Gas® [OTC]; Mylicon® [OTC]; Phazyme® [OTC]; Silain® [OTC]

Synonyms Activated Dimethicone; Activated Methylpolysiloxane

Generic Available Yes: Tablet

Therapeutic Category Antiflatulent

Use Relieve flatulence and functional gastric bloating, and postoperative gas pains; painful distention due to air swallowing, peptic ulcer, diverticulitis, irritable (spastic) colon, and functional dyspepsia

Contraindications Hypersensitivity to drug or components

Mechanism of Action Decreases the surface tension of gas bubbles thereby dispersing and preventing gas pockets in the GI system

Pharmacokinetics Elimination: In feces

Usual Dosage Geriatrics and Adults:
Oral: 40-120 mg after meals and at bedtime as needed, not to exceed 500 mg/day
Drops: 40 mg after meals and at bedtime

Monitoring Parameters Monitor for feelings of relief, decreased pain, bloating

Patient Information Chew tablets thoroughly before swallowing; shake drops well before using

Nursing Implications Shake drops before using; mix with water or other liquids; monitor for decrease in pain, bloating, cramping

Additional Information Drops have small amount of saccharin calcium and sodium benzoate

Special Geriatric Considerations Before treating excess gas or pain due to gas accumulation, a thorough evaluation must be made to determine cause since many bowel diseases may present with flatulence and bloating.

Dosage Forms
Capsule: 125 mg
Drops, oral: 40 mg/0.6 mL (30 mL)
Tablet: 50 mg, 60 mg, 95 mg
Tablet, chewable: 40 mg, 80 mg, 125 mg

Simethicone and Magaldrate see Magaldrate and Simethicone on page 562

Simron® [OTC] see Ferrous Gluconate on page 378

Simvastatin (SIM va stat in)
Brand Names Zocor®
Generic Available No
Therapeutic Category Antilipemic Agent; HMG-CoA Reductase Inhibitor
Use Adjunct to dietary therapy to decrease elevated serum total and LDL cholesterol concentrations in primary hypercholesterolemia
Contraindications Active liver disease or unexplained persistent elevations of LFTs, hypersensitivity to simvastatin or other HMG-CoA reductase inhibitors
Warnings Musculoskeletal effects include myopathy (myalgia and/or muscle weakness accompanied by markedly elevated CK concentrations), rash and/or pruritus; hepatocellular carcinomas have been found in mice taking in excess of 300 times the recommended dose based on body weight
Precautions May elevate aminotransferases; LFTs should be performed before and every 4-6 weeks during the first 12-15 months of therapy and periodically thereafter; serum cholesterol and triglyceride concentrations should be determined prior to and regularly during therapy; use with caution in patients who consume large quantities of alcohol
Adverse Reactions
Central nervous system: Headache, dizziness
Dermatologic: Rash
Gastrointestinal: Flatulence, dyspepsia, abdominal pain and/or cramps diarrhea and/or constipation, nausea
Neuromuscular & skeletal: Myalgia, muscle cramps, myopathy
Ocular: Blurred vision
Overdosage Few cases have been reported; no patients were symptomatic and all recovered without adverse effects
Drug Interactions Increased anticoagulant effect of warfarin, niacin, gemfibrozil, erythromycin, clarithromycin, troleandomycin, itraconazole, ketoconazole, protease inhibitors, and cyclosporine (rhabdomyolysis or myopathy)
Mechanism of Action Simvastatin is a methylated derivative of lovastatin that acts by competitively inhibiting 3-hydroxy-3-methylglutaryl-coenzyme A reductase (HMG-CoA reductase), the enzyme that catalyzes the rate-limiting step in cholesterol biosynthesis
Pharmacokinetics
Absorption: Oral: Although 85% is absorbed following administration, <5% reaches the general circulation due to an extensive first-pass effect
Time to peak concentration: 1.3-2.4 hours
Protein binding: ~95%
Metabolism: Substrate CYP3A4
Elimination: 13% excreted in urine and 60% in feces; the elimination half-life is unknown
In patients with severe renal insufficiency, high systemic serum concentrations may occur
(Continued)

Simvastatin *(Continued)*

Usual Dosage Oral:

    Geriatrics: Start at 5 mg/day as a single bedtime dose; increase as needed every 4 weeks by 5-10 mg; maximum LDL lowering may be achieved with ≤20 mg/day

    Adults: Start with 5-10 mg/day as a single bedtime dose; if LDL is ≤190 mg/dL start with 5 mg; if LDL >190 mg/dL, start with 10 mg/day; increase every 4 weeks as needed; maximum dose: 40 mg/day

Monitoring Parameters Serum cholesterol (total and fractionated), CPK serum concentrations; LFTs before and every 4-6 weeks during the first 12-15 months of therapy and periodically thereafter or LFTs before and every 4-6 weeks during the first 3 months of therapy and then every 6-12 weeks during the next 12 months and periodically thereafter (see Precautions)

Test Interactions Increased ALT, AST, CPK, alkaline phosphatase, bilirubin; altered thyroid function tests

Patient Information Promptly report any unexplained muscle pain, tenderness or weakness, especially if accompanied by malaise or fever; follow prescribed diet; take with meals

Nursing Implications The best effect is seen when administered at night; monitor for symptoms of adverse effects (see Adverse Reactions and Special Geriatric Considerations)

Special Geriatric Considerations Effective and well tolerated in the elderly. The definition of and, therefore, when to treat hyperlipidemia in the elderly is a controversial issue. The National Cholesterol Education Program recommends that all adults 20 years of age and older maintain a plasma cholesterol <200 mg/dL. By this definition, 60% of all elderly would be considered to have a borderline high (200-239 mg/dL) or high (≥240 mg/dL) plasma cholesterol. However, plasma cholesterol has been shown to be a less reliable predictor of coronary heart disease in the elderly. Therefore, it is the authors' belief that pharmacologic treatment be reserved for those who are unable to obtain a desirable plasma cholesterol concentration by diet alone and for whom the benefits of treatment are believed to outweigh the potential adverse effects, drug interactions, and cost of treatment.

Dosage Forms Tablet: 5 mg, 10 mg, 20 mg, 40 mg

References

Bach LA, Cooper ME, O'Brien RC, et al, "The Use of Simvastatin, an HMG-CoA Reductase Inhibitor, in Older Patients With Hypercholesterolemia and Atherosclerosis," *J Am Geriatr Soc,* 1990, 38(1):10-4.

Lintott CJ and Scott RS, "HMG-CoA Reductase Inhibitor Use in the Aged: A Review of Clinical Experience," *Drugs Aging,* 1992, 2(6):518-29.

"Summary of the Second Report of the National Cholesterol Education Program (NCEP) Expert Panel on Detection, Evaluation, and Treatment of High Blood Cholesterol in Adults," *JAMA,* 1993, 269(23):3015-23.

Sinarest® 12 Hour Nasal Solution *see* Oxymetazoline *on page 706*

Sinarest® Nasal Solution [OTC] *see* Phenylephrine *on page 740*

Sinemet® *see* Levodopa and Carbidopa *on page 530*

Sinequan® Oral *see* Doxepin *on page 321*

Sinex® Long-Acting [OTC] *see* Oxymetazoline *on page 706*

Sinumist®-SR Capsulets® *see* Guaifenesin *on page 437*

Sinusol-B® *see* Brompheniramine *on page 129*

Sirdalud® *see* Tizanidine *on page 927*

Skelid® *see* Tiludronate *on page 924*

Sleep-eze 3® Oral [OTC] *see* Diphenhydramine *on page 302*

Sleepinal® [OTC] *see* Diphenhydramine *on page 302*

Sleepwell 2-nite® [OTC] *see* Diphenhydramine *on page 302*

Slo-bid™ *see* Theophylline *on page 902*

Slo-Niacin® [OTC] *see* Niacin *on page 665*

Slo-Phyllin® *see* Theophylline *on page 902*

Slow FE® [OTC] *see* Ferrous Sulfate *on page 379*

Slow-K® *see* Potassium Chloride *on page 763*

Slow-Mag® [OTC] *see* Magnesium Salts (Various Salts) *on page 568*

SMZ-TMP *see* Co-Trimoxazole *on page 253*

Sodium Acid Carbonate *see* Sodium Bicarbonate *on this page*

Sodium Bicarbonate *(SOW dee um bye KAR bun ate)*

Related Information

    I.V. Push Recommended Guidelines *on page 1083*

Brand Names Neut® Injection

Synonyms Baking Soda; NaHCO$_3$; Sodium Acid Carbonate; Sodium Hydrogen Carbonate

Therapeutic Category Alkalinizing Agent, Oral; Alkalinizing Agent, Parenteral; Antacid; Electrolyte Supplement, Oral; Electrolyte Supplement, Parenteral; Sodium Salt

Use Management of metabolic acidosis; antacid; alkalinize urine

Contraindications Alkalosis, hypocalcemia; unknown abdominal pain, inadequate ventilation during cardiopulmonary resuscitation

Warnings Use of I.V. NaHCO$_3$ should be reserved for documented metabolic acidosis and for hyperkalemia-induced cardiac arrest. Routine use in cardiac arrest is not recommended. Avoid extravasation, tissue necrosis can occur due to the hypertonicity of NaHCO$_3$. May cause sodium retention especially if renal function is impaired; not to be used in treatment of peptic ulcer; use with caution in patients with CHF, edema, cirrhosis, or renal failure; attenuation of effects of hyperkalemia.

Adverse Reactions
Cardiovascular: Edema, cerebral hemorrhage
Endocrine & metabolic: Metabolic alkalosis, hypernatremia, hypokalemia, hypocalcemia, intracranial acidosis, increased affinity of hemoglobin for oxygen-reduced pH in myocardia
Gastrointestinal: Gastric distention, flatulence
Local: Tissue necrosis when extravasated

Overdosage Symptoms of overdose include hypocalcemia, hypokalemia, hypernatremia, seizures

Drug Interactions
Decreased effect/serum concentrations of lithium, chlorpropamide, salicylates due to urinary alkalinization
Increased toxicity/serum concentrations of amphetamines, ephedrine, pseudoephedrine, flecainide, quinidine, quinine due to urinary alkalinization

Stability Store injection at room temperature; protect from heat and from freezing; use only clear solutions; incompatible with acids, acidic salts, alkaloid salts, calcium salts, catecholamines, atropine

Mechanism of Action Dissociates to provide bicarbonate ion which neutralizes hydrogen ion concentration and raises blood and urinary pH

Pharmacodynamics
Oral:
Onset of action: Rapid
Duration: of 8-10 minutes
I.V.:
Onset of action: 15 minutes
Duration: 1-2 hours

Pharmacokinetics
Absorption: Oral: Well absorbed
Elimination: Reabsorbed by kidney and <1% excreted by urine

Usual Dosage Geriatrics and Adults:
Cardiac arrest: See Warnings. Patient should be adequately ventilated before administering NaHCO$_3$
HCO$_3$-(mEq) = 0.3 x weight (kg) x base deficit (mEq/L); **routine use of NaHCO$_3$ is not recommended and should be given only after adequate alveolar ventilation has been established and effective cardiac compressions are provided**
I.V.: Initial: 1 mEq/kg/dose one time; maintenance: 0.5 mEq/kg/dose every 10 minutes or as indicated by arterial blood gases
Metabolic acidosis: I.V.: 2-5 mEq/kg/dose over 4-8 hours infusion or calculate dose based on base deficit (re-evaluate acid-base status) mEq NaHCO$_3$ = 0.3 x body weight (kg) x base deficit (mEq/L); administer up to 1 mEq/kg/dose over several minutes or dilute larger doses in maintenance fluids for slow infusion; re-evaluate acid-base status frequently
Maximum daily dose: 200 mEq in adults <60 years and 100 mEq in adults >60 years
Maintenance electrolyte requirements of sodium: Daily requirements: 3-4 mEq/kg/24 hours or 25-40 mEq/1000 kcal/24 hours
Chronic renal failure: Oral: Initiate when plasma HCO$_3$ <15 mEq/L; start with 20-36 mEq/day in divided doses, titrate to bicarbonate concentration of 18-20 mEq/L

Reference Range Therapeutic (sodium): 135-145 mmol/L (SI: 135-145 mmol/L)

Patient Information Avoid chronic use as an antacid (<2 weeks)

Nursing Implications Advise patient of milk-alkali syndrome if use is long-term; observe for extravasation when giving I.V.
(Continued)

Sodium Bicarbonate *(Continued)*

Additional Information May cause sodium retention especially if renal function is impaired; not to be used in treatment of peptic ulcer

Sodium content of injection 50 mL, 8.4%: 1150 mg (50 mEq); each 6 mg of $NaHCO_3$ contains 12 mEq sodium; 1 mEq $NaHCO_3$ = 84 mg; 1 mEq $NaHCO_3$ = 0.3 x body weight (kg) x base deficit (mEq/L)
Each 84 mg of sodium bicarbonate provides 1 mEq of sodium and bicarbonate ions; each gram of sodium bicarbonate provides 12 mEq of sodium and bicarbonate ions

Special Geriatric Considerations Not the antacid of choice for the elderly because of sodium content and potential for systemic alkalosis (see maximum daily dose under Usual Dosage)

Dosage Forms
Injection: 4% (5 mL, 10 mL); 4.2% (1 mL, 5 mL, 10 mL); 5% (500 mL); 7.5% (50 mL); 8.4% (10 mL, 50 mL)
Powder: 120 g, 480 g
Tablet: 300 mg, 324 mg, 600 mg, 648 mg

Sodium Chloride *(SOW dee um KLOR ide)*

Brand Names Adsorbonac® Ophthalmic [OTC]; Afrin® Saline Mist [OTC]; AK-NaCl® [OTC]; Ayr® Saline [OTC]; Breathe Free® [OTC]; Dristan® Saline Spray [OTC]; HuMist® Nasal Mist [OTC]; Muro 128® Ophthalmic [OTC]; Muroptic-5® [OTC]; NāSal™ [OTC]; Nasal Moist® [OTC]; Ocean Nasal Mist [OTC]; Pretz® [OTC]; SalineX® [OTC]; SeaMist® [OTC]

Synonyms NaCl; Normal Saline; Salt

Generic Available Yes

Therapeutic Category Electrolyte Supplement, Oral; Electrolyte Supplement, Parenteral; Lubricant, Ocular; Sodium Salt

Use Prevention of muscle cramps and heat prostration; restoration of sodium ion in hyponatremia; restore moisture to nasal membranes; GU irrigant; reduction of corneal edema; source of electrolytes and water for expansion of the extracellular fluid compartment

Contraindications Hypersensitivity to sodium chloride or any component; hypernatremia, fluid retention

Warnings Sodium toxicity is almost exclusively related to how fast a sodium deficit is corrected; both rate and magnitude are extremely important

Precautions Use with caution in patients with congestive heart failure, renal insufficiency, liver cirrhosis, hypertension

Adverse Reactions
Cardiovascular: Congestive conditions
Endocrine & metabolic: Extravasation, hypervolemia, hypernatremia, dilution of serum electrolytes, overhydration, hypokalemia
Local: Thrombosis, phlebitis, extravasation
Respiratory: Pulmonary edema

Overdosage Symptoms of overdose include nausea, vomiting, diarrhea, abdominal cramps, hypocalcemia, hypokalemia, hypernatremia

Toxicology Hypernatremia is resolved through the use of diuretics and free water replacement

Drug Interactions Decreased serum concentration of lithium

Stability Store injection at room temperature; protect from heat and from freezing; use only clear solutions

Mechanism of Action Principal extracellular cation; functions in fluid and electrolyte balance, osmotic pressure control and water distribution

Pharmacokinetics
Absorption: Oral, I.V.: Rapid
Distribution: Widely distributed
Elimination: Mainly in urine but also in sweat, tears, and saliva

Usual Dosage Geriatrics and Adults:
Heat cramps: Oral: 0.5-1 g with full glass of water, up to 4.8 g/day
Replacement: Determined by laboratory determinations
Nasal: Use as often as needed
Ophthalmic:
Ointment: Apply once daily or more often
Solution: 1-2 drops in affected eye(s) every 3-4 hours
To correct acute, serious hyponatremia: mEq sodium = (desired sodium (mEq/L) - actual sodium (mEq/L) x 0.6 x wt (kg)); for acute correction use 125 mEq/L as the desired serum sodium; acutely correct serum sodium in 5 mEq/L/dose increments; more gradual correction in increments of 10 mEq/L/day is indicated in the asymptomatic patient

Monitoring Parameters I & O, weight, presence or worsening of rales and degree of peripheral edema with infusions, electrolyte levels

Reference Range Serum/plasma concentration: 135-145 mEq/L

Patient Information Blurred vision is common with ophthalmic ointment; may sting eyes when first applied

Nursing Implications I.V. infusion of 3% or 5% sodium chloride should not exceed 100 mL/hour and should be administered via a central line only

Special Geriatric Considerations See Contraindications and Precautions

Dosage Forms

Injection: 0.45% (500 mL, 1000 mL); 0.9% (10 mL, 20 mL, 50 mL, 100 mL, 150 mL, 250 mL, 500 mL, 1000 mL); 3% (500 mL); 5% (500 mL); 20% (250 mL); 23.4% (30 mL, 100 mL)

Injection:
Admixtures: 50 mEq, 100 mEq, 625 mEq
Bacteriostatic: 0.9% (30 mL)

Ointment, ophthalmic: 5% (3.5 g)

Solution:
Irrigation: 0.45% (500 mL, 1000 mL, 1500 mL); 0.9% (150 mL, 250 mL, 500 mL, 1000 mL, 1500 mL, 2000 mL, 4000 mL)
Ophthalmic: 2% (15 mL); 5% (15 mL, 30 mL)

Tablet: 650 mg, 1 g, 2.25 g

Tablet:
Enteric coated: 1 g
Slow release: 600 mg

Sodium Citrate and Citric Acid

(SOW dee um SIT rate & SI trik AS id)

Brand Names Bicitra®; Oracit®

Synonyms Modified Shohl's Solution

Therapeutic Category Alkalinizing Agent, Oral

Use Treatment of metabolic acidosis; alkalinizing agent in conditions where long-term maintenance of an alkaline urine is desirable

Contraindications Severe renal insufficiency, sodium-restricted diet

Warnings Conversion to bicarbonate may be impaired in patients with hepatic failure or in shock

Precautions Use with caution in patients with congestive heart failure, hypertension, pulmonary edema; severe renal impairment

Adverse Reactions

Endocrine & metabolic: Metabolic alkalosis, hyperkalemia
Gastrointestinal: Diarrhea, nausea, vomiting, laxative effect
Genitourinary: Urolithiasis
Neuromuscular & skeletal: Tetany

Overdosage Symptoms of overdose include diarrhea, nausea, vomiting, excessive mental activity

Drug Interactions Other alkylating agents; acts as a urinary alkalinizer which may increase urinary excretion and decrease serum concentrations of chlorpropamide, lithium, methenamine, methotrexate, salicylates, tetracyclines; the converse is true (decreased urinary excretion, increased serum concentrations) for flecainide, mecamylamine, quinidine, and sympathomimetics

Usual Dosage Geriatrics and Adults: Oral: 15-30 mL with water after meals and at bedtime

Monitoring Parameters Blood gas for pH and bicarbonate; serum bicarbonate

Patient Information Palatability is improved by chilling solution, dilute each dose with 1-3 oz of water and follow with additional water (will also minimize laxative effect); take after meals to prevent saline laxative effect

Nursing Implications May be ordered as modified Shohl's solution; dilute with 30-90 mL of chilled water to enhance taste; 1 mL of solution contains 1 mEq sodium and bicarbonate; take after meals

Additional Information 1 mL of solution contains 1 mEq of sodium and is metabolized to form the equivalent of 1 mEq of bicarbonate/mL

Special Geriatric Considerations See Precautions, Usual Dosage, and Additional Information

Dosage Forms Solution, oral: Sodium citrate 500 mg and citric acid 334 mg per 5 mL (15 mL 30 mL, 120 mL, 473 mL, 4000 mL)

Sodium Citrate and Potassium Citrate Mixture
(SOW dee um SIT rate & poe TASS ee um SIT rate MIKS chur)

Brand Names Polycitra®

Therapeutic Category Alkalinizing Agent, Oral

Use Conditions where long-term maintenance of an alkaline urine is desirable as in control and dissolution of uric acid and cystine calculi of the urinary tract

Contraindications Oliguria, azotemia, untreated Addison's disease

Warnings Citrate is converted to bicarbonate in the liver; this conversion may be blocked in patients who are severely ill, in shock, or in hepatic failure

Precautions Use caution in patients with congestive heart failure, hypertension, edema or any condition sensitive to sodium or potassium intake

Adverse Reactions
  Cardiovascular: Cardiac abnormalities
  Endocrine & metabolic: Metabolic alkalosis, calcium levels, hyperkalemia, hypernatremia
  Gastrointestinal: Diarrhea
  Neuromuscular & skeletal: Tetany

Toxicology Treat hyperkalemia

Drug Interactions Potassium-sparing diuretics; will alkalinize the urine which may increase the urinary excretion and decrease serum concentrations of chlorpropamide, lithium, methenamine, methotrexate, salicylate, tetracycline; the converse is true (decreased urinary excretion, increased serum concentrations) for flecainide, mecamylamine, quinidine, and sympathomimetics

Usual Dosage Geriatrics and Adults: Oral: 15-30 mL diluted in water after meals and at bedtime

Monitoring Parameters Blood gas (pH and bicarbonate); serum bicarbonate

Patient Information Palatability is improved by chilling solution, dilute each dose with 1-3 oz of water and follow with additional water; take after meals to prevent saline laxative effect

Nursing Implications Dilute each dose in 30-90 mL of water prior to administration; administer after meals to prevent laxative effect

Special Geriatric Considerations See Precautions, Adverse Reactions, and Usual Dosage

Dosage Forms Syrup: Potassium citrate 550 mg, sodium citrate 500 mg, citric acid 334 mg/5 mL (1 mEq sodium, 1 mEq potassium, 2 mEq bicarbonate/mL)

Sodium Etidronate see Etidronate Disodium on page 362

Sodium Fluoride see Fluoride on page 392

Sodium Hydrogen Carbonate see Sodium Bicarbonate on page 858

Sodium L-Triiodothyronine see Liothyronine on page 539

Sodium Methicillin see Methicillin on page 602

Sodium Nafcillin see Nafcillin on page 648

Sodium Nitroferricyanide see Nitroprusside on page 680

Sodium Nitroprusside see Nitroprusside on page 680

Sodium Phosphate and Potassium Phosphate see Potassium Phosphate and Sodium Phosphate on page 767

Sodium Phosphates (SOW dee um FOS fates)

Brand Names Fleet® Enema [OTC]; Fleet® Phospho®-Soda [OTC]

Generic Available Yes

Therapeutic Category Electrolyte Supplement, Parenteral; Laxative, Saline; Phosphate Salt; Sodium Salt

Use Short-term treatment of constipation, evacuation of the colon for rectal and bowel exams; source of sodium and phosphorus; treatment and prevention of hypophosphatemia

Contraindications Hyperphosphatemia, hypernatremia, hypocalcemia, renal failure, congestive heart failure, abdominal pain, fecal impaction

Warnings Use with caution in patients with renal insufficiency, adrenal insufficiency, CHF, sodium restriction, cirrhosis; phosphate salts may precipitate in the presence of calcium; prolonged and/or excessive use of laxative may result in dependence; rapid I.V. infusion may precipitate hypocalcemia, hypotension, muscular irritability, calcium deposits, renal function deterioration, and hyperkalemia

Precautions Guide replacement therapy by phosphate serum concentrations and limits imposed by changes in sodium

Adverse Reactions
  1% to 10%:
    Cardiovascular: Edema, hypotension

Endocrine & metabolic: Hyperphosphatemia, hypocalcemia, hypernatremia, calcium phosphate precipitation

Gastrointestinal: Nausea, vomiting, diarrhea

Renal: Acute renal failure

Overdosage Symptoms of overdose include tetany, convulsions and neuroexcitability, secondary to the hypocalcemia associated with hyperphosphatemia or hypernatremia; other signs include flacid paralysis, confusion, weakness, cardiac arrhythmias, heart block, and abnormal EKG

Toxicology The dose should be tailored to the patient (aluminum forms an insoluble compound with the phosphate which is excreted in the stool); hypernatremia is treated with loop diuretics and free water replacement; seizures may require diazepam 0.1-0.25 mg/kg; tetany should be treated with I.V. calcium salts; aluminum hydroxide may be administered to adults in doses of 60-200 mL/day; 8-24 capsules (or tablets)/day

Drug Interactions Do not administer with magnesium- and aluminum-containing antacids or sucralfate which can bind with phosphate

Stability Phosphate salts may precipitate when mixed with calcium salts; solubility is improved in amino acid parenteral nutrition solutions; check with a pharmacist to determine compatibility

Mechanism of Action As a laxative, exerts osmotic effect in the small intestine by drawing water into the lumen of the gut, producing distention and promoting peristalsis and evacuation of the bowel; phosphorous participates in bone deposition, calcium metabolism, utilization of B complex vitamins, and as a buffer in acid-base equilibrium

Pharmacodynamics

Onset of action:

Cathartic: 3-6 hours

Rectal: 2-5 minutes

Pharmacokinetics

Absorption: Oral: ~1% to 20%

Elimination:

Oral phosphate: In feces

I.V. phosphate: In urine with over 80% of dose reabsorbed by the kidney

Usual Dosage

Normal requirements elemental phosphorus: Geriatrics and Adults RDA: Oral: 800 mg

I.V. doses should be incorporated into the patient's maintenance I.V. fluids whenever possible; intermittent I.V. infusion should be reserved for severe depletion situations and requires continuous EKG monitoring. It is difficult to determine total body phosphorus deficit due to redistribution into intracellular compartment or bone tissue; (it is recommended that repletion of severe hypophosphatemia (<1 mg/dL in adults) be done via I.V. route since large dose of oral phosphate may cause diarrhea and intestinal absorption may be unreliable). The following dosages are empiric guidelines. **Note:** Doses listed as mmol of phosphate.

Severe hypophosphatemia: Geriatrics and Adults: I.V.: 0.15-0.3 mmol/kg/dose over 12 hours, may repeat as needed to achieve desired serum concentration

Maintenance: Adults: 50-70 mmol/24 hours I.V. or 50-150 mmol/24 hours orally in divided doses **or**

Phosphate maintenance electrolyte requirement in parenteral nutrition: 2 mmol/kg/24 hours or 35 mmol/kcal/24 hours; maximum: 15-30 mmol/24 hours

Laxative (Fleet®): Geriatrics and Adults: Rectal: Contents of one 4.5 oz enema as a single dose, may repeat

Laxative (Fleet® Phospho®-Soda): Oral:

Geriatrics and Adults: 20-30 mL as a single dose

Administration Rate of I.V. infusion should not exceed 0.05 mmol/kg/hour; risks of rapid I.V. infusion include hypocalcemia, hypotension, muscular irritability, calcium deposits, renal function deterioration, and hyperkalemia

With orders for I.V. phosphate, there is considerable confusion associated with the use of millimoles versus milliequivalents to express the phosphate requirement. Because inorganic phosphate exists as monobasic and dibasic anions, with the mixture of valences dependent on pH, ordering by mEq amounts is unreliable and may lead to large dosing errors. In addition, I.V. phosphate is available in the sodium and potassium salt, therefore, the content of these cations must be considered when ordering phosphate. The most reliable method of ordering I.V. phosphate is by millimoles, then specifying the potassium or sodium salt.

(Continued)

Sodium Phosphates *(Continued)*

Contents of one packet should be diluted in 75 mL water before administration; maintain adequate fluid intake

Monitoring Parameters Serum sodium, phosphorus, calcium, renal function, EKG monitor if severe hypophosphatemia

Reference Range Phosphorous serum concentrations; it should be noted that serum concentrations do not accurately reflect intracellular phosphorous concentrations or extent of total body depletion

Adults: 3-4.5 mg/dL

Patient Information May cause diarrhea with the oral preparation; excessive or prolonged use as a laxative may cause dependence

Nursing Implications Most monitor for changes in electrolytes (see Monitoring Parameters); monitor for cardiovascular problems; hypotension, edema, signs of CHF when using parenteral form

Special Geriatric Considerations The use of laxatives should be limited in the elderly since abuse could lead to fluid/electrolyte deficiencies. Since elderly often have reduced renal function, or disease that could predispose them to adverse effects, caution must be used with parenteral sodium phosphate (see Warnings)

Dosage Forms

Enema: Sodium phosphate 6 g and sodium biphosphate 16 g/100 mL (135 mL adult enema unit)

Injection: Phosphate 3 mmol and sodium 4 mEq per mL (5 mL, 10 mL, 15 mL, 30 mL, 50 mL)

Solution, oral: Sodium phosphate 18 g and sodium biphosphate 48 g/100 mL (45 mL, 90 mL, 273 mL)

See table.

	Phosphate (mmol)	Sodium (mEq)	Potassium (mEq)
Oral			
Whole cow's milk	0.29/mL	0.025/mL	0.035/mL
Fleet® Phospho®-Soda	4.15/mL	4.8/mL	None
Intravenous			
Sodium phosphate	3/mL	4/mL	None

References

Lentz RD, Brown BM, and Kjellstrand CM, "Treatment of Severe Hypophosphatemia," *Ann Intern Med*, 1978, 89(6):941-4.

Lloyd CW and Johnson CE, "Management of Hypophosphatemia," *Clin Pharm*, 1988, 7(2):123-8.

Sodium Polystyrene Sulfonate

(SOW dee um pol ee STYE reen SUL fon ate)

Related Information

Antacid Drug Interactions *on page 1096*

Brand Names Kayexalate®; SPS®

Synonyms SPS

Generic Available Yes

Therapeutic Category Antidote, Hyperkalemia; Antidote, Potassium

Use Treatment of hyperkalemia

Contraindications Hypernatremia

Warnings Enema may be prepared with powder and diluted with sorbitol 10% solution or oral solution with 25% sorbitol solution. Enema will reduce the serum potassium faster than oral administration, but the oral route will result in a greater reduction over several hours. In severe hyperkalemia, consider treatment concomitantly with I.V. calcium, sodium bicarbonate, or glucose and insulin; hypokalemia may be precipitated by this agent. Measure serum potassium frequently; loss of magnesium and calcium occurs with polystyrene sulfonate.

Precautions Use with caution in patients with severe congestive heart failure, hypertension, or edema

Adverse Reactions

Endocrine & metabolic: Hypokalemia, hypocalcemia, hypomagnesemia, sodium retention

Gastrointestinal: Anorexia, nausea, vomiting, constipation, intestinal necrosis, gastric irritation, occasionally diarrhea

Overdosage Symptoms of overdose include hypokalemia including cardiac dysrhythmias, confusion, irritability, EKG changes, muscle weakness; irritable confusion may be first sign of hypokalemia

Drug Interactions Cation-donating antacids (eg, magnesium, calcium, aluminum) and saline cathartics should be avoided

Stability Store prepared suspensions at 15°C to 30°C (59°F to 86°F); store repackaged product in refrigerator and use within 14 days; freshly prepared suspensions should be used within 24 hours; do not heat resin suspension

Mechanism of Action Removes potassium by exchanging sodium ions for potassium ions in the intestine before the resin is passed from the body

Pharmacodynamics

Onset of action: Within 2-12 hours

Exchange capacity is ~1 mEq/g *in vivo; in vitro* capacity is 3.1 mEq/g; therefore, a wide range of exchange capacity exists such that close monitoring of serum electrolytes is necessary

Pharmacokinetics Remains in the GI tract to be completely excreted in the feces (primarily as potassium polystyrene sulfonate)

Usual Dosage Geriatrics and Adults:

Oral: 15 g 1-4 times/day

Powder formula: Prepare suspension in a ratio of liquid vehicle to powder of 3-4 mL/g of resin; water, syrup, or sorbitol may be used; sorbitol helps prevent constipation

Rectal: 30-50 g every 6 hours; retention time 30 minutes minimum

Monitoring Parameters Monitor serum electrolytes (potassium, sodium) frequently/24 hours; occasional serum calcium and magnesium is recommended; monitor for constipation and bowel obstruction; EKG monitoring for hypokalemia

Nursing Implications Administer oral (or NG) as ~25% sorbitol solution, never mix in orange juice; enema route is less effective than oral administration; retain enema in colon for at least 30-60 minutes and for several hours, if possible

Additional Information 1 gram of resin binds ~1 mEq of potassium; chilling the oral mixture will increase palatability

Sodium content of 1 g: 31 mg (1.3 mEq)

Special Geriatric Considerations Large doses in elderly may cause fecal impaction and intestinal obstruction; best to administer using sorbitol 70% as vehicle

Dosage Forms

Powder for suspension, oral or rectal: 454 g

Suspension, oral or rectal: 1.25 g/5 mL (60 mL, 120 mL, 200 mL, 480 mL, 500 mL)

Sodium Salicylate *see* Salicylates (Various Salts) *on page 842*

Sodium Sulamyd® Ophthalmic *see* Sulfacetamide Sodium *on page 874*

Sodium Sulfacetamide *see* Sulfacetamide Sodium *on page 874*

Sodium Thiosalicylate *see* Salicylates (Various Salts) *on page 842*

Sodol® *see* Carisoprodol *on page 165*

Solarcaine® Aloe Extra Burn Relief [OTC] *see* Lidocaine *on page 537*

Solfoton® *see* Phenobarbital *on page 737*

Solganal® *see* Aurothioglucose *on page 96*

Solu-Cortef® *see* Hydrocortisone *on page 462*

Solu-Medrol® Injection *see* Methylprednisolone *on page 611*

Solurex® *see* Dexamethasone *on page 274*

Solurex L.A.® *see* Dexamethasone *on page 274*

Soma® *see* Carisoprodol *on page 165*

Soma® Compound *see* Carisoprodol *on page 165*

Soma® Compound with Codeine *see* Carisoprodol *on page 165*

Sominex® Oral [OTC] *see* Diphenhydramine *on page 302*

Somophyllin® *see* Aminophylline *on page 55*

Soprodol® *see* Carisoprodol *on page 165*

Sorbitol (SOR bi tole)

Generic Available Yes

Therapeutic Category Genitourinary Irrigant; Laxative

Use Genitourinary irrigant in transurethral prostatic resection or other transurethral resection or other transurethral surgical procedures; diuretic; humectant; sweetening agent; hyperosmotic laxative; facilitate the passage of sodium polystyrene sulfonate through the intestinal tract

(Continued)

Sorbitol *(Continued)*

Contraindications Anuria

Warnings When used for TURP irrigation, large volumes of fluid may enter systemic circulation. The osmotic diuresis it may induce can affect renal, pulmonary, and cardiac status. Use in diabetics may cause hyperglycemia when absorbed systemically from urethral irrigation.

Precautions Systemic absorption may cause a shift of intracellular fluid to the extracellular space, thus causing or aggravating existing hyponatremia. Systemic absorption may cause significant diuresis to cause or aggravate existing hypovolemia and dehydration.

Adverse Reactions
I.V. infusion:
   Cardiovascular: Edema, hypotension, tachycardia, angina
   Central nervous system: Seizures, vertigo, chills
   Dermatologic: Urticaria
   Endocrine & metabolic: Acidosis, electrolyte loss, dehydration
   Gastrointestinal: Xerostomia, thirst, nausea, vomiting, diarrhea
   Genitourinary: Urinary retention
   Local: Thrombophlebitis
   Ocular: Blurred vision
   Renal: Marked diuresis
Oral:
   Cardiovascular: Hypotension
   Endocrine & metabolic: Dehydration, fluid and electrolyte loss
   Gastrointestinal: Diarrhea, flatulence, abdominal cramps, unpleasant sweet taste

Overdosage Symptoms of overdose include diarrhea, hypotension, dehydration, lethargy

Stability Protect from freezing; avoid storage in temperatures >150°F

Mechanism of Action A polyalcoholic sugar (monosaccharide) with osmotic cathartic actions

Pharmacodynamics Onset of action: ~15-60 minutes

Pharmacokinetics
Absorption: Oral, rectal: Poor
Metabolism: Mainly in the liver to carbon dioxide (70%) and dextrose (30%)
Elimination: In kidneys

Usual Dosage Hyperosmotic laxative (as single dose, at infrequent intervals): Geriatrics and Adults:

Oral: 30-150 mL (as 70% solution)
Rectal enema: 120 mL as 25% to 30% solution
Adjunct to sodium polystyrene sulfonate: 15 mL as 70% solution orally until diarrhea occurs (10-20 mL/2 hours) or 20-100 mL as an oral vehicle for the sodium polystyrene sulfonate resin
When administered with charcoal: Oral: 4.3 mL/kg of 70% sorbitol with 1 g/kg of activated charcoal

Monitoring Parameters Blood pressure, serum electrolytes, number of stools per day; when used as an irrigant in TURP (see Warnings and Precautions)

Patient Information Take with a full glass of water. When used as a cathartic, report failure of laxative effect, dizziness, weakness, and dehydration to physician, pharmacist, or nurse. Contact physician if more than 3-5 stools per day are produced.

Nursing Implications Do not use unless solution is clear (see Monitoring Parameters)

Special Geriatric Considerations Causes for constipation must be evaluated prior to initiating treatment. Nonpharmacological dietary treatment should be initiated before laxative use. Sorbitol is as effective as lactulose but is much less expensive.

Dosage Forms Solution: 3% (1500 mL, 3000 mL); 3.3% (2000 mL)

References
Lederle FA, Busch DL, Mattox KM, et al, "Cost-Effective Treatment of Constipation in the Elderly: A Randomized Double-Blend Comparison of Sorbitol and Lactulose," *Am J Med*, 1990, 89(5):597-601.

Sorbitrate® *see* Isosorbide Dinitrate *on page 503*
Soridol® *see* Carisoprodol *on page 165*

Sotalol *(SOE ta lole)*
Related Information
Beta-Blockers Comparison *on page 1026*

Brand Names Betapace®

Therapeutic Category Antiarrhythmic Agent, Class II; Antiarrhythmic Agent, Class III; Beta-Adrenergic Blocker

Use Treatment of ventricular arrhythmias, prevention of life-threatening arrhythmias, and sudden death postmyocardial infarction

Contraindications Uncompensated congestive heart failure, cardiogenic shock, bradycardia or heart block, pulmonary edema, asthma

Warnings Use with caution in patients with congestive heart failure, peripheral vascular disease, hypokalemia, hypomagnesemia, renal dysfunction, sick sinus syndrome; abrupt withdrawal may result in return of life-threatening arrhythmias; sotalol can provoke new or worsening ventricular arrhythmias

Adverse Reactions

Cardiovascular: Hypotension (especially with higher doses), bradycardia, Raynaud's phenomena

Central nervous system: Dizziness, somnolence, confusion, lethargy, depression, headache

Gastrointestinal: Nausea, vomiting

Local: Skin necrosis after extravasation, phlebitis

Miscellaneous: Diaphoresis, cold extremities

Overdosage Symptoms of overdose include severe hypotension, bradycardia, heart failure and bronchospasm, hypoglycemia

Toxicology Sympathomimetics (eg, epinephrine or dopamine), glucagon or a pacemaker can be used to treat the toxic bradycardia, asystole, and/or hypotension. Initially, fluids may be the best treatment for toxic hypotension. Following GI decontamination, treatment is supportive. Lidocaine should be used for torsade de pointes or other ventricular arrhythmias; magnesium may be helpful; may require isoproterenol or cardioversion.

Drug Interactions Decreased effect/levels with coadministration of aluminum and/or magnesium-containing antacids

Mechanism of Action Has both beta$_1$- and beta$_2$-receptor blocking activity; also passes some type III antiarrhythmic activity

Pharmacokinetics

Absorption: Decreased 20% to 30% by meals

Distribution: Low lipid solubility

Protein binding: Not protein bound

Bioavailability: 90% to 100%

Half-life: 12 hours

Elimination: Unchanged through kidney

Usual Dosage Geriatrics and Adults: Oral: Initial: 80 mg twice daily; may be increased to 240-320 mg/day and up to 480-640 mg/day in patients with life-threatening refractory ventricular arrhythmias; adjust dose every 2-3 days; due to the 12-hour half-life, twice daily dosing is all that is necessary with Cl$_{cr}$ >60 mL/minute (see Additional Information)

Dosing adjustment in renal impairment:

Cl$_{cr}$ >60 mL/minute: Administer every 12 hours

Cl$_{cr}$ 30-60 mL/minute: Administer every 24 hours

Cl$_{cr}$ 10-30 mL/minute: Administer every 36-48 hours

Cl$_{cr}$ <10 mL/minute: Individualize dose

Monitoring Parameters Serum magnesium, potassium, EKG, pulse

Patient Information Seek emergency help if palpitations occur; do not discontinue abruptly or change dose without notifying physician; take on an empty stomach

Nursing Implications Initiation of therapy and dose escalation should be done in a hospital with cardiac monitoring; lidocaine and other resuscitative measures should be available

Additional Information If patients are receiving another antiarrhythmic, it is best to withdraw the agent, with careful monitoring, for at least 2-3 half-lives of the agent if clinical condition allows before initiating sotalol; treatment with sotalol has been initiated in some with patients receiving I.V. lidocaine without problems; if patients are receiving amiodarone, **do not** start sotalol until Q-T interval is normal

Special Geriatric Considerations Since elderly frequently have Cl$_{cr}$ <60 mL/minute, attention to dose, creatinine clearance, and monitoring is important; make dosage adjustments at 3-day intervals or after 5-6 doses at any dosage

Dosage Forms Tablet, as hydrochloride: 80 mg, 120 mg, 160 mg, 240 mg

Span-FF® [OTC] *see Ferrous Fumarate on page 376*

Sparfloxacin (spar FLOKS a sin)

Related Information
Antacid Drug Interactions *on page 1096*

Brand Names Zagam®

Therapeutic Category Antibiotic, Quinolone

Use Treatment of adults with community-acquired pneumonia caused by *C. pneumoniae, H. influenzae, H. parainfluenza, M. catarrhalis, M. pneumoniae* or *S. pneumoniae*; also for treatment of acute bacterial exacerbations of chronic bronchitis caused by *C. pneumoniae, E. cloacae, H. influenzae, H. parainfluenza, K. pneumoniae, M. catarrhalis, S. aureus* or *S. pneumoniae*; offers a potential advantage over other fluoroquinolones due to enhanced activity (particularly against g (+) cocci and anaerobes) and a long half-life, allowing once daily dosing

Contraindications Hypersensitivity to sparfloxacin, any component, or other quinolones

Warnings Not recommended in children <18 years of age, other quinolones have caused transient arthropathy in children; CNS stimulation may occur (tremor, restlessness, confusion, and very rarely hallucinations or seizures); use with caution in patients with known or suspected CNS disorder or renal dysfunction; prolonged use may result in superinfection; if an allergic reaction (itching, urticaria, dyspnea, pharyngeal or facial edema, loss of consciousness, tingling, cardiovascular collapse) occurs, discontinue the drug immediately; use caution to avoid possible photosensitivity reactions during and for several days following fluoroquinolone therapy; pseudomembranous colitis may occur and should be considered in patients who present with diarrhea

Adverse Reactions
Cardiovascular: Dose-related Q-T$_c$ prolongation, torsades de pointes
Central nervous system: Insomnia, agitation, sleep disorders, anxiety, delirium
Dermatologic: Photosensitivity, rash
Gastrointestinal: Diarrhea, abdominal pain, nausea, vomiting
Hematologic: Leukopenia, eosinophilia, anemia
Hepatic: Increased LFTs
Neuromuscular & skeletal: Myalgia, arthralgia

Overdosage Symptoms of overdose include acute renal failure, seizures

Toxicology GI decontamination and supportive care; not removed by peritoneal or hemodialysis

Drug Interactions
Decreased effect: Decreased absorption with antacids containing aluminum, magnesium, and/or calcium (by up to 98% if given at the same time); phenytoin serum concentrations may be reduced by quinolones; antineoplastic agents may also decrease serum concentrations of fluoroquinolones
Increased toxicity/serum concentrations: Quinolones cause increased serum concentrations of caffeine, warfarin, azlocillin, cyclosporine, and theophylline (although one study indicates that sparfloxacin may not affect theophylline metabolism), azlocillin, cimetidine, and probenecid increase quinolone serum concentrations; an increased incidence of seizures may occur with foscarnet

Mechanism of Action Inhibits DNA-gyrase in susceptible organisms; inhibits relaxation of supercoiled DNA and promotes breakage of double-stranded DNA

Pharmacokinetics
Absorption: Slow and erratic
Distribution: V$_d$: 3.6 L/kg; distributes into many tissues, including lung, skin, prostate, and gynecological tissue; CSF penetration is limited
Protein binding: 44%
Metabolism: Hepatic, major metabolite is inactive glucuronide
Half-life: 16-20 hours
Time to peak serum concentration: 3-5 hours
Elimination: 7% to 12% excreted in urine as unchanged drug

Usual Dosage Geriatrics and Adults: Oral:
Loading dose: 2 tablets (400 mg) on day 1
Maintenance: 1 tablet (200 mg)/day for 9 additional days (total 11 tablets)
Dosing adjustment in renal impairment: Cl$_{cr}$ <50 mL/minute: Administer 400 mg on day 1, then 200 mg every 48 hours for a total of 9 days of therapy (total 6 tablets)

Monitoring Parameters Evaluation of organ system functions (renal, hepatic, ophthalmologic, and hematopoietic) is recommended periodically during therapy; the possibility of crystalluria should be assessed; WBC and signs and symptoms of infection

Patient Information May take with or without food; drink with plenty of fluids; avoid exposure to direct sunlight during therapy and for several days following; do not take antacids within 4 hours before or 2 hours after dosing; contact your physician immediately if signs of allergy occur; do not discontinue therapy until your course has been completed; take a missed dose as soon as possible, unless it is almost time for your next dose

Special Geriatric Considerations Adjust dose based on renal function; evaluate patient's drug regimen prior to initiating therapy to avoid or make allowances for possible drug interactions since elderly frequently have diseases requiring medications that can interact with quinolones (see Usual Dosage and Drug Interactions)

Dosage Forms Tablet: 200 mg

Sparine® see Promazine on page 788

Spaslin® see Hyoscyamine, Atropine, Scopolamine, and Phenobarbital on page 472

Spasmoject® Injection see Dicyclomine on page 285

Spasmolin® see Hyoscyamine, Atropine, Scopolamine, and Phenobarbital on page 472

Spasmophen® see Hyoscyamine, Atropine, Scopolamine, and Phenobarbital on page 472

Spasquid® see Hyoscyamine, Atropine, Scopolamine, and Phenobarbital on page 472

Spironazide® see Hydrochlorothiazide and Spironolactone on page 459

Spironolactone (speer on oh LAK tone)

Brand Names Aldactone®

Generic Available Yes

Therapeutic Category Diuretic, Potassium Sparing

Use Management of edema associated with excessive aldosterone excretion; hypertension; primary hyperaldosteronism; hypokalemia; cirrhosis of the liver accompanied by edema or ascites

Unlabeled use: Treatment of hirsutism

Contraindications Renal insufficiency, hypersensitivity to spironolactone or any component, hyperkalemia, patients receiving other potassium-sparing diuretics or potassium supplements

Warnings Spironolactone has been shown to be tumorigenic in toxicity studies using rats at 25-250 times the usual human dose

Precautions Use with caution in patients with dehydration, hepatic disease, hyponatremia; potassium excretion may be decreased in the elderly, increasing the risk of hyperkalemia with the use of spironolactone

Adverse Reactions

Central nervous system: Lethargy, headache, confusion, ataxia

Dermatologic: Rash

Endocrine & metabolic: Hyperkalemia, dehydration, hyponatremia, gynecomastia, hyperchloremic metabolic acidosis, postmenopausal bleeding

Gastrointestinal: Anorexia, nausea, vomiting, diarrhea, cramping, gastric bleeding, ulceration, gastritis

Genitourinary: Inability to achieve or maintain an erection

Overdosage Symptoms of overdose include drowsiness, confusion, clinical signs of dehydration, and electrolyte imbalance

Toxicology Ingestion of large amounts of potassium-sparing diuretics, may result in life-threatening hyperkalemia. This can be treated with I.V. insulin and glucose (dextrose 25% in water), with concurrent I.V. sodium bicarbonate (1 mEq/kg up to 44 mEq/dose). If needed, Kayexalate® oral or rectal solutions in sorbitol may also be used.

Drug Interactions Increased serum potassium concentration with potassium, potassium-sparing diuretics, indomethacin, angiotensin-converting enzymes inhibitors

Drug/Food Interactions Administration of spironolactone with food increases its absorption

Stability Protect from light

Mechanism of Action Competes with aldosterone for receptor sites in the distal renal tubules, increasing sodium, chloride, and water excretion while conserving potassium and hydrogen ions; may block the effect of aldosterone on arteriolar smooth muscle as well

Pharmacokinetics

Protein binding: 91% to 98%

(Continued)

Spironolactone *(Continued)*

Metabolism: In the liver to multiple metabolites, including canrenone (active)

Half-life: 78-84 minutes

Time to peak serum concentrations: Oral: Within 1-3 hours (primarily as the active metabolite)

Elimination: Urinary and biliary

In the elderly, levels of the metabolites were found to be twice as high as in younger patients

Usual Dosage Oral:

Geriatrics: Initial: 25-50 mg/day in 1-2 divided doses increasing by 25-50 mg every 5 days as needed

Adults:

Edema, hypertension, hypokalemia: 25-200 mg/day in 1-2 divided doses

Diagnosis of primary aldosteronism: 100-400 mg/day in 1-2 divided doses

Monitoring Parameters Blood pressure, serum electrolytes, renal function, weight, I & O

Test Interactions May cause false elevation in serum digoxin concentrations measured by RIA

Patient Information Avoid hazardous activity such as driving, until response to drug is known (may cause lethargy or confusion); take with meals or milk; avoid excessive ingestion of foods high in potassium or use of salt substitutes. Take in the morning; take the last dose of multiple doses no later than 6 PM unless instructed otherwise.

Nursing Implications Diuretic effect may be delayed 2-3 days and maximum hypertensive may be delayed 2-3 weeks

Additional Information To reduce delay in onset of effect, a loading dose of 2 or 3 times the daily dose may be administered on the first day of therapy; it is recommended the drug be discontinued several days prior to adrenal vein catheterization; adverse reactions are dose related and usually disappear upon drug withdrawal, except possibly gynecomastia

Special Geriatric Considerations Monitor serum potassium (see Precautions and Pharmacokinetics)

Dosage Forms Tablet: 25 mg, 50 mg, 100 mg

Spironolactone and Hydrochlorothiazide *see* Hydrochlorothiazide and Spironolactone *on page 459*

Spirozide® *see* Hydrochlorothiazide and Spironolactone *on page 459*

Sporanox® *see* Itraconazole *on page 509*

SPS *see* Sodium Polystyrene Sulfonate *on page 864*

SPS® *see* Sodium Polystyrene Sulfonate *on page 864*

S-P-T *see* Thyroid *on page 917*

SSD® AF *see* Silver Sulfadiazine *on page 856*

SSD® Cream *see* Silver Sulfadiazine *on page 856*

Stadol® *see* Butorphanol *on page 138*

Stadol® NS *see* Butorphanol *on page 138*

Stagesic® *see* Hydrocodone and Acetaminophen *on page 461*

Stannous Fluoride *see* Fluoride *on page 392*

Staphcillin® *see* Methicillin *on page 602*

Staticin® Topical *see* Erythromycin, Topical *on page 347*

Stay Trim® Diet Gum [OTC] *see* Phenylpropanolamine *on page 741*

S-T Cort® *see* Hydrocortisone *on page 462*

Stelazine® *see* Trifluoperazine *on page 954*

Sterapred® *see* Prednisone *on page 776*

Stilbestrol *see* Diethylstilbestrol *on page 287*

Stilphostrol® *see* Diethylstilbestrol *on page 287*

Stimate® Nasal *see* Desmopressin Acetate *on page 273*

St Joseph® Adult Chewable Aspirin [OTC] *see* Aspirin *on page 84*

St. Joseph® Cough Suppressant [OTC] *see* Dextromethorphan *on page 278*

St. Joseph® Measured Dose Nasal Solution [OTC] *see* Phenylephrine *on page 740*

Stop® [OTC] *see* Fluoride *on page 392*

Streptase® *see* Streptokinase *on this page*

Streptokinase *(strep toe KYE nase)*

Brand Names Kabikinase®; Streptase®

Therapeutic Category Thrombolytic Agent

Use Thrombolytic agent used in treatment of recent severe or massive deep vein thrombosis, pulmonary emboli, myocardial infarction, and occluded arteriovenous cannulas

Contraindications Hypersensitivity to streptokinase or any component; recent strep infection; active internal bleeding, recent CVA (within 2 months), or intracranial or intraspinal surgery, major surgery within the last 10 days, GI bleeding, recent trauma, severe hypertension

Warnings Avoid I.M. injections

Adverse Reactions

Cardiovascular: Hypotension, arrhythmias, noncardiac pulmonary edema, flushing

Central nervous system: Fever

Dermatologic: Itching, urticaria, angioneurotic edema

Hematologic: Surface bleeding, internal bleeding, cerebral hemorrhage

Neuromuscular & skeletal: Musculoskeletal pain

Respiratory: Bronchospasm

Overdosage Symptoms of overdose include epistaxis, bleeding gums, hematoma, spontaneous ecchymoses, oozing at catheter site

Drug Interactions Increased effect of anticoagulants (discontinue heparin before giving streptokinase), and antiplatelet agents; decreased effect with antifibrinolytic agents (aminocaproic acid)

Stability Keep in refrigerator, use reconstituted solutions within 24 hours; store unopened vials at room temperature

Mechanism of Action Activates the conversion of plasminogen to plasmin by forming a complex exposing plasminogen-activating site and clearing a peptide bond that converts plasminogen to plasmin; plasmin being capable of thrombolysis, by degrading fibrin, fibrinogen and other procoagulant proteins into soluble fragments; effective both outside and within the formed thrombus/embolus

Pharmacodynamics

Onset of effect: Following injection, activation of plasminogen occurs almost immediately

Duration: Fibrinolytic effects last only a few hours, while anticoagulant effects can persist for 12-24 hours

Pharmacokinetics

Half-life: 83 minutes

Elimination: By circulating antibodies and via the reticuloendothelial system

Usual Dosage Geriatrics and Adults: I.V. (best results are realized if used within 5-6 hours of myocardial infarction; antibodies to streptokinase remain 3-6 months after initial dose; use another thrombolytic enzyme (ie, urokinase), if thrombolytic therapy is indicated):

Guidelines for acute myocardial infarction (AMI):

1.5 million units infused over 60 minutes. Monitor for the first few hours for signs of anaphylaxis or allergic reaction. **Infusion should be slowed if blood pressure is lowered by 25 mm Hg or if asthmatic symptoms appear.** Begin heparin 5000-10,000 unit bolus followed by 1000 units/hour approximately 3-4 hours after completion of streptokinase infusion or when PTT is <100 seconds.

Intracoronary infusion (250,000 IU/125 mL): Administer 20,000 IU bolus followed by 2000 IU/minute for 60 minutes; total dose: 140,000 IU

Guidelines for acute pulmonary embolism (APE), DVT, arterial thrombosis, or embolism:

3 million unit dose; administer 250,000 units over 30 minutes followed by 100,000 units/hour for 24-72 hours. Monitor for the first few hours for signs of anaphylaxis or allergic reaction. **Infusion should be slowed if blood pressure is lowered by 25 mm Hg or if asthmatic symptoms appear.** Begin heparin 1000 units/hour approximately 3-4 hours after completion of streptokinase infusion or when PTT is <100 seconds.

Cannula occlusion: 250,000 units into cannula, clamp for 2 hours, then aspirate contents and flush with normal saline

Monitoring Parameters Before therapy, hematocrit, platelet count, PT, APTT, thrombin time (TT), fibrinogen concentration; check PT, APTT, TT, or fibrinogen level every 4 hours after starting therapy

Test Interactions I.V. and intracoronary administration will increase thrombin time, APTT, PT, and decrease fibrinogen and plasminogen levels

Nursing Implications For I.V. or intracoronary use only; monitor for bleeding every 15 minutes for the first hour of therapy; avoid I.M. injections

(Continued)

Streptokinase *(Continued)*

Special Geriatric Considerations Investigators applied analysis to data for patients ≥75 years of age from two large trials studying the impact of streptokinase on patient outcome after acute myocardial infarction; their conclusion was that age alone is not a contraindication to the use of streptokinase and that thrombolytic therapy is cost-effective and is beneficial toward the survival of elderly patients. Additional studies are needed to determine if a weight-adjusted dose will maintain efficacy but decrease adverse events such as stroke.

Dosage Forms Injection: 250,000 units (5 mL, 6.5 mL); 600,000 units (5 mL); 750,000 units (6 mL, 6.5 mL); 1,500,000 units (6.5 mL, 50 mL)

References
Krumholz HM, Pasternak RC, Weinstein MC, et al, "Cost Effectiveness of Thrombolytic Therapy With Streptokinase in Elderly Patients With Suspected Acute Myocardial Infarction," *N Engl J Med,* 1992, 327:7-13.

Streptomycin *(strep toe MYE sin)*

Related Information
Cephalosporins, Aminoglycosides, Macrolides, & Quinolones *on page 1014*

Generic Available Yes

Therapeutic Category Antibiotic, Aminoglycoside; Antitubercular Agent

Use Combination therapy of active tuberculosis; used in combination with other agents for treatment of streptococcal or enterococcal endocarditis, mycobacterial infections, plague, tularemia, and brucellosis

Contraindications Hypersensitivity to streptomycin or any component

Warnings Aminoglycosides are associated with significant nephrotoxicity or ototoxicity; the ototoxicity is directly proportional to the amount of drug given and the duration of treatment; tinnitus or vertigo are indications of vestibular injury and impending bilateral irreversible damage; renal damage is usually reversible

Precautions Use with caution in patients with pre-existing vertigo, tinnitus, hearing loss, neuromuscular disorders, or renal impairment; modify dosage in patients with renal impairment

Adverse Reactions
Cardiovascular: Myocarditis, cardiovascular collapse
Central nervous system: Dizziness, vertigo, ataxia, neuromuscular blockade, headache
Dermatologic: Toxic epidermal necrolysis
Gastrointestinal: Vomiting
Otic: Ototoxicity
Renal: Nephrotoxicity
Miscellaneous: Serum sickness

Overdosage Symptoms of overdose include ototoxicity, nephrotoxicity, and neuromuscular toxicity

Toxicology The treatment of choice following a single acute overdose appears to be the maintenance of good urine output of at least 3 mL/kg/hour. Dialysis is of questionable value in the enhancement of aminoglycoside elimination. If required, hemodialysis is preferred over peritoneal dialysis in patients with normal renal function. Careful hydration may be all that is required to promote diuresis and therefore the enhancement of the drug's elimination.

Drug Interactions
Increased/prolonged effect: Depolarizing and nondepolarizing neuromuscular blocking agents
Increased toxicity: Concurrent use of amphotericin may increase nephrotoxicity

Stability Depending upon manufacturer reconstituted solution remains stable for 2-4 weeks when refrigerated; exposure to light causes darkening of solution without apparent loss of potency

Mechanism of Action Inhibits bacterial protein synthesis by binding directly to the 30S ribosomal subunits causing faulty peptide sequence to form in the protein chain

Pharmacodynamics Bactericidal at an alkaline pH

Pharmacokinetics
Protein binding: 34%; CNS penetration is fair
Half-life: 2-4.7 hours and is prolonged with renal impairment (up to 100 hours)
Time to peak serum concentration: I.M.: Within 1 hour
Elimination: Almost completely (90%) as unchanged drug in urine, with small amounts (1%) excreted in bile, saliva, sweat, and tears

Usual Dosage

Geriatrics: 10 mg/kg/day not to exceed 750 mg/day; dosing interval should be adjusted for renal function; some authors suggest not to administer more than 5 days/week or administer as 20-25 mg/kg/dose twice weekly

Adults: I.M.:

Tuberculosis: 15 mg/kg/day in divided doses every 12 hours, not to exceed 2 g/day

Enterococcal endocarditis: 1 g every 12 hours for 2 weeks, 500 mg every 12 hours for 4 weeks in combination with penicillin

Streptococcal endocarditis: 1 g every 12 hours for 1 week, 500 mg every 12 hours for 1 week

Tularemia: 1-2 g/day in divided doses for 7-10 days or until patient is afebrile for 5-7 days

Plague: 2-4 g/day in divided doses until the patient is afebrile for at least 3 days

Dosage adjustment in renal impairment:

Cl_{cr} 10-50 mL/minute: Administer every 24-72 hours

Cl_{cr} <10 mL/minute: Administer every 72-96 hours

Monitoring Parameters BUN and serum creatinine, hearing (if appropriate); in tuberculosis patients, monitor sputum culture and chest x-ray 2-3 months into treatment and at its completion

Reference Range

Therapeutic: Peak: 20-30 µg/mL; trough: <5 µg/mL

Toxic: Peak: >50 µg/mL; trough: >10 µg/mL

Test Interactions False-positive urine glucose with Benedict's solution

Patient Information Report any unusual symptom

Nursing Implications Inject deep I.M. into large muscle mass; I.V. administration is not recommended; modify dosage in patients with renal insufficiency

Additional Information Eighth cranial nerve damage is usually preceded by high-pitched tinnitus, roaring noises, sense of fullness in ears, or impaired hearing and may persist for weeks after drug is discontinued

Special Geriatric Considerations Streptomycin is indicated for persons from endemic areas of drug-resistant *Mycobacterium tuberculosis* or who are HIV infected; since most older patients acquired the *M. tuberculosis* infection prior to the availability of effective chemotherapy, isoniazid and rifampin are usually effective unless resistant organisms are suspected or the patient is HIV infected; adjust dose interval for renal function

Dosage Forms Injection, as sulfate: 400 mg/mL (2.5 mL)

References

Bass JB Jr, Farer LS, Hopewell PC, et al, "Treatment of Tuberculosis and Tuberculosis Infection in Adults and Children," *Am J Respir Crit Care Med*, 1994, 149(5):1359-74.

Stead WW and Dutt AK, "Tuberculosis: A Special Problem in the Elderly," *Principles of Geriatric Medicine and Gerontology*, 2nd ed, 1990, 522.

Yoshikawa TT, "Tuberculosis in Aging Adults," *J Am Geriatr Soc*, 1992, 40(2):178-87.

Stye® Ophthalmic Ointment [OTC] *see Ocular Lubricant on page 688*

Sublimaze® Injection *see Fentanyl on page 374*

Sucralfate (soo KRAL fate)

Brand Names Carafate®

Synonyms Aluminum Sucrose Sulfate, Basic

Generic Available No

Therapeutic Category Gastrointestinal Agent, Miscellaneous

Use Short-term management of duodenal ulcers

Unlabeled use: Gastric ulcers; maintenance of duodenal ulcers; suspension may be used topically for treatment of stomatitis due to cancer chemotherapy and other causes of esophageal and gastric erosions; GERD, esophagitis; treatment of NSAID mucosal damage; prevention of stress ulcers

Contraindications Hypersensitivity to sucralfate or any component

Warnings Use caution with chronic renal failure, dialysis (aluminum accumulation)

Precautions Successful therapy with sucralfate should not be expected to alter the posthealing frequency of recurrence or the severity of duodenal ulceration

Adverse Reactions

Central nervous system: Dizziness, sleepiness, vertigo, headache

Dermatologic: Rash, pruritus

Gastrointestinal: Constipation, diarrhea, nausea, gastric discomfort, indigestion, xerostomia

Neuromuscular & skeletal: Back pain

(Continued)

Sucralfate (Continued)

Overdosage Risk appears minimal

Toxicology Deferoxamine, traditionally used as an iron chelator, has been shown to increase urinary aluminum output. Deferoxamine chelation of aluminum has resulted in improvements of clinical symptoms and bone histology. Deferoxamine, however, remains an experimental treatment for aluminum poisoning and has a significant potential for adverse effects.

Drug Interactions Cimetidine, digoxin, phenytoin (hydantoins), warfarin, ketoconazole, quinidine, ciprofloxacin, norfloxacin (quinolones), ranitidine, tetracycline, theophylline; because of the potential for sucralfate to alter the absorption of some drugs, separate administration (2 hours before or after) should be considered when alterations in bioavailability are believed to be critical; do not administer antacids within 30 minutes of administration

Note: When given with aluminum-containing antacids, may increase serum/body aluminum concentrations (see Warnings)

Mechanism of Action Forms a complex by binding with positively charged proteins in exudates, forming a viscous paste-like, adhesive substance, when combined with gastric acid adheres to the damaged mucosal area. This selectively forms a protective coating that protects the lining against peptic acid, pepsin, and bile salts.

Pharmacodynamics
Onset of paste formation and ulcer adhesion: within 1-2 hours
Duration of action: Up to 6 hours

Pharmacokinetics
Absorption: Oral: <5% of dose
Metabolism: Not metabolized
Protein binding: Unbound in GI tract to aluminum and sucrose octasulfate
Elimination: Small amounts that are absorbed are excreted in urine as unchanged compounds

Usual Dosage Geriatrics and Adults: Oral: 1 g 4 times/day, 1 hour before meals or food and at bedtime, or alternatively 2 g twice daily; adult treatment is recommended for 4-8 weeks; elderly will often require 12 weeks

Prophylaxis (maintenance): 1 g twice daily (tablets only)
Stomatitis: 2.5-5 mL, swish and spit or swish and swallow 4 times/day

Monitoring Parameters Monitor signs and symptoms of disease process and adverse effects; evaluate by endoscopic examination or x-ray

Patient Information Take 1 hour before meals or on an empty stomach; may allow tablet to disintegrate in ~1 oz of room temperature water and drink the resulting suspension, if unable to swallow tablets whole; do not take within 30 minutes of antacids (before or after)

Nursing Implications Monitor for constipation; administer 2 hours before or after administration of other oral drugs; tablets may be disintegrated in water before administering

Additional Information May decrease gastric emptying; many trials have demonstrated sucralfate is equivalent in efficacy to antacids and H_2 blockers; equivalence of sucralfate suspension to sucralfate tablets has not been established in studies

Special Geriatric Considerations Caution should be used in elderly due to reduced renal function; patients with Cl_{cr} <30 mL/minute may be at risk for aluminum intoxication; due to low side effect profile, this may be an agent of choice in elderly with PUD

Dosage Forms
Suspension, oral: 1 g/10 mL (420 mL)
Tablet: 1 g

Sucrets® Cough Calmers [OTC] see Dextromethorphan on page 278

Sudafed® [OTC] see Pseudoephedrine on page 802

Sudafed® 12 Hour [OTC] see Pseudoephedrine on page 802

Sufedrin® [OTC] see Pseudoephedrine on page 802

Sular® see Nisoldipine on page 674

Sulbactam and Ampicillin see Ampicillin and Sulbactam on page 75

Sulf-10® Ophthalmic see Sulfacetamide Sodium on this page

Sulfacetamide Sodium (sul fa SEE ta mide SOW dee um)

Brand Names AK-Sulf® Ophthalmic; Bleph®-10 Ophthalmic; Cetamide® Ophthalmic; Isopto® Cetamide® Ophthalmic; Ocusulf-10® Ophthalmic; Sebizon® Topical Lotion; Sodium Sulamyd® Ophthalmic; Sulf-10® Ophthalmic

Synonyms Sodium Sulfacetamide

Generic Available Yes

Therapeutic Category Antibiotic, Ophthalmic

Use Treatment and prophylaxis of conjunctivitis due to susceptible organisms; corneal ulcers; adjunctive treatment with systemic sulfonamides for therapy of trachoma

Contraindications Hypersensitivity to sulfacetamide or any component, sulfonamides

Warnings Inactivated by purulent exudates containing PABA; use with caution in patients with severe dry eye; ointment may retard corneal wound healing

Precautions Inactivated by purulent exudates containing PABA; use with caution in severe dry eye; ointment may retard corneal epithelial healing; sulfite in some products may cause hypersensitivity reactions

Adverse Reactions
Central nervous system: Headache, brow ache
Dermatologic: Stevens-Johnson syndrome, exfoliative dermatitis, toxic epidermal necrolysis
Local: Irritation, stinging, burning
Ocular: Blurred vision
Miscellaneous: Hypersensitivity reactions

Drug Interactions Silver, gentamicin (antagonism)

Stability Protect from light; discolored solution should not be used; incompatible with silver and zinc sulfate; sulfacetamide is inactivated by blood or purulent exudates

Mechanism of Action Interferes with bacterial growth by inhibiting bacterial folic acid synthesis through competitive antagonism of PABA

Pharmacokinetics Unknown

Usual Dosage Geriatrics and Adults: Ophthalmic:
Ointment: Apply to lower conjunctival sac 1-4 times/day and at bedtime
Solution: Instill 1-2 drops every 2-3 hours in the lower conjunctival sac during the waking hours and less frequently at night

Monitoring Parameters Response to therapy

Patient Information Eye drops will burn upon instillation; wait at least 10 minutes before using another eye preparation; ointment may sting eyes when first applied and blur vision; do not touch dropper to eye to maintain sterility

Nursing Implications Eye drops will burn upon instillation (especially 30% solution); wait at least 10 minutes before administering another eye preparation

Additional Information Course of therapy is usually short-term; if infection does not clear in 7-10 days, need to reassess

Special Geriatric Considerations Assess whether patient can adequately instill drops or ointment

Dosage Forms
Ophthalmic:
Ointment: 10% (3.5 g)
Solution: 10% (1 mL, 2 mL, 3.75 mL, 5 mL, 15 mL); 15% (2 mL, 15 mL); 30% (5 mL, 15 mL)

Sulfacetamide Sodium and Phenylephrine
(sul fa SEE ta mide SOW dee um & fen il EF rin)

Related Information
Phenylephrine *on page 740*
Sulfacetamide Sodium *on previous page*

Brand Names Vasosulf® Ophthalmic

Therapeutic Category Antibiotic, Ophthalmic; Ophthalmic Agent, Vasoconstrictor

Use Treatment of conjunctivitis, corneal ulcer, other superficial ocular infections due to susceptible micro-organisms

Stability Keep tightly closed; protect from light

Usual Dosage Geriatrics and Adults: Instill 1 or 2 drops into the lower conjunctival sac(s) every 2 or 3 hours during the day, less often at night

Dosage Forms Solution, ophthalmic: Sulfacetamide sodium 15% and phenylephrine hydrochloride 0.125% (5 mL, 15 mL)

Sulfacetamide Sodium and Prednisolone
(sul fa SEE ta mide SOW dee um & pred NIS oh lone)

Related Information
Prednisolone *on page 774*
Sulfacetamide Sodium *on previous page*
(Continued)

Sulfacetamide Sodium and Prednisolone *(Continued)*

Brand Names AK-Cide® Ophthalmic; Blephamide® Ophthalmic; Cetapred® Ophthalmic; Isopto® Cetapred® Ophthalmic; Metimyd® Ophthalmic; Vasocidin® Ophthalmic

Synonyms Prednisolone Acetate and Sodium Sulfacetamide

Therapeutic Category Antibiotic, Ophthalmic; Corticosteroid, Ophthalmic

Use Steroid-responsive inflammatory ocular conditions where infection is present or there is a risk of infection

Contraindications Mycobacteria infections, fungal infections, hypersensitivity to sulfacetamide, prednisolone or any component

Precautions Inactivated by purulent exudates containing PABA; use with caution in severe dry eyes; ointment may retard corneal epithelial healing; sulfite in some products may cause hypersensitivity reactions

Adverse Reactions
Central nervous system: Vertigo, headache
Dermatologic: Stevens-Johnson syndrome, skin atrophy
Endocrine & metabolic: Cushing's syndrome, pituitary-adrenal axis suppression
Local: Irritation, stinging, burning
Ocular: Cataracts, glaucoma

Drug Interactions Silver, gentamicin, vaccines, toxoids

Usual Dosage Geriatrics and Adults:
Ointment: Apply to lower conjunctival sac 1-4 times/day
Solution/Suspension: Instill 1-3 drops every 2-3 hours

Patient Information Shake ophthalmic solution before using; eye drops will burn upon instillation; wait at least 10 minutes before using another eye preparation; ointment may sting eyes when first applied and blur vision; do not touch dropper to eye

Nursing Implications Shake ophthalmic suspension before using

Additional Information The ophthalmic suspension may be used as an otic preparation; usually duration of therapy is short-term; if infection and inflammation does not clear in 7-10 days, need to reassess

Special Geriatric Considerations Assess whether patient can adequately instill drops or ointment

Dosage Forms
Ophthalmic:
Ointment:
Blephamide®: Sodium sulfacetamide 10% and prednisolone acetate 0.2% (3.5 g)
Cetapred®: Sodium sulfacetamide 10% and prednisolone acetate 0.25% (3.5 g)
Metimyd®: Sodium sulfacetamide 10% and prednisolone acetate 0.5% (3.5 g)
Suspension:
Blephamide®: Sodium sulfacetamide 10% and prednisolone acetate 0.2% (2.5 mL, 5 mL, 10 mL)
Isopto® Cetapred®: Sodium sulfacetamide 10% and prednisolone acetate 0.25% (5 mL, 15 mL)
Optimyd®: Sodium sulfacetamide 10% and prednisolone sodium phosphate 0.5% (5 mL)
Vasocidin®: Sodium sulfacetamide 10% and prednisolone acetate 0.25% (5 mL, 10 mL)

Sulfalax® [OTC] *see* Docusate *on page 312*

Sulfamethoxazole *(sul fa meth OKS a zole)*

Brand Names Gantanol®; Urobak®

Generic Available Yes: Tablet

Therapeutic Category Antibiotic, Sulfonamide Derivative

Use Treatment of urinary tract infections, nocardiosis, toxoplasmosis, acute otitis media, and acute exacerbations of chronic bronchitis due to susceptible organisms

Contraindications Porphyria; known hypersensitivity to sulfa drug or any component

Warnings Should not be used for group A beta-hemolytic streptococcal infections

Precautions Maintain adequate fluid intake to prevent crystalluria; use with caution in patients with renal or hepatic impairment, and patients with G-6-PD deficiency

Adverse Reactions
Central nervous system: Dizziness, fever, headache

Dermatologic: Rash, exfoliative dermatitis, Stevens-Johnson syndrome, photosensitivity

Endocrine & metabolic: Folic acid deficiency (rare)

Gastrointestinal: Nausea, vomiting

Hematologic: Granulocytopenia, leukopenia, thrombocytopenia, aplastic anemia, hemolytic anemia

Hepatic: Jaundice

Renal: Acute nephropathy

Miscellaneous: Serum sickness-like reactions

Overdosage
Symptoms of overdose include drowsiness, dizziness, anorexia, abdominal pain, nausea, vomiting, hemolytic anemia, acidosis, jaundice

Drug Interactions
Decreased effect with PABA or PABA metabolites of drugs (ie, procaine, proparacaine, tetracaine)

Increased effect of oral anticoagulants and oral hypoglycemic agents

Stability
Protect from light

Mechanism of Action
Interferes with bacterial growth by inhibiting bacterial folic acid synthesis through competitive antagonism of PABA

Pharmacokinetics
Absorption: Oral: 90%

Protein binding: 70%

Metabolism: Primarily in the liver, with 10% to 20% as the N-acetylated form in the plasma

Half-life: 9-12 hours, prolonged with renal impairment; in elderly, half-life has been reported to be increased while total and renal clearances are decreased

Time to peak serum concentration: Within 3-4 hours

Elimination: Unchanged drug (20%) and its metabolites are excreted in urine

Usual Dosage
Oral:

Geriatrics: Same as adults unless Cl_{cr} <30 mL/minute; see below. Single dose or 3-day dosing has not been shown to be reliable for treating urinary tract infections in the elderly

Adults: 2 g stat, 1 g 2-3 times/day; maximum: 3 g/24 hours

Dosing interval in renal impairment: Cl_{cr} <30 mL/minute: Decrease dose by 50%

Moderately dialyzable (20% to 50%)

Monitoring Parameters
Temperature, WBC, urine analysis and culture, appetite, mental status

Reference Range
Therapeutic: Peak: 100-500 mg/L; Trough: 75-120 mg/L (not routinely monitored)

Test Interactions
Increased cholesterol (S), increased protein, increased uric acid (S)

Patient Information
Report sore throat, mouth sores, unusual bleeding or fever; drink plenty of fluid; avoid aspirin and vitamin C products; complete full course of therapy; wear sunscreen if going out in the sun

Nursing Implications
Shake suspension before administering; watch for signs of adverse reactions

Special Geriatric Considerations
Sulfamethoxazole is an effective anti-infective agent; most prescribers prefer the combination of sulfamethoxazole and trimethoprim for its dual mechanism of action; trimethoprim penetrates the prostate; adjust dose for renal function (see Usual Dosage and Pharmacokinetics)

Dosage Forms
Suspension, oral: 500 mg/5 mL (480 mL)

Tablet: 500 mg

References
Ljungberg B and Nilsson-Ehle I, "Pharmacokinetics of Antimicrobial Agents in the Elderly," *Rev Infect Dis*, 1987, 9(2):250-64.

Varoquaux O, Lajoie D, Gobert C, et al, "Pharmacokinetics of the Trimethoprim-Sulfamethoxazole Combination in the Elderly," *Br J Clin Pharmacol*, 1985, 20:575-81.

Sulfamethoxazole and Trimethoprim *see* Co-Trimoxazole *on page 253*

Sulfasalazine (sul fa SAL a zeen)
Brand Names
Azulfidine®; Azulfidine® EN-tabs®

Synonyms
Salicylazosulfapyridine

Generic Available
Yes

Therapeutic Category
5-Aminosalicylic Acid Derivative; Anti-inflammatory Agent

(Continued)

Sulfasalazine *(Continued)*

Use Management of ulcerative colitis
    Labeled use: Rheumatoid arthritis

Contraindications Hypersensitivity to sulfasalazine, sulfa drugs, or any component; porphyria, GI or GU obstruction; hypersensitivity to salicylates

Precautions Use with caution in patients with renal impairment; impaired hepatic function or urinary obstruction, blood dyscrasias, severe allergies or asthma, or G-6-PD deficiency

Adverse Reactions
Cardiovascular: Vasculitis
Central nervous system: Headache, fever, dizziness
Dermatologic: Rash, toxic epidermal necrolysis, itching, photosensitivity, Stevens-Johnson syndrome
Endocrine & metabolic: Folic acid deficiency, thyroid function disturbance
Gastrointestinal: Nausea, vomiting, diarrhea, anorexia
Genitourinary: Crystalluria
Hematologic: Hemolytic anemia, agranulocytosis, aplastic anemia, granulocytopenia, leukopenia
Hepatic: Hepatitis, jaundice
Renal: Hematuria, interstitial nephritis
Respiratory: Fibrosing alveolitis
Miscellaneous: Orange-yellow discoloration of urine and skin (rare), serum sickness-like reaction

Overdosage Symptoms of overdose include drowsiness, dizziness, anorexia, abdominal pain, nausea, vomiting, hemolytic anemia, acidosis, jaundice

Toxicology Doses of as little as 2-5 g/day may produce toxicity; the aniline radical is responsible for hematologic toxicity; high volume diuresis may aid in elimination and prevention of renal failure

Drug Interactions
Folic acid decreased absorption, digoxin decreased serum concentrations
Iron decreased sulfasalazine absorption
Decreased effect with PABA or PABA metabolites of drugs (ie, procaine, proparacaine, tetracaine); decreased effect of oral anticoagulants and oral hypoglycemic agents

Stability Protect from light; shake suspension well

Mechanism of Action Acts locally in the colon to decrease the inflammatory response and interferes with secretion by inhibiting prostaglandin synthesis

Pharmacokinetics
Absorption: Oral: Up to 33% as unchanged drug from the small intestine
Metabolism: Following absorption, both components are metabolized in the liver
Half-life: 5.7-10 hours; upon administration, the drug is split into sulfapyridine and 5-aminosalicylic acid (5-ASA) in the colon
Time to peak serum concentration:
    5-aminosalicylic acid (active metabolite): Within 1.5-6 hours
    Serum sulfapyridine (active metabolite): 6-24 hours
Elimination: Primary excretion in urine (as unchanged drug, components, and acetylated metabolites)

Usual Dosage Geriatrics and Adults: Oral: 1 g 3-4 times/day, 2 g/day maintenance in divided doses; not to exceed 6 g/day; individualize dose based upon patient's response; start with lower dose, 1-2 g/day, to avoid GI intolerance
    Rheumatoid arthritis: Initial: 500 mg 1-2 times/day increasing to 2 g/day in 2-4 divided doses

Dosing interval in renal impairment:
    Cl$_{cr}$ 10-30 mL/minute: Administer twice daily
    Cl$_{cr}$ <10 mL/minute: Administer once daily

Dosing adjustment in hepatic impairment: Avoid use

Monitoring Parameters Response to therapy, GI complaints

Patient Information Maintain adequate fluid intake; may cause orange-yellow discoloration of urine and skin; take after meals or with food; do not take with antacids; may permanently stain soft contact lenses yellow; avoid prolonged exposure to sunlight (wear sunscreen); do not chew or crush enteric coated tablets

Nursing Implications Shake suspension well; GI intolerance is common during the first few days of therapy; drug commonly imparts an orange-yellow discoloration to urine and skin

Additional Information This drug should be administered after food to reduce GI irritation. Sulfasalazine can be used as a disease-modifying agent

(DMARD) in the treatment of progressive rheumatoid arthritis that has not responded adequately to anti-inflammatory agents.

Special Geriatric Considerations Adjust dose for renal function (see Usual Dosage); see Additional Information

Dosage Forms
Suspension, oral: 250 mg/5 mL (473 mL)
Tablet: 500 mg
Tablet, enteric coated: 500 mg

Sulfatrim® *see Co-Trimoxazole on page 253*

Sulfinpyrazone (sul fin PEER a zone)

Brand Names Anturane®

Generic Available Yes

Therapeutic Category Uric Acid Lowering Agent; Uricosuric Agent

Use Treatment of chronic gouty arthritis and intermittent gouty arthritis

Unlabeled use: Decrease the incidence of sudden death postmyocardial infarction

Contraindications Active peptic ulcers, GI inflammation, blood dyscrasias, hypersensitivity to sulfinpyrazone or any component

Precautions Avoid in patients with a Cl$_{cr}$ <50 mL/minute (sulfinpyrazone loses its effectiveness and may cause acute renal failure); administer with caution to patients with healed peptic ulcers

Adverse Reactions
Cardiovascular: Flushing
Central nervous system: Dizziness, headache
Dermatologic: Rash
Gastrointestinal: Anorexia, nausea, vomiting
Hematologic: Anemia, leukopenia, increased bleeding time (decreased platelet aggregation)
Hepatic: Hepatic necrosis
Genitourinary: Polyuria
Renal: Uric acid stones, nephrotic syndrome

Overdosage Symptoms of overdose include nausea, vomiting, ataxia, respiratory depression, seizures

Toxicology Following GI decontamination, treatment is supportive only

Drug Interactions
Decreased effect of theophylline, verapamil; decreased uricosuric effects with salicylates, niacin
Increased effect of warfarin, tolbutamide
Risk of acetaminophen hepatotoxicity is increased, but therapeutic effects may be reduced

Mechanism of Action Inhibits renal tubular reabsorption of uric acid, thus promoting urinary excretion of uric acid and decreasing blood urate levels; also has antithrombic and platelet inhibitory effects

Pharmacokinetics
Absorption: Oral: Well absorbed
Protein binding: 98% to 99%
Metabolism: Inhibitor CYP2C9; inducer CYP3A4
Half-life: 2.2-3 hours
Elimination: ~50% of dose appears in urine unchanged

Usual Dosage Geriatrics and Adults: Oral: 100-200 mg twice daily increasing to 400 mg twice daily, monitoring uric acid concentrations; decrease to 200 mg/day as a maintenance dose (see Special Geriatric Considerations)

Monitoring Parameters Serum and urinary uric acid; CBC, renal function

Test Interactions Decreased uric acid (S)

Patient Information Take with food or milk; drink adequate fluids; avoid aspirin containing products

Additional Information This drug should only be used when other treatments for hyperuricemia or gout have failed or were not tolerated

Special Geriatric Considerations Since sulfinpyrazone loses its effectiveness when the Cl$_{cr}$ is <50 mL/minute and since many elderly have reduced creatinine clearances, its usefulness in the elderly is limited (see Additional Information)

Dosage Forms
Capsule: 200 mg
Tablet: 100 mg

References
Emmerson BT, "The Management of Gout," *N Engl J Med*, 1996, 334(7):445-51.

Sulfisoxazole (sul fi SOKS a zole)

Brand Names Gantrisin®

Synonyms Sulfisoxazole Acetyl; Sulphafurazole

Therapeutic Category Antibiotic, Sulfonamide Derivative

Use Treatment of urinary tract infections, otitis media, *Chlamydia*; nocardiosis

Contraindications Hypersensitivity to any sulfa drug or any component; porphyria; patients with urinary obstruction

Precautions Use with caution in patients with G-6-PD deficiency (hemolysis may occur), hepatic or renal impairment; dosage modification required in patients with renal impairment; risk of crystalluria should be considered in patients with impaired renal function

Adverse Reactions

Central nervous system: Dizziness, headache, fever, kernicterus

Dermatologic: Rash, Stevens-Johnson syndrome, photosensitivity

Endocrine & metabolic: Folic acid deficiency (rare), thyroid function disturbance

Gastrointestinal: Nausea, vomiting, anorexia, diarrhea

Genitourinary: Crystalluria

Hematologic: Thrombocytopenia, leukopenia, agranulocytosis, aplastic anemia, hemolytic anemia, granulocytopenia

Hepatic: Jaundice, hepatitis, serum sickness-like reactions

Renal: Nephrotoxicity, hematuria

Miscellaneous: Hypersensitivity reactions

Overdosage Symptoms of overdose include drowsiness, dizziness, anorexia, abdominal pain, nausea, vomiting, hemolytic anemia, acidosis, jaundice

Drug Interactions Increased effect of tolbutamide, chlorpropamide, oral anticoagulants (displaced from protein binding sites); PABA (antagonizes the antibacterial activity of sulfas); thiopental

Mechanism of Action Interferes with bacterial growth by inhibiting bacterial folic acid synthesis through competitive antagonism of PABA

Pharmacokinetics

Absorption: Sulfisoxazole acetyl is hydrolyzed in the GI tract to sulfisoxazole which is readily absorbed

Protein binding: 85% to 88%

Metabolism: Metabolized in the liver by acetylation and glucuronide conjugation to inactive compounds

Half-life: 4-7 hours, prolonged with renal impairment

Time to peak serum concentration: Within 2-3 hours

Elimination: Primarily in urine (95% within 24 hours), 40% to 60% as unchanged drug

In a single dose study, absorption and peak serum concentrations were similar in elderly and younger subjects; in the elderly, half-life was prolonged and renal and nonrenal clearance decreased

Usual Dosage

Pelvic inflammatory disease: 500 mg every 6 hours for 21 days; used in combination with ceftriaxone

Chlamydia trachomatis: 500 mg every 6 hours for 10 days

Geriatrics and Adults: Ophthalmic:

Ointment: Instill small amount to affected eye 1-3 times/day and at bedtime

Solution: Instill 1-2 drops to affected eye every 2-3 hours

Geriatrics: 2 g stat, 2-8 g/day every 6 hours; adjust dose for Cl_{cr}; single and 3-day dosing for urinary tract infections in the elderly are not reliable.

Adults: Oral: 2-4 g stat, 4-8 g/day in divided doses every 4-6 hours

Dosing interval in renal impairment:

Cl_{cr} 10-50 mL/minute: Administer every 8-12 hours

Cl_{cr} <10 mL/minute: Administer every 12-24 hours

>50% removed by hemodialysis

Monitoring Parameters Temperature, WBC, urine analysis and culture, appetite, mental status

Reference Range Therapeutic: 5-15 mg/dL; Toxic: >20 mg/dL (not routinely monitored)

Test Interactions False-positive protein in urine; false-positive urine glucose with Clinitest®

Patient Information Take with a glass of water on an empty stomach; avoid prolonged exposure to sunlight (wear sunscreen); report to physician any sore throat, mouth sores, rash, unusual bleeding, or fever; complete full course of therapy

Nursing Implications Administer around-the-clock rather than 4 times/day, 3 times/day, etc (ie, 12-6-12-6, not 9-1-5-9) to promote less variation in peak and trough serum concentrations; maintain adequate fluid intake; watch for signs of adverse reactions

Additional Information Lipo Gantrisin® and Gantrisin® are not to be used interchangeably; routine alkalinization of urine is normally not required

Special Geriatric Considerations Sulfisoxazole is an effective anti-infective agent; most prescribers prefer the combination of sulfamethoxazole and trimethoprim for its dual mechanism of action; trimethoprim penetrates the prostate; adjust dose for renal function

Dosage Forms

Ointment, ophthalmic: 4% (3.75 g)

Solution, ophthalmic: 4% (15 mL)

Syrup, as acetyl: 500 mg/5 mL (480 mL)

Tablet: 500 mg

References

Boisvert A, Barbeau G, and Belanger PM, "Pharmacokinetics of Sulfisoxazole in Young and Elderly Subjects," *Gerontology*, 1984, 30(2):125-31.

Sulfisoxazole Acetyl *see* Sulfisoxazole *on previous page*

Sulfisoxazole and Erythromycin *see* Erythromycin and Sulfisoxazole *on page 346*

Sulindac (sul IN dak)

Brand Names Clinoril®

Generic Available Yes

Therapeutic Category Analgesic, Non-narcotic; Anti-inflammatory Agent; Antipyretic; Nonsteroidal Anti-inflammatory Agent (NSAID), Oral

Use Management of inflammatory disease, rheumatoid disorders; acute gouty arthritis, osteoarthritis, ankylosing spondylitis, acute painful shoulder, bursitis, tendonitis

Contraindications Hypersensitivity to sulindac, any component, aspirin or other nonsteroidal anti-inflammatory drugs (NSAIDs)

Warnings A potentially fatal hypersensitivity has occurred with sulindac; GI toxicity (bleeding, ulceration, perforation); CNS effects may occur (headaches, confusion, depression); hypersensitivity, anaphylactoid reactions (intermittent tolmetin use more often); renal function decline, acute renal insufficiency, interstitial nephritis, dysuria, cystitis, hematuria, nephrotic syndrome, hyperkalemia in acute renal insufficiency, hyponatremia, papillary necrosis, hepatic function impairment; elderly have increased risk for adverse reactions to NSAIDs (see Special Geriatric Considerations)

Precautions Use with caution in patients with congestive heart failure, hypertension, decreased renal or hepatic function, history of GI disease (bleeding or ulcers), or those receiving anticoagulants; perform ophthalmologic evaluation for those who develop eye complaints during therapy (blurred vision, diminished vision, changes in color vision, retinal changes); NSAIDs may mask signs/symptoms of infections; photosensitivity reported

Adverse Reactions

Cardiovascular: Congestive heart failure, angina, hypertension, hypotension, arrhythmias, edema

Central nervous system: Headache, drowsiness, vertigo, dizziness, fatigue, hallucinations, confusion, depression, emotional lability, psychotic behavior, pyrexia

Dermatologic: Rash, urticaria, angioedema, Stevens-Johnson syndrome, exfoliative dermatitis, bruising, petechiae, purpura

Endocrine & metabolic: Hyperglycemia, hypoglycemia, hyperkalemia, gynecomastia, hyponatremia, fluid retention

Gastrointestinal: Dyspepsia, heartburn, nausea, diarrhea, constipation, flatulence, stomatitis, vomiting, abdominal pain, peptic ulcer, GI bleeding, GI perforation, gingival ulcers, pancreatitis, proctitis, paralytic ulcers, colitis, anorexia, weight loss, dry mucous membranes

Genitourinary: Impotence, azotemia

Hematologic: Neutropenia, anemia, agranulocytosis, bone marrow suppression, hemolytic anemia, hemorrhage, inhibition of platelet aggregation

Hepatic: Hepatitis, elevated LFTs, cholestatic jaundice

Neuromuscular & skeletal: Involuntary muscle movements, muscle weakness, tremors, weakness

Ocular: Vision changes

Otic: Tinnitus

Renal: Dysuria, polyuria, pyuria, oliguria, anuria, acute renal failure

Respiratory: Exacerbation of asthma, dyspnea

Miscellaneous: Thirst, diaphoresis

(Continued)

Sulindac *(Continued)*

Overdosage Symptoms include drowsiness, lethargy, disorientation, confusion, dizziness, numbness, paresthesia, nausea, vomiting, gastric irritation, abdominal pain, headache, tinnitus, sweating, blurred vision, muscle twitching, seizures, coma, acute renal failure, increased BUN and serum creatinine, hypotension, tachycardia, and metabolic acidosis

Toxicology Management of a nonsteroidal anti-inflammatory agent (NSAID) intoxication is primarily supportive and symptomatic. Fluid therapy is commonly effective in managing the hypotension that may occur following an acute NSAID overdose, except when this is due to an acute blood loss. Seizures tend to be very short-lived and often do not require drug treatment although recurrent seizures should be treated with I.V. diazepam. Since many of the NSAIDs undergo enterohepatic cycling, multiple doses of charcoal may be needed to reduce the potential for delayed toxicities.

Drug Interactions

DMSO or ASA may decrease sulindac serum concentration

May increase digoxin, methotrexate, and little effect on lithium serum concentrations or may decrease lithium concentrations

Aspirin may decrease NSAID serum concentrations

Other NSAIDs may increase adverse GI effects

Increased prothrombin time with anticoagulants

Decreased antihypertensive effects of ACE inhibitors, beta-blockers, and thiazide diuretics

Effects of loop diuretics may decrease

Increased response to sympathomimetics

Probenecid may increase toxicity of NSAIDs by increase in serum concentrations

Diuretics may increase risk of acute renal insufficiency; azotemia may be enhanced in elderly receiving loop diuretics

Mechanism of Action Inhibits prostaglandin synthesis, acts on the hypothalamus heat-regulating center to reduce fever, blocks prostaglandin synthetase action which prevents formation of the platelet-aggregating substance thromboxane A_2; decreases pain receptor sensitivity. Other proposed mechanisms of action are lysosomal stabilization, inhibition of kinin and leukotriene production, alteration of chemotactic factors, and inhibition of neutrophil activation. This latter mechanism may be the most significant pharmacologic action to reduce inflammation.

Pharmacodynamics

Onset of anti-inflammatory action: Within 7 days

Maximum response: 2-3 weeks

Pharmacokinetics

Absorption: Oral: 90%; sulindac is a prodrug and therefore requires metabolic activation

Protein binding: >90%

Half-life:

Parent: 7 hours

Active metabolite: 18 hours

Requires hepatic metabolism to sulfide metabolite (active) for therapeutic effects

Metabolism: In the liver to sulfone metabolites (inactive)

Time to peak serum concentration: 2-4 hours

Elimination: Principally in urine (50%) with some biliary excretion (25%)

Usual Dosage Geriatrics and Adults: Oral: 150-200 mg twice daily; not to exceed 400 mg/day (see Pharmacodynamics)

Monitoring Parameters Monitor response (pain, range of motion, grip strength, mobility, ADL function), inflammation; observe for weight gain, edema; monitor renal function; observe for bleeding, bruising; evaluate gastrointestinal effects (abdominal pain, bleeding, dyspepsia); mental confusion, disorientation, CBC, serum, creatinine, BUN, liver function tests

Test Interactions Increased chloride (S), increased sodium (S)

Patient Information Serious gastrointestinal bleeding can occur as well as ulceration and perforation. Pain may or may not be present. Avoid aspirin and aspirin-containing products while taking this medication. If gastric upset occurs, take with food, milk, or antacid. If gastric adverse effects persist, contact physician. May cause drowsiness, dizziness, blurred vision, and confusion. Use caution when performing tasks which require alertness (eg, driving). Do not take for more than 3 days for fever or 10 days for pain without physician's advice.

Nursing Implications Observe for edema and fluid retention; monitor blood pressure (see Overdosage, Monitoring Parameters, Patient Information, and Special Geriatric Considerations)

Additional Information Structurally similar to indomethacin but acts like aspirin; associated with the highest (one study) incidence of upper GI bleeds among NSAIDs; safest NSAID for use in mild renal impairment; maximum therapeutic response may not be realized for up to 3 weeks. There are no clinical guidelines to predict which NSAID will give which response in a particular patient. Trials with each must be initiated until response determined. Consider dose, patient convenience, and cost.

Special Geriatric Considerations Elderly are a high-risk population for adverse effects from nonsteroidal anti-inflammatory agents. As much as 60% of elderly who develop GI complications can develop peptic ulceration and/or hemorrhage asymptomatically. The concomitant use of H_2 blockers, omeprazole, and sucralfate is not effective as prophylaxis with the exception of NSAID-induced duodenal ulcers which may be prevented by the use of ranitidine. Misoprostol and proton pump inhibitors are the only agents proven to help prevent the development of NSAID-induced ulcers. Also, concomitant disease and drug use contribute to the risk for GI adverse effects. Use lowest effective dose for shortest period possible. Consider renal function decline with age. Use of NSAIDs can compromise existing renal function especially when Cl_{cr} is ≤30 mL/minute. Tinnitus may be a difficult and unreliable indication of toxicity due to age-related hearing loss or eighth cranial nerve damage. CNS adverse effects such as confusion, agitation, and hallucination are generally seen in overdose or high-dose situations, but elderly may demonstrate these adverse effects at lower doses than younger adults.

Dosage Forms Tablet: 150 mg, 200 mg

References

Brooks PM, Day RO, "Nonsteroidal Anti-inflammatory Drugs - Differences and Similarities," *N Engl J Med*, 1991, 324(24):1716-25.

Clinch D, Banerjee AK, Ostick G, "Absence of Abdominal Pain in Elderly Patients With Peptic Ulcer," *Age Ageing*, 1984, 13(2):120-3.

Clive DM, Stoff JS, "Renal Syndromes Associated With Nonsteroidal Anti-inflammatory Drugs," *N Engl J Med*, 1984, 310(9):563-72.

Graham DY, "Prevention of Gastroduodenal Injury Induced by Chronic Nonsteroidal Anti-inflammatory Drug Therapy," *Gastroenterology*, 1989, 96(2 Pt 2 Suppl):675-81.

Gurwitz JH, Avorn J, Ross-Degnan D, et al, "Nonsteroidal Anti-Inflammatory Drug-Associated Azotemia in the Very Old," *JAMA*, 1990, 264(4):471-5.

Hawkey CJ, Karrasch JA, Szczepaski L, et al, "Omeprazole Compared With Misoprostrol for Ulcers Associated With Nonsteroidal Anti-inflammatory Drugs," *N Engl J Med*, 1998, 338(11):727-34.

Knodel LC, "Preventing NSAID-Induced Ulcers: The Role of Misoprostol," *Consult Pharm*, 1989, 4:37-41.

Pounder R, "Silent Peptic Ulceration: Deadly Silence or Golden Silence?" *Gastroenterology*, 1989, 96:(2 Pt 2 Suppl)626-31.

Yeomans ND, Tulassay Z, Juhasz L, et al, "A Comparison of Omeprazole With Ranitidine for Ulcers Associated With Nonsteroidal Anti-inflammatory Drugs," *N Engl J Med*, 1998, 338(11):719-26.

Sulphafurazole *see* Sulfisoxazole *on page 880*

Sumatriptan Succinate (SOO ma trip tan SUKS i nate)

Brand Names Imitrex®

Therapeutic Category Antimigraine Agent

Use Acute treatment of migraine with or without aura

Unlabeled use: Cluster headaches

Contraindications I.V. use; use in patients with ischemic heart disease or Prinzmetal angina, patients with signs or symptoms of ischemic heart disease, uncontrolled HTN, use with ergotamine derivatives, hypersensitivity to any component, management of hemiplegic or basilar migraine

Warnings Use with caution in elderly, patients with hepatic or renal impairment; may cause mild, transient elevation of blood pressure; may cause coronary vasospasm

Precautions Safety and efficacy in cluster headache not established; chest tightness has been reported commonly but rarely associated with EKG changes

Adverse Reactions

Cardiovascular: Transient elevation of blood pressure may occur

Central nervous system: Dizziness, drowsiness, headache, numbness

Dermatologic: Skin rashes

Gastrointestinal: Abdominal discomfort

Endocrine & metabolic: Hot flashes, polydipsia, dysmenorrhea, dehydration

Local: Injection site reaction, burning sensation

(Continued)

Sumatriptan Succinate *(Continued)*

Neuromuscular & skeletal: Tightness in chest, neck pain, mouth discomfort, jaw discomfort, myalgia, tingling, weakness

Renal: Dysuria, renal calculus

Respiratory: Dyspnea

Miscellaneous: Thirst, hiccups, diaphoresis

Overdosage Symptoms of overdose include tremor, coronary vasospasm, seizures, erythema of extremities, reduced respiratory rate, ataxia, cyanosis, mydriasis, paralysis

Toxicology Treatment is continued monitoring with general supportive care

Drug Interactions Increased toxicity: Ergot-containing drugs

Stability Store at 2°C to 20°C (36°F to 86°F); protect from light

Mechanism of Action Selective agonist for serotonin (5-HT, receptor) in cranial arteries to cause vasoconstriction and reduces sterile inflammation associated with antidromic neuronal transmission correlating with relief of migraine

Pharmacokinetics

Oral:

Bioavailability: 15%; may be markedly increased in patients with liver disease

Half-life: 2.5 hours

Elimination: 37% excreted unchanged

Time to peak serum concentration: 2.5 hours

After S.C. administration:

Distribution: V_d: 50 L

Protein binding: 14% to 21%

Bioavailability: 97%

Half-life:

Distribution: 15 minutes

Terminal: 115 minutes

Time to peak serum concentration: 5-20 minutes

Elimination: In urine unchanged (22%), excreted as indole acetic acid metabolite (38%)

Usual Dosage Geriatrics and Adults:

Oral: 25 mg taken with adequate fluid; maximum recommended single dose is 100 mg; no data to demonstrate increased efficacy with larger doses >25 mg; if insufficient response by 2 hours, may repeat dose to a maximum of 100 mg. Doses may be repeated at 2-hour intervals **not** to exceed 300 mg/day total dose. If headache returns after an initial dose of the injection, additional doses of single tablets (up to 200 mg/day) may be given at intervals of at least 2 hours. If parenteral form is used prior to oral therapy, oral tablets may be used at 2-hour intervals to a maximum of 200 mg/day total dose. No evidence that doses >25 mg result in greater pain relief.

S.C.: 6 mg; a second injection may be administered at least 1 hour after the initial dose, but not more than 2 injections in a 24-hour period (see Special Geriatric Considerations)

Monitoring Parameters Monitor blood pressure, signs and symptoms of coronary vasospasm, response (resolution of migraine)

Patient Information If pain or tightness in chest or throat occurs, notify physician; pain at injection site lasts <1 hour; instruct about dosage maximum

Nursing Implications Do not administer I.V., may cause coronary vasospasm

Special Geriatric Considerations Use cautiously in elderly, particularly since many elderly have cardiovascular disease which would put them at risk for cardiovascular adverse effects; safety and efficacy in elderly (>65 years of age) have not been established; pharmacokinetic disposition is, however, similar to that in young adults

Dosage Forms

Injection: 12 mg/mL (0.5 mL, 2 mL)

Tablet: 25 mg, 50 mg

Sumycin® Oral *see* Tetracycline *on page 900*

Suppress® [OTC] *see* Dextromethorphan *on page 278*

Suprax® *see* Cefixime *on page 178*

Surfak® [OTC] *see* Docusate *on page 312*

Surmontil® *see* Trimipramine *on page 964*

Susano® *see* Hyoscyamine, Atropine, Scopolamine, and Phenobarbital *on page 472*

Sus-Phrine® *see* Epinephrine *on page 336*

Sustaire® *see* Theophylline *on page 902*

Syllact® [OTC] *see* Psyllium *on page 804*

Symadine® *see* Amantadine *on page 49*

Symmetrel® *see* Amantadine *on page 49*

Synacol® CF [OTC] *see* Guaifenesin and Dextromethorphan *on page 439*

Synacort® *see* Hydrocortisone *on page 462*

Synalar® *see* Fluocinolone *on page 391*

Synalar-HP® *see* Fluocinolone *on page 391*

Synalgos® [OTC] *see* Aspirin *on page 84*

Synemol® *see* Fluocinolone *on page 391*

Synthroid® *see* Levothyroxine *on page 534*

Syracol-CF® [OTC] *see* Guaifenesin and Dextromethorphan *on page 439*

Sytobex® *see* Cyanocobalamin *on page 257*

T₃ Sodium *see* Liothyronine *on page 539*

T₃/T₄ Liotrix *see* Liotrix *on page 541*

T₄ *see* Levothyroxine *on page 534*

Tac™-3 *see* Triamcinolone *on page 949*

Tac™-40 *see* Triamcinolone *on page 949*

Tacrine (TAK reen)

Brand Names Cognex® Oral

Synonyms Tetrahydroaminoacrine; THA

Generic Available No

Therapeutic Category Cholinergic Agent; Cholinesterase Inhibitor

Use Treatment of mild to moderate dementia of the Alzheimer's type

Contraindications Patients previously treated with the drug who developed jaundice and in those who are hypersensitive to tacrine or acridine derivatives

Warnings The use of tacrine has been associated with elevations in serum transaminases; serum transaminases (specifically ALT) must be monitored throughout therapy (see Monitoring Parameters for specific guidelines). Use extreme caution in patients with current evidence of a history of abnormal liver function tests; use caution in patients with bladder outlet obstruction, asthma, and sick sinus syndrome (tacrine may cause bradycardia). Tacrine may increase gastric acid secretion, therefore, closely monitor patients at increased risk for developing peptic ulcer disease.

Adverse Reactions

Central nervous system: Ataxia

Gastrointestinal: Diarrhea, nausea, vomiting, dyspepsia, anorexia

Hepatic: Elevated transaminases

Musculoskeletal: Myalgia

Note: In many of the studies comparing tacrine with placebo, there was a high incidence of physical complaints with placebo; overall frequency of adverse effects was 81% with tacrine and 75% with placebo

Toxicology General supportive measures; can cause a cholinergic crisis characterized by severe nausea, vomiting, salivation, sweating, bradycardia, hypotension, collapse, and convulsions; increased muscle weakness is a possibility and may result in death if respiratory muscles are involved

Tertiary anticholinergics, such as atropine, may be used as an antidote for overdosage. I.V. atropine sulfate titrated to effect is recommended; initial dose of 1-2 mg I.V. with subsequent doses based upon clinical response. Atypical increases in blood pressure and heart rate have been reported with other cholinomimetics when coadministered with quaternary anticholinergics such as glycopyrrolate.

Drug Interactions

Decreased effect of anticholinergics and potential decrease in tacrine effect

Increased effect of theophylline, cimetidine, succinylcholine, cholinesterase inhibitors, or cholinergic agonists; increased effect with cimetidine

Mechanism of Action A deficiency of cortical acetylcholine is thought to account for some of the symptoms of Alzheimer's disease; tacrine is a centrally-acting reversible cholinesterase inhibitor; it presumably acts by slowing the degradation of acetylcholine thus elevating acetylcholine levels in the cerebral cortex

Pharmacokinetics

Absorption: Reduced with food

Protein binding: 55%

Metabolism: Extensive by CYP1A2 (substrate inhibitor); saturable at relatively low doses

(Continued)

Tacrine *(Continued)*

Bioavailability, absolute: 17%

Half-life: 2-4 hours

No clinically relevant age-related changes in pharmacokinetics have been found

Usual Dosage Geriatrics and Adults: Initial: 10 mg 4 times/day; may increase by 40 mg/day every 6 weeks; maximum: 160 mg/day; best administered separate from meal times; see table.

Recommended ALT Monitoring and Dose Modification

ALT (SGPT)	Treatment and Monitoring Regimen
<2 x ULN*	Continue treatment according to recommended titration and monitoring schedule
<2 to >3 x ULN	Continue treatment according to recommended titration; monitor ALT weekly until return to normal limits
>3 to <5 x ULN	Reduce the daily dose of tacrine by 40 mg/day; monitor ALT levels weekly; resume dose titration and every other week monitoring when ALT returns to normal limits
>5 x ULN	Stop tacrine therapy; follow ALT levels weekly until within normal limits; may resume tacrine at 40 mg/day

*ULN = upper limit of normal.

Patients with clinical jaundice confirmed by elevated total bilirubin (>3 mg/dL) should not be rechallenged with tacrine

Monitoring Parameters Serum ALT every other week for 16 weeks, then every month for 2 months, and then every 3 months thereafter

Reference Range In clinical trials, serum concentrations >20 ng/mL were associated with a much higher risk of development of symptomatic adverse effects

Patient Information Effect of tacrine therapy is thought to depend upon its administration at regular intervals, as directed; take between meals if possible; if GI upset occurs, may take with meals; inform physician of the emergence of new events or any increase in the severity of existing adverse effects (those that occur upon initiation of therapy or an increase in dose, ie, nausea, vomiting, loose stools, diarrhea; and those that can occur later in therapy, ie, rash, jaundice, very light stools, or black stools); abrupt discontinuation of the drug or a large reduction in total daily dose (≥80 mg/day) may cause a decline in cognitive function and behavioral disturbances; unsupervised increases in the dose may also have serious consequences; do not change dose without consulting physician; be compliant with required liver tests

Nursing Implications See Monitoring Parameters and Usual Dosage

Special Geriatric Considerations Tacrine is not a cure for Alzheimer's disease. At least 25% of patients may not tolerate the drug and only 50% of patients demonstrate some improvement in symptoms or a slowing of deterioration. While worth a trial in mild to moderate dementia of the Alzheimer's type, patients and their families must be counseled about the limitations of the drug and the importance of regular monitoring of liver function tests. No specific dosage adjustments are necessary due to age.

Dosage Forms Capsule, as hydrochloride: 10 mg, 20 mg, 30 mg, 40 mg

References

Crismon ML, "Tacrine: First Drug Approved for Alzheimer's Disease," *Ann Pharmacother*, 1994, 28(6):744-51.

Davis KL, Thal LJ, Gamzu ER, et al, "A Double-Blind, Placebo-Controlled Multicenter Study of Tacrine for Alzheimer's Disease," *N Engl J Med*, 1992, 327(18):1253-9.

Farlow M, Gracon SI, Hershey LA, et al, "A Controlled Trial of Tacrine in Alzheimer's Disease," *JAMA*, 1992, 268(18):2523-9.

Knapp MJ, Knopman DS, Solomon PR, et al, "A 30-Week Randomized Controlled Trial of High-Dose Tacrine in Patients With Alzheimer's Disease," *JAMA*, 1994, 271(13):985-91.

Tagamet® *see* Cimetidine *on page 223*

Tagamet® HB [OTC] *see* Cimetidine *on page 223*

Talwin® *see* Pentazocine *on page 727*

Talwin® NX *see* Pentazocine *on page 727*

Tambocor™ *see* Flecainide *on page 385*

Tamine® [OTC] *see* Brompheniramine and Phenylpropanolamine *on page 130*

Tamoxifen (ta MOKS i fen)

Brand Names Nolvadex®

Generic Available No

Therapeutic Category Antineoplastic Agent, Hormone (Antiestrogen)

Use Palliative or adjunctive treatment of advanced breast cancer

   Unlabeled use: Treatment of mastalgia, gynecomastia, male breast cancer, and pancreatic carcinoma; studies are currently underway to evaluate use of tamoxifen as chemosuppressive therapy in women at high risk for primary breast cancer

Contraindications Hypersensitivity to tamoxifen

Warnings Decreased visual acuity; retinopathy and corneal changes have been reported with use for more than 1 year at doses above recommended; hypercalcemia in patients with bone metastasis; hepatocellular carcinomas have been reported in animal studies; endometrial hyperplasia and polyps have occurred

Precautions Use with caution in patients with leukopenia, thrombocytopenia, and hyperlipidemia

Adverse Reactions

   Cardiovascular: Edema, deep vein thrombosis, pulmonary embolism

   Central nervous system: Depression, headache

   Dermatologic: Rash, pruritus vulvae

   Endocrine & metabolic: Rarely hypercalcemia, hot flashes, fluid retention

   Gastrointestinal: Nausea, vomiting, weight gain, diarrhea, anorexia, abdominal cramps

   Hematologic: Thrombocytopenia, leukopenia

   Hepatic: Increased ALT, bilirubin, and alkaline phosphatase

   Neuromuscular & skeletal: Increased bone and tumor pain may occur at initiation of therapy which indicates a good tumor response and generally subsides rapidly

Overdosage Symptoms of overdose include hypercalcemia, edema

Toxicology General supportive care

Drug Interactions

   Anticoagulants may have increased effect when used with tamoxifen

   Bromocriptine increases serum concentrations of tamoxifen and N-desmethyl tamoxifen; erythromycin, cyclosporine, nifedipine, diltiazem may inhibit metabolism

Mechanism of Action Competitively binds to estrogen receptors on tumors and other tissue targets, producing a nuclear complex that decreases DNA synthesis and inhibits estrogen effects

Pharmacokinetics

   Metabolism: In the liver; substrate CYP1A2, 2A6, 2B6, 2D6, 2E1, 3A4

   Half-life: 7 days

   Time to peak serum concentration: Oral: Within 4-7 hours

   Elimination: In feces, with only small amounts appearing in urine; undergoes enterohepatic recycling

Usual Dosage Geriatrics and Adults: Oral: 10-20 mg twice daily (morning and evening)

Monitoring Parameters Monitor tumor, WBC, platelets

Test Interactions Transient increased serum calcium; T_4 elevations (no clinical evidence of hyperthyroidism)

Patient Information Report any vomiting that occurs after taking dose; women should be advised to notify their physician of vaginal bleeding or itching

Nursing Implications Monitor WBC and platelet counts

Additional Information "Hot flashes" may be countered by Bellergal-S® tablets; increase of bone pain usually indicates a good therapeutic response

   Myelosuppressive effects:

   WBC: Rare

   Platelets: None

   Onset (days): 7-10

   Nadir (days): 14

   Recovery (days): 21

Special Geriatric Considerations Studies have shown tamoxifen to be effective in the treatment of primary breast cancer in elderly women. Comparative studies with other antineoplastic agents in elderly women with breast cancer had more favorable survival rates with tamoxifen. Initiation of hormone (Continued)

Tamoxifen *(Continued)*

therapy rather than chemotherapy is justified for elderly patients with metastatic breast cancer who are responsive. Reduction of mortality and recurrence was greater in those studies that used tamoxifen for ≥2 years than those that use it for <2 years.

Dosage Forms Tablet, as citrate: 10 mg, 20 mg

References

Allan SG, Rodger A, Smyth JF, et al, "Tamoxifen as Primary Treatment of Breast Cancer in Elderly or Frail Patients: A Practical Management," *Br Med J [Clin Res]*, 1985, 290:358.

Taylor SG, Gelman RS, Falkson G, et al, "Combination Chemotherapy Compared to Tamoxifen as Initial Therapy for Stage IV Breast Cancer in Elderly Women," *Ann Intern Med*, 1986, 104:455-61.

Tamsulosin *(tam SOO loe sin)*

Brand Names Flomax™

Therapeutic Category Alpha-Adrenergic Blocking Agent

Use Treatment of signs and symptoms of benign prostatic hyperplasia (BPH); it is **not** indicated for the treatment of hypertension

Contraindications Hypersensitivity to tamsulosin

Warnings Signs and symptoms of orthostasis may occur; potential risk of syncope

Precautions BPH and prostate cancer may cause the same symptoms; carcinoma of the prostate should be ruled out; do not use in combination with other alpha-adrenergic blocking agents

Adverse Reactions

Cardiovascular: Orthostatic hypotension (0.2% to 0.4%), chest pain

Central nervous system: Headache, dizziness, somnolence, insomnia

Endocrine & metabolic: Decreased libido

Gastrointestinal: Diarrhea, nausea

Genitourinary: Ejaculation disturbances

Neuromuscular & skeletal: Back pain, asthenia

Ocular: Amblyopia

Respiratory: Rhinitis, pharyngitis, increased cough, sinusitis

Miscellaneous: Infection

Overdosage Symptoms of overdose include hypotension and headache

Toxicology Keep patient in supine position, consider use of intravenous fluids; if necessary, vasopressors should be used

Drug Interactions Cimetidine significantly decreased the clearance of tamsulosin which resulted in an increase in tamsulosin AUC (44%)

Drug/Food Interactions Taking tamsulosin in a fasting state increased the bioavailability by 30% and the C_{max} by 40% to 70%

Mechanism of Action Selectively blocks alpha$_1$-receptors in the prostate, prostatic capsule, prostatic urethra, and bladder neck; this causes relaxation of the smooth muscle in the bladder neck and prostate, resulting in an improvement in urine flow rate and reductions of symptoms of BPH

Pharmacokinetics

Absorption: >90% under fasting conditions

Protein binding: 94% to 99% to alpha$_1$-glycoprotein

Metabolism: Cytochrome P450 enzymes (specific ones not identified)

Bioavailability: Fasting: 30% increase

Half-life:

Healthy volunteers: 9-13 hours

Target population: 14-15 hours

Geriatrics: Slightly prolonged and AUC is increased by 40%

Elimination: 76% in urine as metabolites

Usual Dosage Geriatrics and Adults: Oral: Initial: 0.4 mg once daily approximately 30 minutes following the same meal each day; if response is inadequate after 2-4 weeks, the dose may be increased to 0.8 mg once daily

Monitoring Parameters Relief of symptoms, blood pressure

Patient Information Take approximately 30 minutes after the same meal each day. Do not chew, crush, or open the capsules. Though the incidence of orthostatic hypotension is minimal, patients should be instructed to rise slowly from a sitting or lying position. May cause dizziness, use caution when driving until you see how the medication affects you.

Nursing Implications Monitor for orthostasis; do not crush or open capsule

Additional Information If therapy with tamsulosin is discontinued or interrupted for several days, restart therapy at the 0.4 mg once daily dose

Special Geriatric Considerations See Pharmacokinetics, Adverse Effects

Dosage Forms Capsule, as hydrochloride: 0.4 mg

Tapazole® see Methimazole on page 603
Taractan® see Chlorprothixene on page 214
Tasmar® see Tolcapone on page 935
TAT see Tetanus Antitoxin on page 897
Tavist® see Clemastine on page 231
Tavist®**-1 [OTC]** see Clemastine on page 231
Tazicef® see Ceftazidime on page 188
Tazidime® see Ceftazidime on page 188
Tazobactam and Piperacillin see Piperacillin and Tazobactam on page 754
TCN see Tetracycline on page 900
Td see Diphtheria and Tetanus Toxoid on page 305
Tear Drop® **Solution [OTC]** see Artificial Tears on page 82
TearGard® **Ophthalmic Solution [OTC]** see Artificial Tears on page 82
Teargen® **Ophthalmic Solution [OTC]** see Artificial Tears on page 82
Tearisol® **Solution [OTC]** see Artificial Tears on page 82
Tears Naturale® **Free Solution [OTC]** see Artificial Tears on page 82
Tears Naturale® **II Solution [OTC]** see Artificial Tears on page 82
Tears Naturale® **Solution [OTC]** see Artificial Tears on page 82
Tears Plus® **Solution [OTC]** see Artificial Tears on page 82
Tears Renewed® **Ophthalmic Ointment [OTC]** see Ocular Lubricant on page 688
Tears Renewed® **Solution [OTC]** see Artificial Tears on page 82
Tebamide® see Trimethobenzamide on page 961
Tega-Vert® **Oral** see Dimenhydrinate on page 300
Tegopen® see Cloxacillin on page 243
Tegretol® see Carbamazepine on page 160
Tegretol-XR® see Carbamazepine on page 160
Tegrin®**-HC [OTC]** see Hydrocortisone on page 462
Telachlor® see Chlorpheniramine on page 208
Teladar® see Betamethasone on page 114
Teldrin® **[OTC]** see Chlorpheniramine on page 208
Temaril® see Trimeprazine on page 960

Temazepam (te MAZ e pam)
Related Information
Antacid Drug Interactions on page 1096
Anxiolytic/Hypnotic Use in Long-Term Care Facilities on page 1099
Benzodiazepines Comparison on page 1024
Federal OBRA Regulations Recommended Maximum Doses - Hypnotics on page 1057

Brand Names Restoril®
Generic Available Yes
Therapeutic Category Benzodiazepine; Hypnotic; Sedative
Use Short-term treatment of insomnia
Restrictions C-IV
Contraindications Hypersensitivity to temazepam or any component, there may be cross-sensitivity with other benzodiazepines; severe uncontrolled pain, pre-existing CNS depression or narrow-angle glaucoma; sleep apnea
Precautions Use with caution in patients with mental impairment, reflex slowing, or the potential for drug dependence
Adverse Reactions
Central nervous system: Drowsiness, dizziness, confusion, sedation, ataxia, headache
Gastrointestinal: Xerostomia, constipation, diarrhea, nausea, vomiting
Neuromuscular & skeletal: Impaired coordination
Ocular: Blurred vision
Respiratory: Decreased respiratory rate, apnea, laryngospasm
Miscellaneous: Physical and psychological dependence with prolonged use
Overdosage Symptoms of overdose include somnolence, confusion, coma, and diminished reflexes
Toxicology Treatment for benzodiazepine overdose is supportive; rarely is mechanical ventilation required

Flumazenil has been shown to selectively block the binding of benzodiazepines to CNS receptors, resulting in a reversal of benzodiazepine-induced sedation; however, its use may not alter the course of overdose
(Continued)

Temazepam *(Continued)*

Drug Interactions
CNS depressants and alcohol may increase CNS adverse effects

Benzodiazepines may decrease the effect of levodopa

Mechanism of Action Depresses all levels of the CNS, including the limbic and reticular formation, probably through the increased action of gamma-aminobutyric acid (GABA), which is a major inhibitory neurotransmitter in the brain

Pharmacodynamics Onset of hypnotic effect: 30 minutes to 1 hour; considered an intermediate-acting benzodiazepine; studies have shown that the elderly are more sensitive to the effects of benzodiazepines as compared to younger adults

Pharmacokinetics
Protein binding: 96%

Metabolism: In the liver

Half-life: 3.5-18.4 hours (mean: 8.8 hours)

Time to peak serum concentrations: Oral: Approximately 1.5 hours

Elimination: 80% to 90% in urine as inactive metabolites

Pharmacokinetics are not significantly affected by aging

Usual Dosage May be taken 30 minutes before the desired onset of sleep

Geriatrics: Initial: 7.5 mg at bedtime; may need to increase to 15 mg

Adults: 15-30 mg at bedtime

Monitoring Parameters Respiratory, cardiovascular and mental status

Reference Range Therapeutic: 26 ng/mL after 24 hours

Patient Information Avoid alcohol and other CNS depressants; may cause daytime drowsiness; avoid activities needing good psychomotor coordination until CNS effects are known; may cause physical or psychological dependence; avoid abrupt discontinuation after prolonged use; may be taken 30 minutes before bedtime

Nursing Implications Provide safety measures (ie, side rails, night light, and call button); remove smoking materials from area; supervise ambulation

Additional Information Causes minimal change in REM sleep patterns; reformulation of the commercial product now allows for a faster onset

Special Geriatric Considerations Because of its lack of active metabolites, temazepam is recommended in the elderly when a benzodiazepine hypnotic is indicated; hypnotic use should be limited to 10-14 days; if insomnia persists, the patient should be evaluated for etiology (see Pharmacodynamics, Usual Dosage)

Dosage Forms Capsule: 7.5 mg, 15 mg, 30 mg

References
Divoll M, Greenblatt DJ, Harmatz JS, et al, "Effect of Age and Gender on Disposition of Temazepam," *J Pharm Sci*, 1981, 70(10):1104-7.

Scharf MB, Berkowitz DV, and Brannen DE, "Effectiveness of Low-Dose Temazepam on Sleep Patterns in Geriatric Insomniac Subjects," *Consult Pharm*, 1993, 8(12):1367-73.

Temovate® *see* Clobetasol *on page 233*

Tempra® **[OTC]** *see* Acetaminophen *on page 16*

Tenex® *see* Guanfacine *on page 443*

Ten-K® *see* Potassium Chloride *on page 763*

Tenormin® *see* Atenolol *on page 88*

Tensilon® *see* Edrophonium *on page 328*

Terazol® Vaginal *see* Terconazole *on page 894*

Terazosin *(ter AY zoe sin)*

Brand Names Hytrin®

Generic Available No

Therapeutic Category Alpha-Adrenergic Blocking Agent, Oral

Use Management of mild to moderate hypertension; treatment of symptomatic benign prostatic hypertrophy (BPH)

Contraindications Hypersensitivity to terazosin, other alpha-adrenergic blockers, or any component

Warnings Can cause marked hypotension and syncope with sudden loss of consciousness with the first few doses. Anticipate a similar effect if therapy is interrupted for a few days, if dosage is increased rapidly, or if another antihypertensive drug is introduced.

Precautions Syncope and postural hypotension frequently occur with the first dose; use with caution in patients with confirmed or suspected coronary artery disease

Adverse Reactions

Cardiovascular: Orthostatic hypotension, syncope, palpitations, tachycardia, edema

Central nervous system: Dizziness, lightheadedness, nightmares, drowsiness, headache

Dermatologic: Rash

Endocrine & metabolic: Fluid retention

Gastrointestinal: Nausea, xerostomia

Genitourinary: Polyuria, incontinence

Neuromuscular & skeletal: Weakness

Respiratory: Nasal congestion

Overdosage Symptoms of overdose include hypotension, drowsiness, and shock

Toxicology Hypotension usually responds to I.V. fluids or Trendelenburg positioning. If unresponsive to these measures the use of a parenteral vasoconstrictor may be required (eg, norepinephrine 0.1-0.2 mcg/kg/minute titrated to response). Treatment is primarily supportive and symptomatic.

Drug Interactions Increased hypotensive effect with diuretics and other antihypertensive agents (especially beta-blockers)

Mechanism of Action An alpha$_1$-specific blocking agent with minimal alpha$_2$ effects; this allows peripheral postsynaptic blockade, with the resultant decrease in arterial tone, while preserving the negative feedback loop which is mediated by the peripheral presynaptic alpha$_2$-receptors

In BPH, terazosin relaxes the smooth muscle of the bladder neck, thus reducing bladder outlet obstruction

Pharmacokinetics

Absorption: Oral: Rapid

Protein binding: 90% to 95%

Metabolism: Extensive in the liver

Half-life: 9.2-12 hours; half-life is not significantly prolonged in elderly

Time to peak: Within 60 minutes

Elimination: In feces (60%) and urine (40%)

Usual Dosage Geriatrics and Adults: Oral:

Hypertension: Initial: 1 mg at bedtime; slowly increase dose to achieve desired blood pressure, up to 20 mg/day; usual dose: 1-5 mg/day

Benign prostatic hypertrophy: Initial: 1 mg at bedtime, increasing as needed; most patients require 10 mg/day; if no response after 4-6 weeks of 10 mg/day, may increase to 20 mg/day

Monitoring Parameters Blood pressure, standing and sitting/supine, urinary symptoms

Patient Information Report any gain of body weight; fainting sometimes occurs after the first dose, take first dose at bedtime; rise from sitting/lying carefully, may cause dizziness

Nursing Implications Syncope may occur usually within 90 minutes of the initial dose; administer initial dose at bedtime; assist patients with ambulation

Special Geriatric Considerations Adverse reactions such as dry mouth and urinary problems can be particularly bothersome in the elderly (see Warnings and Nursing Implications)

Dosage Forms

Capsule: 1 mg, 2 mg, 5 mg, 10 mg

Tablet: 1 mg, 2 mg, 5 mg, 10 mg

Terbinafine, Oral (TER bin a feen, OR al)

Brand Names Lamisil® Oral

Generic Available No

Therapeutic Category Antifungal Agent

Use Treatment of onychomycosis infections of the toenail or fingernail due to dermatophytes

Contraindications Hypersensitivity to terbinafine

Warnings

Symptomatic hepatobiliary dysfunction including cholestatic hepatitis have been reported to occur rarely. Discontinue terbinafine if hepatobiliary dysfunction occurs. Isolated reports of serious skin reactions (ie, Stevens-Johnson syndrome and toxic epidermal necrolysis). Discontinue terbinafine treatment if progressive skin rash occurs.

Terbinafine therapy is not recommended in patients with liver disease or renal impairment (creatinine clearance <50 mL/minute). A decrease in terbinafine clearance by ~50% has been reported. Changes in ocular lens and retina have been reported, clinical significance is unknown. Neutropenia has been

(Continued)

Terbinafine, Oral *(Continued)*

reported. If signs and symptoms of secondary infection occur, obtain a complete blood count. Discontinue therapy if neutrophil count is ≤1000 cells/mm³ and start supportive therapy. Transient decreases in absolute lymphocyte count have been observed. Clinical significance is unknown.

Adverse Reactions

Central nervous system: Headache (>10%)

Dermatologic: Rash, pruritus, urticaria, serious skin reactions (toxic epidermal necrolysis, Stevens-Johnson syndrome)

Gastrointestinal: Diarrhea, dyspepsia, abdominal pain, nausea, flatulence, abnormal taste, hepatobiliary dysfunction

Hematologic: Transient decrease in absolute lymphocyte count neutropenia

Hepatic: Elevated liver enzyme ≥2 times upper limit of normal range, cholestatic hepatitis

Ocular: Visual disturbance, changes in ocular lens and retina

Toxicology No information on human overdosage. Symptomatic and supportive treatment is recommended.

Drug Interactions

Decreases clearance of I.V. administered caffeine

Increases clearance of cyclosporine by 15%

Terbinafine clearance increased by rifampin (100%)

Terbinafine clearance decreased by terfenadine (16%), cimetidine (33%)

Mechanism of Action Terbinafine is a synthetic allylamine derivative which inhibits squalene epoxidase which is a key enzyme in sterol biosynthesis in fungi. The resulting deficiency in ergosterol within the cell wall causes fungi death.

Pharmacokinetics

Absorption: Oral: >70%

Metabolism: Extensive in liver

Bioavailability: ~40% after first-pass effect in the liver

Half-life: 200-400 hours

Time to peak concentration: 2 hours

Elimination: In urine (70%)

Usual Dosage Geriatrics and Adults: Oral:

Fingernail onychomycosis: 250 mg once daily for 6 weeks

Toenail onychomycosis: 250 mg once daily for 12 weeks

Monitoring Parameters Recommend baseline liver function tests, and repeat if therapy exceeds 6 weeks; consider monitoring CBC in patients with known or suspected immunodeficiency receiving terbinafine for more than 6 weeks

Patient Information Use the medication for the recommended treatment time. Nails will not look normal at end of treatment period; wait several months for healthy new nail growth.

Nursing Implications Observe for rashes or any evidence of serious skin reaction (see Warnings)

Additional Information Optimal clinical effect is seen some months after mycological cure and end of treatment due to the time required for healthy nail outgrowth. Mean time to overall success was approximately 10 months for toenails and 4 months for fingernails. When terbinafine taken with food, absorption increased by 20%. Terbinafine appears to be more effective than griseofulvin and at least as effective as itraconazole for the treatment of onychomycosis. Unlike itraconazole, terbinafine does not interact with drugs metabolized by cytochrome P-450 isoenzymes.

Special Geriatric Considerations No specific information on the systemic use of terbinafine in the elderly is available; however, since many elderly will have creatinine clearances <50 mL/minute, this drug is not a drug of choice for elderly with onychomycosis (see Warnings)

Dosage Forms Tablet: 250 mg

References

Brautigam M, Nolting S, Schopf RE, et al, "Randomised Double Blind Comparison of Terbinafine and Itraconazole for Treatment of Toenail Tinea Infection. Seventh Lamisil German Onychomycosis Study Group," *BMJ*, 1995, 311(7010):919-22.

Faergemann J, Anderson C, Hersle K, et al, "Double-Blind, Parallel-Group Comparison of Terbinafine and Griseofulvin the Treatment of Toenail Onychomycosis," *J Am Acad Dermatol*, 1995, 32(5 Pt 1):750-3.

Hofmann H, Brautigam M, Weidinger G, et al, "Treatment of Toenail Onychomycosis. A Randomized, Double-Blind Study With Terbinafine and Griseofulvin. LAGOS II Study Group," *Arch Dermatol*, 1995, 131(8):919-22.

Terbinafine, Topical (TER bin a feen, TOP i kal)
Brand Names Lamisil® Topical
Therapeutic Category Antifungal Agent, Topical
Use Topical antifungal for the treatment of tinea pedis (athlete's foot), tinea cruris (jock itch), and tinea corporis (ring worm)
  Unlabeled use: Cutaneous candidiasis and pityriasis versicolor
Contraindications Hypersensitivity to terbinafine or any component
Warnings For external use only
Adverse Reactions Local: Irritation, burning, itching, dryness
Stability Store at room temperature 5°C to 30°C (41°F to 86°F)
Mechanism of Action Synthetic alkylamine derivative which inhibits squalene epoxidases which is a key enzyme in sterol biosynthesis in fungi to result in a deficiency in ergosterol within fungal cell wall and result in fungal cell death
Pharmacokinetics
  Absorption: Topical: Limited
  Elimination: ~75% of cutaneously absorbed drug excreted in urine; 3.5% of administered dose recovered in urine and feces
Usual Dosage Geriatrics and Adults: Topical:
  Athlete's foot: Apply to affected area twice daily for at least 1 week, not to exceed 4 weeks
  Ringworm and jock itch: Apply to affected area once or twice daily for at least 1 week, not to exceed 4 weeks
Patient Information For external use only; not for oral, ophthalmic, or intravaginal use; if irritation or sensitivity occurs, discontinue use and notify physician
Nursing Implications See Usual Dosage
Special Geriatric Considerations No specific recommendations for use in the elderly; use as recommended in Usual Dosage
Dosage Forms Cream: 1% (15 g, 30 g)

Terbutaline (ter BYOO ta leen)
Related Information
  Asthma Guidelines *on page 1040*
  Inhaled Medications Comparison *on page 1034*
Brand Names Brethaire®; Brethine®; Bricanyl®
Generic Available No
Therapeutic Category Adrenergic Agonist Agent; Beta$_2$-Adrenergic Agonist Agent; Bronchodilator
Use Bronchodilator in reversible airway obstruction and bronchial asthma
Contraindications Hypersensitivity to terbutaline or any component
Warnings Use caution in patients with unstable vasomotor symptoms, diabetes, hyperthyroidism, prostatic hypertrophy, or a history of seizures; also use caution in the elderly and those patients with cardiovascular disorders such as coronary artery disease, arrhythmias, and hypertension
Precautions Excessive or prolonged use may lead to tolerance; paradoxical bronchoconstriction may occur with excessive use, if it occurs, discontinue terbutaline immediately. Deaths have been reported after excessive use of sympathomimetics; though the exact cause is unknown, cardiac arrest after a severe asthmatic crisis is suspected.
Adverse Reactions
  Cardiovascular: Tachycardia, palpitations, elevation or depression of blood pressure
  Central nervous system: Nervousness, CNS stimulation, hyperactivity, insomnia
  Gastrointestinal: GI upset
  Neuromuscular: Tremors (may be more common in the elderly)
Overdosage Symptoms of overdose include hypertension, tachycardia, seizures, angina, hypokalemia, and tachyarrhythmias
Toxicology In cases of overdose, supportive therapy should be instituted, and prudent use of a cardioselective beta-adrenergic blocker (eg, atenolol or metoprolol) should be considered, keeping in mind the potential for induction of bronchoconstriction in an asthmatic individual. Dialysis has not been shown to be of value in the treatment of an overdose with this agent.
Drug Interactions
  Decreased therapeutic effect: Beta-adrenergic blockers (eg, propranolol)
  Increased therapeutic effect: Inhaled ipratropium may increase duration of bronchodilation, nifedipine may increase FEV-1
(Continued)

Terbutaline *(Continued)*

Increased toxicity (cardiovascular): MAO inhibitors, tricyclic antidepressants, sympathomimetic agents (eg, amphetamine, dopamine, dobutamine), inhaled anesthetics (eg, enflurane)

Stability Store injection at room temperature; protect from heat, light, and from freezing; use only clear solutions

Mechanism of Action Relaxes bronchial smooth muscle by action on beta$_2$-receptors with less effect on heart rate (minor beta$_1$ activity)

Pharmacodynamics S.C. doses are more bioavailable and of quicker onset than oral doses

Onset of action:
Oral: Within 30-45 minutes
Inhalation: 5-30 minutes
S.C.: Within 6-15 minutes
Duration of action:
Oral: 4-8 hours
Inhalation: 3-6 hours
S.C.: 1.5-4 hours

Pharmacokinetics
Protein binding: 25%
Metabolism: In the liver to inactive sulfate conjugates
Half-life: 11-16 hours
Elimination: In urine

Usual Dosage Geriatrics and Adults:
Oral: 2.5-5 mg/dose every 8 hours; maintenance: do not exceed 15 mg/24 hours
Inhalation: 2 puffs every 4-6 hours
S.C.: 0.25 mg/dose repeated in 15-30 minutes for one time only; a total dose of 0.5 mg should not be exceeded within a 4-hour period. **Note:** Side effects to S.C. dose are similar to epinephrine in severity.

Monitoring Parameters Pulmonary function, blood pressure, pulse

Patient Information Do not exceed recommended dosage; rinse mouth with water following each inhalation to help with dry throat and mouth. Follow specific instructions accompanying inhaler. If more than one inhalation is necessary, wait at least 1 full minute between inhalations. May cause nervousness, restlessness, insomnia - if these effects continue after dosage reduction, notify physician. Also notify physician if palpitations, tachycardia, chest pain, muscle tremors, dizziness, headache, flushing, or if breathing difficulty persists.

Nursing Implications Parenteral form is only for S.C. use. Before using, the inhaler must be shaken well; assess lung sounds, pulse, and blood pressure before administration and during peak of medication; observe patient for wheezing after administration, if this occurs, call physician.

Special Geriatric Considerations Oral terbutaline should be avoided in the elderly due to the increased incidence of adverse effects as compared to the inhaled form. Elderly patients may find it useful to utilize a spacer device when using the metered dose inhaler. Difficulty in using the inhaler often limits its effectiveness.

Dosage Forms
Terbutaline sulfate:
Aerosol, oral: 0.2 mg/actuation (10.5 g)
Injection: 1 mg/mL (1 mL)
Tablet: 2.5 mg, 5 mg

Terconazole *(ter KONE a zole)*

Brand Names Terazol® Vaginal

Synonyms Triaconazole

Therapeutic Category Antifungal Agent, Vaginal

Use Local treatment of vulvovaginal candidiasis

Adverse Reactions
Central nervous system: Headache
Dermatologic: Urticaria, rash
Local: Irritation, burning, itching
Neuromuscular & skeletal: Myalgia

Mechanism of Action Exact mechanism of action is unknown; it is proposed that terconazole disrupts fungal cell wall permeability

Pharmacokinetics Absorption: Extent of systemic absorption after vaginal administration may be dependent on the presence of a uterus; 5% to 8% in women who had a hysterectomy versus 12% to 16% in nonhysterectomized women

Usual Dosage Geriatrics and Adults: One applicatorful in vagina at bedtime for 7 consecutive days

Monitoring Parameters Response to treatment

Patient Information Follow directions included with products; complete full course of therapy; notify physician if irritating; use sanitary napkin to protect clothing

Nursing Implications Watch for local irritation; assist patient in administration, if necessary

Special Geriatric Considerations Assess patient's ability to self-administer, may be difficult in patients with arthritis or limited range of motion

Dosage Forms
Cream, vaginal: 0.4% (45 g); 0.8% (20 g)
Suppository, vaginal: 80 mg (3s)

References
Drug Facts and Comparisons, St Louis, MO: 1989, 528-9.

Terramycin® I.M. Injection *see Oxytetracycline on page 709*
Terramycin® Oral *see Oxytetracycline on page 709*
Tesamone® Injection *see Testosterone on this page*
Tessalon® Perles *see Benzonatate on page 109*
Testoderm® Transdermal System *see Testosterone on this page*
Testopel® Pellet *see Testosterone on this page*

Testosterone (tes TOS ter one)

Brand Names Androderm® Transdermal System; Andro-L.A.® Injection; Andropository® Injection; Delatest® Injection; Delatestryl® Injection; depAndro® Injection; Depotest® Injection; Depo®-Testosterone Injection; Duratest® Injection; Durathate® Injection; Everone® Injection; Histerone® Injection; Tesamone® Injection; Testoderm® Transdermal System; Testopel® Pellet

Synonyms Aqueous Testosterone

Generic Available Yes

Therapeutic Category Androgen

Use Male hypogonadism, inoperable breast cancer; also used as androgen replacement therapy in the treatment of delayed male puberty

Restrictions C-III

Contraindications Severe renal or cardiac disease, benign prostatic hypertrophy with obstruction, undiagnosed genital bleeding, males with carcinoma of the breast or prostate; hypersensitivity to testosterone or any component

Warnings Has both androgenic and anabolic activity, the anabolic action may enhance hypoglycemia

Precautions May cause hypercalcemia in women with breast cancer, monitor for hepatotoxicity; may cause urethral obstruction in patients with BPH

Adverse Reactions
Cardiovascular: Flushing, edema
Central nervous system: Excitation, aggressive behavior, sleeplessness, anxiety, mental depression, headache
Dermatologic: Acne (>10%), hirsutism (increase in pubic hair growth)
Endocrine & metabolic: Menstrual problems (amenorrhea) (>10%), virilism (>10%), breast soreness (>10%), gynecomastia, hypercalcemia, hypoglycemia
Gastrointestinal: Nausea, vomiting, GI irritation
Genitourinary: Epididymitis (>10%), priapism (>10%), bladder irritability (>10%), prostatic hypertrophy, prostatic carcinoma, impotence, testicular atrophy
Hematologic: Leukopenia, suppression of clotting factors, polycythemia
Hepatic: Hepatic dysfunction, cholestatic hepatitis, hepatic necrosis
Miscellaneous: Hypersensitivity reactions

Drug Interactions Cytochrome P-450 3A enzyme substrate
Insulin: Increased effect of insulin
Cyclosporine: Increased risk of toxicity
Warfarin: Increased hypoprothrombinemic effect

Mechanism of Action Principal endogenous androgen responsible for promoting the growth and development of the male sex organs and maintaining secondary sex characteristics in androgen-deficient males

Pharmacokinetics
Protein binding: 98% (to transcortin and albumin)
Metabolism: In the liver; substrate CYP3A4, 3A5-7
(Continued)

Testosterone *(Continued)*

Half-life: 10-100 minutes

Elimination: In urine (90%) and feces via bile (6%)

Usual Dosage Adults:

Inoperable breast cancer: I.M.:

Enanthate or cypionate salt: 200-400 mg every 2-4 weeks

Aqueous suspension: 50-100 mg 3 times/week

Hypogonadism: Male:

I.M.:

Testosterone or testosterone propionate: 10-25 mg 2-3 times/week

Testosterone cypionate or enanthate: 50-400 mg every 2-4 weeks

Postpubertal cryptorchism: Testosterone or testosterone propionate: 10-25 mg 2-3 times/week

Topical: Transdermal:

Testoderm®: Initial: 6 mg/day system applied daily applied on scrotal skin. If scrotal area is inadequate, start with a 4 mg/day system. Transdermal system should be worn for 22-24 hours. Determine total serum testosterone after 3-4 weeks of daily application. If patients have not achieved desired results after 6-8 weeks of therapy, another form of testosterone replacement therapy should be considered.

Androderm®: 2 systems every night (leave on for 24 hours). Do **not** apply to scrotum. Apply to clean, dry area on back, abdomen, upper arms, or thighs. Rotate sites. After confirming testosterone serum concentrations, dosage may be increased to 3 systems or decreased to 1 system nightly.

Dosing adjustment/comments in hepatic disease: Reduce dose

Monitoring Parameters Periodic liver function tests

Reference Range Testosterone, urine: Male: 100-1500 ng/24 hours; Female: 100-500 ng/24 hours

Test Interactions May cause a decrease in creatinine and creatine excretion and an increase in the excretion of 17-ketosteroids, thyroid function tests

Patient Information Virilization may occur in female patients; report menstrual irregularities; male patients report persistent penile erections; all patients should report persistent GI distress, diarrhea, or jaundice. Instruct on proper placement of transdermal patch (see Usual Dosage).

Nursing Implications Warm injection to room temperature and shaking vial will help redissolve crystals that have formed after storage; administer by deep I.M. injection into the upper outer quadrant of the gluteus maximus. Testoderm® should be applied on clean, dry, scrotal skin. Dry-shave scrotal hair for optimal skin contact. Do not use chemical depilatories. Androderm® should **not** be applied to scrotum.

Additional Information

Testosterone (aqueous): Andro®, Histerone®, Tesanone®

Testosterone cypionate: Andro-Cyp®, Andronate®, Depotest®, Depo®-Testosterone, Duratest®

Testosterone enanthate: Andro-L.A.®, Andropository®, Delatestryl®, Durathate®, Everone®, Testrin® P.A.

Testosterone propionate: Testex®

Special Geriatric Considerations Elderly males treated with androgens may be at increased risk of developing prostatic hypertrophy and prostatic carcinoma; increase in libido may occur

Dosage Forms

Injection:

Aqueous suspension: 25 mg/mL (10 mL, 30 mL); 50 mg/mL (10 mL, 30 mL); 100 mg/mL (10 mL, 30 mL)

In oil, as cypionate: 100 mg/mL (1 mL, 10 mL); 200 mg/mL (1 mL, 10 mL)

In oil, as enanthate: 100 mg/mL (5 mL, 10 mL); 200 mg/mL (5 mL, 10 mL)

In oil, as propionate: 50 mg/mL (10 mL, 30 mL); 100 mg/mL (10 mL, 30 mL)

Pellet: 75 mg (1 pellet per vial)

Transdermal system:

Androderm®: 2.5 mg/day

Testoderm®: 4 mg/day; 6 mg/day

References

Cunningham GR, Cordero E, and Thornby JI, "Testosterone Replacement With Transdermal Therapeutic Systems. Physiological Serum Testosterone and Elevated Dihydrotestosterone Levels," *JAMA*, 1989, 261(17):2525-30.

Ruch W and Jenny P, "Priapism Following Testosterone Administration for Delayed Male Puberty," *Am J Med*, 1989, 86(2):256.

Testred® *see* Methyltestosterone *on page 613*

Tetanus and Diphtheria Toxoid *see* Diphtheria and Tetanus Toxoid *on page 305*

Tetanus Antitoxin (TET a nus an tee TOKS in)
Synonyms TAT
Therapeutic Category Antitoxin
Use Tetanus prophylaxis or treatment of active tetanus only when tetanus immune globulin (TIG) is not available; may be given concomitantly with tetanus toxoid adsorbed when immediate treatment is required, but active immunization is desirable
Contraindications Patients sensitive to equine-derived preparations
Warnings Tetanus antitoxin is not the same as tetanus immune globulin
Adverse Reactions
Dermatologic: Skin eruptions, erythema, urticaria
Local: Local pain, numbness
Neuromuscular & skeletal: Arthralgia
Miscellaneous: Anaphylaxis, serum sickness may develop up to several weeks after injection in 10% of patients
Stability Refrigerate
Mechanism of Action Solution of concentrated globulins containing antitoxic antibodies obtained from horse serum after immunization against tetanus toxin
Pharmacodynamics Protection from antitoxin lasts 15 days; this time is decreased in individuals who have received horse serum injections
Usual Dosage Geriatrics and Adults:
Prophylaxis (perform equine serum sensitivity tests): I.M., S.C.: >30 kg: 3000-5000 units
Treatment: Inject 10,000-40,000 units into wound; administer 40,000-100,000 units I.V.; preferable to administer part of I.V. dose I.M. or into wound (see Additional Information)
Nursing Implications All patients should have sensitivity testing prior to starting therapy with tetanus antitoxin
Additional Information Tetanus immune globulin (Hyper-Tet®) is the preferred tetanus immunoglobulin for the treatment of active tetanus
Special Geriatric Considerations Tetanus is a rare disease in U.S. with <100 cases annually; 66% of cases occur in persons >50 years of age; protective tetanus and diphtheria antibodies decline with age; it is estimated that <50% of elderly are protected.

Elderly are at risk because:
Many lack proper immunization maintenance
Higher case fatality ratio
Immunizations are not available from childhood
Indications for vaccination:
Primary series with combined tetanus-diphtheria (Td) should be given to all elderly lacking a clean history of vaccination
Boosters should be given at 10-year intervals; earlier for wounds
Elderly are more likely to require tetanus immune globulin with infection of tetanus due to lower antibody titer
Dosage Forms Injection, equine: Not less than 400 units/mL in 5000 and 20,000 unit vials

Tetanus Immune Globulin, Human
(TET a nus i MYUN GLOB yoo lin, HYU man)
Related Information
Immunization Guidelines *on page 1058*
Brand Names Hyper-Tet®
Synonyms TIG
Therapeutic Category Immune Globulin
Use Passive immunization against tetanus
Contraindications Hypersensitivity to tetanus immune globulin, thimerosal, or any immune globulin product or component; patients with IgA deficiency; I.V. administration
Warnings Have epinephrine 1:1000 available for anaphylactic reactions; do not administer I.V.
Precautions TIG is preferred over tetanus antitoxin for passive immunity; tetanus antitoxin should only be used when TIG is unavailable due to high risk of adverse effects (ie, serum sickness); skin testing should not be done
Adverse Reactions
Central nervous system: Fever (mild), lethargy
(Continued)

Tetanus Immune Globulin, Human *(Continued)*

Dermatologic: Urticaria, angioedema
Gastrointestinal: Nausea
Local: Pain, tenderness, erythema
Neuromuscular & skeletal: Muscle stiffness, myalgia
Respiratory: Chest tightness
Miscellaneous: Anaphylaxis reaction

Drug Interactions Never administer tetanus toxoid and TIG in same syringe (toxoid will be neutralized); toxoid should be administered at a separate site

Stability Refrigerate at 2°C to 8°C (36°F to 46°F)

Mechanism of Action If given at time of injury, it will not interfere with primary immune response to tetanus toxoid given at a separate site

Pharmacokinetics Half-life (tetanus toxoids): 3.5-4.5 weeks

Usual Dosage Geriatrics and Adults: I.M.:
Prophylaxis of tetanus: 250 units
Treatment of tetanus: 3000-6000 units

Monitoring Parameters Monitor for hypersensitivity reactions

Patient Information Be aware of adverse reactions

Nursing Implications Do not administer I.V.

Additional Information Tetanus immune globulin is preferred over tetanus antitoxin for treatment of active tetanus

Special Geriatric Considerations Tetanus is a rare disease in U.S. with <100 cases annually; 66% of cases occur in persons >50 years of age; protective tetanus and diphtheria antibodies decline with age; it is estimated that <50% of elderly are protected.

Elderly are at risk because:
Many lack proper immunization maintenance
Higher case fatality ratio
Immunizations are not available from childhood
Indications for vaccination:
Primary series with combined tetanus-diphtheria (Td) should be given to all elderly lacking a clear history of vaccination
Boosters should be given at 10-year intervals; earlier for wounds
Elderly are more likely to require tetanus immune globulin with infection of tetanus due to lower antibody titer

Dosage Forms Injection: 250 units

Tetanus Toxoid, Adsorbed *(TET a nus TOKS oyd, ad SORBED)*

Related Information
Immunization Guidelines *on page 1058*

Therapeutic Category Toxoid

Use Active immunity against tetanus

Contraindications Hypersensitivity to tetanus toxoid or any component; acute respiratory infections or other active infections

Warnings Not equivalent to tetanus toxoid fluid; the tetanus toxoid adsorbed is the preferred toxoid for immunization; do not use to treat active tetanus infections or use for immediate prophylaxis; allergic reactions, have epinephrine 1:1000 available for anaphylactic reactions

Precautions Avoid use in patients who receive immunosuppressive therapy or have immunodeficiency diseases; do not administer I.V.

Adverse Reactions
Cardiovascular: Flushing, tachycardia, hypotension, local edema
Central nervous system: Malaise and transient fever, rarely neurological disturbances (radial nerve paralysis, dysphagia), chills
Dermatologic: Urticaria, rash, pruritus
Local: Redness, warmth, induration, tenderness
Neuromuscular & skeletal: Generalized aches, pains
Miscellaneous: Arthus-type hypersensitivity reactions have occurred rarely in patients >25 years of age and who have received multiple booster doses

Drug Interactions If primary immunization is started in individuals receiving an immunosuppressive agent, serologic testing may be needed to ensure adequate antibody response; chloramphenicol may interfere with response

Stability Refrigerate, do not freeze

Mechanism of Action Boosters are necessary every 10 years: 0.5 mL

Usual Dosage Geriatrics and Adults: I.M.: 0.5 mL in deltoid or midlateral thigh muscles; primary immunization requires 2 injections 4-8 weeks apart; administer a third injection 6-12 months after second injection; boosters every 10 years

Patient Information Be aware of adverse reactions

Nursing Implications Inject intramuscularly in the area of the vastus lateralis (midthigh laterally) or deltoid

Additional Information Routine booster doses are recommended only every 10 years

Special Geriatric Considerations Tetanus is a rare disease in U.S. with <100 cases annually; 66% of cases occur in persons >50 years of age; protective tetanus and diphtheria antibodies decline with age; it is estimated that <50% of elderly are protected.

Elderly are at risk because:
  Many lack proper immunization maintenance
  Higher case fatality ratio
  Immunizations are not available from childhood
Indications for vaccination:
  Primary series with combined tetanus-diphtheria (Td) should be given to all elderly lacking a clean history of vaccination
  Boosters should be given at 10-year intervals; earlier for wounds
  Elderly are more likely to require tetanus immune globulin with infection of tetanus due to lower antibody titer

Dosage Forms Injection: Adsorbed: Tetanus 5 Lf units per 0.5 mL dose (0.5 mL, 5 mL); tetanus 10 Lf units per 2.5 mL dose (5 mL)

References
Bentley DW, "Vaccinations," *Clin Geriatr Med*, 1992, 8(4):745-60.
Gardner P and Schaffner W, "Immunization of Adults," *N Engl J Med*, 1993, 328(17):1252-8.

Tetanus Toxoid, Fluid (TET a nus TOKS oyd, FLOO id)

Related Information
  Immunization Guidelines *on page 1058*

Synonyms Tetanus Toxoid Plain

Therapeutic Category Toxoid

Use Active immunization against tetanus in adults

Contraindications Prior hypersensitivity reactions, neurological signs or symptoms after prior administrations; respiratory infections or other active infections or use for immediate prophylaxis; allergic reactions, have epinephrine 1:1000 available to treat anaphylactic reactions

Warnings For primary immunization, tetanus toxoid, absorbed is preferred; do not use to treat active infections

Precautions Concomitant immunosuppressive therapy, allergic reactions; do not administer I.V.

Adverse Reactions
  Cardiovascular: Flushing, tachycardia, hypotension, local edema
  Central nervous system: Malaise and transient fever, chills, rarely neurological disturbances (radial nerve paralysis, dysphagia)
  Dermatologic: Urticaria, rash, pruritus
  Local: Redness, warmth, induration, tenderness
  Neuromuscular & skeletal: Generalized aches, pains
  Miscellaneous: Arthus-type hypersensitivity reactions have occurred rarely in patients >25 years of age and who have received multiple booster doses

Reactions rarely occur in patients receiving tetanus toxoid fluid intradermally

Drug Interactions If primary immunization is started in individuals receiving an immunosuppressive agent, serologic testing may be needed to ensure adequate antibody response; chloramphenicol may interfere with response

Stability Refrigerate, do not freeze

Usual Dosage Geriatrics and Adults: Inject 3 doses of 0.5 mL I.M. or S.C. at 4- to 8-week intervals with fourth dose given only 6-12 months after third dose; boosters every 10 years

Patient Information A nodule may be palpable at the injection site for a few weeks; be aware of adverse reactions

Nursing Implications Must not be used I.V.

Additional Information Tetanus toxoid, adsorbed is preferred for all basic immunizing and recall reactions because of more persistent antitoxin titer induction

Special Geriatric Considerations Tetanus is a rare disease in U.S. with <100 cases annually; 66% of cases occur in persons >50 years of age; protective tetanus and diphtheria antibodies decline with age; it is estimated that <50% of elderly are protected.

Elderly are at risk because:
  Many lack proper immunization maintenance
  Higher case fatality ratio
(Continued)

Tetanus Toxoid, Fluid *(Continued)*

Immunizations are not available from childhood
Indications for vaccination:
Primary series with combined tetanus-diphtheria (Td) should be given to all
elderly lacking a clean history of vaccination
Boosters should be given at 10-year intervals; earlier for wounds
Elderly are more likely to require tetanus immune globulin with infection of
tetanus due to lower antibody titer

Dosage Forms Injection: Fluid: Tetanus 4 Lf units per 0.5 mL dose (7.5 mL);
tetanus 5 Lf units per 0.5 mL dose (0.5 mL, 7.5 mL)

References
Gardner P and Schaffner W, "Immunization of Adults," *N Engl J Med*, 1993, 328(17):1252-8.

Tetanus Toxoid Plain *see* Tetanus Toxoid, Fluid *on previous page*

Tetracycline *(tet ra SYE kleen)*

Related Information
Antacid Drug Interactions *on page 1096*
Penicillins, Penicillin-Related Antibiotics, & Other Antibiotics *on page 1010*
Regimens Used to Treat *Helicobacter pylori* and Ulcers *on page 1033*

Brand Names Achromycin® Ophthalmic; Achromycin® Topical; Achromycin®
V Oral; Nor-tet® Oral; Panmycin® Oral; Sumycin® Oral; Topicycline® Topical

Synonyms TCN

Therapeutic Category Acne Products; Antibacterial, Topical; Antibiotic,
Ophthalmic; Antibiotic, Tetracycline Derivative; Antibiotic, Topical

Use Treatment of susceptible bacterial infections of both gram-positive and
gram-negative organisms; also some unusual organisms including *Mycoplasma*, *Chlamydia*, and *Rickettsia*; may also be used for acne, exacerbations
of chronic bronchitis; treatment of gonorrhea and syphilis in patients that are
allergic to penicillin; treatment of Lyme disease

Contraindications Hypersensitivity to tetracycline or any component

Warnings Photosensitivity reaction may occur with this drug; avoid prolonged
exposure to sunlight or tanning equipment; wear sunscreen

Precautions Outdated drug can cause nephropathy, throw away any unused
medication

Adverse Reactions
Central nervous system: Pseudotumor cerebri, fever
Dermatologic: Rash, photosensitivity
Gastrointestinal: Nausea, vomiting, diarrhea, stomatitis, glossitis, antibiotic-
associated pseudomembranous colitis
Hepatic: Hepatotoxicity
Neuromuscular & skeletal: Injury to growing bones and teeth
Renal: Renal damage, Fanconi-like syndrome
Miscellaneous: Hypersensitivity reactions, candidal superinfection

Overdosage Symptoms of overdose include photosensitivity, nausea,
anorexia, diarrhea

Drug Interactions Calcium-, magnesium-, or aluminum-containing antacids
and sodium bicarbonate (decreased tetracyclic absorption); iron, methoxyflurane, zinc, penicillins, cimetidine (decreased dissolution), oral anticoagulants,
lithium (increased or decreased serum concentrations)

Drug/Food Interactions Do not take with food, take 1 hour before or 2 hours
after meals

Stability Outdated tetracyclines have caused a Fanconi-like syndrome; reconstituted I.M. solution is stable for 24 hours at room temperature

Mechanism of Action Inhibits bacterial protein synthesis by binding with the
30S and possibly the 50S ribosomal subunit(s) of susceptible bacteria; may
also cause alterations in the cytoplasmic membrane

Pharmacodynamics Bacteriostatic

Pharmacokinetics
Absorption:
Oral: 75%
I.M.: Poor with <60% of dose absorbed (the I.M. route is reserved for
situations where oral therapy is not feasible)
Protein binding: 65%
Half-life: Normal renal function: 8-11 hours
Time to peak serum concentration: Oral: Within 2-4 hours
Elimination: Primary route of elimination is the kidney, with 60% of a dose
excreted as unchanged drug in urine; small amount appears in bile

Usual Dosage See manufacturer's and CDC's specific dosing recommendations by indication

Geriatrics and Adults:
  Oral: 250-500 mg/dose every 6-12 hours
  Ophthalmic:
    Suspension: Instill 1-2 drops 2-4 times/day
    Ointment: Instill every 2-12 hours
  I.M.: 250-300 mg/day divided every 8-12 hours
  I.V.: 250-500 mg every 12 hours; maximum: 500 mg every 6 hours
  Slightly dialyzable (5% to 20%)
Administration Do not administer I.M. injection I.V., or I.V. injection I.M. (specific products available for each). I.V. should be infused over at least 2 hours
Monitoring Parameters Temperature, WBC, cultures and sensitivity (if applicable), appetite, mental status
Reference Range Therapeutic: Not established; Toxic: >16 µg/mL
Test Interactions False-negative urine glucose with Clinistix®
Patient Information Take 1 hour before or 2 hours after meals with adequate amounts of fluid; avoid prolonged exposure to sunlight or sunlamps; avoid taking antacids, iron, or dairy products with tetracyclines
Nursing Implications See Administration
Additional Information Use of tetracycline in animal feed has caused emergence of resistant organisms

  Tetracycline: Achromycin® V oral suspension, Sumycin® syrup, Tetralan® syrup
  Tetracycline hydrochloride: Achromycin® injection, Achromycin® V capsule, Nor-tet® capsule, Panmycin® capsule, Robitet® capsule, Sumycin® capsule and tablet, Teline® capsule, Tetracyn® capsule, Tetralan® capsule
Special Geriatric Considerations The role of tetracycline has decreased because of the emergence of resistant organisms. Doxycycline is the tetracycline of choice when one is indicated because of its better GI absorption, less interactions with divalent cations, longer half-life, and the fact that the majority is cleared by nonrenal mechanisms.
Dosage Forms
  Tetracycline hydrochloride:
    Capsule: 100 mg, 250 mg, 500 mg
    Ointment:
      Ophthalmic: 1% [10 mg/mL] (3.5 g)
      Topical: 3% [30 mg/mL] (14.2 g, 30 g)
    Solution, topical: 2.2 mg/mL (70 mL)
    Suspension:
      Ophthalmic: 1% [10 mg/mL] (0.5 mL, 1 mL, 4 mL)
      Oral: 125 mg/5 mL (60 mL, 480 mL)
    Tablet: 250 mg, 500 mg
References
Yoshikawa TT, "Antimicrobial Therapy for the Elderly Patient," *J Am Geriatr Soc*, 1990, 38(12):1353-72.

Tetrahydroaminoacrine *see* Tetracrine *on page 885*

Tetrahydrozoline (tet ra hye DROZ a leen)

Brand Names Collyrium Fresh® Ophthalmic [OTC]; Eyesine® Ophthalmic [OTC]; Geneye® Ophthalmic [OTC]; Mallazine® Eye Drops [OTC]; Murine® Plus Ophthalmic [OTC]; Optigene® Ophthalmic [OTC]; Tetrasine® Ophthalmic [OTC]; Tetrasine® Extra Ophthalmic [OTC]; Tyzine® Nasal; Visine® Ophthalmic [OTC]; Visine® Extra Ophthalmic [OTC]
Synonyms Tetryzoline
Generic Available Yes
Therapeutic Category Adrenergic Agonist Agent; Adrenergic Agonist Agent, Ophthalmic; Decongestant, Nasal; Nasal Agent, Vasoconstrictor; Ophthalmic Agent, Vasoconstrictor; Vasoconstrictor, Nasal; Vasoconstrictor, Ophthalmic
Use Symptomatic relief of nasal congestion and conjunctival congestion
Contraindications Narrow-angle glaucoma, patients receiving MAO inhibitors, known hypersensitivity to tetrahydrozoline
Warnings Discontinue use prior to the use of anesthetics which sensitize the myocardium to the systemic effects of sympathomimetics
Precautions Use caution in patients with hypertension, diabetes, thyroid disorders, heart disease, and asthma
Adverse Reactions
  Cardiovascular: Tachycardia, palpitations, increased blood pressure, heart rate
  (Continued)

Tetrahydrozoline *(Continued)*

Central nervous system: Headache
Local: Stinging, sneezing
Neuromuscular & skeletal: Tremors
Ocular: Blurred vision
Miscellaneous: Diaphoresis

Overdosage Symptoms of overdose include CNS depression, hypothermia, bradycardia, cardiovascular collapse, coma

Toxicology Following initiation of essential overdose management, toxic symptoms should be treated. The patient should be kept warm and monitored for alterations in vital functions. Seizures commonly respond to diazepam (5-10 mg I.V. bolus in adults every 15 minutes if needed up to a total of 30 mg) or to phenytoin or phenobarbital.

Drug Interactions MAO inhibitors can cause an exaggerated adrenergic response if taken concurrently or within 21 days of discontinuing MAO inhibitors; beta-blockers can cause hypertensive episodes and increased risk of intracranial hemorrhage; anesthetics

Mechanism of Action Stimulates alpha-adrenergic receptors in the arterioles of the conjunctiva and the nasal mucosa to produce vasoconstriction

Pharmacodynamics
Onset of action: Intranasal: Decongestant effects occur within 4-8 hours
Duration: Ophthalmic vasoconstriction lasts 2-3 hours

Pharmacokinetics Absorption: Topical: Systemic absorption sometimes occurs

Usual Dosage Geriatrics and Adults:
Nasal congestion: Instill 2-4 drops or 3-4 sprays of 0.1% solution to the nasal mucosa every 3-6 hours as needed
Conjunctival congestion: Instill 1-2 drops in each eye 2-4 times/day

Administration See Patient Information and package instructions

Monitoring Parameters Blood pressure, heart rate, symptom response

Patient Information Remove contact lenses before using in eye; do not use >72 hours; consult physician of changes in vision or visual acuity occur; do not exceed recommended dose or duration to avoid rebound congestion

Nursing Implications Do not use for longer than 3-4 days without direct physician supervision

Special Geriatric Considerations Use with caution in patients with cardiovascular disease (see Precautions and Usual Dosage)

Dosage Forms
Tetrahydrozoline hydrochloride:
Solution:
Nasal: 0.05% (15 mL), 0.1% (30 mL, 473 mL)
Ophthalmic: 0.05% (15 mL)

Tetrasine® Extra Ophthalmic [OTC] *see* Tetrahydrozoline *on previous page*

Tetrasine® Ophthalmic [OTC] *see* Tetrahydrozoline *on previous page*

Tetryzoline *see* Tetrahydrozoline *on previous page*

T-Gen® *see* Trimethobenzamide *on page 961*

T-Gesic® *see* Hydrocodone and Acetaminophen *on page 461*

THA *see* Tacrine *on page 885*

Thalitone® *see* Chlorthalidone *on page 217*

Theo-24® *see* Theophylline *on this page*

Theobid® *see* Theophylline *on this page*

Theochron® *see* Theophylline *on this page*

Theoclear-80® *see* Theophylline *on this page*

Theoclear® L.A. *see* Theophylline *on this page*

Theo-Dur® *see* Theophylline *on this page*

Theolair™ *see* Theophylline *on this page*

Theophylline *(thee OF i lin)*

Related Information
Asthma Guidelines *on page 1040*
Serum Drug Concentrations Commonly Monitored: Guidelines *on page 1114*

Brand Names Aerolate III®; Aerolate JR®; Aerolate SR®; Aquaphyllin®; Asmalix®; Bronkodyl®; Elixomin®; Elixophyllin®; Lanophyllin®; Quibron®-T; Quibron®-T/SR; Respbid®; Slo-bid™; Slo-Phyllin®; Sustaire®; Theo-24®;

Theobid®; Theochron®; Theoclear-80®; Theoclear® L.A.; Theo-Dur®; Theo-lair™; Theo-Sav®; Theospan®-SR; Theostat-80®; Theovent®; Theo-X®; T-Phyl®; Uni-Dur®; Uniphyl®

Generic Available Yes

Therapeutic Category Bronchodilator; Theophylline Derivative

Use Bronchodilator in reversible bronchospasm due to asthma, chronic bronchitis, and emphysema

Contraindications Hypersensitivity to xanthines; peptic ulcer, uncontrolled seizure disorders, uncontrolled arrhythmias

Warnings May precipitate or worsen pre-existing arrhythmias

Precautions Use with caution in patients with peptic ulcer, hyperthyroidism, hypertension, and patients with compromised cardiac function; hepatic function, esophageal reflux disease, alcoholism, and elderly

Adverse Reactions Adverse reactions are uncommon at serum theophylline concentrations <20 mcg/mL

Cardiovascular: Palpitations, sinus tachycardia, extrasystoles, hypotension, ventricular arrhythmias, flushing

Central nervous system: Irritability, restlessness, fever, headache, insomnia, seizures

Endocrine & metabolic: Hyperglycemia

Gastrointestinal: Nausea, vomiting, esophageal reflux, diarrhea, hematemesis, rectal bleeding, epigastric pain

Neuromuscular & skeletal: Tremors, muscle twitching

Renal: Proteinuria, diuresis

Respiratory: Tachypnea, respiratory arrest

Overdosage Symptoms of overdose include tachycardia, extrasystoles, nausea, vomiting, anorexia, tonic-clonic seizures, insomnia, circulatory failure; agitation, irritability, headache

Toxicology If seizures have not occurred, induce vomiting; ipecac syrup is preferred. Do not induce emesis in the presence of impaired consciousness. Repeated doses of charcoal have been shown to be effective in enhancing the total body clearance of theophylline. Do not repeat charcoal doses if an ileus is present. Charcoal hemoperfusion may be considered if the serum theophylline concentrations exceed 40 mcg/mL, the patient is unable to tolerate repeat oral charcoal administrations, or if severe toxic symptoms are present. Clearance with hemoperfusion is better than clearance from hemodialysis. Administer a cathartic, especially if sustained release agents are used. Phenobarbital administered prophylactically may prevent seizures.

Drug Interactions

Changes in diet may affect the elimination of theophylline; theophylline may decrease the effects of phenytoin, lithium, and neuromuscular blocking agents

Theophylline increases the excretion of lithium; theophylline may have synergistic toxicity with sympathomimetics

Cimetidine, ranitidine, allopurinol, beta-blockers (nonspecific), erythromycin, clarithromycin, influenza virus vaccine, corticosteroids, ephedrine, quinolones, thyroid hormones, oral contraceptives, amiodarone, troleandomycin, clindamycin, fluvoxamine, zileuton, tacrine, carbamazepine, isoniazid, loop diuretics, and lincomycin may increase theophylline serum concentrations

Cigarette and marijuana smoking, rifampin, ritonavir, barbiturates, hydantoins, ketoconazole, sulfinpyrazone, sympathomimetics, isoniazid,

Factors Reported to Affect Theophylline Serum Concentrations

Decreased Theophylline Concentration	Increased Theophylline Concentration
Smoking (cigarettes, marijuana)	Hepatic cirrhosis
High protein/low carbohydrate diet	Cor pulmonale
Charcoal broiled beef	CHF
Phenytoin	Fever/viral illness
Phenobarbital	Propranolol
Carbamazepine	Allopurinol (>600 mg/d)
Rifampin	Erythromycin
I.V. isoproterenol	Cimetidine
	Troleandomycin
	Ciprofloxacin
	Oral contraceptives

(Continued)

Theophylline (Continued)

loop diuretics, carbamazepine, and aminoglutethimide may decrease theophylline serum concentrations

Tetracyclines enhance toxicity and benzodiazepine's action may be antagonized; see table.

Stability Store injection at room temperature; protect from heat and from freezing; use only clear solutions

Stability of parenteral admixture at room temperature (25°C): 30 days

Stability of parenteral admixture at refrigeration temperature (4°C): Do not refrigerate

Mechanism of Action Causes bronchodilatation, diuresis, CNS and cardiac stimulation, and gastric acid secretion by blocking phosphodiesterase which increases tissue concentrations of cyclic adenine monophosphate (cAMP) which in turn promotes catecholamine stimulation of lipolysis, glycogenolysis, and gluconeogenesis and induces release of epinephrine from adrenal medulla cells. Other proposed mechanisms include inhibition of extracellular adenosine, stimulation of endogenous catecholamines, antagonism of PGE_2 and $PGE_{2\alpha}$, mobilization of intracellular calcium, and increased sensitivity of beta-adrenergic receptors in reactive airways.

Pharmacokinetics

Absorption: Oral: Up to 100%, depending upon the formulation used

Distribution: V_d: 0.45 L/kg

Metabolism: In the liver by demethylation; substrate CYP1A2

Half-life: Varies from 3-15 hours in healthy adults (nonsmokers); 4-5 hours in smokers (1-2 packs/day); see table.

Half-life (h)	Patient Population
7-9	Normal healthy geriatrics/adults
18-24	Severe congestive heart failure
29	Cirrhosis

Time to peak plasma concentration: 1-2 hours, 4 hours for sustained release

Elimination: In urine; adults excrete 10% in urine as unchanged drug

Usual Dosage See aminophylline for I.V. doses

Geriatrics and Adults:

Initial dosage recommendation: Loading dose (to achieve a serum concentration of about 10 mcg/mL; loading doses should be given using a rapidly absorbed oral product **not** a sustained release product):

If no theophylline has been administered in the previous 24 hours: 4-6 mg/kg theophylline

If theophylline has been administered in the previous 24 hours: Administer ½ loading dose; 2-3 mg/kg theophylline can be given in emergencies when serum concentrations are not available

On the average, for every 1 mg/kg theophylline given, blood concentrations will rise 2 mcg/mL

Maintenance dose: See table.

Maintenance Dose for Acute Symptoms

Population Group	Oral Theophylline (mg/kg/day)	I.V. Aminophylline
Healthy nonsmoking adults (including elderly patients)	10 (not to exceed 900 mg/day)	0.5 mg/kg/hour
Cardiac decompensation, cor pulmonale, and/or liver dysfunction	5 (not to exceed 400 mg/day)	0.25 mg/kg/hour

*For continuous I.V. infusion divide total daily dose by 24 = mg/kg/hour.

Oral:

Nonsustained release: 16-20 mg/kg/day divided into 4 doses/day

Sustained release: 9-13 mg/kg/day divided into 2-3 doses/day

These recommendations, based on mean clearance rates for age or risk factors, were calculated to achieve a serum concentration of 10 mcg/mL. In healthy adults, a slow-release product can be used (9-13 mg/kg in divided dose). The total daily dose can be divided every 8-12 hours. Geriatrics should be started with a 25% reduction.

Use ideal body weight for obese patients

Dose should be adjusted further based on serum concentrations. Guidelines for obtaining theophylline serum concentrations are shown in the table.

Guidelines for Obtaining Theophylline Serum Concentrations

Dosage Form	Time to Draw Level
I.V. bolus	30 min after end of 30 min infusion
I.V. continuous infusion	12-24 h after initiation of infusion
P.O. liquid, fast-release tab	Peak: 1 h postdose after at least 1 day of therapy Trough: Just before a dose after at least one day of therapy
P.O. slow-release product	Peak: 4 h postdose after at least 1 day of therapy Trough: Just before a dose after at least one day of therapy

Monitoring Parameters Heart rate, CNS effects (insomnia, irritability); respiratory rate (COPD patients often have resting controlled respiratory rates in low 20's)

Reference Range
Sample size: 0.5-1 mL serum (red top tube)
Therapeutic: 10-20 µg/mL; Toxic: >20 µg/mL; some patients may have adequate clinical response with serum concentrations from 5-10 µg/mL
Timing of serum samples: If toxicity is suspected, obtain a concentration any time during a continuous I.V. infusion, or 2 hours after an oral dose; if lack of therapeutic is affected, draw a trough immediately before the next oral dose or intermittent I.V. dose

Test Interactions May elevate uric acid serum concentrations

Patient Information Oral preparations should be taken with a full glass of water; avoid drinking or eating large quantities of caffeine-containing beverages or food; take at regular intervals; take sustained release tablets whole; sustained release capsule forms may be opened and sprinkled on soft foods; do not chew beads; take with food if GI upset occurs; notify physician if nausea, vomiting, insomnia, nervousness, irritability, palpitations, seizures occur; do not change from one brand to another without consulting physician and pharmacist; do not change doses without consulting your physician

Nursing Implications Administer oral and I.V. administration around-the-clock rather than 4 times/day, 3 times/day, etc (ie, 12-6-12-6, not 9-1-5-9) to promote less variation in peak and trough serum concentrations; do not crush sustained release drug products; do not crush enteric coated drug product; monitor vital signs, serum concentrations, and CNS effects (insomnia, irritability); encourage patient to drink adequate fluids (2 L/day) to decrease mucous viscosity in airways

Additional Information Saliva levels are approximately equal to 60% of plasma concentrations. Charcoal-broiled foods may increase elimination, reducing half-life by 50%; cigarette smoking may require an increase of dosage by 50% to 100%. Because different salts of theophylline have different theophylline content, various salts are equivalent. The following are percent content of theophylline for various salts:
Theophylline anhydrous: 100%
Theophylline monohydrate: 91%
Aminophylline anhydrous: 86%
Oxtriphylline: 64%
Most preparations are now labeled with actual milligram content delivered by the particular product.
Theophylline immediate release tablet/capsule: Bronkodyl®, Elixophyllin®, Quibron®-T, Slo-Phyllin®-T, Somophyllin®-T, Theolair™
Theophylline liquid: Accurbron®, Aerolate®, Aquaphyllin®, Asmalix®, Elixicon®, Elixophyllin®, Lixolin®, Theon®
Theophylline timed release capsule: Aerolate III®, Aerolate JR®, Aerolate SR®, Elixophyllin® SR, Lodrane®, Slo-bid™ Gyrocaps®, Slo-Phyllin® Gyrocaps®, Somophyllin®-CRT, Theobid®, Theoclear® L.A., Theophyl-SR®, Theospan®-SR, Theospan®-SR
Theophylline timed release tablet: Constant-T®, Duraphyl™, LaBID®, Quibron®-T/S, Respbid®, Sustaire®, Theochron®, Theo-Dur®, Theolair™-SR, Theo-Time®, Uniphyl®

Special Geriatric Considerations Although there is a great intersubject variability for half-lives of methylxanthines (2-10 hours), elderly as a group have slower hepatic clearance. Therefore, use lower initial doses and monitor
(Continued)

Theophylline *(Continued)*

closely for response and adverse reactions. Additionally, elderly are at greater risk for toxicity due to concomitant disease (eg, CHF, arrhythmias), and drug use (eg, cimetidine, ciprofloxacin, etc) (see Precautions and Drug Interactions).

Dosage Forms

Capsule:
Immediate release: 100 mg, 200 mg
Sustained release (8-12 hours): 50 mg, 60 mg, 65 mg, 75 mg, 100 mg, 125 mg, 130 mg, 200 mg, 250 mg, 260 mg, 300 mg
Timed release:
12 hours: 50 mg, 75 mg, 125 mg, 130 mg, 200 mg, 250 mg, 260 mg
24 hours: 100 mg, 200 mg, 300 mg
Solution, oral: 80 mg/15 mL (15 mL, 30 mL, 500 mL); 150 mg/15 mL (480 mL)
Tablet: 125 mg, 250 mg
Tablet:
Immediate release: 100 mg, 125 mg, 200 mg, 250 mg, 300 mg
Sustained release: 100 mg, 200 mg, 300 mg
Timed release:
8-12 hours: 100 mg, 200 mg, 250 mg, 300 mg
8-24 hours: 100 mg, 200 mg, 250 mg, 300 mg, 500 mg
12-24 hours: 100 mg, 200 mg, 300 mg
24 hours: 400 mg

References

Kearney TE, Manoguerra AS, Curtis GP, et al, "Theophylline Toxicity and the Beta-Adrenergic System," *Ann Intern Med*, 1985, 102(6):766-9.

Mahler DA, Barlow PB, and Matthay RA, "Chronic Obstructive Pulmonary Disease," *Clin Geriatr Med*, 1986, 2(2):285-312.

Upton RA, "Pharmacokinetic Interactions Between Theophylline and Other Medication (Part I)," *Clin Pharmacokinet*, 1991, 20(1):66-80.

Weinberger M and Hendeles L, "Theophylline in Asthma," *N Engl J Med*, 1996, 334(21):1380-8.

Theophylline Ethylenediamine *see* Aminophylline *on page 55*

Theo-Sav® *see* Theophylline *on page 902*

Theospan®-SR *see* Theophylline *on page 902*

Theostat-80® *see* Theophylline *on page 902*

Theovent® *see* Theophylline *on page 902*

Theo-X® *see* Theophylline *on page 902*

Thera-Flur® *see* Fluoride *on page 392*

Thera-Flur-N® *see* Fluoride *on page 392*

Theralax® [OTC] *see* Bisacodyl *on page 121*

Thermazene® *see* Silver Sulfadiazine *on page 856*

Thiamazole *see* Methimazole *on page 603*

Thiamilate® *see* Thiamine *on this page*

Thiamine *(THYE a min)*

Brand Names Thiamilate®

Synonyms Aneurine Hydrochloride; Thiaminium Chloride Hydrochloride; Vitamin B₁

Generic Available Yes

Therapeutic Category Vitamin, Water Soluble

Use Treatment or prophylaxis of thiamine deficiency including beriberi, Wernicke's encephalopathy syndrome, and peripheral neuritis associated with pellagra, alcoholic patients with altered sensorium; various genetic metabolic disorders; parenteral use for patients in whom the oral route is not possible, impaired gastrointestinal absorption

Contraindications Hypersensitivity to thiamine or any component

Warnings Use with caution with parenteral route (especially I.V.) of administration since sensitivity reactions can occur; death has resulted from I.V. use. Use intradermal test for patients who are suspected of sensitivity. Thiamine-deficient patients may experience a sudden onset or worsening of Wernicke's encephalopathy following glucose administration, therefore, thiamine should be given before or along with glucose. Thiamine deficiency alone is rare and patients should be evaluated for multiple vitamin deficiencies.

Adverse Reactions

Cardiovascular: Cardiovascular collapse and death, cyanosis
Central nervous system: Warmth, restlessness
Dermatologic: Rash, angioedema, angioneurotic edema, pruritus, urticaria
Gastrointestinal: Nausea, tightness in the throat
Hematologic: Hemorrhage

Neuromuscular & skeletal: Paresthesia, weakness
Respiratory: Pulmonary edema

Stability Protect oral dosage forms from light; **incompatible** with alkaline or neutral solutions and with oxidizing or reducing agents (see Additional Information)

Mechanism of Action An essential coenzyme in carbohydrate metabolism by combining with adenosine triphosphate to form thiamine pyrophosphate

Pharmacokinetics
Absorption:
Oral: Adequate
I.M.: Rapid and complete
Elimination: Renally as unchanged drug, and as pyrimidine after body storage sites become saturated

Usual Dosage Geriatrics and Adults:
Recommended daily allowance:
Male: 1-1.5 mg
Female: 1.1 mg
Thiamine deficiency (beriberi): 5-30 mg/dose I.M. or I.V. 3 times/day (if critically ill); then orally 5-30 mg/day in single or divided doses 3 times/day for 1 month
Wernicke's encephalopathy: Initial: 100 mg I.V., then 50-100 mg/day I.M. or I.V. until consuming a regular, balanced diet
Dietary supplement depends on caloric or carbohydrate content of the diet: Recommended intake of thiamine: 0.5 mg/1000 Kcal
Note: The above doses can be found in multivitamin preparations; see Additional Information
Metabolic disorders: Oral: 10-20 mg/day (dosages up to 4 g/day in divided doses have been used)

Administration Parenteral form may be administered by I.M. or slow I.V. injection

Reference Range Therapeutic: 1.6-4 mg/dL

Test Interactions False-positive for uric acid using the phosphotungstate method and for urobilinogen using the Ehrlich's reagent; large doses may interfere with the spectrophotometric determination of serum theophylline concentration

Patient Information Dietary sources include legumes, pork, beef, whole grains, yeast, fresh vegetables; a deficiency state can occur in as little 3 weeks following total dietary absence

Nursing Implications Single vitamin deficiency is rare; look for other deficiencies; parenteral (I.M.) use may produce tenderness and an induration at the site of injection

Additional Information Thiamine (vitamin B_1) is unstable in alkaline or neutral solutions, therefore, do not mix with carbonates, citrates, barbiturates. Also, any solution containing sulfites is incompatible with thiamine. Recommended thiamine intake is 0.5 mg/1000 Kcal.

Special Geriatric Considerations No special recommendations are necessary; elderly are treated the same as younger adults; see Usual Dosage and Warnings

Dosage Forms
Thiamine hydrochloride:
Injection: 100 mg/mL (1 mL, 2 mL, 10 mL, 30 mL); 200 mg/mL (30 mL); preloaded syringes available
Tablet: 50 mg, 100 mg, 250 mg, 500 mg
Tablet, enteric coated: 20 mg

References

Doyon S and Roberts JR, "Reappraisal of the "Coma Cocktail": Dextrose, Flumazenil, Naloxone, and Thiamine," *Emerg Med Clin North Am*, 1994, 12(2):301-16.

Hoffman RS and Goldfrank LR, "The Poisoned Patient With Altered Consciousness. Controversies in the Use of a 'Coma Cocktail'," *JAMA*, 1995, 274(7):562-9.

Petrie WM and Ban TA, "Vitamins in Psychiatry. Do They Have a Role?" *Drugs*, 1985, 30(1):58-65.

Proebstle TM, Gall H, and Jugert FK, "Specific IgE and IgG Serum Antibodies to Thiamine Associated With Anaphylactic Reaction," *J Allergy Clin Immunol*, 1995, 95(5 Pt 1):1059-60.

Reuler JB, Girard DE, and Cooney TG, "Current Concepts: Wernicke's Encephalopathy," *N Engl J Med*, 1985, 312(16):1035-39.

Stephen JM, Grant R, and Veh CS, "Anaphylaxis From Administration of Intravenous Thiamine," *Am J Emerg Med*, 1992, 10(1):61-3.

Van Haecke P, Ramaekers D, Vanderwegen L, et al, "Thiamine-Induced Anaphylactic Shock," *Am J Emerg Med*, 1995, 13(3):371-2.

Wrenn KD, Murphy F, and Slovis CM, "A Toxicity Study of Parenteral Thiamine Hydrochloride," *Ann Emerg Med*, 1989, 18(8):867-70.

Thiaminium Chloride Hydrochloride *see* Thiamine *on previous page*

Thiethylperazine (thye eth il PER a zeen)

Related Information
Antacid Drug Interactions *on page 1096*

Brand Names Torecan®

Generic Available No

Therapeutic Category Antiemetic; Phenothiazine Derivative

Use Relief of nausea and vomiting

Unlabeled use: Treatment of vertigo

Contraindications Comatose states, hypersensitivity to thiethylperazine or any component; cross-sensitivity to other phenothiazines may exist, severe CNS depression; do not administer I.V.

Warnings parenterally; extended release capsules and injection contain benzyl alcohol; injection also contains sulfites which may cause allergic reaction

Tardive dyskinesia: Prevalence rate may be 40% in elderly; elderly women especially at risk; embarrassment from dyskinesias may lead to greater social isolation; development of the syndrome and the irreversible nature are proportional to duration and total cumulative dose over time. May be reversible if diagnosed early in therapy; intermittent use of antipsychotics (not proven use) helps decrease total cumulative dose.

EPS: Extrapyramidal reactions are more common in elderly with up to 50% developing these reactions after age 60. These reactions may be more common in dementia patients. Drug-induced **Parkinson's syndrome** occurs often. Discontinuation usually resolves symptoms but may take weeks to months (12+) to clear. **Akathisia** is the most common EPS reaction in elderly. The symptoms of motor restlessness are difficult to diagnose in demented elderly; increased nervousness, assertiveness, restlessness with constant movement may indicate this adverse event. Consider decreasing dose if antipsychotic to treat as well as diagnose problem; usually see this reaction within 2-3 months of initiating antipsychotic drug.

Anticholinergic effects: These side effects most common with low potency antipsychotics (eg, thioridazine, chlorpromazine). CNS toxicity occurs more frequently and severely in elderly; increased confusion, memory loss, psychotic behavior, and agitation frequently occur as a consequence of anticholinergic effects to antipsychotic agents. Peripheral anticholinergic action troublesome to elderly; most peripheral anticholinergic effects last only 2-3 weeks (see Adverse Reactions).

Orthostatic hypotension: More common with low potency agents (eg, thioridazine, chlorpromazine, and clozapine) but of concern with all antipsychotic agents; orthostasis due to alpha-receptor blockade by antipsychotic agents. Elderly present many risk factors for orthostatic hypotension: blunted baroreceptor reflexes, decreased vascular tone, decreased vascular volume, and possible presence of cardiac diseases which result in decreased cardiac output.

Sedation: Common side effect with antipsychotic therapy; should not be used as a hypnotic unless insomnia is associated with target behavior symptoms treated with antipsychotic medications (see Special Geriatric Considerations). Anecdotal reports suggesting antipsychotic sedation in nonpsychotic patients is extremely unpleasant due to feelings of depersonalization, derealization, and dysphoria. Due to the long duration of action with antipsychotic drugs, these reactions may last up to 24 hours and result in decreased daytime function.

Cardiac toxicity: Life-threatening arrhythmias have occurred at therapeutic doses of antipsychotics. Thioridazine more commonly demonstrates EKG changes than other antipsychotics; suggested to use high potency antipsychotic agents (ie, haloperidol) in patients with cardiac conduction defects.

Precautions Use with caution in patients with cardiovascular disease, seizures, narrow-angle glaucoma, and Parkinson's disease; benefits of therapy must be weighed against risks

Adverse Reactions

Cardiovascular: Hypotension (especially with I.V. use), orthostatic hypotension, tachycardia, arrhythmias, abnormal T waves with prolonged ventricular repolarization

Central nervous system: Sedation, drowsiness, restlessness, anxiety, extrapyramidal reactions, pseudoparkinsonian signs and symptoms, tardive dyskinesia, neuroleptic malignant syndrome, seizures, altered central temperature regulation

Dermatologic: Hyperpigmentation, pruritus, rash, photosensitivity

Endocrine & metabolic: Amenorrhea, galactorrhea, gynecomastia

Gastrointestinal: GI upset, xerostomia (problem for denture users), constipation, adynamic ileus, weight gain

Genitourinary: Urinary retention, overflow incontinence, priapism, sexual dysfunction (up to 60%), impotence

Hematologic: Agranulocytosis, leukopenia (usually in patients with large doses for prolonged periods), thrombocytopenia, hemolytic anemia, eosinophilia

Hepatic: Cholestatic jaundice (rare)

Ocular: Retinal pigmentation, blurred vision

Miscellaneous: Anaphylactoid reactions

Overdosage Symptoms of overdose include deep sleep, coma, extrapyramidal symptoms, abnormal involuntary muscle movements, hypotension

Toxicology Following initiation of essential overdose management, toxic symptom treatment and supportive treatment should be initiated. Hypotension usually responds to I.V. fluids or Trendelenburg positioning. If unresponsive to these measures, use of a parenteral inotrope may be required (eg, norepinephrine 0.1-0.2 mcg/kg/minute titrated to response); avoid epinephrine for thiethylperazine-induced hypotension. Seizures commonly respond to diazepam (I.V. 5-10 mg bolus in adults every 15 minutes if needed up to a total of 30 mg; I.V. 0.25-0.4 mg/kg/dose up to a total of 10 mg in children) or to phenytoin or phenobarbital. Critical cardiac arrhythmias often respond to I.V. phenytoin (15 mg/kg up to 1 g), while other antiarrhythmics can be used. Neuroleptics often cause extrapyramidal symptoms especially in elderly (eg, dystonic reactions) requiring management with diphenhydramine 1-2 mg/kg up to a maximum of 50 mg I.M. or I.V. slow push followed by a maintenance dose for 48-72 hours. When these reactions are unresponsive to diphenhydramine, benztropine mesylate I.V. 1-2 mg may be effective. These agents are generally effective within 2-5 minutes.

Drug Interactions

Alcohol may increase CNS sedation

Anticholinergic agents may decrease pharmacologic effects; increase anticholinergic side effects; may enhance tardive dyskinesia

Aluminum salts may decrease absorption of phenothiazines

Anorexiants with phenothiazines may decrease the effects of amphetamines and their congeners

Barbiturates may decrease phenothiazine serum concentrations

Bromocriptine may have decreased efficacy when administered with phenothiazines

Guanethidine's hypotensive effect is decreased by phenothiazines

Lithium administration with phenothiazines may increase disorientation

Meperidine and phenothiazine coadministration increases sedation and hypotension

Methyldopa administration with phenothiazine (trifluoperazine) may significantly increase blood pressure

Norepinephrine, epinephrine have decreased pressor effect when administered with chlorpromazine; therefore, be aware of possible decreased effectiveness or when any phenothiazine is used

Phenytoin serum concentrations may increase or decrease with phenothiazines; tricyclic antidepressants may have increased serum concentrations with concomitant administration with phenothiazines

Propranolol administered with phenothiazines may increase serum concentrations of both drugs

Tricyclic antidepressants may have serum concentrations increased by phenothiazines

Valproic acid may have increased half-life when administered with phenothiazines (chlorpromazine)

Stability Store suppositories below 25°C (77°F) in foil

Mechanism of Action Blocks postsynaptic mesolimbic dopaminergic D_1 and D_2 receptors in the brain; exhibits a strong alpha-adrenergic blocking and anticholinergic effect; depresses the release of hypothalamic and hypophyseal hormones; believed to depress the reticular activating system thus affecting basal metabolism, body temperature, wakefulness, vasomotor tone, and emesis

Pharmacodynamics

Onset of antiemetic effect: Within 30 minutes

Duration of action: ~4 hours

Usual Dosage Geriatrics and Adults:

Oral, I.M., rectal: 10 mg 1-3 times/day as needed

(Continued)

Thiethylperazine *(Continued)*

I.V. and S.C. routes of administration are not recommended (see Additional Information)

Hemodialysis: Not dialyzable (0% to 5%)

Dosing comments in hepatic impairment: Use with caution

Administration Inject I.M. deeply into large muscle mass, patient should be lying down and remain so for at least 1 hour after administration

Monitoring Parameters Orthostatic blood pressures; tremors, gait changes, abnormal movement in trunk, neck, buccal area, or extremities; monitor target behaviors for which the agent is given

Test Interactions False-positives for phenylketonuria, amylase, uroporphyrins, urobilinogen; possible false-negative pregnancy urinary test

Patient Information May cause drowsiness, impair judgment and coordination; may cause photosensitivity; avoid excessive sunlight; notify physician of involuntary movements or feelings of restlessness

Nursing Implications Assist with ambulation, observe for extrapyramidal symptoms (see Monitoring Parameters)

Additional Information Tablets contain tartrazine and sorbitol

Special Geriatric Considerations Elderly are more likely to experience extrapyramidal reactions than younger adults. Dystonic reactions are possible but seen more often in younger adults. Confusion is also possible in elderly (see Warnings).

Dosage Forms

Thiethylperazine maleate:
Injection: 5 mg/mL (2 mL)
Suppository, rectal: 10 mg
Tablet: 10 mg

References

Khanderia U, "Recurrent Dystonic Reactions Induced by Thiethylperazine," *Drug Intell Clin Pharm*, 1985, 19(7-8):550-1.
Sulkava R, "Thiethylperazine and Tardive Dyskinesia," *Acta Neurol Scand*, 1984, 70(5):364-72.

Thioridazine *(thye oh RID a zeen)*

Related Information

Antacid Drug Interactions *on page 1096*
Antipsychotic Agents Comparison *on page 1023*
Antipsychotic Medication Guidelines *on page 1076*
Federal OBRA Regulations Recommended Maximum Doses - Antipsychotics *on page 1056*

Brand Names Mellaril®; Mellaril-S®

Generic Available Yes

Therapeutic Category Antipsychotic Agent; Neuroleptic Agent; Phenothiazine Derivative

Use Management of manifestations of psychotic disorders; depressive neurosis; alcohol withdrawal; nausea and vomiting; nonpsychotic symptoms associated with dementia in elderly, Tourette's syndrome; Huntington's chorea; spasmodic torticollis and Reye's syndrome (see Special Geriatric Considerations)

Contraindications Severe CNS depression, hypersensitivity to thioridazine or any component; cross-sensitivity to other phenothiazines may exist; avoid use in patients with narrow-angle glaucoma, blood dyscrasias, severe liver or cardiac disease; subcortical brain damage; circulatory collapse; severe hypotension or hypertension

Warnings

Tardive dyskinesia: Prevalence rate may be 40% in elderly; elderly women especially at risk; embarrassment from dyskinesias may lead to greater social isolation; development of the syndrome and the irreversible nature are proportional to duration and total cumulative dose over time. May be reversible if diagnosed early in therapy; intermittent use of antipsychotics (not proven use) helps decrease total cumulative dose.

EPS: Extrapyramidal reactions are more common in elderly with up to 50% developing these reactions after age 60. These reactions may be more common in dementia patients. Drug-induced **Parkinson's syndrome** occurs often. Discontinuation usually resolves symptoms but may take weeks to months (12+) to clear. **Akathisia** is the most common EPS reaction in elderly. The symptoms of motor restlessness are difficult to diagnose in demented elderly; increased nervousness, assertiveness, restlessness with constant movement may indicate this adverse event. Consider decreasing dose if antipsychotic to treat as well as diagnose problem; usually see this reaction within 2-3 months of initiating antipsychotic drug.

Anticholinergic effects: These side effects most common with low potency antipsychotics (eg, thioridazine, chlorpromazine). CNS toxicity occurs more frequently and severely in elderly; increased confusion, memory loss, psychotic behavior, and agitation frequently occur as a consequence of anticholinergic effects to antipsychotic agents. Peripheral anticholinergic action troublesome to elderly; most peripheral anticholinergic effects last only 2-3 weeks (see Adverse Reactions).

Orthostatic hypotension: More common with low potency agents (eg, thioridazine, chlorpromazine, and clozapine) but of concern with all antipsychotic agents; orthostasis due to alpha-receptor blockade by antipsychotic agents. Elderly present many risk factors for orthostatic hypotension: blunted baroreceptor reflexes, decreased vascular tone, decreased vascular volume, and possible presence of cardiac diseases which result in decreased cardiac output.

Sedation: Common side effect with antipsychotic therapy; should not be used as a hypnotic unless insomnia is associated with target behavior symptoms treated with antipsychotic medications (see Special Geriatric Considerations). Anecdotal reports suggesting antipsychotic sedation in nonpsychotic patients is extremely unpleasant due to feelings of depersonalization, derealization, and dysphoria. Due to the long duration of action with antipsychotic drugs, these reactions may last up to 24 hours and result in decreased daytime function.

Cardiac toxicity: Life-threatening arrhythmias have occurred at therapeutic doses of antipsychotics. Thioridazine more commonly demonstrates EKG changes than other antipsychotics; suggested to use high potency antipsychotic agents (ie, haloperidol) in patients with cardiac conduction defects.

Precautions Use with caution in patients with severe cardiovascular disorder, seizures, and Parkinson's disease; benefits of therapy must be weighed against risks

Adverse Reactions

Cardiovascular: Orthostatic hypotension, tachycardia, arrhythmias, abnormal T waves with prolonged ventricular repolarization

Central nervous system: Sedation, drowsiness, restlessness, anxiety, extrapyramidal reactions, pseudoparkinsonian signs and symptoms, tardive dyskinesia, neuroleptic malignant syndrome, seizures, altered central temperature regulation

Dermatologic: Hyperpigmentation, pruritus, rash, photosensitivity

Endocrine & metabolic: Amenorrhea, galactorrhea, gynecomastia

Gastrointestinal: GI upset, xerostomia (problem for denture users), constipation, adynamic ileus, weight gain

Genitourinary: Urinary retention, overflow incontinence, priapism, impotence, sexual dysfunction (up to 60%)

Hematologic: Agranulocytosis, leukopenia (usually in patients with large doses for prolonged periods), thrombocytopenia, hemolytic anemia, eosinophilia

Hepatic: Cholestatic jaundice (rare)

Ocular: Retinal pigmentation, blurred vision

Miscellaneous: Anaphylactoid reactions

Overdosage Symptoms of overdose include deep sleep, coma, extrapyramidal symptoms, abnormal involuntary muscle movements, hypotension or hypertension; agitation, restlessness, fever, hypothermia or hyperthermia, seizures, cardiac arrhythmias, EKG changes

Toxicology Following initiation of essential overdose management, toxic symptom treatment and supportive treatment should be initiated. Hypotension usually responds to I.V. fluids or Trendelenburg positioning. If unresponsive to these measures the use of a parenteral inotrope may be required (eg, norepinephrine 0.1-0.2 mcg/kg/minute titrated to response). Do not use epinephrine. Seizures commonly respond to diazepam (I.V. 5-10 mg bolus in adults every 15 minutes if needed up to a total of 30 mg) or to phenytoin or phenobarbital. Also critical cardiac arrhythmias often respond to I.V. phenytoin (15 mg/kg up to 1 g), while other antiarrhythmics can be used. Neuroleptics often cause extrapyramidal symptoms (eg, dystonic reactions) requiring management with diphenhydramine 1-2 mg/kg up to a maximum of 50 mg I.M. or I.V. slow push followed by a maintenance dose for 48-72 hours. When these reactions are unresponsive to diphenhydramine, benztropine mesylate I.V. 1-2 mg may be effective. These agents are generally effective within 2-5 minutes.

(Continued)

Thioridazine *(Continued)*

Drug Interactions

Alcohol may increase CNS sedation

Anticholinergic agents may decrease pharmacologic effects; increase anticholinergic side effects; may enhance tardive dyskinesia

Aluminum salts may decrease absorption of phenothiazines

Barbiturates may decrease phenothiazine serum concentrations

Bromocriptine may have decreased efficacy when administered with phenothiazines

Guanethidine's hypotensive effect is decreased by phenothiazines

Lithium administration with phenothiazines may increase disorientation

Meperidine and phenothiazine coadministration increases sedation and hypotension

Methyldopa administration with phenothiazine (trifluoperazine) may significantly increase blood pressure

Norepinephrine, epinephrine have decreased pressor effect when administered with chlorpromazine; therefore, be aware of possible decreased effectiveness or when any phenothiazine is used

Phenytoin serum concentrations may increase or decrease with phenothiazines; tricyclic antidepressants may have increased serum concentrations with concomitant administration with phenothiazines

Propranolol administered with phenothiazines may increase serum concentrations of both drugs

Valproic acid may have increased half-life when administered with phenothiazines (chlorpromazine)

Stability Protect all dosage forms from light, clear or slightly yellow solutions may be used; should be dispensed in amber or opaque vials/bottles. Solutions may be diluted or mixed with fruit juices or other liquids but must be administered immediately after mixing; do not prepare bulk dilutions or store bulk dilutions.

Mechanism of Action Blocks postsynaptic mesolimbic dopaminergic D_1 and D_2 receptors in the brain; exhibits a strong alpha-adrenergic blocking and anticholinergic effect, depresses the release of hypothalamic and hypophyseal hormones; believed to depress the reticular activating system thus affecting basal metabolism, body temperature, wakefulness, vasomotor tone, and emesis

Pharmacokinetics

Absorption: May be affected by the inherent anticholinergic action on the gastrointestinal tissue causing variable absorption. Absorption from tablets is erratic with less variation seen with solutions. These agents are widely distributed in tissues with CNS concentrations exceeding that of plasma due to their lipophilic characteristics.

Protein binding: Antipsychotic agents are bound 90% to 99% to plasma proteins; highly bound to brain and lung tissue and other tissues with a high blood perfusion.

Metabolism: Substrate and inhibitor CYP2D6

Time to peak concentration: Oral: 2-4 hours

Elimination: Occurs through hepatic metabolism (oxidation) where numerous active metabolites are produced; active metabolites excreted in urine; elimination half-lives of antipsychotics ranges from 20-40 hours which may be extended in elderly due to decline in oxidative hepatic reactions (phase I) with age.

The biologic effect of a single dose persists for 24 hours. When the patient has accommodated to initial side effects (sedation), once daily dosing is possible due to the long half-life of antipsychotics.

Steady-state plasma concentrations are achieved in 4-7 days; therefore, if possible, do not make dose adjustments more than once in a 7-day period. Due to the long half-lives of antipsychotics, as needed (prn) use is ineffective since repeated doses are necessary to achieve therapeutic tissue concentrations in the CNS.

Usual Dosage Oral:

Geriatrics (nonpsychotic patient; dementia behavior): Initial: 10-25 mg 1-2 times/day; increase at 4- to 7-day intervals by 10-25 mg/day; increase dose intervals (qd, bid, etc) as necessary to control response or side effects. Maximum daily dose: 400 mg; gradual increases (titration) may prevent some side effects or decrease their severity.

Adults: Psychoses: Initial: 50-100 mg 3 times/day with gradual increments as needed and tolerated; maximum daily dose: 800 mg/day in 2-4 divided doses

Not dialyzable (0% to 5%)

Monitoring Parameters Orthostatic blood pressures; tremors, gait changes, abnormal movement in trunk, neck, buccal area, or extremities; monitor target behaviors for which the agent is given

Reference Range Therapeutic: 1.0-1.5 µg/mL (SI: 2.7-4.1 µmol/L); Toxic: >10 µg/mL (SI: >27 µmol/L)

Test Interactions False-positives for phenylketonuria, urinary amylase, uroporphyrins, urobilinogen

Patient Information Oral concentrate must be diluted in 2-4 oz of liquid (water, fruit juice, carbonated drinks, milk, or pudding); do not take antacid within 1 hour of taking drug; avoid alcohol; avoid excess sun exposure (use sun block); may cause drowsiness, rise slowly from recumbent position; use of supportive stockings may help prevent orthostatic hypotension

Nursing Implications Dilute the oral concentrate with water or juice before administration; avoid skin contact with oral suspension or solution; may cause contact dermatitis; monitor orthostatic blood pressures 3-5 days after initiation of therapy or a dose increase; observe for tremor and abnormal movement or posturing (extrapyramidal symptoms)

Additional Information Oral formulations may cause stomach upset; may cause thermoregulatory changes

Thioridazine: Mellaril-S® oral suspension

Thioridazine hydrochloride: Mellaril® oral solution and tablet

Special Geriatric Considerations See Warnings.

Many elderly patients receive antipsychotic medications for inappropriate nonpsychotic behavior. Before initiating antipsychotic medication, the clinician should investigate any possible reversible cause; any stress or stress from any disease can cause acute "confusion" or worsening of baseline nonpsychotic behavior. Most commonly acute changes in behavior are due to increases in drug dose or addition of new drug to regimen; fluid electrolyte loss; infections; and changes in environment.

Any changes in disease status in any organ system can result in behavior changes.

In the treatment of agitated, demented, elderly patients, authors of meta-analysis of controlled trials of the response to the traditional antipsychotics (phenothiazines, butyrophenones) have concluded that the use of neuroleptics results in a response rate of 18%. Clearly neuroleptic therapy for behavior control should be limited with frequent attempts to withdraw the agent given for behavior control.

Dosage Forms

Thioridazine hydrochloride:

Concentrate, oral: 30 mg/mL (120 mL); 100 mg/mL (3.4 mL, 120 mL)

Suspension, oral: 25 mg/5 mL (480 mL); 100 mg/5 mL (480 mL)

Tablet: 10 mg, 15 mg, 25 mg, 50 mg, 100 mg, 150 mg, 200 mg

References

Peabody CA, Warner MD, Whiteford HA, et al, "Neuroleptics and the Elderly," *J Am Geriatr Soc*, 1987, 35(3):233-8.

Risse SC and Barnes R, "Pharmacologic Treatment of Agitation Associated With Dementia," *J Am Geriatr Soc*, 1986, 34(5):368-76.

Saltz BL, Woerner MG, Kane JM, et al, "Prospective Study of Tardive Dyskinesia Incidence in the Elderly," *JAMA*, 1991, 266(17):2402-6.

Seifert RD, "Therapeutic Drug Monitoring: Psychotropic Drugs," *J Pharm Pract*, 1984, 6:403-16.

Thiothixene (thye oh THIKS een)

Related Information

Antacid Drug Interactions *on page 1096*
Antipsychotic Agents Comparison *on page 1023*
Antipsychotic Medication Guidelines *on page 1076*
Federal OBRA Regulations Recommended Maximum Doses - Antipsychotics *on page 1056*

Brand Names Navane®

Synonyms Tiotixene

Generic Available Yes

Therapeutic Category Antipsychotic Agent; Neuroleptic Agent; Phenothiazine Derivative

Use Management of psychotic disorders; nonpsychotic symptoms associated with dementia in elderly, Tourette's syndrome, Huntington's chorea

Contraindications Hypersensitivity to thiothixene or any component; cross-sensitivity with other phenothiazines may exist; avoid use in patients with narrow-angle glaucoma, bone marrow suppression, severe liver or cardiac disease; subcortical brain damage; circulatory collapse, severe hypotension or hypertension

(Continued)

Thiothixene (Continued)

Warnings

Tardive dyskinesia: Prevalence rate may be 40% in elderly; elderly women especially at risk; embarrassment from dyskinesias may lead to greater social isolation; development of the syndrome and the irreversible nature are proportional to duration and total cumulative dose over time. May be reversible if diagnosed early in therapy; intermittent use of antipsychotics (not proven use) helps decrease total cumulative dose.

EPS: Extrapyramidal reactions are more common in elderly with up to 50% developing these reactions after age 60. These reactions may be more common in dementia patients. Drug-induced **Parkinson's syndrome** occurs often. Discontinuation usually resolves symptoms but may take weeks to months (12+) to clear. **Akathisia** is the most common EPS reaction in elderly. The symptoms of motor restlessness are difficult to diagnose in demented elderly; increased nervousness, assertiveness, restlessness with constant movement may indicate this adverse event. Consider decreasing dose if antipsychotic to treat as well as diagnose problem; usually see this reaction within 2-3 months of initiating antipsychotic drug.

Anticholinergic effects: These side effects most common with low potency antipsychotics (eg, thioridazine, chlorpromazine). CNS toxicity occurs more frequently and severely in elderly; increased confusion, memory loss, psychotic behavior, and agitation frequently occur as a consequence of anticholinergic effects to antipsychotic agents. Peripheral anticholinergic action troublesome to elderly; most peripheral anticholinergic effects last only 2-3 weeks (see Adverse Reactions).

Orthostatic hypotension: More common with low potency agents (eg, thioridazine, chlorpromazine, and clozapine) but of concern with all antipsychotic agents; orthostasis due to alpha-receptor blockade by antipsychotic agents. Elderly present many risk factors for orthostatic hypotension: blunted baroreceptor reflexes, decreased vascular tone, decreased vascular volume, and possible presence of cardiac diseases which result in decreased cardiac output.

Sedation: Common side effect with antipsychotic therapy; should not be used as a hypnotic unless insomnia is associated with target behavior symptoms treated with antipsychotic medications (see Special Geriatric Considerations). Anecdotal reports suggesting antipsychotic sedation in nonpsychotic patients is extremely unpleasant due to feelings of depersonalization, derealization, and dysphoria. Due to the long duration of action with antipsychotic drugs, these reactions may last up to 24 hours and result in decreased daytime function.

Cardiac toxicity: Life-threatening arrhythmias have occurred at therapeutic doses of antipsychotics. Thioridazine more commonly demonstrates EKG changes than other antipsychotics; suggested to use high potency antipsychotic agents (ie, haloperidol) in patients with cardiac conduction defects.

Precautions Watch for hypotension when administering I.M. or I.V.; use with caution in patients with cardiovascular disease, seizures, and Parkinson's disease; benefits of therapy must be weighed against risks of therapy

Adverse Reactions

Cardiovascular: Orthostatic hypotension, tachycardia, arrhythmias, abnormal T waves with prolonged ventricular repolarization

Central nervous system: Sedation, drowsiness, restlessness, anxiety, extrapyramidal reactions, pseudoparkinsonian signs and symptoms, tardive dyskinesia, neuroleptic malignant syndrome, seizures, altered central temperature regulation

Dermatologic: Hyperpigmentation, pruritus, rash, photosensitivity

Endocrine & metabolic: Amenorrhea, galactorrhea, gynecomastia

Gastrointestinal: GI upset, xerostomia (problem for denture users), constipation, adynamic ileus, weight gain

Genitourinary: Urinary retention, overflow incontinence, priapism, impotence, sexual dysfunction (up to 60%)

Hematologic: Agranulocytosis, leukopenia (usually in patients with large doses for prolonged periods), thrombocytopenia, hemolytic anemia, eosinophilia

Hepatic: Cholestatic jaundice (rare)

Ocular: Retinal pigmentation, blurred vision

Miscellaneous: Anaphylactoid reactions

EKG changes, retinal pigmentation are more common than with chlorpromazine

Overdosage Symptoms of overdose include deep sleep, coma, extrapyramidal symptoms, abnormal involuntary muscle movements, hypotension or hypertension; agitation, restlessness, fever, hypothermia or hyperthermia, seizures, cardiac arrhythmias, EKG changes

Toxicology Following initiation of essential overdose management, toxic symptom treatment and supportive treatment should be initiated. Hypotension usually responds to I.V. fluids or Trendelenburg positioning. If unresponsive to these measures the use of a parenteral inotrope may be required (eg, norepinephrine 0.1-0.2 mcg/kg/minute titrated to response). Do not use epinephrine. Seizures commonly respond to diazepam (I.V. 5-10 mg bolus every 15 minutes if needed up to a total of 30 mg) or to phenytoin or phenobarbital. Also critical cardiac arrhythmias often respond to I.V. phenytoin (15 mg/kg up to 1 g), while other antiarrhythmics can be used. Neuroleptics often cause extrapyramidal symptoms (eg, dystonic reactions) requiring management with diphenhydramine 1-2 mg/kg up to a maximum of 50 mg I.M. or I.V. slow push followed by a maintenance dose for 48-72 hours. When these reactions are unresponsive to diphenhydramine, benztropine mesylate I.V. 1-2 mg may be effective. These agents are generally effective within 2-5 minutes.

Drug Interactions

Alcohol may increase CNS sedation

Anticholinergic agents may decrease pharmacologic effects; increase anticholinergic side effects; may enhance tardive dyskinesia

Aluminum salts may decrease absorption of phenothiazines

Barbiturates may decrease phenothiazine serum concentrations

Bromocriptine may have decreased efficacy when administered with phenothiazines

Guanethidine's hypotensive effect is decreased by phenothiazines

Lithium administration with phenothiazines may increase disorientation

Meperidine and phenothiazine coadministration increases sedation and hypotension

Methyldopa administration with phenothiazine (trifluoperazine) may significantly increase blood pressure

Norepinephrine, epinephrine have decreased pressor effect when administered with chlorpromazine; therefore, be aware of possible decreased effectiveness or when any phenothiazine is used

Phenytoin serum concentrations may increase or decrease with phenothiazines; tricyclic antidepressants may have increased serum concentrations with concomitant administration with phenothiazines

Propranolol administered with phenothiazines may increase serum concentrations of both drugs

Valproic acid may have increased half-life when administered with phenothiazines (chlorpromazine)

Stability I.M. solution is stable for 12 months at room temperature; reconstituted powder is stable for 48 hours at room temperature

Mechanism of Action Blocks postsynaptic mesolimbic dopaminergic D_1 and D_2 receptors in the brain; exhibits a strong alpha-adrenergic blocking and anticholinergic effect; depresses the release of hypothalamic and hypophyseal hormones; believed to depress the reticular activating system thus affecting basal metabolism, body temperature, wakefulness, vasomotor tone, and emesis

Pharmacokinetics

Absorption: May be affected by the inherent anticholinergic action on the gastrointestinal tissue causing variable absorption. Absorption from tablets is erratic with less variation seen with solutions. These agents are widely distributed in tissues with CNS concentrations exceeding that of plasma due to their lipophilic characteristics.

Protein binding: Antipsychotic agents are bound 90% to 99% to plasma proteins; highly bound to brain and lung tissue and other tissues with a high blood perfusion.

Metabolism: Extensive in the liver

Half-life: >24 hours with chronic use

Time to peak serum concentration: Oral: 2-4 hours

Elimination: Occurs through hepatic metabolism (oxidation) where numerous active metabolites are produced; active metabolites excreted in urine; elimination half-lives of antipsychotics ranges from 20-40 hours which may be extended in elderly due to decline in oxidative hepatic reactions (phase I) with age.

(Continued)

Thiothixene *(Continued)*

The biologic effect of a single dose persists for 24 hours. When the patient has accommodated to initial side effects (sedation), once daily dosing is possible due to the long half-life of antipsychotics.

Steady-state plasma concentrations are achieved in 4-7 days; therefore, if possible, do not make dose adjustments more than once in a 7-day period. Due to the long half-lives of antipsychotics, as needed (prn) use is ineffective since repeated doses are necessary to achieve therapeutic tissue concentrations in the CNS.

Usual Dosage

Geriatrics (nonpsychotic patients, dementia behavior): Initial: 1-2 mg 1-2 times/day; increase dose at 4- to 7-day intervals by 1-2 mg/day; increase dosing intervals (bid, tid, etc) as necessary to control response or side effects; maximum daily dose: 30 mg; gradual increases in dose may prevent some side effects or decrease their severity

Adults:
Oral: Initial: 2 mg 3 times/day, up to 20-30 mg/day; maximum: 60 mg/day
I.M.: 4 mg 2-4 times/day, increase dose gradually; usual: 16-20 mg/day; maximum: 30 mg/day; change to oral dose as soon as able

Not dialyzable (0% to 5%)

Monitoring Parameters
Orthostatic blood pressures; tremors, gait changes, abnormal movement in trunk, neck, buccal area, or extremities; monitor target behaviors for which the agent is given

Reference Range
Serum concentration: 2-57 ng/mL; concentrations do not always correspond to response and are controversial; dose to response for efficacy and safety

Test Interactions
Increased cholesterol (S), increased glucose; decreased uric acid (S)

Patient Information
Oral concentrate must be diluted in 2-4 oz of liquid (water, fruit juice, carbonated drinks, milk, or pudding); do not take antacid within 1 hour of taking drug; avoid alcohol; avoid excess sun exposure (use sun block); may cause drowsiness, rise slowly from recumbent position; use of supportive stockings may help prevent orthostatic hypotension

Nursing Implications
Store injection in the refrigerator; injection for intramuscular use only; dilute the oral concentrate with water or juice before administration; avoid skin contact with oral suspension or solution; may cause contact dermatitis; monitor orthostatic blood pressures 3-5 days after initiation of therapy or a dose increase; observe for tremor and abnormal movement or posturing (extrapyramidal symptoms)

Special Geriatric Considerations
See Warnings.

Many elderly patients receive antipsychotic medications for inappropriate nonpsychotic behavior. Before initiating antipsychotic medication, the clinician should investigate any possible reversible cause; any stress or stress from any disease can cause acute "confusion" or worsening of baseline nonpsychotic behavior. Most commonly acute changes in behavior are due to increases in drug dose or addition of new drug to regimen; fluid electrolyte loss; infections; and changes in environment.

Any changes in disease status in any organ system can result in behavior changes.

In the treatment of agitated, demented, elderly patients, authors of meta-analysis of controlled trials of the response to the traditional antipsychotics (phenothiazines, butyrophenones) in controlling agitation have concluded that the use of neuroleptics results in a response rate of 18%. Clearly neuroleptic therapy for behavior control should be limited with frequent attempts to withdraw the agent given for behavior control.

Dosage Forms
Capsule: 1 mg, 2 mg, 5 mg, 10 mg, 20 mg
Thiothixene hydrochloride:
Concentrate, oral: 5 mg/mL (30 mL, 120 mL)
Injection: 2 mg/mL (2 mL)
Powder for injection: 5 mg/mL (2 mL)

References
Peabody CA, Warner MD, Whiteford HA, et al, "Neuroleptics and the Elderly," *J Am Geriatr Soc*, 1987, 35(3):233-8.

Risse SC and Barnes R, "Pharmacologic Treatment of Agitation Associated With Dementia," *J Am Geriatr Soc*, 1986, 34(5):368-76.

Saltz BL, Woerner MG, Kane JM, et al, "Prospective Study of Tardive Dyskinesia Incidence in the Elderly," *JAMA*, 1991, 266(17):2402-6.

Seifert RD, "Therapeutic Drug Monitoring: Psychotropic Drugs," *J Pharm Pract*, 1984, 6:403-16.

Thorazine® *see* Chlorpromazine *on page 209*
Thyrar® *see* Thyroid *on this page*

Thyroid (THYE royd)
Brand Names Armour® Thyroid; S-P-T; Thyrar®; Thyroid Strong®
Synonyms Desiccated Thyroid; Thyroid Extract; Thyroid USP
Generic Available Yes
Therapeutic Category Thyroid Hormone; Thyroid Product
Use Replacement or supplemental therapy in hypothyroidism; pituitary TSH suppressants (thyroid nodules, thyroiditis, multinodular goiter, thyroid cancer), thyrotoxicosis, diagnostic suppression tests
Contraindications Recent myocardial infarction or thyrotoxicosis, uncomplicated by hypothyroidism; uncorrected adrenal insufficiency, hypersensitivity to active or extraneous constituents
Warnings Ineffective for weight reduction; high doses may produce serious or even life-threatening toxic effects particularly when used with some anorectic drugs; use cautiously in patients with pre-existing cardiovascular disease (angina, CHD), elderly since they may be more likely to have compromised cardiovascular function
Precautions Patients with angina pectoris or other cardiovascular disease; adrenal insufficiency, myxedema, diabetes mellitus and insipidus may have symptoms exaggerated or aggravated; thyroid replacement requires periodic assessment of thyroid status; TSH is the most reliable guide for evaluating adequacy of thyroid replacement dosage. TSH may be elevated during the first few months of thyroid replacement despite patients being clinically euthyroid. In cases where T_4 remains low and TSH is within normal limits, an evaluation of "free" (unbound) T_4 is needed to evaluate further increase in dosage. Chronic hypothyroidism predisposes patients to coronary artery disease.

Adverse Reactions
Cardiovascular: Palpitations, tachycardia, cardiac arrhythmias
Central nervous system: Nervousness, headache, insomnia, fever
Dermatologic: Alopecia
Gastrointestinal: Weight loss, increased appetite, diarrhea, abdominal cramps, vomiting
Neuromuscular & skeletal: Excessive bone loss with overtreatment (excess thyroid replacement), tremors
Miscellaneous: Heat intolerance, diaphoresis

Overdosage Chronic excessive use results in signs and symptoms of hyperthyroidism, weight loss, nervousness, sweating, tachycardia, insomnia, heat intolerance, palpitations, vomiting, psychosis, fever, seizures, angina, arrhythmias, and CHF in those predisposed

Toxicology Reduce dose or temporarily discontinue therapy; normal hypothalamic-pituitary-thyroid axis will return to normal in 6-8 weeks; serum T_4 levels do not correlate well with toxicity; in massive acute ingestion, reduce GI absorption, administer general supportive care; treat CHF with digitalis glycosides; excessive adrenergic activity (tachycardia) require propranolol 1-3 mg I.V. over 10 minutes or 80-160 mg orally/day; fever may be treated with acetaminophen

Drug Interactions
Cholestyramine and colestipol decrease the effect of orally administered thyroid replacement
Estrogens increase TBG, thereby decreasing effect of thyroid replacement
Anticoagulants may increase action
Beta-blocker effect is decreased when patients become euthyroid
Serum digitalis concentrations are reduced in hyperthyroidism or when hypothyroid patients are converted to a euthyroid state
Theophylline serum concentrations decrease when hypothyroid patients converted to a euthyroid state

Mechanism of Action The primary active compound is T_3 (triiodothyronine), which may be converted from T_4 (thyroxine) and then circulates throughout the body; exact mechanism of action is unknown; however, it is believed the thyroid hormone exerts its many metabolic effects through control of DNA transcription and protein synthesis; involved in normal metabolism, growth, and development; promotes gluconeogenesis, increases utilization and mobilization of glycogen stores and stimulates protein synthesis, increases basal metabolic rate

Pharmacodynamics
Onset of therapeutic effects: May be seen in 3-5 days
Maximum effects: 4-6 weeks may be required for any given dose
(Continued)

Thyroid (Continued)

Pharmacokinetics

Absorption: T_4 is 48% to 79% absorbed; T_3 is 95% absorbed; desiccated thyroid contains thyroxine, liothyronine, and iodine (primarily bound); following absorption thyroxine is largely converted to liothyronine

Protein binding: 99% (bound to albumin, thyroxine-binding globulin, and thyroxin-binding prealbumin)

Metabolism: Liothyronine is metabolized in the liver, kidneys, and other tissues to inactive compounds

Half-life:

Liothyronine: 1-2 days

Thyroxine: 6-7 days

Elimination: In urine as conjugated forms

Usual Dosage Geriatrics and Adults (see Additional Information): Initial: 15-30 mg; increase with 15 mg increments every 2-4 weeks; use 15 mg in patients with cardiovascular disease or myxedema. Maintenance dose: Usually 60-120 mg/day; monitor TSH and clinical symptoms.

Thyroid cancer: Requires larger amounts than replacement therapy

Monitoring Parameters T_4, TSH, heart rate, blood pressure, clinical signs of hypo- and hyperthyroidism; TSH is the most reliable guide for evaluating adequacy of thyroid replacement dosage. TSH may be elevated during the first few months of thyroid replacement despite patients being clinically euthyroid. In cases where T_4 remains low and TSH is within normal limits, an evaluation of "free" (unbound) T_4 is needed to evaluate further increase in dosage.

Reference Range

TSH 0.4-10 (for those ≥80 years) mIU/L

T_4: 4-12 µg/dL (51-154 mmol:/L)

T_3 (RIA) (total T_3): 80-230 ng/dL (1.2-3.5 mmol/L)

T_4 free (Free T_4): 0.7-1.8 ng/dL (9-23 pmol/L)

Test Interactions Increased calcium (S); many drugs may have effects on thyroid function tests; para-aminosalicylic acid, aminoglutethimide, amiodarone, barbiturates, carbamazepine, chloral hydrate, clofibrate, colestipol, corticosteroids, danazol, diazepam, estrogens, ethionamide, fluorouracil, I.V. heparin, insulin, lithium, methadone, methimazole, mitotane, nitroprusside, oxyphenbutazone, phenylbutazone, PTU, perphenazine, phenytoin, propranolol, salicylates, sulfonylureas, and thiazides

Patient Information Do not change brands without physician's knowledge; report immediately to physician any chest pain, increased pulse, palpitations, heat intolerance, excessive sweating; do not stop use without physician's advice; replacement therapy will be for life; take as a single dose before breakfast

Nursing Implications Monitor pulse rate and blood pressure (see Precautions, Adverse Reactions, Toxicology, Monitoring Parameters, Special Geriatric Considerations)

Additional Information Equivalent levothyroxine dose: Thyroid USP 60 mg = levothyroxine 0.05-0.06 mg; liothyronine: 15-37.5 mcg; liotrix: 60 mg

Special Geriatric Considerations Desiccated thyroid contains variable amounts of T_3, T_4, and other triiodothyronine compounds which are more likely to cause cardiac signs and symptoms due to fluctuating levels; should avoid use in elderly for this reason; many clinicians consider levothyroxine to be the drug of choice

Dosage Forms Tablet: 15 mg, 30 mg, 60 mg, 120 mg, 180 mg, 300 mg

References

Helfand M and Crapo LM, "Monitoring Therapy in Patients Taking Levothyroxine," *Ann Intern Med*, 1990, 113(6):450-4.

Johnson DG and Campbell S, "Hormonal and Metabolic Agents," *Geriatric Pharmacology*, Bressler R and Katz MD, eds, New York, NY: McGraw-Hill, 1993, 427-50.

Sanders LR, "Pituitary, Thyroid, Adrenal and Parathyroid Diseases in the Elderly," *Geriatric Medicine*, 1990, 475-87.

Sawin CT, Geller A, Hershman JM, et al, "The Aging Thyroid. The Use of Thyroid Hormone in Older Persons," *JAMA*, 1989, 261(18):2653-5.

Watts NB, "Use of a Sensitive Thyrotropin Assay for Monitoring Treatment With Levothyroxine," *Arch Intern Med*, 1989, 149(2):309-12.

Thyroid Extract see Thyroid on previous page

Thyroid Strong® see Thyroid on previous page

Thyroid USP see Thyroid on previous page

Thyrolar® see Liotrix on page 541

Tiagabine (tye AJ a bene)

Brand Names Gabitril®

Therapeutic Category Anticonvulsant

Use Adjunctive therapy in adults and children 12 years and older in the treatment of partial seizures

Contraindications Patients who have demonstrated hypersensitivity to the drug or any of its agreements

Warnings Anticonvulsants should not be discontinued abruptly because of the possibility of increasing seizure frequency; clinical studies were carried out that demonstrated an increase in seizure frequency upon abrupt withdrawal; tiagabine should be withdrawn gradually to minimize the potential of increased seizure frequency, unless safety concerns require a more rapid withdrawal; decrease dose in liver disease; potential to exacerbate impaired cognitive function

Adverse Reactions All adverse effects are dose related

Central nervous system: Dizziness, headache, somnolence, CNS depression, memory disturbance, ataxia

Neuromuscular & skeletal: Tremors, weakness

Drug Interactions The clearance of tiagabine is affected by the co-administration of hepatic enzyme inducing antiepilepsy drugs; tiagabine is cleared more rapidly in patients who have been treated with carbamazepine, phenytoin, primidone, and phenobarbital than in patients who have not received these drugs

Mechanism of Action The exact mechanism by which tiagabine exerts antiseizure activity is not definitively known; however, *in vitro* experiments demonstrate that it enhances the activity of gamma aminobutyric acid (GABA), the major neuroinhibitory transmitter in the nervous system; it is thought that binding to the GABA uptake carrier inhibits the uptake of GABA into presynaptic neurons, allowing an increased amount of GABA to be available to postsynaptic neurons; based on *in vitro* studies, tiagabine does not inhibit the uptake of dopamine, norepinephrine, serotonin, glutamate, or choline

Pharmacokinetics

Absorption: Rapid (within 1 hour); food prolongs absorption

Protein binding: 96%

Half-life: 6.7 hours

Elimination: Oral: 25% of dose recovered in urine, 63% in feces

Usual Dosage Geriatrics and Adults: Oral: Starting dose is 4 mg, once daily; the total daily dose may be increased in 4 mg increments beginning the second week of therapy; thereafter, the daily dose may be increased by 4-8 mg/day until clinical response is achieved, up to a maximum of 32 mg/day; the total daily dose at higher dosages should be given in divided doses, 2-4 times/day

Monitoring Parameters Seizure frequency

Reference Range Maximal plasma concentration after a 24 mg/dose: 552 ng/mL

Patient Information Contact physician if dizziness, headache, mood changes, stomach pain, memory difficulties, or excessive sedation occur

Special Geriatric Considerations No special recommendations are made for elderly; dose according to response; see Usual Dosage

Dosage Forms Tablet, as hydrochloride: 4 mg, 12 mg, 16 mg, 20 mg

References

Patsalos PN and Sander JW, "Newer Antiepileptic Drugs: Towards an Improved Risk-Benefit Ratio," *Drug Saf*, 1994, 11(1):37-67.

Tiamate® *see Diltiazem on page 298*

Tiazac® *see Diltiazem on page 298*

Ticar® *see Ticarcillin on this page*

Ticarcillin (tye kar SIL in)

Related Information

I.V. Medication Recommendations *on page 1080*

Brand Names Ticar®

Synonyms Ticarcillin Disodium

Therapeutic Category Antibiotic, Penicillin

Use Treatment of susceptible infections such as septicemia, acute and chronic respiratory tract infections, skin and soft tissue infections, and urinary tract infections due to susceptible strains of *Pseudomonas*, *Proteus*, and *Escherichia coli* and *Enterobacter*

(Continued)

Ticarcillin *(Continued)*

Contraindications Hypersensitivity to ticarcillin or any component or penicillins

Precautions Use with caution in patients with congestive heart failure due to high sodium load (~6 mEq/g); dosage modification required in patients with impaired renal and/or hepatic function; use with caution in patients with a history of cephalosporin allergy

Adverse Reactions

Central nervous system: Seizures, headache, confusion, sedation, fever

Dermatologic: Rash

Endocrine & metabolic: Hypernatremia, hypokalemia, metabolic alkalosis

Gastrointestinal: Diarrhea, stomatitis

Hematologic: Inhibition of platelet aggregation, eosinophilia, leukopenia, neutropenia, bleeding diathesis, hemolytic anemia, positive Coombs' test, decreased hemoglobin and hematocrit

Hepatic: Elevated AST, hepatitis

Local: Thrombophlebitis

Renal: Acute interstitial nephritis

Miscellaneous: Allergic reactions, Jarisch-Herxheimer reactions

Overdosage Symptoms of overdose include neuromuscular hypersensitivity, seizure

Toxicology Many beta-lactam-containing antibiotics have the potential to cause neuromuscular hyperirritability or convulsive seizures. Hemodialysis may be helpful to aid in the removal of the drug from the blood, otherwise most treatment is supportive or symptom directed.

Drug Interactions Aminoglycosides, bacteriostatic agents

Increased duration of neuromuscular blockers

Increased/prolonged serum concentration with probenecid

Stability Reconstituted solution is stable for 72 hours at room temperature and 14 days when refrigerated; for I.V. infusion in NS or D_5W solution is stable for 72 hours at room temperature, 14 days when refrigerated or 30 days when frozen; after freezing, thawed solution is stable for 72 hours at room temperature or 14 days when refrigerated; incompatible with aminoglycosides

Mechanism of Action Interferes with bacterial cell wall synthesis during active multiplication causing cell death and resultant bactericidal activity against susceptible bacteria

Pharmacokinetics

Absorption: I.M.: 86%

Protein binding: 45% to 65%

Half-life: 66-72 minutes, prolonged with renal impairment and/or hepatic impairment

Time to peak serum concentration: I.M.: Within 30-75 minutes

Elimination: Almost entirely in urine as unchanged drug and its metabolites with small amounts excreted in feces (3.5%); CNS distribution is low and increased when the meninges are inflamed

Usual Dosage Ticarcillin is generally given I.M. only for the treatment of uncomplicated urinary tract infections.

Geriatrics: I.V.: 3 g every 4-6 hours; adjust dosing interval for renal impairment

Adults: I.V.: 1-4 g every 4-6 hours

Dosing interval in renal impairment: I.V.:

Cl_{cr} >60 mL/minute: Administer 3 g every 4 hours

Cl_{cr} 30-60 mL/minute: Administer 2 g every 4 hours

Cl_{cr} 10-30 mL/minute: Administer 2 g every 8 hours

Cl_{cr} <10 mL/minute: Administer 2 g every 12 hours

Cl_{cr} <10 mL/minute with hepatic dysfunction: Administer 2 g every 24 hours

Peritoneal dialysis: Administer 3 g every 12 hours

Hemodialysis: Administer 2 g every 12 hours; follow each dialysis with 3 g

Moderately dialyzable (20% to 50%)

Administration Administer 1 hour apart from aminoglycosides; do not administer I.M.

Monitoring Parameters Temperature, WBC, respiratory rate; cultures and sensitivity (if applicable), mental status, appetite

Test Interactions False-positive urinary or serum protein

Nursing Implications See Administration

Additional Information Sodium content of 1 g: 5.2 to 6.5 mEq; normally used with other antibiotics (ie, aminoglycosides)

Special Geriatric Considerations When used as empiric therapy or for documented pseudomonal pneumonia, it is best to combine with an aminoglycoside such as gentamicin or tobramycin; high sodium may limit use in patients with congestive heart failure; adjust dose for renal function (see Precautions)

Dosage Forms Powder for injection, as disodium: 1 g, 3 g, 6 g, 20 g, 30 g

References

Brogden RN, Heel RC, Speight TM, et al, "Ticarcillin: A Review of Its Pharmacological Properties and Therapeutic Efficacy," *Drugs*, 1980, 20(5):325-52.

Yoshikawa TT, "Antimicrobial Therapy for the Elderly Patient," *J Am Geriatr Soc*, 1990, 38(12):1353-72.

Ticarcillin and Clavulanate Potassium

(tye kar SIL in & klav yoo LAN ate poe TASS ee um)

Related Information

I.V. Medication Recommendations *on page 1080*

Penicillins, Penicillin-Related Antibiotics, & Other Antibiotics *on page 1010*

Brand Names Timentin®

Synonyms Ticarcillin and Clavulanic Acid

Therapeutic Category Antibiotic, Penicillin

Use Treatment of infections of lower respiratory tract, urinary tract, skin and skin structures, bone and joint, and septicemia caused by susceptible organisms. Clavulanate expands activity of ticarcillin to include beta-lactamase producing strains of *S. aureus*, *H. influenzae*, *Enterobacteriaceae*, *Pseudomonas*, *Klebsiella*, *Citrobacter*, and *Serratia*

Contraindications Known hypersensitivity to ticarcillin, clavulanate, and any penicillin

Precautions Use with caution and modify dosage in patients with renal impairment; use with caution in patients with congestive heart failure due to high sodium load (~6 mEq/g); use with caution in patients with cephalosporin allergy

Adverse Reactions

Central nervous system: Seizures, headache, confusion, sedation, fever

Dermatologic: Rash

Endocrine & metabolic: Hypernatremia, hypokalemia, metabolic alkalosis

Gastrointestinal: Diarrhea, stomatitis

Hematologic: Inhibition of platelet aggregation, eosinophilia, leukopenia, decreased hemoglobin and hematocrit, prolongation of bleeding time, positive Coombs' test

Hepatic: Elevated AST, hepatitis

Local: Thrombophlebitis

Renal: Acute interstitial nephritis

Miscellaneous: Hypersensitivity reactions, Jarisch-Herxheimer reactions

Toxicology Many beta-lactam-containing antibiotics have the potential to cause neuromuscular hyperirritability or convulsive seizures. Hemodialysis may be helpful to aid in the removal of the drug from the blood, otherwise most treatment is supportive or symptom directed.

Drug Interactions Aminoglycosides, bacteriostatic agents

Increased duration of neuromuscular blockers

Increased/prolonged serum concentration with probenecid

Stability Reconstituted solution is stable for 6 hours at room temperature and 72 hours when refrigerated; for I.V. infusion in NS is stable for 24 hours at room temperature, 7 days when refrigerated, or 30 days when frozen; after freezing, thawed solution is stable for 8 hours at room temperature; for I.V. infusion in D₅W solution is stable for 24 hours at room temperature, 3 days when refrigerated, or 7 days when frozen; after freezing, thawed solution is stable for 8 hours at room temperature; darkening of drug indicates loss of potency of clavulanate potassium; incompatible with sodium bicarbonate, aminoglycosides

Mechanism of Action Ticarcillin interferes with bacterial cell wall synthesis during active multiplication causing cell death and resultant bactericidal activity against susceptible bacteria; clavulanic acid prevents degradation of ticarcillin by binding to the active site on beta-lactamase

Pharmacokinetics

Distribution: Low concentrations of ticarcillin distribute into the CSF and increase when meninges are inflamed

Protein binding:

Ticarcillin: 45% to 65%

Clavulanic acid: 9% to 30%

Metabolism: Clavulanic acid is metabolized in the liver

(Continued)

Ticarcillin and Clavulanate Potassium *(Continued)*

Half-life:
Clavulanate: 66-90 minutes
Ticarcillin: 66-72 minutes in patients with normal renal function
Clavulanic acid does not affect the clearance of ticarcillin
Elimination: 45% of clavulanic acid is excreted unchanged in urine, whereas 60% to 90% of ticarcillin is excreted unchanged in urine
Removed by hemodialysis

Usual Dosage I.V.:
Geriatrics (based on ticarcillin): 3 g every 4-6 hours; adjust for renal function
Adults: 3.1 g (ticarcillin 3 g plus clavulanic acid 0.1 g) every 4-6 hours; maximum: 18-24 g/day; for urinary tract infections: 3.1 g every 6-8 hours

Dosing interval in renal impairment:
Cl_{cr} >60 mL/minute: Administer 3 g every 4 hours
Cl_{cr} 30-60 mL/minute: Administer 2 g every 4 hours
Cl_{cr} 10-30 mL/minute: Administer 2 g every 8 hours
Cl_{cr} <10 mL/minute: Administer 2 g every 12 hours

Dosing interval in hepatic/renal impairment: Cl_{cr} <10 mL/minute: Administer 2 g every 24 hours

Administration Infuse over 30 minutes; do not administer I.M.

Monitoring Parameters Temperature, WBC, respiratory rate; culture and sensitivity (if applicable), mental status, appetite

Test Interactions Positive Coombs' test, false-positive urinary proteins

Nursing Implications See Administration

Additional Information Usually given for at least for 2 days after symptoms have disappeared

Special Geriatric Considerations When used as empiric therapy or for a documented pseudomonal pneumonia, it is best to combine with an aminoglycoside such as gentamicin or tobramycin; high sodium content may limit use in patients with congestive heart failure; adjust dose for renal function (see Precautions)

Dosage Forms Powder for injection: Ticarcillin disodium 3 g and clavulanic acid 0.1 g per g (3.1 g)

Ticarcillin and Clavulanic Acid *see* Ticarcillin and Clavulanate Potassium *on previous page*

Ticarcillin Disodium *see* Ticarcillin *on page 919*

Ticlid® *see* Ticlopidine *on this page*

Ticlopidine *(tye KLOE pi deen)*

Brand Names Ticlid®

Generic Available No

Therapeutic Category Antiplatelet Agent

Use Reduction of risk of thrombotic stroke (fatal or nonfatal) in patients who have experienced stroke precursors or have had a completed thrombotic stroke

Unlabeled use (more study needed): Intermittent claudication, chronic arterial occlusion, subarachnoid hemorrhage, open heart surgery, coronary artery bypass grafts, stent implantation, and primary glomerulonephritis. **Note:** Because of the risk of neutropenia occurring with ticlopidine, reserve its use for those patients intolerant to aspirin.

Contraindications Hypersensitivity to ticlopidine; presence of hematopoietic disorders (ie, neutropenia, thrombocytopenia); hemostatic disorders; active pathological bleeding (ie, peptic ulcer or intracranial bleeding); severe liver impairment

Warnings Neutropenia, sometimes severe (ANC <450 neutrophils/mm³), has been experienced by 0.9% to 2.4% of patients in two large clinical trials. The drop in ANC was in the first 3 weeks to 3 months of treatment. Discontinuation of the drug may be necessary; neutrophil counts should return to baseline in 1-3 weeks (see Monitoring Parameters).

Thrombocytopenia (platelet count <80,000 cells/mm³) is rare, but can occur alone or in conjunction with neutropenia. If confirmed by clinical evaluation and laboratory findings, discontinue therapy. Rare case of pancytopenia and thrombotic thrombocytopenia purpura have been reported. Total cholesterol and triglyceride concentrations may be increased while the lipoprotein subfraction ratios remain unchanged.

Discontinue anticoagulant or fibrinolytic drug therapy before starting ticlopidine. Ticlopidine is not recommended for patients with severe hepatic disease and has not been studied in patients with severe renal function impairment. A dosage adjustment (decrease) may be necessary or the drug stopped if hemorrhagic or hematopoietic complications arise.

Precautions An increased risk of bleeding may be present in patients undergoing a surgical procedure who experience trauma or who have certain pathological conditions. When possible, discontinue ticlopidine 10-14 days prior to elective surgery. Prolonged bleeding time can be reversed in 2 hours following 20 mg I.V. methylprednisolone; oral steroids are also effective; platelet transfusion is another option.

Adverse Reactions

Dermatologic: Rash (>5%), pruritus, purpura

Gastrointestinal: Diarrhea, nausea, dyspepsia, GI pain vomiting, flatulence, anorexia

Hematologic: Bleeding disorders, neutropenia

Hepatic: Abnormal liver function tests (alkaline phosphatase and transaminase)

Overdosage In one case of intentional overdose, the only abnormalities reported were increased bleeding time and increased ALT.

Toxicology See Warnings and Precautions

Drug Interactions

Antacids decreased bioavailability

Cimetidine decreased ticlopidine clearance

Aspirin increased antiplatelet aggregation effects, coadministration is not recommended

Digoxin small decreased digoxin plasma concentrations

Theophylline increased half-life by ~50%

Mechanism of Action Ticlopidine is an inhibitor of platelet function with a mechanism which is different from other antiplatelet drugs. Ticlopidine results in a time and dose-dependent inhibition of platelet aggregation and release of granule constituents; this is accomplished through inhibition of ADP-induced platelet fibrinogen binding and further platelet-platelet interactions which are irreversible for life of the platelet. The drug significantly increases bleeding time. This effect may not be solely related to ticlopidine's effects on platelets. The prolongation of the bleeding time caused by ticlopidine is further increased by the addition of aspirin in *ex vivo* experiments. Although many metabolites of ticlopidine have been found, none have been shown to account for *in vivo* activity. The effect on platelet function is irreversible for the life of the platelet.

Pharmacodynamics

Onset of action: Within 6 hours

Peak effects: Oral: Achieved after 3-5 days of therapy

Because the duration of inhibition of platelet function corresponds to the normal life span of the platelet, these effects usually reverse 1-2 weeks after stopping the drug

Pharmacokinetics

Absorption: Following administration, 80% to 90% absorbed from GI tract with an average peak plasma steady-state concentration of 0.9 mg/mL ~2 hours after a 250 mg dose

Protein binding: 98% bound to plasma proteins, primarily albumin and lipoproteins, with ≤15% bound to alpha$_1$-acid glycoprotein

Metabolism: Metabolized in the liver extensively, principally by N-dealkylation and oxidation of the thiophene ring; four metabolites have been identified in humans

Half-life: 12-36 hours increasing to 4-5 days after continuous dosing; clearance decreases in older subjects; mean area under the serum concentration time curve was 2-3 times that in younger adults and trough concentrations were twice as high as compared to younger adults; at steady-state there were no significant differences in time to peak or elimination half-life between young and elderly subjects, but the average plasma concentration in the elderly was twice that of the younger group. It is unknown whether these differences are due to increased absorption, decreased clearance, or a change in plasma protein binding.

Elimination: <1% excreted unchanged in urine

Usual Dosage Oral:

Geriatrics: 250 mg twice daily with food; dosage in the elderly has not been determined; however, in two large clinical trials, the average age of subjects was 63 and 66 years; a dosage decrease may be necessary if bleeding abnormalities develop

Adults: 250 mg twice daily with food

Stent implantation: 250 mg twice daily

Dosing in renal or hepatic impairment: Not established

(Continued)

Ticlopidine *(Continued)*

Monitoring Parameters Signs of bleeding; CBC with differential every 2 weeks starting the second week through the third month of treatment; more frequent monitoring is recommended for patients whose absolute neutrophil counts have been consistently declining or are 30% less than baseline values. Liver function tests (alkaline phosphatase and transaminases) should be performed in the first 4 months of therapy if liver dysfunction is suspected.

Reference Range Serum concentrations do not correlate with clinical anti-platelet activity

Test Interactions Increased alkaline phosphatase, increased ALT, AST, slight increased bilirubin, decreased neutrophils

Patient Information Possibility of signs and symptoms of neutropenia, thrombocytopenia, and abnormal bleeding; comply with biweekly blood tests; report any symptoms of infection such as fever, chills, sore throat; report unusual bleeding; tell all physicians and dentists that you are on ticlopidine; take with food to minimize GI complaints

Nursing Implications Monitor for signs of bleeding, infection; administer with food

Special Geriatric Considerations Because of the risk of neutropenia and its relative expense as compared with aspirin, ticlopidine should only be used in patients with a documented intolerance to aspirin (see Pharmacokinetics and Usual Dosage).

Dosage Forms Tablet, as hydrochloride: 250 mg

References

Ito MK, Smith AR, and Lee ML, "Ticlopidine: A New Platelet Aggregation Inhibitor," *Clin Pharm,* 1992, 11(7):603-17.

Schömig A, Neumann, FJ, Kastrati A, et al, "A Randomized Comparison of Antiplatelet and Anticoagulant Therapy After the Placement of Coronary-Artery Stents," *N Engl J Med,* 1996, 334(17):1084-9.

Shah J, Teitelbaum P, Molony B, et al, "Single and Multiple Dose Pharmacokinetics of Ticlopidine in Young and Elderly Subjects," *Br J Clin Pharmacol,* 1991, 32:761-4.

Teitelbaum P, Gabzuda TG, Koretz SH, et al, "Pharmacokinetics of Ticlopidine Hydrochloride in Young and Old Normal Adult Subjects Following Single and Multiple Dosing," *J Pharm Sci,* 1987, 76:S99.

Ticon® *see* Trimethobenzamide *on page 961*

TIG *see* Tetanus Immune Globulin, Human *on page 897*

Tigan® *see* Trimethobenzamide *on page 961*

Tilade® Inhalation Aerosol *see* Nedocromil Sodium *on page 658*

Tiludronate *(tye LOO droe nate)*

Brand Names Skelid®

Therapeutic Category Bisphosphonate Derivative

Use Paget's disease of the bone

Contraindications Hypersensitivity to tiludronate; not for use in patients whose creatinine clearance is <30 mL/minute

Warnings May cause dysphasia, esophagitis, esophageal ulcer, or gastric ulcer

Adverse Reactions
Cardiovascular: Edema, chest pain
Central nervous system: Headache, somnolence, tinnitus, dizziness
Dermatologic: Rash
Endocrine: Hyperparathyroidism
Gastrointestinal: Diarrhea, nausea, vomiting, flatulence
Genitourinary: Renal impairment

Drug Interactions Avoid administration of all drugs within 2 hours pre- and postdose

Drug/Food Interactions Food decreases bioavailability

Mechanism of Action As a bisphosphonate, it may inhibit enzyme secretion by osteoclasts or osteoblast stimulation of osteoclasts

Pharmacodynamics Initial response in Paget's disease: 2 days to 1 month

Pharmacokinetics
Bioavailability: 4% to 8%
Distribution: 90% bound to plasma proteins, bone
Half-life: 43-150 hours
Elimination: Kidney (60%)

Usual Dosage Geriatrics and Adults: Oral: 400 mg (2 tablets) [tiludronic acid] daily for 3 months

Dosing adjustment in renal impairment: Cl_{cr} <30 mL/minute: Avoid
Dosing adjustment in hepatic impairment: No adjustment necessary

Monitoring Parameters Alkaline phosphatase, urinary hydroxyproline, adjusted calcium, serum osteocalcin

Patient Information Take with 6-8 ounces of plain water; do not take other medications or food for 2 hours before or after dose; do not double dose if a dose is missed

Nursing Implications Administer with 6-8 ounces of plain water; avoid food and other medications for 2 hours pre- and postdose

Additional Information Three months of treatment is recommended; because of bioavailability problems, tiludronate should not be taken with beverages other than water or within 2 hours of food, calcium or mineral supplements, aspirin, or indomethacin; aluminum- or magnesium-containing antacids should be taken at least 2 hours after tiludronate

Special Geriatric Considerations No dose adjustment necessary

Dosage Forms Tablet, as disodium: 240 mg [tiludronic acid 200 mg]; dosage is expressed in terms of tiludronic acid.

Timentin® *see* Ticarcillin and Clavulanate Potassium *on page 921*

Timolol (TYE moe lole)

Related Information

Beta-Blockers Comparison *on page 1026*
Glaucoma Drug Therapy Comparison *on page 1032*

Brand Names Betimol® Ophthalmic; Blocadren® Oral; Timoptic® Ophthalmic; Timoptic-XE® Ophthalmic

Therapeutic Category Beta-Adrenergic Blocker; Beta-Adrenergic Blocker, Ophthalmic

Use

Ophthalmic: Treatment of elevated intraocular pressure such as glaucoma or ocular hypertension

Oral: Treatment of hypertension and angina and reduce mortality following myocardial infarction, hypertrophic subaortic stenosis, and prophylaxis of migraine; treatment of the postmyocardial infarction patient

Contraindications Uncompensated congestive heart failure, cardiogenic shock, bradycardia or heart block, bronchial asthma, severe chronic obstructive pulmonary disease or history of asthma; hypersensitivity to beta-blocking agents

Warnings Severe CNS, cardiovascular and respiratory adverse effects have been seen following ophthalmic use; patients with a history of asthma, congestive heart failure, bradycardia, hyperthyroidism, or cerebral insufficiency appear to be at a higher risk; use cautiously in diabetes mellitus

Precautions Some products contain sulfites which can cause allergic reactions; diminished response over time; may increase muscle weaknesses; use with a miotic in angle-closure glaucoma; similar to other beta-blockers; use with caution in patients with decreased renal or hepatic function (dosage adjustment required); abrupt withdrawal of drug should be avoided; discontinuation should be accomplished over a 2-week tapering

Adverse Reactions

Cardiovascular: Bradycardia, arrhythmias, hypotension, syncope, congestive heart failure

Central nervous system: Dizziness, headache, confusion, mental depression, nightmares

Dermatologic: Rash

Endocrine: Blocks signs or symptoms of hypoglycemia

Gastrointestinal: Diarrhea, nausea

Ocular: Irritation, conjunctivitis, keratitis, visual disturbances, blepharitis

Respiratory: Bronchospasm, wheezing, dyspnea

Other adverse effects similar to other beta-blockers, alopecia, weakness

Overdosage Symptoms of overdose include severe hypotension, bradycardia, heart failure and bronchospasm

Toxicology Sympathomimetics (eg, epinephrine or dopamine), glucagon or a pacemaker can be used to treat the toxic bradycardia, asystole, and/or hypotension; initially, fluids may be the best treatment for toxic hypotension. For ophthalmic product, flush eye(s) with water or normal saline. Not significantly dialyzable.

Drug Interactions May cause bradycardia and asystole when also giving verapamil; has caused sinus bradycardia in one patient also taking quinidine; controversial when used with epinephrine; nonsteroidal anti-inflammatory agents, salicylates, sympathomimetics, thyroid hormones, insulins, lidocaine, calcium channel blockers, nifedipine, catecholamine-depleting drugs, clonidine, disopyramide, prazosin, theophylline, cimetidine
(Continued)

Timolol *(Continued)*

Mechanism of Action Blocks both beta$_1$-adrenergic and beta$_2$-adrenergic receptors, reduces intraocular pressure by most likely reducing aqueous humor production or possibly outflow; reduces blood pressure by blocking adrenergic receptors and decreasing sympathetic outflow, produces a negative chronotropic and inotropic activity through an unknown mechanism

Pharmacodynamics

Onset of action: Oral: Following administration hypotensive effects occur within 15-45 minutes

Peak effect: Within 30-150 minutes

Duration: ~4 hours; intraocular effects persist for 24 hours after ophthalmic instillation

Pharmacokinetics

Protein binding: 60%

Metabolism: Extensive in the liver; extensive first-pass effect; substrate CYP2D6

Half-life: 2-2.7 hours; half-life prolonged with reduced renal function

Elimination: Urinary (15% to 20% as unchanged drug)

Usual Dosage Geriatrics and Adults:

Ophthalmic: Initial:

Gel: Invert container and shake once; instill 1 drop once daily

Solution, 0.25%: Instill 1 drop twice daily; increase to 0.5% solution if response not adequate; decrease to 1 drop/day if controlled; do not exceed 1 drop twice daily of 0.5% solution

Oral:

Hypertension: Initial: 10 mg twice daily, increase gradually every 7 days, usual dosage: 20-40 mg/day in 2 divided doses; maximum: 60 mg/day

Prevention of myocardial infarction: 10 mg twice daily initiated within 1-4 weeks after infarction

Migraine: Initial: 10 mg twice daily; increase to maximum of 30 mg/day

Monitoring Parameters Intraocular pressure, heart rate, blood pressure, respiratory rate, funduscopic exam, visual field tests

Test Interactions Increased cholesterol (S), elevated glucose

Patient Information May sting on instillation; do not touch dropper to eye; visual acuity may be decreased after administration; distance vision may be altered; assess patient's or caregiver's ability to administer; apply gentle pressure to lacrimal sac during and immediately following instillation (1 minute) to avoid systemic absorption; stop drug if breathing difficulty occurs; administer other ophthalmics at least 10 minutes before the gel

Nursing Implications Monitor for signs of congestive heart failure, hypotension, respiratory difficulty (bronchospasm); use cautiously in diabetics receiving hypoglycemic agents; teach proper instillation of eye drops; administer other ophthalmics at least 10 minutes before the gel (see Monitoring Parameters)

Additional Information Does not cause night blindness

Special Geriatric Considerations Due to alterations in the beta-adrenergic autonomic nervous system, beta-adrenergic blockade may result in less hemodynamic response than seen in younger adults. Studies indicate that despite decreased sensitivity to the chronotropic effects of beta blockade with age, there appears to be an increased myocardial sensitivity to the negative inotropic effect during stress (ie, exercise). Controlled trials have shown the overall response rate for propranolol to be only 20% to 50% in elderly populations. Therefore, all beta-adrenergic blocking drugs may result in a decreased response as compared to younger adults.

Dosage Forms

Solution, ophthalmic, as hemihydrate (Betimol®): 0.25% (2.5 mL, 5 mL, 10 mL, 15 mL); 0.5% (2.5 mL, 5 mL, 10 mL, 15 mL)

Timolol maleate:

Gel, ophthalmic (Timoptic-XE®): 0.25% (2.5 mL, 5 mL); 0.5% (2.5 mL, 5 mL)

Solution, ophthalmic (Timoptic®): 0.25% (2.5 mL, 5 mL, 10 mL, 15 mL); 0.5% (2.5 mL, 5 mL, 10 mL, 15 mL)

Solution, ophthalmic, as maleate, preservative free, single use (Timoptic® OcuDose®): 0.25%, 0.5%

Tablet (Blocadren®): 5 mg, 10 mg, 20 mg

References

Kligman EW and Higbee MD, "Drug Therapy for Hypertension in the Elderly," *J Fam Pract*, 1989, 28(1):81-7.

Levison SP, "Treating Hypertension in the Elderly," *Clin Geriatr Med*, 1988, 4(1):1-12.

Passo MS, Palmer EA, and Van Buskirk EM, "Plasma Timolol in Glaucoma Patients," *Ophthalmology*, 1984, 91(11):1361-3.

Vestal RE, Wood AJ, and Shand DG, "Reduced Beta-Adrenoceptor Sensitivity in the Elderly," *Clin Pharmacol Ther*, 1979, 26(2):181-6.

Yin FC, Raizes, GS, Guarnieri T, et al, "Age-Associated Decrease in Ventricular Response to Haemodynamic Stress During Beta-Adrenergic Blockade," *Br Heart J*, 1978, 40(12):1349-55.

Timoptic® Ophthalmic *see* Timolol *on page 925*

Timoptic-XE® Ophthalmic *see* Timolol *on page 925*

Tinactin® [OTC] *see* Tolnaftate *on page 939*

Tinactin® for Jock Itch [OTC] *see* Tolnaftate *on page 939*

Tindal® *see* Acetophenazine *on page 22*

Tine Test *see* Tuberculin Purified Protein Derivative *on page 971*

Tine Test PPD *see* Tuberculin Purified Protein Derivative *on page 971*

Ting® [OTC] *see* Tolnaftate *on page 939*

Tioconazole (tye oh KONE a zole)
Brand Names Vagistat-1® Vaginal [OTC]

Generic Available No

Therapeutic Category Antifungal Agent, Imidazole Derivative; Antifungal Agent, Vaginal

Use Local treatment of vulvovaginal candidiasis

Contraindications Known hypersensitivity to tioconazole

Warnings Not effective when applied to the scalp; may interact with condoms and vaginal contraceptive diaphragms; avoid these products for 3 days following treatment

Adverse Reactions Genitourinary: Vulvar/vaginal burning; vulvar itching, soreness, edema, or discharge; polyuria

Mechanism of Action A 1-substituted imidazole derivative with a broad antifungal spectrum against a wide variety of dermatophytes and yeasts, usually at a concentration ≤6.25 mg/L; has been demonstrated to be at least as active *in vitro* as other imidazole antifungals. *In vitro*, tioconazole has been demonstrated 2-8 times as potent as miconazole against common dermal pathogens including *Trichophyton mentagrophytes*, *T. rubrum*, *T. erinacei*, *T. tonsurans*, *Microsporum canis*, *Microsporum gypseum*, and *Candida albicans*. Both agents appear to be similarly effective against *Epidermophyton floccosum*.

Pharmacokinetics

Absorption: Intravaginal: Following application small amounts of drug are absorbed systemically (25%) within 2-8 hours; therapeutic levels persist for 3-5 days after single dose

Half-life: 21-24 hours

Elimination: Urine and feces in approximate equal amounts

Usual Dosage Geriatrics and Adults: Vaginal: Insert 1 applicatorful in vagina, just prior to bedtime, as a single dose; therapy may extend to 7 days

Patient Information Insert high into vagina; contact physician if itching or burning continues; Vagistat-1 may interact with condoms and vaginal contraceptive diaphragms (ie, weaken latex); do not rely on these products for 3 days following treatment

Dosage Forms Cream, vaginal: 6.5% with applicator (4.6 g)

Tiotixene *see* Thiothixene *on page 913*

Titralac® Plus Liquid [OTC] *see* Calcium Salts (Oral) *on page 152*

Tizanidine (tye ZAN i deen)
Brand Names Zanaflex®

Synonyms Sirdalud®

Therapeutic Category Alpha$_2$-Adrenergic Agonist Agent

Use Skeletal muscle relaxant used for treatment of muscle spasticity

Unlabeled use: Has been shown to be effective for tension headaches, low back pain and trigeminal neuralgia in a limited number of trials

Contraindications Previous hypersensitivity to tizanidine

Warnings Reduce dose in patients with liver or renal disease; use with caution in patients with hypotension or cardiac disease as this agent's alpha$_2$-adrenergic action produces hypotension

Liver disease: Tizanidine may cause hepatocellular damage; reversible with drug discontinuation. Three deaths have been reported from liver damage

Sedation: Sedation is a common side effect reported in multiple-dose studies

Hallucinations/psychotic symptoms have been associated with tizanidine use

Renal impairment: Use with caution in patients with reduced renal function since clearance is reduced

Elderly: Use tizanidine with caution since clearance is decreased fourfold

(Continued)

Tizanidine *(Continued)*

Precautions Monitor liver function tests (see Monitoring Parameters); dose-related retinal degeneration and corneal opacities have been reported in animal studies; no such reports in humans

Adverse Reactions

Cardiovascular: Hypotension, bradycardia, syncope, vasodilation, palpitations, ventricular extrasystoles, angina, heart failure, myocardial infarction, pulmonary embolus

Central nervous system: Sedation, daytime drowsiness, somnolence, fatigue, dizziness, anxiety, nervousness, insomnia, psychotic-like symptoms, visual hallucinations, delusions, migraine headache, emotional lability, seizures, vertigo, abnormal dreams, agitation, euphoria, stupor, dysautonomia, dementia symptoms, neuropathy

Dermatologic: Pruritus, skin rash, dry skin, acne, exfoliative dermatitis, urticaria, herpes infections, skin ulcers (1%), ecchymosis, petechia, purpura

Endocrine & metabolic: Hypothyroidism, adrenal insufficiency, hyperglycemia, hypokalemia, hyponatremia, hyperlipidemia

Gastrointestinal: Xerostomia, nausea, vomiting, dyspepsia, constipation, diarrhea, abdominal pain, dysphagia, fecal impaction, flatulence, hepatitis, melena, hematemesis, intestinal obstruction, weight loss

Genitourinary: Urinary frequency, pyelonephritis, urinary retention, uterine fibroids, vaginitis

Hematologic: Anemia, leukopenia, leukocytosis, thrombocythemia, thrombocytopenia

Hepatic: Elevation of liver enzymes, hepatoma, hepatic failure

Local: Phlebitis

Neuromuscular & skeletal: Muscle weakness, tremor, myasthenia, back pain, arthralgia, bursitis, arthritis, paresthesia, neuralgia, hemiplegia

Ocular: Glaucoma, eye pain, optic neuritis, retinal hemorrhage, visual field defects, iritis, keratitis, optic atrophy

Otic: Ear pain, tinnitus

Renal: kidney stones, glucosuria, hematuria, albuminuria

Respiratory: Sinusitis, bronchitis

Miscellaneous: Diaphoresis, moniliasis, sepsis

Overdosage Symptoms of overdose include dry mouth, bradycardia, hypotension

Toxicology Lavage (within 2 hours of ingestion) with activated charcoal; benzodiazepines for seizure control; atropine can be given for treatment of bradycardia; flumazenil has been used to reverse coma successfully; forced diuresis is not helpful; multiple dosing of activated charcoal may be helpful. Following attempts to enhance drug elimination, hypotension should be treated with I.V. fluids and/or Trendelenburg positioning.

Drug Interactions

Increased effect: Oral contraceptives

Increased toxicity: Additive hypotensive effects may be seen with diuretics, other alpha adrenergic agonists, or antihypertensives; CNS depression with alcohol, baclofen or other CNS depressants

Drug/Food Interactions Food increases maximum concentration by 33% and shortens time to peak by 40 minutes; extent of absorption is not affected

Mechanism of Action An alpha$_2$-adrenergic agonist agent which decreases excitatory input to alpha motor neurons; an imidazole derivative chemically-related to clonidine, which acts as a centrally acting muscle relaxant with alpha$_2$-adrenergic agonist properties; presumably decreases spasticity by increasing presynaptic inhibition of motor neurons

Pharmacodynamics

Peak effect: 1-2 hours

Duration: 3-6 hours

Pharmacokinetics

Distribution: V_d: 204 L/kg

Metabolism: Some liver metabolism

Bioavailability: 98%; absolute bioavailability after first-pass effect: 40%

Half-life: 4-8 hours

Albumin binding: 3%

Time to peak serum concentration: 1-5 hours

Usual Dosage Geriatrics and Adults: Oral: Usual initial dose: 4 mg, may increase by 2-4 mg as needed for satisfactory reduction of muscle tone every 6-8 hours to a maximum of 3 doses in any 24-hour period; maximum dose: 36 mg/day (see Additional Information)

Dosing adjustment in renal/hepatic impairment: Cl$_{cr}$ <25 mL/minute: Reduce dosage 50%

Monitoring Parameters Monitor liver function (aminotransferases) at baseline, 1, 3, 6 months and then periodically thereafter

Patient Information May cause hypotension, sedation, impaired coordination which affects operating hazardous machinery (ie, automobiles); other CNS depressants will be additive to sedation of tizanidine

Nursing Implications Monitor for orthostatic hypotension; monitor LFTs and for positive response

Additional Information Single doses of 8 mg reduce muscle tone for a period of several hours; the effect peaks in 1-2 hours and lasts 3-6 hours; effects are dose-related, however, it is prudent to start at lower doses as above

Special Geriatric Considerations Since elderly commonly have renal function <30 mL/minute creatinine clearance, creatinine clearance should be estimated before dosing this medication. Low doses should be started initially because of the possibility of CNS effects (see Adverse Reactions and Warnings).

Dosage Forms Tablet: 4 mg

TMP *see* Trimethoprim *on page 962*

TMP-SMZ *see* Co-Trimoxazole *on page 253*

TobraDex® *see* Tobramycin and Dexamethasone *on page 931*

Tobramycin (toe bra MYE sin)
Related Information
Aminoglycoside Dosing Guidelines *on page 1009*
Cephalosporins, Aminoglycosides, Macrolides, & Quinolones *on page 1014*
I.V. Medication Recommendations *on page 1080*
Serum Drug Concentrations Commonly Monitored: Guidelines *on page 1114*
Tobramycin and Dexamethasone *on page 931*
Brand Names AKTob® Ophthalmic; Nebcin® Injection; Tobrex® Ophthalmic
Therapeutic Category Antibiotic, Aminoglycoside; Antibiotic, Ophthalmic
Use Treatment of documented or suspected *Pseudomonas aeruginosa* infection; infection with a nonpseudomonal enteric bacillus which is more sensitive to tobramycin than gentamicin based on susceptibility tests; empiric therapy in cystic fibrosis and immunocompromised patients; topically used to treat superficial ophthalmic infections caused by susceptible bacteria
Contraindications Hypersensitivity to tobramycin or other aminoglycosides
Warnings
Not intended for long-term therapy due to toxic hazards associated with extended administration; pre-existing renal insufficiency, vestibular or cochlear impairment, myasthenia gravis, hypocalcemia, conditions which depress neuromuscular transmission

I.M. & I.V.: Aminoglycosides are associated with significant nephrotoxicity or ototoxicity; the ototoxicity is directly proportional to the amount of drug given and the duration of treatment; tinnitus or vertigo are indications of vestibular injury and impending irreversible bilateral deafness; nephrotoxicity is associated with trough concentrations >2 mcg/mL and is usually reversible

Precautions Use with caution in patients with renal impairment; pre-existing auditory or vestibular impairment; and in patients with neuromuscular disorders; dosage modification required in patients with impaired renal function
Adverse Reactions
Central nervous system: Fever
Dermatologic: Allergic contact dermatitis, rash
Gastrointestinal: Diarrhea, pseudomembranous colitis
Local: Thrombophlebitis
Neuromuscular & skeletal: Neuromuscular blockade
Ocular: Lacrimation, itching, edema of the eyelid, keratitis
Otic: Ototoxicity
Renal: Nephrotoxicity
Overdosage Symptoms of overdose include ototoxicity, nephrotoxicity, and neuromuscular toxicity
Toxicology The treatment of choice following a single acute overdose appears to be the maintenance of good urine output of at least 3 mL/kg/hour. Dialysis is of questionable value in the enhancement of aminoglycoside elimination. If required, hemodialysis is preferred over peritoneal dialysis in patients with normal renal function. Careful hydration may be all that is
(Continued)

Tobramycin (Continued)

required to promote diuresis and therefore the enhancement of the drug's elimination.

Drug Interactions
Increased/prolonged effect: Depolarizing and nondepolarizing neuromuscular blocking agents
Increased toxicity: Concurrent use of amphotericin, vancomycin, or loop diuretics may increase nephrotoxicity

Stability Reconstituted solution is stable for 24 hours at room temperature and 96 hours when refrigerated; incompatible with penicillins

Mechanism of Action Interferes with bacterial protein synthesis by binding to 30S and 50S ribosomal subunits resulting in a defective bacterial cell membrane

Pharmacokinetics
Absorption: I.M.: Rapid and complete
Distribution: V_d: 0.2-0.3 L/kg
Half-life: 2-3 hours, directly dependent upon glomerular filtration rate; half-life (impaired renal function): 5-70 hours
Time to peak serum concentration:
I.M.: Within 30-60 minutes
I.V.: Within 30 minutes
Elimination: With normal renal function, about 90% to 95% of dose is excreted in urine within 24 hours
The pharmacokinetics of the aminoglycosides are heterogeneous in the elderly. It is best to assume that clearance is reduced and half-life prolonged in the elderly, while volume of distribution is usually unchanged. The establishment of each patient's pharmacokinetic parameters is important for proper dosing in order to achieve an optimal therapeutic benefit and minimize the risks of toxicity. Following I.M. administration, the time to peak serum concentration was delayed in the elderly.

Usual Dosage Dosage should be based on an estimate of ideal body weight
Geriatrics:
I.M., I.V.: 1.5-5 mg/kg/day in 1-2 divided doses
I.V.: Once daily or extended interval: 5-7 mg/kg/dose given every 24, 36, or 48 hours based on Cl_{cr} (see Dosing Adjustment in Renal Impairment) (see Special Geriatric Considerations)
Adults: I.M., I.V.: 3-5 mg/kg/day in 3 divided doses or as indicated by adjustment for renal function
Renal dysfunction: 2 mg/kg (2-3 serum concentration measurements should be obtained after the initial dose to measure the half-life in order to determine the frequency of subsequent doses)

Dosage adjustment in renal impairment:
Cl_{cr} ≥60 mL/minute: Administer every 24 hours
Cl_{cr} 40-59 mL/minute: Administer every 36 hours
Cl_{cr} 20-39 mL/minute: Administer every 48 hours
Cl_{cr} <20 mL/minute: Individualize dose
Dialyzable (50% to 100%)
Ophthalmic: Instill 1-2 drops every 4 hours; apply ointment 2-3 times/day; for severe infections apply ointment every 3-4 hours, or 2 drops every 30-60 minutes initially, then reduce to less frequent intervals

Monitoring Parameters Draw peak concentrations 30 minutes after the end of a 30-minute infusion; the trough is drawn just before the next dose; urine output; serum BUN and creatinine, signs and symptoms of infection; culture and sensitivities

Reference Range
Therapeutic:
Peak: 5-10 µg/mL (SI: 11-21 µmol/L)
Trough: 1-1.5 µg/mL (SI: 2-3 µmol/L)
Once daily or extended interval: Trough: <0.5 µg/mL
Toxic:
Peak: >12 µg/mL (SI: >21 µmol/L)
Trough: >2 µg/mL (SI: >9 µmol/L)

Test Interactions Increased protein; decreased magnesium

Patient Information Report symptoms of superinfection; for eye drops - no other eye drops 5-10 minutes before or after tobramycin

Nursing Implications Eye solutions: Allow 5 minutes between application of "multiple-drop" therapy; with I.M. or I.V. treatment, obtain drug serum concentrations after the third dose

Additional Information Should not be mixed with other drugs

Special Geriatric Considerations The aminoglycosides are an important therapeutic intervention for susceptible organisms and as empiric therapy in seriously ill patients. Their use is not without risk of toxicity; however, these risks can be minimized if initial dosing is adjusted for estimated renal function and appropriate monitoring is performed. High dose, once daily aminoglycosides have been advocated as an alternative to traditional dosing regimens. Once daily or extended interval dosing is as effective and may be safer than traditional dosing. Interval must be adjusted for renal function. See Pharmacokinetics and Usual Dosage.

Dosage Forms
Tobramycin sulfate:
Injection: 10 mg/mL (2 mL); 40 mg/mL (1.5 mL, 2 mL)
Ophthalmic:
Ointment: 0.3% (3.5 g)
Solution: 0.3% (5 mL)
Powder for injection: 40 mg/mL (1.2 g); 30 mg/mL (1.2 g)

References
Bauer LA and Blouin RA, "Influence of Age on Tobramycin. Pharmacokinetics in Patients With Normal Renal Function," *Antimicrob Agents Chemother*, 1981, 20:587-9.

Matzke GR, Jameson JJ, and Halstenson CE, "Gentamicin Disposition in Young and Elderly Patients With Various Degrees of Renal Function," *J Clin Pharmacol*, 1987, 27(3):216-20.

Mayer PR, Brown CH, Carter RA, et al, "Intramuscular Tobramycin Pharmacokinetics in Geriatric Patients," *Drug Intell Clin Pharm*, 1986, 20:611-5.

Nicolau DP, Freeman CD, Belliveau PP, et al, "Experience With a Once-Daily Aminoglycoside Program Administered to 2184 Adult Patients," *Antimicrob Agents Chemother*, 1995, 39(3):650-5.

Preston SL and Briceland LL, "Single Daily Dosing of Aminoglycosides," *Pharmacotherapy*, 1995, 15(3):297-316.

Zaske DE, Irvine P, Strand LM, et al, "Wide Interpatient Variations in Gentamicin Dose Requirements for Geriatric Patients," *JAMA*, 1982, 248(23):3122-6.

Tobramycin and Dexamethasone
(toe bra MYE sin & deks a METH a sone)

Brand Names TobraDex®

Synonyms Dexamethasone and Tobramycin

Generic Available No

Therapeutic Category Antibiotic, Ophthalmic; Corticosteroid, Ophthalmic

Use Treatment of external ocular infection caused by susceptible gram-negative bacteria and steroid responsive inflammatory conditions of the palpebral and bulbar conjunctiva, lid, cornea, and anterior segment of the globe

Contraindications Known hypersensitivity to tobramycin or dexamethasone, most viral diseases of the cornea, fungal diseases, use after uncomplicated removal of a corneal foreign body

Adverse Reactions
Dermatologic: Allergic contact dermatitis
Ocular: Delayed wound healing, lacrimation, itching eyes, edema of eyelid, keratitis, increased intraocular pressure, glaucoma, cataract formation

Overdosage Symptoms of overdose include punctate keratitis, erythema, increased lacrimation, edema, lid itching

Toxicology Flush eye with copious amounts of fluid at low pressure for 15 minutes

Drug Interactions Refer to individual monographs for Dexamethasone and Tobramycin

Mechanism of Action Refer to individual monographs for Dexamethasone and Tobramycin

Pharmacokinetics
Absorption: Into the aqueous humor
Time to peak serum concentration: 1-2 hours after instillation in the cornea and aqueous humor

Usual Dosage Geriatrics and Adults: Ophthalmic: Instill 1-2 drops of solution every 4 hours; apply ointment 2-3 times/day; for severe infections apply ointment every 3-4 hours, or solution 2 drops every 30-60 minutes initially, then reduce to less frequent intervals

Monitoring Parameters Relief of symptoms

Patient Information Shake well before using; tilt head back, place medication in conjunctival sac and close eyes, apply light finger pressure on lacrimal sac for 1 minute following instillation, notify physician if condition fails to improve or worsens. Do not touch dropper to eye.

Nursing Implications Wash hands before and after administering

Special Geriatric Considerations Assess patient's ability to correctly self-administer eye drops
(Continued)

Tobramycin and Dexamethasone *(Continued)*

Dosage Forms
Ointment, ophthalmic: Tobramycin 0.3% and dexamethasone 0.1% (3.5 g)
Suspension, ophthalmic: Tobramycin 0.3% and dexamethasone 0.1% (2.5 mL, 5 mL)

Tobrex® Ophthalmic *see* Tobramycin *on page 929*

Tocainide (toe KAY nide)
Brand Names Tonocard®
Generic Available No
Therapeutic Category Antiarrhythmic Agent, Class I-B
Use Suppress and prevent symptomatic life-threatening ventricular arrhythmias
Unlabeled use: Trigeminal neuralgia

Contraindications Second or third degree A-V block, hypersensitivity to tocainide or any component

Warnings Agranulocytosis, bone marrow suppression, leukopenia, neutropenia, aplastic anemia, thrombocytopenia, septicemia, septic shock; fatalities secondary to blood dyscrasias; pulmonary fibrosis, interstitial pneumonitis, fibrosing alveolitis, pneumonia, and pulmonary edema; may cause or exacerbate pre-existent arrhythmias; sudden death; use cautiously in patients with heart failure or poor cardiac reserve and in patients with renal or hepatic impairment

Precautions May exacerbate some arrhythmias; use with caution in congestive heart failure patients; administer with caution in patients with pre-existing bone marrow failure or cytopenia

Adverse Reactions
Cardiovascular: Hypotension, bradycardia, tachycardia, palpitations
Central nervous system: Vertigo, dizziness, confusion, hallucinations, nervousness, anxiety
Dermatologic: Rash, skin lesions
Gastrointestinal: Nausea, vomiting, diarrhea
Hematologic: Agranulocytosis, anemia, leukopenia, neutropenia
Neuromuscular & skeletal: Tremors, paresthesia
Ocular: Blurred vision
Otic: Tinnitus
Respiratory: Respiratory arrest
Miscellaneous: Diaphoresis

Overdosage Symptoms of overdose include convulsions, confusion, altered mood, ataxia, paresthesia, congestive heart failure, cardiopulmonary depression; tremor may indicate maximum tolerable dose; also see GI side effects

Toxicology Toxicity is similar to that of lidocaine, but the effects are longer in duration. Bradycardia and asystole may be difficult to control with standard therapeutic agents. Temporary pacemaker insertion may be required. Provide general supportive care; gastric lavage and charcoal administration may be effective; treat seizures with I.V. diazepam or barbiturates.

Drug Interactions
Cimetidine decreases absorption of tocainide
Metoprolol, rifampin, allopurinol increases half-life of tocainide

Mechanism of Action Suppresses automaticity of conduction tissue, by increasing electrical stimulation threshold of ventricle, HIS-Purkinje system, and spontaneous depolarization of the ventricles during diastole by a direct action on the tissues; blocks both the initiation and conduction of nerve impulses by decreasing the neuronal membrane's permeability to sodium ions, which results in inhibition of depolarization with resultant blockade of conduction

Pharmacokinetics
Absorption: Oral: Extensive, 99% to 100%
Distribution: V_d: 1.62-3.2 L/kg
Protein binding: 10% to 20%
Metabolism: Metabolized in the liver to inactive metabolites; first-pass effect is negligible
Half-life: 11-14 hours, prolonged with renal and hepatic impairment with half-life increased to 23-27 hours
Time to peak serum concentration: Within 30-160 minutes
Elimination: In urine (40% to 50% as unchanged drug)

Usual Dosage Geriatrics and Adults: Initial dose: 400 mg every 8 hours; increase to 1200-1800 mg/day in 3 divided doses; do not exceed 2400 mg/day; patients with hepatic and renal dysfunction may be controlled with doses

<1200 mg/day; may be given in 2 divided doses if tolerated; food results in slower absorption and a 40% decrease in maximum serum concentration, but extent of absorption is unaltered

Moderately dialyzable (20% to 50%)

Monitoring Parameters Guide dose by clinical effect and EKG monitoring; periodically monitor CBC and liver function tests; monitor for tremor

Reference Range Therapeutic: 5-12 µg/mL (SI: 22-52 µmol/L)

Test Interactions Abnormal LFTs observed at initiation of drug

Patient Information Report any unusual bleeding, cough, tremor, palpitations, rash, bruising, chills, fever, sore throat, or any breathing difficulties; may cause drowsiness, nausea, vomiting, and diarrhea; notify physician if these adverse reactions persist or are severe; may take with food

Additional Information Known as "oral lidocaine"

Special Geriatric Considerations Tocainide may cause confusion; tremor indicates potential toxicity and should not be mistaken for age related changes; renal and phase I liver metabolism changes with age may affect clearance; monitor closely since half-life may be prolonged

Dosage Forms Tablet, as hydrochloride: 400 mg, 600 mg

References
Fenster PE and Nolan PE, "Antiarrhythmic Drugs," *Geriatric Pharmacology*, Bressler R and Katz MD, eds, New York, NY: McGraw-Hill, 1993, 6:105-49.

Tofranil® *see* Imipramine *on page 480*

Tofranil-PM® *see* Imipramine *on page 480*

Tolazamide (tole AZ a mide)

Related Information

Antacid Drug Interactions *on page 1096*

Brand Names Tolinase®

Therapeutic Category Antidiabetic Agent; Hypoglycemic Agent, Oral; Sulfonylurea Agent

Use Adjunct to diet for the management of mild to moderately severe, stable, noninsulin-dependent (type II) diabetes mellitus

Contraindications Therapy of type 1 diabetes, hypersensitivity to sulfonylureas, diabetes complicated by ketoacidosis

Warnings False-positive response has been reported in patients with liver disease, severe malnutrition, acute pancreatitis, renal dysfunction

Adverse Reactions

Central nervous system: Headache, dizziness

Dermatologic: Rash, urticaria, photosensitivity

Endocrine & metabolic: Hypoglycemia

Gastrointestinal: Anorexia, nausea, vomiting, diarrhea, constipation, heartburn, epigastric fullness

Hematologic: Aplastic anemia, hemolytic anemia, bone marrow suppression, thrombocytopenia, granulocytosis

Renal: Diuretic effect

Overdosage Symptoms of overdose include low blood sugar, tingling of lips and tongue, nausea, yawning, confusion, agitation, tachycardia, sweating, convulsions, stupor, and coma

Toxicology Intoxications with sulfonylureas can cause hypoglycemia and are best managed with glucose administration (oral for milder hypoglycemia or by injection in more severe forms)

Drug Interactions Monitor patient closely; large number of drugs interact with sulfonylureas including salicylates, anticoagulants, H_2 antagonists, TCA, MAO inhibitors, beta-blockers, thiazides; increase hypoglycemic effect with metformin

Mechanism of Action Stimulates insulin release from the pancreatic beta cells; reduces glucose output from the liver; insulin sensitivity is increased at peripheral target sites

Pharmacodynamics

Onset of action: Oral: Following administration, effects occur within 4-6 hours

Duration: 10-24 hours

Pharmacokinetics

Protein binding: >98% ionic/nonionic

Metabolism: Extensive in the liver to one active and three inactive metabolite

Half-life: 7 hours

Elimination: Renal

Usual Dosage Geriatrics and Adults: Oral: Initial: 100 mg/day; increase at 2- to 4-week intervals; maximum dose: 1000 mg; administer as a single or twice daily dose (doses >500 mg/day twice daily)

(Continued)

Tolazamide *(Continued)*

Administration See Nursing Implications

Monitoring Parameters Fasting blood glucose; hemoglobin A₁c, or fructosamine

Reference Range Fasting blood glucose: Geriatrics: 100-150 mg/dL; Adults: 80-140 mg/dL

Test Interactions Decreased prothrombin time, decreased sodium (S)

Patient Information Tablets may be crushed; take drug at the same time each day; avoid alcohol; recognize signs and symptoms of hypoglycemia; avoid hypoglycemia, eat regularly, do not skip meals; carry a quick sugar source; medical alert bracelet

Nursing Implications Patients who are anorexic or NPO may need to have their dose held to avoid hypoglycemia

Additional Information Transferring a patient from one sulfonylurea to another does not require a priming dose; doses >1000 mg/day normally does not improve diabetic control

Special Geriatric Considerations Has not been studied in older patients, however, except for drug interactions it appears to have a safe profile and decline in renal function does not affect its pharmacokinetics. How "tightly" a geriatric patient's blood glucose should be controlled is controversial; however, a fasting blood sugar of <150 mg/dL is now an acceptable end point. Such a decision should be based on the patient's functional and cognitive status, how well they recognize hypoglycemic or hyperglycemic symptoms, and how to respond to them and their other disease states.

Dosage Forms Tablet: 100 mg, 250 mg, 500 mg

Tolbutamide *(tole BYOO ta mide)*

Related Information

Antacid Drug Interactions *on page 1096*

Brand Names Orinase® Diagnostic Injection; Orinase® Oral

Generic Available Yes

Therapeutic Category Antidiabetic Agent; Hypoglycemic Agent, Oral; Sulfonylurea Agent

Use Adjunct to diet for the management of mild to moderately severe, stable, noninsulin-dependent (type II) diabetes mellitus

Contraindications Diabetes complicated by ketoacidosis, therapy of type 1 diabetes, hypersensitivity to sulfonylureas

Precautions False-positive response has been reported in patients with liver disease, severe malnutrition, acute pancreatitis

Adverse Reactions

Cardiovascular: Venospasm

Central nervous system: Headache, dizziness

Dermatologic: Skin rash, urticaria, photosensitivity

Endocrine & metabolic: Hypoglycemia, SIADH

Gastrointestinal: Constipation, diarrhea, heartburn, anorexia, epigastric fullness

Hematologic: Aplastic anemia, hemolytic anemia, bone marrow suppression, thrombocytopenia, leukopenia

Local: Thrombophlebitis

Otic: Tinnitus

Miscellaneous: Hypersensitivity reaction, disulfiram-like reactions

Overdosage Symptoms of overdose include low blood sugar, tingling of lips and tongue, nausea, yawning, confusion, agitation, tachycardia, sweating, convulsions, stupor, and coma

Drug Interactions

Increased effects with salicylates, probenecid, MAO inhibitors, chloramphenicol, insulin, phenylbutazone, antidepressants, metformin, H₂ antagonists, and others

Hypoglycemic effects may be decreased by beta-blockers, cholestyramine, hydantoins, thiazides, rifampin, and others

Ethanol may decrease the half-life of tolbutamide

Stability Use within 1 hour following reconstitution

Mechanism of Action Stimulates insulin release from the pancreatic beta cells; reduces glucose output from the liver; insulin sensitivity is increased at peripheral target sites, suppression of glucagon may also contribute

Pharmacodynamics

Onset of hypoglycemic effect: 1 hour

Duration: 6-24 hours; no apparent change in response with age

Pharmacokinetics
Half-life, plasma: 4-25 hours
Protein binding: 95% to 97% (principally to albumin) ionic/nonionic
Metabolism/Elimination: Hepatic metabolism to hydroxymethyltolbutamide (mildly active) and carboxytolbutamide (inactive) both rapidly excreted renally, less 2% excreted in urine unchanged; metabolism does not appear to be affected by age
Increased plasma concentrations and volume of distribution secondary to decreased albumin concentrations and less protein binding have been reported

Usual Dosage Oral:
Geriatrics: Initial: 250 mg 1-3 times/day; usual: 500-2000 mg; maximum: 3 g/day
Adults: Initial: 500-1000 mg 1-3 times/day; usual dose should not be more than 2 g/day
Not dialyzable (0% to 5%)

Administration See Nursing Implications

Monitoring Parameters Fasting blood glucose, hemoglobin A_{1c}, or fructosamine

Reference Range Fasting blood glucose: Geriatrics: 100-150 mg/dL; Adults: 80-140 mg/dL

Test Interactions Increased protein; decreased prothrombin time, decreased sodium (S); false-positive proteinuria

Patient Information Fast the night before the test

Nursing Implications Patients who are anorexic or NPO may need to have their dose held to avoid hypoglycemia

Special Geriatric Considerations Because of its low potency and short duration, it is a useful agent in the elderly if drug interactions can be avoided (see Pharmacodynamics and Pharmacokinetics). How "tightly" a geriatric patient's blood glucose should be controlled is controversial; however, a fasting blood sugar <150 mg/dL is now an acceptable end point. Such a decision should be based on the patient's functional and cognitive status, how well they recognize hypoglycemic or hyperglycemic symptoms, and how to respond to them and their other disease states.

Dosage Forms Tablet, as sodium: 250 mg, 500 mg

References
Miller AK, Adir J, and Vestal RE, "Effect of Age on the Pharmacokinetics of Tolbutamide in Man," *Pharmacologist*, 1977, 19:128.
Miller AK, Adir J, and Vestal RE, "Tolbutamide Binding to Plasma Proteins of Young and Old Human Subjects," *J Pharm Sci*, 1978, 67(8):1192-3.

Tolcapone (TOLE ka pone)

Brand Names Tasmar®

Therapeutic Category Anti-Parkinson's Agent

Use Adjunct to levodopa and carbidopa for the treatment of signs and symptoms of idiopathic Parkinson's disease

Contraindications Patients who have experienced hypersensitivity reactions to tolcapone or other ingredients

Warnings It is not recommended that patients receive tolcapone concomitantly with nonselective MAO inhibitors (see Drug Interactions). Selegiline is a selective MAO-B inhibitor and can be taken with tolcapone.

Precautions Patients receiving tolcapone are predisposed to orthostatic hypotension. Inform the patient and explain methods to manage the symptoms. Patients may experience diarrhea, most commonly 6-12 weeks after tolcapone is started. Diarrhea is sometimes associated with anorexia. Patients may experience hallucinations shortly after starting therapy, most commonly within the first 2 weeks. Hallucinations may diminish or resolve with a decrease in the levodopa dose. Hallucinations commonly accompany confusion and sometimes insomnia or excessive dreaming. Tolcapone may exacerbate or induce dyskinesia. Lowering the levodopa dose may help. Use tolcapone with caution in patients with severe renal or hepatic failure. Elevations in liver enzymes have been reported. In about half of the cases, the enzymes returned to normal while on tolcapone.

Adverse Reactions
Cardiovascular: Orthostasis, hypotension, chest pain, syncope
Central nervous system: Sleep disorder, excessive dreaming, headache, dizziness, somnolence, confusion, hallucination, fatigue
Gastrointestinal: Nausea, anorexia, diarrhea, vomiting, constipation, dry mouth, dyspepsia, abdominal pain, flatulence
Genitourinary: Urine discoloration
(Continued)

Tolcapone *(Continued)*

Hepatic: Increased liver enzymes

Neuromuscular & skeletal: Dyskinesia, dystonia, muscle cramps, hyperkinesia, stiffness, arthritis

Respiratory: Dyspnea

<1% (Limited to important or life-threatening symptoms):

Cardiovascular: Bradycardia, coronary artery disorder, heart arrest, angina pectoris, myocardial infarct, myocardial ischemia, arteriosclerosis, thrombosis, hypertension, vasodilation

Central nervous system: Amnesia, extrapyramidal syndrome, manic reaction, cerebrovascular accident, psychosis, myoclonus, delirium, encephalopathy, meningitis

Dermatologic: Cellulitis

Endocrine & metabolic: Hypercholesteremia

Gastrointestinal: Gastrointestinal hemorrhage, colitis, duodenal ulcer

Genitourinary: Uterine hemorrhage

Hematologic: Anemia, leukemia, thrombocytopenia

Hepatic: Cholecystitis

Neuromuscular & skeletal: Neuralgia, hemiplegia

Renal: Hematuria

Respiratory: Bronchitis, epistaxis, hyperventilation

Miscellaneous: Allergic reaction

Drug Interactions

Theoretically, nonselective MAO inhibitors (phenelzine and tranylcypromine) taken with tolcapone may inhibit the major metabolism pathways for catecholamines which may result in excessive adverse effects possibly due to levodopa accumulation. Concomitant therapy is not recommended.

Tolcapone increases the AUC and elimination half-life of levodopa but does not alter the C_{max} or T_{max}

Drug/Food Interactions Tolcapone taken with food within 1 hour before or 2 hours after the dose, decreases bioavailability by 10% to 20%

Mechanism of Action A reversible inhibitor of catechol-O-methyltransferase (COMT). COMT is a major route of metabolism for levodopa. When tolcapone is taken with levodopa, the pharmacokinetics of levodopa are altered, resulting in more sustained levodopa serum concentration compared to when levodopa is taken alone.

Pharmacokinetics

Absorption: Rapid

Distribution: V_d: 9 L

Protein binding: >99.0%

Metabolism: By glucuronidation

Bioavailability: Oral: 65%

Half-life: 2-3 hours

Time to peak serum: Within 2 hours

Elimination: In urine and feces (40%)

Usual Dosage Geriatrics and Adults: Oral: Initial: 100 mg 3 times/day; may be increased to 200 mg 3 times/day; always given as an adjunct to levodopa/carbidopa. The first dose of the day should be given with the first dose of the day of levodopa/carbidopa, and then administer the next 2 doses 6 and 12 hours later.

Note: Many patients will require a decrease in levodopa dosage to avoid increased dopaminergic side effects

Dosing adjustment in renal impairment: Generally, no adjustment necessary; however, in patients with severe renal failure, treat with caution and do not exceed 100 mg 3 times/day

Dosing adjustment in hepatic impairment: Dose should be reduced in patients with cirrhotic liver disease since unbound drug increases by ~50%. Patients with severe liver failure should be treated with caution and receive doses no higher than 100 mg 3 times/day.

Monitoring Parameters Blood pressure, symptoms of Parkinson's, liver enzymes monthly for first 3 months, then every 6 weeks for the next 3 months; discontinue therapy if greater than 5 times upper limit of normal

Nursing Implications Monitor for effectiveness, orthostasis

Special Geriatric Considerations No specific data in geriatric patients, but based on the pharmacokinetic profile, no dosage adjustment appears necessary. See Warnings, Monitoring Parameters.

Dosage Forms Tablet: 100 mg, 200 mg

Tolectin® *see* Tolmetin *on next page*

Tolectin® DS *see* Tolmetin *on this page*
Tolinase® *see* Tolazamide *on page 933*

Tolmetin (TOLE met in)
Related Information
Antacid Drug Interactions *on page 1096*
Brand Names Tolectin®; Tolectin® DS
Generic Available No
Therapeutic Category Analgesic, Non-narcotic; Anti-inflammatory Agent; Antipyretic; Nonsteroidal Anti-inflammatory Agent (NSAID), Oral
Use Treatment of rheumatoid arthritis and osteoarthritis, juvenile rheumatoid arthritis, sunburn, mild to moderate pain
Contraindications Known hypersensitivity to tolmetin, any component, aspirin, or other nonsteroidal anti-inflammatory drugs (NSAIDs)
Warnings Anaphylactoid reactions have been reported in patients with intermittent use and aspirin sensitivity; GI toxicity (bleeding, ulceration, perforation); CNS effects may occur (headaches, confusion, depression); hypersensitivity, anaphylactoid reactions (intermittent tolmetin use more often); renal function decline, acute renal insufficiency, interstitial nephritis, dysuria, cystitis, hematuria, nephrotic syndrome, hyperkalemia in acute renal insufficiency, hyponatremia, papillary necrosis, hepatic function impairment; elderly have increased risk for adverse reactions to NSAIDs (see Special Geriatric Considerations)
Precautions Use with caution in patients with congestive heart failure, hypertension, decreased renal or hepatic function, history of GI disease (bleeding or ulcers), or those receiving anticoagulants; perform ophthalmologic evaluation for those who develop eye complaints during therapy (blurred vision, diminished vision, changes in color vision, retinal changes); NSAIDs may mask signs/symptoms of infections; photosensitivity reported
Adverse Reactions
Cardiovascular: Congestive heart failure, angina, hypertension, hypotension, arrhythmias, edema

Central nervous system: Headache, drowsiness, vertigo, dizziness, fatigue, hallucinations, confusion, depression, emotional lability, psychotic behavior, pyrexia

Dermatologic: Rash, urticaria, angioedema, Stevens-Johnson syndrome, exfoliative dermatitis, bruising, petechiae, purpura

Endocrine & metabolic: Hyperglycemia, hypoglycemia, hyperkalemia, gynecomastia, hyponatremia, fluid retention

Gastrointestinal: Dyspepsia, heartburn, nausea, diarrhea, constipation, flatulence, stomatitis, vomiting, abdominal pain, peptic ulcer, GI bleeding, GI perforation, gingival ulcers, pancreatitis, proctitis, paralytic ulcers, colitis, anorexia, weight loss, dry mucous membranes

Genitourinary: Impotence, azotemia

Hematologic: Neutropenia, anemia, agranulocytosis, bone marrow suppression, hemolytic anemia, hemorrhage, inhibition of platelet aggregation

Hepatic: Hepatitis, elevated LFTs, cholestatic jaundice

Neuromuscular & skeletal: Involuntary muscle movements, muscle weakness, tremors, weakness

Ocular: Vision changes

Otic: Tinnitus

Renal: Dysuria, polyuria, pyuria, oliguria, anuria, acute renal failure

Respiratory: Exacerbation of asthma, dyspnea

Miscellaneous: Thirst, diaphoresis
Overdosage Symptoms include drowsiness, lethargy, disorientation, confusion, dizziness, numbness, paresthesia, nausea, vomiting, gastric irritation, abdominal pain, headache, tinnitus, sweating, blurred vision, muscle twitching, seizures, coma, acute renal failure, increased BUN and serum creatinine, hypotension, tachycardia, and metabolic acidosis
Toxicology Management of a nonsteroidal anti-inflammatory agent (NSAID) intoxication is primarily supportive and symptomatic. Fluid therapy is commonly effective in managing the hypotension that may occur following an acute NSAID overdose, except when this is due to an acute blood loss. Seizures tend to be very short-lived and often do not require drug treatment although recurrent seizures should be treated with I.V. diazepam. Since many of the NSAIDs undergo enterohepatic cycling, multiple doses of charcoal may be needed to reduce the potential for delayed toxicities.
Drug Interactions
May increase digoxin, methotrexate, and lithium serum concentrations
Aspirin or other salicylates may decrease NSAID serum concentrations
(Continued)

Tolmetin *(Continued)*

Other NSAIDs may increase adverse GI effects

Increased prothrombin time with anticoagulants

Decreased antihypertensive effects of ACE inhibitors, beta-blockers, and thiazide diuretics

Effects of loop diuretics may decrease

Increased response to sympathomimetics

Probenecid may increase toxicity of NSAIDs by increase in serum concentrations

Diuretics may increase risk of acute renal insufficiency

Azotemia may be enhanced in elderly receiving loop diuretics

Mechanism of Action Inhibits prostaglandin synthesis, acts on the hypothalamus heat-regulating center to reduce fever, blocks prostaglandin synthetase action which prevents formation of the platelet-aggregating substance thromboxane A_2; decreases pain receptor sensitivity. Other proposed mechanisms of action for salicylate anti-inflammatory action are lysosomal stabilization, inhibition of kinin and leukotriene production, alteration of chemotactic factors, and inhibition of neutrophil activation. This latter mechanism may be the most significant pharmacologic action to reduce inflammation.

Pharmacodynamics

Onset of analgesic action: 0.5-1 hour

Duration: 4-6 hours

Onset of anti-inflammatory action: Within 7 days; Maximum benefit: 1-2 weeks

Pharmacokinetics

Absorption: Oral: Well absorbed

Protein binding: >90%

Half-life: 1-2 hours

Time to peak serum concentration: Within 30-60 minutes

Usual Dosage Geriatrics and Adults: Oral: 200-400 mg 3 times/day; usual dose: 600 mg to 1.8 g/day; maximum: 2 g/day

Monitoring Parameters Monitor response (pain, range of motion, grip strength, mobility, ADL function), inflammation; observe for weight gain, edema; monitor renal function; observe for bleeding, bruising; evaluate gastrointestinal effects (abdominal pain, bleeding, dyspepsia); mental confusion, disorientation, CBC, serum, creatinine, BUN, liver function tests

Test Interactions Increased protein

Patient Information Serious gastrointestinal bleeding can occur as well as ulceration and perforation. Pain may or may not be present. Avoid aspirin and aspirin-containing products while taking this medication. If gastric upset occurs, take with food, milk, or antacid. If gastric adverse effects persist, contact physician. May cause drowsiness, dizziness, blurred vision, and confusion. Use caution when performing tasks which require alertness (eg, driving). Do not take for more than 3 days for fever or 10 days for pain without physician's advice.

Nursing Implications Assess audiometric and ophthalmic exam before, during, and after treatment (see Overdosage, Patient Information, Monitoring Parameters, and Special Geriatric Considerations)

Additional Information Only NSAID affected by food/milk, which decreases total bioavailability by 16%. If GI upset occurs with tolmetin, take with antacids other than sodium bicarbonate. Each 200 mg of tolmetin contains 0.8 mEq of sodium. There are no clinical guidelines to predict which NSAID will give response in a particular patient. Trials with each must be initiated until response determined. Consider dose, patient convenience, and cost.

Special Geriatric Considerations Elderly are a high-risk population for adverse effects from nonsteroidal anti-inflammatory agents. As much as 60% of elderly can develop peptic ulceration and/or hemorrhage asymptomatically. The concomitant use of H_2 blockers, omeprazole, and sucralfate is not effective as prophylaxis with the exception of NSAID-induced duodenal ulcers which may be prevented by the use of ranitidine. Misoprostol and proton pump inhibitors are the only agents proven to help prevent the development of NSAID-induced ulcers. Also, concomitant disease and drug use contribute to the risk for GI adverse effects. Use lowest effective dose for shortest period possible. Consider renal function decline with age. Use of NSAIDs can compromise existing renal function especially when Cl_{cr} is ≤30 mL/minute. Tinnitus may be a difficult and unreliable indication of toxicity due to age-related hearing loss or eighth cranial nerve damage. CNS adverse effects such as confusion, agitation, and hallucination are generally seen in overdose or high dose situations, but elderly may demonstrate these adverse effects at lower doses than younger adults.

Dosage Forms
Tolmetin sodium:
Capsule (Tolectin® DS): 400 mg
Tablet (Tolectin®): 200 mg, 600 mg

References
Brooks PM, Day RO, "Nonsteroidal Anti-inflammatory Drugs - Differences and Similarities," *N Engl J Med*, 1991, 324(24):1716-25.

Clinch D, Banerjee AK, Ostick G, "Absence of Abdominal Pain in Elderly Patients With Peptic Ulcer," *Age Ageing*, 1984, 13:120-3.

Clive DM, Stoff JS, "Renal Syndromes Associated With Nonsteroidal Anti-inflammatory Drugs," *N Engl J Med*, 1984, 310(9):563-72.

Graham DY, "Prevention of Gastroduodenal Injury Induced by Chronic Nonsteroidal Anti-inflammatory Drug Therapy," *Gastroenterology*, 1989, 96(2 Pt 2 Suppl):675-81.

Gurwitz JH, Avorn J, Ross-Degnan D, et al, "Nonsteroidal Anti-inflammatory Drug-Associated Azotemia in the Very Old," *JAMA*, 1990, 264(4):471-5.

Hawkey CJ, Karrasch JA, Szczepaski L, et al, "Omeprazole Compared With Misoprostrol for Ulcers Associated With Nonsteroidal Anti-inflammatory Drugs," *N Engl J Med*, 1998, 338(11):727-34.

Knodel LC, "Preventing NSAID-Induced Ulcers: The Role of Misoprostol," *Consult Pharm*, 1989, 4:37-41.

Pounder R, "Silent Peptic Ulceration: Deadly Silence or Golden Silence?" *Gastroenterology*, 1989, 96(2 Pt 2 Suppl):626-31.

Yeomans ND, Tulassay Z, Juhasz L, et al, "A Comparison of Omeprazole With Ranitidine for Ulcers Associated With Nonsteroidal Anti-inflammatory Drugs," *N Engl J Med*, 1998, 338(11):719-26.

Tolnaftate (tole NAF tate)

Brand Names Absorbine® Antifungal [OTC]; Absorbine® Jock Itch [OTC]; Absorbine Jr.® Antifungal [OTC]; Aftate® for Athlete's Foot [OTC]; Aftate® for Jock Itch [OTC]; Blis-To-Sol® [OTC]; Breezee® Mist Antifungal [OTC]; Dr Scholl's Athlete's Foot [OTC]; Dr Scholl's Maximum Strength Tritin [OTC]; Genaspor® [OTC]; NP-27® [OTC]; Quinsana Plus® [OTC]; Tinactin® [OTC]; Tinactin® for Jock Itch [OTC]; Ting® [OTC]; Zeasorb-AF® Powder [OTC]

Generic Available Yes

Therapeutic Category Antifungal Agent, Topical

Use Treatment of tinea pedis, tinea cruris, tinea corporis, tinea manuum, tinea versicolor infections

Contraindications Known hypersensitivity to tolnaftate; nail and scalp infections

Warnings Cream is not recommended for nail or scalp infections; keep from eyes; if no improvement within 4 weeks, treatment should be discontinued. Usually not effective alone for the treatment of infections involving hair follicles or nails.

Adverse Reactions
Dermatologic: Pruritus, contact dermatitis
Local: Irritation, stinging

Mechanism of Action Distorts the hyphae and stunts mycelial growth in susceptible fungi

Pharmacodynamics Onset of action: Response may be seen 24-72 hours after initiation of therapy

Usual Dosage Geriatrics and Adults: Topical: Wash and dry affected area; apply 1-3 drops of solution or a small amount of cream or powder and rub into the affected areas 2-3 times/day for 2-4 weeks

Monitoring Parameters Resolution of skin infection

Patient Information Avoid contact with the eyes; apply to clean dry area; consult the physician if a skin irritation develops or if the skin infection worsens or does not improve after 10 days of therapy; does not stain skin or clothing

Nursing Implications Itching, burning, and soreness are usually relieved within 24-72 hours

Additional Information Usually not effective alone for the treatment of infections involving hair follicles or nails

Special Geriatric Considerations No specific recommendations for use in the elderly

Dosage Forms
Aerosol, topical:
Liquid: 1% (59.2 mL, 90 mL, 118.3 mL, 120 mL)
Powder: 1% (90 g, 100 g, 105 g, 150 g)
Cream: 1% (15 g, 30 g)
Gel, topical: 1% (15 g)
Powder, topical: 1% (45 g, 56.7 g, 67.5 g, 70.9 g, 90 g)
(Continued)

Tolnaftate *(Continued)*

Solution, topical: 1% (10 mL, 15 mL)

Tolu-Sed® DM [OTC] *see* Guaifenesin and Dextromethorphan *on page 439*

Tonocard® *see* Tocainide *on page 932*

Topamax® *see* Topiramate *on this page*

Topicycline® Topical *see* Tetracycline *on page 900*

Topiramate *(toe PYE ra mate)*

Related Information

Antiepileptic Drug Interactions Comparison *on page 1022*

Brand Names Topamax®

Therapeutic Category Anticonvulsant, Miscellaneous

Use Adjunctive therapy for partial onset seizures in adults; topiramate has also been granted orphan drug status for the treatment of Lennox-Gastaut syndrome

Contraindications Patients with a known hypersensitivity to any components of this drug

Warnings Avoid abrupt withdrawal of topiramate therapy, it should be withdrawn slowly to minimize the potential of increased seizure frequency; the risk of kidney stones is about 2-4 times that of the untreated population; the risk of this event may be reduced by increasing fluid intake; use cautiously in patients with hepatic or renal impairment; topiramate produces CNS adverse events with psychomotor slowing (affecting speech primarily) and CNS symptoms of fatigue and somnolence; these effects are not dose related

Precautions Kidney stones were seen at a two- to fourfold increase from an untreated population; kidney stones may be explained by topiramate's weak carbonic anhydrase inhibition which increases urinary pH. To help prevent stone formation, have patient increase fluid intake. Paresthesia can occur with topiramate use, again an effect possibly of the weak carbonic anhydrase inhibition

Adverse Reactions

Cardiovascular: Chest pain, edema, bradycardia, arrhythmias, palpitations, bundle branch block, hypotension, hypertension, A-V block, angina, atrial fibrillation

Central nervous system: Fatigue, dizziness, ataxia, somnolence, confusion, psychomotor slowing, nervousness, memory difficulties, speech problems, difficulty concentrating, depression, language problems, abnormal coordination, agitation, hypoesthesia, mood changes, aggressive reaction, apathy, emotional lability, depersonalization, hypokinesia, vertigo, stupor, grand mal seizures, hyperkinesia, hypertonia, insomnia, hallucinations, psychosis, euphoria, dysphoria, paranoia, paranoid reaction, delirium, abnormal dreams, manic reaction, abnormal EEG, coma

Dermatologic: Rash, pruritus, acne, alopecia, folliculitis, dry skin, eczema, skin discoloration, photosensitivity, seborrhea, chloasma, abnormal hair texture, abnormal nails

Endocrine & metabolic: Hot flashes, hypoglycemia, hyperglycemia, increased libido, hypokalemia, dehydration, elevated alkaline phosphatase, acidosis, hypocalcemia, hyponatremia, hypercholesterolemia, decreased libido, mastodynia, menorrhagia, breast discharge, hypophosphatemia (see Miscellaneous)

Gastrointestinal: Dyspepsia, abdominal pain, anorexia, constipation, xerostomia, gingivitis, weight loss, diarrhea, nausea, vomiting, gingival hyperplasia, stomatitis, gastritis, salivation, dysphagia, melena, gastroesophageal reflux, esophagitis, tongue edema, increased appetite, flatulence, eructation, loss of taste

Genitourinary: Hematuria, leukorrhea, vaginitis, UTIs, urinary frequency, urinary incontinence, dysuria, ejaculation dysfunction, urinary retention, nocturia, polyuria, oliguria, albuminuria

Hematologic: Leukopenia

Neuromuscular & skeletal: Paresthesia, tremor, myalgia, weakness, back pain, leg pain, rigors, leg cramps

Ocular: Nystagmus, diplopia, eye pain, photophobia, abnormal accommodation, cataract, corneal opacities, color blindness, myopia, mydriasis, iritis, strabismus

Otic: Decreased hearing, hyperacusis

Renal: Nephrolithiasis, increased serum creatinine

Respiratory: Upper respiratory infections, pharyngitis, sinusitis, epistaxis, dyspnea, bronchospasm, laryngismus, asthma

Miscellaneous: Flu-like symptoms, diaphoresis, hiccups

Overdosage Most likely to see central nervous system, ocular, GI effects (see Adverse Reactions)

Toxicology Activated charcoal has not been shown to adsorb topiramate and is therefore not recommended; hemodialysis can remove drug, however, most cases do not require removal and instead is best treated with supportive measures

Drug Interactions
Decreased effect: Phenytoin can decrease topiramate levels by as much as 48%, carbamazepine reduces it by 40% and valproic acid reduces topiramate by 14%; digoxin levels and norethindrone blood concentrations are decreased when coadministered with topiramate
Increased toxicity: Concomitant administration with other CNS depressants will increase its sedative effects; coadministration with other carbonic anhydrase inhibitors may increase the chance of nephrolithiasis

Mechanism of Action Mechanism is not fully understood, it is thought to decrease seizure frequency by blocking sodium channels in neurons, enhancing GABA activity and by blocking glutamate activity

Pharmacokinetics
Absorption: Well absorbed; unaffected by food
Protein binding: 13% to 17%
Metabolism: Minimal, less than 5% of metabolites are active
Bioavailability: 80%
Half-life: Mean: 21 hours in adults with a normal renal function
Time to peak serum concentration: ~2-4 hours
Elimination: Primarily eliminated unchanged in the urine (70%)
Dialyzable: ~30%

Usual Dosage
Geriatrics and Adults: Initial: 50 mg/day; titrate by 50 mg/day at 1-week intervals to target dose of 200 mg twice daily; usual maximum dose: 1600 mg/day; see table

Recommended Titration Rate

Week	AM Dose (mg)	PM Dose (mg)
1	none	50
2	50	50
3	50	100
4	100	100
5	100	150
6	150	150
7	150	200
8	200	200

Dosing adjustment in renal impairment: Cl_{cr} <70 mL/minute: Administer 50% dose and titrate more slowly

Dosing adjustment in hepatic impairment: Clearance may be minimally reduced (see Special Geriatric Considerations)

Monitoring Parameters Monitor for CNS effects, seizure control

Patient Information Advise patient to maintain adequate fluid intake (8-10 eight oz glasses of fluid/day); patients should be warned of somnolence, dizziness, confusion, and difficulty concentrating on tasks such as driving; warn about driving or operating hazardous machinery; patients must be advised not to break tablets due to their bitter taste; patients can take with or without meals

Nursing Implications Monitor for CNS side effects, nystagmus; do not crush or break tablets due to bitter taste

Special Geriatric Considerations Since drug is renally excreted and most elderly will have creatinine clearance <70 mL/minute, doses must be reduced 50% and titrated more slowly. Obtain a serum creatinine and calculate creatinine clearance prior to starting therapy. Follow the recommended titration schedule and adjust time intervals to meet patient's needs.

Dosage Forms Tablet: 25 mg, 100 mg, 200 mg

Toprol XL® see Metoprolol on page 619

TOPV see Poliovirus Vaccine, Live, Trivalent, Oral on page 761

Toradol® Injection see Ketorolac Tromethamine on page 517

Toradol® Oral see Ketorolac Tromethamine on page 517

Torecan® see Thiethylperazine on page 908

Tornalate® *see* Bitolterol *on page 125*

Torsemide (TOR se mide)
Related Information
I.V. Push Recommended Guidelines *on page 1083*
Brand Names Demadex®
Generic Available No
Therapeutic Category Diuretic, Loop
Use Management of edema associated with congestive heart failure and hepatic or renal disease; used alone or in combination with antihypertensives in treatment of hypertension
Contraindications Hypersensitivity to torsemide or any component; allergy to sulfonamides may result in cross-hypersensitivity to torsemide
Warnings Loop diuretics are potent diuretics, excess amounts can lead to profound diuresis with fluid and electrolyte loss; close medical supervision and dose evaluation is required, particularly in the elderly
Adverse Reactions
Cardiovascular: Hypotension
Central nervous system: Dizziness, headache, encephalopathy
Dermatologic: Rash, photosensitivity
Endocrine & metabolic: Hyperglycemia, hypokalemia, hypochloremia, hyponatremia
Gastrointestinal: Cramps, nausea, vomiting
Genitourinary: Azotemia
Hepatic: Alteration of liver function test results
Neuromuscular & skeletal: Weakness
Otic: Impaired hearing
Renal: Decreased uric acid excretion, increased serum creatinine
Overdosage Symptoms of overdose include electrolyte depletion, volume depletion, hypotension, dehydration, circulatory collapse
Toxicology Following GI decontamination, treatment is supportive; hypotension responds to fluids and Trendelenburg position; replace electrolytes as necessary
Drug Interactions
Decreased effect: Indomethacin, other NSAIDs
Increased hypotensive effect: Other antihypertensives
Increased level of lithium
Increased risk of ototoxicity: Aminoglycosides, other loop diuretics, vancomycin
When given with digoxin, diuretic-induced hypokalemia increases the risk of digoxin toxicity
Mechanism of Action Inhibits reabsorption of sodium and chloride in the ascending loop of Henle and distal renal tubule, interfering with the chloride-binding cotransport system, thus causing increased excretion of water, sodium, chloride, magnesium, and calcium
Pharmacodynamics
Onset of diuresis: 30-60 minutes
Peak effect: 1-4 hours
Duration: ~6 hours
Pharmacokinetics
Absorption: Oral: Rapid
Protein binding: Plasma: ~97% to 99%
Metabolism: Hepatic by cytochrome P-450, 80%
Bioavailability: 80% to 90%
Half-life: 2-4; 7-8 hours in cirrhosis (dose modification appears unnecessary)
Elimination: 20% excreted unchanged in urine
Usual Dosage Geriatrics and Adults:
Oral: 5-10 mg once daily; if ineffective, may double dose until desired effect is achieved; in the treatment of hypertension, if 10 mg is insufficient, add an additional antihypertensive agent
I.V.: 10-20 mg/dose repeated in 2 hours as needed with a doubling of the dose with each succeeding dose until desired diuresis is achieved
Continues to be effective in patients with cirrhosis, no apparent change in dose is necessary
Administration Administer the I.V. dose slowly over 2 minutes
Monitoring Parameters Blood pressure, both standing and sitting/supine, serum electrolytes, weight, I & O; in high doses, monitor auditory function
Patient Information May be taken with food or milk; rise slowly from a lying or sitting position to minimize dizziness, lightheadedness or fainting; also use

extra care when exercising, standing for long periods of time, and during hot weather; take in the morning

Nursing Implications Be alert to complaints about hearing difficulty; check patient for orthostasis (see Monitoring Parameters)

Additional Information 10-20 mg torsemide is approximately equivalent to:
Furosemide 40 mg
Bumetanide 1 mg

Special Geriatric Considerations Dosage adjustment in the elderly appears unnecessary; usual starting dose should be 5 mg

Dosage Forms
Injection: 10 mg/mL (2 mL, 5 mL)
Tablet: 5 mg, 10 mg, 20 mg, 100 mg

Totacillin® see Ampicillin on page 73

Totacillin®-N see Ampicillin on page 73

Touro Ex® see Guaifenesin on page 437

t-PA see Alteplase on page 40

T-Phyl® see Theophylline on page 902

Tramadol (TRA ma dole)

Brand Names Ultram®

Generic Available No

Therapeutic Category Analgesic, Non-narcotic

Use Management of moderate to moderately severe pain

Contraindications Previous hypersensitivity to tramadol or any components; concurrent use of monoamine oxidase inhibitors; acute alcohol intoxication; concurrent use of hypnotics, centrally-acting analgesics, opioids, or psychotropic drugs

Warnings Elderly patients and patients with chronic respiratory disorders may be at greater risk of adverse events; liver disease; patients with myxedema, hypothyroidism, or hypoadrenalism should use tramadol with caution and at reduced dosages; may enhance the risk of seizures in patients with epilepsy

Precautions Respiratory depression may occur when large doses of tramadol are used with anesthetic medication or alcohol. Use with caution in patients with increased intracranial pressure or head injury; not recommended for patients who are dependent on opioids; may cause drug dependence of the mu-opioid type and may potentially be abused.

Adverse Reactions
Cardiovascular: Palpitations, vasodilation, syncope, orthostatic hypotension, tachycardia, hypertension, myocardial ischemia
Central nervous system: Dizziness, headache, somnolence, stimulation, restlessness, confusion, coordination disturbance, sleep disorder, seizures, cognitive dysfunction, hallucinations
Dermatologic: Pruritus, rash, urticaria
Gastrointestinal: Nausea, diarrhea, constipation, vomiting, dyspepsia, xerostomia, anorexia
Genitourinary: Urinary retention/frequency, menopausal symptoms, dysuria
Neuromuscular & skeletal: Tremor, weakness
Ocular: Visual disturbance
Respiratory: Respiratory depression
Miscellaneous: Diaphoresis

Overdosage Symptoms of overdose include CNS and respiratory depression, gastrointestinal cramping, constipation, seizures

Toxicology Naloxone 2 mg I.V. with repeat administration as needed up to 18 mg; naloxone will reverse some, but not all symptoms of overdosage; general supportive treatment is also recommended

Drug Interactions
Decreased effects: Carbamazepine (decreases half-life by 33% to 50%) (may need up to twice the recommended dose of tramadol)
Increased toxicity: Monoamine oxidase inhibitors (seizures); quinidine (inhibits cytochrome P4502D6, thereby increases tramadol serum concentrations); cimetidine (tramadol half-life increased 20% to 25%); CYP2D6 inhibitors, such as the SSRIs and quinidine may inhibit tramadol's metabolism to its active metabolite (decreased analgesic effect)

Mechanism of Action Binds to mu-opioid receptors in the CNS causing inhibition of ascending pain pathways, altering the perception of and response to pain; also inhibits the reuptake of norepinephrine and serotonin, which also modifies the ascending pain pathway

Pharmacodynamics
Onset of analgesia: Within 1 hour
(Continued)

943

Tramadol *(Continued)*

Peak effect: 2-3 hours

Duration of effect: 3-7 hours

Pharmacokinetics

Absorption: Rapid; T_{max}: 2 hours

Protein binding: 20%

Metabolism: Extensive to 11 metabolites, of which only one is active; 90% of tramadol and metabolites eliminated renally (30% of dose eliminated as unchanged drug); substrate CYP2D6

Bioavailability: 75% (mean)

Half-life:

Parent drug: 6.3 hours

Active metabolite: 7.4 hours

Note: In subjects >75 years of age, peak serum concentrations were slightly elevated and the half-life was slightly prolonged (7 hours); no significant changes in the 65-75 year age group were noted as compared to younger adults

Usual Dosage Oral:

Geriatrics >75 years: 50-100 mg every 4-6 hours not to exceed 300 mg/day; see dosing in renal impairment

Adults: 50-100 mg every 4-6 hours, not to exceed 400 mg/day

Dosing interval in renal impairment: Cl_{cr} <30 mL/minute: Dosage interval should be extended to 12 hours with a maximum daily dose of 200 mg

Note: In patients with cirrhosis, the recommended dose is 50 mg every 12 hours

Administration Can be given without regard to food

Monitoring Parameters Monitor patient for pain, respiratory rate, and signs of tolerance and, therefore, abuse potential; monitor blood pressure and pulse rate, especially in patients on higher doses

Reference Range 100-300 ng/mL; however, serum concentration monitoring is not required

Test Interactions Creatinine increase, elevated liver enzymes, proteinuria, hemoglobin decrease

Patient Information Avoid driving or operating machinery until the effect of drug wears off; tramadol has not been fully evaluated for its abuse potential, report cravings to your physician immediately

Nursing Implications See Monitoring Parameters

Special Geriatric Considerations One study in the elderly found that tramadol 50 mg was similar in efficacy as acetaminophen 300 mg with codeine 30 mg (see Pharmacokinetics and Usual Dosage)

Dosage Forms Tablet, as hydrochloride: 50 mg

References

Rauck RL, Ruoff GE, and McGillen, "Comparison of Tramadol and Acetaminophen With Codeine for Long-Term Pain Management in Elderly Patients," *Curr Ther Res*, 1994, 556:1417-31.

Trandate® *see* Labetalol *on page 520*

Trandolapril *(tran DOE la pril)*

Related Information

ACE Inhibitors Comparison *on page 1019*

Brand Names Mavik®

Generic Available No

Therapeutic Category Angiotensin-Converting Enzyme (ACE) Inhibitors

Use Management of hypertension alone or in combination with other antihypertensive agents

Unlabeled use: As a class, ACE inhibitors are recommended in the treatment of systolic congestive heart failure

Contraindications Hypersensitivity to trandolapril, other ACE inhibitors, in patients with a history of angioedema related to previous treatment with an ACE inhibitor, or any component

Warnings Neutropenia, agranulocytosis, angioedema, decreased renal function (hypertension, renal artery stenosis, CHF), hepatic dysfunction (elimination, activation), proteinuria, first-dose hypotension (hypovolemia, CHF, dehydrated patients at risk, eg, diuretic use, elderly), elderly (due to renal function changes)

Precautions Use with caution and modify dosage in patients with renal impairment; use with caution in patients with collagen vascular disease, CHF, hypovolemia, valvular stenosis, hyperkalemia (>5.7 mEq/L), anesthesia

Adverse Reactions

Cardiovascular: Tachycardia, chest pain, palpitations, orthostatic blood pressure changes, syncope, heart failure, hypotension, angioedema, cardiogenic shock

Central nervous system: Headache, fatigue, dizziness, malaise, vertigo, somnolence, ataxia, nervousness, insomnia, fever

Dermatologic: Rash, pruritus, alopecia, exfoliative dermatitis, urticaria, photosensitivity

Endocrine & metabolic: Hyperkalemia

Gastrointestinal: Dysgeusia, abdominal pain, nausea, vomiting, diarrhea, anorexia, constipation, xerostomia, ageusia, glossitis

Genitourinary: Oliguria, impotence, decreased libido

Hematologic: Neutropenia, agranulocytosis

Hepatic: Hepatitis

Neuromuscular & skeletal: Arthritis, arthralgia, myalgia, paresthesias

Ocular: Blurred vision

Otic: Tinnitus

Renal: Oliguria, increase in BUN, increased serum creatinine, proteinuria, worsening renal failure

Respiratory: Chest pain, chronic cough (nonproductive, persistent - more frequent in women)

Miscellaneous: Diaphoresis

Overdosage Symptoms include hypertension, vertigo, dizziness

Toxicology Following initiation of essential overdose management, toxic symptom treatment and supportive treatment should be initiated. Hypotension usually responds to I.V. fluids or Trendelenburg positioning. If unresponsive to these measures, the use of a parenteral inotrope may be required (eg, norepinephrine 0.1-0.2 mcg/kg/minute titrated to response). Seizures commonly respond to diazepam (I.V. 5-10 mg bolus in adults every 15 minutes if needed up to a total of 30 mg) or to phenytoin or phenobarbital.

Drug Interactions

ACE inhibitors (trandolapril) and potassium-sparing diuretics may cause additive hyperkalemic effect

ACE inhibitors (trandolapril) and indomethacin or nonsteroidal anti-inflammatory agents may cause reduced antihypertensive response to ACE inhibitors (trandolapril)

Allopurinol and trandolapril may cause neutropenia

Antacids and ACE inhibitors may decrease absorption of ACE inhibitors

Phenothiazines and ACE inhibitors may increase ACE inhibitor effect

Probenecid and ACE inhibitors (trandolapril) may increase ACE inhibitors (trandolapril) levels

Rifampin and ACE inhibitors (trandolapril) may decrease ACE inhibitor effect

Digoxin and ACE inhibitors may increase serum digoxin concentrations

Lithium and ACE inhibitors may increase lithium serum concentrations

Tetracycline and ACE inhibitors (trandolapril) may decrease tetracycline absorption (up to 37%)

Food decreases trandolapril absorption; rate, but not extent, of ramipril and fosinopril is reduced by concomitant administration with food; food does not reduce absorption of enalapril, lisinopril, or benazepril; trandolapril has a decreased rate and extent (25% to 30%) of absorption when taken with a high fat meal

Mechanism of Action Trandolapril is an angiotensin-converting enzyme (ACE) inhibitor which prevents the formation of angiotensin II from angiotensin I. Trandolapril must undergo enzymatic hydrolysis, mainly in liver, to its biologically active metabolite, trandolaprilat. A CNS mechanism may also be involved in the hypotensive effect as angiotensin II increases adrenergic outflow from the CNS. Vasoactive kallikrein's may be decreased in conversion to active hormones by ACE inhibitors, thus, reducing blood pressure.

Pharmacodynamics

Peak reduction in blood pressure: 6 hours postdose

Peak concentrations: 6 hours

Trandolaprilat (active metabolite) is very lipophilic in comparison to other ACE inhibitors which may contribute to its prolonged duration of action (72 hours after a single dose)

Pharmacokinetics

Absorption: Rapid

Metabolism: Hydrolyzed, mainly in liver, to the active metabolite, trandolaprilat

Half-life: 24 hours

(Continued)

Trandolapril (Continued)

Elimination: As metabolites in urine; reduce dose in renal failure; creatinine clearances ≤30 mL/minute result in accumulation of active metabolite

Usual Dosage Geriatrics and Adults:

Non-Black patients: 0.5-1 mg for those not receiving diuretics, 0.5 mg for those receiving diuretics; increase dose at 0.5-1 mg increments at 1- to 2-week intervals; maximum dose: 4 mg/day

Black patients: Initiate doses of 1-2 mg; maximum dose: 4 mg/day

Congestive heart failure: Initial: 0.5-1 mg/day; titrate dose slowly over several weeks to a "target dose" of 4 mg once daily; do not exceed 4 mg/day

Dosing adjustment in renal impairment: Cl_{cr} ≤30 mL/minute: Administer lowest doses

Monitoring Parameters Serum potassium, renal function, serum creatinine, BUN, CBC

Test Interactions Increased serum potassium

Patient Information Do not discontinue medication without advice of physician; notify physician if sore throat, swelling, palpitations, cough, chest pains, difficulty swallowing, swelling of face, eyes, tongue, lips, hoarseness, sweating, vomiting, or diarrhea occurs; may cause dizziness, lightheadedness during first few days; may also cause changes in taste perception; do not use salt substitutes containing potassium without consulting a physician

Nursing Implications May cause depression in some patients; discontinue if angioedema of the face, extremities, lips, tongue, or glottis occurs; watch for hypotensive effects within 1-3 hours of first dose or new higher dose (see Precautions and Special Geriatric Considerations)

Additional Information Patients taking diuretics are at risk for developing hypotension on initial dosing; to prevent this, discontinue diuretics 2-3 days prior to initiating trandolapril; may restart diuretics if blood pressure is not controlled by trandolapril alone

Special Geriatric Considerations Due to frequent decreases in glomerular filtration (also creatinine clearance) with aging, elderly patients may have exaggerated responses to ACE inhibitors; differences in clinical response due to hepatic changes are not observed. ACE inhibitors may be preferred agents in elderly patients with CHF and diabetes mellitus. Diabetic proteinuria is reduced and insulin sensitivity is enhanced. In general, the side effect profile is favorable in elderly and causes little or no CNS confusion; use lowest dose recommendations initially. Adjust for renal function.

Dosage Forms Tablet: 1 mg, 2 mg, 4 mg

References

Bevan EG, McInnes GT, Aldigier JC, et al, "Effect of Renal Function on the Pharmacokinetics and Pharmacodynamics of Trandolapril," *Br J Clin Pharmacol*, 1993, 35(2):128-35.

Conen H and Brunner HR, "Pharmacologic Profile of Trandolapril, A New Angiotensin-Converting Enzyme Inhibitor," *Am Heart J*, 1993, 125(5 Pt 2):1525-31.

Zannad F, "Trandolapril: How Does It Differ From Other Angiotensin-Converting Enzyme Inhibitors?" *Drugs*, 1993, 46(Suppl 2):172-81.

Transamine Sulphate see Tranylcypromine on this page

Transdermal-NTG® Patch see Nitroglycerin on page 677

Transderm-Nitro® Patch see Nitroglycerin on page 677

Transderm Scop® Patch see Scopolamine on page 850

Trans-Ver-Sal® AdultPatch [OTC] see Salicylic Acid on page 845

Trans-Ver-Sal® PediaPatch [OTC] see Salicylic Acid on page 845

Trans-Ver-Sal® PlantarPatch [OTC] see Salicylic Acid on page 845

Tranxene® see Clorazepate on page 241

Tranylcypromine (tran il SIP roe meen)

Related Information

Antidepressant Medication Guidelines on page 1075

Brand Names Parnate®

Synonyms Transamine Sulphate

Generic Available No

Therapeutic Category Antidepressant, Monoamine Oxidase Inhibitor

Use Symptomatic treatment of depressed patients refractory to or intolerant to tricyclic antidepressants or electroconvulsive therapy

Contraindications Uncontrolled hypertension, known hypersensitivity to tranylcypromine, pheochromocytoma, congestive heart failure - patients <16 years of age, severe renal or hepatic impairment

Warnings Hypertensive crisis within several hours of ingestion of a contraindicated substance (tyramine-containing product)

Adverse Reactions
Cardiovascular: Hypotension, edema, hypertensive crises
Central nervous system: Drowsiness, hyperexcitability, insomnia
Dermatologic: Skin rash
Gastrointestinal: Xerostomia, constipation, weight gain
Genitourinary: Urinary retention, impotence
Hepatic: Hepatotoxicity (rare)
Ocular: Blurred vision
Miscellaneous: Diaphoresis, lupus-like reaction

Overdosage Symptoms of overdose include tachycardia, palpitations, muscle twitching, seizures, headache

Toxicology Competent supportive care is the most important treatment for an overdose with a monoamine oxidase (MAO) inhibitor. Both hypertension or hypotension can occur with intoxication. Hypotension may respond to I.V. fluids or vasopressors and hypertension usually responds to an alpha-adrenergic blocker (or phentolamine 5 mg I.V.) or nifedipine 10 mg; do not use parenteral reserpine. While treating the hypertension, care is warranted to avoid sudden drops in blood pressure, since this may worsen the MAO inhibitor toxicity. Muscle irritability and seizures often respond to diazepam, while hyperthermia is best treated antipyretics and cooling blankets. Cardiac arrhythmias are best treated with phenytoin or procainamide.

Drug Interactions
Decreased effect of antihypertensives
Increased toxicity with disulfiram (seizures), fluoxetine and other serotonin-active agents (eg, paroxetine, sertraline), TCAs (cardiovascular instability), meperidine (cardiovascular instability), phenothiazine (hypertensive crisis), sympathomimetics (hypertensive crisis), sumatriptan (hypothetical), CNS depressants, levodopa (hypertensive crisis), dextroamphetamine (psychosis)
Note: Many of these drug interactions can occur weeks after the MAO inhibitor has been stopped

Drug/Food Interactions Tyramine-containing foods (eg, aged foods) (see Warnings and Patient Information)

Mechanism of Action Inhibits the enzymes monoamine oxidase A and B which are responsible for the intraneuronal metabolism of norepinephrine and serotonin and increasing their availability to postsynaptic neurons; decreased firing rate of the locus ceruleus, reducing norepinephrine concentration in the brain; agonist effects of serotonin

Pharmacodynamics Onset of therapeutic effect: 2-3 weeks are required of continued dosing to obtain full effect

Pharmacokinetics
Half-life: 90-190 minutes
Time to peak serum concentration: Oral: Within 2 hours
Elimination: In urine

Usual Dosage Geriatrics and Adults: Oral: 10 mg twice daily, increase to a maximum of 20-40 mg/day after 2 weeks

Administration Administer second dose before 4 PM to avoid insomnia

Monitoring Parameters Blood pressure, heart rate, diet, mood and depressive symptoms, weight

Reference Range Inhibition of platelet monoamine oxidase (≥80%) correlated with clinical response

Test Interactions Decreased glucose

Patient Information Tablets may be crushed; avoid alcohol; do not discontinue abruptly; avoid foods high in tyramine (eg, cheese [except cottage, ricotta, and cream], smoked or pickled fish, beef or chicken liver, dried sausage, fava or broad bean pods, yeast, vitamin supplements); change positions slowly; discuss list of drugs and foods to avoid with pharmacist or physician; take second dose no later than 4 PM to avoid insomnia

Nursing Implications Assist with ambulation during initiation of therapy (see Administration, Monitoring Parameters, and Drug Interactions)

Additional Information Has a more rapid onset of therapeutic effect than other MAO inhibitors, but causes more severe hypertensive reactions

Special Geriatric Considerations The MAO inhibitors are effective and generally well tolerated by older patients; it is their potential interactions with tyramine- or tryptophan-containing foods (see Warnings) and other drugs (see Drug Interactions), and their effect on blood pressure that have limited their use. The MAO inhibitors are usually reserved for patients who do not tolerate or respond to the traditional "cyclic" or "second generation" antidepressants. Tranylcypromine is the preferred MAO inhibitor because its enzymatic-blocking effects are more rapidly reversed. The brain activity of (Continued)

Tranylcypromine *(Continued)*

monoamine oxidase increases with age and even more so in patients with Alzheimer's disease. Therefore, the MAO inhibitors may have an increased role in patients with Alzheimer's disease who are also depressed.

Dosage Forms Tablet, as sulfate: 10 mg

References

Georgotas A, Friedman E, McCarthy M, et al, "Resistant Geriatric Depression and Therapeutic Response to Monoamine-Oxidase Inhibitors," *Biol Psychiatry*, 1983, 18:195-205.

Goff DC and Jenike MA, "Treatment-Resistant Depression in the Elderly," *J Am Geriatr Soc*, 1986, 34(1):63-70.

Jenike MA, "MAO Inhibitors as Treatment for Depressed Patients With Primary Degenerative Dementia (Alzheimer's Disease)," *Am J Psychiatry* 1985, 142:763.

Trazodone *(TRAZ oh done)*

Related Information

Antidepressant Agents Comparison *on page 1021*

Antidepressant Medication Guidelines *on page 1075*

Federal OBRA Regulations Recommended Maximum Doses - Antidepressants *on page 1056*

Serum Drug Concentrations Commonly Monitored: Guidelines *on page 1114*

Brand Names Desyrel®

Therapeutic Category Antidepressant

Use Treatment of depression

Unlabeled uses: Trazodone 50 mg twice daily with tryptophan 500 mg twice daily for aggressive behavior; panic disorders; cocaine withdrawal

Contraindications Hypersensitivity to trazodone, nefazodone, or any component

Warnings Monitor closely and use with extreme caution in patients with cardiac disease or arrhythmias

Precautions Cardiovascular effects may warrant EKG prior to initiation of treatment

Adverse Reactions Possesses fewer anticholinergic and cardiac adverse effects than tricyclic antidepressants

Cardiovascular: Postural hypotension (5%), arrhythmias

Central nervous system: Drowsiness (20% to 50%), sedation, dizziness, headache, insomnia, confusion, agitation, seizures, rarely extrapyramidal reactions

Gastrointestinal: Xerostomia (15% to 30%), constipation, nausea, vomiting

Genitourinary: Prolonged priapism (1:6000), urinary retention (rare)

Hepatic: Hepatitis

Neuromuscular & skeletal: Weakness

Ocular: Blurred vision

Overdosage Symptoms of overdose include drowsiness, vomiting, hypotension, tachycardia, incontinence, coma

Toxicology Following initiation of essential overdose management, toxic symptoms should be treated. Ventricular arrhythmias often respond to phenytoin 15-20 mg/kg with concurrent systemic alkalinization (sodium bicarbonate 0.5-2 mEq/kg I.V.). Arrhythmias unresponsive to this therapy may respond to lidocaine 1 mg/kg I.V. followed by a titrated infusion. Physostigmine (1-2 mg I.V. slowly) may be indicated in reversing cardiac arrhythmias that are due to vagal blockade or for anticholinergic effects. Seizures usually respond to diazepam I.V. boluses (5-10 mg, up to 30 mg). If seizures are unresponsive or recur, phenytoin or phenobarbital may be required.

Drug Interactions Trazodone may antagonize the antihypertensive effects of clonidine and methyldopa; may increase the serum concentrations of phenytoin or digoxin; effects may be additive with other CNS depressants; fluoxetine may increase trazodone serum concentration; may decrease the effect of anticoagulants; unknown if interactions occur with MAO inhibitors, best to avoid

Mechanism of Action Traditionally believed to increase the synaptic concentration of serotonin in the central nervous system by inhibition of its reuptake by the presynaptic neuronal membrane. However, additional receptor effects have been found including desensitization of adenyl cyclase, down regulation of beta-adrenergic receptors, and down regulation of serotonin receptors

Pharmacodynamics Onset of therapeutic effects: May take 1-3 weeks to appear; 5-HT only

Pharmacokinetics

Protein binding: 85% to 95%

Metabolism: In the liver; substrate CYP2D6

Half-life: 4-7.5 hours, 2 compartment kinetics
  Elimination: Geriatrics: 11.6 hours, nearly twice that of younger patients
Time to peak serum concentration: Oral: Within 30-100 minutes, prolonged in the presence of food (up to 2.5 hours)
Elimination: Primarily in urine and secondarily in feces

Usual Dosage Oral:
Geriatrics: 25-50 mg at bedtime with 25-50 mg/day dose increase every 3 days for inpatients and weekly for outpatients, if tolerated; usual dose: 75-150 mg/day in 3 divided doses where practical (eg, dose of 75 mg/day as above should be divided into 2-3 doses; see Pharmacokinetics)
Adults: Initial: 150 mg/day in 3 divided doses (may increase by 50 mg/day every 3-7 days); maximum: 600 mg/day

Monitoring Parameters Blood pressure, pulse, target symptoms

Reference Range Therapeutic: 0.5-2.5 µg/mL (SI: 1-6 µmol/L); not well established

Patient Information Take shortly after a meal or light snack, can be given as bedtime dose if drowsiness occurs; avoid alcohol; be aware of possible photosensitivity reaction; may cause painful erections; avoid sudden changes of position

Nursing Implications Use side rails on bed if administered to the elderly; observe patient's activity and compare with admission behaviors; sitting and standing blood pressure and pulse

Additional Information Therapeutic effects may take up to 4 weeks to occur; therapy is normally maintained for several months after optimum response is reached to prevent recurrence of depression

Special Geriatric Considerations Very sedating, but little anticholinergic effects

Dosage Forms Tablet, as hydrochloride: 50 mg, 100 mg, 150 mg, 300 mg

References
Bayer AJ, Pathy MSJ, and Ankier SI, "Pharmacokinetic and Pharmacodynamic Characteristics of Trazodone in the Elderly," *Br J Clin Pharmacol*, 1983, 16:371-6.
Gerson SC, Plotkin DA, and Jarvik LF, "Antidepressant Drug Studies, 1964-1986: Empirical Evidence for Aging Patients," *J Clin Psychopharmacol*, 1988, 8(5):311-21.

Trecator®-SC *see Ethionamide on page 359*

Trendar® [OTC] *see Ibuprofen on page 475*

Trental® *see Pentoxifylline on page 728*

Triacet® *see Triamcinolone on this page*

Triaconazole *see Terconazole on page 894*

Triam-A® *see Triamcinolone on this page*

Triamcinolone (trye am SIN oh lone)
Related Information
  Antacid Drug Interactions *on page 1096*
  Asthma Guidelines *on page 1040*
  Corticosteroids Comparison, Topical *on page 1030*
  Estimated Comparative Daily Dosages for Inhaled Corticosteroids *on page 1045*
  Inhaled Medications Comparison *on page 1034*

Brand Names Amcort®; Aristocort®; Aristocort® A; Aristocort® Forte; Aristocort® Intralesional; Aristospan® Intra-Articular; Aristospan® Intralesional; Atolone®; Azmacort™; Delta-Tritex®; Flutex®; Kenacort®; Kenaject-40®; Kenalog®; Kenalog-10®; Kenalog-40®; Kenalog® H; Kenalog® in Orabase®; Kenonel®; Nasacort®; Nasacort® AQ; Tac™-3; Tac™-40; Triacet®; Triam-A®; Triam Forte®; Triderm®; Tri-Kort®; Trilog®; Trilone®; Tristoject®

Synonyms Triamcinolone, Oral

Generic Available Yes

Therapeutic Category Adrenal Corticosteroid; Anti-inflammatory Agent; Corticosteroid, Inhalant; Corticosteroid, Systemic; Corticosteroid, Topical (Medium Potency); Corticosteroid, Topical (High Potency)

Use
Topical: Inflammatory dermatoses responsive to steroids. Inhalation: Control of bronchial asthma and related bronchospastic conditions
Systemic: Adrenocortical insufficiency, rheumatic disorders, allergic states, respiratory diseases, systemic lupus erythematosus, and other diseases requiring anti-inflammatory or immunosuppressive effects

Contraindications Known hypersensitivity to triamcinolone; systemic fungal infections; serious infections, except septic shock or tuberculous meningitis; primary treatment of acute episodes of asthma

Warnings Fatalities have occurred due to adrenal insufficiency in asthmatic patients during and after transfer from systemic corticosteroids to aerosol
(Continued)

Triamcinolone *(Continued)*

steroids; several months may be required for recovery from this syndrome; during this period, aerosol steroids do **not** provide the increased systemic steroid requirement needed to treat patients having trauma, surgery or infections

Precautions Use with caution in patients with hypothyroidism, cirrhosis, nonspecific ulcerative colitis and patients at increased risk for peptic ulcer disease; do not use occlusive dressings on weeping or exudative lesions and general caution with occlusive dressings should be observed; discontinue if skin irritation or contact dermatitis should occur; do not use in patients with decreased skin circulation; avoid the use of high potency steroids on the face

Adverse Reactions

Cardiovascular: Hypertension, edema, accelerated atherogenesis, facial edema

Central nervous system: Euphoria, mental changes, headache, vertigo, seizures, psychoses, pseudotumor cerebri

Dermatologic: Folliculitis, hypertrichosis, acneiform eruption dermatitis, maceration, skin atrophy, acne, impaired wound healing, hirsutism, itching, hypopigmentation, hyperpigmentation, striae, miliaria, telangiectasia

Endocrine & metabolic: Growth suppression, Cushing's syndrome, pituitary-adrenal axis suppression, alkalosis, glucose intolerance, hypokalemia, postmenopausal bleeding, hot flashes

Gastrointestinal: Peptic ulcer, nausea, vomiting, pancreatitis, oral candidiasis, dry throat, xerostomia

Local: Burning, irritation

Neuromuscular & skeletal: Muscle weakness, osteoporosis, fractures, aseptic necrosis of femoral and humeral heads, steroid myopathy

Ocular: Cataracts, glaucoma

Respiratory: Hoarseness, wheezing, cough

Miscellaneous: Increased susceptibility to infection

Toxicology When consumed in excessive quantities for prolonged periods, systemic hypercorticism and adrenal suppression may occur; in those cases, discontinuation and withdrawal of the corticosteroid should be done judiciously

Drug Interactions

Steroids decrease the effect of anticholinesterases, isoniazid, salicylates, insulin, oral hypoglycemics

Decreased effect: Barbiturates, phenytoin, rifampin

Increased effect (hypokalemia) of potassium-depleting diuretics

Increased risk of digoxin toxicity (due to hypokalemia)

Increased effect: Estrogens, ketoconazole

Mechanism of Action Decreases inflammation by suppression of migration of polymorphonuclear leukocytes and reversal of increased capillary permeability; suppresses the immune system by reducing activity and volume of the lymphatic system; suppresses adrenal function at high doses

Pharmacodynamics Duration of action: Oral: 8-12 hours

Pharmacokinetics

Time to peak serum concentration: I.M.: Within 8-10 hours

Half-life, biologic: 18-36 hours

Usual Dosage

Geriatrics and Adults:

Topical: Apply thin film 2-3 times/day

Triamcinolone Dosing

	Acetonide	Diacetate	Hexacetonide
Intrasynovial	2.5-40 mg	5-40 mg	
Intralesional	2.5-40 mg	5-48 mg	Up to 0.5 mg/sq inch affected area
Sublesional	1-30 mg	5-48 mg	Up to 0.5 mg/sq inch affected area
Systemic I.M.	2.5-60 mg/d	~40 mg/wk	20-100 mg
Intra-articular		5-40 mg	2-20 mg average
large joints	5-15 mg		10-20 mg
small joints	2.5-5 mg		2-6 mg
Tendon sheaths	10-40 mg		
Intradermal	1 mg/site		

Oral inhalation: 2 inhalations 3-4 times/day, not to exceed 16 inhalations/day

Intra-articularly, intrasynovially, intralesionally: 2.5-40 mg, dose may be repeated when signs and symptoms recur

Intra-articularly: 2-20 mg every 3-4 weeks as hexacetonide

Intralesionally, sublesionally (as acetonide): Up to 1 mg per injection site and may be repeated one or more times weekly; multiple sites may be injected if they are 1 cm or more apart, not to exceed 30 mg

Geriatrics: Systemically use the lowest effective daily dose

Adults:

Oral: 4-48 mg/day

I.M.: Average dose: 40 mg once weekly

See table.

Monitoring Parameters Blood pressure, blood glucose, electrolytes

Test Interactions Increases amylase (S), cholesterol (S), glucose, protein, sodium (S); decreases calcium (S), potassium (S), thyroxine (S)

Patient Information Report any change in body weight; do not discontinue or decrease the drug without contacting your physician; carry an identification card or bracelet advising that you are on steroids; may take with meals to decrease GI upset; take single daily dose in the morning; apply topical preparations in a thin layer. For the inhaler, follow instructions that accompany the product and do not exceed the recommended dose; notify physician if any signs of infection occur.

Nursing Implications Evaluate clinical response and mental status; may mask signs and symptoms of infection; inject I.M. dose deep in large muscle mass, avoid deltoid; avoid S.C. dose; apply topical products sparingly, do not occlude area unless desired; once daily doses should be given in the morning

Additional Information Systemic absorption may occur after topical application; 16 mg triamcinolone is equivalent to 100 mg cortisone (no mineralocorticoid activity)

Triamcinolone acetonide, aerosol: Azmacort™

Triamcinolone acetonide, parenteral: Cenocort®, Cinonide®, Kenalog® injection, Triam-A®, Tri-Kort®, Trilog®

Triamcinolone diacetate, oral: Aristocort® syrup, Kenacort® syrup

Triamcinolone diacetate, parenteral: Aristocort® intralesional, Amcort®, Aristocort® Forte, Cenocort® Forte, Triamolone®, Trilone®, Trisoject®

Triamcinolone hexacetonide: Aristospan®

Triamcinolone, oral: Aristocort® tablet, Kenacort® tablet

Special Geriatric Considerations Because of the risk of adverse effects, systemic corticosteroids should be used cautiously in the elderly, in the smallest possible dose, and for the shortest possible time. Azmacort™ (metered dose inhaler) comes with its own spacer device attached and may be easier to use in older patients.

Dosage Forms

Aerosol:

Oral inhalation: 100 mcg/metered spray (2 oz)

Topical, as acetonide: 0.2 mg/2 second spray (23 g, 63 g)

Cream, as acetonide: 0.025% (15 g, 60 g, 80 g, 240 g, 454 g); 0.1% (15 g, 30 g, 60 g, 80 g, 90 g, 120 g, 240 g); 0.5% (15 g, 20 g, 30 g, 240 g)

Injection, as acetonide: 10 mg/mL (5 mL); 40 mg/mL (1 mL, 5 mL, 10 mL)

Injection, as diacetate: 25 mg/mL (5 mL); 40 mg/mL (1 mL, 5 mL, 10 mL)

Injection, as hexacetonide: 5 mg/mL (5 mL); 20 mg/mL (1 mL, 5 mL)

Lotion, as acetonide: 0.025% (60 mL); 0.1% (15 mL, 60 mL)

Ointment, oral: 0.1% (5 g)

Ointment, topical, as acetonide: 0.025% (15 g, 30 g, 60 g, 80 g, 120 g, 454 g); 0.1% (15 g, 30 g, 60 g, 80 g, 120 g, 240 g, 454 g); 0.5% (15 g, 20 g, 30 g, 240 g)

Syrup: 2 mg/5 mL (120 mL); 4 mg/5 mL (120 mL)

Tablet: 1 mg, 2 mg, 4 mg, 8 mg

Triamcinolone and Nystatin see Nystatin and Triamcinolone on page 687 see Nystatin and Triamcinolone on page 687

Triamcinolone, Oral see Triamcinolone on page 949 see Triamcinolone on page 949

Triam Forte® see Triamcinolone on page 949 see Triamcinolone on page 949

Triaminic® AM Decongestant Formula [OTC] see Pseudoephedrine on page 802 see Pseudoephedrine on page 802

Triamterene (trye AM ter een)

Brand Names Dyrenium®

Generic Available No

Therapeutic Category Diuretic, Potassium Sparing

(Continued)

Triamterene *(Continued)*

Use Alone or in combination with other diuretics to treat edema and hypertension; decreases potassium excretion caused by kaliuretic diuretics

Contraindications Hyperkalemia, renal impairment, hypersensitivity to triamterene or any component; do not administer to patients receiving spironolactone or amiloride

Precautions Use with caution in patients with severe hepatic encephalopathy and in patients with diabetes. Potassium excretion may be decreased in the elderly, increasing the risk of hyperkalemia with the use of triamterene.

Adverse Reactions

Endocrine & metabolic: Hyperkalemia, electrolyte imbalance (decreased sodium, decreased magnesium, decreased bicarbonate, increased chloride, possibility of metabolic acidosis), hyperuricemia

Gastrointestinal: Nausea, vomiting, diarrhea

Genitourinary: Slight prerenal azotemia, slight alkalinization of urine

Hematologic: Blood dyscrasias

Hepatic: Abnormal liver function

Renal: Nephrolithiasis

Miscellaneous: Allergic reactions have been reported

Overdosage Symptoms of overdose include drowsiness, confusion, clinical signs of dehydration, electrolyte imbalance, and hypotension

Toxicology Ingestion of large amounts of potassium-sparing diuretics, may result in life-threatening hyperkalemia. This can be treated with I.V. insulin and glucose (dextrose 25% in water), with concurrent I.V. sodium bicarbonate (1 mEq/kg up to 44 mEq/dose). If needed, Kayexalate® oral or rectal solutions in sorbitol may also be used.

Drug Interactions

Increased risk of hyperkalemia if given together with amiloride, spironolactone, angiotensin-converting enzyme (ACE) inhibitors, NSAIDs

Increased toxicity of amantadine (possibly by decreasing its renal excretion)

Mechanism of Action Interferes with potassium/sodium exchange in the distal tubule

Pharmacodynamics

Onset of action: Within 2-4 hours

Duration: 7-9 hours

Pharmacokinetics

Absorption: Oral: Unreliably absorbed

Time to peak serum concentration: One study found that peak serum concentrations in elderly were approximately twice those in younger patients

Usual Dosage Oral (when used alone; decrease total daily dose when combined with other diuretics or antihypotensives):

Geriatrics: Initial: 50 mg/day; maximum: 100 mg/day in 1-2 divided doses

Adults: 100-300 mg/day in 1-2 divided doses; maximum: 300 mg/day

Monitoring Parameters Blood pressure, serum electrolytes, renal function, weight, I & O

Test Interactions Interferes with fluorometric assay of quinidine

Patient Information Take in the morning; take the last dose of multiple doses no later than 6 PM unless instructed otherwise; take after meals; notify physician if weakness, headache or nausea occurs; avoid excessive ingestion of food high in potassium or use of salt substitute; may increase blood glucose; may impart a blue fluorescent color to urine

Nursing Implications Observe for hyperkalemia in geriatric patients and in patients with renal insufficiency; assess weight and I & O daily to determine weight loss

Special Geriatric Considerations Monitor serum potassium (see Precautions)

Dosage Forms Capsule: 50 mg, 100 mg

Triamterene and Hydrochlorothiazide *see Hydrochlorothiazide and Triamterene on page 460*

Triavil® *see Amitriptyline and Perphenazine on page 62*

Triazolam *(trye AY zoe lam)*

Related Information

Antacid Drug Interactions *on page 1096*

Anxiolytic/Hypnotic Use in Long-Term Care Facilities *on page 1099*

Benzodiazepines Comparison *on page 1024*

Federal OBRA Regulations Recommended Maximum Doses - Hypnotics *on page 1057*

Brand Names Halcion®

Generic Available No

Therapeutic Category Benzodiazepine; Hypnotic; Sedative

Use Short-term treatment of insomnia

Restrictions C-IV

Contraindications Hypersensitivity to triazolam, or any component, cross-sensitivity with other benzodiazepines may occur; severe uncontrolled pain; pre-existing CNS depression; narrow-angle glaucoma; sleep apnea

Warnings Abrupt discontinuance may precipitate withdrawal or rebound insomnia; anterograde amnesia has occurred with triazolam, generally it occurred with doses of 0.5 mg but it has also been reported with lower doses

Precautions Has potential for drug dependence and abuse; use with caution in patients with a potential for drug dependence

Adverse Reactions

Central nervous system: Drowsiness, ataxia, anterograde amnesia, confusion, dizziness, agitation, hallucinations, nightmares, headache

Gastrointestinal: Xerostomia, nausea, vomiting, constipation

Hepatic: Cholestatic jaundice

Neuromuscular & skeletal: Impaired coordination

Respiratory: Decreased respiratory rate, apnea, laryngospasm

Miscellaneous: Physical and psychological dependence may occur with prolonged use

Overdosage Symptoms of overdose include somnolence, confusion, coma, and diminished reflexes

Toxicology Treatment for benzodiazepine overdose is supportive; rarely is mechanical ventilation required

Flumazenil has been shown to selectively block the binding of benzodiazepines to CNS receptors, resulting in a reversal of benzodiazepine-induced sedation; however, its use may not alter the course of overdose

Drug Interactions

Increased toxicity: CNS depressants, alcohol; macrolides may increase the bioavailability of triazolam; nefazodone, protease inhibitors, SSRIs may inhibit triazolam metabolism

Decreased effect: Benzodiazepines may decrease the effect of levodopa

Mechanism of Action Benzodiazepines appear to potentiate the effects of GABA and other inhibitory neurotransmitters by binding to specific benzodiazepine-receptor sites in various areas of the CNS

Pharmacodynamics Hypnotic effects:

Onset of action: Within 15-30 minutes

Duration: 6-7 hours; studies have shown that the elderly are more sensitive to the effects of benzodiazepines as compared to younger adults

Pharmacokinetics

Distribution: V_d: 0.8-1.8 L/kg

Protein binding: 89%

Metabolism: Extensive in the liver; substrate CYP3A4

Half-life: 1.7-5 hours

Elimination: In urine as unchanged drug and metabolites; triazolam clearance is lower in elderly

Note: In elderly, peak plasma concentrations and AUC are increased

Usual Dosage Oral:

Geriatrics: 0.0625-0.125 mg at bedtime

Adults: 0.125-0.25 mg at bedtime

Monitoring Parameters Respiratory, cardiovascular and mental status

Patient Information Avoid alcohol and other CNS depressants; may cause drowsiness; avoid activities needing good psychomotor coordination until CNS effects are known; may cause physical or psychological dependence; avoid abrupt discontinuation after prolonged use; **for short-term use only; do not exceed prescribed dose**

Nursing Implications Provide safety measures (ie, side rails, night light, call button); remove smoking materials from area; supervise ambulation

Additional Information Onset of action is rapid, patient should take triazolam right before going to bed

Special Geriatric Considerations Due to the higher incidence of CNS adverse reactions and its short half-life, this benzodiazepine is not a drug of first choice; for short-term only (see Warnings, Pharmacodynamics, and Pharmacokinetics)

Dosage Forms Tablet: 0.125 mg, 0.25 mg

References

Greenblatt DJ, Harmatz JS, Shapiro L, et al, "Sensitivity to Triazolam in the Elderly," *N Engl J Med*, 1991, 324(24):1691-8.

Triban® *see* Trimethobenzamide *on page 961*

Tribavirin *see* Ribavirin *on page 828*

Trichloroacetaldehyde Monohydrate *see* Chloral Hydrate *on page 200*

Tricosal® *see* Choline Magnesium Trisalicylate *on page 221*

Triderm® *see* Triamcinolone *on page 949*

Tridil® Injection *see* Nitroglycerin *on page 677*

Triethanolamine Polypeptide Oleate-Condensate
(trye eth a NOLE a meen pol i PEP tide OH lee ate-KON den sate)

Brand Names Cerumenex® Otic

Generic Available No

Therapeutic Category Otic Agent, Cerumenolytic

Use Removal of ear wax (cerumen)

Contraindications Perforated tympanic membrane or otitis media, hypersensitivity to product or any component

Warnings Avoid undue exposure to peridural skin during administration and the flushing out of ear canal; discontinue if sensitization or irritation occurs

Adverse Reactions Local: Localized dermatitis, mild erythema and pruritus, severe eczematoid reactions involving the external ear and periauricular tissue

Mechanism of Action Emulsifies and disperses accumulated cerumen

Pharmacodynamics Onset of effect: Produces slight disintegration of very hard ear wax by 24 hours

Usual Dosage Geriatrics and Adults: Otic: Fill ear canal, insert cotton plug; allow to remain 15-30 minutes; flush ear with lukewarm water as a single treatment; if a second application is needed for unusually hard impactions, repeat the procedure

Monitoring Parameters Evaluate hearing before and after instillation of medication

Patient Information For external use in the ear only; warm to body temperature before using to improve effect; avoid touching dropper to any surface; hold ear lobe up and back; lie on your side or tilt the affected ear up for ease of administration; fill ear canal, let stand for 15-30 minutes, then flush

Nursing Implications Warm solution to body temperature before using; avoid undue exposure of the drug to the periauricular skin

Special Geriatric Considerations Avoid contact with hearing aids

Dosage Forms Solution, otic: 6 mL, 12 mL

Trifluoperazine (trye floo oh PER a zeen)
Related Information

Antacid Drug Interactions *on page 1096*

Antipsychotic Agents Comparison *on page 1023*

Antipsychotic Medication Guidelines *on page 1076*

Federal OBRA Regulations Recommended Maximum Doses - Antipsychotics *on page 1056*

Brand Names Stelazine®

Generic Available Yes

Therapeutic Category Antianxiety Agent; Antipsychotic Agent; Neuroleptic Agent; Phenothiazine Derivative

Use Management of manifestations of psychotic disorders; depressive neurosis; alcohol withdrawal; nausea and vomiting; nonpsychotic symptoms associated with dementia in elderly; Tourette's syndrome; Huntington's chorea; spasmodic torticollis and Reye's syndrome (see Special Geriatric Considerations)

Contraindications Hypersensitivity to trifluoperazine or any component, cross-sensitivity with other phenothiazines may exist; avoid use in patients with narrow-angle glaucoma, bone marrow suppression, severe liver or cardiac disease; subcortical brain damage; circulatory collapse, severe hypotension or hypertension

Warnings

Tardive dyskinesia: Prevalence rate may be 40% in elderly; elderly women especially at risk; embarrassment from dyskinesias may lead to greater social isolation; development of the syndrome and the irreversible nature are proportional to duration and total cumulative dose over time. May be reversible if diagnosed early in therapy; intermittent use of antipsychotics (not proven use) helps decrease total cumulative dose.

EPS: Extrapyramidal reactions are more common in elderly with up to 50% developing these reactions after age 60. These reactions may be more common in dementia patients. Drug-induced **Parkinson's syndrome** occurs often. Discontinuation usually resolves symptoms but may take weeks to months (12+) to clear. **Akathisia** is the most common EPS reaction in elderly. The symptoms of motor restlessness are difficult to diagnose in demented elderly; increased nervousness, assertiveness, restlessness with constant movement may indicate this adverse event. Consider decreasing dose if antipsychotic to treat as well as diagnose problem; usually see this reaction within 2-3 months of initiating antipsychotic drug.

Anticholinergic effects: These side effects most common with low potency antipsychotics (eg, thioridazine, chlorpromazine). CNS toxicity occurs more frequently and severely in elderly; increased confusion, memory loss, psychotic behavior, and agitation frequently occur as a consequence of anticholinergic effects to antipsychotic agents. Peripheral anticholinergic action troublesome to elderly; most peripheral anticholinergic effects last only 2-3 weeks (see Adverse Reactions).

Orthostatic hypotension: More common with low potency agents (eg, thioridazine, chlorpromazine, and clozapine) but of concern with all antipsychotic agents; orthostasis due to alpha-receptor blockade by antipsychotic agents. Elderly present many risk factors for orthostatic hypotension: blunted baroreceptor reflexes, decreased vascular tone, decreased vascular volume, and possible presence of cardiac diseases which result in decreased cardiac output.

Sedation: Common side effect with antipsychotic therapy; should not be used as a hypnotic unless insomnia is associated with target behavior symptoms treated with antipsychotic medications (see Special Geriatric Considerations). Anecdotal reports suggesting antipsychotic sedation in nonpsychotic patients is extremely unpleasant due to feelings of depersonalization, derealization, and dysphoria. Due to the long duration of action with antipsychotic drugs, these reactions may last up to 24 hours and result in decreased daytime function.

Cardiac toxicity: Life-threatening arrhythmias have occurred at therapeutic doses of antipsychotics. Thioridazine more commonly demonstrates EKG changes than other antipsychotics; suggested to use high potency antipsychotic agents (ie, haloperidol) in patients with cardiac conduction defects.

Precautions Use with caution in patients with cardiovascular disease, seizures, and Parkinson's disease; benefits of therapy must be weighed against risks

Adverse Reactions

Cardiovascular: Hypotension (especially with I.V. use), orthostatic hypotension, tachycardia, arrhythmias, abnormal T waves with prolonged ventricular repolarization

Central nervous system: Sedation, drowsiness, restlessness, anxiety, extrapyramidal reactions, pseudoparkinsonian signs and symptoms, tardive dyskinesia, neuroleptic malignant syndrome, seizures, altered central temperature regulation

Dermatologic: Hyperpigmentation, pruritus, rash, photosensitivity

Endocrine & metabolic: Amenorrhea, galactorrhea, gynecomastia

Gastrointestinal: GI upset, xerostomia (problem for denture users), constipation, adynamic ileus, weight gain

Genitourinary: Urinary retention, overflow incontinence, priapism, impotence, sexual dysfunction (up to 60%)

Hematologic: Agranulocytosis, leukopenia (usually in patients with large doses for prolonged periods), thrombocytopenia, hemolytic anemia, eosinophilia

Hepatic: Cholestatic jaundice (rare)

Ocular: Blurred vision, retinal pigmentation is more common than with chlorpromazine

Miscellaneous: Anaphylactoid reactions

Overdosage Symptoms of overdose include deep sleep, coma, extrapyramidal symptoms, abnormal involuntary muscle movements, hypotension or hypertension; agitation, restlessness, fever, hypothermia or hyperthermia, seizures, cardiac arrhythmias, EKG changes

Toxicology Following initiation of essential overdose management, toxic symptom treatment and supportive treatment should be initiated. Hypotension usually responds to I.V. fluids or Trendelenburg positioning. If unresponsive to these measures the use of a parenteral inotrope may be required (eg, norepinephrine 0.1-0.2 mcg/kg/minute titrated to response). Do not use epinephrine. Seizures commonly respond to diazepam (I.V. 5-10 mg bolus every 15 minutes if needed up to a total of 30 mg) or to phenytoin or phenobarbital. Also critical cardiac arrhythmias often respond to I.V. phenytoin (15

(Continued)

Trifluoperazine *(Continued)*

mg/kg up to 1 g), while other antiarrhythmics can be used. Neuroleptics often cause extrapyramidal symptoms (eg, dystonic reactions) requiring management with diphenhydramine 1-2 mg/kg up to a maximum of 50 mg I.M. or I.V. slow push followed by a maintenance dose for 48-72 hours. When these reactions are unresponsive to diphenhydramine, benztropine mesylate I.V. 1-2 mg may be effective. These agents are generally effective within 2-5 minutes.

Drug Interactions

Alcohol may increase CNS sedation

Anticholinergic agents may decrease pharmacologic effects; increase anticholinergic side effects; may enhance tardive dyskinesia

Aluminum salts may decrease absorption of phenothiazines

Barbiturates may decrease phenothiazine serum concentrations

Bromocriptine may have decreased efficacy when administered with phenothiazines

Guanethidine's hypotensive effect is decreased by phenothiazines

Lithium administration with phenothiazines may increase disorientation

Meperidine and phenothiazine coadministration increases sedation and hypotension

Methyldopa administration with phenothiazine (trifluoperazine) may significantly increase blood pressure

Norepinephrine, epinephrine have decreased pressor effect when administered with chlorpromazine; therefore, be aware of possible decreased effectiveness or when any phenothiazine is used

Phenytoin serum concentrations may increase or decrease with phenothiazines; tricyclic antidepressants may have increased serum concentrations with concomitant administration with phenothiazines

Propranolol administered with phenothiazines may increase serum concentrations of both drugs

Valproic acid may have increased half-life when administered with phenothiazines (chlorpromazine)

Stability Store injection at room temperature; protect from heat and from freezing; protect all dosage forms from light, clear or slightly yellow solutions may be used; should be dispensed in amber or opaque vials/bottles. Solutions may be diluted or mixed with fruit juices or other liquids but must be administered immediately after mixing; do not prepare bulk dilutions or store bulk dilutions.

Mechanism of Action Blocks postsynaptic mesolimbic dopaminergic D_1 and D_2 receptors in the brain; exhibits a strong alpha-adrenergic blocking and anticholinergic effect, depresses the release of hypothalamic and hypophyseal hormones; believed to depress the reticular activating system thus affecting basal metabolism, body temperature, wakefulness, vasomotor tone, and emesis

Pharmacokinetics

Absorption: May be affected by the inherent anticholinergic action on the gastrointestinal tissue causing variable absorption. Absorption from tablets is erratic with less variation seen with solutions. These agents are widely distributed in tissues with CNS concentrations exceeding that of plasma due to their lipophilic characteristics.

Protein binding: Antipsychotic agents are bound 90% to 99% to plasma proteins; highly bound to brain and lung tissue and other tissues with a high blood perfusion.

Half-life: >24 hours with chronic use

Time to peak concentration: Oral: 2-4 hours

Elimination: Occurs through hepatic metabolism (oxidation) where numerous active metabolites are produced; active metabolites excreted in urine; elimination half-lives of antipsychotics ranges from 20-40 hours which may be extended in elderly due to decline in oxidative hepatic reactions (phase I) with age.

Biologic effect of a single dose persists for 24 hours. When the patient has accommodated to initial side effects (sedation), once daily dosing is possible due to the long half-life of antipsychotics.

Steady-state plasma concentrations are achieved in 4-7 days; therefore, if possible, do not make dose adjustments more than once in a 7-day period. Due to the long half-lives of antipsychotics, as needed (prn) use is ineffective since repeated doses are necessary to achieve therapeutic tissue concentrations in the CNS.

Usual Dosage Oral:

Geriatrics (nonpsychotic patients, dementia behavior): Initial: 0.5-1 mg 1-2 times/day; increase dose at 4- to 7-day intervals by 0.5-1 mg/day; increase dosing intervals (bid, tid, etc) as necessary to control response or side effects; maximum daily dose: 40 mg; gradual increases (titration) may prevent some side effects or decrease their severity

I.M.: Initial: 1 mg every 4-6 hours; increase at 1 mg increments; do not exceed 6 mg/day

Adults:

Psychoses:

Outpatients: 1-2 mg twice daily

Hospitalized or well supervised patients: Initial dose: 2-5 mg twice daily with optimum response in the 15-20 mg/day range; do not exceed 40 mg/day

Anxiety: 1-2 mg twice daily; maximum: 6 mg/day; therapy for anxiety should not exceed 12 weeks

I.M.: 1-2 mg every 4-6 hours; do not exceed 6 mg/day

Not dialyzable (0% to 5%)

Monitoring Parameters Orthostatic blood pressures; tremors, gait changes, abnormal movement in trunk, neck, buccal area, or extremities; monitor target behaviors for which the agent is given

Test Interactions Increased cholesterol (S), increased glucose; decreased uric acid (S)

Patient Information Oral concentrate must be diluted in 2-4 oz of liquid (water, fruit juice, carbonated drinks, milk, or pudding); do not take antacid within 1 hour of taking drug; avoid alcohol; avoid excess sun exposure (use sun block); may cause drowsiness, rise slowly from recumbent position; use of supportive stockings may help prevent orthostatic hypotension

Nursing Implications Administer I.M. injection deep in upper outer quadrant of buttock; watch for hypotension when administering I.M. or I.V.; dilute the oral concentrate with water or juice before administration; avoid skin contact with oral solution; may cause contact dermatitis; monitor orthostatic blood pressures 3-5 days after initiation of therapy or a dose increase; observe for tremor and abnormal movement or posturing (extrapyramidal symptoms)

Additional Information Do not exceed 6 mg/day for longer than 12 weeks when treating anxiety; drug-induced agitation, jitteriness, or insomnia may be confused with original anxious or psychotic symptoms

Special Geriatric Considerations See Warnings. Elderly are more susceptible to hypotension and neuromuscular reactions.

Many elderly patients receive antipsychotic medications for inappropriate nonpsychotic behavior. Before initiating antipsychotic medication, the clinician should investigate any possible reversible cause; any stress or stress from any disease can cause acute "confusion" or worsening of baseline nonpsychotic behavior. Most commonly acute changes in behavior are due to increases in drug dose or addition of new drug to regimen; fluid electrolyte loss; infections; and changes in environment.

Any changes in disease status in any organ system can result in behavior changes

In the treatment of agitated, demented, elderly patients, authors of meta-analysis of controlled trials of the response to the traditional antipsychotics (phenothiazines, butyrophenones) in controlling agitation have concluded that the use of neuroleptics results in a response rate of 18%. Clearly neuroleptic therapy for behavior control should be limited with frequent attempts to withdraw the agent given for behavior control.

Dosage Forms

Trifluoperazine hydrochloride:

Concentrate, oral: 10 mg/mL (60 mL)

Injection: 2 mg/mL (10 mL)

Tablet: 1 mg, 2 mg, 5 mg, 10 mg

References

Peabody CA, Warner MD, Whiteford HA, et al, "Neuroleptics and the Elderly," *J Am Geriatr Soc*, 1987, 35(3):233-8.

Risse SC and Barnes R, "Pharmacologic Treatment of Agitation Associated With Dementia," *J Am Geriatr Soc*, 1986, 34(5):368-76.

Saltz BL, Woerner MG, Kane JM, et al, "Prospective Study of Tardive Dyskinesia Incidence in the Elderly," *JAMA*, 1991, 266(17):2402-6.

Seifert RD, "Therapeutic Drug Monitoring: Psychotropic Drugs," *J Pharm Pract*, 1984, 6:403-16.

Trifluorothymidine *see* Trifluridine *on next page*

Trifluridine (trye FLURE i deen)
Brand Names Viroptic® Ophthalmic
Synonyms F₃T; Trifluorothymidine
Generic Available No
Therapeutic Category Antiviral Agent, Ophthalmic
Use Treatment of primary keratoconjunctivitis and recurrent epithelial keratitis caused by herpes simplex virus types I and II
Contraindications Known hypersensitivity to trifluridine or any component
Warnings Mild local irritation of conjunctival and cornea may occur when instilled but usually transient effects
Adverse Reactions
Local: Burning, stinging
Ocular: Palpebral edema, epithelial keratopathy, keratitis, stromal edema, increased intraocular pressure
Miscellaneous: Hypersensitivity reactions, hyperemia
Stability Refrigerate at 2°C to 8°C (36°F to 46°F); storage at room temperature may result in a solution altered pH which could result in ocular discomfort upon administration and/or decreased potency
Mechanism of Action Interferes with viral replication by incorporating into viral DNA in place of thymidine, inhibiting thymidylate synthetase resulting in the formation of defective proteins
Pharmacokinetics Absorption: Ophthalmic instillation: Systemic absorption is negligible, while corneal penetration is adequate
Usual Dosage Geriatrics and Adults: Instill 1 drop into affected eye every 2 hours while awake, to a maximum of 9 drops/day, until re-epithelialization of corneal ulcer occurs; then use 1 drop every 4 hours for another 7 days; do **not** exceed 21 days of treatment; if improvement has not taken place in 7-14 days, consider another form of therapy
Monitoring Parameters Ophthalmologic exam (test for corneal staining with fluorescein or rose bengal)
Patient Information Notify physician if improvement is not seen after 7 days, condition worsens, or if irritation occurs; do not discontinue without notifying the physician, do not exceed recommended dosage
Special Geriatric Considerations Assess ability to self-administer
Dosage Forms Solution, ophthalmic: 1% (7.5 mL)

Trihexy® *see* Trihexyphenidyl *on this page*

Trihexyphenidyl (trye heks ee FEN i dil)
Brand Names Artane®; Trihexy®
Synonyms Benzhexol Hydrochloride
Generic Available Yes: Tablet
Therapeutic Category Anticholinergic Agent; Anti-Parkinson's Agent
Use Adjunctive treatment of Parkinson's disease; also used in treatment of drug-induced extrapyramidal effects and acute dystonic reactions
Contraindications Hypersensitivity to trihexyphenidyl or any component, patients with narrow-angle glaucoma; pyloric or duodenal obstruction, stenosing peptic ulcers; bladder neck obstructions; achalasia; myasthenia gravis
Precautions Use with caution in hot weather or during exercise. Elderly patients frequently develop increased sensitivity and require strict dosage regulation - side effects may be more severe in elderly patients with atherosclerotic changes. Use with caution in patients with tachycardia, cardiac arrhythmias, hypertension, hypotension, prostatic hypertrophy (especially in the elderly) or any tendency toward urinary retention, liver or kidney disorders and obstructive disease of the GI or GU tract. May exacerbate mental symptoms and precipitate a toxic psychosis when used to treat extrapyramidal reactions resulting from phenothiazines. When given in large doses or to susceptible patients, may cause weakness and inability to move particular muscle groups. Anticholinergic agents can aggravate tardive dyskinesia caused by neuroleptic agents.
Adverse Reactions
Cardiovascular: Tachycardia
Central nervous system: Drowsiness, nervousness, hallucinations, memory loss, coma (**the elderly may be at increased risk for confusion and hallucinations**)
Gastrointestinal: Nausea, vomiting, constipation, dryness of mouth
Genitourinary: Urinary hesitancy or retention
Ocular: Blurred vision, mydriasis

Miscellaneous: Heat intolerance

Overdosage Symptoms of overdose include CNS depression, confusion, nervousness, hallucinations, dizziness, blurred vision, nausea, vomiting, hyperthermia

Toxicology Anticholinergic toxicity is caused by strong binding of the drug to cholinergic receptors. Cholinesterase inhibitors reduce acetylcholinesterase, the enzyme that breaks down acetylcholine and thereby allows acetylcholine to accumulate and compete for receptor binding with the offending anticholinergic. For anticholinergic overdose with severe life-threatening symptoms, physostigmine 1-2 mg S.C. or I.V., slowly may be given to reverse these effects.

Drug Interactions

Decreased effect of levodopa (decreased absorption), metoclopramide, cisapride

Increased toxicity (central anticholinergic syndrome): Narcotic analgesics, phenothiazines, and other antipsychotics, tricyclic antidepressants, some antihistamines, quinidine, disopyramide

Antagonistic effect: Tacrine, donepezil

Mechanism of Action Thought to act by blocking excess acetylcholine at cerebral synapses; many of its effects are due to its pharmacologic similarities with atropine

Pharmacodynamics Peak effects: Within 60 minutes

Pharmacokinetics

Half-life: 5.6-10.2 hours

Time to peak serum concentrations: Oral: Within 60-90 minutes

Elimination: Primarily in urine

Usual Dosage Geriatrics and Adults:

Parkinsonism: 1 mg on first day, increase by 2 mg every 3-5 days as needed until a total of 6-10 mg/day (in 3-4 divided doses) is reached. If the patient is on concomitant levodopa therapy, the daily dose is reduced to 1-2 mg 3 times/day.

Drug-induced extrapyramidal reaction: 1 mg on first day, increase as needed; usual range: 5-15 mg/day in 3-4 divided doses

Monitoring Parameters Symptoms of EPS, Parkinson's, pulse, anticholinergic effects (ie, CNS, bowel and bladder function)

Patient Information Take after meals or with food if GI upset occurs; do not discontinue drug abruptly; notify physician if adverse GI effects, rapid or pounding heartbeat, confusion, eye pain, rash, fever or heat intolerance occurs. Observe caution when performing hazardous tasks or those that require alertness such as driving, as may cause drowsiness. Avoid alcohol and other CNS depressants. May cause dry mouth - adequate fluid intake or hard sugar-free candy may relieve. Difficult urination or constipation may occur - notify physician if effects persist; may increase susceptibility to heat stroke

Nursing Implications Tolerated best if given in 3 daily doses and with food; high doses may be divided into 4 doses, at meal times and at bedtime

Additional Information Incidence and severity of side effects are dose related; patients may be switched to sustained-action capsules when stabilized on conventional dosage forms

Special Geriatric Considerations Anticholinergic agents are generally not well tolerated in the elderly (confusion, constipation, urinary retention) and their use should be avoided when possible (see Precautions and Adverse Reactions). In the elderly, anticholinergic agents should not be used as prophylaxis against extrapyramidal symptoms.

Dosage Forms

Trihexyphenidyl hydrochloride:

Capsule, sustained release: 5 mg

Elixir: 2 mg/5 mL (480 mL)

Tablet: 2 mg, 5 mg

References

Feinberg M, "The Problems of Anticholinergic Adverse Effects in Older Patients," *Drugs Aging*, 1993, 3(4):335-48.

Trimeprazine (trye MEP ra zeen)

Related Information
Antacid Drug Interactions *on page 1096*

Brand Names Temaril®

Synonyms Alimenazine Tartrate; Trimeprazine Tartrate

Generic Available No

Therapeutic Category Antihistamine; Phenothiazine Derivative

Use Perennial and seasonal allergic rhinitis and other allergic symptoms including urticaria

Contraindications Hypersensitivity to trimeprazine or any component, narrow-angle glaucoma, bladder neck obstruction, symptomatic prostatic hypertrophy, asthmatic attacks, and stenosing peptic ulcer

Warnings Antihistamines are more likely to cause dizziness, excessive sedation, syncope, toxic confusion states, and hypotension in the elderly. Phenothiazine side effects (especially EPS) are more prone to develop in the elderly.

Precautions Use with caution in patients with cardiovascular disease, impaired liver function, asthma, sleep apnea, seizures, hypertensive crisis; avoid in patients with Reye's syndrome

Adverse Reactions
Cardiovascular: Postural hypotension

Central nervous system: Drowsiness, confusion, fatigue, excitation, extrapyramidal reactions with high doses

Dermatologic: Photosensitivity

Gastrointestinal: Xerostomia, constipation, increased appetite

Genitourinary: Urinary hesitancy or retention

Ocular: Blurred vision

Respiratory: Thickening of bronchial secretions

Overdosage Symptoms of overdose include deep sleep, coma, extrapyramidal symptoms, abnormal involuntary muscle movements, hypo- or hypertension

Toxicology Following initiation of essential overdose management, toxic symptom treatment and supportive treatment should be initiated. Hypotension usually responds to I.V. fluids or Trendelenburg positioning. If unresponsive to these measures the use of a parenteral vasopressor may be required (eg, norepinephrine 0.1-0.2 mcg/kg/minute titrated to response). Seizures commonly respond to diazepam (I.V. 5-10 mg bolus every 15 minutes if needed up to a total of 30 mg, I.V.) or to phenytoin or phenobarbital. Also critical cardiac arrhythmias often respond to I.V. phenytoin (15 mg/kg up to 1 g), while other antiarrhythmics can be used. Neuroleptics often cause extrapyramidal symptoms (eg, dystonic reactions) requiring management with diphenhydramine 1-2 mg/kg up to a maximum of 50 mg I.M. or I.V. slow push followed by a maintenance dose for 48-72 hours. When these reactions are unresponsive to diphenhydramine, benztropine mesylate I.V. 1-2 mg may be effective. These agents are generally effective within 2-5 minutes. Cholinesterase inhibitors including physostigmine, neostigmine, pyridostigmine, and edrophonium may be useful in treating life-threatening anticholinergic symptoms. Physostigmine 1-2 mg I.V., slowly may be given to reverse these effects.

Drug Interactions Increased effect/toxicity: CNS depressants, MAO inhibitors, alcohol

Mechanism of Action Blocks postsynaptic mesolimbic dopaminergic receptors in the brain; exhibits a strong alpha-adrenergic blocking effect and depresses the release of hypothalamic and hypophyseal hormones; competes with histamine for the H_1-receptor; reduces stimuli to the brainstem reticular system

Pharmacokinetics
Absorption: Well absorbed

Metabolism: Extensively hepatically metabolized largely to n-desalkyl metabolites

Bioavailability: Tablet: ~70%; the sustained release capsules give closely comparable serum and urinary levels

Half-life, elimination: 4.78 hours mean

Time to peak serum concentration:
Syrup: 3.5 hours
Tablet: 4.5 hours

Usual Dosage Oral:
Geriatrics: 2.5 mg twice daily
Adults: 2.5 mg 4 times/day (capsule: 5 mg every 12 hours)

Not dialyzable (0% to 5%)

Monitoring Parameters Relief of symptoms, mental status, blood pressure, EPS

Patient Information May cause drowsiness; avoid CNS depressants and alcohol

Additional Information Toxic manifestations normally appear between 4-10 weeks of therapy

Special Geriatric Considerations Because trimeprazine is a phenothiazine (and can, therefore, cause side effects such as extrapyramidal symptoms), it is not considered an antihistamine of choice in the elderly (see Warnings)

Dosage Forms
Capsule, extended release: 5 mg
Syrup: 2.5 mg/5 mL
Tablet: 2.5 mg

Trimeprazine Tartrate *see* Trimeprazine *on previous page*

Trimethobenzamide (trye meth oh BEN za mide)

Brand Names Arrestin®; Pediatric Triban®; Tebamide®; T-Gen®; Ticon®; Tigan®; Triban®; Trimazide®

Generic Available No

Therapeutic Category Antiemetic

Use Control of nausea and vomiting (especially for long-term antiemetic therapy)

Contraindications Hypersensitivity to trimethobenzamide, benzocaine, similar local analgesics, or any component

Precautions Use in patients with acute vomiting should be **avoided**; electrolyte imbalance, gastroenteritis, dehydration, encephalitis, and CNS side effects have occurred when used in acute febrile illness

Adverse Reactions
Cardiovascular: Hypotension (especially with I.M. administration), coma
Central nervous system: Drowsiness, sedation, EPS symptoms, dizziness, seizures, convulsions, depression, disorientation (confusion), headache
Gastrointestinal: Diarrhea
Hematologic: Blood dyscrasias
Hepatic: Jaundice
Neuromuscular & skeletal: Opisthotonos, muscle cramps
Ocular: Blurred vision
Miscellaneous: Hypersensitivity skin reactions

Overdosage Symptoms of overdose include hypotension, seizures, CNS depression

Toxicology Following initiation of essential overdose management, toxic symptom treatment and supportive treatment should be initiated. Hypotension usually responds to I.V. fluids or Trendelenburg positioning. If unresponsive to these measures, the use of a parenteral inotrope may be required (eg, norepinephrine 0.1-0.2 mcg/kg/minute titrated to response). Seizures commonly respond to diazepam (I.V. 5-10 mg bolus every 15 minutes if needed up to a total of 30 mg) or to phenytoin or phenobarbital. Also critical cardiac arrhythmias often respond to I.V. phenytoin (15 mg/kg up to 1 g), while other antiarrhythmics can be used. Neuroleptics often cause extrapyramidal symptoms (eg, dystonic reactions) requiring management with diphenhydramine 1-2 mg/kg up to a maximum of 50 mg I.M. or I.V. slow push followed by a maintenance dose for 48-72 hours. When these reactions are unresponsive to diphenhydramine, benztropine mesylate I.V. 1-2 mg may be effective. These agents are generally effective within 2-5 minutes.

Stability Store injection at room temperature; protect from heat and from freezing; use only clear solutions

Mechanism of Action Acts centrally to inhibit the medullary chemoreceptor trigger zone; direct impulses to the vomiting center are not inhibited

Pharmacodynamics
Onset of antiemetic effects:
Oral: Within 10-40 minutes
I.M.: Within 15-35 minutes
Duration of action: Effects can persist for 3-4 hours

Usual Dosage Geriatrics and Adults:
Oral: 250 mg 3-4 times/day
I.M., rectal: 200 mg 3-4 times/day

Monitoring Parameters See Adverse Reactions

Patient Information May cause drowsiness

Nursing Implications Use only clear solution

(Continued)

Trimethobenzamide *(Continued)*

Additional Information Note: Less effective than phenothiazines but may be associated with fewer side effects; rectal is ~60% absorbed

Special Geriatric Considerations No specific data for use in elderly have been established; as with any drug which has EPS adverse effects and possibility of confusion, caution should be used when administering to elderly (see Adverse Reactions)

Dosage Forms

Trimethobenzamide hydrochloride:
Capsule: 100 mg, 250 mg
Injection: hydrochloride: 100 mg/mL (2 mL, 20 mL)
Suppository, rectal: 100 mg, 200 mg

Trimethoprim *(trye METH oh prim)*

Brand Names Proloprim®; Trimpex®

Synonyms TMP

Therapeutic Category Antibiotic, Miscellaneous

Use Treatment of uncomplicated urinary tract infections due to susceptible organisms (*Escherichia coli, Proteus mirabilis, Klebsiella pneumoniae, Enterobacter* sp, and coagulase-negative *Staphylococcus* sp); acute exacerbations of chronic bronchitis

Contraindications Hypersensitivity to trimethoprim or any component, megaloblastic anemia due to folate deficiency

Precautions Use with caution in patients with impaired renal or hepatic function or with possible folate deficiency

Adverse Reactions

Central nervous system: Fever
Dermatologic: Rash (3% to 7%), pruritus, exfoliative dermatitis
Gastrointestinal: Nausea, vomiting, epigastric distress
Hematologic: Thrombocytopenia, neutropenia, leukopenia, megaloblastic anemia
Hepatic: Increased LFTS, cholestatic jaundice
Renal: Increased BUN and serum creatinine

Overdosage Symptoms of overdose include bone marrow suppression, nausea, vomiting, confusion, dizziness

Toxicology

Acute toxicity: Gastric lavage and supportive measures; acidification of urine increases renal elimination; hemodialysis is moderately effective
Chronic toxicity: Stop drug; administer leucovorin 3-6 mg I.M. daily or 5-15 mg/day orally for 3 days or until normal hematopoiesis resumes

Drug Interactions Phenytoin increased serum concentration

Mechanism of Action Inhibits folic acid reduction to tetrahydrofolate, and thereby inhibits microbial growth

Pharmacokinetics

Absorption: Oral: Readily and extensively
Protein binding: 42% to 46%
Metabolism: Partially in the liver
Half-life: 8-14 hours, prolonged with renal impairment
Time to peak serum concentration: Within 1-4 hours
Elimination: Significantly in urine (60% to 80% as unchanged drug); in elderly, the area under the curve and peak concentration have been reported to be greater compared to younger subjects

Usual Dosage Geriatrics and Adults: Oral: 100 mg every 12 hours or 200 mg every 24 hours for 10 days; longer treatment periods may be necessary for prostatitis (ie, 4-16 weeks)

Dosing interval in renal impairment:
Cl_{cr} 15-30 mL/minute: Administer 50 mg every 12 hours
Cl_{cr} <15 mL/minute: Not recommended
Moderately dialyzable (20% to 50%)

Monitoring Parameters Obtain culture and sensitivity results; repeat after treatment has concluded

Reference Range Therapeutic: Peak: 5-15 mg/L; Trough: 2-8 mg/L

Patient Information Complete full course of treatment; notify physician if sore throat, bleeding, or fever develops

Nursing Implications Watch for signs of bone marrow suppression such as fever, sore throat, or bleeding; tablets can be crushed

Special Geriatric Considerations Trimethoprim is often used in combination with sulfamethoxazole; it can be used alone in patients who are allergic to sulfonamides; adjust dose for renal function (see Pharmacokinetics and Usual Dosage).

Dosage Forms Tablet: 100 mg, 200 mg

References

Varoquaux O, Lajoie D, Gobert C, et al, "Pharmacokinetics of the Trimethoprim-Sulfamethoxazole Combination in the Elderly," *Br J Clin Pharmacol*, 1985, 20:575-81.

Trimethoprim and Sulfamethoxazole *see Co-Trimoxazole on page 253*

Trimetrexate Glucuronate

(tri me TREKS ate gloo KYOOR oh nate)

Brand Names Neutrexin™ Injection

Therapeutic Category Antibiotic, Miscellaneous

Use Alternative therapy for the treatment of moderate-to-severe *Pneumocystis carinii* pneumonia (PCP) in immunocompromised patients, including patients with acquired immunodeficiency syndrome (AIDS), who are intolerant of, or are refractory to, co-trimoxazole therapy or for whom co-trimoxazole is contraindicated

Contraindications Previous hypersensitivity to trimetrexate or methotrexate, severe existing myelosuppression

Warnings Must be administered with concurrent leucovorin to avoid potentially serious or life-threatening toxicities; leucovorin therapy must extend for 72 hours past the last dose of trimetrexate; use with caution in patients with mild myelosuppression, severe hepatic or renal dysfunction, hypoproteinemia, hypoalbuminemia, or previous extensive myelosuppressive therapies

Adverse Reactions

Central nervous system: Seizures, fever

Dermatologic: Rash

Gastrointestinal: Stomatitis, nausea, vomiting

Hematologic: Neutropenia, thrombocytopenia, anemia

Hepatic: Elevated liver function tests

Neuromuscular & skeletal: Peripheral neuropathy

Renal: Increased serum creatinine

Miscellaneous: Flu-like illness, hypersensitivity reactions

Drug Interactions

Decreased effect of pneumococcal vaccine

Increased toxicity (infection rates) of yellow fever vaccine

Stability Reconstituted I.V. solution is stable for 24 hours at room temperature or 7 days when refrigerated; intact vials should be refrigerated at 2°C to 8°C

Mechanism of Action Exerts an antimicrobial effect through potent inhibition of the enzyme dihydrofolate reductase (DHFR)

Pharmacokinetics

Distribution: V_d: 0.62 L/kg

Metabolism: Extensive in the liver

Half-life: 15-17 hours

Usual Dosage Geriatrics and Adults: I.V.: 45 mg/m² once daily over 60 minutes for 21 days; it is necessary to reduce the dose in patients with liver dysfunction, although no specific recommendations exist

Administration Reconstituted solution should be filtered (0.22 µM) prior to further dilution; final solution should be clear, hue will range from colorless to pale yellow; trimetrexate forms a precipitate instantly upon contact with chloride ion or leucovorin, therefore it should not be added to solutions containing sodium chloride or other anions; trimetrexate and leucovorin solutions **must** be administered separately; intravenous lines should be flushed with at least 10 mL of D_5W between trimetrexate and leucovorin

Monitoring Parameters Check and record patient's temperature daily

Laboratory tests:

Hematology, CBC with differential (absolute neutrophil counts (ANC)), platelets

Renal functions (serum creatinine, BUN)

Hepatic function (ALT, AST, alkaline phosphatase)

Patient Information Report promptly any fever, rash, flu-like symptoms, numbness or tingling in the extremities, nausea, vomiting, abdominal pain, mouth sores, increased bruising or bleeding, black tarry stools

Nursing Implications Notify primary physician if there is:

Fever ≥103°F

Generalized rash

Seizures

Bleeding from any site

Uncontrolled nausea/vomiting

Laboratory abnormalities which warrant dose modification

(Continued)

Trimetrexate Glucuronate *(Continued)*

Any other clinical adverse event or laboratory abnormality occurring in therapy which is judged as serious for that patient or which causes unexplained effects or concern

Initiate "Bleeding Precautions" for platelet counts ≤50,000/mm³

Initiate "Infection Control Measures" for absolute neutrophil counts (ANC) ≤1000/mm³

Additional Information Not a vesicant; methotrexate derivative

Special Geriatric Considerations No specific recommendations are available for the elderly; use with caution in patients with liver dysfunction (see Usual Dosage)

Dosage Forms Powder for injection: 25 mg

Trimipramine (trye MI pra meen)
Related Information
Antidepressant Agents Comparison *on page 1021*
Antidepressant Medication Guidelines *on page 1075*
Federal OBRA Regulations Recommended Maximum Doses - Antidepressants *on page 1056*

Brand Names Surmontil®

Therapeutic Category Antidepressant, Tricyclic

Use Treatment of various forms of depression, often in conjunction with psychotherapy

Unlabeled use: Peptic ulcer disease, chronic urticaria, angioedema, and nocturnal pruritus

Contraindications Narrow-angle glaucoma

Warnings To avoid cholinergic crisis do not discontinue abruptly in patients receiving long-term high dose therapy; some oral preparations contain tartrazine and injection contains sulfites both of which can cause allergic reactions

Precautions Use with caution in patients with cardiovascular disease, conduction disturbances, seizure disorders, urinary retention, hyperthyroidism or those receiving thyroid replacement; an EKG prior to the start of therapy is advised

Adverse Reactions
Cardiovascular: Postural hypotension, arrhythmias, tachycardia, sudden death
Central nervous system: Sedation, fatigue, insomnia, anxiety, impaired cognitive function, seizures have occurred occasionally, dizziness, headache
Gastrointestinal: Xerostomia, constipation, increased appetite, dysgeusia
Genitourinary: Urinary retention
Hematologic: Agranulocytosis, eosinophilia, may cause alterations in bleeding time
Hepatic: Jaundice
Neuromuscular & skeletal: Tremors, weakness
Ocular: Blurred vision, increased intraocular pressure
Miscellaneous: Allergic reactions

Overdosage Symptoms of overdose include agitation, confusion, hallucinations, urinary retention, hypothermia, hypotension, tachycardia

Toxicology Following initiation of essential overdose management, toxic symptoms should be treated. Ventricular arrhythmias often respond to phenytoin 15-20 mg/kg with concurrent systemic alkalinization (sodium bicarbonate 0.5-2 mEq/kg I.V.). Arrhythmias unresponsive to this therapy may respond to lidocaine 1 mg/kg I.V. followed by a titrated infusion. Physostigmine (1-2 mg I.V. slowly) may be indicated in reversing cardiac arrhythmias that are due to vagal blockade or for anticholinergic effects. Seizures usually respond to diazepam I.V. boluses (5-10 mg, up to 30 mg). If seizures are unresponsive or recur, phenytoin or phenobarbital may be required.

Drug Interactions
May decrease or reverse effects of guanethidine and clonidine
May increase effects of CNS depressants, adrenergic agents, anticholinergic agents
With MAO inhibitors, hyperpyrexia, tachycardia, hypertension, seizures and death may occur; similar interactions as with other tricyclics may occur

Stability Solutions stable at a pH of 4-5; turns yellowish or reddish on exposure to light. Slight discoloration does not affect potency; marked discoloration is associated with loss of potency. Capsules stable for 3 years following date of manufacture.

Mechanism of Action Traditionally believed to increase the synaptic concentration of serotonin and/or norepinephrine in the central nervous system by inhibition of their reuptake by the presynaptic neuronal membrane. However, additional receptor effects have been found including desensitization of adenyl cyclase, down regulation of beta-adrenergic receptors, and down regulation of serotonin receptors.

Pharmacodynamics Onset of therapeutic effects: May take 1-3 weeks to appear; serotonin greater than norepinephrine

Pharmacokinetics
Protein binding: 95%
Metabolism: Undergoes significant first-pass metabolism metabolized in the liver; substrate CYP2D6
Half-life: 20-26 hours
Time to peak: Oral: Therapeutic plasma concentrations occur within 6 hours
Elimination: In urine

Usual Dosage Oral:
Geriatrics: Initial: 25 mg at bedtime, increase by 25 mg/day every 3 days for inpatients and weekly for outpatients, as tolerated, to a maximum of 100 mg/day
Adults: 50 mg/day as a single bedtime dose; maximum dose: 200 mg/day outpatients; 300 mg/day inpatients

Chronic urticaria, angioedema, nocturnal pruritus: 50 mg/day

Monitoring Parameters Blood pressure, pulse, target symptoms

Test Interactions Elevated glucose

Patient Information To prevent dizziness, avoid abrupt changes of position, may cause dry mouth, dizziness, blurred vision, constipation, sedation

Nursing Implications Monitor sitting and standing blood pressure and pulse

Additional Information May cause alterations in bleeding time

Special Geriatric Considerations Similar to doxepin in its side effect profile; has not been well studied in the elderly; very anticholinergic and, therefore, not considered a drug of first choice in the elderly when selecting an antidepressant. Data from a clinical trial comparing fluoxetine to tricyclics suggest that fluoxetine is significantly less effective than nortriptyline in hospitalized elderly patients with unipolar major affective disorder, especially those with melancholia and concurrent cardiovascular diseases.

Dosage Forms Capsule, as maleate: 25 mg, 50 mg, 100 mg

References
Roose SP, Glassman AH, Attia E, et al, "Comparative Efficacy of Selective Serotonin Reuptake Inhibitors and Tricyclics in the Treatment of Melancholia," *Am J Psychiatry*, 1994, 151(12):1735-9.

Trimox® see Amoxicillin on page 67

Trimpex® see Trimethoprim on page 962

Triofed® Syrup [OTC] see Triprolidine and Pseudoephedrine on next page

Triostat™ Injection see Liothyronine on page 539

Tripelennamine (tri pel EN a meen)

Brand Names PBZ®; PBZ-SR®

Generic Available No

Therapeutic Category Antihistamine, H₁ Blocker

Use Perennial and seasonal allergic rhinitis and other allergic symptoms including urticaria, vasomotor rhinitis, allergic conjunctivitis, angioedema, allergic reactions to administration of blood in blood products, dermographism, adjunctive therapy in anaphylaxis therapy

Contraindications Hypersensitivity to tripelennamine or any component

Warnings Use with caution in patients with narrow-angle glaucoma, bladder neck obstruction, symptomatic prostate hypertrophy, sleep apnea, asthmatic attacks, and stenosing peptic ulcer

Precautions Tripelennamine has less anticholinergic action than many antihistamines. However, elderly are susceptible to anticholinergic action and should be used cautiously in patients predisposed to constipation, urinary retention, history of asthma, hyperthyroidism, hypertension, increased ocular pressure, and cardiovascular disease. Antihistamines cause, initially, drowsiness and put patients at risk when operating hazardous machinery or driving; photosensitivity may occur.

Adverse Reactions
Cardiovascular: Edema, palpitations, hypotension, bradycardia, tachycardia, extrasystoles
Central nervous system: Slight to moderate drowsiness, headache, fatigue, nervousness, restlessness, dizziness, depression, sedation, lassitude,
(Continued)

Tripelennamine *(Continued)*

paradoxical excitement, insomnia, confusion, seizures, euphoria, hallucinations, disorientation, disturbing dreams, vertigo

Dermatologic: Angioedema, photosensitivity, rash

Gastrointestinal: Appetite increase, weight gain, nausea, diarrhea, abdominal pain, xerostomia, dry mouth

Genitourinary: Urinary retention, urinary frequency

Hematologic: Thrombocytopenia, agranulocytosis, pancytopenia, hemolytic anemia

Hepatic: Hepatitis

Neuromuscular & skeletal: Arthralgia, myalgia, paresthesia, tremor

Ocular: Blurred vision

Otic: Tinnitus

Respiratory: Thickening of bronchial secretions, pharyngitis, wheezing, bronchospasm, epistaxis

Overdosage Symptoms of overdose include CNS stimulation or depression; flushed skin, mydriasis, ataxia, athetosis, dry mouth

Toxicology There is no specific treatment for an antihistamine overdose, however, most of its clinical toxicity is due to anticholinergic effects. For anticholinergic overdose with severe life-threatening symptoms, physostigmine 1-2 mg (0.5 or 0.02 mg/kg for children) I.V., slowly may be given to reverse these effects.

Drug Interactions Increased effect/toxicity with alcohol, CNS depressants, MAO inhibitors

Mechanism of Action Competes with histamine for H_1-receptor sites on effector cells in the gastrointestinal tract, blood vessels, and respiratory tract

Pharmacodynamics

Onset of antihistaminic effect: Within 15-30 minutes

Duration: 4-6 hours (up to 8 hours with PBZ-SR®)

Pharmacokinetics

Metabolism: Almost completely in the liver

Elimination: In urine

Usual Dosage Geriatrics and Adults: Oral: 25-50 mg every 4-6 hours, extended release tablets 100 mg morning and evening up to 100 mg every 8 hours (see Special Geriatric Considerations)

Monitoring Parameters Monitor for control of allergy symptoms and observe for sedation, confusion, urinary retention, constipation

Patient Information Swallow whole, do not crush or chew extended release tablets; urinary hesitancy can be reduced if patient voids just prior to taking drug; may cause drowsiness; avoid alcohol, may impair coordination and judgment

Nursing Implications Raise bed rails, institute safety measures, assist with ambulation

Special Geriatric Considerations Elderly are more likely to experience dizziness, syncope, confusion, hypotension, sedation, and paradoxical excitation than younger adults. Anticholinergic effects may cause constipation, urinary retention, and confusion. However, tripelennamine has lower anticholinergic effects than most antihistamines with the exception of second generation antihistamines.

Dosage Forms

Tripelennamine hydrochloride:

Tablet: 25 mg, 50 mg

Tablet, extended release: 100 mg

References

Monforte JR, Gault R, Smialek J, et al, "Toxicological and Pathological Findings in Fatalities Involving Pentazocine and Tripelennamine," *J Forensic Sci*, 1983, 28(1):90-101.

Yeh SY, Todd GD, Johnson RE, et al, "The Pharmacokinetics of Pentazocine and Tripelennamine," *Clin Pharmacol Ther*, 1986, 39(6):669-76.

Triposed® Syrup [OTC] *see* Triprolidine and Pseudoephedrine *on this page*

Triposed® Tablet [OTC] *see* Triprolidine and Pseudoephedrine *on this page*

Triprolidine and Pseudoephedrine

(trye PROE li deen & soo doe e FED rin)

Related Information

Pseudoephedrine *on page 802*

Brand Names Actagen® Syrup [OTC]; Actagen® Tablet [OTC]; Allercon® Tablet [OTC]; Allerfrin® Syrup [OTC]; Allerfrin® Tablet [OTC]; Allerphed Syrup [OTC]; Aprodine® Syrup [OTC]; Aprodine® Tablet [OTC]; Cenafed® Plus

Tablet [OTC]; Genac® Tablet [OTC]; Silafed® Syrup [OTC]; Triofed® Syrup [OTC]; Triposed® Syrup [OTC]; Triposed® Tablet [OTC]

Synonyms Pseudoephedrine and Triprolidine

Generic Available Yes

Therapeutic Category Antihistamine/Decongestant Combination

Use Temporary relief of nasal congestion, running nose, sneezing, itching of nose or throat and itchy, watery eyes due to common cold, hay fever or other upper respiratory allergies

Contraindications Narrow-angle glaucoma, bladder neck obstruction, asthmatic attacks, stenosing peptic ulcer, MAO inhibitor therapy, hypertension, coronary artery disease, hypersensitivity to pseudoephedrine, triprolidine or any component

Precautions Use with caution in patients with high blood pressure, heart disease, diabetes, asthma, thyroid disease, or prostatic hypertrophy

Adverse Reactions

Cardiovascular: Tachycardia, palpitations, arrhythmias

Central nervous system: Nervousness, excitability, dizziness, insomnia, drowsiness, headache

Gastrointestinal: Nausea, vomiting, xerostomia

Genitourinary: Dysuria

Neuromuscular & skeletal: Tremors

Respiratory: Thickening of bronchial secretions

Overdosage Symptoms of overdose include hallucinations, CNS depression, seizures, death

Toxicology

There is no specific antidote for pseudoephedrine intoxication and the bulk of the treatment is supportive

Hyperactivity and agitation usually respond to reduced sensory input, however with extreme agitation haloperidol (2-5 mg I.M. for adults) may be required

Hyperthermia is best treated with external cooling measures, or when severe or unresponsive, muscle paralysis with pancuronium may be needed

Hypertension is usually transient and generally does not require treatment unless severe. For diastolic blood pressures >110 mm Hg, a nitroprusside infusion should be initiated.

Seizures usually respond to diazepam I.V. and/or phenytoin maintenance regimens

Drug Interactions

Decreased effect: Beta-blockers, methyldopa

Increased toxicity/effect: Tricyclic antidepressants, MAO inhibitors (increased blood pressure), sympathomimetics

Usual Dosage Geriatrics and Adults:

Capsule, extended release: 1 capsule every 12 hours

Syrup: 10 mL

Tablet: 1 tablet 3-4 times/day; maximum: 4 tablets/day

Monitoring Parameters Relief of symptoms, blood pressure, pulse

Test Interactions Increased amylase, increased lipase

Patient Information Do not exceed recommended dosage; do not crush or chew extended release capsule

Nursing Implications Do not crush extended release capsule

Special Geriatric Considerations Use with caution in patients with cardiovascular disease; the anticholinergic action of triprolidine may cause confusion, constipation, or urinary retention in elderly (see Contraindications and Precautions); also see Pseudoephedrine monograph

Dosage Forms

Capsule: Triprolidine hydrochloride 2.5 mg and pseudoephedrine hydrochloride 60 mg

Capsule, extended release: Triprolidine hydrochloride 5 mg and pseudoephedrine hydrochloride 120 mg

Syrup: Triprolidine hydrochloride 1.25 mg and pseudoephedrine hydrochloride 30 mg per 5 mL

Tablet: Triprolidine hydrochloride 2.5 mg and pseudoephedrine hydrochloride 60 mg

TripTone® Caplets® [OTC] see Dimenhydrinate on page 300

Tri-Statin® II Topical see Nystatin and Triamcinolone on page 687

Tristoject® see Triamcinolone on page 949

Trocal® [OTC] see Dextromethorphan on page 278

Troglitazone (TROE gli to zone)

Brand Names Rezulin®

Therapeutic Category Antidiabetic Agent; Antihyperglycemic Agent; Hypoglycemic Agent, Oral

Use Type 2 diabetes: For use in patients with type 2 diabetes currently on insulin therapy whose hyperglycemia is inadequately controlled (Hb A_{1c} >8.5%) despite insulin therapy >30 units/day given as multiple injections; either monotherapy or combination therapy with sulfonylureas as an adjunct to diet and exercise

Contraindications Hypersensitivity to troglitazone or any component

Warnings Patients with New York Heart Association (NYHA) Class III and IV cardiac status were not studied during clinical trials. Heart enlargement without microscopic changes has been observed in rodents at exposures exceeding 14 times the AUC of the 400 mg human dose. Caution is advised during the administration of troglitazone to patients with NYHA Class III or IV cardiac status.

During all clinical studies, a total of 20 troglitazone-treated patients were withdrawn from treatment because of liver function test abnormalities. Two of the 20 patients developed reversible jaundice. Both had liver biopsies that were consistent with an idiosyncratic drug reaction.

Patients on troglitazone who develop jaundice or whose laboratory results indicate liver injury should stop taking the drug. Approximately 2% of patients can expect to stop taking the drug because of elevated liver enzymes.

Because of its mechanism of action, troglitazone is active only in the presence of insulin. Therefore, do not use in type 1 diabetes or for the treatment of diabetic ketoacidosis.

Patients receiving troglitazone in combination with insulin may be at risk for hypoglycemia, and a reduction in the dose of insulin may be necessary. Hypoglycemia has not been observed during the administration of troglitazone as monotherapy and would not be expected based on the mechanism of action.

Across all clinical studies, hemoglobin declined by 3% to 4% in troglitazone-treated patients compared with 1% to 2% with placebo. White blood cell counts also declined slightly in troglitazone-treated patients compared with those treated with placebo. These changes occurred within the first 4-8 weeks of therapy. Serum concentrations stabilized and remained unchanged for ≤ 2 years of continuing therapy. These changes may be due to the dilutional effects of increased plasma volume and have not been associated with any significant hematologic clinical effects.

Adverse Reactions

Cardiovascular: Peripheral edema

Central nervous system: Headache, pain, dizziness

Gastrointestinal: Nausea, diarrhea, pharyngitis

Genitourinary: Urinary tract infection

Hepatic: Mild, reversible increases in aminotransferase enzymes, jaundice

Neuromuscular & skeletal: Neck pain, weakness

Respiratory: Rhinitis

Miscellaneous: Infection

Drug Interactions Cytochrome P-4503A4 enzyme inducer

Decreased effects: Cholestyramine: Concomitant administration of cholestyramine with troglitazone reduces the absorption of troglitazone by 70%; **co-administration of cholestyramine and troglitazone is not recommended**

Increased toxicity: Sulfonylureas (glyburide): Co-administration of troglitazone with glyburide may further decrease plasma glucose concentration

Mechanism of Action Thiazolidinedione antidiabetic agent that lowers blood glucose by improving target cell response to insulin, without increasing pancreatic insulin secretion. It has a unique mechanism of action that is dependent on the presence of insulin for activity. Troglitazone decreases hepatic glucose output and increases insulin-dependent glucose disposal in skeletal muscle and possible liver and adipose tissue.

Pharmacokinetics

Absorption: Food increases absorption by 30% to 85%

Distribution: V_d: 10.5-26.5 L/kg

Protein binding: >99% to serum albumin

Metabolism: Extensive; troglitazone does induce cytochrome P-4503A4 metabolism; the inhibitory effect on P-450 isozymes (especially 3A4, 2C9, and 2C19) is believed to not be clinically important and associated with troglitazone concentrations of 11 mcg/mL. **Note:** Serum concentrations of 1-3 mcg/mL are obtained at 600 mg/day of troglitazone (ie, the maximum adult dosage).

Bioavailability: Absolute

Half-life, plasma elimination: 16-34 hours

Time to peak plasma concentrations: 2-3 hours

Elimination: 85% in feces and 3% in urine

Usual Dosage Geriatrics and Adults: Oral (take with meals):

Continue the current insulin dose upon initiation of troglitazone therapy.

Initiate therapy at 200 mg once daily in patients on insulin therapy. For patients not responding adequately, increase the dose after 2-4 weeks. The usual dose is 400 mg/day; maximum recommended dose: 600 mg/day.

It is recommended that the insulin dose be decreased by 10% to 25% when fasting plasma glucose concentrations decrease to <120 mg/dL in patients receiving concomitant insulin and troglitazone. Individualize further adjustments based on glucose-lowering response.

As monotherapy: Initial: 400 or 600 mg once daily; increase to 600 mg/day if inadequate response to 400 mg/day after 6-8 weeks; for patients with inadequate response to 600 mg/day, alternative therapeutic options should be pursued

In combination with sulfonylureas: Initiate troglitazone at 200 mg once daily; continue sulfonylurea at its current dose; the dose of troglitazone can be increased by 200 mg every 2-4 weeks to a maximum of 600 mg/day

Dosing adjustment/comments in renal impairment: Dose adjustment is not necessary

Dosing adjustment in hepatic impairment: Use with caution in patients with hepatic disease

Monitoring Parameters Fasting blood glucose, hemoglobin A_{1c}, and fructosamine. Serum transaminase levels should be checked routinely within the first 1-2 months of therapy, then every 3 months during the first year of treatment, and periodically thereafter. Additionally, liver function tests should be performed on any patient on troglitazone who develops symptoms of liver dysfunction, such as nausea, vomiting, abdominal pain, fatigue, loss of appetite, or dark urine.

Reference Range Target range: Adults:

Fasting blood glucose: 100-150 mg/dL

Glycosylated hemoglobin: <7%

Patient Information

Notify physician if symptoms of liver dysfunction such as nausea, vomiting, abdominal pain, fatigue, loss of appetite, or dark urine occur

Take troglitazone with meals. If the dose is missed at the usual meal, take it at the next meal. If the dose is missed on one day, do not double the dose the following day.

It is important to adhere to dietary instructions and to have blood glucose and glycosylated hemoglobin tested regularly. During periods of stress such as fever, trauma, infection or surgery, insulin requirements may change and patients should seek the advice of their physician.

When using combination therapy with insulin, explain the risks of hypoglycemia, its symptoms, treatment and predisposing conditions to patients and their family members.

Nursing Implications Patients who are NPO may need to have their dose held to avoid hypoglycemia

Special Geriatric Considerations Steady-state pharmacokinetics of troglitazone and metabolites in healthy elderly subjects were comparable to those seen in young adults (see Usual Dosage)

Dosage Forms Tablet: 200 mg, 300 mg, 400 mg

Trovafloxacin/Alatrofloxacin

(TROE va flox a sin/a lat roe FLOX a sin)

Related Information

Antacid Drug Interactions *on page 1096*

Brand Names Trovan™

Synonyms Alatrofloxacin/Trovafloxacin

Generic Available No

Therapeutic Category Antibiotic, Quinolone

Use Treatment of nosocomial pneumoniae; community-acquired pneumoniae; acute bacterial exacerbation of chronic bronchitis; acute bacterial sinusitis; complicated intra-abdominal infections, including postsurgical infections; gynecological and pelvic infections; prophylaxis of infection associated with (Continued)

Trovafloxacin/Alatrofloxacin *(Continued)*

elective colorectal surgery, vaginal and abdominal hysterectomy; complicated and uncomplicated skin and skin structure infections, uncomplicated UTI caused by *E. coli*; chronic bacterial prostatitis caused by *E. coli*, *E. faecalis*, or *S. epidermidis*; uncomplicated urethral gonorrhea in men and endocervical and rectal gonorrhea in women; cervicitis due to *C. trachomatis*; pelvic inflammatory disease caused by *N. gonorrhoeae* or *C. trachomatis*. Trovafloxacin has demonstrated activity against *E. coli*, *P. aeruginosa*, *H. influenzae*, *S. aureus*, *K. pneumoniae*, *H. parainfluenzae*, *B. fragilis*, viridans group streptococci, *Peptostreptococcus* sp or *Prevotella* sp, *E. faecalis*, *S. agalactiae*, *G. vaginalis*, *S. pyogenes*, *P. mirabilis*, *S. epidermidis*, *N. gonorrhoeae*, and *C. trachomatis*.

Contraindications History of hypersensitivity to trovafloxacin, alatrofloxacin, quinolone antimicrobial agents, or any other components of these products

Warnings May alter GI flora resulting in pseudomembranous colitis due to *Clostridium difficile*; use with caution in patients with seizure disorders or severe cerebral atherosclerosis; discontinue if skin rash or pain, inflammation, or rupture of a tendon occurs; photosensitivity; CNS stimulation may occur which may lead to tremor, restlessness, confusion, hallucinations, paranoia, depression, nightmares, insomnia, or lightheadedness

Adverse Reactions
Central nervous system: Dizziness, lightheadedness, headache
Dermatologic: Rash, pruritus
Gastrointestinal: Nausea, vomiting, diarrhea, abdominal pain
Genitourinary: Vaginitis
Hepatic: Increased liver function tests
Local: Injection site reaction, pain or inflammation

Drug Interactions Oral bioavailability decreased when given with aluminum- or magnesium-containing antacids, sucralfate, iron, concomitant intravenous morphine, calcium carbonate, and omeprazole; increases caffeine serum concentrations

Stability I.V. alatrofloxacin, when diluted, is physically and chemically stable for up to 7 days when refrigerated or up to 3 days at room temperature stored in glass or PVC-type plastic containers

Mechanism of Action Inhibition of DNA gyrase and topoisomerase IV; bactericidal

Pharmacokinetics
Distribution: Concentration in most tissues greater than plasma or serum
Protein binding: 76%
Metabolism: Hepatic conjugation
Bioavailability: 88%
Half-life: 9-12 hours
Elimination: 50% excreted unchanged (43% feces, 6% urine)
Pharmacokinetics unaffected by age

Usual Dosage Geriatrics and Adults:
Oral: 100-200 mg/day; total duration of therapy and dose depend on indication
I.V. (alatrofloxacin): 300 mg followed by 200 mg/day
  Dosing adjustment in renal impairment: No adjustment needed
  Dosing adjustment in mild/moderate cirrhosis:
    I.V.: In normal hepatic function, dose is 300 mg; in chronic hepatic disease, adjust dose to 200 mg
    Oral or I.V.: In normal hepatic function, dose is 200 mg; in chronic hepatic disease, adjust dose to 100 mg
  Dosing adjustment in severe cirrhosis: No dosing guidelines

Monitoring Parameters Signs and symptoms of infection; mental status

Patient Information Take without regard to meals; take at least 2 hours before or after taking tablet formulation; may cause lightheadedness and/or dizziness which may be minimized by taking at bedtime or with food; discontinue and contact physician if you experience musculoskeletal pains or rash; avoid excessive sunlight or artificial ultraviolet light; complete entire course of treatment

Nursing Implications I.V. formulation should be infused over 60 minutes by direct infusion or through a Y-type infusion set. If I.V. line is to be used for administering other medications, flush line before and after infusion of alatrofloxacin with compatible solution. Oral form may be given without regard to meals. Separate administration of tablets from antacids, iron, magnesium-, or aluminum-containing products by at least 2 hours. I.V. morphine should be given ≥2 hours after oral trovafloxacin when taken in the fasting state and ≥4 hours when taken with food.

Additional Information For more information on trovafloxacin, see package insert from Pfizer, 1998

Special Geriatric Considerations No dose adjustment for age or renal function. According to the manufacturer, trovafloxacin was well tolerated by patients ≥65 years of age in clinical trials; see Usual Dosage.

Dosage Forms

Injection, as mesylate (alatrofloxacin): 5 mg/mL (40 mL, 60 mL)

Tablet, as mesylate (trovafloxacin): 100 mg, 200 mg

References

Haria M and Lamb HA, "Trovafloxacin," *Drugs*, 1997, 54(3):435-45.

Trovan™ *see* Trovafloxacin/Alatrofloxacin *on page 969*

Truphylline® *see* Aminophylline *on page 55*

Trusopt® *see* Dorzolamide *on page 318*

Trypsin, Balsam Peru, and Castor Oil

(TRIP sin, BAL sam pe RUE , & KAS tor oyl)

Brand Names Granulex

Generic Available Yes

Therapeutic Category Protectant, Topical; Topical Skin Product

Use Treatment of decubitus ulcers, varicose ulcers, debridement of eschar, dehiscent wounds and sunburn

Warnings Do not spray on fresh arterial clots; avoid contact with eyes

Adverse Reactions Local: Itching or stinging may be associated with initial application

Mechanism of Action Trypsin is an enzymatic debriding agent. Peruvian balsam is a capillary bed stimulant and may have mild bactericidal action. Castor oil may improve epithelialization and act as a protective barrier.

Usual Dosage Geriatrics and Adults: Apply a minimum of twice daily or as often as necessary

Monitoring Parameters Size of the ulcer, skin integrity

Patient Information Avoid contact with eyes; for external use only; shake well before spraying

Nursing Implications Clean wound prior to application and at each redressing; shake well before spraying; hold can upright ~12" from area to be treated

Special Geriatric Considerations Preventive skin care should be instituted in all older patients at high risk for decubitus ulcers. Practical experience with Granulex has found that it is not as effective in debriding wounds as compared to other enzymatic products. Therefore, Granulex may be more appropriately used on stage 1 and 2 decubiti.

Dosage Forms Aerosol, topical: Trypsin 0.1 mg, balsam Peru 72.5 mg, and castor oil 650 mg per 0.82 mL (60 g, 120 g)

References

Chamberlain TM, Cali TJ, Cuzzell J, et al, "Assessment and Management of Pressure Sores in Long-Term Care Facilities," *Consult Pharm*, 1992, 7(12):1328-40.

TST *see* Tuberculin Purified Protein Derivative *on this page*

T-Stat® Topical *see* Erythromycin, Topical *on page 347*

Tuberculin Purified Protein Derivative

(too BER kyoo lin PURE eh fide PRO teen dah RIV ah tiv)

Related Information

Immunization Guidelines *on page 1058*

Brand Names Aplisol®; Aplitest®; Tine Test PPD; Tubersol®

Synonyms Mantoux; PPD; Tine Test; TST; Tuberculin Skin Test

Generic Available No

Therapeutic Category Diagnostic Agent, Skin Test

Use Skin test in diagnosis of tuberculosis, cell-mediated immunodeficiencies

Contraindications Tuberculin positive reactions; 250 TU strength should not be used for initial testing

Warnings Do not administer I.V. or S.C.; epinephrine (1:1000) should be available to treat possible allergic reactions; skin test responsiveness may be suppressed during and after (up to 6 months) viral infections, vaccinations with live viral vaccines, and patients with tuberculosis, severe bacterial infections, malnutrition, malignant diseases or immunosuppression

Precautions Do not apply on hairy areas without adequate subcutaneous tissue or on acneiform skin; use extreme caution in patients with perceived

(Continued)

Tuberculin Purified Protein Derivative *(Continued)*

active tuberculosis; positive test does not confirm diagnosis and further diagnostic procedures should be performed

Adverse Reactions
Dermatologic: Ulceration, necrosis
Local: Vesiculation, pain

Drug Interactions Reaction may be suppressed in patients receiving systemic corticosteroids, aminocaproic acid, or within 4-6 weeks following immunization with live or inactivated viral vaccines

Stability Refrigerate

Mechanism of Action Tuberculosis results in individuals becoming sensitized to certain antigenic components of the M tuberculosis organism. Culture extracts called tuberculins are contained in tuberculin skin test preparations. Upon intracutaneous injection of these culture extracts, a classic delayed (cellular) hypersensitivity reaction occurs. This reaction is characteristic of a delayed course (peak occurs >24 hours after injection, induration of the skin secondary to cell infiltration, and occasional vesiculation and necrosis). Delayed hypersensitivity reactions to tuberculin may indicate infection with a variety of nontuberculosis mycobacteria, or vaccination with the live attenuated mycobacterial strain of M bovis vaccine, BCG, in addition to previous natural infection with M tuberculosis.

Pharmacodynamics
Onset of action: Delayed hypersensitivity reactions to tuberculin usually occur within 5-6 hours following injection
Peak effect: Becomes maximal at 48-72 hours
Duration: Reactions subside over a few days

Usual Dosage Geriatrics and Adults: Intradermal: 0.1 mL about 4" below elbow; use $\frac{1}{4}$" to $\frac{1}{2}$" or 26- or 27-gauge needle; significant reactions are ≥5 mm in diameter

Interpretation of induration: Positive: ≥10 mm; inconclusive: 5-9 mm; negative: <5 mm

Administration Administer intradermally; avoid subcutaneous injections

Monitoring Parameters Monitor for induration (48-72 hours), ulcerations, necrosis, vesiculations

Patient Information Return to physician or nurse for reaction interpretation at 48-72 hours

Nursing Implications Test dose: 0.1 mL intracutaneously; store in refrigerator; examine site at 48-72 hours after administration; whenever tuberculin is administered, a record should be made of the administration technique (Mantoux method, disposable multiple-puncture device), tuberculin used (OT or PPD), manufacturer and lot number of tuberculin used, date of administration, date of test reading, and the size of the reaction in millimeters (mm)

Special Geriatric Considerations Due to changes in the immune system with age, skin-test response may be delayed or reduced in magnitude; therefore when testing, use a 2-step test procedure; repeat test 2-4 weeks after reading first test dose; this elicits a "booster effect"

Dosage Forms
Injection:
First test strength: 1 TU/0.1 mL (1 mL)
Intermediate test strength: 5 TU/0.1 mL (1 mL, 5 mL, 10 mL)
Second test strength: 250 TU/0.1 mL (1 mL)
Tine: 5 TU each test

References
Dutt AK and Stead WW, "Tuberculosis," *Clin Geriatr Med*, 1992, 8(4):761-75.

Tussi-Organidin® NR *see* Guaifenesin and Codeine *on page 438*
Tusstat® Syrup *see* Diphenhydramine *on page 302*
Twice-A-Day® Nasal [OTC] *see* Oxymetazoline *on page 706*
Twilite® Oral [OTC] *see* Diphenhydramine *on page 302*
Tylenol® [OTC] *see* Acetaminophen *on page 16*
Tylenol® Extended Relief [OTC] *see* Acetaminophen *on page 16*
Tylenol® With Codeine *see* Acetaminophen and Codeine *on page 18*
Tylox® *see* Oxycodone and Acetaminophen *on page 705*
Typhim Vi® *see* Typhoid Vaccine *on this page*

Typhoid Vaccine (TYE foid vak SEEN)
Related Information
Immunization Guidelines *on page 1058*
Brand Names Typhim Vi®; Vivotif Berna™ Oral
Synonyms Typhoid Vaccine Live Oral Ty21a
Therapeutic Category Vaccine, Inactivated Bacteria
Use Promotes active immunity to typhoid fever for patients exposed to typhoid carrier or foreign travel to typhoid fever endemic area
Contraindications Acute respiratory or other active infections, previous sensitivity to typhoid vaccine or enteric coated capsule; immunosuppressed patients
Precautions Immune deficiency conditions; vaccine does not protect all recipients
Adverse Reactions
Central nervous system: Malaise, headache, fever
Local: Tenderness, erythema, induration
Neuromuscular & skeletal: Myalgia
Overdosage No symptoms noted with oral capsule; can cause *S. typhi* shedding
Drug Interactions Simultaneous administration with other vaccines which cause local or systemic adverse effects should be avoided
Stability Refrigerate at 2°C to 8°C (36°F to 46°F); do not freeze; not viable at room temperature
Mechanism of Action >70% effective
Usual Dosage Geriatrics and Adults:
S.C.: 0.5 mL; repeat dose in 4 weeks (total immunization is 2 doses); booster: 0.5 mL S.C. or 0.1 mL intradermally at 3-year intervals
Primary immunization: Oral: 1 capsule on alternate days (every other day) for a total of 4 capsules; take 1 hour after meals with cold or lukewarm water
Booster: Repeat at 5-year intervals; use same schedule as for primary immunization (4 capsules)
Patient Information Oral capsule should be taken 1 hour before a meal with cold or lukewarm drink; systemic adverse effects may persist for 1-2 days
Nursing Implications Doses of vaccine are different between S.C. and intradermal; S.C. injection only should be used
Additional Information If >3 years elapse after vaccination, only booster is needed; do not need to repeat primary vaccination
Special Geriatric Considerations Vaccinating elderly is often overlooked; if no record of immunization can be recalled, repeat primary series
Dosage Forms
Capsule, enteric coated
Injection: 1.5 mL
References
Gardner P and Schaffner W, "Immunization of Adults," *N Engl J Med*, 1993, 328(17):1252-8.

Typhoid Vaccine Live Oral Ty21a *see* Typhoid Vaccine *on this page*
Tyzine® Nasal *see* Tetrahydrozoline *on page 901*
UCB-P071 *see* Cetirizine *on page 199*
U-Cort™ *see* Hydrocortisone *on page 462*
Ultracef® *see* Cefadroxil *on page 173*
Ultralente® *see* Insulin Preparations *on page 488*
Ultram® *see* Tramadol *on page 943*
Ultrase® MT12 *see* Pancrelipase *on page 712*
Ultrase® MT20 *see* Pancrelipase *on page 712*
Ultra Tears® Solution [OTC] *see* Artificial Tears *on page 82*
Ultravate™ *see* Halobetasol *on page 445*
Unasyn® *see* Ampicillin and Sulbactam *on page 75*
Uni-Ace® [OTC] *see* Acetaminophen *on page 16*

Uni-Bent® Cough Syrup *see* Diphenhydramine *on page 302*

Uni-Dur® *see* Theophylline *on page 902*

Unipen® Injection *see* Nafcillin *on page 648*

Unipen® Oral *see* Nafcillin *on page 648*

Uniphyl® *see* Theophylline *on page 902*

Uni-Pro® [OTC] *see* Ibuprofen *on page 475*

Uni-tussin® [OTC] *see* Guaifenesin *on page 437*

Uni-tussin® DM [OTC] *see* Guaifenesin and Dextromethorphan *on page 439*

Univasc® *see* Moexipril *on page 633*

Urabeth® *see* Bethanechol *on page 117*

Urea Peroxide *see* Carbamide Peroxide *on page 162*

Urecholine® *see* Bethanechol *on page 117*

Urex® *see* Methenamine *on page 601*

Urispas® *see* Flavoxate *on page 384*

Uri-Tet® Oral *see* Oxytetracycline *on page 709*

Urobak® *see* Sulfamethoxazole *on page 876*

Urodine® *see* Phenazopyridine *on page 734*

Urogesic® *see* Phenazopyridine *on page 734*

Urokinase (yoor oh KIN ase)

Brand Names Abbokinase®

Generic Available No

Therapeutic Category Thrombolytic Agent

Use Thrombolytic agent used in treatment of recent severe or massive deep vein thrombosis, pulmonary emboli, myocardial infarction, and occluded arteriovenous cannulas; more expensive than streptokinase; not useful on thrombi over 1 week old

Contraindications Hypersensitivity to urokinase or any component; active internal bleeding; CVA (within 2 months); brain carcinoma, bacterial endocarditis, anticoagulant therapy, intracranial or intraspinal surgery, surgery or trauma within past 10 days

Warnings Use with caution in patients with severe hypertension, recent L.P., patients receiving I.M. administration of medications, patients with trauma or surgery in the last 10 days

Adverse Reactions

Cardiovascular: Hypotension, arrhythmias

Central nervous system: Headache, chills

Dermatologic: Angioneurotic edema, rash

Gastrointestinal: Nausea, vomiting

Hematologic: Bleeding at sites of percutaneous trauma, anemia

Ocular: Periorbital swelling, eye hemorrhage

Respiratory: Bronchospasm, epistaxis

Miscellaneous: Anaphylaxis, diaphoresis

Overdosage Symptoms of overdose include epistaxis, bleeding gums, hematoma, spontaneous ecchymoses, oozing at catheter site

Toxicology In case of overdose, stop infusion, reverse bleeding with blood products that contain clotting factors

Drug Interactions Increased toxicity (increased bleeding) with anticoagulants, antiplatelet drugs, aspirin, indomethacin, dextran, clopidogrel

Stability Store in refrigerator; reconstitute by gently rolling and tilting; do not shake; contains no preservatives, should not be reconstituted until immediately before using, discard unused portion; stable at room temperature for 24 hours after reconstitution

Mechanism of Action Promotes thrombolysis by directly activating plasminogen to plasmin, which degrades fibrin, fibrinogen, and other procoagulant plasma proteins

Pharmacodynamics

Onset of action: I.V.: Fibrinolysis occurs rapidly

Duration: 4 or more hours

Pharmacokinetics

Half-life: 10-20 minutes

Elimination: Cleared by the liver with a small amount excreted in urine and bile

Usual Dosage Geriatrics and Adults:

Deep vein thrombosis: I.V.: Loading: 4400 units/kg over 10 minutes, then 4400 units/kg/hour for 12 hours

Myocardial infarction: Intracoronary: 750,000 units over 2 hours (6000 units/minute over up to 2 hours)

Occluded I.V. catheters:
5000 units (use only Abbokinase® Open Cath) in each lumen over 1-2 minutes, leave in lumen for 1-4 hours, then aspirate; may repeat with 10,000 units in each lumen if 5000 units fails to clear the catheter; **do not infuse into the patient**; volume to instill into catheter is equal to the volume of the catheter

I.V. infusion: 200 units/kg/hour in each lumen for 12-48 hours at a rate of at least 20 mL/hour

Dialysis patients: 5000 units is administered in each lumen over 1-2 minutes; leave urokinase in lumen for 1-2 days, then aspirate

Clot lysis (large vessel thrombi): Loading: I.V.: 4400 units/kg over 10 minutes, increase to 6000 units/kg/hour; maintenance: 4400-6000 units/kg/hour adjusted to achieve clot lysis or patency of affected vessel; doses up to 50,000 units/kg/hour have been used. **Note:** Therapy should be initiated as soon as possible after diagnosis of thrombi and continued until clot is dissolved (usually 24-72 hours).

Acute pulmonary embolism: Three treatment alternatives: 3 million unit dosage

Alternative 1: 12-hour infusion: 4400 units/kg (2000 units/lb) bolus over 10 minutes followed by 4400 units/kg/hour (2000 units/lb); begin heparin 1000 units/hour approximately 3-4 hours after completion of urokinase infusion or when PTT is <100 seconds

Alternative 2: 2-hour infusion: 1 million unit bolus over 10 minutes followed by 2 million units over 110 minutes; begin heparin 1000 units/hour approximately 3-4 hours after completion of urokinase infusion or when PTT is <100 seconds

Alternative 3: Bolus dose only: 15,000 units/kg over 10 minutes; begin heparin 1000 units/hour approximately 3-4 hours after completion of urokinase infusion or when PTT is <100 seconds

Administration Use 0.22 or 0.45 micron filter during I.V. therapy

Monitoring Parameters CBC, reticulocyte count, platelet count, DIC panel (fibrinogen, plasminogen, FDP, D-dimer, PT, PTT), thrombosis panel (AT-III, protein C), urinalysis, ACT

Special Geriatric Considerations No specific recommendations for elderly when using this agent; studies of similar agents have demonstrated that age is not a contraindication for use

Dosage Forms
Powder for injection: 250,000 units (5 mL)
Powder for injection, catheter clear: 5000 units (1 mL)

Uro-KP-Neutral® *see* Potassium Phosphate and Sodium Phosphate *on page 767*

Ursodeoxycholic Acid *see* Ursodiol *on this page*

Ursodiol (ER soe dye ole)

Brand Names Actigall™
Synonyms Ursodeoxycholic Acid
Generic Available No
Therapeutic Category Gallstone Dissolution Agent
Use Gallbladder stone dissolution in patients with radiolucent, noncalcified stones <20 mm in greatest diameter with an increased risk for surgical removal; safety beyond 2 years use is not established
Contraindications Not to be used with cholesterol, radiopaque, bile pigment stones, or stones larger than 20 mm in diameter; allergy to bile acids; chronic liver disease; patients who have very good reason for cholecystectomy for diseases which require this procedure (eg, cholangitis, biliary obstruction, gallstones, pancreatitis, etc)
Warnings Gallbladder stone dissolution may take several months of therapy; complete dissolution may not occur and recurrence of stones within 5 years has been observed in 50% of patients; use with caution in patients with a nonvisualizing gallbladder and those with chronic liver disease
Precautions Patients who develop abnormal liver tests during therapy should be closely monitored for worsening gallstone disease; discontinue if liver function tests persist in elevation
Adverse Reactions
Central nervous system: Fatigue, headache, depression, sleep difficulties
Dermatologic: Pruritus, rash, urticaria, dry skin, thinning hair
Gastrointestinal: Nausea, vomiting, dyspepsia, metallic taste, abdominal pain, biliary pain, constipation, cholecystitis, flatulence
Neuromuscular & skeletal: Myalgia, arthralgia, backache
Respiratory: Cough, rhinitis
(Continued)

Ursodiol *(Continued)*

Miscellaneous: Diaphoresis

Overdosage Symptoms of overdose predominantly include diarrhea

Toxicology No specific therapy for diarrhea and for overdose; administer general supportive care

Drug Interactions Decreased effect with aluminum-containing antacids, cholestyramine, colestipol, clofibrate, oral contraceptives (estrogens)

Mechanism of Action Decreases the cholesterol content of bile and bile stones by reducing the secretion of cholesterol from the liver and the fractional reabsorption of cholesterol by the intestines

Pharmacokinetics

Metabolism: Undergoes extensive enterohepatic recycling; following hepatic conjugation and biliary secretion, the drug is hydrolyzed to active ursodiol, where it is recycled or transformed to lithocholic acid by colonic microbial flora

Half-life: 100 hours

Elimination: In feces via bile

Usual Dosage Geriatrics and Adults: Oral: 8-10 mg/kg/day in 2-3 divided doses; use beyond 24 months is not established; obtain ultrasound images at 6-month intervals for the first year of therapy; 30% of patients have stone recurrence after dissolution

Monitoring Parameters ALT, AST at initiation, 1 and 3 months and every 6 months thereafter, sonogram

Patient Information Frequent blood work necessary to follow drug effects; report any persistent nausea, vomiting, abdominal pain

Nursing Implications See Adverse Reactions and Special Geriatric Considerations

Special Geriatric Considerations No specific clinical studies in elderly; would recommend starting at lowest recommended dose with scheduled monitoring

Dosage Forms Capsule: 300 mg

Vagistat-1® Vaginal [OTC] *see* Tioconazole *on page 927*

Valacyclovir (val ay SYE kloe veer)

Related Information

Acyclovir *on page 26*

Brand Names Valtrex®

Therapeutic Category Antiviral Agent, Oral

Use Treatment of herpes zoster (shingles) in immunocompetent patients

Contraindications Hypersensitivity to acyclovir

Precautions Use with caution in patients with pre-existing renal disease or in those receiving nephrotoxic drugs concurrently

Adverse Reactions

Cardiovascular: Tachycardia, vasodilatation

Central nervous system: Fever, fatigue

Dermatologic: Pruritus

Gastrointestinal: Nausea, vomiting, diarrhea

Hematologic: Bone marrow suppression, thrombotic thrombocytopenia

Neuromuscular & skeletal: Myalgia

Ophthalmic: Eye pain, photophobia

Overdosage Symptoms of overdose include elevated serum creatinine, renal failure

Toxicology In the event of an overdose, sufficient urine flow must be maintained to avoid drug precipitation within the renal tubules. Hemodialysis has resulted in up to 60% reductions in serum acyclovir levels.

Drug Interactions

Probenecid increases acyclovir bioavailability, terminal half-life may be increased and renal clearance may be decreased

Zidovudine increases drowsiness and lethargy

Mechanism of Action A prodrug of acyclovir containing a l-valine ester which is hydrolyzed in the intestine and/or liver to acyclovir (see Acyclovir monograph)

Pharmacokinetics Valacyclovir is undetectable in the plasma; peak acyclovir concentrations appear in 2 hours

Usual Dosage Geriatrics and Adults: Oral: 1000 mg 3 times/day for 7 days

Dosing interval in renal impairment:

Cl_{cr} >50 mL/minute: Administer 100% of dose every 8 hours

Cl_{cr} 30-49 mL/minute: Administer 100% of dose every 12 hours

Cl$_{cr}$ 10-29 mL/minute: Administer 100% of dose every 24 hours

Cl$_{cr}$ <10 mL/minute: Administer 50% of dose every 24 hours

Monitoring Parameters Urinalysis, BUN, serum creatinine, liver enzymes, CBC

Patient Information Contagious only when viral shedding is occurring; avoid sexual intercourse when lesions are visible; recurrences tend to appear within 3 months of original infection; acyclovir is **not** a cure

Nursing Implications Maintain adequate hydration of patient; check infusion site for phlebitis, rotate site to prevent phlebitis

Additional Information See Acyclovir monograph for complete information

Special Geriatric Considerations More convenient dosing and increased bioavailability, without increasing side effects, make valacyclovir a favorable choice compared to acyclovir; has been shown to accelerate resolution of postherpetic pain (see Usual Dosage and Acyclovir monograph)

Dosage Forms Caplets: 500 mg

References

Beutner KR, Friedman DJ, Forszpaniak C, et al, "Valacyclovir Compared With Acyclovir for Improved Therapy for Herpes Zoster in Immunocompetent Adults," *Antimicrob Agents Chemother*, 1995, 39(7):1546-53.

Valergen® Injection *see* Estradiol *on page 350*

Valisone® *see* Betamethasone *on page 114*

Valium® Injection *see* Diazepam *on page 279*

Valium® Oral *see* Diazepam *on page 279*

Valproate Semisodium *see* Valproic Acid and Derivatives *on this page*

Valproate Sodium *see* Valproic Acid and Derivatives *on this page*

Valproic Acid *see* Valproic Acid and Derivatives *on this page*

Valproic Acid and Derivatives
(val PROE ik AS id & dah RIV ah tives)

Related Information

Antiepileptic Drug Interactions Comparison *on page 1022*

Serum Drug Concentrations Commonly Monitored: Guidelines *on page 1114*

Brand Names Depacon®; Depakene®; Depakote®

Synonyms Dipropylacetic Acid; Divalproex Sodium; DPA; 2-Propylpentanoic Acid; 2-Propylvaleric Acid; Valproate Semisodium; Valproate Sodium; Valproic Acid

Generic Available Yes

Therapeutic Category Anticonvulsant, Miscellaneous

Use Management of simple and complex absence seizures; mixed seizure types; myoclonic and generalized tonic-clonic (grand mal) seizures; may be effective in partial seizures; treatment of bipolar affective disorder; migraine prophylaxis; complex partial seizures either as single or adjunctive therapy; Depacon® is indicated as a temporary intravenous alternative when oral administration is not possible

Unlabeled use: Treatment of atypical absence, myoclonic, and grand mal seizures; incontinence following ileoanal anastomosis; aggressive behavior associated with dementia

Contraindications Hypersensitivity to valproic acid or derivatives or any component; hepatic dysfunction and hepatic disease

Warnings Hepatic failure resulting in fatalities has occurred in patients; monitor patients closely for appearance of malaise, loss of seizure control, weakness, facial edema, anorexia, jaundice and vomiting; hepatotoxicity has been reported after 3 days to 6 months of therapy

Precautions May cause severe thrombocytopenia, bleeding; hyperammonemia in absence of abnormal LFTs or mental changes may occur; valproic acid may interact with other anticonvulsants (see Drug Interactions); carcinogenicity reported in animals (fibrosarcoma, pulmonary adenomas), but no such data in humans

Adverse Reactions

Cardiovascular: Peripheral edema

Central nervous system: Drowsiness, ataxia, irritability, confusion, restlessness, sedation, hyperactivity, headache, malaise, dizziness, depression, psychosis, aggression

Dermatologic: Alopecia, transient alopecia, erythema multiforme, rash, bruising

Endocrine & metabolic: Hyperammonemia, abnormal thyroid tests, parotid gland edema

(Continued)

Valproic Acid and Derivatives *(Continued)*

Gastrointestinal: Nausea, vomiting, indigestion, diarrhea, abdominal cramps, constipation, anorexia, weight loss, weight gain, pancreatitis

Hematologic: Thrombocytopenia, prolongation of bleeding time, leukopenia, eosinophilia, bone marrow suppression, hemorrhage

Hepatic: Transient elevated liver enzymes, liver failure, lymphocytosis

Neuromuscular & skeletal: Asterixis, dysarthria, incoordination, weakness, tremors

Ocular: Diplopia, "spots before eyes"

Overdosage Symptoms of overdose include coma, deep sleep, motor restlessness, asterixis, visual hallucinations

Toxicology Supportive treatment is necessary; naloxone has been used to reverse CNS depressant effects, but may block action of other anticonvulsants

Drug Interactions

Valproic acid may displace phenytoin and diazepam from protein binding sites. Aspirin may displace valproic acid from protein binding sites which may result in toxicity. Valproic acid may significantly increase phenobarbital serum concentrations in patients receiving phenobarbital or primidone. Valproic acid may inhibit the metabolism of phenytoin.

Felbamate may increase valproic acid serum concentrations and cause valproic acid toxicity. Lamotrigine decreases valproic acid serum concentrations; however, lamotrigine serum concentration can increase by a factor of 2 (increased lamotrigine).

Phenobarbital, primidone, phenytoin, and carbamazepine may decrease serum concentrations of valproic acid

Food may delay absorption but does not affect extent absorbed

Valproic acid increases clozapine's serum concentrations

Mechanism of Action Causes increased availability of gamma-aminobutyric acid (GABA), an inhibitory neurotransmitter, to brain neurons or may enhance the action of GABA or mimic its action at postsynaptic receptor sites; valproate may also inhibit catabolism of GABA; potentiate postsynaptic GABA response, have direct membrane stabilization effect possibly by effecting potassium channel operation

Pharmacokinetics

Protein binding: 80% to 90% (dose dependent)

Metabolism: Extensive in the liver; substrate 2C19

Half-life (adults): 8-17 hours, increased half-life in patients with liver disease

Time to peak serum concentration: Oral: Within 1-4 hours; 3-5 hours after divalproex (enteric coated)

Elimination: 2% to 3% excreted unchanged in urine

Usual Dosage Geriatrics and Adults:

Oral: Initial: 10-15 mg/kg/day in 1-3 divided doses; increase by 5-10 mg/kg/day at weekly intervals until therapeutic levels are achieved; maintenance: 30-60 mg/kg/day in 2-3 divided doses; twice daily administration most frequent (see Additional Information)

I.V.: Administer as a 60 minute infusion (≤20 mg/min) with the same frequency as oral products; switch patient to oral products as soon as possible

Rectal: Dilute syrup 1:1 with water for use as a retention enema; loading dose: 17-20 mg/kg one time; maintenance: 10-15 mg/kg/dose every 8 hours

Not dialyzable (0% to 5%)

Monitoring Parameters Monitor serum concentrations; observe for side effects and obtain LFTs and CBC during first 6 months of therapy

Reference Range

Therapeutic: 50-100 µg/mL (SI: 350-690 µmol/L); Toxic: >200 µg/mL (SI: >1390 µmol/L); Bipolar: 50-125 µg/mL

Seizure control may improve at levels >100 µg/mL (SI: 690 µmol/L), but toxicity may occur at levels of 100-150 µg/mL (SI: 690-1040 µmol/L)

Test Interactions False-positive result for urine ketones; possible alterations in thyroid function tests

Patient Information Take with food or milk; do not chew, break or crush the tablet or capsule; do not administer with carbonated drinks; report any sore throat, fever, or fatigue

Nursing Implications Do not crush enteric coated drug product or capsules (see Monitoring Parameters)

Additional Information Tremors may indicate overdosage. The most frequent side effects to valproic acid use are anorexia, vomiting, and nausea;

taking doses with meals or changing to the enteric coated product may reduce these side effects

Sodium content of valproate sodium syrup (5 mL): 23 mg (1 mEq)

Divalproex sodium: Depakote®

Valproate sodium: Depakene® syrup

Valproic acid: Depakene® capsule

Special Geriatric Considerations No specific data available for use in elderly (see Warnings and Additional Information)

Dosage Forms

Valproic acid as divalproex sodium:

Capsule, sprinkle (Depakote® Sprinkle®): 125 mg

Tablet, delayed release (Depakote®): 125 mg, 250 mg, 500 mg

Valproic acid as sodium valproate:

Injection (Depacon®): 100 mg/mL (5 mL)

Syrup (Depakene®): 250 mg/5 mL (5 mL, 50 mL, 480 mL)

Capsule, as valproic acid (Depakene®): 250 mg

References

Dreifuss FE, Santilli N, Langer DH, et al, "Valproic Acid Hepatic Fatalities: A Retrospective Review," *Neurology*, 1987, 37(3):379-85.

Mazure CM, Druss BG, and Cellar JS, "Valproate Treatment of Older Psychotic Patients With Organic Mental Syndromes and Behavioral Dyscontrol," *J Am Geriatr Soc*, 1992, 40(9):914-6.

Mellow AM, Solano-Lopez C, and Davis S, "Sodium Valproate in the Treatment of Behavioral Disturbance in Dementia," *J Geriatr Psychiatry Neurol*, 1993, 6(4):205-9.

Valsartan (val SAR tan)

Brand Names Diovan®

Generic Available No

Therapeutic Category Angiotensin II Antagonists

Use Alone or in combination with other antihypertensive agents in treating essential hypertension; may have an advantage over losartan due to minimal metabolism requirements and consequent use in mild to moderate hepatic impairment

Unlabeled use: Treatment of heart failure

Contraindications Hypersensitivity to valsartan or any components, severe hepatic insufficiency, biliary cirrhosis or biliary obstruction, primary hyperaldosteronism, bilateral renal artery stenosis

Warnings Use extreme caution with concurrent administration of potassium-sparing diuretics or potassium supplements, in patients with mild-moderate hepatic dysfunction (adjust dose), in those who may be sodium/water depleted (eg, on high-dose diuretics), and in the elderly; avoid use in patients with congestive heart failure, unilateral renal artery stenosis, aortic/mitral valve stenosis, coronary artery disease, or hypertrophic cardiomyopathy

Precautions Elevations of liver function tests frequently occur, including serum bilirubin; serum creatinine and BUN may be increased; decreases in hemoglobin and hematocrit (>20%); serum potassium increases of greater than 20% observed in 4% of patients

Adverse Reactions Similar incidence to placebo; independent of race, age, and gender

Cardiovascular: Edema, chest pain, tachycardia

Central nervous system: Headache, dizziness, drowsiness, ataxia, insomnia, fatigue, anxiety/nervousness

Dermatologic: Rash

Endocrine & metabolic: Decreased libido

Gastrointestinal: Diarrhea, abdominal pain, nausea, abnormal taste, dyspepsia, heartburn

Hematologic: Neutropenia, anemia

Hepatic: Increased LFTs

Neuromuscular & skeletal: Arthralgia, pain, muscle cramps, myalgia

Renal: Polyuria, increased creatinine

Respiratory: Cough (2.6%), upper respiratory infection, rhinitis, sinusitis, nasal congestion, pharyngitis

Overdosage Symptoms are hypotension, tachycardia, bradycardia from vagal response

Toxicology Treatment is symptomatic (eg, fluids) and supportive

Drug Interactions

Decreased effect: Phenobarbital, ketoconazole, troleandomycin

Increased effect: Cimetidine

Drug/Food Interactions Food decreases rate of absorption and decreases C_{max} by 50% and AUC by 40%

(Continued)

Valsartan *(Continued)*

Mechanism of Action As a prodrug, valsartan produces direct antagonism of the angiotensin II (AT2) receptors, unlike the angiotensin-converting enzyme inhibitors. It displaces angiotensin II from the AT1 receptor and produces its blood pressure lowering effects by antagonizing AT1-induced vasoconstriction, aldosterone release, catecholamine release, arginine vasopressin release, water intake, and hypertrophic responses. This action results in more efficient blockade of the cardiovascular effects of angiotensin II and fewer side effects than the ACE inhibitors.

Pharmacokinetics

Distribution: V_d: 17 L (adults)

Protein binding: 94% to 97%

Metabolism: Metabolized to an inactive metabolite

Bioavailability: 23%

Half-life: 6 hours

Time to peak serum concentration: 2 hours (maximal effect: 4-6 hours)

Elimination: 13% and 83% excreted as unchanged drug in urine and feces, respectively

Usual Dosage Geriatrics and Adults: 80 mg/day; may be increased to 320 mg if needed (antihypertensive effect seen in 1-2 weeks with maximal effects observed in 4-6 weeks); see Additional Information

Dosing adjustment in renal impairment: No dosage adjustment necessary if Cl_{cr} >10 mL/minute

Dosing adjustment in hepatic impairment (mild - moderate): ≤80 mg/day

Dialysis: Not significantly removed

Monitoring Parameters Baseline and periodic electrolyte panels, renal and liver function tests, urinalysis; symptoms of hypotension or hypersensitivity; monitor blood pressure and pulse

Patient Information Do not stop taking this medication unless instructed by a physician; take a missed dose as soon as possible unless it is almost time for your next dose; call your physician immediately if you have symptoms of allergy or develop side effects including headache and dizziness

Nursing Implications Monitor initial doses for hypotension; stress need for adequate fluid intake (see Warnings and Precautions)

Additional Information Increasing dose beyond 80 mg/day has less antihypertensive effect than the addition of a diuretic to the 80 mg/day dose

Special Geriatric Considerations No dosage adjustment is necessary when initiating angiotensin II receptor antagonists in elderly. In clinical studies, no differences between younger adults and elderly were demonstrated.

Dosage Forms Capsule: 80 mg, 160 mg

References

Munger MA and Furniss SM, "Angiotensin II Receptor Blockers: Novel Therapy for Heart Failure?" *Pharmacotherapy*, 1996, 16(2 Pt 2):59S-68S.

Valtrex® *see Valacyclovir on page 976*

Vamate® *see Hydroxyzine on page 470*

Vancenase® AQ Inhaler *see Beclomethasone on page 105*

Vancenase® Nasal Inhaler *see Beclomethasone on page 105*

Vanceril® Oral Inhaler *see Beclomethasone on page 105*

Vancocin® *see Vancomycin on this page*

Vancoled® *see Vancomycin on this page*

Vancomycin (van koe MYE sin)

Related Information

I.V. Medication Recommendations *on page 1080*

Penicillins, Penicillin-Related Antibiotics, & Other Antibiotics *on page 1010*

Prevention of Bacterial Endocarditis *on page 1062*

Serum Drug Concentrations Commonly Monitored: Guidelines *on page 1114*

Brand Names Lyphocin®; Vancocin®; Vancoled®

Generic Available Yes

Therapeutic Category Antibiotic, Miscellaneous

Use Treatment of patients with the following infections or conditions: treatment of infections due to documented or suspected methicillin-resistant *S. aureus* or beta-lactam resistant coagulase negative *Staphylococcus*; treatment of serious or life-threatening infections (ie, endocarditis, meningitis) due to documented or suspected staphylococcal or streptococcal infections in patients who are allergic to penicillins and/or cephalosporins; empiric therapy of infections associated with central lines, VP shunts, vascular grafts, prosthetic heart valves; treatment of febrile granulocytopenic patient who has not responded after 48 hours to antibiotic treatment directed at gram-negative rod infections; used orally for staphylococcal enterocolitis or for antibiotic-associated pseudomembranous colitis produced by *C. difficile*

Contraindications Hypersensitivity to vancomycin or any component; avoid in patients with previous hearing loss

Precautions Use with caution in patients with renal impairment or those receiving other nephrotoxic or ototoxic drugs; dosage modification required in patients with impaired renal function; vancomycin-resistant enterococci and coagulase-negative staphylococci have been reported, the CDC has guidelines on the use of vancomycin to reduce resistance (see References)

Adverse Reactions

Cardiovascular: Tachycardia, hypotension

Central nervous system: Fever, chills

Dermatologic: Erythema multiforme-like reaction with intense pruritus, rash involving face, neck, upper trunk, urticaria, macular skin rash, back and upper arms (red neck or red man syndrome)

Gastrointestinal: Nausea (oral), bitter taste

Hematologic: Neutropenia, eosinophilia, thrombocytopenia

Local: Phlebitis

Otic: Ototoxicity

Renal: Nephrotoxicity

Toxicology There is no specific therapy for an overdosage with vancomycin. Care is symptomatic and supportive in nature. Peritoneal filtration and hemofiltration have been shown to reduce the serum concentration of vancomycin.

Drug Interactions Anesthetic agents, aminoglycosides (may increase risk of nephrotoxicity and ototoxicity), nondepolarizing muscle relaxants

Stability After the oral or parenteral solution is reconstituted, refrigerate and discard after 14 days; after further dilution, the parenteral solution is stable, at room temperature, for 24 hours

Mechanism of Action Inhibits bacterial cell wall synthesis by blocking glycopeptide polymerization through binding tightly to D-alanyl-D-alanine portion of cell wall precursor; also inhibits RNA synthesis

Pharmacokinetics

Absorption:

Oral: Poor

I.M.: Erratic

Protein binding: 10%

Half-life: Biphasic: Terminal: Adults: 5-11 hours, half-life prolonged significantly with reduced renal function

Time to peak serum concentration: I.V.: Within 45-65 minutes

Elimination: As unchanged drug in urine (80% to 90%); oral doses are excreted primarily in feces

Geriatrics: Volume of distribution has been reported to be decreased 44% while total clearance decreased by 23% and the terminal half-life increased to 12 hours

Usual Dosage Initial dosage recommendation: I.V.:

Geriatrics: Best to individualize therapy; dose (mg/kg/24 hours) = (0.227 x Cl_{cr}) + 5.67

Cl_{cr} male: (140 - age) x IBW (kg) divided by 72 x serum creatinine

Cl_{cr} female: Cl_{cr} male x 0.85

The calculated dose should be divided and given as specified in the following dosing intervals based upon Cl_{cr}:

Cl_{cr} >65 mL/minute: Administer every 8 hours

Cl_{cr} 40-65 mL/minute: Administer every 12 hours

Cl_{cr} 20-39 mL/minute: Administer every 24 hours

Cl_{cr} 10-19 mL/minute: Administer every 48 hours

Not dialyzable (0% to 5%)

Adults: With normal renal function: 0.5 g every 6 hours or 1 g every 12 hours

Renal dysfunction, end stage renal disease, or on dialysis: 10-20 mg/kg; subsequent dosages and frequency of administration are best determined by measurement of serum concentrations and assessment of renal insufficiency

Geriatrics and Adults: Intrathecal: 20 mg/day

C. difficile colitis: Geriatrics and Adults: Oral: 125-500 mg every 6-8 hours for 7-10 days; no dosage adjustment necessary for renal impairment

(Continued)

Vancomycin *(Continued)*

Monitoring Parameters Peak and trough vancomycin serum concentrations, serum BUN and creatinine, hearing, culture and sensitivity results, I.V. site; signs of Red Man's syndrome

Reference Range
Therapeutic:
Depends on MIC of organism being treated, usually peak: 20-40 µg/mL (SI: 14-27 µmol/L)
Trough: 5-10 µg/mL (SI: 3.4-6.8 µmol/L)
Toxic: >80 µg/mL (SI: >54 µmol/L)

Patient Information Report pain at infusion site, dizziness, fullness or ringing in ears with I.V. use; nausea or vomiting with oral use

Nursing Implications Obtain serum concentrations after the third dose; peaks are obtained 30 minutes to 3 hours after the completion of a 1-hour infusion; troughs are obtained just before the next dose; slow I.V. infusion rate to ≥2 hours if maculopapular rash appears on face, neck, trunk, and upper extremities; dosage modification required in patients with impaired renal function; do not administer antidiarrheal products to patients on oral vancomycin; do not give I.M.

Additional Information Vancomycin should not be used first line in *C. difficile*-induced diarrhea; to prevent resistance, it should be saved for patients who do not respond to metronidazole

Special Geriatric Considerations As a result of age-related changes in renal function and volume of distribution, accumulation and toxicity are a risk in the elderly (see Pharmacokinetics and Adverse Reactions); hence, careful monitoring and dosing adjustment is necessary

Dosage Forms
Vancomycin hydrochloride:
Capsule: 125 mg, 250 mg
Powder for oral solution: 1 g, 10 g
Powder for injection: 500 mg, 1 g, 2 g, 5 g, 10 g

References
Centers for Disease Control and Prevention, "Recommendations for Preventing the Spread of Vancomycin Resistance - Recommendations of the Hospital Infection Control Practice Advisory Committee (HICPAC)," *MMWR Morb Mortal Wkly Rep* 1995, 44(RR-12):1-9.
Cutler NR, Narang PK, Lesko LJ, et al, "Vancomycin Disposition: The Importance of Age," *Clin Pharmacol Ther*, 1984, 36(6):803-10.
Rodvold KA, Blum RA, Fischer JH, et al, "Vancomycin Pharmacokinetics in Patients With Various Degrees of Renal Function," *Antimicrob Agents Chemother*, 1988, 32(6):848-52.

Vantin® *see* Cefpodoxime *on page 186*
Vaponefrin® *see* Epinephrine *on page 336*

Varicella-Zoster Immune Globulin (Human)
(var i SEL a- ZOS ter i MYUN GLOB yoo lin HYU man)

Related Information
Immunization Guidelines *on page 1058*

Synonyms VZIG

Therapeutic Category Immune Globulin

Use Passive immunization of susceptible immunodeficient patients after exposure to varicella

Contraindications Allergic response to gamma globulin or anti-immunoglobulin; sensitivity to thimerosal; persons with IgA deficiency; do not administer to patients with thrombocytopenia or coagulopathies

Warnings Do not administer I.V.; caution in patients with sensitivity to human immunoglobulin preparations

Precautions Skin test should not be performed to determine if patient is sensitive to agent

Adverse Reactions
Cardiovascular: Local edema
Central nervous system: Lethargy, fever, chills
Dermatologic: Urticaria, angioedema
Gastrointestinal: Nausea
Local: Pain, redness
Neuromuscular & skeletal: Muscle stiffness, tenderness, myalgia
Respiratory: Chest tightness

Drug Interactions Live virus vaccines; do not administer immune globulin within 3 months of immunization

Stability Refrigerate at 2°C to 8°C (36°F to 46°F)

Usual Dosage I.M. (do not inject I.V.): Administer by deep injection in the gluteal muscle or in another large muscle mass. Inject 125 units/10 kg (22

pounds); maximum dose: 625 units (5 vials); minimum dose: 125 units; do not administer fractional doses.

Patient Information Be aware of adverse reactions

Nursing Implications Administer as soon as possible after presumed exposure; do not inject I.V.; administer by deep I.M. injection into gluteal muscle or other large muscle; administer entire contents of each vial (see Usual Dosage)

Special Geriatric Considerations VZIG provides passive immunity for those susceptible to varicella; neoplastic disease, immunosuppressed elderly, or institutionalized who are exposed to other patients with varicella; CDC provides specific guidelines for use. Age is the most important risk factor for reactivation of varicella zoster; persons <50 years of age have incidence of 2.5 cases per 1000, whereas those 60-79 have 6.5 cases per 1000 and those >80 years have 10 cases per 1000

Dosage Forms Injection: 125 units of antibody in single dose vials

Vascor® see Bepridil on page 112

Vasocidin® Ophthalmic see Sulfacetamide Sodium and Prednisolone on page 875

VasoClear® Ophthalmic [OTC] see Naphazoline on page 653

Vasocon-A® [OTC] Ophthalmic see Naphazoline and Antazoline on page 654

Vasocon Regular® Ophthalmic see Naphazoline on page 653

Vasodilan® see Isoxsuprine on page 507

Vasopressin (vay soe PRES in)

Brand Names Pitressin® Injection

Synonyms ADH; Antidiuretic Hormone; 8-Arginine Vasopressin

Therapeutic Category Antidiuretic Hormone Analog; Hormone, Posterior Pituitary

Use Treatment of diabetes insipidus; prevention and treatment of postoperative abdominal distention; differential diagnosis of diabetes insipidus

Unlabeled use: Adjunct in the treatment of GI hemorrhage and esophageal varices

Contraindications Hypersensitivity to vasopressin or any component; chronic nephritis with nitrogen retention

Warnings I.V. infiltration may lead to severe vasoconstriction and localized tissue necrosis; also gangrene of extremities, tongue, and ischemic colitis

Precautions Use with caution in patients with seizure disorders, migraine, asthma, vascular disease, renal disease, cardiac disease (may precipitate anginal pain or myocardial infarction)

Adverse Reactions

Cardiovascular: Pounding in the head, increased blood pressure, bradycardia, arrhythmias, venous thrombosis, vasoconstriction with higher doses, angina, cardiac arrest

Central nervous system: Vertigo, fever

Dermatologic: Urticaria

Endocrine & metabolic: Water intoxication

Gastrointestinal: Abdominal cramps, nausea, vomiting, flatus

Neuromuscular & skeletal: Tremors

Respiratory: Wheezing

Miscellaneous: Diaphoresis

Overdosage Symptoms of overdose include drowsiness, weight gain, confusion, listlessness

Toxicology Restrict fluids and withdraw vasopressin until polyuria; may require treatment with osmotic diuretics or furosemide

Drug Interactions Lithium, epinephrine, demeclocycline, heparin, and alcohol block antidiuretic activity to varying degrees; carbamazepine, chlorpropamide, phenformin, urea and fludrocortisone potentiate antidiuretic response

Stability Store injection at room temperature; protect from heat and from freezing; use only clear solutions

Mechanism of Action Increases cyclic adenosine monophosphate (cAMP) which increases water permeability at the renal tubule resulting in decreased urine volume and increased osmolality; causes peristalsis by directly stimulating the smooth muscle in the GI tract

Pharmacodynamics

Nasal:

Onset of action: 1 hour

Duration: 3-8 hours

(Continued)

Vasopressin *(Continued)*

Parenteral: Duration of action:
Aqueous: 2-8 hours
Tannate: 24-72 hours

Pharmacokinetics Destroyed by trypsin in GI tract, must be administered parenterally or intranasally

Nasal:
Metabolism: In the liver and kidneys
Half-life: 15 minutes
Elimination: In urine
Parenteral:
Metabolism: Most of dose is metabolized by liver and kidney
Half-life: 10-20 minutes
Elimination: 5% of S.C. dose (aqueous) is excreted unchanged in urine after 4 hours

Usual Dosage Geriatrics and Adults:

Diabetes insipidus:
I.M., S.C. (tannate form): Highly variable dosage; titrated based upon serum and urine sodium and osmolality in addition to fluid balance and urine output: 5-10 units 2-4 times/day as needed
Continuous infusion: Initial: 0.5 milliunit/kg/hour (0.0005 unit/kg/hour); titrate up to 2 milliunits/kg/hour; maximum: 10 milliunits/kg/hour

Abdominal distention: I.M.: 5 units stat, 10 units every 3-4 hours
GI hemorrhage: I.V. continuous infusion: Initial: 0.2-0.4 unit/minute, then titrate dose as needed

Monitoring Parameters EKG, serum and urine sodium, urine output, fluid input and output, urine specific gravity, urine and serum osmolality

Reference Range Plasma: 0-2 pg/mL (SI: 0-2 ng/L) if osmolality <285 mOsm/L; 2-12 pg/mL (SI: 2-12 ng/L) if osmolality >290 mOsm/L

Test Interactions Decreased sodium (S)

Patient Information If nausea, abdominal cramping, or blanching of the skin occurs, take 1-2 glasses of water with each dose

Nursing Implications Before withdrawing a dose, vasopressin tannate in oil should be shaken thoroughly to obtain a uniform suspension; vasopressin tannate in oil must not be administered I.V.; monitor fluid I & O; watch for signs of I.V. infiltration and gangrene

Special Geriatric Considerations Elderly patients should be cautioned not to increase their fluid intake beyond that sufficient to satisfy their thirst in order to avoid water intoxication and hyponatremia; under experimental conditions, the elderly have shown to have a decreased responsiveness to vasopressin with respect to its effects on water homeostasis

Dosage Forms
Injection: 20 units/mL (0.5 mL, 1 mL)
Injection, as tannate (in oil): 5 units/mL (1 mL)

References
Lindeman RD, Lee TD Jr, Yiengst MJ, et al, "Influence of Age, Renal Disease, Hypertension, Diuretics, and Calcium on the Antidiuretic Responses to Suboptimal Infusions of Vasopressin," *J Lab Clin Med*, 1966, 68(2):206-23.
Miller JH and Shock NW, "Age Differences in the Renal Tubular Response to Antidiuretic Hormone," *J Gerontol*, 1953, 8:446-50.

Vasosulf® Ophthalmic *see* Sulfacetamide Sodium and Phenylephrine *on page 875*

Vasotec® I.V. *see* Enalapril *on page 329*

Vasotec® Oral *see* Enalapril *on page 329*

V-Cillin K® *see* Penicillin V Potassium *on page 725*

Veetids® *see* Penicillin V Potassium *on page 725*

Velosef® *see* Cephradine *on page 198*

Velosulin® Human *see* Insulin Preparations *on page 488*

Veltane® *see* Brompheniramine *on page 129*

Venlafaxine *(VEN la faks een)*

Related Information
Antidepressant Agents Comparison *on page 1021*
Antidepressant Medication Guidelines *on page 1075*

Brand Names Effexor®

Therapeutic Category Antidepressant

Use Treatment of depression

Contraindications Hypersensitivity to venlafaxine or any component; patients receiving MAO inhibitors within the past 14 days; MAO inhibitors should not be initiated within 7 days of discontinuing venlafaxine

Precautions Sustained hypertension (increased diastolic blood pressure) which is dose related, reduced clearance in persons with impaired renal or hepatic impairment; use with caution in patients with a history of mania, history of seizures; taper dose when discontinuing after therapy of 1 week or longer

Adverse Reactions

Cardiovascular: Hypertension, tachycardia

Central nervous system: Headache, somnolence, dizziness, insomnia, nervousness, anxiety

Gastrointestinal: Nausea, xerostomia, constipation, anorexia, diarrhea, vomiting

Genitourinary: Abnormal ejaculation/orgasm, impotence (men)

Neuromuscular & skeletal: Tremors, weakness

Ocular: Blurred vision

Miscellaneous: Diaphoresis

Overdosage Symptoms of overdosage include somnolence, convulsions, coma, mild sinus tachycardia

Toxicology In overdose, maintain adequate airway and oxygenation and other supportive measures and symptomatic treatment; removal of venlafaxine from the gastrointestinal tract may be achieved with activated charcoal, emesis, or gastric lavage; hemodialysis, hemoperfusion, exchange transfusion, and forced diuresis will not remove substantial amounts of venlafaxine due to its large volume of distribution; monitor cardiac rhythm and vital signs

Drug Interactions Cimetidine reduced the clearance of venlafaxine and increased its serum concentration; MAO inhibitors (see Precautions)

Mechanism of Action Venlafaxine and metabolite o-desmethylvenlafaxine inhibit the reuptake of serotonin and norepinephrine and weakly inhibit the reuptake of dopamine

Pharmacodynamics Onset of action: 1-3 weeks; 5-HT = NE

Pharmacokinetics

Absorption: 92% to 100%; not affected by food

Distribution: V_d: 7.5 L/kg

Protein binding, plasma: 27% to 30%

Metabolism: Major active metabolite o-desmethylvenlafaxine (OVD); 2 less active metabolites; metabolic pathway (first-pass) are saturable; substrate CYP2D6, 3A4; inhibitor CYP2D6

Peak concentration: 1.8-3 hours

Half-life (prolonged in renal and hepatic impairment):

Venlafaxine: 5 hours

OVD: 11 hours

Elimination: 1% to 10% excreted unchanged in urine; 30% OVD, 26% conjugated OVD, and 27% other metabolites

Not readily dialyzed

Usual Dosage When discontinuing this medication, it is imperative to taper the dose; if venlafaxine is used >6 weeks, the dose should be tapered over 2 weeks when discontinuing its use

Geriatrics: No specific recommendations, but may be best to start lower at 25-50 mg twice daily and increase as tolerated by 25 mg/dose

Adults: Oral: 75 mg/day, administered in 2 or 3 divided doses, taken with food; dose may be increased to 150 mg/day up to 225-375 mg/day

Dosing adjustment in renal impairment: Reduce dose by 25% in mild-moderate impairment (Cl_{cr} 10-70 mL/minute); reduce dose by 50% and hold dose until a dialysis in dialysis patients

Dosing adjustment in hepatic impairment: Reduce dose by 50% or more

Administration May be administered with food; if switching from a MAO inhibitor to venlafaxine, allow 2 weeks "washout" period before starting venlafaxine; allow 7 days "washout" if switching venlafaxine therapy to a MAO inhibitor

Monitoring Parameters Signs and symptoms of depression, weight; blood pressure

Reference Range Not established

Test Interactions Increase in serum cholesterol (mean: 3 mg/dL)

Patient Information Use caution when driving or operating machinery; advise physician and pharmacist of any changes or additions in drug therapy; avoid alcohol; notify physician of rash or any other adverse event; may cause dry mouth, increased blood pressure

(Continued)

Venlafaxine *(Continued)*

Nursing Implications See Monitoring Parameters

Special Geriatric Considerations Has not been studied exclusively in the elderly, however, its low anticholinergic activity, minimal sedation, and hypotension makes this a potentially valuable antidepressant in treating elderly with depression. No dose adjustment is necessary for age alone, additional studies are necessary; adjust dose for renal function in elderly (see Usual Dosage).

Dosage Forms Tablet: 25 mg, 37.5 mg, 50 mg, 75 mg, 100 mg

Venoglobulin®-I *see* Immune Globulin *on page 482*

Ventolin® *see* Albuterol *on page 29*

Ventolin® Rotocaps® *see* Albuterol *on page 29*

Verapamil *(ver AP a mil)*

Related Information

Calcium Channel Blocking Agents Comparison *on page 1027*
I.V. Push Recommended Guidelines *on page 1083*

Brand Names Calan®; Calan® SR; Covera-HS®; Isoptin®; Isoptin® SR; Verelan®

Synonyms Iproveratril Hydrochloride

Generic Available Yes

Therapeutic Category Antianginal Agent; Antiarrhythmic Agent, Class IV; Calcium Channel Blocker

Use Angina (vasospastic, chronic stable, and unstable), hypertension; I.V. for supraventricular tachyarrhythmias (PSVT, atrial fibrillation, atrial flutter)

Unlabeled use: Migraine headache, cardiomyopathy, incontinence

Contraindications Sinus bradycardia; advanced heart block; ventricular tachycardia; cardiogenic shock, hypotension, congestive heart failure; hypersensitivity to verapamil or any component, hypersensitivity to calcium channel blockers and adenosine; atrial fibrillation or flutter associated with accessory conduction pathways; not to be given within a few hours of I.V. beta-blocking agents

Warnings Monitor EKG and blood pressure closely in patients receiving I.V. therapy; hypotension, congestive heart failure; cardiac conduction defects, PVCs, idiopathic hypertrophic subaortic stenosis; may cause platelet inhibition; do not abruptly withdraw (chest pain); hepatic dysfunction, renal function impairment, increased angina, decreased neuromuscular transmission with Duchenne's muscular dystrophy; increased intracranial pressure with cranial tumors; elderly may have greater hypotensive effect

The FDA's Cardiovascular and Renal Drug Advisory Committee reviewed current data regarding the risk of heart attacks in patients treated with calcium channel blockers and determined that as a class, the calcium channel antagonists are safe; however, they warned that short-acting nifedipine could increase the risk of myocardial infarction in some patients. The committee was in agreement with a statement issued September, 1995 by the National Heart Lung, and Blood Institute of the National Institute of Health, that warned that short-acting nifedipine should be used with great caution especially at higher doses.

Precautions Sick sinus syndrome, severe left ventricular dysfunction, congestive heart failure, hepatic or renal impairment, hypertrophic cardiomyopathy (especially obstructive), concomitant therapy with beta-blockers or digoxin, edema

Adverse Reactions

Cardiovascular: Hypotension, bradycardia, first, second, or third degree A-V block, worsening heart failure, palpitations, congestive heart failure, myocardial infarction, angina, tachycardia, peripheral edema

Central nervous system: Dizziness, headache, fatigue, seizures (occasionally with I.V. use), lightheadedness, psychotic symptoms, insomnia

Gastrointestinal: Constipation (more of a problem in elderly), nausea, abdominal discomfort, diarrhea, xerostomia

Genitourinary: Urinary incontinence

Hepatic: Increase in hepatic enzymes

Neuromuscular & skeletal: Paresthesia, weakness

Ocular: Blurred vision

Respiratory: May precipitate insufficiency of respiratory muscle function in Duchenne muscular dystrophy

Miscellaneous: Gingival swelling and inflammation

Overdosage Symptoms of overdose include heartblock, hypotension, asystole, nausea, weakness, dizziness, drowsiness, confusion and slurred speech; profound bradycardia and occasionally hyperglycemia

Toxicology Ipecac-induced emesis can hypothetically worsen calcium antagonist toxicity, since it can produce vagal stimulation. The potential for seizures precipitously following acute ingestion of large doses of a calcium antagonist may also contraindicate the use of ipecac. Supportive and symptomatic treatment, including I.V. fluids and Trendelenburg positioning, should be initiated as intoxication may cause hypotension. Although calcium (calcium chloride I.V. 1-2 g over 5-10 minutes with repeats as needed) has been used as an "antidote" for acute intoxications, there is limited experience to support its routine use and should be reserved for those cases where definite signs of myocardial depression are evident. Heart block may respond to isoproterenol, glucagon, atropine and/or calcium although a temporary pacemaker may be required.

Drug Interactions

Increased cardiovascular adverse effects with beta-adrenergic blocking agents, digoxin, quinidine, and disopyramide

Verapamil may increase serum concentrations of digoxin, quinidine, carbamazepine, prazosin, and cyclosporine necessitating a decrease in dosage

Phenobarbital, rifabutin, and rifampin may decrease verapamil serum concentrations by increased hepatic metabolism

Erythromycin, itraconazole, ketoconazole, protease inhibitors, and other CYP3A4 inhibitors may decrease verapamil's metabolism

Avoid combination with disopyramide, discontinue disopyramide 48 hours before starting therapy, do not restart until 24 hours after verapamil has been discontinued

May interfere with lithium control

May increase pharmacologic action of theophylline

Stability Store injection at room temperature; protect from heat and from freezing; use only clear solutions; compatible in solutions of pH of 3-6, but may precipitate in solutions having a pH of ≥6

Mechanism of Action Inhibits calcium ion from entering the "slow channels" or select voltage-sensitive areas of vascular smooth muscle and myocardium during depolarization; produces a relaxation of coronary vascular smooth muscle and coronary vasodilation; increases myocardial oxygen delivery in patients with vasospastic angina

Pharmacodynamics

Duration:

Oral: 6-8 hours; elderly have greater hypotensive effect than younger adults

I.V.: 10-20 minutes

Peak effects:

Oral (nonsustained tablets): 2 hours

I.V.: 1-5 minutes

Pharmacokinetics

Protein binding: 90%

Metabolism: In the liver; extensive first-pass effect; substrate CYP1A2, 3A4

Bioavailability: Oral: 20% to 30%

Half-life (single dose) (adults): 2-8 hours, increased up to 12 hours with multiple dosing; elderly have increased half-life: 7-8 hours; increased half-life with hepatic cirrhosis

Elimination: 70% in urine (3% to 4% as unchanged drug), and 16% in feces

Usual Dosage Geriatrics and Adults:

Oral: 120-480 mg/24 hours divided 3-4 times/day

Sustained release:

Geriatrics: 120 mg/day; adjust dose after 24 hours by increases of 120 mg/day; when switching from immediate release forms, total daily dose may remain the same. Controlled onset: initiate therapy with 180 mg in the evening; titrate upward as needed to obtain desired response and avoiding adverse effects.

Adults: 240 mg/day

I.V.: 5-10 mg (0.075-0.15 mg/kg); may repeat 10 mg (0.15 mg/kg) 15-30 minutes after the initial dose if needed and if patient tolerated initial dose

Not dialyzable (0% to 5%)

Monitoring Parameters Heart rate, blood pressure, signs and symptoms of congestive heart failure

Reference Range Therapeutic: 50-200 ng/mL (SI: 100-410 nmol/L) for parent; under normal conditions norverapamil concentration is the same as parent drug; Toxic: >90 µg/mL

(Continued)

987

Verapamil *(Continued)*

Patient Information Sustained release products should be taken with food and not crushed or chewed; limit caffeine intake; avoid alcohol; notify physician if angina pain is not reduced when taking this drug, irregular heartbeat, shortness of breath, swelling, dizziness, constipation, nausea, or hypotension occur; do not stop therapy without advice of physician

Nursing Implications Help patient with ambulation; monitor blood pressure closely; administer around-the-clock rather than 4 times/day, 3 times/day, etc (ie, 12-6-12-6, not 9-1-5-9) to promote less variation in peak and trough serum concentrations; I.V. rate of infusion is over 2 minutes; do not crush sustained release drug product

Additional Information Incidence of adverse reactions is most common with I.V. administration; discontinue disopyramide 48 hours before starting therapy, do not restart therapy until 24 hours after verapamil has been discontinued

Special Geriatric Considerations Elderly may experience a greater hypotensive response; constipation may be more of a problem in elderly; calcium channel blockers are no more effective in elderly than other therapies; however, they do not cause significant CNS effects which is an advantage over some antihypertensive agents; generic verapamil products which are bioequivalent in young adults may not be bioequivalent in elderly; use generics cautiously (see Pharmacodynamics)

Dosage Forms

Verapamil hydrochloride:

Capsule, sustained release (Verelan®): 120 mg, 180 mg, 240 mg, 360 mg

Injection: 2.5 mg/mL (2 mL, 4 mL)

Isoptin®: 2.5 mg/mL (2 mL, 4 mL)

Tablet: 40 mg, 80 mg, 120 mg

Calan®, Isoptin®: 40 mg, 80 mg, 120 mg

Tablet, sustained release: 180 mg, 240 mg

Calan® SR, Isoptin® SR: 120 mg, 180 mg, 240 mg

Covera-HS®: 180 mg, 240 mg

References

Carter BL, Noyes MA, and Demmler RW, "Differences in Serum Concentrations of and Responses to Generic Verapamil in the Elderly," *Pharmacotherapy*, 1993, 13(4):359-68.

Verazinc® Oral [OTC] *see* Zinc Sulfate *on page 995*

Verelan® *see* Verapamil *on page 986*

Vergon® [OTC] *see* Meclizine *on page 574*

Vermizine® *see* Piperazine *on page 755*

Versed® *see* Midazolam *on page 626*

Vexol® *see* Rimexolone *on page 834*

Vibramycin® Injection *see* Doxycycline *on page 322*

Vibramycin® Oral *see* Doxycycline *on page 322*

Vibra-Tabs® *see* Doxycycline *on page 322*

Vicks® 44E [OTC] *see* Guaifenesin and Dextromethorphan *on page 439*

Vicks® DayQuil® Allergy Relief 4 Hour Tablet [OTC] *see* Brompheniramine and Phenylpropanolamine *on page 130*

Vicks Formula 44® [OTC] *see* Dextromethorphan *on page 278*

Vicks® Formula 44® Pediatric Formula [OTC] *see* Dextromethorphan *on page 278*

Vicks® Pediatric Formula 44E [OTC] *see* Guaifenesin and Dextromethorphan *on page 439*

Vicks Sinex® Nasal Solution [OTC] *see* Phenylephrine *on page 740*

Vicodin® *see* Hydrocodone and Acetaminophen *on page 461*

Vicodin® ES *see* Hydrocodone and Acetaminophen *on page 461*

Vicodin® HP *see* Hydrocodone and Acetaminophen *on page 461*

Vidarabine *(vye DARE a been)*

Brand Names Vira-A® Ophthalmic

Synonyms Adenine Arabinoside; Ara-A; Arabinofuranosyladenine

Generic Available No

Therapeutic Category Antiviral Agent, Ophthalmic

Use Treatment of acute keratoconjunctivitis and epithelial keratitis due to herpes simplex virus; definitive diagnosis of herpes simplex conjunctivitis should be made before instituting ophthalmic therapy

Contraindications Hypersensitivity to vidarabine or any component

Adverse Reactions

Local: Burning, lacrimation, pain

Ocular: Keratitis, photophobia, foreign body sensation, uveitis, stromal edema, blurred vision

Mechanism of Action Inhibits viral DNA synthesis by blocking DNA polymerase

Usual Dosage Geriatrics and Adults: Ophthalmic: Keratoconjunctivitis: Instill ½" of ointment in lower conjunctival sac 5 times/day every 3 hours while awake until complete re-epithelialization has occurred, then twice daily for an additional 7 days

Patient Information Do not use eye make-up when on this medication for ophthalmic infection; use sunglasses if photophobic reaction occurs; may cause blurred vision; notify physician if improvement not seen after 7 days or if condition worsens

Special Geriatric Considerations Assess ability to self-administer ophthalmic ointment; no specific recommendations for use in the elderly (see Usual Dosage)

Dosage Forms Ointment, ophthalmic, as monohydrate: 3% [30 mg/g = 28 mg/g base] (3.5 g)

Videx® Oral *see Didanosine on page 286*

Viokase® *see Pancrelipase on page 712*

Viosterol *see Ergocalciferol on page 340*

Vira-A® Ophthalmic *see Vidarabine on previous page*

Virazole® *see Ribavirin on page 828*

Virilon® *see Methyltestosterone on page 613*

Viroptic® Ophthalmic *see Trifluridine on page 958*

Visine® Extra Ophthalmic [OTC] *see Tetrahydrozoline on page 901*

Visine® L.R. Ophthalmic [OTC] *see Oxymetazoline on page 706*

Visine® Ophthalmic [OTC] *see Tetrahydrozoline on page 901*

Visken® *see Pindolol on page 751*

Vistacon-50® *see Hydroxyzine on page 470*

Vistaquel® *see Hydroxyzine on page 470*

Vistaril® *see Hydroxyzine on page 470*

Vistazine® *see Hydroxyzine on page 470*

Vita-C® [OTC] *see Ascorbic Acid on page 82*

Vitamin B$_1$ *see Thiamine on page 906*

Vitamin B$_3$ *see Niacin on page 665*

Vitamin B$_3$ *see Niacinamide on page 666*

Vitamin B$_6$ *see Pyridoxine on page 807*

Vitamin B$_{12}$ *see Cyanocobalamin on page 257*

Vitamin B$_{12}$ *see Hydroxocobalamin on page 466*

Vitamin C *see Ascorbic Acid on page 82*

Vitamin D$_2$ *see Ergocalciferol on page 340*

Vitamin K$_1$ *see Phytonadione on page 747*

Vitrasert® *see Ganciclovir on page 419*

Vivactil® *see Protriptyline on page 801*

Viva-Drops® Solution [OTC] *see Artificial Tears on page 82*

Vivelle® Transdermal *see Estradiol on page 350*

Vivotif Berna™ Oral *see Typhoid Vaccine on page 973*

V-Lax® [OTC] *see Psyllium on page 804*

Volmax® *see Albuterol on page 29*

Voltaren® Ophthalmic *see Diclofenac on page 281*

Voltaren® Oral *see Diclofenac on page 281*

Voltaren-XR® Oral *see Diclofenac on page 281*

VZIG *see Varicella-Zoster Immune Globulin (Human) on page 982*

Warfarin *(WAR far in)*

Related Information

American Geriatrics Society Current Standards of Practice - Oral Anticoagulation for Older Adults *on page 1069*

Anticoagulant Therapy Guidelines *on page 1069*

Serum Drug Concentrations Commonly Monitored: Guidelines *on page 1114*

Brand Names Coumadin®

Generic Available Yes: Tablet

Therapeutic Category Anticoagulant

(Continued)

Warfarin *(Continued)*

Use Prophylaxis and treatment of venous thrombosis, pulmonary embolism and thromboembolic disorders; atrial fibrillation with embolism and as an adjunct in the prophylaxis of systemic embolism after myocardial infarction.

Unlabeled use: Prevention of recurrent transient ischemic attacks and to reduce risk of recurrent myocardial infarction

Contraindications Hypersensitivity to warfarin or any component; severe liver or kidney disease; open wounds; uncontrolled bleeding; GI ulcers; neurosurgical procedures; malignant hypertension

Warnings Concomitant use with vitamin K may decrease anticoagulant effect; monitor carefully; concomitant use with ethacrynic acid, indomethacin, mefenamic acid, phenylbutazone, or aspirin increases warfarin's anticoagulant effect and may cause severe GI irritation

Precautions Do not switch brands once desired therapeutic response has been achieved

Adverse Reactions

Central nervous system: Fever

Dermatologic: Skin lesions, alopecia

Gastrointestinal: Anorexia, nausea, vomiting, diarrhea

Hematologic: Hemorrhage

Respiratory: Hemoptysis

Overdosage Symptoms of overdose include internal or external hemorrhage, hematuria

Toxicology Avoid emesis and lavage to avoid the possible trauma and incidental bleeding. When a large or chronic ingestion occurs vitamin K_1 (phytonadione) should be administered 10-15 mg I.M./I.V.; when hemorrhaging occurs whole blood or plasma transfusions can help control bleeding by replacing clotting factors

Drug Interactions Amiodarone, metronidazole, anabolic steroids, chloral hydrate, clofibrate, disulfiram, nonsteroidal anti-inflammatory agents, chloramphenicol, cimetidine, salicylates, streptokinase, urokinase, sulfonamides, ketoconazole, sucralfate, phenylbutazone, quinolones, corticosteroids, SSRIs, zileuton, erythromycin, omeprazole, isoniazid, phenytoin may increase the effects of warfarin; alcohol, cholestyramine, sucralfate, barbiturates, trazodone, carbamazepine, rifampin, and estrogens may decrease the effects of warfarin; caution must be observed when any drug is added to or deleted from the therapeutic regimen of a patient receiving warfarin

Mechanism of Action Interferes with hepatic synthesis of vitamin K-dependent coagulation factors (II, VII, IX, X)

Pharmacodynamics

Onset of action: Following rapid oral absorption, anticoagulation effects occur within 36-72 hours

Peak effect: Within 5-7 days; the elderly are more sensitive to the effects of warfarin and usually respond to a lower mg/day dose

Pharmacokinetics

Metabolism: In the liver; substrate CYP1A2, 2C9, 2C18, 2A6, 3A4

Half-life: 42 hours, highly variable among individuals

The pharmacokinetics of warfarin have not been shown to be altered by aging

Usual Dosage

Oral:

Geriatrics: Usual maintenance dose: 2-5 mg/day

Adults: 5-15 mg/day for 2-5 days, then adjust dose according to results of prothrombin time; usual maintenance dose range: 2-10 mg/day

I.V.: Geriatrics and Adults (administer as a slow bolus injection): 2-5 mg/day

Monitoring Parameters Prothrombin time (PT), PT ratio, international normalization ratio (INR); stool guaiac for blood; hemoglobin, hematocrit

Reference Range See Appendix for tables on oral anticoagulation for older adults

Patient Information Do not take with food; report any signs of bleeding; avoid hazardous activities; use soft tooth brush; urine may turn red/orange; carry Medi-Alert® ID identifying drug usage; consult physician and dentist before dental procedures; be sure of other drugs (aspirin and alcohol) and foods to avoid; report any bleeding, red or dark urine, red or tarry black stools to physician at once

Nursing Implications Avoid all I.M. injections; monitor patient for signs and symptoms of bleeding

Special Geriatric Considerations Before committing an elderly patient to long-term anticoagulation therapy, their risk for bleeding complications secondary to falls, drug interactions, living situation, and cognitive status should be considered. The risk for bleeding complications decreases with the duration of therapy and has been associated with increased age. See Appendix for tables on oral anticoagulation for older adults and see Drug Interactions, Pharmacodynamics, and Usual Dosage.

Dosage Forms
Warfarin sodium:
  Powder for injection, lyophilized: 2 mg
  Tablet: 1 mg, 2 mg, 2.5 mg, 4 mg, 5 mg, 7.5 mg, 10 mg

References
Gurwitz JH, Avorn J, Ross-Degnan D, et al, "Aging and the Anticoagulant Response to Warfarin Therapy," *Ann Intern Med*, 1992, 116(11):901-4.

Redwood M, Taylor C, Bain BJ, et al, "The Association of Age With Dosage Requirement for Warfarin," *Age Ageing*, 1991, 20(3):217-20.

Shepherd AM, Hewick DS, Moreland TA, et al, "Age as a Determinant of Sensitivity to Warfarin," *Br J Clin Pharmacol*, 1977, 4(3):315-20.

Wart-Off® [OTC] see Salicylic Acid *on page 845*

4-Way® Long Acting Nasal Solution [OTC] see Oxymetazoline *on page 706*

Wellbutrin® see Bupropion *on page 134*

Wellbutrin® SR see Bupropion *on page 134*

Westcort® see Hydrocortisone *on page 462*

Westrim® LA [OTC] see Phenylpropanolamine *on page 741*

White Mineral Oil see Mineral Oil *on page 628*

Wigraine® see Ergotamine *on page 343*

40 Winks® [OTC] see Diphenhydramine *on page 302*

Wycillin® see Penicillin G Procaine *on page 723*

Wydase® Injection see Hyaluronidase *on page 455*

Wygesic® see Propoxyphene and Acetaminophen *on page 796*

Wymox® see Amoxicillin *on page 67*

Wytensin® see Guanabenz *on page 440*

Xalatan® see Latanoprost *on page 527*

Xanax® see Alprazolam *on page 37*

Xero-Lube® [OTC] see Saliva Substitute *on page 846*

X-Prep® Liquid [OTC] see Senna *on page 853*

Xylocaine® see Lidocaine *on page 537*

Xylometazoline (zye loe met AZ oh leen)

Related Information
Antacid Drug Interactions *on page 1096*

Brand Names Otrivin® [OTC]

Generic Available Yes

Therapeutic Category Adrenergic Agonist Agent; Decongestant, Nasal; Nasal Agent, Vasoconstrictor; Sympathomimetic

Use Symptomatic relief of nasal and nasopharyngeal mucosal congestion

Contraindications Known hypersensitivity to xylometazoline hydrochloride, narrow-angle glaucoma, patients receiving MAO inhibitors

Warnings Excessive use may cause rebound congestion or chemical rhinitis; use with caution in patients with hypertension, diabetes, cardiovascular or coronary artery disease, hyperthyroidism, long-standing bronchial asthma

Adverse Reactions
Cardiovascular: Palpitations
Central nervous system: Drowsiness, dizziness, seizures, headache
Ocular: Blurred vision, ocular irritation, photophobia
Miscellaneous: Diaphoresis

Overdosage Symptoms of overdose include CNS depression, hypothermia, bradycardia, cardiovascular collapse, coma, respiratory depression, apnea

Toxicology Following initiation of essential overdose management, toxic symptoms should be treated. The patient should be kept warm and monitored for alterations in vital functions. Seizures commonly respond to diazepam (5-10 mg I.V. bolus in adults every 15 minutes if needed up to a total of 30 mg) or to phenytoin or phenobarbital. Apnea may respond to naloxone.

Drug Interactions Increased toxicity: MAO inhibitors

Mechanism of Action Stimulates alpha-adrenergic receptors in the arterioles of the conjunctiva and the nasal mucosa to produce vasoconstriction

Pharmacodynamics
Onset of action: Intranasal: Local vasoconstriction occurs within 5-10 minutes
Duration: 5-6 hours
(Continued)

Xylometazoline *(Continued)*

Usual Dosage Geriatrics and Adults: Instill 2-3 drops or sprays (0.1%) in each nostril every 8-10 hours

Monitoring Parameters Blood pressure in hypertensive patients

Patient Information Do not exceed recommended dosage; do not use for more than 4 consecutive days; if symptoms persist, drug should be discontinued and a physician consulted; notify physician of insomnia, tremor, or irregular heartbeat; burning, stinging, or drying of the nasal mucosa may occur

Special Geriatric Considerations Evaluate the patient's ability to self-administer; use with caution in patients with cardiovascular disease

Dosage Forms Solution, nasal, as hydrochloride: 0.05% [0.5 mg/mL] (20 mL); 0.1% [1 mg/mL] (15 mL, 20 mL)

Yellow Fever Vaccine (YEL oh FEE ver vak SEEN)

Related Information

Immunization Guidelines *on page 1058*

Brand Names YF-VAX®

Generic Available No

Therapeutic Category Vaccine, Live Virus

Use Selected persons traveling or living in areas where yellow fever infection exists. Some countries require a valid international Certification of Vaccination showing receipt of vaccine; if a pregnant woman is to be vaccinated only to satisfy an international requirement, efforts should be made to obtain a waiver letter.

Contraindications Sensitivity to egg or chick embryo protein; any form of immunodeficiency

Warnings Do not use in any immunodeficient patient (contains live virus); do not administer to patients hypersensitive to egg or chicken protein. Do intradermal testing in patients in whom this is suspected or questionable.

Precautions Do not vaccinate within 8 weeks following blood or plasma transfusion

Adverse Reactions

Central nervous system: Fever, malaise (usually appearing 7-14 days after vaccination), headache, encephalitis in very young infants (rare)

Neuromuscular & skeletal: Myalgia

Miscellaneous: Anaphylaxis (even with no history of hypersensitivity)

Drug Interactions Administer yellow fever vaccine at least 1 month apart from other live virus vaccines; defer vaccination for 8 weeks following blood, plasma, or immune globulin

Stability Yellow fever vaccine is shipped with dry ice; do not use vaccine unless shipping case contains some dry ice upon arrival; maintain vaccine continuously at a temperature between 0°C to 5°C (32°F to 41°F); use within 60 minutes after reconstitution. Sterilize and discard unused reconstituted vaccine after 1 hour. Shelf life is 12 months.

Usual Dosage Geriatrics and Adults: S.C.: One dose of 0.5 mL 10 days to 10 years before travel, booster every 10 years; reconstitute only diluent supplied; will be opalescent and light orange when mixed; let mixture stand for 1-2 minutes before administering; avoid vigorous shaking

Monitoring Parameters Monitor for adverse effects which may be seen 7-14 days after vaccination

Patient Information Immunity develops by the tenth day and **WHO** requires revaccination every 10 years to maintain travelers' vaccination certificates

Nursing Implications Sterilize and discard all unused rehydrated vaccine and containers after 1 hour; avoid vigorous shaking; administer S.C.

Additional Information Federal law requires that the date of administration, the vaccine manufacturer, lot number of vaccine, and the administering person's name, title and address be entered into the patient's permanent medical record; the World Health Organization (WHO) requires revaccination every 10 years to maintain traveler's vaccination certificates

Special Geriatric Considerations No special considerations except in patients with immunodeficient diseases

Dosage Forms Injection: Not less than 5.04 Log_{10} Plaque Forming Units (PFU) per 0.5 mL

YF-VAX® *see Yellow Fever Vaccine on this page*

Yodoxin® *see Iodoquinol on page 494*

Zafirlukast (za FIR loo kast)

Related Information

    Asthma Guidelines *on page 1040*

Brand Names Accolate®

Generic Available No

Therapeutic Category Leukotriene Receptor Antagonist

Use Prophylaxis and chronic treatment of asthma

Contraindications Hypersensitivity to zafirlukast or any of its inactive ingredients

Warnings The clearance of zafirlukast is reduced in patients with stable alcoholic cirrhosis such that the C_{max} and AUC are approximately 50% to 60% greater than those of normal adults.

Zafirlukast is not indicated for use in the reversal of bronchospasm in an acute asthma attacks, including status asthmaticus. Therapy, however, can be continued during acute exacerbations of asthma.

An increased proportion of zafirlukast patients reported respiratory infections during clinical trials.

Use cautiously and monitor closely in patients with hepatic impairment; clearance is reduced

Precautions A single report of symptomatic hepatitis has been published

Adverse Reactions

    Central nervous system: Headache (12.9%), dizziness, pain, fever, asthenia

    Gastrointestinal: Nausea, diarrhea, abdominal pain, vomiting, dyspepsia

    Neuromuscular & skeletal: Myalgia, weakness

Overdosage There is no experience to date with zafirlukast overdose in humans

Toxicology Use supportive treatment measures

Drug Interactions Cytochrome P-450 2C9 and 3A4 isoenzyme inhibitor

    Decreased effect:

        Erythromycin: Coadministration with zafirlukast decreases bioavailability by 40%

        Terfenadine: Coadministration of zafirlukast with terfenadine results in a decrease in the mean C_{max} and AUC of zafirlukast

        Theophylline: Coadministration of zafirlukast with liquid theophylline preparations decreased mean plasma concentrations of zafirlukast by 30%

    Increased effect: Aspirin: Coadministration of zafirlukast with aspirin results in mean increased plasma concentrations of zafirlukast by 45%

    Increased toxicity: Warfarin: Coadministration of zafirlukast with warfarin results in significant increase in prothrombin time (PT). Closely monitor prothrombin times of patients on oral warfarin anticoagulant therapy and zafirlukast, and adjust anticoagulant dose accordingly.

Drug/Food Interactions Food decreases bioavailability of zafirlukast

Stability Store tablets at room temperature (20°C to 25°C; 68°F to 77°F); protect from light and moisture; dispense in original airtight container

Mechanism of Action Zafirlukast is a selectively and competitive leukotriene-receptor antagonist (LTRA) of leukotriene D4 and E4 (LTD4 and LTE4), components of slow-reacting substance of anaphylaxis (SRSA). Cysteinyl leukotriene production and receptor occupation have been shown to be an integral part of asthma, including airway edema, smooth muscle constriction and altered cellular activity associated with the inflammatory process, which contribute to the pathophysiology of asthma.

Pharmacokinetics

    Absorption: Food reduces bioavailability by 40%

    Protein binding: >99%, predominantly albumin

    Metabolism: extensively metabolized by liver via CYP2C9 enzyme pathway; inhibitor CYP2C9, 3A4

    Half-life: 10 hours

    Time to peak serum concentration: 3 hours

    Elimination: Urinary excretion (10%) and feces

Usual Dosage Geriatrics and Adults: Oral: 20 mg twice daily

    Dosing adjustment in renal impairment: There are no apparent differences in the pharmacokinetics between renally impaired patients and normal subjects

    Dosing adjustment in hepatic impairment: In patients with hepatic impairment, there is a greater C_{max} and AUC compared to normal subjects

Administration Take at least 1 hour before or 2 hours after a meal

Monitoring Parameters Monitor pulmonary function tests and symptomatic effects

(Continued)

Zafirlukast *(Continued)*

Patient Information Do not use to treat acute episodes of asthma. Do not increase or decrease the dose without consulting your physician.

Special Geriatric Considerations No specific data for elderly; in clinical trials, the AUC and C_{max} were increased and clearance was decreased. However, no apparent change in dose needed.

Dosage Forms Tablet: 20 mg

Zileuton *(zye LOO ton)*

Related Information
Asthma Guidelines *on page 1040*

Brand Names Zyflo®

Generic Available No

Therapeutic Category Leukotriene Receptor Antagonist

Use Prophylaxis and chronic treatment of asthma in adults

Contraindications Active liver disease or transaminase elevations greater than or equal to three times the upper limit of normal (≥3 x ULN), hypersensitivity to zileuton or any of its active ingredients

Warnings Elevations of liver function tests may occur during therapy. Evaluation of continuation of therapy should be considered. Follow LFTs closely if a rise is noted. Use with caution in patients who consume quantities of alcohol or have a past history of liver disease. Zileuton is not indicated for use in the reversal of bronchospasm in acute asthma attacks. Zileuton can be continued during acute exacerbations of asthma.

Precautions Monitor LFTs once per month for first 3 months of therapy; every 2-3 months thereafter for first year and periodically thereafter

Adverse Reactions
Cardiovascular: Chest pain
Central nervous system: Headache (24.6%), pain, dizziness, fever, insomnia, malaise, nervousness, somnolence, asthenia
Gastrointestinal: Dyspepsia, nausea, abdominal pain, constipation, flatulence, vomiting
Hematologic: Low white blood cell count, lymphadenopathy
Hepatic: ALT elevation (12%)
Neuromuscular & skeletal: Myalgia, arthralgia, weakness
Ocular: Conjunctivitis

Overdosage Human experience is limited. No deaths occurred, but nephritis was reported in dogs at an oral dose of 1,000 mg/kg. During a clinical study, one patient took 6-9 g in a single dose; vomiting occurred and the patient recovered without incident.

Toxicology Treat symptomatically; institute supportive measures as required. If indicated, achieve elimination of unabsorbed drug by emesis or gastric lavage; observe usual precautions to maintain the airway. Zileuton is **not** removed by dialysis.

Drug Interactions Zileuton is a cytochrome P-450 1A2, 2C9 and 3A4 enzyme substrate
Increased toxicity:
Propranolol: Doubling of propranolol AUC and consequent increased beta-blocker activity
Terfenadine: Decrease in clearance of terfenadine leading to increase in AUC
Theophylline: Doubling of serum theophylline concentrations - reduce theophylline dose and monitor serum theophylline concentrations closely.
Warfarin: Clinically significant increases in prothrombin time (PT) - monitor PT closely

Mechanism of Action Specific inhibitor of 5-lipoxygenase and therefore results in inhibition of leukotriene (LTB1, LTC1, LTD1 and LTE1) formation. Leukotrienes induce numerous biological effects including augmentation of neutrophil and eosinophil migration, neutrophil and monocyte aggregation, leukocyte adhesion, increased capillary permeability and smooth muscle contraction, which contribute to edema, inflammation, increased mucus secretion and bronchoconstriction in patients with asthma.

Pharmacokinetics

Absorption: Oral: Rapidly absorbed

Distribution: 1.2 L/kg

Protein binding: 93%

Metabolism: Several metabolites in plasma and urine; metabolized by the cytochrome P-450 isoenzymes 1A2, 2C9 and 3A4

Half-life: 2.5 hours

Time to peak serum concentration: 1.7 hours

Elimination: Predominantly via metabolism

Dialyzable: Not removed (>0.5%)

Usual Dosage

Geriatrics and Adults: Oral: 600 mg 4 times/day with meals and at bedtime

Dosing adjustment in renal impairment: Dosing adjustment is not necessary in renal impairment, renal failure, or for dialysis

Dosing adjustment in hepatic impairment: Contraindicated in patients with active liver disease

Administration Can be administered without regard to meals (ie, with or without food)

Monitoring Parameters Evaluate hepatic transaminases at initiation of and during therapy with zileuton. Monitor serum ALT before treatment begins, once-a-month for the first 3 months, every 2-3 months for the remainder of the first year, and periodically thereafter for patients receiving long-term zileuton therapy. If liver dysfunction develops or transaminases increase to >5 times the ULN, discontinue therapy and follow transaminase concentrations until within normal limits.

Patient Information Do not use to treat acute episodes of asthma. When taking zileuton, do not increase or decrease the dose unless instructed by a physician.

While using zileuton, seek medical attention if short-acting bronchodilators are needed more often than usual or if more than the maximum number of inhalations of short-acting bronchodilator treatment prescribed for a 24-period are needed.

The most serious side effect of zileuton is elevation of liver enzymes. If patients experience signs or symptoms of liver dysfunction (right upper quadrant pain, nausea, fatigue, lethargy, pruritus, jaundice, or "flu-like" symptoms), contact a physician immediately.

Nursing Implications This is not a bronchodilator; do not use to treat acute bronchospastic events. Monitor liver function tests closely; observe for signs and symptoms of liver side effects.

Special Geriatric Considerations No differences in the pharmacokinetics found between younger adults and elderly; no dosage adjustments necessary. However, monitor liver effects closely as with any patient regardless of age.

Dosage Forms Tablet: 600 mg

Zinacef® Injection see Cefuroxime on page 193

Zincate® Oral see Zinc Sulfate on this page

Zinc Sulfate (zingk SUL fate)

Brand Names Eye-Sed® Ophthalmic [OTC]; Orazinc® Oral [OTC]; Verazinc® Oral [OTC]; Zincate® Oral

Generic Available Yes

Therapeutic Category Mineral, Oral; Trace Element, Parenteral

Use Zinc supplement (oral and parenteral); may improve wound healing in those who are deficient (pressure sores)

Contraindications Hypersensitivity to any component

Warnings Do not use undiluted by direct injection into a peripheral vein because of potential for phlebitis, tissue irritation and potential to increase renal loss of minerals from a bolus injection

Adverse Reactions

Central nervous system: Restlessness, dizziness

Gastrointestinal: Nausea, vomiting, gastric ulcers, diarrhea

(Continued)

Zinc Sulfate *(Continued)*

Overdosage Symptoms of overdose include profuse sweating, decreased consciousness, blurred vision, tachycardia, hypothermia, hyperamylasemia, hypotension, pulmonary edema, diarrhea, vomiting, jaundice, oliguria; impaired lymphocyte and polymorphonuclear leukocyte function and a decrease in high density lipoproteins has been reported with excessive supplementation in healthy persons

Toxicology Emesis should be instituted following ingestion of zinc sulfate except when there is evidence of mucosal burns, instead dilute rapidly with milk or water. Calcium disodium edetate or dimercaprol can be very effective at binding zinc. Supportive care should always be instituted.

Drug Interactions Decreased effect of penicillamine and iron; decreased absorption of some fluoroquinolones, tetracyclines, and iron

Drug/Food Interactions Bran products, dairy products reduce zinc absorption

Stability Store oral liquid (injectable used orally) in refrigerator

Mechanism of Action Provides for normal growth and tissue repair, is a cofactor for more than 70 enzymes; ophthalmic astringent and weak antiseptic due to precipitation of protein and clearing mucus from outer surface of the eye

Pharmacokinetics
Absorption: Zinc and its salts are poorly absorbed from the gastrointestinal tract (20% to 30%)
Elimination: In feces with only traces appearing in urine

Usual Dosage Geriatrics and Adults: Oral: Zinc deficiency: 110-220 mg zinc sulfate (25-50 mg elemental zinc)/dose 3 times/day

Monitoring Parameters Skin integrity

Reference Range Serum: 50-150 µg/dL (<20 µg/dL as solid test with dermatitis followed by alopecia)

Patient Information Take with food if GI upset occurs, but avoid foods high in calcium, phosphorous or phytate (high fiber foods)

Nursing Implications Administer with food if GI upset occurs; avoid foods high in calcium or phosphorus; injection must be diluted before use; refrigerate suspension

Additional Information Zinc acetate can be used as an alternative to zinc sulfate in patients who cannot tolerate the gastrointestinal irritant effects of the sulfate salt

Special Geriatric Considerations May be useful to promote wound healing in patients with pressure sores

Dosage Forms
Capsule: 110 mg, 220 mg
Injection: 1 mg/mL (10 mL, 30 mL); 4 mg/mL (10 mL); 5 mg/mL (5 mL, 10 mL)
Solution, ophthalmic: 0.217% (15 mL)
Tablet: 66 mg, 200 mg

Zithromax™ *see* Azithromycin *on page 101*

Zocor® *see* Simvastatin *on page 857*

Zofran® *see* Ondansetron *on page 694*

Zolicef® *see* Cefazolin *on page 175*

Zoloft™ *see* Sertraline *on page 854*

Zolpidem *(zole Pl dem)*

Related Information
Anxiolytic/Hypnotic Use in Long-Term Care Facilities *on page 1099*

Brand Names Ambien™

Generic Available No

Therapeutic Category Hypnotic; Sedative

Use Short-term treatment of insomnia

Restrictions C-IV

Warnings Closely monitor elderly or debilitated patients for impaired cognitive or motor performance

Precautions Administer with caution to depressed patients; tolerance and withdrawal symptoms are not seen, but caution should be used in patients with a history of drug dependence

Adverse Reactions
Central nervous system: Headache, drowsiness, dizziness
Gastrointestinal: Nausea, diarrhea
Neuromuscular & skeletal: Myalgia

Overdosage Symptoms of overdose include impairment of consciousness, coma

Toxicology Treatment for zolpidem overdose is supportive. Monitor for hypotension and CNS depression; flumazenil may be useful in reversing the hypnotic effects.

Drug Interactions Increased effect/toxicity with alcohol, CNS depressants

Mechanism of Action Structurally dissimilar to benzodiazepines, however, has much or all of its actions explained by its effects on benzodiazepine (BZD) receptors, especially the omega-1 receptor; retains hypnotic and much of the anxiolytic properties of the BZD, but has reduced effects on skeletal muscle and seizure threshold.

Pharmacodynamics
Onset of action: 30 minutes
Duration: 6-8 hours

Pharmacokinetics
Absorption: Rapid
Protein binding: 92%
Metabolism: Hepatic to inactive metabolites
Half-life: 2-2.6 hours, in cirrhosis increased to 9.9 hours; in elderly, maximum AUC and half-life are increased

Usual Dosage Oral (duration of therapy should be limited to 7-10 days):
Geriatrics: 5 mg immediately before bedtime
Adults: 10 mg immediately before bedtime; maximum dose: 10 mg
Dosing adjustment in hepatic impairment: Decrease dose to 5 mg
Not dialyzable

Monitoring Parameters Mental status

Reference Range 80-150 ng/mL

Patient Information Avoid alcohol and other CNS depressants while taking this medication; for fastest onset, take on an empty stomach; may cause daytime drowsiness

Nursing Implications Patients may require assistance with ambulation; lower doses in the elderly are usually effective; institute safety measures; administer on an empty stomach

Additional Information Zolpidem causes less disturbances in sleep stages as compared to benzodiazepines; time spent in sleep stages 3 and 4 are maintained; zolpidem decreases sleep latency

Special Geriatric Considerations In doses >5 mg, there was subjective evidence of impaired sleep on the first post-treatment night; there have been few reports of increased hypotension and/or falls in the elderly with this drug; can be considered a drug of choice in the elderly when a hypnotic is indicated (see Pharmacokinetics and Additional Information)

Dosage Forms Tablet, as tartrate: 5 mg, 10 mg

References
Salva P and Costa J, "Clinical Pharmacokinetics and Pharmacodynamics of Zolpidem. Therapeutic Implications," *Clin Pharmacokinet*, 1995, 29(3):142-53.
Simcox DA, "Zolpidem-Associated Falls," *Consult Pharm*, 1995, 10:1378-80.

Zonalon® Topical Cream see Doxepin on page 321

ZORprin® see Aspirin on page 84

Zostrix® [OTC] see Capsaicin on page 155

Zostrix-® HP [OTC] see Capsaicin on page 155

Zosyn™ see Piperacillin and Tazobactam on page 754

Zovirax® see Acyclovir on page 26

Zyban® see Bupropion on page 134

Zydone® see Hydrocodone and Acetaminophen on page 461

Zyflo® see Zileuton on page 994

Zyloprim® see Allopurinol on page 35

Zymase® see Pancrelipase on page 712

Zymenol® [OTC] see Mineral Oil on page 628

Zyprexa® see Olanzapine on page 689

Zyrtec™ see Cetirizine on page 199

APPENDIX TABLE OF CONTENTS

APPENDIX TABLE OF CONTENTS *(Continued)*

ABBREVIATIONS & SYMBOLS
COMMONLY USED IN MEDICAL ORDERS

Abbreviation	From	Meaning
µg		microgram
µmol		micromole
°C		degrees Celsius (Centigrade)
<		less than
>		greater than
≤		less than or equal to
≥		greater than or equal to
aa, aa	ana	of each
ABG		arterial blood gas
ac	ante cibum	before meals or food
ACE		angiotensin-converting enzyme
ACLS		adult cardiac life support
ad	ad	to, up to
a.d.	aurio dextra	right ear
ADH		antidiuretic hormone
ad lib	ad libitum	at pleasure
AED		antiepileptic drug
a.l.	aurio laeva	left ear
ALL		acute lymphoblastic leukemia
ALT		alanine aminotransferase (was SGPT)
AM	ante meridiem	morning
AML		acute myeloblastic leukemia
amp		ampul
amt		amount
ANA		antinuclear antibodies
ANC		absolute neutrophil count
ANL		acute nonlymphoblastic leukemia
aq	aqua	water
aq. dest.	aqua destillata	distilled water
APTT		activated partial thromboplastin time
a.s.	aurio sinister	left ear
ASA (class I-IV)		classification of surgical patients according to their baseline health (eg, healthy ASA I and II or increased severity of illness ASA III or IV)
ASAP		as soon as possible
AST		aspartate aminotransferase (was SGOT)
a.u.	aures utrae	each ear
A-V		atrial-ventricular
bid	bis in die	twice daily
bm		bowel movement
BMT		bone marrow transplant
bp		blood pressure
BSA		body surface area
BUN		blood urea nitrogen
c	cong	gallon
c̄	cum	with
cal		calorie
cAMP		cyclic adenosine monophosphate
cap	capsula	capsule
CBC		complete blood count
cc		cubic centimeter
CHF		congestive heart failure
CI		cardiac index
Cl$_{cr}$		creatinine clearance
cm		centimeter
CNS		central nervous system
comp	compositus	compound
cont		continue
COPD		chronic obstructive pulmonary disease
CSF		cerebral spinal fluid

ABBREVIATIONS & SYMBOLS COMMONLY USED IN MEDICAL ORDERS *(Continued)*

Abbreviation	From	Meaning
CT		computed tomography
CVA		cerebral vascular accident
CVP		central venous pressure
d	dies	day
D_5W		dextrose 5% in water
$D_5\frac{1}{2}NS$		dextrose 5% in sodium chloride 0.45%
$D_{10}W$		dextrose 10% in water
d/c		discontinue
DIC		disseminated intravascular coagulation
dil	dilue	dilute
disp	dispensa	dispense
div	divide	divide
DNA		deoxyribonucleic acid
dtd	dentur tales doses	give of such a dose
DVT		deep vein thrombosis
EEG		electroencephalogram
EKG		electrocardiogram
elix, el	elixir	elixir
emp		as directed
ESR		erythrocyte sedimentation rate
E.T.		endotracheal
et	et	and
ex aq		in water
f, ft	fac, fiat, fiant	make, let be made
FDA		Food and Drug Administration
FEV_1		forced expiratory volume
FVC		forced vital capacity
g	gramma	gram
G-6-PD		glucose-6-phosphate dehydrogenase
GA		gestational age
GABA		gamma-aminobutyric acid
GE		gastroesophageal
GI		gastrointestinal
gr	granum	grain
gtt	gutta	a drop
GU		genitourinary
h	hora	hour
HIV		human immunodeficiency virus
HPLC		high performance liquid chromatography
hs	hora somni	at bedtime
IBW		ideal body weight
ICP		intracranial pressure
IgG		immune globulin G
I.M.		intramuscular
INR		international normalized ratio
I.O.		intraosseous
I & O		input and output
IOP		intraocular pressure
I.T.		intrathecal
I.V.		intravenous
IVH		intraventricular hemorrhage
IVP		intravenous push
JRA		juvenile rheumatoid arthritis
kcal		kilocalorie
kg		kilogram
L		liter
LDH		lactate dehydrogenase
LE		lupus erythematosus
liq	liquor	a liquor, solution
LP		lumbar puncture
M	misce	mix
MAO		monoamine oxidase

Abbreviation	From	Meaning
MAP		mean arterial pressure
mcg		microgram
m. dict	more dictor	as directed
mEq		milliequivalent
mg		milligram
MI		myocardial infarction
min		minute
mixt	mixtura	a mixture
mL		milliliter
mm		millimeter
mo		month
mOsm		milliosmols
MRI		magnetic resonance image
ND		nasoduodenal
NF		National Formulary
ng		nanogram
NG		nasogastric
NMDA		n-methyl-d-aspartate
nmol		nanomole
no.	numerus	number
noc	nocturnal	in the night
non rep	non repetatur	do not repeat, no refills
NPO		nothing by mouth
NSAID		nonsteroidal anti-inflammatory drug
O, Oct	octarius	a pint
o.d.	oculus dexter	right eye
o.l.	oculus laevus	left eye
O.R.		operating room
o.s.	oculus sinister	left eye
OTC		over-the-counter (nonprescription)
o.u.	oculo uterque	each eye
PALS		pediatric advanced life support
pc, post cib	post cibos	after meals
PCA		postconceptional age
PCP		*Pneumocystis carinii* pneumonia
PCWP		pulmonary capillary wedge pressure
PDA		patent ductus arteriosus
per		through or by
PM	post meridiem	afternoon or evening
PNA		postnatal age
P.O.	per os	by mouth
P.R.	per rectum	rectally
prn	pro re nata	as needed
PSVT		paroxysmal supraventricular tachycardia
PT		prothrombin time
PTT		partial thromboplastin time
PUD		peptic ulcer disease
pulv	pulvis	a powder
PVC		premature ventricular contraction
q		every
qd		every day
qh	quiaque hora	every hour
qid	quater in die	four times a day
qod		every other day
qs	quantum sufficiat	a sufficient quantity
qs ad		a sufficient quantity to make
qty		quantity
qv	quam volueris	as much as you wish
Rx	recipe	take, a recipe
RAP		right atrial pressure
rep	repetatur	let it be repeated
$\bar{s}$	sine	without
S-A		sino-atrial
sa	secundum artem	according to art
sat	sataratus	saturated

ABBREVIATIONS & SYMBOLS COMMONLY USED IN MEDICAL ORDERS *(Continued)*

Abbreviation	From	Meaning
S.C.		subcutaneous
S_{cr}		serum creatinine
SIADH		syndrome of inappropriate antidiuretic hormone
sig	signa	label, or let it be printed
S.L.		sublingual
SLE		systemic lupus erythematosus
sol	solutio	solution
solv		dissolve
$\overline{ss}$, ss	semis	one-half
sos	si opus sit	if there is need
stat	statim	at once, immediately
supp	suppositorium	suppository
SVR		systemic vascular resistance
SVT		supraventricular tachycardia
SWI		sterile water for injection
syr	syrupus	syrup
tab	tabella	tablet
tal		such
tid	ter in die	three times a day
tr, tinct	tinctura	tincture
trit		triturate
tsp		teaspoonful
TT		thrombin time
u.d., ut dict	ut dictum	as directed
ung	unguentum	ointment
USAN		United States Adopted Names
USP		United States Pharmacopeia
UTI		urinary tract infection
V_d		volume of distribution
V_{dss}		volume of distribution at steady-state
v.o.		verbal order
w.a.		while awake
x3		3 times
x4		4 times
y		year

BODY SURFACE AREA

Cautionary note: With increased age, height may decrease due to kyphotic changes which may make the surface area in the nomogram inaccurate. Since obtaining height in elderly is rather difficult and/or inacurate, some clinicians use: $BSA = 0.06 (BW_{kg}^{0.805})$

BODY SURFACE AREA OF ADULTS

HEIGHT	BODY SURFACE AREA	WEIGHT
CM 200 — 79 IN	2.80 M²	KG 150 — 330 LB
78	2.70	145 / 320
195 — 77		140 / 310
76	2.60	135 / 300
190 — 75		130 / 290
74	2.50	
185 — 73		125 / 280
72	2.40	120 / 270
180 — 71	2.30	115 / 260
175 — 70, 69		250
68	2.20	110 / 240
170 — 67		105 / 230
66	2.10	100 / 220
165 — 65		
64	2.00	95 / 210
160 — 63	1.95	
62	1.90	90 / 200
155 — 61	1.85	85 / 190
60	1.80	
150 — 59	1.75	80 / 180
58	1.70	75 / 170
145 — 57	1.65	70 / 160
56	1.60	
140 — 55	1.55	/ 150
54	1.50	65 / 140
135 — 53	1.45	60 / 130
52	1.40	
130 — 51	1.35	55 / 120
50	1.30	
125 — 49	1.25	50 / 110
48	1.20	/ 105
120 — 47	1.15	45 / 100
46	1.10	/ 95
115 — 45		40 / 90
44	1.05	/ 85
110 — 43	1.00	/ 80
42		35 / 75
105 — 41	0.95	
40	0.90	/ 70
CM 100 — 30 IN	0.86 M²	KG 30 / 66 LB

A straight edge is placed from the patient's height in the left column to his weight in the right column and this intersection on the body surface area column indicates his body surface area.

From the formula of Du Bois and Du Bois, *Arch Intern Med*, 17, 863 (1916): $S = W^{0.425} \times H^{0.725} \times 71.84$ or $\log S = \log W \times .425 + \log H^7 \times 0.725 + 1.8564$ (S = body surface in cm^2, W^7 = weight in kg, H = height in cm)

CALCULATIONS

Ideal Body Weight

Adults (18 years and older)

IBW (male) = 50 + (2.3 x height in inches over 5 feet)

IBW (female) = 45.5 + (2.3 x height in inches over 5 feet)

*IBW is in kg.

Millimoles and Millequivalents

Definitions

mole	=	gram molecular weight of a substance (aka molar weight)
millimole (mM)	=	milligram molecular weight of a substance (a millimole is 1/1000 of a mole)
equivalent weight	=	gram weight of a substance which will combine with or replace 1 gram (1 mole) of hydrogen; an equivalent weight can be determined by dividing the molar weight of a substance by its ionic valence
milliequivalent (mEq)	=	milligram weight of a substance which will combine with or replace 1 milligram (1 millimole) of hydrogen (a milliequivalent is 1/1000 of an equivalent)

Calculations

moles	=	$\dfrac{\text{weight of a substance (grams)}}{\text{molecular weight of that substance (grams)}}$
millimoles	=	$\dfrac{\text{weight of a substance (milligrams)}}{\text{molecular weight of that substance (milligrams)}}$
equivalents	=	moles x valence of ion
milliequivalents	=	millimoles x valence of ion
moles	=	$\dfrac{\text{equivalents}}{\text{valence of ion}}$
millimoles	=	$\dfrac{\text{milliequivalents}}{\text{valence of ion}}$
millimoles	=	moles x 1000
milliequivalents	=	equivalents x 1000

Note: Use of equivalents and milliequivalents is valid only for those substances which have fixed ionic valences (eg, sodium, potassium, calcium, chlorine, magnesium bromine, etc). For substances with variable ionic valences (eg, phosphorous), a reliable equivalent value cannot be determined. In these instances, one should calculate millimoles (which are fixed and reliable) rather than milliequivalents.

Milliequivalent Conversions

Approximate Milliequivalents — Weights of Selected Ions

Salt	mEq/g Salt	Mg Salt/mEq
Calcium carbonate [$CaCO_3$]	20	50
Calcium chloride [$CaCl_2 \cdot 2H_2O$]	14	74
Calcium gluceptate [$Ca(C_7H_{13}O_8)_2$]	4	245
Calcium gluconate [$Ca(C_6H_{11}O_7)_2 \cdot H_2O$]	5	224
Calcium lactate [$Ca(C_3H_5O_3)_2 \cdot 5H_2O$]	7	154
Magnesium gluconate [$Mg(C_6H_{11}O_7)_2 \cdot H_2O$]	5	216
Magnesium oxide [MgO]	50	20
Magnesium sulfate [$MgSO_4$]	17	60
Magnesium sulfate [$MgSO_4 \cdot 7H_2O$]	8	123
Potassium acetate [$K(C_2H_3O_2)$]	10	98
Potassium chloride [KCl]	13	75
Potassium citrate [$K_3(C_6H_5O_7) \cdot H_2O$]	9	108
Potassium iodide [KI]	6	166
Sodium acetate [$Na(C_2H_3O_2)$]	12	82
Sodium acetate [$Na(C_2H_3O_2) \cdot 3H_2O$]	7	136
Sodium bicarbonate [$NaHCO_3$]	12	84
Sodium chloride [$NaCl$]	17	58
Sodium citrate [$Na_3(C_6H_5O_7) \cdot 2H_2O$]	10	98
Sodium iodine [NaI]	7	150
Sodium lactate [$Na(C_3H_5O_3)$]	9	112
Zinc sulfate [$ZnSO_4 \cdot 7H_2O$]	7	144

Valences and Approximate Weights of Selected Ions

Substance	Electrolyte	Valence	Ionic Wt
Calcium	Ca^{++}	2	40
Chloride	Cl^-	1	35.5
Magnesium	Mg^{++}	2	24
Phosphate	PO_4^{---}	3	95*
	HPO_4^{--}	2	96
	$H_2PO_4^-$	1	97
Potassium	K^+	1	39
Sodium	Na^+	1	23
Sulfate	SO_4^{--}	2	96*

*The atomic weight of phosphorus is 31, and of sulfur is 32.

CONVERSIONS

Apothecary-Metric Exact Equivalents

1 gram (g)	=	15.43 grains	0.1 mg	=	1/600 gr
1 milliliter (mL)	=	16.23 minims	0.12 mg	=	1/500 gr
1 grain (gr)	=	64.8 milligrams	0.15 mg	=	1/400 gr
1 fluid ounce (fl. oz)	=	29.57 mL	0.2 mg	=	1/300 gr
1 pint (pt)	=	473.2 mL	0.3 mg	=	1/200 gr
1 ounce (oz)	=	28.35 grams	0.4 mg	=	1/150 gr
1 pound (lb)	=	453.6 grams	0.5 mg	=	1/120 gr
1 kilogram (kg)	=	2.2 pounds	0.6 mg	=	1/100 gr
1 quart (qt)	=	946.4 mL	0.8 mg	=	1/80 gr
			1 mg	=	1/65 gr

Apothecary-Metric Approximate Equivalents*

Liquids			Solids		
1 teaspoonful	=	5 mL	1/4 grain	=	15 mg
1 tablespoonful	=	15 mL	1/2 grain	=	30 mg
			1 grain	=	60 mg
			1 1/2 grain	=	100 mg
			5 grains	=	300 mg
			10 grains	=	600 mg

*Use exact equivalents for compounding and calculations requiring a high degree of accuracy.

Pounds-Kilograms

1 pound = 0.45359 kilograms
1 kilogram = 2.2 pounds

Temperature

Celsius to Fahrenheit = (°C x 9/5) + 32 = °F
Fahrenheit to Celsius = (°F - 32) x 5/9 = °C

AMINOGLYCOSIDES

Aminoglycoside Dosing Guidelines

Aminoglycosides	Usual Loading Dose (mg/kg)	Expected Peak Serum Levels (mcg/mL)
Tobramycin Gentamicin	1.5-2	4-10
Amikacin Kanamycin	5-7.5	15-30

Percentage of Loading Dose Required* for Dosage Interval Selected

Cl_{cr} (mL/min)	Half-Life (h)	8 h %	12 h %	24 h %
90	3.1	84		
80	3.4	80	91	
70	3.9	76	88	
60	4.5	71	84	
50	5.3	65	79	
40	6.5		72	92
30	8.4		63	86
25	9.9		57	81
20	11.9			75
17	13.6			70
15	15.1			67
12	17.9			61
10*	20.4			56
7	25.9			47
5	31.5			41
2	46.8			30
0	69.3			21

*Sarubbi FA and Hull JH, "Amikacin Serum Concentrations: Predictions of Levels and Dosage Guidelines," *Ann Intern Med*, 1978, 89:612-8.

Patients >65 years of age should not receive initial aminoglycoside maintenance dosing more often than every 12 hours.

PENICILLINS, PENICILLIN-RELATED ANTIBIOTICS, AND OTHER ANTIBIOTICS

KEY TO TABLE

- **A** Recommended drug therapy
- **B** Alternate drug therapy
- **C** Organism is usually or always sensitive to this agent
- **D** Organism portrays variable sensitivity to this agent
- (Blank) This drug should not be used for this organism or insufficient data is available

GRAM-POSITIVE AEROBES

Class	Drug	Listeria monocytogenes	Corynebacterium jeikeium	Corynebacterium sp.	Streptococcus, Viridans Group	Streptococcus pneumoniae	Streptococcus bovis (Group D)	Enterococcus sp. (Group D)	Streptococcus agalactiae (Group B)	Streptococcus pyogenes (Group A)	Staphylococcus epidermidis: Methicillin-Resistant	Staphylococcus epidermidis: Methicillin-Susceptible	Staphylococcus aureus: Methicillin-Resistant	Staphylococcus aureus: Methicillin-Susceptible
Penicillins	Amoxicillin				C	C	C		C	C				
	Ampicillin	A			C	C	C	A	C	C				
	Penicillin G	A	B	B	A	A	A	A	A	A				
	Penicillin V				C	C	C	C	C	C				
	Azlocillin													
	Mezlocillin				D	C	D	D	C	C				
	Piperacillin				D	C	D	C	C	C				
	Ticarcillin				D	C	D		C	C				
	Cloxacillin				D						D	A		A
	Dicloxacillin				D						D	A		A
	Methicillin				D						D	A		A
	Nafcillin				D						D	A		A
	Oxacillin				D						D	A		A
Penicillin-Related Antibiotics	Amoxicillin/Clavulanate	C			C	C	C	C	C	C		C		C
	Ampicillin/Sulbactam	C			C	C	C	C	C	C		C		C
	Ticarcillin/Clavulanate				C	C	C	D	C	C		C		C
	Aztreonam													
	Imipenem/Cilastatin				C	C	C	D	C	C		C		C
	Piperacillin/Tazobactam				C	C	C	C	C	C		C		C
Other Antibiotics	Chloramphenicol	C					B	D						
	Clindamycin				D	D	C	D	C	C		B		B
	Co-trimoxazole	B				C					B	C	B	C
	Metronidazole													
	Rifampin			D							A	C	A	C
	Sulfonamides													
	Tetracyclines	C				C	C		C				A	D
	Vancomycin	D	A		B	B	B	B	B	B	A	B	A	B
UTI Agents	Indanyl Carbenicillin							D						
	Nitrofurantoin							D						

Penicillins, Penicillin-Related Antibiotics & Other Antibiotics

KEY TO TABLE

- **A** Recommended drug therapy
- **B** Alternate drug therapy
- **C** Organism is usually or always sensitive to this agent
- **D** Organism portrays variable sensitivity to this agent
- (Blank) This drug should not be used for this organism or insufficient data is available

GRAM-NEGATIVE AEROBES — Enteric bacilli / Cocci

Class	Drug	Yersinia enterocolitica	Shigella sp.	Serratia sp.	Salmonella sp.	Providencia sp.	Proteus sp.	Proteus mirabilis	Klebsiella pneumoniae	Escherichia coli	Enterobacter sp.[1]	Citrobacter sp.[1]	Neisseria meningitidis	Neisseria gonorrhoeae	Moraxella (Branhamella) catarrhalis
Penicillin	Amoxicillin				B			A		C			C	D	
Penicillin	Ampicillin		A		B			A		A			C	D	
Penicillin	Penicillin G												A	D	
Penicillin	Penicillin V													D	
Penicillin	Azlocillin														
Penicillin	Mezlocillin			A		B	B	C	B	C	A	A		D	
Penicillin	Piperacillin			A		B	B	C	B	C	A	A		D	
Penicillin	Ticarcillin			A		B	B	C	D	C	A	A		D	
Penicillin	Cloxacillin														
Penicillin	Dicloxacillin														
Penicillin	Methicillin														
Penicillin	Nafcillin														
Penicillin	Oxacillin														
Penicillin-Related Antibiotics	Amoxicillin/Clavulanate				C			C	C	C			C	C	A
Penicillin-Related Antibiotics	Ampicillin/Sulbactam	C			C			C	C	C			C	C	C
Penicillin-Related Antibiotics	Ticarcillin/Clavulanate	C		A	C	C	B	C	B	C	A	A	C	C	C
Penicillin-Related Antibiotics	Aztreonam	C		B	C	C	C	C	B	C	A	C		C	C
Penicillin-Related Antibiotics	Imipenem/Cilastatin	B	B	C	B	B	C	B	C	B	B	B	D	C	C
Penicillin-Related Antibiotics	Piperacillin/Tazobactam	C		A	C	C	B	C	B	C	A	A	C	C	C
Other Antibiotics	Chloramphenicol	C		B							C		B		
Other Antibiotics	Clindamycin														
Other Antibiotics	Co-trimoxazole	C	A	C	B	A	C	B	C	A	C	C			A
Other Antibiotics	Metronidazole														
Other Antibiotics	Rifampin												D		
Other Antibiotics	Sulfonamides			C		C			C	C	C		D		
Other Antibiotics	Tetracyclines	C	C						C	C		D	C	B	C
Other Antibiotics	Vancomycin														
UTI Agents	Indanyl Carbenicillin			C		C	C	C	C	C	C				
UTI Agents	Nitrofurantoin								C	C	C	C			

[1] *Citrobacter freundii, Citrobacter diversus, Enterobacter cloacae* and *Enterobacter aerogenes* often have significantly different antibiotic sensitivity patterns. Speciation and susceptibility testing are particularly important

PENICILLINS, PENICILLIN-RELATED ANTIBIOTICS, AND OTHER ANTIBIOTICS (Continued)

Penicillins, Penicillin-Related Antibiotics & Other Antibiotics

KEY TO TABLE

- **A** Recommended drug therapy
- **B** Alternate drug therapy
- **C** Organism is usually or always sensitive to this agent
- **D** Organism portrays variable sensitivity to this agent
- ☐ (Blank) This drug should not be used for this organism or insufficient data is available

GRAM-NEGATIVE AEROBES — Other bacilli

Category	Drug	Vibrio cholerae	Xanthomonas maltophilia	Pseudomonas aeruginosa	Pasteurella multocida	Legionella pneumophila	Haemophilus influenzae	Gardnerella vaginalis	Francisella tularensis	Campylobacter jejuni	Brucella sp.	Bordetella pertussis	Alcaligenes	Acinetobacter sp.
Penicillin	Amoxicillin				C		B	C						
	Ampicillin				C		B	B		D				
	Penicillin G				A									
	Penicillin V				C									
	Azlocillin													
	Mezlocillin			A	C		D							A
	Piperacillin			A	C		D							A
	Ticarcillin			A	C		D							A
	Cloxacillin													
	Dicloxacillin													
	Methicillin													
	Nafcillin													
	Oxacillin													
Penicillin-Related Antibiotics	Amoxicillin/Clavulanate				B		B	B	C					C
	Ampicillin/Sulbactam				B		C	C	C					C
	Ticarcillin/Clavulanate		B	A	C		C							A
	Aztreonam			C			C							B
	Imipenem/Cilastatin			A			C							B
	Piperacillin/Tazobactam			A	C		C							A
Other Antibiotics	Chloramphenicol		C		C		B		A	C	C			
	Clindamycin							C		C				
	Co-trimoxazole	A	A				A	B				B	A	
	Metronidazole							A						
	Rifampin					A	D			D	A			
	Sulfonamides				C			C			C			
	Tetracyclines	A			C		C	C		B		A	C	
	Vancomycin													
UTI Agents	Indanyl Carbenicillin			D										C
	Nitrofurantoin													

Penicillins, Penicillin-Related Antibiotics & Other Antibiotics

KEY TO TABLE

A — Recommended drug therapy

B — Alternate drug therapy

C — Organism is usually or always sensitive to this agent

D — Organism portrays variable sensitivity to this agent

(Blank) This drug should not be used for this organism or insufficient data is available

		Treponema pallidum	Leptospira sp.	Borrelia burgdorferi (Lyme disease)	Rickettsia sp.	Ureaplasma urealyticum	Mycoplasma pneumoniae	Chlamydia trachomatis	Chlamydia pneumoniae (TWAR)	Chlamydia psittaci	Bacteroides sp. (Gram−)	Streptococcus, anaerobic (Gram+)	Clostridium perfringens	Clostridium difficile²
Penicillin	Amoxicillin			B							D	C	D	
	Ampicillin			B							C	C	D	
	Penicillin G	A	A	B							C	A	A	
	Penicillin V	C	C	B							C	C	C	
	Azlocillin													
	Mezlocillin										C	C	C	
	Piperacillin										C	C	C	
	Ticarcillin										C	C	C	
	Cloxacillin													
	Dicloxacillin													
	Methicillin													
	Nafcillin													
	Oxacillin													
Penicillin-Related Antibiotics	Amoxicillin/Clavulanate										C	C	C	
	Ampicillin/Sulbactam										C	C	C	
	Ticarcillin/Clavulanate										C	C	C	
	Aztreonam													
	Imipenem/Cilastatin										C	C	B	
	Piperacillin/Tazobactam										C	C	C	
Other Antibiotics	Chloramphenicol				A						C	C	C	D
	Clindamycin										A	B	B	
	Co-trimoxazole													
	Metronidazole										A	D	A	A
	Rifampin													
	Sulfonamides							D						
	Tetracyclines	B	B	A	A	A	A	A	B	B	D	C	C	
	Vancomycin											B		B
UTI Agents	Indanyl Carbenicillin													
	Nitrofurantoin													

² Vancomycin is effective orally only.

CEPHALOSPORINS, AMINOGLYCOSIDES, MACROLIDES, AND QUINOLONES

KEY TO TABLE

- **A** Recommended drug therapy
- **B** Alternate drug therapy
- **C** Organism is usually or always sensitive to this agent
- **D** Organism portrays variable sensitivity to this agent
- (Blank) This drug should not be used for this organism or insufficient data is available

GRAM-POSITIVE AEROBES

		Bacilli			Cocci									
		Listeria monocytogenes	Corynebacterium jeikeium	Corynebacterium sp.	Streptococcus, Viridans Group	Streptococcus pneumoniae	Streptococcus bovis (Group D)	Enterococcus sp. (Group D)	Streptococcus agalactiae (Group B)	Streptococcus pyogenes (Group A)	Staphylococcus epidermidis: Methicillin-Resistant	Staphylococcus epidermidis: Methicillin-Susceptible	Staphylococcus aureus: Methicillin-Resistant	Staphylococcus aureus: Methicillin-Susceptible
1st Generation	Cefadroxil				B	B	C		B	B		B		B
	Cefazolin				B	B	C		B	B		B		B
	Cephalexin				B	B	C		B	B		B		B
	Cephalothin				B	B	C		B	B		B		B
	Cephapirin				B	B	C		B	B		B		B
	Cephradine				B	B	C		B	B		B		B
2nd Generation and others	Cefaclor				C	C	C		C	C		D		D
	Cefamandole				C	C	C		C	C		C		C
	Cefmetazole				C	C	C		C	C		D		D
	Cefonicid				C	C	C		C	C		D		D
	Cefotetan				C	C	C		C	C		D		D
	Cefoxitin				C	C	C		C	C		D		D
	Cefpodoxime Proxetil				C	C	C		C	C		D		D
	Cefprozil				C	C	D		C	C				D
	Ceftibuten					D			C	C				
	Cefuroxime				C	C	C		C	C		D		D
	Cefuroxime Axetil				C	C			C	C		C		C
	Loracarbef				C	C	D		C	C		C		C
3rd Generation	Cefepime				C	C			C	C		C		C
	Cefixime				D	D			C	C				
	Cefoperazone				D	D	C		C	C		D		D
	Cefotaxime				D	D	C		C	C		D		D
	Ceftazidime				D		D		D	D				
	Ceftizoxime				D	D	C		C	C		D		D
	Ceftriaxone				C	C	C		C	C		D		D
Aminoglycosides	Amikacin	C	C					D	D					
	Gentamicin	A	B		A			D	A		A	D	A	D
	Netilmicin	C	C						C					
	Streptomycin							D	C					
	Tobramycin	C	C					D						D
Macrolides	Azithromycin	C			C	C			C	C				C
	Clarithromycin	C			C	C			C	C				C
	Dirithromycin	C			C	C			C	C				C
	Erythromycin	C	C	A	C	B			B	B				C
Quinolones	Lomefloxacin		D		D	D	D	D	D	D	D	D	D	D
	Ciprofloxacin		D		D	D	D	D	D	D	D	D	D	D
	Norfloxacin										D	D		
	Ofloxacin			D	D	D	D	D	D	D	D	D	D	D

Cephalosporins, Aminoglycosides, Macrolides & Quinolones

KEY TO TABLE

- **A** Recommended drug therapy
- **B** Alternate drug therapy
- **C** Organism is usually or always sensitive to this agent
- **D** Organism portrays variable sensitivity to this agent
- ☐ (Blank) This drug should not be used for this organism or insufficient data is available

GRAM-NEGATIVE AEROBES — Other bacilli

Class	Drug	Vibrio cholerae	Xanthomonas maltophilia	Pseudomonas aeruginosa	Pasteurella multocida	Legionella pneumophila	Haemophilus influenzae	Haemophilus ducreyi	Gardnerella vaginalis	Francisella tularensis	Campylobacter jejuni	Brucella sp.	Bordetella pertussis	Alcaligenes	Acinetobacter sp.
1st Generation	Cefadroxil						D								
	Cefazolin						D								
	Cephalexin						D								
	Cephalothin						D								
	Cephapirin						D								
	Cephradine						D								
2nd Generation and others	Cefaclor						B								
	Cefamandole				C		B								
	Cefmetazole				D		C								
	Cefonicid						C								
	Cefotetan				D		C								
	Cefoxitin				D		C		D						
	Cefpodoxime Proxetil						B								
	Cefprozil						B								
	Ceftibuten														
	Cefuroxime						B								
	Cefuroxime Axetil				D		B								
	Loracarbef						B								
3rd Generation	Cefepime														
	Cefixime						A								D
	Cefoperazone		D	D	C		A	C							D
	Cefotaxime			D	C		C	C							A
	Ceftazidime		D	A			C	C							A
	Ceftizoxime			D	C		C								A
	Ceftriaxone			D	C		A	D							A
Aminoglycosides	Amikacin		C	A			C			C					C
	Gentamicin		C	A			C			A	C	C			C
	Netilmicin		C	A			C					C			C
	Streptomycin									A		C			
	Tobramycin		C	A			C								C
Macrolides	Azithromycin				D	B	C	C			C		C		
	Clarithromycin				D	B	C				C		C		
	Dirithromycin														
	Erythromycin				D	A		C			C	A	A		
Quinolones	Lomefloxacin	C	C	D	C		C	C	D		B	C			D
	Ciprofloxacin	C	B	A	C	B	C	B	C	C	B	C			C
	Norfloxacin			C								B			D
	Ofloxacin	C	B	D	C	C	C	C	C	C	B	C			C

CEPHALOSPORINS, AMINOGLYCOSIDES, MACROLIDES, AND QUINOLONES (Continued)

Cephalosporins, Aminoglycosides, Macrolides & Quinolones

KEY TO TABLE

A — Recommended drug therapy

B — Alternate drug therapy

C — Organism is usually or always sensitive to this agent

D — Organism portrays variable sensitivity to this agent

(Blank) This drug should not be used for this organism or insufficient data is available

Group	Drug	Treponema pallidum	Leptospira sp.	Borrelia burgdorferi (lyme disease)	Rickettsia sp.	Mycoplasma pneumoniae	Ureaplasma urealyticum	Chlamydia trachomatis	Chlamydia pneumoniae (TWAR)	Chlamydia psittaci	Bacteroides sp., anaerobic (Gram -)	Streptococcus, anaerobic (Gram +)	Clostridium perfringens	Clostridium difficile [2]
1st Generation	Cefadroxil											B		
	Cefazolin											B		
	Cephalexin											B		
	Cephalothin											B		
	Cephapirin											B		
	Cephradine											B		
2nd Generation and others	Cefaclor													
	Cefamandole													
	Cefmetazole										C	C	C	
	Cefonicid													
	Cefotetan										B	C	C	
	Cefoxitin										B	C	C	
	Cefpodoxime Proxetil													
	Cefprozil													
	Ceftibuten													
	Cefuroxime											C	C	
	Cefuroxime Axetil													
	Loracarbef													
3rd Generation	Cefepime													
	Cefixime													
	Cefoperazone													D
	Cefotaxime				C						D	C	C	
	Ceftazidime													D
	Ceftizoxime				C						D	C	C	
	Ceftriaxone	C		A								C		
Aminoglycosides	Amikacin													
	Gentamicin													
	Netilmicin													
	Streptomycin													
	Tobramycin													
Macrolides	Azithromycin	D		C		B	C	C	C	C			D	D
	Clarithromycin	D		D		B	C	C	C	C			D	D
	Dirithromycin					C	C	C	C	C			D	D
	Erythromycin	D		C		A	A	A	A	A			D	D
Quinolones	Lomefloxacin					D	D	D						
	Ciprofloxacin					D	D	D	D					
	Norfloxacin													
	Ofloxacin					D	D	D	C					

[2] Vancomycin is effective orally only.

Cephalosporins, Aminoglycosides, Macrolides & Quinolones

KEY TO TABLE

A	Recommended drug therapy
B	Alternate drug therapy
C	Organism is usually or always sensitive to this agent
D	Organism portrays variable sensitivity to this agent
(Blank)	This drug should not be used for this organism or insufficient data is available

GRAM-NEGATIVE AEROBES

Class	Drug	*Yersinia enterocolitica*	*Shigella sp.*	*Salmonella sp.*	*Providencia sp.*	*Proteus vulgaris*	*Proteus mirabilis*	*Klebsiella pneumoniae*	*Escherichia coli*	*Enterobacter sp.*[1]	*Citrobacter sp.*[1]	*Neisseria meningitidis*	*Neisseria gonorrhoeae*	*Moraxella (Branhamella) catarrhalis*
1st Generation	Cefadroxil							A	A	B				D
1st Generation	Cefazolin							A	A	B				D
1st Generation	Cephalexin							A	A	B				D
1st Generation	Cephalothin							A	A	B				D
1st Generation	Cephapirin							A	A	B				D
1st Generation	Cephradine							A	A	B				D
2nd Generation and others	Cefaclor							C	A	B			C	B
2nd Generation and others	Cefamandole						D	C	A	B			C	B
2nd Generation and others	Cefmetazole	D	C	C		C	D	C	A	B			C	B
2nd Generation and others	Cefonicid							C	A	B			C	B
2nd Generation and others	Cefotetan	C	C	C		C	D	C	A	B			C	B
2nd Generation and others	Cefoxitin			D		C	D	C	A	B			C	B
2nd Generation and others	Cefpodoxime Proxetil							C	A	B			C	B
2nd Generation and others	Cefprozil	C						C	D	B			C	B
2nd Generation and others	Ceftibuten													
2nd Generation and others	Cefuroxime	C	C				D	C	A	B			C	B
2nd Generation and others	Cefuroxime Axetil							C	A	B		C	C	B
2nd Generation and others	Loracarbef							C	C	B			C	B
3rd Generation	Cefepime					A								
3rd Generation	Cefixime		C	C				C	C	A	A		C	B
3rd Generation	Cefoperazone		B	A	A	A	A	C	A	A	A			B
3rd Generation	Cefotaxime	A	B	A	A	A	A	C	A	A	A	B	C	B
3rd Generation	Ceftazidime		B	A	A	A	A	C	A	A	A			B
3rd Generation	Ceftizoxime	A	B	A	A	A	A	C	A	A	A	B	C	B
3rd Generation	Ceftriaxone	A	B	A	A	A	A	C	A	A	A	B	A	B
Aminoglycosides	Amikacin	A		C	C	C	C	C	C	C	C			
Aminoglycosides	Gentamicin	A	D	C	D	D	C	C	C	C	C			
Aminoglycosides	Netilmicin	A	D	C	D	D	C	C	C	C	C			
Aminoglycosides	Streptomycin				D									
Aminoglycosides	Tobramycin	A		C	D	D	C	C	C	C	C			
Macrolides	Azithromycin												C	C
Macrolides	Clarithromycin												C	C
Macrolides	Dirithromycin													
Macrolides	Erythromycin												D	C
Quinolones	Lomefloxacin	C	C	C	C	C	C	C	C	C	C	D	C	C
Quinolones	Ciprofloxacin	C	B	C	B	C	C	C	C	C	C	C	A	C
Quinolones	Norfloxacin	C	C	C	C	C	C	C	C	C	C		C	
Quinolones	Ofloxacin	C	C	C	C	C	C	C	C	C	C	C	A	C

[1] *Citrobacter freundii, Citrobacter diversus, Enterobacter cloacae* and *Enterobacter aerogenes* often have significantly different antibiotic sensitivity patterns. Speciation and susceptibility testing are particularly important

CREATININE CLEARANCE ESTIMATING METHODS IN PATIENTS WITH STABLE RENAL FUNCTION

The following formulas provide an acceptable estimate of the patient's creatinine clearance except when:

a. patient's serum creatinine is changing rapidly (either up or down)

b. patients are markedly emaciated

In these situations (a and b above), certain assumptions have to be made.

a. In patients with rapidly rising serum creatinines (ie, >0.5-0.7 mg/dL/ day), it is best to assume that the patient's creatinine clearance is probably <10 mL/minute.

b. In emaciated patients, although their actual creatinine clearance is less than their calculated creatinine clearance (because of decreased creatinine production), it is not possible to easily predict how much less. Many clinicians advocate using a serum creatinine value of "1" in the calculations for estimating creatinine clearance when emaciated patients' serum creatinine is less than normal range.

Adults (18 years and older)

Method 1: (Cockroft DW and Gault MH, *Nephron*, 1976, 16:31-41)

Estimated creatinine clearance (Cl_{cr}) (mL/min):

$$\text{Male} = \frac{(140 - \text{age}) \text{ IBW (kg)}}{72 \times \text{serum creatinine}}$$

$$\text{Female} = \text{Estimated } Cl_{cr} \text{ male} \times 0.85$$

Note: The use of the patient's ideal body weight (IBW) is recommended for the above formula except when the patient's actual body weight is less than ideal. Use of the IBW is especially important in obese patients.

Method 2: (Jelliffe RW, *Ann Intern Med*, 1973, 79:604)

Estimated creatinine clearance (Cl_{cr}) (mL/min/1.73 m²):

$$\text{Male} = \frac{98 - 0.8 (\text{age} - 20)}{\text{serum creatinine}}$$

$$\text{Female} = \text{Estimated } Cl_{cr} \text{ male} \times 0.90$$

ACE INHIBITORS*

ACE Inhibitors Comparison

	Benazepril (Lotensin®)	Captopril (Capoten®)	Enalapril (Vasotec®)	Enalaprilat (Vasotec®)	Fosinopril (Monopril®)	Lisinopril (Prinvil®, Zestril®)	Moexipril (Univasc®)	Quinapril (Accupril®)	Ramipril (Altace™)	Trandolapril (Mavik®)
Route	P.O.	P.O.	P.O.	I.V.	P.O.	P.O.	P.O.	P.O.	P.O.	P.O.
Dosage forms (mg)	5 10 20 40	12.5 25 50 100	2.5 5 10 20	1.25 mg/mL	10 20	2.5 5.0 10 20 40	7.5 15	5 10 20 40	1.25 2.5 5 10	1 2 4
Usual geriatric starting dose (mg)	5-10	12.5-25	2.5-5	0.625-1.25 mg over 5 min	5-10	2.5-5	3.75-7.5	2.5-5	2.5-5	0.5-1
Dosing interval	qd	tid	qd	q6h over 5 min	qd	qd	qd	qd	qd	qd
Indications and starting dose (adult) HTN	10 mg qd 5 mg qd#	12.5-25 mg bid-tid	5 mg qd 2.5 mg qd#	x	10 mg qd	10 mg qd 5 mg qd#	7.5 mg qd 3.75 mg qd•	10 mg qd 5 mg qd¶	2.5 mg qd 1.25 mg qd•	1 mg nonblack patient 2 mg black patient
CHF (target dose)	20 mg	50 mg tid	10 mg bid		20-40 mg qd	20 mg qd	7.5-30 mg qd	20 mg bid,	5 mg bid•	4 mg qd
Protein binding	>95%	25%-30%		50%-60%	~95%	—	~50%	<97%	~73% ramipril 56% ramiprilat	
Active metabolites	Benazeprilat		Enalaprilat		Fosinoprilat		Moexiprilat	Quinaprilat	Ramiprilat	
Half-life normal renal function (h)	10-11†	<2	1.3	11	12†	12	2-9 (moexiprilat)	2	13-17	
Half-life impaired renal function (h)	Prolonged	3.5-32	No data	Prolonged	Prolonged	Prolonged	Prolonged	Prolonged	Prolonged	

ACE INHIBITORS* (Continued)

ACE Inhibitors Comparison (continued)

	Benazepril (Lotensin[9])	Captopril (Capoten[9])	Enalapril (Vasotec[9])	Enalaprilat (Vasotec[9])	Fosinopril (Monopril[‡])	Lisinopril (Prinivil, Zestril[9])	Moexipril (Univasc[9])	Quinapril (Accupril[9])	Ramipril (Altace[9])	Trandolapril (Mavik[9])
Elimination Total	No data	>95% urine	94% urine and feces	No data	50% urine 50% feces	No data	13% urine 53% feces	60% urine 37% feces	60% urine 40% feces	
Unchanged	Trace	40%-50% urine	54% urine (40% enalapril)	>90% urine	Negligible	100% urine§	1% urine 1% feces	Trace	<2§	
Incidence of side effects										
Cough	1.9-3.4	0.5-2	1.3-2.2		2.2	2.9-4.5	6.1	2	12	
Angioedema	0.5	0.1	0.2		≤1	0.1	<1	0.1	0.3	
Rash	x	4-7	1.3-1.4		≤1	1.5	1.6	x	x	
Headache	5	0.5-2	1.8-5.2		3.2	5.3	>1	5.6	5.4	
Dizziness	3.3	0.5-2	4.3-7.9		1.6	6.3	4.3	3.9	2.2	
Chest pain		1	2.1		≤1	1.3	>1	x	<1	
Hypotension	0.3	x	6.7		≤1	1.2-5	0.5	x	0.5	
Diarrhea		0.5-2	1.4-2.1		1.5	3.2	3.1	x	<1	

*All doses listed are oral and assume patient is **not** on a diuretic. See specific drug monograph for dosing concurrently with diuretics to avoid adverse reactions.

†Half-life accumulates after multiple dosing.

‡Fosinoprilat, after I.V. administration.

§Time frame undefined.

¶Cl$_{cr}$ 30-60 mL/min.

#Cl$_{cr}$ 10-30 mL/min.

•Cl$_{cr}$ <40 mL/min.

x — reported, no incidence given.

ANTIDEPRESSANT AGENTS

Antidepressant Agents Comparison

Drug	Class	Therapeutic Drug Conc (ng/mL)	Anticholinergic Side Effects	Sedation	Orthostatic Hypotension	Usual Adult Daily Dose (mg)
Amitriptyline	TCA	100-250	++++	++++	++	75-300
Amoxapine	TCA	20-100*	+++	++	+	150-600
Bupropion	Aminoketone	50-100†	++	++	+	225-450
Clomipramine	TCA	330-800*†	+++	+++	++	100-250
Desipramine	TCA	115-160	+	+	+	75-300
Doxepin	TCA	>110	++	+++	++	75-300
Fluoxetine	SSRI	*†	+/-	+/-	+/-	20-80
Fluvoxamine	SSRI	-	(-)	(-/+)	(-)	20-80
Imipramine	TCA	150-250†	++	++	+++	75-300
Maprotiline	Tetracyclic	*	++	++	+	75-225
Nefazodone	Phenylpiperazine	Not established	Insufficient comparisons to score			300-500
Nortriptyline	TCA	50-150	++	++	+	75-300
Paroxetine	SSRI	-	(-)	+/-	(-)	10-50
Protriptyline	TCA	100-200	+++	+	+	15-60
Sertraline	SSRI	-	(-)	+/-	-	50-200
Trazodone	Triazolopyridine	900-2100*	+	++	++	150-600
Trimipramine	TCA	Not established	++	+++	++	75-300
Venlafaxine	Phenylethylamine	-	(-)	(-)	(-)	75-325

TCA = tricyclic antidepressant.

*Drug concentration in the serum correlates poorly with clinical response.

†Levels represent a combination of parent compound and active metabolites.

ANTIEPILEPTIC DRUG INTERACTIONS

Antiepileptic Drug Interactions Comparison

Added Drug	CURRENT THERAPY							
	Gapapentin	Lamotrigine	Carbamazepine	Phenytoin	Felbamate	Valproic Acid	Phenobarbital	Topiramate
Carbamazepine	No change	↓	—	→	↓	↓	Unknown	↓
Phenytoin	No change	↓	→↓ (cbz) ↑ (cbz epoxide)	—	↓	⇅	⇅	↓
Felbamate	Unknown	Unknown	↑ (cbz epoxide)	↑	—	↑	↑	Unknown
Valproic acid	No change	↑	↑ (ratio of cbz epoxide to parent drug*)	⇅ (total) ↑ (free fraction)	No significant change	—	↑	→
Phenobarbital	No change	→	→	⇅ or no change	Unknown	Unknown	—	Unknown
Lamotrigine	Unknown	—	No change†	No change	Unknown	Unknown	Unknown	Unknown
Gabapentin	—	Unknown	No change	No change	Unknown	No change	No change	Unknown
Topiramate	Unknown	Unknown	No change	↑ or no change	Unknown	↓	No change	—

Note: If the current therapy is held constant and one of the drugs listed below is added, this chart indicates what changes to expect in the current drug serum concentrations.

↑ = increased concentrations of current drug.

↓ = decreased concentrations of current drug.

⇅ = the interaction has been reported to produce variable results.

*The effect of valproic acid on carbamazepine blood levels is not clearly established, although an increase in the ratio of active 10, 11 epoxide metabolite to parent compound is a consistent finding.

†Limited clinical data suggest there is a higher incidence of dizziness, diplopia, ataxia, and blurred vision in patients receiving carbamazepine with lamotrigine than in patients receiving other enzyme-inducing AEDs with lamotrigine. The mechanism of this interaction is unclear.

Please see full prescribing information for Neurontin® and Dilantin®.

ANTIPSYCHOTIC AGENTS

Antipsychotic Agents Comparison

Antipsychotic Agent	Equivalent Dosages (approx) (mg)	Usual Adult Daily Maintenance Dose (mg)	Sedation (Incidence)	Extrapyramidal Side Effects	Anticholinergic Side Effects	Cardiovascular Side Effects	Orthostatic Hypotension
Acetophenazine	20	60-120	Moderate	High	Low	Low	Low
Chlorpromazine	100	200-1000	High	Moderate	Moderate	Moderate/high	High
Chlorprothixene	100	75-600	High	Moderate	Moderate	Low/moderate	Moderate
Clozapine	50	50-400	High	Low	High	High	High
Fluphenazine	2	5-40	Low	High	Low	Low	Low
Haloperidol	2	5-40	Low	High	Low	Low	Low
Loxapine	10	25-100	Moderate	High	Low	Low	Moderate
Mesoridazine	50	30-400	High	Low	High	Moderate	Moderate
Molindone	15	25-100	Low	High	Low	Low	Low
Olanzapine	5	10-15	Moderate	Low	Moderate	Low	Low
Perphenazine	10	16-48	Low	High	Low	Low	Low
Pimozide	0.3-0.5	1-10	Moderate	High	Moderate	Low	Low
Promazine	200	40-1200	Moderate	Moderate	High	Moderate	Moderate
Quetiapine	50	300-400	Moderate	Low	Low	Low	Low
Risperidone	-	4-16	Low	None/low	Low	Low	Low
Thioridazine	100	200-800	High	Low	High	Moderate/high	High
Thiothixene	5	5-40	Low	Moderate	Low	Low/moderate	Low
Trifluoperazine	5	10-40	Low	High	Low	Low	Low

BENZODIAZEPINES

Benzodiazepines Comparison

	Peak Blood Concentration (oral)	Protein Binding %	Major Active Metabolite	t$\frac{1}{2}$ (parent) Adults	t$\frac{1}{2}$* (metabolite) Adults	Adult Oral Dosage Range	Geriatric Oral Dosage Range
Anxiolytic							
Alprazolam (Xanax®)	1-2 h	80	No	12-15 h	—	0.75-4 mg/d	0.25-0.75 mg/d
Chlordiazepoxide (Librium®)	2-4 h	90-98	Yes	5-30 h	24-96 h	15-100 mg/d	10-20 mg/d†
Clorazepate (Tranxene®)	1 h	ND‡	Yes	Not significant	50-100 h	15-60 mg/d	7.5-15 mg/d†
Diazepam (Valium®)	1-2 h	98	Yes	20-50 h	50-100 h	6-40 mg/d	1-5 mg/d†
Halazepam (Paxipam®)	1-3 h	ND‡	Yes	14 h	50-100 h	60-160 mg/d	20-40 mg/d
Lorazepam (Ativan®)	0.5-3 h	85	No	10-20 h	—	2-6 mg/d	0.5-2 mg/d
Oxazepam (Serax®)	2-4 h	86-99	No	5-20 h	—	30-120 mg/d	10-30 mg/d
Prazepam (Centrax®)	6 h	ND‡	Yes	1 h	50-100 h	20-60 mg/d	10-15 mg/d†
Sedative/Hypnotic							
Estazolam (ProSom™)	2 h	93	No	10-24 h	—	1-2 mg	0.5-1 mg
Flurazepam (Dalmane®)	0.5-2 h	97	Yes	Not significant	40-114 h	15-30 mg	15 mg†
Quazepam (Doral®)	2 h	>95	Yes	25-41 h	40-114 h	7.5-15 mg	7.5 mg†

Benzodiazepines Comparison (continued)

	Peak Blood Concentration (oral)	Protein Binding %	Major Active Metabolite	t½ (parent) Adults	t½* (metabolite) Adults	Adult Oral Dosage Range	Geriatric Oral Dosage Range
Temazepam (Restoril®)	2-3 h	96	No	9.5-12 h	—	7.5-30 mg	7.5-15 mg
Triazolam (Halcion®)	0.5-2 h	89-94	No	1.7-5 h	—	0.125-0.5 mg	0.0625-0.125 mg
Miscellaneous							
Clonazepam (Klonopin®)	1-2 h	86	No	18-50 h	—	1.5-20 mg/d	0.5-1.5 mg/d

* = significant metabolite.

†Not recommended for use in geriatric patients.

‡No specific data available, but all benzodiazepines are highly protein bound.

Abstracted from Micromedex, Inc.

BETA-BLOCKERS

Beta-Blockers Comparison

Agent	Adrenergic Receptor Blocking Activity	Lipid Solubility	Half-life (h)	Primary (Secondary) Route of Elimination	Starting Oral Daily Dose
Acebutolol (Sectral®)	beta$_1$	Low	3-4	Hepatic (renal)	400 mg
Atenolol (Tenormin®)	beta$_1$	Low	6-9*	Renal (hepatic)	50 mg
Betaxolol (Kerlone®)	beta$_1$	Low	14-22	Hepatic (renal)	20 mg
Bisoprolol (Zebeta®)	beta$_1$	Low	9-12	Renal/hepatic	2.5-5 mg
Carteolol (Cartrol®)	beta$_1$ beta$_2$	Low	6	Renal (biliary)	15 mg
Carvedilol (Coreg®)	beta$_1$ beta$_2$	Moderate	7-10	Hepatic	16.5 mg
Esmolol (Brevibloc®)	beta$_1$	Low	0.15	Red blood cell	NA
Labetalol (Trandate®, Normodyne®)	alpha$_1$ beta$_1$ beta$_2$	Moderate	5.5-8	Renal (hepatic)	200 mg
Metoprolol (Lopressor®)	beta$_1$	Moderate	3-7	Hepatic/renal	50 mg
Nadolol (Corgard®)	beta$_1$ beta$_2$	Low	20-24	Renal	320 mg
Penbutolol (Levatol®)	beta$_1$ beta$_2$	High	5	Hepatic (renal)	20 mg
Pindolol (Visken®)	beta$_1$ beta$_2$	Moderate	3-4†	Hepatic/renal	20 mg
Propranolol (Inderal®, various)	beta$_1$ beta$_2$	High	3-5	Hepatic	80 mg
Propranolol long-acting (Inderal-LA®)	beta$_1$ beta$_2$	High	9-18	Hepatic	80 mg
Sotalol (Betapace®)	beta$_1$ beta$_2$	Low	7-18	Renal (hepatic)	80 mg
Timolol (Blocadren®)	beta$_1$ beta$_2$	Low to moderate	4	Hepatic (renal)	20 mg

*Half-life increased to 16-27 hours in creatinine clearances of 15-35 mL/minute and >27 hours in Cl_{cr} <15 mL/minute.

†Half-life variable: 7-15 hours.

Note: All beta$_1$ selective agents will inhibit beta$_2$ receptors at higher doses. For specific geriatric information, see individual monographs.

CALCIUM CHANNEL BLOCKING AGENTS

Calcium Channel Blocking Agents Comparison

	Amlodipine	Bepridil	Diltiazem	Felodipine	Isradipine	Nicardipine	Nifedipine	Nimodipine	Nisoldipine	Verapamil
Absorption (%)	—	99-100	40	99-100	90-95	35	60-75	13	ND	20-35
Protein binding	93	>99	High	>99	95	Very high	Very high	Very high	>99%	High
Half-life	30-50 h	24 h	6-8 h	11-16 h	8 h	2-4 h	5 h	1-2 h	7-12 h	Oral: 1 dose: 2.8-7.4 h; Rep dose: 4.5-12 h; I.V. (biphasic): Short phase: 4 min; Long phase: 2-5 h
Onset of action	—	60 min	Oral: 60 min	2-5 h	2 h	20 min	Oral: 10-20 min	20 min	ND	Oral: 30 min; I.V.: 1-5 min
Peak	6-12 h	2-3 h	Oral: 2-3 h	2.5-5 h	1.5 h	0.5-2 h	Oral: 0.5-6 h	<1 h	6-12 h	Oral: 1-2.2 h; Oral, ext release: 5-7 h; I.V.: 2 h
Duration of action	—	24 h	Ext release: 12 h; Tablet: 6-8 h	24 h	12 h	8 h	12-24 h	4-6 h	ND	Oral, ext release: 24 h; Tablet: 8-10 h; I.V.: 2 h
Elimination	Hepatic 90% Renal 10%	Hepatic/ biliary almost 100%	Biliary/renal 96%-98% (2%-4% unchanged)	Hepatic 99% Renal <0.5%	Hepatic/ biliary 100%	Renal 60% Biliary/ fecal 35%	Renal 80% Biliary/fecal 20%	Renal 60% Biliary/fecal 35%	Hepatic 5% major urinary metabolites	Renal 70% Biliary/fecal 9%-16%
Actions										
contractility	←	→	→	←	0	→	←	←	0	↓↓
heart rate	±	→	→	←	±	←	←	←	0	→
cardiac output	←	0	←	←	←	↑↑	←	←	0	↓↑

CALCIUM CHANNEL BLOCKING AGENTS *(Continued)*

Calcium Channel Blocking Agents Comparison *(continued)*

	Amlodipine	Bepridil	Diltiazem	Felodipine	Isradipine	Nicardipine	Nifedipine	Nimodipine	Nisoldipine	Verapamil
peripheral vascular resistance	↓↓↓	↓	↓	↓↓↓	↓↓↓	↓↓↓	↓↓↓	↓↓	↓↓↓	↓↓
Side effects										
constipation	-	+	+	+	-	-	+	-	(-)	+
dizziness	+	++	+	++	++	+	++	+	++	+
flushing	++	-	+	++	+	++	++	-	+	-
headache	++	++	+	++	++	+	++	+	++	+
nausea	+	++	+	+	+	+	++	+	+	+

++ = most frequent

+ = less frequent

- = rare

± = negligible effect

0 = no effect

CORTICOSTEROIDS

Corticosteroids Comparison, Systemic

Corticosteroids, Systmeic

Relative Potencies and Equivalent Doses of Corticosteroids
(Glucocorticoid potency compared to hydrocortisone "mg" for "mg" basis)

Compound	Glucocor-ticoid Potency	Mineralo-corticoid Potency	Equivalent Dose (mg)	Duration* of Action
Cortisone (Cortone®)	0.8	++	25	S
Injection: 50 mg/mL susp				
Tablet: 5 mg				
Dexamethasone (Decadron®, Dexone®, Hexadrol®)	25-30	0	0.75	L
Elixir: 0.5 mg/5 mL				
Injection: 4 mg/mL				
Intensol: 1 mg/mL				
Tablet: 0.25 mg, 0.5 mg, 0.75 mg, 1 mg, 1.5 mg, 2 mg, 4 mg				
Fludrocortisone (Florinef®)	10	+++++		I
Tablet: 0.1 mg				
Hydrocortisone (Cortef®)	1	++	20	S
Injection: 50 mg/mL				
Suspension: 10 mg/5 mL				
Tablet: 5 mg, 10 mg, 20 mg				
Methylprednisolone (Medrol®, Solu-Medrol®, Depo-Med-rol®)	5	0	4	I
Injection: 40 mg, 125 mg, 500 mg, 1 g				
Injection, susp: 80 mg/mL				
Tablet: 2 mg, 4 mg, 16 mg, 24 mg				
Prednisolone (Delta-Cortef®, Prelone® Syrup, Pediapred®)	4	+	5	I
Liquid: 5 mg/5 mL				
Syrup: 15 mg/5 mL				
Tablet: 5 mg				
Prednisone (Deltasone®, Liq-uid Pred®, Orasone®)	4	+	5	I
Liquid: 5 mg/5 mL				
Tablet: 1 mg, 2.5 mg, 5 mg, 10 mg, 20 mg, 50 mg				

*S = Short, 8-12 hours biologic activity.
I = Intermediate, 12-36 hours biologic activity.
L = Long, 36-54 hours biologic activity.

CORTICOSTEROIDS *(Continued)*

The following topical corticosteroid preparations are grouped in order of potency.

Corticosteroids Comparison, Topical

Drug/Dosage Form	Brand Name
I Super Potency	
Clobetasol propionate 0.05% cream and ointment	Temovate®
Betamethasone dipropionate 0.05% cream and ointment	Diprolene®
Halobetasol propionate 0.05% cream and ointment	Ultravate™
Diflorasone diacetate 0.05% (optimized) ointment	Psorcon®
II Higher Potency	
Amcinonide 0.1% ointment	Cyclocort®
Betamethasone dipropionate 0.05% (optimized) cream	Diprolene® AF
Betamethasone dipropionate 0.05% ointment	Diprosone®, Maxivate®
Mometasone furoate 0.1% ointment	Elocon®
Diflorasone diacetate 0.05% ointment	Florone®, Maxiflor®
Halcinonide 0.1% cream	Halog®
Fluocinonide 0.05% ointment	Lidex®
Fluocinonide 0.05% cream	Lidex®
Desoximetasone 0.05% gel	Topicort®
Desoximetasone 0.25% cream	Topicort®
Desoximetasone 0.25% ointment	Topicort®
Fluocinonide 0.05% gel	Lidex®
III High Potency	
Triamcinolone acetonide 0.5% ointment	Aristocort®, Kenalog®
Fluticasone propionate 0.005% ointment	Cutivate™
Amcinonide 0.1% cream	Cyclocort®
Amcinonide 0.1% lotion	Cyclocort®
Betamethasone dipropionate 0.05% cream	Diprosone®, Maxivate®
Diflorasone diacetate 0.05% cream	Florone®, Maxiflor®
Fluocinonide 0.05% cream	Lidex®-E
Betamethasone valerate 0.01% ointment	Valisone®
IV Midpotency	
Triamcinolone acetonide 0.1% ointment	Aristocort®, Kenalog®
Flurandrenolide 0.05% ointment	Cordran®
Mometasone furoate 0.1% cream	Elocon®
Fluocinolone acetonide 0.025% ointment	Synalar®
Hydrocortisone valerate 0.2% ointment	Westcort®
V Midpotency	
Flurandrenolide 0.05% cream	Cordran®
Fluticasone propionate 0.05% cream	Cutivate™
Betamethasone dipropionate 0.05% lotion	Diprosone®
Triamcinolone acetonide 0.1% lotion	Aristocort®, Kenalog®
Hydrocortisone butyrate 0.1% cream	Locoid®
Fluocinolone acetonide 0.025% cream	Synalar®
Betamethasone valerate 0.1% cream	Valisone®
Hydrocortisone valerate 0.2% cream	Westcort®
VI Low Potency	
Alclometasone dipropionate 0.05% ointment	Aclovate®
Alclometasone dipropionate 0.05% cream	Aclovate®
Triamcinolone acetonide 0.1% cream	Aristocort®, Kenalog®
Fluocinolone acetonide 0.025% cream	Synalar®
Fluocinolone acetonide 0.01% solution	Synalar®

Corticosteroids Comparison, Topical *(continued)*

Drug/Dosage Form	Brand Name
Betamethasone valerate 0.1% lotion	Valisone®
Desonide 0.05% cream	DesOwen®, Tridesilon®
VII Lowest Potency	
Hydrocortisone acetate	Hytone®
Dexamethasone phosphate	Decaderm®

GLAUCOMA DRUG THERAPY

Glaucoma Drug Therapy Comparison

	Ophthalmic Agent	Strengths Available	Reduces Aqueous Humor Production	Increases Aqueous Humor Outflow	Average Duration of Action
Mydriatics	**Sympathomimetics**				
	Dipivefrin	0.1%	Significant	Moderate	12 h
	Epinephrine	0.25%–2%	Significant	Moderate	18 h
	Beta-blockers				
	Betaxolol	0.5%	Significant	Some activity	12 h
	Levobunolol	0.5%	Significant	Some activity	18 h
	Metipranolol	0.3%	Significant	Some activity	18 h
Miscellaneous	Timolol	0.25%–0.5%	Significant	Some activity	18 h
	Carbonic Anhydrase Inhibitors				
	Acetazolamide	125–250 mg	Significant	No data	10 h
	Dorzalamide	2%	Significant	No data	8–12 h
	Methazolamide	50 mg	Significant	No data	14 h
	Cholinesterase Inhibitors				
	Demecarium	0.125%–0.25%	No data	Significant	7 d
	Echothiophate	0.03%–0.25%	No data	Significant	2 wk
	Isoflurophate	0.025%	No data	Significant	2 wk
Miotics	Physostigmine	0.25%–0.5%	No data	Significant	24 h
	Direct-Acting				
	Acetylcholine	1%	Some activity	Significant	14 min
	Carbachol	0.75%–3%	Some activity	Significant	8 h
	Pilocarpine	0.25%–10%	Some activity	Significant	5 h

*All miotic drugs significantly affect accommodation.

REGIMENS USED TO TREAT
HELICOBACTER PYLORI
AND ULCERS

There has been a lot of discussion in the medical literature about eradicating *Helicobacter pylori* bacteria as a method of treating ulcers. The National Institutes of Health Consensus Statement now recognizes the value of eradicating *H. pylori* as an appropriate method of treating ulcers.

There are a variety of regimens being tried. There is not any one "right" regimen. Depending on who you talk with or which article you read, you will get a slightly different version of the regimen. Regimens include two, three, or four agents. It is important to pay attention to which drugs are used in each combination. The agents are not necessarily interchangeable. Treatment is usually given for 2 weeks; however, some physicians may prescribe only 1 week of combination therapy, followed by up to 4 weeks of the acid blocker. The following table lists the most common regimens used today.

Drug 1	Drug 2	Drug 3	Drug 4	Duration	Efficacy
Bismuth* 2 tablets qid	Metronidazole 250 mg tid/qid	Tetracycline† 500 mg qid	Omeprazole 20 mg bid	1-2 wk	94%-98%
Bismuth* 2 tablets qid	Metronidazole 250 mg tid/qid	Tetracycline† 500 mg qid		1-2 wk	77%-82%‡
Bismuth* 2 tablets qid	Metronidazole 250 mg tid	Amoxicillin 500 mg tid/qid		1 wk or 2 wk	75%-81% 80%-94%
Bismuth* 2 tablets qid	Clarithromycin 500 mg tid	Tetracycline† 500 mg qid		1-2 wk	>90%
Bismuth* 2 tablets qid	Clarithromycin 500 mg tid	Amoxicillin 500 mg qid		1-2 wk	>90%
Bismuth* 2 tablets qid	Clarithromycin 500 mg tid	Omeprazole 20 mg bid		8 days§	80%
Metronidazole 500 mg bid	Omeprazole 20 mg bid	Clarithromycin 500 mg bid		1-2 wk	87%-91%
Amoxicillin 1 g bid	Omeprazole 20 mg bid	Clarithromycin 500 mg bid		1-2 wk	80%-95%
Amoxicillin 1 g bid	Omeprazole 20 mg bid	Metronidazole 500 mg bid		1-2 wk	77%-86%
Amoxicillin 500 mg tid	Omeprazole 40 mg daily			2 wk	54%-79%
Amoxicillin 500 mg qid	Clarithromycin 500 mg tid			2 wk	>90%
Amoxicillin 750 mg tid	Metronidazole 500 mg tid			2 wk	>85%
Clarithromycin 500 mg tid	Omeprazole 40 mg daily			2 wk	64%-83%
Clarithromycin 500 mg tid	RBC (Tritec)¶ 400 mg bid			2 wk	74%-84%
Clarithromycin 500 mg tid	Amoxicillin 1 g bid	Lansoprazole 30 mg bid		2 wk	86%-92%

*Bismuth subsalicylate (*Pepto-Bismol®* Regular Strength).

†See attachment for a discussion of the efficacy of giving *Pepto-Bismol* and tetracycline together.

‡*Helidac Therapy* (in which the bismuth and tetracycline are taken together) also includes an H_2 blocker.

§Bismuth and clarithyromycin for 1 week plus omeprazole for 8 days.

¶Ranitidine bismuth citrate.

Adapted from Soll AH, "Practice Parameters Committee of the American College of Gastroenterology. Medical Treatment of Peptic Ulcer Disease," *JAMA*, 1996, 275:622-9.

INHALED MEDICATIONS

Inhaled Medications Comparison

Agent	Indications	Onset	Duration	Frequency	Comments
Anticholinergics					
Ipratropium bromide (Atrovent®)	Bronchospasm associated with COPD		6 h	2 puffs qid	Additive bronchodilating effects used with α-, β₂-adrenergic agonists
Bronchodilators					
Albuterol (Proventil®, Proventil® HFA, Ventolin®)	Prevent exercise-induced bronchospasm; relief and prevention of bronchospasm	5 min	6-8 h	2 puffs q4-6h	
Bitolterol mesylate (Tornalate®)	Prevent and treat bronchial asthma and reversible bronchospasm	5 min	8 h	2 puffs q8h	Contains a high alcohol content that may irritate the airway
Epinephrine (Bronkaid® Mist, Primatene® Mist)	Acute paroxysms of bronchial asthma; treatment of postintubation and infectious croup	1-5 min	Individualize dosing		OTC; shorter-acting and less effective than prescription β-agonists
Ipratropium bromide and albuterol sulfate (Combivent®)	Patients with chronic obstructive pulmonary disease (COPD) on a regular aerosol bronchodilator who continue to have evidence of bronchospasm and who require a second bronchodilator			2 puffs qid	Additional doses may be administered; however, total doses should not exceed 12 in 24 hours
Isoetharine HCl (Bronkometer)	Bronchial asthma and reversible bronchospasm with bronchitis and emphysema	5 min	1-3 h	1-2 puffs q4h	May cause cardiac stimulation
Isoproterenol (Medihaler-ISO®)	Bronchospasm associated with acute/chronic bronchial asthma, pulmonary emphysema, bronchitis, bronchiectasis	2-5 min	1-2 h	1-2 puffs q4-6h	May cause cardiac stimulation; may cause saliva to turn pinkish-red
Isoproterenol HCl and phenylephrine bitartrate (Duo-Medihaler®)	Bronchospasm with acute/chronic bronchial asthma; reversible bronchospasm with emphysema and bronchitis	2-5 min	4-6 h	1-2 puffs q4-6h	May cause cardiac stimulation
Metaproterenol sulfat (Alupent®, Metaprel®)	Bronchial asthma and reversible bronchospasm; acute asthmatic attacks in children ≥6 years of age	5-30 min	4-6 h	2-3 puffs q3-4h (max 12 puffs/d)	Contraindicated in patients with arrhythmias; should not be used with other β-adrenergic aerosol inhalers because of additive effects

Inhaled Medications Comparison *(continued)*

Agent	Indications	Onset	Duration	Frequency	Comments
Pirbuterol acetate (Maxair™)	Prevent and reverse bronchospasm with reversible bronchospasm	Within 5 min	4-6 h	2 puffs q4-6h	
Salmeterol (Serevent®)	Long-term maintenance treatment of asthma and prevention of bronchospasm in patients >12 years of age	20 min	12 h	2 puffs q12h	Not meant to relieve acute asthmatic symptoms
Terbutaline sulfate (Brethaire®)	Bronchial asthma and reversible bronchospasm with bronchitis or emphysema	5-30 min	6-8 h	2 puffs q4-6h	
Corticosteroids*					
Beclomethasone dipropionate (Beclovent®, Vanceril®)	Bronchial asthma		6-8 h	2 puffs q6-8h	Coughing and wheezing are more common
Dexamethasone Na phosphate (Decadron® phosphate respihaler)	Bronchial asthma		6-8 h	3 puffs q6-8h (max 12 puffs/d)	
Flunisolide (AeroBid®)	Bronchial asthma		12 h	2 puffs bid (max 4 puffs bid)	
Triamcinolone acetonide (Azmacort™)	Bronchial asthma		6-8 h	2 puffs q6-8h (max 16 puffs/d)	Asthma should be reasonably stable before Azmacort™ treatment
Miscellaneous					
Cromolyn (Intal®)	Severe bronchial asthma; prevent exercise-induced bronchospasm		6 h	2 puffs qid	Only useful in prophylaxis; has low toxicity and is as effective as theophylline in many patients
Nedocromil sodium (Tilade®)	Mild to moderate bronchial asthma		6 h	2 puffs qid	Must be taken regularly for benefit — even during symptom-free periods

*Not indicated for rapid relief of bronchospasm. Dysphonia and oral candidiasis can occur. Long-term use is associated with cataract formation.

NARCOTIC AGONISTS

Narcotic Agonist Comparative Pharmacology

Drug	Analgesic	Antitussive	Constipation	Respiratory Depression	Sedation	Emesis	Physical Dependence
Phenanthrenes							
Codeine	+	+++	+	+	+	+	+
Hydrocodone	+	+++		+			+
Hydromorphone	++	+++	+	++	+	+	++
Levorphanol	++	++	++	++	++	+	++
Morphine	++	+++	++	++	++	++	++
Oxycodone	++	+++	++	++	++	++	++
Oxymorphone	++	+	++	+++		+++	+++
Phenylpiperidines							
Fentanyl	++			+			
Meperidine	++	+	+	++	+	+	++
Diphenylheptanes							
Methadone	++	++	++	++	+	+	+
Propoxyphene	+			+	+	+	+

Pharmacokinetics of Narcotic Agonist Analgesics

Drug	Onset (min)	Peak (h)	Duration (h)	Adult ½ (h)	Average Dosing Interval (h)		Equianalgesic Doses* (mg)	
							I.M.	P.O.
Buprenorphine†	15	1	4-8	2-3	6		0.3	NA
Butorphanol†	<10	0.5-1	3-5	2.5-3.5	3	(3-6)	2-3	NA
Codeine	15-30	0.5-1	4-6	3-4	3	(3-6)	120	200
Fentanyl	7-8	ND	1-2	1.5-6	1	(0.5-2)	0.1	NA
Hydrocodone	ND	ND	4-6	3.3-4.4			ND	ND
Hydromorphone	15-30	0.5-1	4-6	2-4	4	(3-6)	1.5	7.5
Levorphanol	30-90	0.5-1	4-8	12-16	12		2	4
Meperidine	10-45	0.5-1	2-4	3-4	3	(2-4)	75	300
Methadone	30-60	0.5-1	4-6 (acute) >8 (chronic)	15-30	8	(6-12)	10	20
Morphine	15-60	0.5-1	3-6	2-4	4	(3-6)	10	60
Nalbuphine†	<15	1	3-6	5		3-6	10	NA
Oxycodone (P.O.)	15-30	0.5-1	4-6	3-4	4	(3-6)	NA	30
Oxymorphone	5-15	0.5-1	3-6	ND		4-6	1	10‡
Pentazocine†	15-20	0.25-1	3-4	2-3	3	(3-6)	30	150
Propoxyphene (P.O.)	30-60	2-2.5	4-6	3.5-15	6	(4-8)	ND	130§-200¶

ND = no data available. NA = not applicable.

*Based on acute, short-term use. Chronic administration may alter pharmacokinetics and decrease the oral parenteral dose ratio. The morphine oral-parenteral ratio decreases to ~1.5-2.5:1 upon chronic dosing.

†Has partial antagonist activity.

‡Rectal.

§HCl salt.

¶Napsylate salt.

SOME POTENTIAL PHOTOSENSITIZING AGENTS

The following table lists agents that may increase sensitivity to ultraviolet light resulting in a phototoxic or photoallergic reaction.

Acne Medications
Benzoyl peroxide (Benzagel®)
Isotretinoin (Accutane®)
Tretinoin (Retin-A™)

Anticancer Agents
Dacarbazine (DTIC-Dome®)
Fluorouracil (Efudex®, Fluoroplex®)
Interferon beta-1b (Betaseron®)
Methotrexate (Mexate®, Trexan®)
Procarbazine (Matulane®)
Vinblastine (Velban®)

Antidepressants
Amitriptyline (Elavil®)
Amoxapine (Asendin®)
Desipramine (Norpramin®, Perto-frane®)
Doxepin (Adapin®, Sinequan®)
Fluvoxamine® (Luvox®)
Imipramine (Tofranil®)
Isocarboxazid (Marplan®)
Maprotiline (Ludiomil®)
Nortriptyline (Aventyl®, Pamelor®)
Paroxetine (Paxil™)
Protriptyline (Vivactil®)
Sertraline (Zoloft®)
Trimipramine (Surmontil®)
Venlafaxine (Effexor®)

Antihistaminess
Astemizole (Hismanal®)
Cyproheptadine (Periactin®)
Dicyclomine hydrochloride (Bentyl®)
Diphenhydramine (Benadryl®)
Loratadine (Claritin®)
Terfenadine (Seldane®/Seldane-D®)

Antihyperlipidemics
Clofibrate (Astromid-S®)
Colestipolhydrochloride (Colestid®)

Antimicrobials
Azithromycin (Zithromax®)
Cinoxacin (Cinobac®)
Ciprofloxacin (Cipro™)
Co-trimoxazole (Bactrim™, Septra®)
Demeclocycline hydrochloride (Declo-mycin®)
Doxycycline (Vibramycin®)
Griseofulvin (Fulvicin-U/F®, Gris-PEG®)
Lomefloxacin (Maxaquin®)
Methacycline (Rondomycin®)
Minocycline (Minocin®)
Nalidixic acid (NegGram®)
Norfloxacin (Noroxin®)
Ofloxacin (Floxin®)
Olsalazine (Dipentum®)
Oxytetracycline (Terramycin®)
Sparfloxacin (Zagam®)
Sulfacytine (Renoquid®)
Sulfadoxine/pyrimethamine (Fansidar®)
Sulfamethazine (Neotrizine®)

Sulfamethizole (Thiosulfil®)
Sulfamethoxazole (Gantanol®)
Sulfasalazine (Azulfidine®)
Sulfisoxazole (Gantrisin®)
Tetracycline (Achromycin®)

Antiparasitic
Bithionol (Bitin®)
Chloroquine (Aralen®)
Pyrvinium pamoate (Povan®)
Quinine

Antipsychotic Agents
Chlorpromazine (Thorazine®)
Chlorprothixene (Taractan®)
Fluphenazine (Permitil®, (Prolixin®)
Haloperidol (Haldol®)
Perphenazine (Trilafon®)
Piperacetazine (Quide®)
Prochlorperazine (Compazine®)
Promethazine (Phenergan®)
Risperidone (Risperdal®)
Thioridazine (Mellaril®)
Thiothixene (Navane®)
Trifluoperazine (Stelazine®)
Triflupromazine (Vesprin®)
Trimeprazine (Temaril®)

Antiseizure
Carbamazepine (Tegretol®)
Felbamate (Felbatol®)
Paramethadione (Paradione®)
Phenytoin (Dilantin®)
Topiramate (Cinobac®)
Trimethadione (Topamax®)
Valproic acid (Depakene®, Depakote®)

Diuretics
Acetazolamide (Diamox®)
Amiloride (Midamor®)
Chlorothiazide (Diuril®)
Cyclothiazide (Anhydron®)
Furosemide (Lasix®)
HCTZ (HydroDIURIL®)
Methyclothiazide (Aquatensen®, (Enduron®)
Metolazone (Diulo®, Zaroxolyn®)
Triamterene/HCTZ (Dyazide®, Maxzide®)

Hypoglycemics
Acetohexamide (Dymelor®)
Chlorpropamide (Diabinese®)
Glipizide (Glucotrol®)
Glyburide (Diaβeta®, Micronase®, Glynase®)
Tolazamide (Tolinase®)
Tolbutamide (Orinase®)

NSAIDs
Carprofen (Rimadyl®)
Diclofenac (Cataflam®, Voltaren®)
Etodolac (Lodine®)
Ketoprofen (Orudis®)
Naproxen (Naprosyn®)

Phenylbutazone (Butazolidin®)
Piroxicam (Feldene®)
Sulindac (Clinoril®)

Others
Amiodarone (Cordarone®)
Atorvastatin (Lipitor®)
Benzocaine (Americaine®, Dermoplast®, Solarcaine®)
Captopril (Capoten® (possibly all ACE inhibitors)
Chlordiazepoxide (Librium®)
DES (diethylstilbestrol)
Diltiazem (Cardizem®)
Disopyramide (Norpace®)
Enalapril (Vaseretic®, Vasotec®)
Estazolam (ProSom™)

Estrogen (Premarin®)
Fluvastatin (Lescol®)
Gold sodium thiomalate (Myochrysine®)
Hexachlorophene (PhisoHex®)
Lovastatin (Mevacor®)
Oral contraceptives (Ortho-Novum™, Norinyl®, etc)
PABA (para-aminobenzoic acid)
Pravastatin (Pravachol®)
Quinidine sulfate and gluconate
Saquinavir (Invirase®)
Selegiline (Eldepryl®)
Simvastatin (Zocor®)
Zolpidem (Ambien®)

ASTHMA GUIDELINES

Expert Panel Report II: Guidelines for the Diagnosis and Management of Asthma

Stepwise Approach for Managing Asthma in Adults and Children >5 Years of Age: Classify Severity

Goals of Asthma Treatment

- Prevent chronic and troublesome symptoms (eg, coughing or breathlessness in the night, in the early morning, or after exertion)
- Maintain (near) "normal" pulmonary function
- Maintain normal activity levels (ie, exercise and other physical activity)
- Prevent recurrent exacerbations of asthma and minimize the need for emergency department visits or hospitalizations
- Provide optimal pharmacotherapy with minimal or no adverse effects
- Meet patients' and families' expectations of and satisfaction with asthma care

Clinical Features Before Treatment*

Symptoms**	Night-time Symptoms	Lung Function
STEP 4: Severe Persistent		
• Continual symptoms • Limited physical activity • Frequent exacerbations	Frequent	• FEV_1/PEF ≤60% predicted • PEF variability >30%
STEP 3: Moderate Persistent		
• Daily symptoms • Daily use of inhaled short-acting beta$_2$-agonist • Exacerbations affect activity • Exacerbations ≥2 times/week may last days	>1 time/week	• FEV_1/PEF >60% - <80% predicted • PEF variability >30%
STEP 2: Mild Persistent		
• Symptoms >2 times/week but <1 time/day • Exacerbations may affect activity	>2 times/month	• FEV_1/PEF ≥80% predicted • PEF variability 20% - 30%
STEP 1: Mild Intermittent		
• Symptoms ≤2 times/week • Asymptomatic and normal PEF between exacerbations • Exacerbations brief (from a few hours to a few days); intensity may vary	≤2 times/month	• FEV_1/PEF ≥80% predicted • PEF variability ≤20%

*The presence of one of the features of severity is sufficient to place a patient in that category. An individual should be assigned to the most severe grade in which any feature occurs. The characteristics noted in this figure are general and may overlap because asthma is highly variable. Furthermore, an individual's classification may change over time.

**Patients at any level of severity can have mild, moderate, or severe exacerbations. Some patients with intermittent asthma experience severe and life-threatening exacerbations separated by long periods of normal lung function and no symptoms.

Stepwise Approach for Managing Asthma in Adults and Children >5 Years of Age: Treatment

(Preferred treatments are in **bold** print)

Long-Term Control	Quick Relief	Education
STEP 4: Severe Persistent		
Daily medications: • **Anti-inflammatory: Inhaled corticosteroid (high dose) and** • Long-acting bronchodilator: Either **long-acting inhaled beta$_2$-agonist**, sustained-release theophylline, or long-acting beta$_2$-agonist tablets **and** • Corticosteroid tablets or syrup long term (2 mg/kg/day, generally do not exceed 60 mg per day).	• Short-acting bronchodilator: **Inhaled beta$_2$-agonists** as needed for symptoms. • Intensity of treatment will depend on severity of exacerbation; see "Managing Exacerbations" • Use of short-acting inhaled beta$_2$-agonists on a daily basis, or increasing use, indicates the need for additional long-term control therapy.	Steps 2 and 3 actions plus: • Refer to individual education/counseling
STEP 3: Moderate Persistent		
Daily medication: • Either – **Anti-inflammatory: Inhaled corticosteroid (medium dose)** or – **Inhaled corticosteroid (low-medium dose)** and add a long-acting bronchodilator, especially for night-time symptoms: Either **long-acting inhaled beta$_2$-agonist**, sustained-release theophylline, or long-acting beta$_2$-agonist tablets. • If needed – Anti-inflammatory: **Inhaled corticosteroids (medium-high dose) and** – **Long-acting bronchodilator,** especially for nighttime symptoms; either **long-acting inhaled beta$_2$-agonist,** sustained release theophylline, or long-acting beta$_2$-agonist tablets.	• Short-acting bronchodilator: **Inhaled beta$_2$-agonists** as needed for symptoms. • Intensity of treatment will depend on severity of exacerbation; see "Managing Exacerbations." • Use of short-acting inhaled beta$_2$-agonists on a daily basis, or increasing use, indicates the need for additional long-term control therapy.	Step 1 actions plus: • Teach self-monitoring • Refer to group education if available • Review and update self-management plan
STEP 2: Mild Persistent		
One daily medication: • **Anti-inflammatory:** Either **inhaled corticosteroid** (low doses) or **cromolyn or nedocromil** (children usually begin with a trial of cromolyn or nedocromil). • Sustained-release theophylline to serum concentration of 5-15 mcg/mL is an alternative, but not preferred, therapy. Zafirlukast or zileuton may also be considered for patients ≥12 years of age, although their position in therapy is not fully established.	• Short-acting bronchodilator: **Inhaled beta$_2$-agonists** as needed for symptoms. • Intensity of treatment will depend on severity of exacerbation; see "Managing Exacerbations." •Use of short-acting inhaled beta$_2$-agonists on a daily basis, or increasing use, indicates the need for additional long-term control therapy.	Step 1 actions plus: • Teach self-monitoring • Refer to group education if available • Review and update self-management plan
STEP 1: Mild Intermittent		
No daily medication needed.	• Short-acting bronchodilator: **Inhaled beta$_2$-agonists** as needed for symptoms. • Intensity of treatment will depend on severity of exacerbation; see "Managing Exacerbations" • Use of short-acting inhaled beta$_2$-agonists more than 2 times/week may indicate the need to initiate long-term control therapy	• Teach basic facts about asthma • Teach inhaler/spacer/holding chamber technique • Discuss roles of medications •Develop self-management plan • Develop action plan for when and how to take rescue actions, especially for patients with a history of severe exacerbations • Discuss appropriate environmental control measures to avoid exposure to known allergens and irritants

ASTHMA GUIDELINES *(Continued)*

↓ **Step down**
Review treatment every 1-6 months; a gradual stepwise reduction in treatment may be possible.

↑**Step up**
If control is not maintained, consider step up. First, review patient medication technique, adherence, and environmental control (avoidance of allergens or other factors that contribute to asthma severity.)

Notes:

- **The stepwise approach presents general guidelines to assist clinical decision making; it is not intended to be a specific prescription. Asthma is highly variable; clinicians should tailor specific medication plans to the needs and circumstances of individual patients.**

- Gain control as quickly as possible; then decrease treatment to the least medication necessary to maintain control. Gaining control may be accomplished by either starting treatment at the step most appropriate to the initial severity of the condition or starting at a higher level of therapy (eg, a course of systemic corticosteroids or higher dose of inhaled corticosteroids).

- A rescue course of systemic corticosteroids may be needed at any time and at any step.

- Some patients with intermittent asthma experience severe and life-threatening exacerbations separated by long periods of normal lung function and no symptoms. This may be especially common with exacerbations provoked by respiratory infections. A short course of systemic corticosteroids is recommended.

- At each step, patients should control their environment to avoid or control factors that make their asthma worse (eg, allergens, irritants); this requires specific diagnosis and education.

Management of Asthma Exacerbations: Home Treatment*

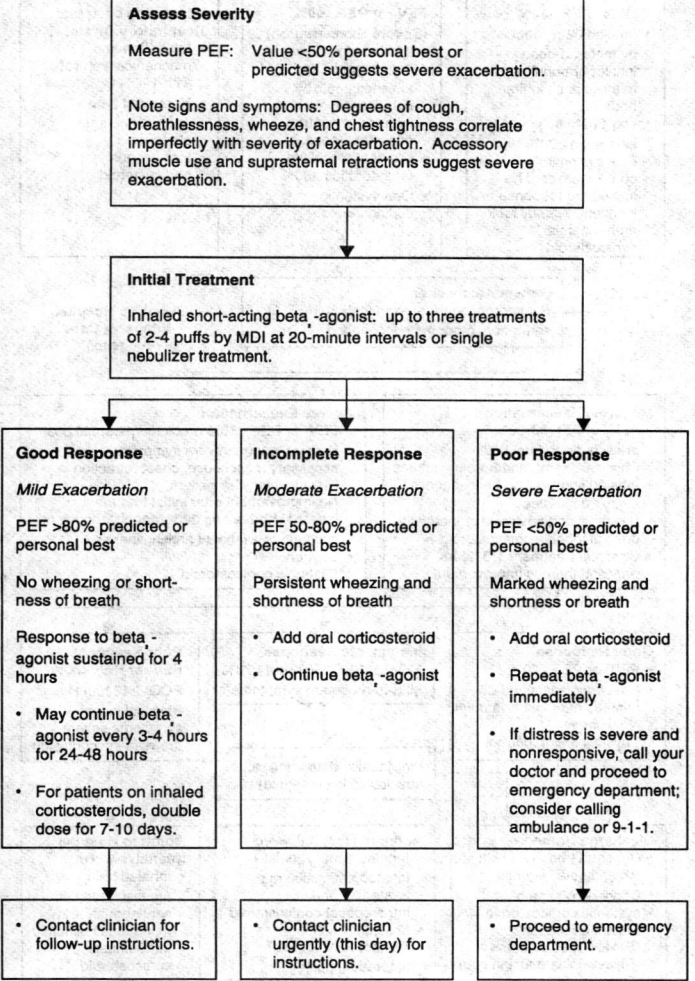

Assess Severity

Measure PEF: Value <50% personal best or predicted suggests severe exacerbation.

Note signs and symptoms: Degrees of cough, breathlessness, wheeze, and chest tightness correlate imperfectly with severity of exacerbation. Accessory muscle use and suprasternal retractions suggest severe exacerbation.

Initial Treatment

Inhaled short-acting beta-agonist: up to three treatments of 2-4 puffs by MDI at 20-minute intervals or single nebulizer treatment.

Good Response

Mild Exacerbation

PEF >80% predicted or personal best

No wheezing or shortness of breath

Response to beta-agonist sustained for 4 hours

- May continue beta-agonist every 3-4 hours for 24-48 hours

- For patients on inhaled corticosteroids, double dose for 7-10 days.

Incomplete Response

Moderate Exacerbation

PEF 50-80% predicted or personal best

Persistent wheezing and shortness of breath

- Add oral corticosteroid

- Continue beta-agonist

Poor Response

Severe Exacerbation

PEF <50% predicted or personal best

Marked wheezing and shortness or breath

- Add oral corticosteroid

- Repeat beta-agonist immediately

- If distress is severe and nonresponsive, call your doctor and proceed to emergency department; consider calling ambulance or 9-1-1.

- Contact clinician for follow-up instructions.

- Contact clinician urgently (this day) for instructions.

- Proceed to emergency department.

* Patients at high risk of asthma-related death should receive immediate clinical attention after initial treatment. Additional therapy may be required.

ASTHMA GUIDELINES *(Continued)*

Management of Asthma Exacerbations: Emergency Department and Hospital-Based Care

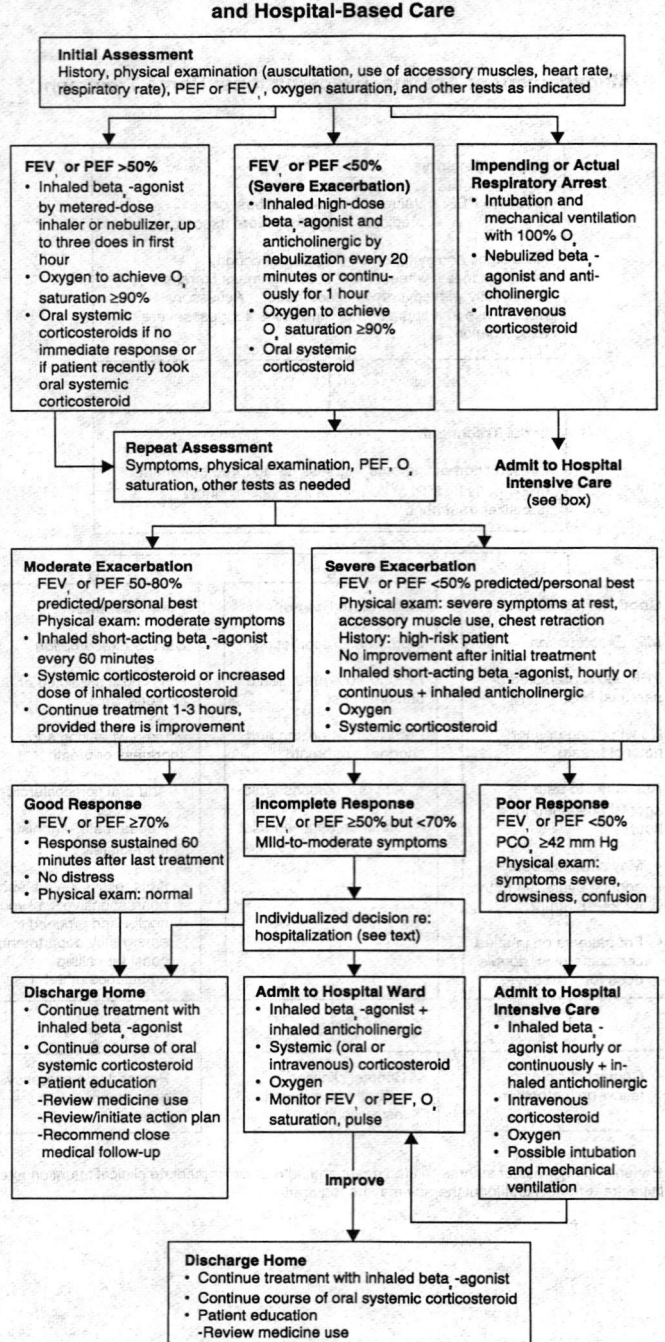

Initial Assessment
History, physical examination (auscultation, use of accessory muscles, heart rate, respiratory rate), PEF or FEV₁, oxygen saturation, and other tests as indicated

FEV₁ or PEF >50%
- Inhaled beta₂-agonist by metered-dose inhaler or nebulizer, up to three doses in first hour
- Oxygen to achieve O₂ saturation ≥90%
- Oral systemic corticosteroids if no immediate response or if patient recently took oral systemic corticosteroid

FEV₁ or PEF <50% (Severe Exacerbation)
- Inhaled high-dose beta₂-agonist and anticholinergic by nebulization every 20 minutes or continuously for 1 hour
- Oxygen to achieve O₂ saturation ≥90%
- Oral systemic corticosteroid

Impending or Actual Respiratory Arrest
- Intubation and mechanical ventilation with 100% O₂
- Nebulized beta₂-agonist and anti-cholinergic
- Intravenous corticosteroid

Repeat Assessment
Symptoms, physical examination, PEF, O₂ saturation, other tests as needed

Admit to Hospital Intensive Care (see box)

Moderate Exacerbation
FEV₁ or PEF 50-80% predicted/personal best
Physical exam: moderate symptoms
- Inhaled short-acting beta₂-agonist every 60 minutes
- Systemic corticosteroid or increased dose of inhaled corticosteroid
- Continue treatment 1-3 hours, provided there is improvement

Severe Exacerbation
FEV₁ or PEF <50% predicted/personal best
Physical exam: severe symptoms at rest, accessory muscle use, chest retraction
History: high-risk patient
No improvement after initial treatment
- Inhaled short-acting beta₂-agonist, hourly or continuous + inhaled anticholinergic
- Oxygen
- Systemic corticosteroid

Good Response
- FEV₁ or PEF ≥70%
- Response sustained 60 minutes after last treatment
- No distress
- Physical exam: normal

Incomplete Response
FEV₁ or PEF ≥50% but <70%
Mild-to-moderate symptoms

Poor Response
FEV₁ or PEF <50%
PCO₂ ≥42 mm Hg
Physical exam: symptoms severe, drowsiness, confusion

Individualized decision re: hospitalization (see text)

Discharge Home
- Continue treatment with inhaled beta₂-agonist
- Continue course of oral systemic corticosteroid
- Patient education
  - Review medicine use
  - Review/initiate action plan
  - Recommend close medical follow-up

Admit to Hospital Ward
- Inhaled beta₂-agonist + inhaled anticholinergic
- Systemic (oral or intravenous) corticosteroid
- Oxygen
- Monitor FEV₁ or PEF, O₂ saturation, pulse

Admit to Hospital Intensive Care
- Inhaled beta₂-agonist hourly or continuously + inhaled anticholinergic
- Intravenous corticosteroid
- Oxygen
- Possible intubation and mechanical ventilation

Improve

Discharge Home
- Continue treatment with inhaled beta₂-agonist
- Continue course of oral systemic corticosteroid
- Patient education
  - Review medicine use
  - Review/initiate action plan
  - Recommend close medical follow-up

ESTIMATED COMPARATIVE DAILY DOSAGES FOR INHALED CORTICOSTEROIDS

Children

Drug	Low Dose	Medium Dose	High Dose
Beclomethasone dipropionate 42 mcg/puff 84 mcg/puff	84-336 mcg (2-8 puffs)	336-672 mcg (8-16 puffs)	>672 mcg (>16 puffs)
Budesonide Turbuhaler 200 mcg/dose	100-200 mcg	200-400 mcg (1-2 inhalations – 200 mcg)	>400 mcg (>2 inhalations – 200 mcg)
Flunisolide 250 mcg/puff	500-750 mcg (2-3 puffs)	1000-1250 mcg (4-5 puffs)	>1250 mcg (>5 puffs)
Fluticasone Metered dose inhaler: 44, 110, 220 mcg/puff	88-176 mcg (2-4 puffs – 44 mcg)	176-440 mcg (4-10 puffs – 44 mcg) or (2-4 puffs – 110 mcg)	>440 mcg (>4 puffs – 110 mcg)
Dry powder inhaler: 50, 100, 250 mcg/dose	(2-4 inhalations – 50 mcg)	(2-4 inhalations – 100 mcg)	(>4 inhalations – 100 mcg)
Triamcinolone acetonide 100 mcg/puff	400-800 mcg (4-8 puffs)	800-1200 mcg (8-12 puffs)	>1200 mcg (>12 puffs)

Adults

Drug	Low Dose	Medium Dose	High Dose
Beclomethasone dipropionate 42 mcg/puff	168-504 mcg (4-12 puffs – 42 mcg)	504-840 mcg (12-20 puffs – 42 mcg)	>840 mcg (>20 puffs – 42 mcg)
84 mcg/puff	(2-6 puffs – 84 mcg)	(6-10 puffs – 84 mcg)	(>10 puffs – 84 mcg)
Budesonide Turbuhaler 200 mcg/dose	200-400 mcg (1-2 inhalations)	400-600 mcg (2-3 inhalations)	>600 mcg (>3 inhalations)
Flunisolide 250 mcg/puff	500-1000 mcg (2-4 puffs)	1000-2000 mcg (4-8 puffs)	>2000 mcg (>8 puffs)
Fluticasone Metered dose inhaler: 44, 110, 220 mcg/puff	88-264 mcg (2-6 puffs – 44 mcg) or (2 puffs – 110 mcg)	264-660 mcg (2-6 puffs – 110 mcg)	>660 mcg (>6 puffs – 110 mcg) or (>3 puffs – 220 mcg)
Dry powder inhaler: 50, 100, 250 mcg/dose	(2-6 inhalations – 50 mcg)	(3-6 inhalations – 100 mcg)	(>6 inhalations – 100 mcg)
Triamcinolone acetonide 100 mcg/puff	400-1000 mcg (4-10 puffs)	1000-2000 mcg (10-20 puffs)	>2000 mcg (>20 puffs)

ASTHMA GUIDELINES *(Continued)*

Notes:

- **The most important determinant of appropriate dosing is the clinician's judgment of the patient's response to therapy.** The clinician must monitor the patient's response on several clinical parameters and adjust the dose accordingly. The stepwise approach to therapy emphasizes that once control of asthma is achieved, the dose of mediation should be carefully titrated to the minimum dose required to maintain control, thus reducing the potential for adverse effect.

- The reference point for the range in the dosages for children is data on the safety on inhaled corticosteroids in children, which, in general, suggest that the dose ranges are equivalent to beclomethasone dipropionate 200-400 mcg/day (low dose), 400-800 mcg/day (medium dose), and >800 mcg/day (high dose).

- Some dosages may be outside package labeling.

- Metered-dose inhaler (MDI) dosages are expressed as the actuator dose (the amount of drug leaving the actuator and delivered to the patient), which is the labeling required in the United States. This is different from the dosage expressed as the valve dose (the amount of drug leaving the valve, all of which is not available to the patient), which is used in many European countries and in some of the scientific literature. Dry powder inhaler (DPI) doses (eg, Turbuhaler) are expressed as the amount of drug in the inhaler following activation.

ESTIMATED CLINICAL COMPARABILITY OF DOSES FOR INHALED CORTICOSTEROIDS

Data from *in vitro* and in clinical trials suggest that the different inhaled corticosteroid preparations are not equivalent on a per puff or microgram basis. However, it is entirely clear what implications these differences have for dosing recommendations in clinical practice because there are few data directly comparing the preparations. Relative dosing for clinical comparability is affected by differences in topical potency, clinical effects at different doses, delivery device, and bioavailability. The Expert Panel developed recommended dose ranges for different preparations based on available data and the following assumptions and cautions about estimating relative doses needed to achieve comparable clinical effect.

- **Relative topical potency using human skin blanching**

  - Standard test for determining relative topical anti-inflammatory potency is the topical vasoconstriction (MacKenzie skin blanching) test.

  - The MacKenzie topical skin blanching test correlates with binding affinities and binding half-lives for human lung corticosteroid receptors (see following table) (Dahlberg, et al, 1984; Hogger and Rohdewald 1994).

  - The relationship between relative topical anti-inflammatory effect and clinical comparability in asthma management is not certain. However, recent clinical trials suggest that different *in vitro* measures of anti-inflammatory effect is not certain. However, recent clinical trials suggest that different in vitro measures of anti-inflammatory effect correlate with clinical efficacy (Barnes and Pedersen 1993; Johnson 1996; Kamada, et al, 1996; Ebden, et al, 1986; Leblanc, et al, 1994; Gustaffson, et al, 1993; Lundback, et al, 1993; Barnes, et al, 1993; Fabbri, et al, 1993; Langdon and Capsey, 1994; Ayres, et al, 1995; Rafferty, et al, 1985; Bjorkander, et al, 1982, Stiksa, et al, 1982; Willey, et al, 1982.)

Medication	Topical Potency (Skin Blanching)*	Corticosteroid Receptor Binding Half-Life	Receptor Binding Affinity
Beclomethasone dipropionate (BDP)	600	7.5 hours	13.5
Budesonide (BUD)	980	5.1 hours	9.4
Flunisolide (FLU)	330	3.5 hours	1.8
Fluticasone propionate (FP)	1200	10.5 hours	18.0
Triamcinolone acetonide (TAA)	330	3.9 hours	3.6

*Numbers are assigned in reference to dexamethasone, which has a value of "1" in the MacKenzie test.

- **Relative doses to achieve similar clinical effects**
  - Clinical effects are evaluated by a number of outcome parameters (eg, changes in spirometry, peak flow rates, symptom scores, quick-relief beta$_2$-agonist use, frequency of exacerbations, airway responsiveness).
  - The daily dose and duration of treatment may affect these outcome parameters differently (eg, symptoms and peak flow may improve at lower doses and over a shorter treatment time than bronchial reactivity) (van Essen-Zandvliet, et al, 1992; Haahtela, et al, 1991)
  - Delivery systems influence comparability. For example, the delivery device for budesonide (Turbuhaler) delivers approximately twice the amount of drug to the airway as the MDI, thus enhancing the clinical effect (Thorsson, et al, 1994); Agertoft and Pedersen, 1993).
  - Individual patients may respond differently to different preparations, as noted by clinical experience.
  - Clinical trials comparing effects in reducing symptoms and improving peak expiratory flow demonstrate:
  - BDP amd BUD achieved comparable effects at similar microgram doses by MDI (Bjorkander, et al, 1982; Ebden, et al, 1986; Rafferty, et al, 1985).
  - BDP achieved effects similar to twice the dose of TAA on a microgram basis.

Reference
National Asthma Education and Prevention Program, February 1997

OSTEOPOROSIS MANAGEMENT QUICK REFERENCE

PREVALENCE

Osteoporosis effects 25 million Americans of which 80% are women. 27% of American women >80 years of age have osteopenia and 70% of American women >80 years of age have osteoporosis.

CONSEQUENCES

1.3 million bone fractures annually (low impact/nontraumatic) and pain, pulmonary insufficiency, decreased quality of life, and economic costs; >250,000 hip fractures per year with a 20% mortality rate.

RISK FACTORS

Advanced age, female, chronic renal disease, hyperparathyroidism, Cushing's disease, hypogonadism/anorexia, hyperprolactinemia, cancer, large and prolonged dose heparin or glucocorticoids, anticonvulsants, hyperthyroidism (current or history, or excessive thyroid supplements), sedentary, excessive exercise, early menopause, oopherectomy without hormone replacement, excessive aluminum-containing antacid, smoking, methotrexate.

DIAGNOSIS/MONITORING

DXA bone density, history of fracture (low impact or nontraumatic), compressed vertebrae, decreased height, hump-back appearance. Osteomark™ urine assay measures bone breakdown fragments and may help assess therapy response earlier than DXA but diagnostic value is uncertain as Osteomark™ doesn't reveal extent of bone loss. Bone markers may be tested to evaluate effectiveness of antiresorptive urine therapy.

OSTEOPOROSIS PREVENTION

1. Adequate dietary calcium (eg, dairy products)

2. Vitamin D (eg, fortified dairy products, cod, fatty fish)

3. Weight-bearing exercise (eg, walking) as tolerated

4. Calcium supplement of 1000-1500 mg <u>elemental</u> calcium daily (divided in 500 mg increments); women >65 years on estrogen replacement therapy supplement 1000 mg <u>elemental</u> calcium; women >65 not receiving estrogens and men >55 years supplement 1500 mg <u>elemental</u> calcium. To minimize constipation add fiber and start with 500 mg/day for several months, then increase to 500 mg twice daily taken at different times than fiber. Chewable and liquid products are available. Calcium carbonate is given tihe food to enhance bioavailability. Calcium citrate may be given without regards to meals.

   - Contraindications: Hypercalcemia, ventricular fibrillation
   - Side effects: Constipation, anorexia
   - Drug interactions: Fiber, tetracycline, iron supplement, minerals

5. Vitamin D Supplement: 400-800 units daily (often satisfied by 1-2 multivitamins or fortified milk) in addition to calcium or a combined calcium and vitamin D supplement and/or >15 minutes direct sunlight/day. Some elderly, especially with significant renal or liver disease can't metabolize (activate) vitamin D and require calcitriol 0.25 mcg orally twice daily or adjusted per serum calcium level, the active form of vitamin D; can check 1,25 OH vitamin D level to confirm need for calcitriol.

   - Contraindications: Hypercalcemia (weakness, headache, drowsiness, nausea, diarrhea), hypercalciuria and renal stones
   - Side effects (uncommon): Hypercalcemia (see above)
   - Monitor 24-hour urine and serum calcium if using >1000 units/day

6. Estrogen: Especially useful if bone density <80% of average plus symptoms of estrogen deficiency or cardiac disease. Bone density increases over 1-2 years then plateaus. This is considered 1st line therapy unless contraindicated due to medicinal history (see below) or patient preference to avoid HRT (hormone replacement therapy).

- Contraindications: Pregnancy, breast or estrogen-dependent cancer, undiagnosed abnormal genital bleeding, active thrombophlebitis, or history of thromboembolism during previous estrogen or oral contraceptive therapy or pregnancy. Pretreatment mammogram, gynecological exam are advised along with routine breast exam because of a possibly increased risk of breast cancer with long-term use.

- Dose: Conjugated estrogen of 0.625 mg/day or its equivalent (continuous therapy preferred).

- Side effects: Vaginal spotting/bleeding, nausea, vomiting, breast tenderness/enlargement, amenorrheic with extended use.
Initiate therapy slowly (side effects are more common and severe in women without estrogen for many years). Administer with medroxyprogesterone acetate (MPA) 2.5-5 mg daily in women with uterus (unopposed estrogen can cause endometrial cancer). MPA can increase vaginal bleeding, increase weight, edema, mood changes.

- Drug Interactions: May increase corticosteroid effect, monitor for need to decrease corticosteroid dose.

OSTEOPOROSIS TREATMENT

1. Calcium, vitamin D, exercise, and estrogen: As above

2. Alendronate (Fosamax®): Consider if patient is intolerant of, or refuses estrogen or it is contraindicated, especially if severe osteoporosis (ie, ≥2.5 standard deviations below average young adult bone density, T-score, or history of low impact or nontraumatic fracture). Increasing bone density of hip and spine observed for at least 3 years (ie, no plateau as seen with estrogen).

   - Contraindications: Hypocalcemia, not advised if existing gastrointestinal disorders (eg, esophageal disorders such as reflux, sensitive stomach).

   - Dose: 10 mg once daily (treatment dose for osteoporosis; not recommended if creatinine clearance <35 mL/minute) before breakfast on an empty stomach with 6-8 ounces tap water (not mineral water, coffee, or juice) and remain upright or raise head of bed for bedridden patients at least 30 degree angle for at least 30 minutes (otherwise may cause ulcerative esophagitis) before eating or drinking. Osteopenia: 5 mg per day for prevention.

   Therapy with calcium and vitamin D is advised, but must be given at a different time of day then alendronate.

   - Side effects (well tolerated): Difficulty swallowing, heartburn, abdominal discomfort, nausea (GI side effects increase with aspirin products), arthralgia/myalgia, constipation, diarrhea, headache, esophagitis.

   - Drug interactions: None known to date.

3. Etidronate: Not FDA approved for postmenopausal osteoporosis and can decrease the quality of bone formation, therefore, change to alendronate.

4. Calcitonin (nasal; Miacalcin): Indicated if estrogen refused, intolerant, or contraindicated. Potential analgesic effect.

   - Contraindications: Hypersensitivity to salmon protein or gelatin diluent; 1 spray (200 units) into 1 nostril daily (alternate right and left nostril daily); 5 days on and 2 days off is also effective; alternate day administration not effective. If use only for pain, can decrease dose once pain is controlled.

   - Side effects (few): Nasal dryness and irritation (periodically inspect); adequate dietary or supplemental calcium + vitamin D is essential.

   Subcutaneous route (100 units daily): Many side effects (eg, nausea, flushing, anorexia) and the discomfort/inconvenience of injection.

5. Fall prevention: Minimize psychoactive and cardiovascular drugs (monitor BP for orthostasis), give diuretics early in the day, environmental safety check.

	% Calcium	Elemental Calcium	Brand
Calcium Gluconate	9% elemental	500 mg = 45 mg	Various
Calcium Glubionate	6.5% elemental	1.8 g = 115 g/5 mL	Neo-Calglucon®

OSTEOPOROSIS MANAGEMENT QUICK REFERENCE
(Continued)

	% Calcium	Elemental Calcium	Brand
Calcium Lactate	13% elemental	325 mg = 42.25 mg	Various
Calcium Citrate	21% elemental	950 mg = 200 mg	Citrical®
		Effervescent tabs 2376 mg = 500 mg	Citrical Liquitab®
Calcium Acetate	25% elemental	1000 mg = 250 mg 667 mg = 169 mg	Phos-Ex 250® Phos-Lo®
Tricalcium Phosphate	39% elemental	1565.2 mg = 600 mg	Posture®
Calcium Carbonate	40% elemental	1.2 g = 500 mg 1.2 g/5 mL = 500 mg 1.5 g = 600 mg	TUMS® Oscal-500®oral suspension Caltrate 600®

References

Ashworth L, "Focus on Alendronate. A Nonhormonal Option for the Treatment of Osteoporosis in Postmenopausal Women," *Formulary*, 1996, 31:23-30.

Johnson SR, "Should Older Women Use Estrogen Replacement," *J Am Geriatr Soc*, 1996, 44:89-90.

Liberman UA, Weiss SR, and Brool J, "Effect of Oral Alendronate on Bone-Mineral Density and the Incidence of Fracture in Postmenopausal Osteoporosis," *N Engl J Med*, 1995, 333:1437-43.

"New Drugs for Osteoporosis," *Med Lett Drugs Ther*, 1996, 38:1-3.

NIH Consensus Development Panel on Optimal Calcium Intake, *JAMA*, 1994, 272:1942-8.

PCA Osteoporosis Prevention and Treatment Video-Teleconference (March 1, April 2 and 3, 1996).

PARKINSON'S DISEASE MANAGEMENT

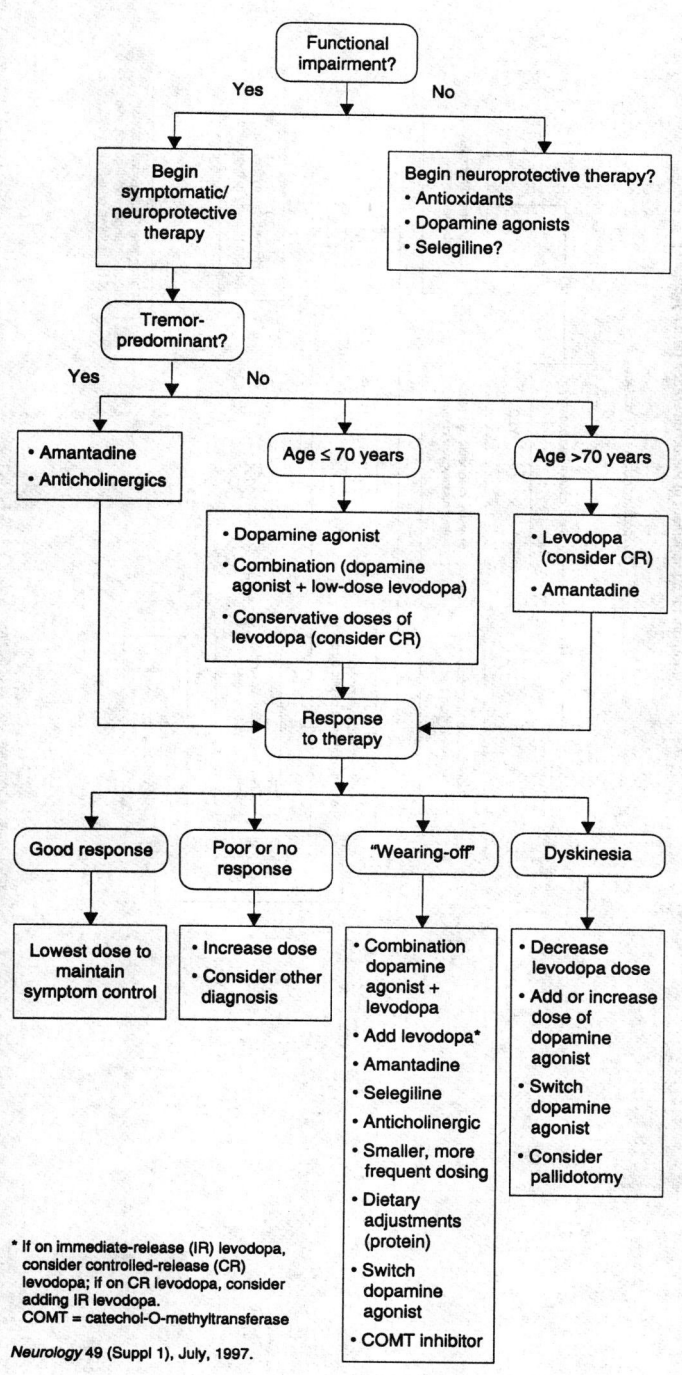

* If on immediate-release (IR) levodopa, consider controlled-release (CR) levodopa; if on CR levodopa, consider adding IR levodopa.
COMT = catechol-O-methyltransferase

Neurology 49 (Suppl 1), July, 1997.

PEPTIC ULCER CARE

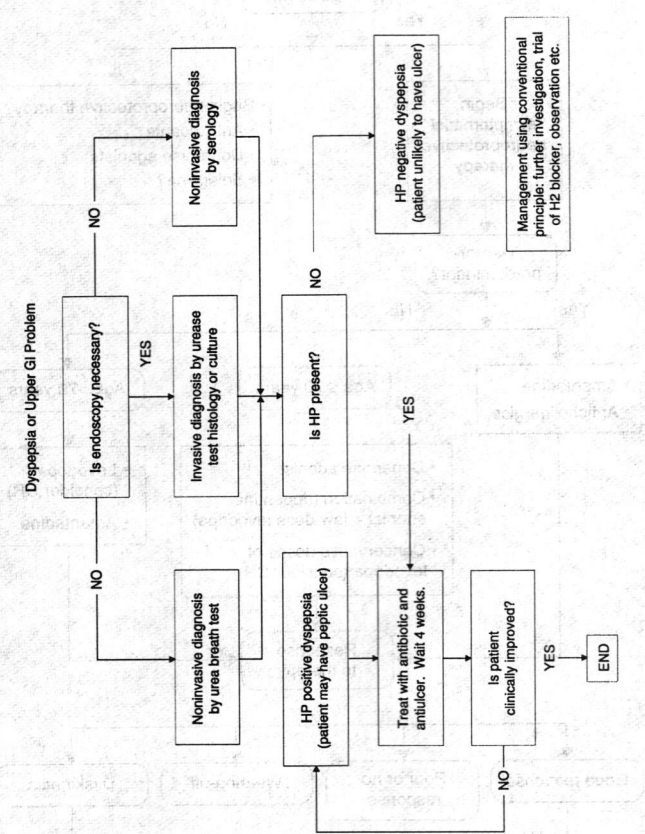

Algorithm for Management of Peptic Ulceration (and Dyspepsia)

Dyspepsia or Upper GI Problem

Is endoscopy necessary?

NO → Noninvasive diagnosis by urea breath test → HP positive dyspepsia (patient may have peptic ulcer) → Treat with antibiotic and antiulcer. Wait 4 weeks. → Is patient clinically improved? → YES → END

YES → Invasive diagnosis by urease test histology or culture → Is HP present?

NO → Noninvasive diagnosis by serology

YES → Treat with antibiotic and antiulcer. Wait 4 weeks.

Is HP present? NO → HP negative dyspepsia (patient unlikely to have ulcer) → Management using conventional principle: further investigation, trial of H2 blocker, observation etc.

Is patient clinically improved? NO → (back to HP positive dyspepsia)

Barry J. Marshall, *American Journal of Gastroenterology*, Vol. 89, No. 8, 1994.

PHARMACOLOGICAL MANAGEMENT OF PATIENTS WITH HEART FAILURE

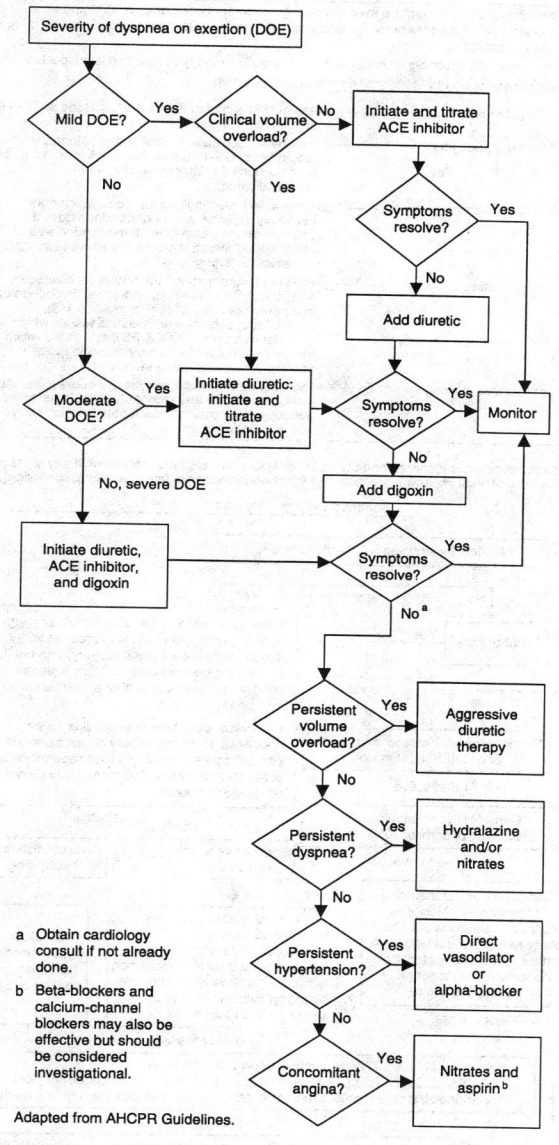

a   Obtain cardiology consult if not already done.

b   Beta-blockers and calcium-channel blockers may also be effective but should be considered investigational.

Adapted from AHCPR Guidelines.

TREATMENT OPTIONS FOR CONSTIPATION

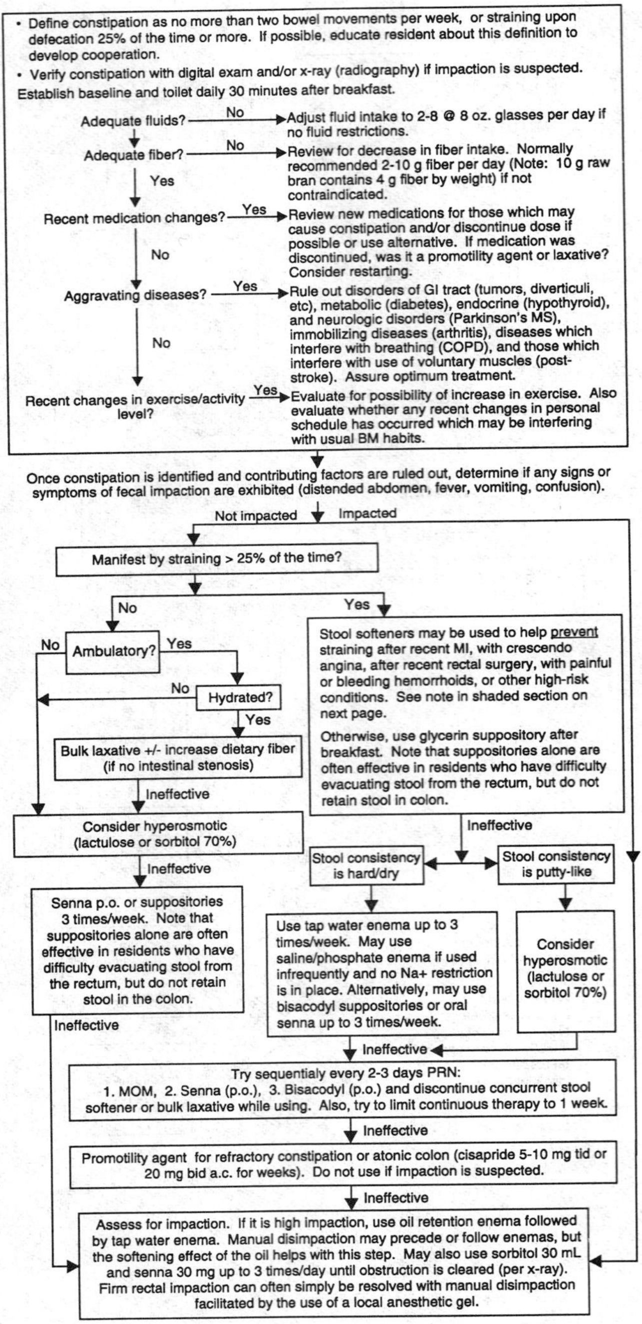

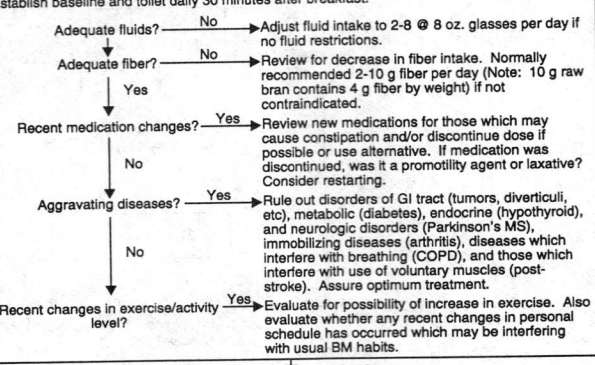

- Define constipation as no more than two bowel movements per week, or straining upon defecation 25% of the time or more. If possible, educate resident about this definition to develop cooperation.
- Verify constipation with digital exam and/or x-ray (radiography) if impaction is suspected. Establish baseline and toilet daily 30 minutes after breakfast.

Adequate fluids? —**No**→ Adjust fluid intake to 2-8 @ 8 oz. glasses per day if no fluid restrictions.

Adequate fiber? —**No**→ Review for decrease in fiber intake. Normally recommended 2-10 g fiber per day (Note: 10 g raw bran contains 4 g fiber by weight) if not contraindicated.

↓ **Yes**

Recent medication changes? —**Yes**→ Review new medications for those which may cause constipation and/or discontinue dose if possible or use alternative. If medication was discontinued, was it a promotility agent or laxative? Consider restarting.

↓ **No**

Aggravating diseases? —**Yes**→ Rule out disorders of GI tract (tumors, diverticuli, etc), metabolic (diabetes), endocrine (hypothyroid), and neurologic disorders (Parkinson's MS), immobilizing diseases (arthritis), diseases which interfere with breathing (COPD), and those which interfere with use of voluntary muscles (post-stroke). Assure optimum treatment.

↓ **No**

Recent changes in exercise/activity level? —**Yes**→ Evaluate for possibility of increase in exercise. Also evaluate whether any recent changes in personal schedule has occurred which may be interfering with usual BM habits.

Once constipation is identified and contributing factors are ruled out, determine if any signs or symptoms of fecal impaction are exhibited (distended abdomen, fever, vomiting, confusion).

Not impacted ← ↓ → **Impacted**

Manifest by straining > 25% of the time?

No ↓ | **Yes** ↓

No ← Ambulatory? **Yes** →

No ← Hydrated? →

↓ **Yes**

Bulk laxative +/- increase dietary fiber (if no intestinal stenosis)

↓ Ineffective

Consider hyperosmotic (lactulose or sorbitol 70%)

↓ Ineffective

Senna p.o. or suppositories 3 times/week. Note that suppositories alone are often effective in residents who have difficulty evacuating stool from the rectum, but do not retain stool in the colon.

↓ Ineffective

(Impacted branch, right column):

Stool softeners may be used to help <u>prevent</u> straining after recent MI, with crescendo angina, after recent rectal surgery, with painful or bleeding hemorrhoids, or other high-risk conditions. See note in shaded section on next page.

Otherwise, use glycerin suppository after breakfast. Note that suppositories alone are often effective in residents who have difficulty evacuating stool from the rectum, but do not retain stool in colon.

↓ Ineffective

Stool consistency is hard/dry ← → Stool consistency is putty-like

Use tap water enema up to 3 times/week. May use saline/phosphate enema if used infrequently and no Na+ restriction is in place. Alternatively, may use bisacodyl suppositories or oral senna up to 3 times/week.

Consider hyperosmotic (lactulose or sorbitol 70%)

↓ Ineffective

Try sequentially every 2-3 days PRN:
1. MOM, 2. Senna (p.o.), 3. Bisacodyl (p.o.) and discontinue concurrent stool softener or bulk laxative while using. Also, try to limit continuous therapy to 1 week.

↓ Ineffective

Promotility agent for refractory constipation or atonic colon (cisapride 5-10 mg tid or 20 mg bid a.c. for weeks). Do not use if impaction is suspected.

↓ Ineffective

Assess for impaction. If it is high impaction, use oil retention enema followed by tap water enema. Manual disimpaction may precede or follow enemas, but the softening effect of the oil helps with this step. May also use sorbitol 30 mL and senna 30 mg up to 3 times/day until obstruction is cleared (per x-ray). Firm rectal impaction can often simply be resolved with manual disimpaction facilitated by the use of a local anesthetic gel.

One should expect gradual rather than immediate results from a newly instituted laxative regimen. Additionally, nondrug interventions should be maintained during pharmacologic treatment of constipation as this is one of the cornerstones of long-term management.

Constipating Drugs

Anticholinergics (antiparkinsons)
Antihistamines
Opiates
MAOIs
Tricyclic Antidepressants
Aluminum
Calcium (supplements & antacids)
Iron
Phenothiazines
Diuretics
Clonidine
Guanabenz
Guanfacine
Disopyramide
Irritant laxatives (with cathartic colon)
Anticonvulsants

Opioid-Induced Constipation

Stimulant laxatives such as senna or bisacodyl in combination with a stool softener such as docusate sodium often serve as an effective first-line regimen. Senna p.o. up to 4 tablets 2-3 times/day may be needed. Next, bisacodyl tablets p.o. at bedtime and up to 2-3 times/day if needed. If desired, use docusate to augment the effect of one or both medications, especially if stool is hard. If impaction can be ruled out, use bisocodyl suppository followed by fleet enema (if needed). If impaction is suspected, see last step of pathway.

Stool Softeners

Stool softeners have no laxative action and are not helpful in alleviating chronic constipation and may cause fecal incontinence. Short-term use is appropriate to minimize straining caused by hard stools following rectal surgery or recent MI or when defecation causes hemorrhoidal pain, rectal bleeding, crescendo angina, or other high risk condition.

Saline Laxatives

Regular use of saline laxatives is not recommended because their risks outweigh the benefits of the laxative. Saline laxatives are only indicated for acute bowel evacuation for diagnostic procedures. Also, note that use of Milk of Magnesia in renally impaired residents can result in Mg^{++} toxicity (hypotension, muscle weakness, EKG changes, CNS changes).

Combination Laxatives

Use of products containing two or more laxatives is not advised because of a lack of documented therapeutic benefit over use of a single ingredient. Additionally, risks may outweigh benefits.

References

Alessi CA and Henderson CT, "Constipation and Fecal Impaction in the Long-Term Care Patient," *Clin Geriatr Med*, 1988; 4:571-88.

Burke C, "Avoiding Problems of GI Dysmotility in Patients Treated for Chronic Pain," *ASCP* 1995 Symposia Highlights, 7-8.

Castle SC, "Constipation: Endemic in the Elderly," *Med Clin N Am* 1989; 73:1497.

Harari D, Gurwitz JH, and Minaker KL, "Constipation in the Elderly," *JAGS*, 1993; 41:1130-40.

Izard MW and Ellison FS, "Treatment of Drug Induced Constipation with a Purified Senna Derivative," *Conn Med*, 1962; 26:589.

Lange RL and DiPiro JT, *Pharmacotherapy*, 2nd ed, Norwalk, CT: Appleton & Lange, 1993.

Maguire LC, Yon JL, and Miller E, "Prevention of Narcotic-Induced Constipation," *N Eng J Med*, 1981; 305:1651.

Rousseau P, "Managing Constipation in the Elderly Population," *Fam Practice Recertification*, 1990; 12:76-95.

Szurszewski JH, Holt PR, and Schuster M, "Proceedings of a Workshop Entitled Neuromuscular Function and Dysfunction of the Gastrointestinal Tract in Aging," *Dig Dis Sci*, 1989; 34:1135.

Wrenn K, "Fecal Impaction," *N Engl J Med*, 1989; 321:658-61.

FEDERAL OBRA REGULATIONS RECOMMENDED MAXIMUM DOSES

Antidepressants

Drug	Brand Name	Usual Max Daily Dose for Age ≥65	Usual Max Daily Dose
Amitriptyline	Elavil®	150 mg	300 mg
Amoxapine	Asendin®	200 mg	400 mg
Desipramine	Norpramin®, Pertofrane®	150 mg	300 mg
Doxepin	Adapin®, Sinequan®	150 mg	300 mg
Imipramine	Tofranil®	150 mg	300 mg
Maprotiline	Ludiomil®	150 mg	300 mg
Nortriptyline	Aventyl®, Pamelor®	75 mg	150 mg
Protriptyline	Vivactil®	30 mg	60 mg
Trazodone	Desyrel®	300 mg	600 mg
Trimipramine	Surmontil®	150 mg	300 mg

Antipsychotics

Drug	Brand Name	Usual Max Daily Dose for Age ≥65	Usual Max Daily Dose	Daily Oral Dose for Residents With Organic Mental Syndromes
Acetophenazine	Tindal®	150 mg	300 mg	20 mg
Chlorpromazine	Thorazine®	800 mg	1600 mg	75 mg
Chlorprothixene	Taractan®	800 mg	1600 mg	75 mg
Clozapine	Clozaril®	25 mg	450 mg	50 mg
Fluphenazine	Prolixin®	20 mg	40 mg	4 mg
Haloperidol	Haldol®	50 mg	100 mg	4 mg
Loxapine	Loxitane®	125 mg	250 mg	10 mg
Mesoridazine	Serentil®	250 mg	500 mg	25 mg
Molindone	Moban®	112 mg	225 mg	10 mg
Perphenazine	Trilafon®	32 mg	64 mg	8 mg
Promazine	Sparine®	50 mg	500 mg	150 mg
Risperidone	Risperdal®	1 mg	16 mg	4 mg
Thioridazine	Mellaril®	400 mg	800 mg	75 mg
Thiothixene	Navane®	30 mg	60 mg	7 mg
Trifluoperazine	Stelazine®	40 mg	80 mg	8 mg
Trifluopromazine	Vesprin®	100 mg	20 mg	–

Anxiolytics*

Drug	Brand Name	Usual Daily Dose for Age ≥65	Usual Daily Dose for Age ≤65
Alprazolam	Xanax®	2 mg	4 mg
Chlorazepate	Tranxene®	30 mg	60 mg
Chlordiazepoxide	Librium®	40 mg	100 mg
Diazepam	Valium®	20 mg	60 mg
Halazepam	Paxipam®	80 mg	160 mg
Lorazepam	Ativan®	3 mg	6 mg
Meprobamate	Miltown®	600 mg	1600 mg
Oxazepam	Serax®	60 mg	90 mg
Prazepam	Centrax®	30 mg	60 mg

*Note: HCFA-OBRA guidelines strongly urge clinicians not to use barbiturates, glutethimide, and ethchlorvynol due to their side effects, pharmacokinetics, and addiction potential in the elderly. Also, HCFA discourages use of long-acting benzodiazepines in the elderly.

Hypnotics
(Should not be used for more than 10 continuous days*)

Drug	Brand Name	Usual Max Single Dose for Age ≥65	Usual Max Single Dose
Alprazolam	Xanax®	0.25 mg	1.5 mg
Amobarbital	Amytal®	105 mg	300 mg
Butabarbital	Butisol®	100 mg	200 mg
Chloral hydrate	Noctec®	750 mg	1500 mg
Chloral hydrate	Various	500 mg	1000 mg
Diphenhydramine	Benadryl®	25 mg	50 mg
Ethchlorvynol	Placidyl®	500 mg	1000 mg
Flurazepam	Dalmane®	15 mg	30 mg
Glutethimide	Doriden®	500 mg	1000 mg
Halazepam	Paxipam®	20 mg	40 mg
Hydroxyzine	Atarax®	50 mg	100 mg
Lorazepam	Ativan®	1 mg	2 mg
Methprylon	Noludar®	200 mg	400 mg
Oxazepam	Serax®	15 mg	30 mg
Pentobarbital	Nembutal®	100 mg	200 mg
Secobarbital	Seconal®	100 mg	200 mg
Temazepam	Restoril®	15 mg	30 mg
Triazolam	Halcion®	0.125 mg	0.5 mg

*Note: HCFA-OBRA guidelines strongly urge clinicians not to use barbiturates, glutethimide, and ethchlorvynol due to their side effects, pharmacokinetics, and addiction potential in the elderly. Also, HCFA discourages use of long-acting benzodiazepines in the elderly and also discourages the use of diphenhydramine and hydroxyzine.

IMMUNIZATION GUIDELINES

Table 1. Dosage and Administration Guidelines for Vaccines Available in the United States

Vaccine	Dosage	Route of Administration	Type
DT	0.5 mL	I.M.	Toxoids
Td	0.5 mL	I.M.	Toxoids
DTP, DTPa	0.5 mL	I.M.	Diphtheria and tetanus toxoids with killed *B. pertussis* organisms
Haemophilus b conjugate vaccine	0.5 mL	I.M.	
ProHIBit® (PRP-D), manufactured by Connaught Laboratories	0.5 mL	I.M.	Polysaccharide (diphtheria toxoid conjugate)
HibTITER® (HbOC)†, manufactured by Praxis Biologicals	0.5 mL	I.M.	Oligosaccharide (diphtheria CRM_{197} protein conjugate)
Hepatitis B,¶		I.M., S.C. in individuals at risk of hemorrhage	Yeast recombinant-derived inactivated viral antigen
Geriatrics and Adults			
Recombivax HB® (MSD)	10 mcg (1 mL)		
Engerix-B® (SKF)	20 mcg (1 mL)		
Dialysis patients and immunosuppressed patients			
Recombivax HB® (MSD)	>11 y, 40 mcg (2 mL); use special dialysis formulation and give as two 1 mL doses at different sites		
Engerix-B® (SKF)	>11 y, 40 mcg (2 mL); give as two 1 mL doses at different sites		
Influenza			
Geriatrics and Adults	0.5 mL (1 dose)	Only one dose needed for annual updates	Inactivated virus subvirion (split) (contraindicated in patients allergic to chicken eggs)
Measles	0.5 mL	S.C.	Live virus (contraindicated in patients with anaphylactic allergy to neomycin)
High-risk areas: 2 doses (first at 12 months with MMR; second dose as above)			
Meningococcal	0.5 mL	S.C.	Polysaccharide
MMR•	0.5 mL	S.C.	Live virus
MR	0.5 mL	S.C.	Live virus
Mumps	0.5 mL	S.C.	Live virus
Pneumococcal polyvalent	0.5 mL (≥2 y)	I.M. or S.C. (I.M. preferred)	Polysaccharide
Poliovirus (OPV) trivalent	0.5 mL	Oral	Live virus
Poliovirus (IPV),**†† trivalent	0.5 mL	S.C.	Inactivated virus

Table 1. Dosage and Administration Guidelines for Vaccines Available in the United States *(continued)*

Vaccine	Dosage	Route of Administration	Type
Rabies	1 mL	I.M.‡‡, I.D.§§	Inactivated virus
Rubella	0.5 mL (≥12 mo)¶¶	S.C.	Live virus
Tetanus (adsorbed)##	0.5 mL	I.M.	Toxoid
Tetanus (fluid)	0.5 mL	I.M., S.C.	Toxoid
Yellow fever	0.5 mL••	S.C.	Live attenuated virus

†The conjugate (HbCV) vaccine is preferred over the polysaccharide (HbPV) vaccine.

¶Engerix-B® — an alternate schedule for postexposure prophylaxis or more rapid induction using four doses at 0, 1, 2, and 12 months can be used.

**The primary series consists of 3 doses. The first two doses should be administered at an interval of 8 weeks. The third dose should be given at least 6 and preferably 12 months after the second dose. When polio vaccine is given to persons >18 years, IPV should be given.

•See measles.

††IPV is indicated for unimmunized or partially immunized patients with compromised immunity; HIV infection; unimmunized adults or adults at future risk of exposure to poliomyelitis; household contacts of an immunodeficient individual.

‡‡I.M. injection can be given into the deltoid muscle. Repeat doses are given on days 3, 7, 14, and 28 postexposure.

§§For pre-exposure prophylaxis against rabies for high-risk individuals, 1 mL I.M. or 0.1 mL intradermal is administered on days 0, 7, and 21 (or 28). Both I.M. and I.D. dosage forms are available.

¶¶As MMR in a two-dose schedule.

##Adsorbed preferred to fluid toxoid because of longer lasting immunity.

••9 months of age living in or traveling to endemic areas. Contraindicated in patients who have had an anaphylactic reaction to eggs.

Note: For each vaccine, check the manufacturer's package insert for specific product information since preparations may change from time to time.

Reference

ACIP, General Recommendations on Immunization, *MMWR*, 1989, 38:205-14, 219-27.

Table 2. Guidelines for Spacing Live and Killed Antigen Administration

Antigen Combinations	Recommended Minimum Interval Between Doses
≥2 killed antigens	None. May be given simultaneously or at any interval between doses.
Killed and live antigens	None. May be given simultaneously or at any interval between doses. (Exception: Concurrent administration of cholera and yellow fever vaccines should be avoided. Separate these vaccines by at least 3 weeks.)
≥2 live antigens	4 weeks minimum interval if not administered simultaneously. (Recent receipt of OPV is not a contraindication to MMR.) Vaccines associated with systemic reactions (cholera and parenteral typhoid or influenza and DTP in young children) should be given on separate occasions.

IMMUNIZATION GUIDELINES *(Continued)*

Table 3. Passive Immunization Agents — Immune Globulins

Immune Globulin	Dosage	Route
Hepatitis B (H-BIG®)		I.M.
percutaneous inoculation	0.06 mL/kg/dose (within 24 hours) (5 mL max)	
perinatal	0.5 mL/dose (within 12 hours of birth)	
sexual exposure	0.06 mL/kg/dose (within 14 days of contact) (5 mL max)	
Immune globulin (IG)		I.M.*
hepatitis A prophylaxis	0.02 mL/kg/dose (as soon as possible or within 2 weeks after exposure) (single exposure)	
	0.06 mL/kg/dose (>3 months or continuous exposure) repeat every 4-6 months	
hepatitis B	0.06 mL/kg/dose (H-BIG should be used)	
hepatitis C	0.06 mL/kg/dose (percutaneous exposure)	
measles†	0.25 mL/kg/dose (max 15 mL/dose) (within 6 days of exposure)	
	0.5 mL/kg/dose (max 15 mL/dose) (immunocompromised children)	
Rabies‡	20 IU/kg/dose (within 3 days)	
Tetanus (serious, contaminated, wounds; <3 previous tetanus vaccine doses)	250-500 units/dose	I.M.
Varicella-zoster (VZIG)	Within 48 hours but not later than 96 hours after exposure	I.M.¶
	0-10 kg 125 units = 1 vial	
	10.1-20 kg 250 units = 2 vials	
	20.1-30 kg 375 units = 3 vials	
	30.1-40 kg 500 units = 4 vials	
	>40 kg 625 units = 5 vials	

*Deep I.M. in the gluteal region for large doses only. Deltoid muscle or the anterolateral aspect of the thigh are preferred sites for injection. No greater than 5 mL/site in adults; maximum dose: 20 mL at one time.

†IG prophylaxis may not be indicated in a patient who has received IGIV within 3 weeks of exposure.

‡½ of dose used to infiltrate the wound with the remaining ½ of dose given I.M. Rabies immune globulin is not recommended in previously HDCV immunized patients.

¶No greater than 2.5 mL of VZIG/one injection site. Doses >2.5 mL should be divided and administered at different sites.

Table 4. Guidelines for Spacing the Administration of Immune Globulin (IG) Preparations and Vaccines

Immunobiologic Combinations	Recommended Minimum Interval Between Doses
Simultaneous Administration	
IG and killed antigen	None. May be given simultaneously at different sites or at any time between doses.
IG and live antigen	Should generally not be given simultaneously. If unavoidable to do so, give at different sites and revaccinate or test for seroconversion in 3 months. Example: MMR should not be given to patients who have received immune globulin within the previous 3 months.

Nonsimultaneous Administration		
First	**Second**	
IG	Killed antigen	None
Killed antigen	IG	None
IG	Live antigen	6 weeks, and preferably 3 months
Live antigen	IG	2 weeks

*The live virus vaccines, OPV and yellow fever are exceptions to these recommendations. Either vaccine may be administered simultaneously or any time before or after IG without significantly decreasing antibody response.

PREVENTION OF BACTERIAL ENDOCARDITIS

Recommendations by the American Heart Association
(*JAMA*, 1997, 277:1794-801)

Consensus Process - The recommendations were formulated by the writing group after specific therapeutic regimens were discussed. The consensus statement was subsequently reviewed by outside experts not affiliated with the writing group and by the Science Advisory and Coordinating Committee of the American Heart Association. These guidelines are meant to aid practitioners but are not intended as the standard of care or as a substitute for clinical judgment.

Table 1. Cardiac Conditions*

Endocarditis Prophylaxis Recommended
High-risk Category
Prosthetic cardiac valves, including bioprosthetic and homograft valves
Previous bacterial endocarditis
Complex cyanotic congenital heart disease (eg, single ventricle states, transposition of the great arteries, tetralogy of Fallot)
Surgically constructed systemic pulmonary shunts or conduits
Moderate-risk Category
Most other congenital cardiac malformations (other than above and below)
Acquired valvar dysfunction (eg, rheumatic heart disease)
Hypertrophic cardiomyopathy
Mitral valve prolapse with valvar regurgitation and/or thickened leaflets
Endocarditis Prophylaxis Not Recommended
Negligible-risk Category (no greater risk than the general population)
Isolated secundum atrial septal defect
Surgical repair of atrial septal defect, ventricular septal defect, or patent ductus arteriosus (without residua beyond 6 months)
Previous coronary artery bypass graft surgery
Mitral valve prolapse without valvar regurgitation†
Physiologic, functional, or innocent heart murmurs
Previous Kawasaki disease without valvar dysfunction
Previous rheumatic fever without valvar dysfunction
Cardiac pacemakers (intravascular and epicardial) and implanted defibrillators

*This table lists selected conditions but is not meant to be all-inclusive.

†Individuals who have a mitral valve prolapse associated with thickening and/or redundancy of the valve leaflets may be at increased risk for bacterial endocarditis, particularly men who are 45 years of age or older.

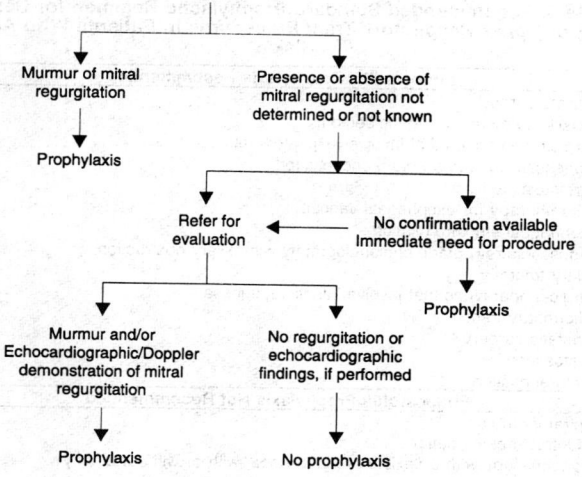

Patient With Suspected Mitral Valve Prolapse

Table 2. Dental Procedures and Endocarditis Prophylaxis

Endocarditis Prophylaxis Recommended*
Dental extractions
Periodontal procedures including surgery, scaling and root planing, probing, and recall maintenance
Dental implant placement and reimplantation of avulsed teeth
Endodontic (root canal) instrumentation or surgery only beyond the apex
Subgingival placement of antibiotic fibers or strips
Initial placement of orthodontic bands but not brackets
Intraligamentary local anesthetic injections
Prophylactic cleaning of teeth or implants where bleeding is anticipated

Endocarditis Prophylaxis Not Recommended
Restorative dentistry† (operative and prosthodontic) with or without retraction cord‡
Local anesthetic injections (nonintraligamentary)
Intracanal endodontic treatment; post placement and buildup
Placement of rubber dams
Postoperative suture removal
Placement of removable prosthodontic or orthodontic appliances
Taking of oral impressions
Fluoride treatments
Taking of oral radiographs
Orthodontic appliance adjustment
Shedding of primary teeth

*Prophylaxis is recommended for patients with high- and moderate-risk cardiac conditions
†This includes restoration of decayed teeth (filling cavities) and replacement of missing teeth.
‡Clinical judgment may indicate antibiotic use in selected circumstances that may create significant bleeding.

PREVENTION OF BACTERIAL ENDOCARDITIS *(Continued)*

Table 3. Recommended Standard Prophylactic Regimen for Dental, Oral, or Upper Respiratory Tract Procedures in Patients Who Are at Risk*

Endocarditis Prophylaxis Recommended

Respiratory tract
   Tonsillectomy and/or adenoidectomy
   Surgical operations that involve respiratory mucosa
   Bronchoscopy with a rigid bronchoscope
Gastrointestinal tract*
   Sclerotherapy for esophageal varices
   Esophageal stricture dilation
   Endoscopic retrograde cholangiography with biliary obstruction
   Biliary tract surgery
   Surgical operations that involve intestinal mucosa
Genitourinary tract
   Prostatic surgery
   Cystoscopy
   Urethral dilation

Endocarditis Prophylaxis Not Recommended

Respiratory tract
   Endotracheal intubation
   Bronchoscopy with a flexible bronchoscope, with or without biopsy†
   Tympanostomy tube insertion
Gastrointestinal tract
   Transesophageal echocardiography†
   Endoscopy with or without gastrointestinal biopsy†
Genitourinary tract
   Vaginal hysterectomy†
   Vaginal delivery†
   Cesarean section
   In uninfected tissues:
      Urethral catheterization
      Uterine dilatation and curettage
      Therapeutic abortion
      Sterilization procedures
      Insertion or removal of intrauterine devices
Other
   Cardiac catheterization, including balloon angioplasty
   Implanted cardiac pacemakers, implanted defibrillators, and coronary stents
   Incision or biopsy or surgically scrubbed skin
   Circumcision

*Prophylaxis is recommended for high-risk patients, optional for medium-risk patients
†Prophylaxis is optional for high-risk patients

Table 4. Prophylactic Regimens for Dental, Oral, Respiratory Tract, or Esophageal Procedures

Situation	Agent	Regimen* Adults
Standard general prophylaxis	Amoxicillin	2 g 1 h before procedure
Unable to take oral medications	Ampicillin	2 g I.M./I.V. within 30 min before procedure
Allergic to penicillin	Clindamycin or	600 mg 1 h before procedure
	Cephalexin† or cefadroxil† or	2 g 1 h before procedure
	Azithromycin or clarithromycin	500 mg 1 h before procedure
Allergic to penicillin and unable to take oral medications	Clindamycin or	600 mg 30 min before procedure
	Cefazolin†	1 g within 30 min before procedure

*Total children's dose should not exceed adult dose

†Cephalosporins should not be used in individuals with immediate-type hypersensitivity reaction (urticaria, angioedema, or anaphylaxis) to penicillins

Table 5. Prophylactic Regimens for Genitourinary/Gastrointestinal (Excluding Esophageal) Procedures*

Situation	Agents*	Regimen† Adults
High-risk‡ patients	Ampicillin plus gentamicin	Ampicillin 2 g I.M. or I.V. plus gentamicin 1.5 mg/kg (not to exceed 120 mg) within 30 min of starting the procedure; 6 h later, ampicillin 1 g I.M./I.V. or amoxicillin 1 g orally
High-risk‡ patients allergic to ampicillin/amoxicillin	Vancomycin plus gentamicin	Vancomycin 1 g I.V. over 1-2 h plus gentamicin 1.5 mg/kg I.M./I.V. (not to exceed 120 mg); complete injection/infusion within 30 min of starting the procedure
Moderate-risk§ patients	Amoxicillin or ampicillin	Amoxicillin 2 g orally 1 h before procedure, or ampicillin 2 g I.M./I.V within 30 min of starting the procedure
Moderate-risk§ patients allergic to ampicillin/amoxicillin	Vancomycin	Vancomycin 1 g I.V. over 1-2 h; complete infusion within 30 min of starting the procedure

*Total children's dose should not exceed adult dose

†No second dose of vancomycin or gentamicin is recommended

‡High-risk: Patients are those who have prosthetic valves, a previous history of endocarditis (even in the absence of other heart disease, complex cyanotic congenital heart disease, or surgically constructed systemic pulmonary shunts or conduits.

§Moderate-risk: Individuals with certain other underlying cardiac defects. Congenital cardiac conditions include the following uncorrected conditions: Patent ductus arteriosus, ventricular septal defect, primum atrial septal defect, coarctation of the aorta, and bicuspid aortic valve. Acquired valvar dysfunction and hypertrophic cardiomyopathy are also moderate risk conditions.

NORMAL LABORATORY VALUES FOR ADULTS

CHEMISTRY

Chemistry, Routine
Albumin	3.5-5.0 g/dL
Bilirubin, conjugated	0-0.2 mg/dL
Bilirubin, total	0.2-1.2 mg/dL
Blood urea nitrogen	8-23 mg/dL
Calcium	8.4-10.3 mg/dL
Creatinine	0.5-1.2 mg/dL
Glucose	65-110 mg/dL
Phosphorus	2.8-4.5 mg/dL
Protein, total	6.0-8.0 g/dL
Uric acid	
male	3.5-7.2 mg/dL
female	2.6-6.5 mg/dL

Electrolytes
Chlorides	100-110 mEq/L
CO_2	23-31 mEq/L
Potassium	3.5-5.0 mEq/L
Sodium	136-146 mEq/L
Anion gap	5-14 mEq/L

Enzymes
Alk phos	
male	34-110 units/L
female	24-100 units/L
ALT	5-35 units/L
AST	5-35 units/L
CPK	
male	0-206 units/L
female	0-175 units/L
LDH	50-200 units/L

Thyroid Function
FTI (free thyroxine index)	4.5-12.0
T_3 resin uptake	25%-35%
T_3 (tri-iodothyronine)	70-200 ng/dL
T_4 (thyroxine)	4.0-11.0 µg/dL
TSH	0.4-6 µIU/L

Others
Ammonia, plasma	20-60 µg/dL
Amylase, serum	44-128 units/L
Calcium, ionized	4.6-5.2 mg/dL
Cholesterol	140-230 mg/dL
Iron, serum	50-170 µg/dL
Lactate, serum	1.4-3.9 mEq/L
Lipase	10-208 units/L
Magnesium	1.5-2.5 mg/dL
Oncotic pressure	22-28 mm Hg
Osmolality	280-300 mOsm/kg
Serum ferritin	
male	25-400 ng/mL
female	10-150 ng/mL
TIBC	270-390 µg/dL
Triglycerides	50-150 mg/dL

HEMATOLOGY

Hematocrit	
male	40%-52%
female	35%-47%
Hemoglobin	
male	13.5-17.5 g/dL
female	11.5-16.0 g/dL
MCH	27-34 pg
MCHC	32%-36%
MCV	82-100 fL
Platelet count	150-450 x 10^3/mm³
RBC count	
male	4.5-5.9 x 10^6/mm³
female	4.0-4.9 x 10^6/mm³
RDW	11.5-14.5
Reticulocyte count	0.5%-1.5%
Sed rate (Westergren)	
male	0-10 mm/h
female	0-20 mm/h
WBC count	4.5-11.0 10^3/mm³
WBC differential	
Bands	2%-8%
Basophils	0%-2%
Eosinophils	0%-4%
Lymphocytes	20%-45%
Monocytes	2%-8%
Neutrophils	40%-70%

BLOOD GASES

	Arterial	Venous
Base excess	-3.0 to +3.0 mEq/L	-5.0 to +5.0 mEq/L
HCO_3	18-25 mEq/L	18-25 mEq/L
O_2 saturation	90%-98%	60%-85%
pCO_2	34-45 mm Hg	35-52 mm Hg
pH	7.35-7.45	7.32-7.42
pO_2	80-95 mm Hg	30-48 mm Hg
TCO_2	23-29 mEq/L	24-30 mEq/L

NORMAL LABORATORY VALUES FOR ADULTS
(Continued)

Weight/Volume Equivalents

1 mg/dL = 10 mcg/mL   1 ppm = 1 mg/L

1 mg/dL = 1 mg%   1 mcg/mL = 1 mg/L

The effects of aging on laboratory parameters have not been fully elucidated. While some alterations in values have been associated with increased age, no reference values have been established for the elderly. The following changes may be seen in elderly patients:

Alkaline phosphatase	↑
Albumin	↓
Uric acid	↑ (possible)
Creatinine clearance	↓
BUN	↑
ESR	↑
WBC	↓
Mg^{++}	↓
2-hour postprandial blood glucose	↑
Hemoglobin	↓
Urine specific gravity	↓

References

Cavalieri TA, Chopra A, and Bryman PN, "When Outside the Norm Is Normal: Interpreting Lab Data in the Aged," *Geriatrics*, 1992, 47(5):66-70.

Fraser CG, "Age-related Changes in Laboratory Test Results, Clinical Implications," *Drugs & Aging*, 1993, 3(3):246-57.

Hodkinson HM, "Alterations of Laboratory Findings," *Principles of Geriatric Medicine and Gerontology*, 2nd ed, Hazzard WR, Andres R, Bierman EL, et al, eds, New York, NY: McGraw-Hill, 1990, 241-6.

Kelso T, "Laboratory Values in the Elderly, Are They Different?" *Emer Med Clin N Am*, 1990, 8(2):241-54.

ANTICOAGULANT THERAPY GUIDELINES

This information, for the use of heparin and warfarin in adults, was obtained from a review of current literature. This information is intended to optimize therapeutic anticoagulation by minimizing patient bleeding risks, decreasing the time required for titration to achieve a desired level of anticoagulation, and promoting efficient use of laboratory tests.

Initiation of Intravenous Heparin Therapy Treatment of Venous Thrombosis and Pulmonary Embolism*

Monitoring	Dosing
Check baseline aPTT, PT/INR, CBC	Bolus 80 units/kg I.V. Initial drip 18 units/kg/hour I.V.
Check CBC with platelet count every 3 days, aPTT 6 hours post bolus and 6 hours after each dosing adjustment. When two consecutive aPTTs are therapeutic, monitor aPTT every 24 hours and readjust heparin drip as needed.	Refer to nomogram below

aPTT*(s)	Dosing
<35	80 units/kg bolus, increase drip 4 units/kg/hour
35-45	40 units/kg bolus, increase drip 2 units/kg/hour
46-70	No change
71-90	Reduce drip by 2 units/kg/hour
>90	Stop infusion 1 hour, reduce drip by 3 units/kg/hour

aPTT — activated partial thromboplastin time; PT/INR — prothrombin time/International Normalized Ratio; CBC — complete blood count and platelet count; s — seconds; kg — kilogram

*It is recommended that each lab perform an *in vitro* heparin titration curve to establish the therapeutic range for a specific aPTT reagent which is equivalent to a heparin concentration of 0.2-0.4 units/mL. Thus, the therapeutic range will vary depending upon the aPTT reagent in use.

AMERICAN GERIATRICS SOCIETY CURRENT STANDARDS OF PRACTICE

Oral Anticoagulant Standards of Practice for Older Adults

Thromboembolic Disorder	INR	Duration	Clinical Comments
Venous Thromboembolism			
Prophylaxis (high risk surgery)	2.0-3.0	≤3 mo or until ambulatory	Alternatives include low molecular weight heparin or adjusted dose heparin.
Treatment: single episode (DVT or PE)	2.0-3.0	3-6 mo	Recurrent DVT or PE requires indefinite anticoagulation.
Prevention of Systemic Embolism			
Atrial fibrillation (AF)	2.0-3.0	Indefinite	Anticoagulation is not indicated in patients <60 y with no associated CV disease. If warfarin is contraindicated, consider ASA.
AF: cardioversion	2.0-3.0	3 wk prior; 4 wk postsinus rhythm	Consider indefinite anticoagulation in patients who do not cardiovert.
Acute myocardial infarction (high risk)	2.0-3.0	≤3 mo	High risk patients for mural thrombosis and systemic embolism (SE); otherwise, ASA.
Cardiomyopathy	2.0-3.0	Indefinite	Consider patient with ejection fraction ≤25% and high risk for SE.

ANTICOAGULANT THERAPY GUIDELINES *(Continued)*

Oral Anticoagulant Standards of Practice for Older Adults *(continued)*

Thromboembolic Disorder	INR	Duration	Clinical Comments
Recurrent systemic embolism	2.0-3.0	Indefinite	Criteria for "recurrence" events, temporal and etiologic relationships.
Tissue heart valves	2.0-3.0	3 mo	ASA is second-line alternative
Valvular heart disease	2.0-3.0	Indefinite	Consider only patients with a history of SE, AF, or left atrium diameter >5.5 cm. If recurrent embolism occurs, add ASA.
Mechanical prosthetic valves	2.5-3.5	Indefinite	If recurrent embolism occurs, add ASA or dipyridamole. If high bleeding risk, INR 2.0-3.0 ± ASA.

Initially developed by Gordon J Vanscoy, PharmD, MBA, University of Pittsburgh Medical Center, Drug Information and Pharmacoepidemiology Center

Revised for Geriatric Population by Laurie Jacobs, MD and the American Geriatrics Society Clinical Practice Committee. For further information call the AGS at (212) 308-1414.

Modified from *Chest*, 1992, 102(4s):303s-539s and *West J Med*, 1989, 151(414-29).

A complete statement on the AGS standards is scheduled for publication in September 1996. See *J Am Geriatrics Soc*, 1996, 44(9).

Abbreviations:

ASA = aspirin

DVT = deep vein thrombosis

PE = pulmonary embolism

AF = atrial fibrillation

CV = cardiovascular

SE = systemic embolism

Dosing Oral Anticoagulants

Dosing Approach	Warfarin Dose		
	Day 1*	Day 2†	Day 3‡
Aggressive	5-7.5 mg	5-7.5 mg	2.5-7.5 mg
Nonaggressive§	2.5-5 mg	2.5-5 mg	2.5-5 mg

*Therapeutic APTT obtained (eg, begin warfarin on day 1 of heparin therapy).

†Check INR.

‡Check INR daily until stable/therapeutic, then three times in first week, two times in second week, weekly for 4 weeks, then monthly.

§Rapid anticoagulation not required (eg, chronic stable AF) or if there is a bleeding risk.

Reversal of Oral Anticoagulant Effect: Nonbleeding*

INR	Vitamin K Dose†	Route	Comments
6-10‡	0.5-1.0 mg	P.O., S.C.	P.O absorption may be unpredictable in the elderly.
10-20	3.0-5.0 mg	S.C., I.V.	Check INR in 6-12 hours; repeat if necessary.
>20	5.0-10.0 mg	S.C., I.V.	Check INR in 6 hours; repeat if necessary.

*For alternative recommendations, see the table, Managing Prolongations of the INR (American College of CHEST Physicians Consensus Conference Recommendations) at the end of this section.

†I.V. route may produce anaphylactic reaction; only Aqua Mephyton may be given I.V.

‡Holding warfarin may be considered.

Reversal of Oral Anticoagulant Effect: Bleeding

Extent of Bleeding	Warfarin Dose	Vitamin K	Fresh Frozen Plasma
Minor bleeding	Reduce	Withhold warfarin or 1 mg (P.O., S.C.) if INR >4.5	–
Severe bleeding	Stop	5 mg I.V.*	Consider
Life-threatening bleeding	Stop	10 mg I.V.*	Yes

*I.V. route may produce anaphylactic reaction; only Aqua Mephyton may be given I.V.

INITIATION OF ORAL ANTICOAGULATION WITH WARFARIN

The dosing of warfarin must be individualized according to the patient's response to the drug as indicated by the PT/INR. Use of a large loading dose may increase the incidence of hemorrhagic and other complications, does not offer more rapid protection against thrombus formation, and is not recommended. Low initiation doses (eg, 2-5 mg/day) are recommended for elderly and/or debilitated patients and patients with potential for increased responsiveness to warfarin.

Step 1: Obtain baseline PT/INR
Begin therapy with warfarin with a dose of 2-5 mg per day with dosage adjustment based on the results of PT/INR determinations.

For patients on heparin: Since the anticoagulant effect of warfarin is delayed, heparin is preferred initially for rapid anticoagulation. Conversion to warfarin may begin concomitantly with heparin therapy or may be delayed 3-6 days. When warfarin has produced the desired therapeutic range, INR, or prothrombin time, heparin may be discontinued.

Step 2: Day that the PT/INR is stabilized in the therapeutic range: Check PT/INR daily. Adjust warfarin dose based on the results of PT/INR determinations.

Patients stabilized in the therapeutic range: Intervals between subsequent PT/INR determinations should be based upon the physician's judgement of the patient's reliability and response to warfarin in order to maintain the individual within the therapeutic range. Acceptable intervals for PT/INR determinations are normally with the range of 1-4 weeks after a stable dosage has been determined. Most patients are satisfactorily maintained on warfarin at a dose of 2-10 mg daily.

MONITORING — THE INTERNATIONAL NORMALIZED RATIO (INR)

Because PT results are very dependent on the thromboplastin reagent used, a system of standardizing the prothrombin time in oral anticoagulant therapy was introduced by the World Health Organization in 1983. It is based upon determination of an INR, which is equivalent to the PT ratio one would obtain if a sensitive reference thromboplastin were used for the PT.

- Thromboplastin sensitivity is determined by the manufacturer and is expressed as an International Sensitivity Index (ISI)

- The INR can be calculated as **INR = (Observed PT ratio)^{ISI}**

- The calculation of the INR from the PT ratio is usually performed by the laboratory

Reminder

- Be aware of potential drug interactions and other factors that may affect INR (refer to prescribing information for warfarin)

- Patient/staff education about warfarin is an important part of therapy. Effective therapeutic levels with minimal complications are in part dependent upon cooperative and well-instructed patients who communicate effectively with their physician. Various warfarin patient educational guides are available to health professionals on request.

ANTICOAGULANT THERAPY GUIDELINES *(Continued)*

DRUG INTERACTIONS WITH WARFARIN

Numerous factors, alone or in combination, including travel, changes in diet, environment, physical state, and medication may influence response of the patient to anticoagulants. It is generally good practice to monitor the patient's response with additional PT/INR determinations in the period immediately after discharge from the hospital, and whenever other medications are initiated, discontinued, or taken irregularly. The following factors are listed for reference; however, other factors may also affect the anticoagulant response.

The following factors, alone or in combination, may be responsible for INCREASED PT/INR response:

Exogenous Factors:
Potential drug interactions with warfarin are listed below by drug class. For specific drugs in these classes that have been reported to interact, see full prescribing information for warfarin.

adrenergic stimulants, central
alcohol abuse reduction preparations
analgesics
anesthetics, inhalation
antiarrhythmics†
antibiotics†
    aminoglycosides (oral)
    cephalosporins, parenteral
    macrolides
    metronidazole
    miscellaneous
        penicillins (intravenous high-dose)
    quinolones (fluoroquinolones)
    sulfonamides, long-acting
    tetracyclines
anticoagulants
anticonvulsants†
antidepressants†
antimalarial agents
antineoplastics†
antiparasitic/antimicrobials
antiplatelet drugs/effects
antithyroid drugs†
beta-adrenergic blockers
bromelains
cholelitholytic agents

diabetes agents, oral
diuretics†
fungal medications, systemic†
gastrointestinal, ulcerative colitis agents
gout treatment agents
hemorrheologic agents
hepatotoxic drugs
hyperglycemic agents
hypertensive emergency agents
hypnotics†
hypolipidemics†
monoamine oxidase inhibitors
narcotics, prolonged
NSAIDs
psychostimulants
pyrazolones
salicylates
steroids, adrenocortical†
steroids, anabolic (17-alkyl testosterone derivatives)
thrombolytics
thyroid drugs†
tuberculosis agents†
uricosuric agents
vaccines
vitamin E

Also: Other medications affecting blood elements which may modify hemostasis, dietary deficiencies, prolonged hot weather, unreliable PT/INR determinations.

†Increased and decreased PT/INR responses have been reported.

The following factors, alone or in combination, may be responsible for DECREASED PT/INR response:

Exogenous Factors
Potential drug interactions with warfarin are listed below by drug class. For specific drugs in these classes that have been reported to interact, see full prescribing information for warfarin.

adrenal cortical steroid inhibitors
antacids
antianxiety agents
antiarrhythmics†
antibiotics†
anticonvulsants†
antidepressants†
antihistamines
antineoplastics†
antipsychotic medications
antithyroid drugs†
barbiturates

diuretics†
enteral nutritional supplements
fungal medications, systemic†
gastric acidity and peptic ulcer agents†
hypnotics†
hypolipidemics†
immunosuppressives
oral contraceptives, estrogen-containing
steroids, adrenocortical†
thyroid drugs†
tuberculosis agents†
vitamin K

Also: Diet high in vitamin K and unreliable PT/INR determinations
†Increased and decreased PT/INR responses have been reported.

Because a patient may be exposed to a combination of the above factors, the net effect of warfarin on PT/INR response may be unpredictable. More frequent PT/INR monitoring is therefore advisable. Medications of unknown interaction with coumarins are best regarded with caution. When these medications are started or stopped, more frequent PT/INR monitoring is advisable.

It has been reported that concomitant administration of warfarin and ticlopidine may be associated with cholestatic hepatitis.

Effect on Other Drugs: Coumarins may also affect the action of other drugs. Hypoglycemic agents (chlorpropamide and tolbutamide) and anticonvulsants (phenytoin and phenobarbital) may accumulate in the body as a result of interference with either their metabolism or excretion.

THERAPY WITH WARFARIN

Warfarin is indicated for the prophylaxis and/or treatment of venous thrombosis and its extension, and pulmonary embolism.

Warfarin is indicated for the prophylaxis and/or treatment of the thromboembolic complications associated with atrial fibrillation and/or cardiac valve replacement.

Warfarin is indicated to reduce the risk of death, recurrent myocardial infarction, and thromboembolic events such as stroke or systemic embolization after myocardial infarction.

The benefits of oral anticoagulant therapy in reducing the occurrence of thromboembolic events in patients with atrial fibrillation has been confirmed by a number of major clinical trials. A pooled analysis of five major clinical trials demonstrated a 68% risk reduction of thromboembolic stroke in patients receiving warfarin (INR 2.0-3.0). The annual rate of major hemorrhage was 1.0% for the control group and 1.3% for the warfarin group.

Warfarin is contraindicated in:

- Patients where the risk of hemorrhage outweighs the potential clinical benefits of therapy
- Pregnancy
- Alcoholism/drug abuse
- Unsupervised dementia/psychosis

Treatment Algorithm for Thromboembolic Stroke Prevention in Patients with Atrial Fibrillation

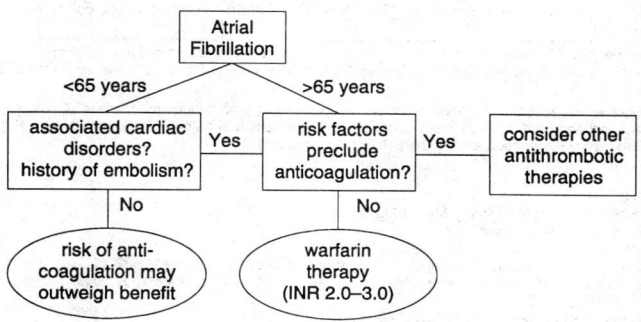

ANTICOAGULANT THERAPY GUIDELINES (Continued)

Managing Prolongations of the INR
American College of CHEST Physicians
Consensus Conference Recommendations*

INR	Symptoms	Recommendation
Above therapeutic range but <6	No bleeding; rapid reversal not indicated for reasons of surgical intervention	Omit next few doses of warfarin and commence at a lower dose when INR is in therapeutic range.
6-10	No bleeding or when rapid reversal is required for elective surgery	Administer subcutaneously 1.0-2.0 mg vitamin K_1†; expect reduction in INR in 8 hours, many patients will be in therapeutic range in 24 hours. If INR still too high in 24 hours, an additional dose of 0.5 mg can be given. Resume warfarin at lower dose when INR returns to the desired range.
>10	No bleeding	Administer subcutaneously 3.0 mg vitamin K_1; expect reduction in INR in 6 hours; check INR in 6 hours and repeat vitamin K_1 if necessary.
>20	Serious bleeding or major warfarin overdose	Administer subcutaneously 10.0 mg vitamin K_1 and supplement with fresh plasma transfusion or prothrombin complex concentrate depending on the urgency of the situation. Check INR every 6 hours; vitamin K_1 may have to be repeated every 12 hours.
	Life-threatening bleeding/ serious warfarin overdose	Administer subcutaneously prothrombin complex concentrate supplemented with 10 mg vitamin K_1 to be repeated as necessary depending on the INR. It is not usually necessary to give vitamin K_1 for the immediate reversal if prothrombin complex concentrates containing factor VII are used.

Use of high doses of vitamin K_1 (10.0-15.0) may cause resistance to warfarin for up to a week. Heparin can be given until the patient becomes responsive to warfarin.

*For alternative recommendations, see the table, Reversal of Oral Anticoagulant Effect: Nonbleeding (American Geriatrics Society Current Standards of Practice) at the beginning of this section.

†Please see recommendations accompanying vitamin K_1 preparations prior to use. A risk of hepatitis and other viral diseases is associated with the use of these blood products. See Full Prescribing Information for Coumadin® (warfarin sodium).

References

Raschke RA, et al, Ann Intern Med, 1993, 119:874-81.
Coumadin® package insert.
Petersen P, et al, Lancet, 1989, 1(8631):175-9.
Stroke Prevention in Atrial Fibrillation Investigators, Circulation, 1991, 84(2):527-39.
The Boston Area Anticoagulation Trial for Atrial Fibrillation Investigators, N Engl J Med, 1990, 323(22):1505-11.
Connolly S, et al, JACC, 1991, 18(2):349-55.
Ezekowitz MD, et al, N Engl J Med, 1992, 327(20):1406-12.
Stroke Prevention in Atrial Fibrillation Investigations, Lancet, 1994, 343:687-91.
Atrial Fibrillation Investigators, Ann Intern Med, 1994, 154:1449-57.
Hirsh J, et al, Chest, 1995, 108(4-Suppl): 231S-46S.

ANTIDEPRESSANT MEDICATION GUIDELINES

The under diagnosis and under treatment of depression in nursing homes has been documented in a *Journal of the American Medical Association* paper entitled "Depression and Mortality in the Nursing home" (*JAMA*, February 27, 1991, 265(8)). HCFA continues to support the accurate identification and treatment of depression in nursing homes.

The surveyor should not urge a facility to use behavioral monitoring charts (eg, documenting quantitatively (number of episodes) and objectively (eg, withdrawn behavior such as staying in their room, refusal to speak, etc)) when antidepressant drugs are used in nursing homes. Such charts are promoted in the interpretative guidelines for antipsychotic and benzodiazepine and other anxiolytic/sedative drugs, but **not** for antidepressant drugs. These charts may be helpful for monitoring the effects of antidepressant drugs in nursing homes, but they may place additional paperwork burden on the facility and thus act as a deterrent to the appropriate diagnosis and treatment of this condition.

The following is a list of commonly used antidepressant drugs.

Generic Name	Brand Name
Amitriptyline*	Elavil®
Amoxapine	Asendin®
Bupropion	Wellbutrin®
Clomipramine*	Anafranil®
Desipramine	Norpramin®, Pertofrane®
Doxepin*	Sinequan®
Imipramine*	Tofranil
Fluoxetine	Prozac®
Fluvoxamine	Luvox®
Isocarboxazid*	Marplan®
Maprotiline	Ludiomil®
Mirtazapine	Remeron®
Nefazodone	Serzone®
Nortriptyline	Aventyl®, Pamelor®
Paroxetine	Paxil™
Phenelzine*	Nardil®
Protriptyline	Vivactil®
Sertraline	Zoloft™
Tranylcypromine*	Parnate®
Trazodone	Desyrel®
Trimipramine*	Surmontil®
Venlafaxine	Effexor®

*These are not necessarily drugs of choice for depression in the elderly. They are listed here only in the event of their potential use.

ANTIPSYCHOTIC MEDICATION GUIDELINES

Appropriate indications for use of antipsychotic medications are outlined in the Health Care Finance Administration's Omnibus Reconciliation Act (OBRA) of 1987. These regulations require that antipsychotics be used to treat specific conditions (listed below) and not solely for behavior control.

Approved indications include:

- acute psychotic episode
- atypical psychosis
- brief reactive psychosis
- delusional disorder
- Huntington's disease
- psychotic mood disorder (including manic depression and depression with psychotic features)
- schizo-affective disorder
- schizophrenia
- schizophrenic form disorder
- Tourette's disease
- short-term (7 days) for hiccups, nausea, vomiting, or pruritus
- organic mental syndrome with psychotic or agitated features:

    - behaviors are quantitatively and objectively documented
    - behaviors must be **persistent**
    - behaviors are not caused by preventable reasons
    - patient presents a danger to self or others
    - continuous crying or screaming if this impairs functional status
    - psychotic symptoms (hallucinations, paranoia, delusions) which cause resident distress or impaired functional capacity

"Clinically contraindicated" means that a resident with a "specific condition" who has had a history of recurrence of psychotic symptoms (eg, delusions, hallucinations) which have been stabilized with a maintenance dose of an antipsychotic drug without incurring significant side effects (eg, tardive dyskinesia) **should not receive gradual dose reductions**. In residents with organic mental syndromes (eg, dementia, delirium), "clinically contraindicated" means that a gradual dose reduction has been attempted **twice** in 1 year and that attempt resulted in the return of symptoms for which the drug was prescribed to a degree that a cessation in the gradual dose reduction, or a return to previous dose levels was necessary.

If the medication is being used outside the guidelines, the physician must provide justification why the continued use of the drug and the dose of the drug is clinically appropriate.

Antipsychotics should not be used if one or more of the following is/are the **only** indication:

- wandering
- poor self care
- restlessness
- impaired memory
- anxiety
- depression (without psychotic features)
- insomnia
- unsociability
- indifference to surroundings
- fidgeting
- nervousness
- uncooperativeness
- agitated behaviors which do **not** represent danger to the resident or others

Selection of an antipsychotic agent should be based on the side effect profile since all antipsychotic agents are equally effective at equivalent doses. Coadministration of two or more antipsychotics does not have any pharmacological basis or clinical advantage and increases the potential for side effects. See Antipsychotic Agents table in Comparison Charts.

DOSING GUIDELINES

1.   Daily dosages should be equal to or less than those listed below, unless documentation exists to support the need for higher doses to maintain or improve functional status.

Generic	Brand	Daily Dose for Patients With Organic Mental Syndrome
Acetophenazine	Tindal®	20 mg
Chlorpromazine	Thorazine®	75 mg
Chlorprothixene	Taractan®	75 mg
Clozapine	Clozaril®	50 mg
Fluphenazine	Prolixin®	4 mg
Haloperidol	Haldol®	4 mg
Loxapine	Loxitane®	10 mg
Mesoridazine	Serentil®	25 mg
Molindone	Moban®	10 mg
Olanzapine	Zyprexa®	
Perphenazine	Trilafon®	8 mg
Pimozide	Orap™	
Prochlorperazine	Compazine®	10 mg
Promazine	Sparine®	150 mg
Risperidone	Risperdal®	4 mg
Thioridazine	Mellaril®	75 mg
Thiothixene	Navane®	7 mg
Trifluoperazine	Stelazine®	8 mg

2.   The dose of prochlorperazine may be exceeded for short-term (up to 7 days) for treatment of nausea and vomiting. Residents with nausea and vomiting secondary to cancer or cancer chemotherapy can also be treated with higher doses for longer periods of time.

3.   The residents must receive adequate monitoring for significant side effects such as tardive dyskinesia, postural hypotension, cognitive-behavioral impairment, akathisia, and parkinsonism.

4.   Gradual dosage reductions are to be attempted twice in 1 year if prescribed for OMS. If symptoms for which the drug has been prescribed return and both reduction attempts have proven unsuccessful, the physician may indicate further reductions are clinically contraindicated.

5.   "Clinically contraindicated" means that a resident **need not undergo** a "gradual dose reduction" or "behavioral interventions" if:

   •   The resident has a "specific condition" and has a history of recurrence of psychotic symptoms (eg, delusions, hallucinations), which have been stabilized with a maintenance dose of an antipsychotic drug without incurring significant side effects.

   •   The resident has organic mental syndrome (now called "delirium, dementia, and amnestic and other cognitive disorders" by DSM IV) and has had a gradual dose reduction attempted **twice** in 1 year and that attempt resulted in the return of symptoms for which the drug was prescribed to a degree that a cessation in the gradual dose reduction, or a return to previous dose reduction was necessary.

   •   The resident's physician provides a justification why the continued use of the drug and the dose of the drug is clinically appropriate. This justification should include: a) a diagnosis, but not simply a diagnostic label or code, but the description of symptoms, b) a discussion of the differential psychiatric and medical diagnosis (eg, why the resident's behavioral symptom is thought to be a result of a dementia with associated psychosis and/or agitated behaviors, and not the result of an unrecognized painful medical condition or a psychosocial or environmental stressor), c) a description of the justification for the choice of a particular treatment, or treatments, and d) a discussion of why the present dose is necessary to manage the symptoms of the resident. This information need not

ANTIPSYCHOTIC MEDICATION GUIDELINES *(Continued)*

necessarily be in the physician's progress notes, but must be a part of the resident's clinical record.

Examples of evidence that would support a justification of why a drug is being used outside these guidelines but in the best interests of the resident may include, but are not limited to the following.

1. A physician's note indicating for example, that the dosage, duration, indication, and monitoring are clinically appropriate, **and the reasons why they are clinically appropriate**; this note should demonstrate that the physician has carefully considered the risk/benefit to the resident in using drugs outside the guidelines.

2. A medical or psychiatric consultation or evaluation (eg, Geriatric Depression Scale) that confirms the physician's judgment that use of a drug outside the guidelines is in the best interest of the resident.

3. Physician, nursing, or other health professional documentation indicating that the resident is being monitored for adverse consequences or complications of the drug therapy.

4. Documentation confirming that previous attempts at dosage reduction have been unsuccessful.

5. Documentation (including MDS documentation) showing resident's subjective or objective improvement, or maintenance of function while taking the medication.

6. Documentation showing that a resident's decline or deterioration is evaluated by the interdisciplinary team to determine whether a particular drug, or a particular dose, or duration of therapy, may be the cause.

7. Documentation showing why the resident's age, weight, or other factors would require a unique drug dose or drug duration, indication, or monitoring.

8. Other evidence you may deem appropriate.

HCFA GUIDELINES FOR UNNECESSARY DRUGS IN LONG-TERM CARE FACILITIES

Procedures: §483.25(1)(1)

Consider drug therapy "unnecessary" only after determining that the facility's use of the drug is

- in excessive dose (including duplicate drug therapy)
- for excessive duration
- without adequate monitoring
- without adequate indications of use
- in the presence of adverse consequences which indicate the dose should be reduced or discontinued, or
- any combination of the reasons above

Allow the facility the opportunity to provide a rationale for the use of drugs prescribed outside the preceding guidelines. The facility may not justify the use of a drug prescribed outside the proceeding guidelines solely on the basis of "the doctor ordered it." This justification would render the regulation meaningless. The rationale must be based on sound risk-benefit analysis of the resident's symptoms and potential adverse effects of the drug.

Examples of evidence that would support a justification of why a drug is being used outside these guidelines but in the best interests of the resident may include, but are not limited to:

- a physician's note indicating for example, that the dosage, duration, indication, and monitoring are clinically appropriate, **and the reasons why they are clinically appropriate**; this note should demonstrate that the physician has carefully considered the risk/benefit to the resident in using drugs outside the guidelines

- a medical or psychiatric consultation or evaluation (eg, geriatric depression scale) that confirms the physician's judgment that use of a drug outside the guidelines is in the best interest of the resident

- physician, nursing, or other health professional documentation indicating that the resident is being monitored for adverse consequences or complications of the drug therapy

- documentation confirming that previous attempts at dosage reduction have been unsuccessful

- documentation (including MDS documentation) showing resident's subjective or objective improvement, or maintenance of function while taking the medication

- documentation showing that a resident's decline or deterioration is evaluated by the interdisciplinary team to determine whether a particular drug, or a particular dose, or duration of therapy, may be the cause

- documentation showing why the resident's age, weight, or other factors would require a unique drug dose or drug duration, indication, monitoring, and

- other evidence the survey team may deem appropriate

If the survey team determines that there is a deficiency in the use of antipsychotics, cite the facility under either the "unnecessary drug" regulation or the "antipsychotic drug" regulation, but not both.

Note: The unnecessary drug criterion of "adequate indications for use" does not simply mean that the **physician's order** must include a reason for using the drug (although such order writing is encouraged). It means that the **resident** lacks a valid clinical reason for use of the drug as evidenced by the survey team's evaluation of some, but not necessarily all, of the following: resident assessment, plan of care, reports of significant change, progress notes, laboratory reports, professional consults, drug orders, observation and interview of the resident, and other information.

PARENTERAL THERAPY RECOMMENDATIONS/GUIDELINES

I.V. Medication Recommendations

Medication	Strength/Solution	Ref Exp	Infusion Time	Filtered	Comments
ALL MEDICATIONS HAVE A 24-HOUR ROOM TEMPERATURE EXPIRATION UNLESS NOTED IN COMMENT SECTION.					
Acyclovir (Zovirax®)	500 mg in 100 mL NS or D_5W 1000 mg in 250 mL NS or D_5W	24 h after nurse admix	60 min	Yes	May precipitate upon refrigeration, but resolves at room temperature
Amikacin (Amikin®)	All strengths in 100 mL NS or D_5W	30 d	60 min	Yes	Monitor serum levels
Aminophylline	Various strengths in NS or D_5W	48 h	0.25 mg/min	Yes	May place in volumes ranging from 250-1000 mL
Amphotericin B (Fungizone®)	All strengths in 500 mL D_5W	7 d	6 h Protect from light	No	Incompatible in NS (may use a 5 micron filter)
Ampicillin	500 mg - 1 g in 50 mL NS >1 g in 100 mL NS	3 d	15-30 min	Yes	Incompatible in D_5W
Ampicillin/ sulbactam (Unasyn®)	All strengths in 100 mL NS only	3 d	30-60 min	Yes	Incompatible in D_5W
Aztreonam (Azactam®)	500 mg - 1 g in 50 mg NS or D_5W 1 g in 100 mg NS or D_5W	7 d	30-60 min	Yes	
Cefamandole (Mandol®)	500 mg - 1 g in 50 mL NS or D_5W >1 g in 100 mL NS or D_5W	4 d	30-60 min	Yes	
Cefazolin (Ancef®, Kefzol®)	500 mg - 1 g in 50 mL NS or D_5W >1 g in 100 mL NS or D_5W	7 d	30-60 min	Yes	
Cefepime (Maxipime®)	0-1 g in 50 mL NS or D_5W >1 g in 100 mL NS or D_5W	7 d	30-60 min	Yes	
Cefonicid (Monocid®)	500 mg in 50 mL NS or D_5W 1 g in 100 mL NS or D_5W	3 d	30-60 min	Yes	
Cefoperazone (Cefobid®)	1 g in 50 mL NS or D_5W >1 g in 100 mL NS or D_5W	5 d	30-60 min	Yes	
Cefotaxime (Claforan®)	All strengths in 100 mL NS or D_5W	5 d	30-60 min	Yes	
Cefotetan (Cefotan®)	1 g in 50 mL NS or D_5W >1 g in 100 mL NS or D_5W	4 d	30 min	Yes	
Cefoxitin (Mefoxin®)	1 g in 50 mL NS or D_5W >1 g in 100 mL NS or D_5W	7 d	30-60 min	Yes	
Ceftazidime (Fortaz®, Tazidime®)	1 g in 50 mL NS or D_5W >1 g in 100 mL NS or D_5W	7 d	30-60 min	Yes	
Ceftizoxime (Cefizox®)	1 g in 50 mL NS or D_5W >1 g in 100 mL NS or D_5W	7 d	30-60 min	Yes	
Ceftriaxone (Rocephin®)	1 g in 50 mL NS or D_5W >1 g in 100 mL NS or D_5W	10 d	30-60 min	Yes	
Cefuroxime (Zinacef®)	750 mg - 1.5 g in 100 mL NS or D_5W	7 d	30-60 min	Yes	I.V. equivalent to Ceftin®

I.V. Medication Recommendations *(continued)*

Medication	Strength/Solution	Ref Exp	Infusion Time	Filtered	Comments
Cimetidine (Tagamet®)	300 mg in 50 mL NS or D₅W >300 mg in 100 mL NS or D₅W	7 d	15-30 min	Yes	Incompatible with aminophylline and barbiturates
Ciprofloxacin (Cipro™)	200 mg in 100 mL NS or D₅W 400 mg in 250 mL NS or D₅W	14 d	60 min	Yes	Do not exceed 2 mg/mL concentration
Clindamycin (Cleocin®)	300-900 mg in 100 mL NS or D₅W	30 d	30 mg/min	Yes	
Dobutamine (Dobutrex®)	250 mg in 250 mL NS or D₅W 500 mg in 500 mL NS or D₅W	7 d	2.5-10 mcg/kg/min	Yes	May exhibit a pink color with no loss in potency
Doxycycline (Vibramycin®)	50-100 mg in 250 mL NS or D₅W	3 d	60 min	Yes	Protect from light; causes phlebitis
Erythromycin	500 mg in 250 mL NS 1 g in 500 mL NS	24 h after nurse admix	60 min	Yes	Incompatible in D₅W
Famotidine (Pepcid®)	20-40 mg in 50 mL NS or D₅W	14 d	15-30 min	Yes	
Fluconazole (Diflucan®)	200 mg in 100 mL Viaflex® bag 400 mg in 200 mL Viaflex® bag	Mfg expired	60 min 120 min	Yes	Maximum rate is 200 mg/h
Foscarnet (Foscavir®)	24 mg/mL for central line mixed in 0-500 mL Viaflex® bag	14 d	Must use I.V. pump at rate ordered	Yes	Must dilute with D₅W or NS to 12 mg/mL for peripheral adm
Ganciclovir (Cytovene®)	0-500 mg in 100 mL NS or D₅W	7 d	60 min	Yes	Use procedures for cytotoxic agents
Gentamicin (Garamycin®)	All strengths in 100 mL NS or D₅W	30 d	60 min	Yes	Monitor serum levels
Heparin	All strengths in NS or D₅W	7 d	As directed by physician	Yes	Can be compounded in volumes from 250-1000 mL
Imipenem/ cilastatin (Primaxin®)	500 mg in 100 mL NS 1 g in 250 mL NS	48 h	30-60 min 60 min	No	Incompatible in D₅W
Iron dextran (InFed™)	All strengths in 500 mL NS	72 h	1-6 h	No	Must give 0.5 mL test dose; incompatible in D₅W
Levofloxacin (Levaquin®)	0-500 mg in 100 ml NaCl or D₅W	14 d	Not < 60 min	Yes	Stable 72 hours at 77° in compatible I.V. solution. Final dilution 5mg/ml
Methicillin (Staphcillin®)	500 mg - 1 g in 100 mL NS or D₅W	4 d	30-60 min	Yes	Only stable at room temperature for 8 hours
Methyldopa (Aldomet®)	250-500 mg in 100 mL D₅W	72 h	30-60 min	Yes	24-hour stability in NS
Metoclopramide (Reglan®)	>10 mg in 50 mL NS or D₅W	48 h	15-30 min Protect from light	Yes	Only make IVPB for doses that exceed 10 mg
Metronidazole (Flagyl®)	500 mg in 100 mL NS RTU	Mfg	60 min	Yes	Incompatible in D₅W; do not refrigerate
Mezlocillin (Mezlin®)	1-4 g in 100 mL NS or D₅W	7 d	30-60 min	Yes	
Nafcillin (Nafcil™, Unipen®)	<2 g in 50 mL NS or D₅W >2 g in 100 mL NS or D₅W	7 d	15-30 min	Yes	
Ofloxacin (Floxin®)	200 mg in 50 mL D₅W RTU 400 mg in 100 mL D₅W RTU	Mfg	60 mg	Yes	May use 10 or 20 mL vials to admix with 14-day exp
Penicillin G	2-4 million units in 100 mL D₅W	7 d	15-30 min	Yes	May use NS, but PCN is more stable in nonalkaline pH

PARENTERAL THERAPY
RECOMMENDATIONS/GUIDELINES *(Continued)*

I.V. Medication Recommendations *(continued)*

Medication	Strength/Solution	Ref Exp	Infusion Time	Filtered	Comments
Piperacillin (Pipracil®)	1-4 g in 100 mL NS or D₅W	7 d	30-60 min	Yes	
Piperacillin/ tazobactam (Zosyn™)	2.25-4.5 g in 100 mL NS or D₅W	7 d	30-60 min	Yes	
Potassium chloride	0-40 mEq/L in NS or D₅W and various solutions	14 d	At rate ordered by physician	Yes	**Do not give undiluted KCl by direct I.V. injection**
Ranitidine (Zantac®)	50 mg in 50 mL NS or D₅W	14 d	30 min	Yes	
Ticarcillin (Ticar®)	1-3 g in 50 mL NS or D₅W	72 h	30-60 min	Yes	
Ticarcillin/ clavulanate (Timentin®)	3.1 g in 100 mL NS	7 d	30-60 min	Yes	72-hour stability in D₅W
Tobramycin (Nebcin®)	All strengths in 100 mL NS or D₅W	30 d	60 min	Yes	Monitor serum levels
Trimethoprim/ sulfamethoxazole (Bactrim™)	80/400 mg SS or 160/ 800 mg DS in 250 mL D₅W	6 h after admix	60-90 min	Yes	Incompatible in NS Protect from light
Vancomycin (Vancocin®, Vancoled®)	0-500 mg in 100 mL NS or D₅W 500 mg - 1.5 g in 250 mL NS or D₅W >1.5 g in 500 mL NS or D₅W	7 d	90 min 120 min	Yes	Monitor serum levels; red-neck or red-man syndrome if administration too rapid

NS = normal saline.

*Ref Exp = Refrigerator expiration.

I.V. Push Recommended Guidelines

Medication	Rate of Administration	Considerations
Acetazolamide (Diamox®)	250-500 mg/min	Pain on injection
Aminophylline	25 mg/min	Continuous I.V. infusion preferred
Atropine sulfate	0.5 mg/min	
Benztropine (Cogentin®)	No restrictions	
Bretylium (Bretylol®)	5 mg/kg over 1-2 min	
Bumetanide (Bumex®)	Given slowly, over 1-2 min	
Butorphanol (Stadol®)	1 mg over 1 min	
Calcium gluconate	1.5-2 mL/min	
Chlordiazepoxide (Librium®)	50-100 mg given slowly over 1 min	Dilute with sterile H_2O for injection
Chlorpromazine (Thorazine®)	1 mg/mL given at 1 mg/min	
Codeine phosphate	5 mg/min over 3-5 min	Causes respiratory depression
Dexamethasone (Decadron®)	Diluted with 10 mL NS over 3-5 min	Burning and tingling after administration
Dextrose 50%	20-50 mL slowly at 3 mL/min	Administer into large peripheral or CVC
Diazepam (Valium®)	5 mg/mL given at 5 mg/min	**Do not dilute!!!**
Diazoxide (Hyperstat®)	15 mg/mL; must be infused within 30 sec	
Digoxin (Lanoxin®)	500 mcg/mL given over 5 min	Pain on injection
Diltiazem (Cardizem®)	Over 2 min	Causes hypotension
Diphenhydramine (Benadryl®)	10 mg/min	
Droperidol (Inapsine®)	Slowly over 5-10 min	
Epinephrine (Adrenalin®)	0.1 mg/min	Diluted 1:10,000=0.1 mg/mL
Famotidine (Pepcid®)	10 mg/min	Dilute 20 mg to 5-10 mL with NS
Fosphenytoin (Cerebyx®)	100-150 mg PE/min not to exceed 150 mg PE/min	**Flush with NS before and after administration; EKG monitoring**
Furosemide (Lasix®)	80 mg over 1-2 min	High dose not >4 mg/min
Glucagon	1 mg/mL at rate of 1 mg/min	Admix with diluent supplied
Haloperidol (Haldol®)	5 mg over 1 min	
Heparin sodium	1000-10,000 units/over 1 min maximum	
Hydrocortisone (Solu-Cortef®)	50 mg/min (30 sec up to 10 min)	
Hydromorphone (Dilaudid®)	Slowly over 3-5 min	Causes respiratory depression
Insulin regular	5-30 units over 1 min	Only use regular insulin
Iron dextran (InFed™)	Give undiluted at 1 mL/min	Give test dose of 0.5 mL for first administration
Ketorolac (Toradol®)	15 mg/mL or 30 mg/mL over 1 min	
Labetalol (Normodyne®)	20 mg over 2 min	
Levothyroxine (Synthroid®)	Over 3-5 min or 50 mcg/min	
Lorazepam (Ativan®)	Rate should not exceed 2 mg/min	May be given diluted or undiluted
Meperidine (Demerol®)	10 mg/mL given slowly over 3-5 min	Causes respiratory depression
Methylprednisolone	Over 1 to several min	For higher doses give by IVPB

PARENTERAL THERAPY
RECOMMENDATIONS/GUIDELINES *(Continued)*

I.V. Push Recommended Guidelines *(continued)*

Medication	Rate of Administration	Considerations
Metoclopramide (Reglan®)	10 mg/2 mL over 1-2 min	>10 mg give IVPB
Note: When using a glass ampul, withdraw with a filter needle then change to a regular needle for administration.		
Metoprolol (Lopressor®)	Given over 1 min	
Morphine sulfate	Given slowly over 4-5 min	Dilute in 4-5 mL NS or sterile H₂O
Nalbuphine (Nubain®)	10 mg over 2-5 min	
Naloxone (Narcan®)	0.4-2 mg over 15 seconds	May repeat dose every 3-6 hours
Ondansetron (Zofran®)	4 mg given over 2-5 min	Doses >4 mg give IVPB
Phenobarbital	60 mg/min	
Procainamide (Pronestyl®)	20 mg/min	
Prochlorperazine (Compazine®)	1 mg/mL given at 5 mg/min	
Promethazine (Phenergan®)	25 mg/mL given at 25 mg/min	Concentration not >25 mg/mL
Propranolol (Inderal®)	1 mg/min	
Protamine sulfate	10 mg/mL very slowly over 1-3 min	Use for heparin overdose
Ranitidine (Zantac®)	Give over 5 min	Dilute to 20 mL with NS
Sodium bicarbonate	Rapidly over 1-2 min	
Torsemide (Demadex®)	Administer over 2 min	Oral dose and I.V. dose therapeutically equivalent
Verapamil (Isoptin®, Calan®)	2.5-10 mg over 3 min	

Note: When using a glass ampul, withdraw with a filter needle then change to a regular needle for administration.

PHARMACOTHERAPY OF URINARY INCONTINENCE

Incontinence Type	Drug Class	Drug Therapy	Adverse Effects and Precautions	Comments
Urge incontinence	Anticholinergic agents	Oxybutynin (2.5-5 mg bid-qid), propantheline (7.5-30 mg at least tid), dicyclomine (10-20 mg tid)	Dry mouth, visual disturbances, constipation, dry skin, confusion	Anticholinergics are the first-line drug therapy (oxybutynin is preferred); propantheline is a second-line therapy
	Tricyclic antidepressants (TCAs)	Imipramine, desipramine, nortriptyline (25-100 mg/day)	Anticholinergic effects (as above), orthostatic hypotension and cardiac dysrhythmia	TCAs are generally reserved for patients with an additional indication (eg, depression, neuralgia) at an initial dose of 10-25 mg 1-3 times/day
Stress incontinence	Alpha-adrenergic agonists	Phenylpropanolamine (PPA) in sustained-release form (25-100 mg bid), pseudoephedrine (15-60 mg tid)	Anxiety, insomnia, agitation, respiratory difficulty, sweating, cardiac dysrhythmia, hypertension, tremor; should not be used in obstructive syndromes and/or hypertension	PPA (preferred) or pseudoephedrine are first-line therapy for women with no contraindication (notably hypertension)
Stress or combined urge/stress incontinence	Estrogen replacement agents	Conjugated estrogens (0.3-0.625 mg/day orally or 1 g vaginal cream at bedtime)	Should not be used if suspected or confirmed breast or endometrial cancer, active or past thromboembolism with past oral contraceptive, estrogen, or pregnancy; headache, spotting, edema, breast tenderness, possible depression	Estrogen (oral or vaginal) is an adjunctive therapy for postmenopausal women as it augments alpha-agonists such as PPA or pseudoephedrine
			Give progesterone with estrogen if uterus is present; pretreatment/periodic mammogram, gynecologic, breast exam advised	Progestin (eg, medroxyprogesterone 2.5-10 mg/day) continuously or intermittently
	Imipramine (10-25 mg tid)		May worsen cardiac conduction abnormalities, postural hypotension, anticholinergic effects	Combined oral or vaginal estrogen and PPA in postmenopausal women if single drug is inadequate; imipramine is an alternative therapy when first-line therapy is inadequate

PHARMACOTHERAPY OF URINARY INCONTINENCE
(Continued)

(continued)

Incontinence Type	Drug Class	Drug Therapy	Adverse Effects and Precautions	Comments
Overflow	Alpha-adrenergic antagonists	Terazosin (1 mg at bedtime with first dose in supine position and increase by 1 mg every 4 days to 5 mg/day)	Postural hypotension, dizziness, vertigo, heart palpitations, edema, headache, anticholinergic effects	Possible benefit in men with obstructive symptoms of benign prostatic hyperplasia; monitor postural vital signs with first dose/each dose increase; may worsen female stress incontinence
		Doxazosin (1 mg at bedtime with first dose in supine position and increase by 1 mg every 7–14 days to 5 mg/day)	Same as terazosin (may be smaller incidence of hypotension)	Same as terazosin

"Urinary Incontinence," *Clinical Practice Guideline*, 1996, American Medical Directors Association, reprinted with permission. For more information call 1-800-876-2632.

TREATMENT OF TUBERCULOSIS AND TUBERCULOSIS INFECTION IN ADULTS

TREATMENT OF TUBERCULOSIS

A 6-month regimen consisting of isoniazid, rifampin, and pyrazinamide given for 2 months followed by isoniazid and rifampin for 4 months is the preferred treatment for patients with fully susceptible organisms who adhere to treatment. Ethambutol (or streptomycin in patients unable to be monitored for visual acuity) should be included in the initial regimen until the results of drug susceptibility studies are available, unless there is little possibility of drug resistance (ie, there is <4% primary resistance to isoniazid in the community, and the patient has had no previous treatment with antituberculosis medications, is not from a country with a high prevalence of drug resistance, and has no known exposure to a drug-resistant case). This four-drug, 6-month regimen is effective even when the infecting organism is resistant to INH. This recommendation applies to both HIV-infected and uninfected persons. However, in the presence of HIV infection, it is critically important to assess the clinical and bacteriologic response. If there is evidence of a slow or suboptimal response, therapy should be prolonged as judged on a case-by-case basis.

Alternatively, a 9-month regimen of isoniazid and rifampin is acceptable for persons who cannot or should not take pyrazinamide. Ethambutol (or streptomycin in patients unable to be monitored for visual acuity) should also be included until the results of drug susceptibility studies are available, unless there is little possibility of drug resistance. If INH resistance is demonstrated, rifampin and ethambutol should be continued for a minimum of 12 months.

Consideration should be given to treating all patients with directly observed therapy (DOT).

Multiple-drug-resistant tuberculosis (ie, resistance to at least isoniazid and rifampin) presents difficult treatment problems. Treatment must be individualized and based on susceptibility studies. In such cases, consultation with an expert in tuberculosis is recommended.

Extrapulmonary tuberculosis should be managed according to the principles and with the drug regimens outlines for pulmonary tuberculosis.

A 4-month regimen of isoniazid and rifampin is acceptable therapy for adults who have active tuberculosis and who are sputum-smear and culture negative, if there is little possibility of drug resistance.

The major determination of the outcome of treatment is patient adherence to the drug regimen. Careful attention should be paid to measures designed to foster adherence and to ensure that patients take the drugs as prescribed. The use of fixed drug combinations may enhance patient adherence and may reduce the risk of inappropriate monotherapy, and it may prevent the development of secondary drug resistance. For this reason, the use of such fixed drug combinations is strongly encouraged in adults. Virtually all the treatment regimens may be given intermittently if directly observed, thus assuring adherence.

TREATMENT OF TUBERCULOSIS INFECTION

Preventive therapy with isoniazid given for 6-12 months is effective in decreasing the risk of future tuberculosis in adults with tuberculosis infection demonstrated by a positive tuberculin skin test reaction. The appropriate criterion for defining a positive skin test reaction depends on the population being tested. For adults with HIV infection, close contacts of infectious cases, and those with fibrotic lesions on chest radiograph, a reaction ≥5 mm is considered positive. For other at-risk adults, a reaction ≥10 mm is positive. Persons who are not likely to be infected with *Mycobacterium tuberculosis* should generally not be skin tested. If a skin test is performed on a person without a defined risk factor for tuberculosis infection, ≥15 mm is positive.

Persons with a positive skin test and any of the following risk factors should be considered for preventive therapy regardless of age: persons with HIV infection, persons at risk for HIV infection with unknown HIV status; close contacts of sputum-positive persons with newly diagnosed infectious tuberculosis; newly infected persons (recent skin test convertors); and persons with medical conditions reported to increase the risk of tuberculosis (ie, diabetes mellitus, adrenocorticosteroid therapy and other immunosuppressive therapy, intravenous drug

TREATMENT OF TUBERCULOSIS AND TUBERCULOSIS INFECTION IN ADULTS *(Continued)*

users, hematologic and reticuloendothelial malignancies, end-stage renal disease, and clinical conditions associated with rapid weight loss or chronic undernutrition). In some circumstances, persons with negative skin tests should also be considered for preventive therapy. These include children who are close contacts of infectious cases and anergic HIV-infected adults at increased risk of tuberculosis. Tuberculin-positive adults with abnormal chest films that show fibrotic lesions likely representing old healed tuberculosis and adults with silicosis should usually receive 4-month multidrug chemotherapy although 12 months of isoniazid preventive therapy is an acceptable alternative.

Persons who are known to be HIV-infected and who are contacts of patients with infectious tuberculosis should be carefully evaluated for evidence of tuberculosis. If there are no findings suggestive of current tuberculosis, preventive therapy with isoniazid should be given. Because HIV-infected contacts are not managed in the same way as those who are not HIV-infected, HIV testing is recommended if there are known or suspected risk factors for acquisition of HIV infection.

In the absence of any of the above risk factors, persons younger than 35 years of age with a positive skin test in the following high incidence groups should also be considered for preventive therapy; foreign-born persons from high-prevalence countries; medically underserved low-income persons from high-prevalence populations (especially African-Americans, Hispanics, and Native Americans); and residents of facilities for long-term care (eg, correctional institutions, nursing homes, and mental institutions).

Twelve months of preventive therapy is recommended for adults and children with HIV infection and other conditions associated with immunosuppression. Persons without HIV infection should receive at least 6 months of preventive therapy.

In patients who have a positive tuberculin skin test and either silicosis or a chest radiograph demonstrating old fibrotic lesions, and who have no evidence of active tuberculosis, acceptable regimens include 4 months of isoniazid plus rifampin or 12 months of isoniazid, providing that infection with drug-resistant organisms is judged to be unlikely.

In persons younger than 35 years of age, routine monitoring for adverse effects of isoniazid should consist of a monthly symptom review. For persons 35 years of age and older, hepatic enzymes should be measures prior to starting isoniazid and monitored monthly throughout treatment, in addition to monthly symptom reviews. Other factors associated with an increased risk of hepatitis include daily use of alcohol, chronic liver disease, and injection drug use. There is also evidence to suggest that postpubertal African-American and Hispanic women are at greater risk for hepatitis. Certain medications taken concurrently with isoniazid may increase the risk of hepatitis or drug interactions. More careful monitoring should be considered in these groups, possibly including more frequent laboratory monitoring.

Persons who are presumed to be infected with isoniazid-resistant organisms should be treated with rifampin rather than with isoniazid.

As with treatment of tuberculosis, the key to success of preventive therapy is patient adherence to the prescribed regimen. Although not evaluated in clinical studies, directly observed, twice-weekly preventive therapy may be used for at-risk adults and children who cannot or will not reliably self-administer therapy.

Adapted from *Am J Respir Crit Care Med*, Vol 149, 1994, 1359-74.

SKIN TESTS FOR DELAYED HYPERSENSITIVITY

Candida 1:100
> Dose = 0.1 mL intradermally
> Can be used as a control antigen

Coccidioidin 1:100
> Dose = 0.1 mL intradermally
> (apply with PPD **and** a control antigen)
> Mercury derivative used as a preservative for spherulin

Histoplasmin 1:100
> Dose = 0.1 mL intradermally
> (yeast derived)

Multitest CMI (*Candida,* diphtheria toxoid, tetanus toxoid, *Streptococcus,* old tuberculin, *Trichophyton, Proteus* antigen, and negative control)
> Press loaded unit into the skin with sufficient pressure to puncture the skin and allow adequate penetration of all points

Mumps 40 cfu per mL
> Dose = 0.1 mL intradermally
> (contraindicated in patients allergic to eggs, egg products, or thimerosal)

Purified Protein Derivative 5 TU (PPD Mantoux Tuberculin)
> Dose = 0.1 mL intradermally
> A positive immune response is 5 mm or more of induration; tuberculin positive patients must have an induration of 10 mm or more

Tetanus Toxoid 1:5
> Dose = 0.1 mL intradermally
> Can be used as a control antigen

Tine Test
> Indication: Survey and screen for exposure to tuberculosis (grasp forearm firmly; stretch the skin of the volar surface tightly; apply the tines to the selected site; press for at least 1 second so that a circular halo impression is left on the skin)

General Information

1. Intradermal skin tests should be injected in the flexor surface of the forearm.

2. A pale wheal 6-10 mm in diameter should form over the needle tip as soon as the injection is administered. If no bleb forms, the injection must be repeated.

3. Space skin tests at least 2 inches apart to prevent reactions from overlapping.

4. Read skin tests for diameter of induration and presence of erythema at 24, 48, and 72 hours. After injection, maximal responses usually occur at 48 hours. Maximal responses to mumps or coccidioidin may occur at 24 hours.

5. False-negative results may occur in patients with malnutrition, viral infections, febrile illnesses, immunodeficiency disorders, severe disseminated infections, uremia, patients who have received immunosuppressive therapy (steroids, antineoplastic agents), patients who have received a recent live attenuated virus vaccine (MMR, measles), or subdermal injection of the antigen.

6. False-positive results may occur in patients sensitive to ingredients in the skin test solution such as thimerosal, due to cross sensitivity between similar antigens, or with improper interpretation of skin test.

7. Side effects are pain, blisters, extensive erythema and necrosis at the injection site.

    *Emergency equipment and epinephrine should be readily available to treat severe allergic reactions that may occur.

8. With initial PPD skin testing, the elderly frequently exhibit anergy; therefore, the 2-step PPD is recommended. For example, if initial PPD is negative, repeat test with 5 TU PPD 2-4 weeks later.

SKIN TESTS FOR DELAYED HYPERSENSITIVITY
(Continued)

Recommended Interpretation of Skin Test Reactions

Reaction	Local Reaction	
	After Intradermal Injections of Antigens	After Dinitrochlorobenzene
1+	Erythema >10 mm and/or induration >1-5 mm	Erythema and/or induration covering <½ area of dose site
2+	Induration 6-10 mm	Induration covering >½ area of dose site
3+	Induration 11-20 mm	Vesiculation and induration at dose site or spontaneous flare at days 7-14 at the site
4+	Induration >20 mm	Bulla or ulceration at dose site or spontaneous flare at days 7-14 at the site

References

Ahmed AR and Blose DA, "Delayed-Type Hypersensitivity Skin Testing, A Review," *Arch Dermatol*, 1983, 119:934-45.

Delafuente JC, Meuleman JR, and Nelson RC, "Anergy Testing in Nursing Home Residents," *J Am Geriatr Soc*, 1988, 36:733-5.

Gordon EG, Krouse HA, Kinney JL, et al, "Delayed Cutaneous Hypersensitivity in Normals: Choice of Antigens and Comparison to *in vitro* Assays of Cell-Mediated Immunity," *J Allergy Clin Immunol*, 1983, 72:487-94.

Sokal JE, "Measurement of Delayed Skin-Test Responses," *N Engl J Med*, 1975, 293:501-2.

OVERDOSE AND TOXICOLOGY INFORMATION

Drug or Drug Class	Signs/Symptoms	Treatment/Comments
Acetaminophen 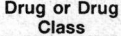	Generally asymptomatic	Assess severity of ingestion; adult doses ≥140 mg/kg are thought to be toxic. Obtain serum concentration ≥4 hours postingestion and use acetaminophen nomogram to evaluate need for acetylcysteine. Gastric decontamination within 2-4 hours after ingestion. May administer activated charcoal for one dose, this may decrease absorption of acetylcysteine if given within 1 hour of acetylcysteine. For unknown ingested quantities and for significant ingestion give acetylcysteine orally (diluted 1:4 with juice or carbonated beverage); initial: 140 mg/kg then give 70 mg/kg every 4 hours for 17 doses.
Alpha-adrenergic blocking agents	Hypotension, drowsiness	Give activated charcoal, additional treatment if symptomatic; use I.V. fluids, dopamine, or norepinephrine to treat hypotension. Epinephrine may worsen hypotension due to beta effects.
Aminoglycosides	Ototoxicity, nephrotoxicity, neuromuscular toxicity	Hemodialysis or peritoneal dialysis may be useful in patients with decreased renal function; calcium may reverse the neuromuscular toxicity.
Anticholinergics, antihistamines	Coma, hallucinations, delirium, tachycardia, dry skin, urinary retention, dilated pupils	For life-threatening arrhythmias or seizures. Adults: 2 mg/dose physostigmine, may repeat 1-2 mg in 20 minutes and give 1-4 mg slow I.V. over 5-10 minutes if signs and symptoms recur (relatively contraindicated if QRS >0.1 msec).
Anticholinesterase agents	Nausea, vomiting, diarrhea, miosis, CNS depression, excessive salivation, excessive sweating, muscle weakness	Suction oral secretions, decontaminate skin, atropinize patient; atropine dose must be individualized. Adults: Initial atropine dose: 1 mg; titrate dose upward; pralidoxime (2-PAM) may need to be added for moderate to severe intoxications.
Barbiturates	Respiratory depression, circulatory collapse, bradycardia, hypotension, hypothermia, slurred speech, confusion, coma	Repeated oral doses of activated charcoal given every 3-6 hours will increase clearance. Adults: 30-60 g. Assure GI motility, adequate hydration, and renal function. Urinary alkalinization with I.V. sodium bicarbonate will increase renal elimination of longer-acting barbiturates (eg, phenobarbital).

OVERDOSE AND TOXICOLOGY INFORMATION *(Continued)*

Benzodiazepines	Respiratory depression, apnea (after rapid I.V.), hypoactive reflexes, hypotension, slurred speech, unsteady gait, coma	Dialysis is of limited value; support blood pressure and respiration until symptoms subside. Flumazenil: Initial dose: 0.2 mg given I.V. over 30 seconds. If further response is desired after 30 seconds, give 0.3 mg over another 30 seconds. Further doses of 0.5 mg can be given over 30 seconds at 1-minute intervals up to a total of 3 mg.
Beta-adrenergic blockers	Hypotension, bronchospasm, bradycardia, hypoglycemia, seizures	Activated charcoal; treat symptomatically; glucagon, atropine, isoproterenol, dobutamine, or cardiac pacing may be needed to treat bradycardia, conduction defects, or hypotension.
Carbamazepine	Dizziness, drowsiness, ataxia, involuntary movements, opisthotonos, seizures, nausea, vomiting, agitation, nystagmus, coma, urinary retention, respiratory depression, tachycardia, arrhythmias	Use supportive therapy, general poisoning management as needed; use repeated oral doses of activated charcoal given every 3-6 hours to decrease serum concentrations; charcoal hemoperfusion may be needed; treat hypotension with I.V. fluids, dopamine, or norepinephrine, monitor EKG; diazepam may control convulsions but may exacerbate respiratory depression.
Cardiac glycosides	Hyperkalemia may develop rapidly and result in life-threatening cardiac arrhythmias, progressive bradyarrhythmias, second or third degree heart block unresponsive to atropine, ventricular fibrillation, asystole	Obtain serum drug level, induce emesis or perform gastric lavage; give activated charcoal to reduce further absorption; atropine may reverse heart block, digoxin immune Fab (digoxin specific antibody fragments) is used in serious cases, each 40 mg of digoxin immune Fab binds with 0.6. mg of digoxin.
Heparin	Severe hemorrhage	1 mg of protamine sulfate will neutralize approximately 90 units of heparin sodium (bovine) or 115 units of heparin sodium (porcine) or 100 units of heparin calcium (porcine).
Hydantoin derivatives	Nausea, vomiting, nystagmus, slurred speech, ataxia, coma	Gastric lavage or emesis; repeated oral doses of activated charcoal may increase clearance of phenytoin. Use 0.5-1 g/kg (30-60 g/dose) activated charcoal every 3-6 hours until nontoxic serum concentration is obtained; assure adequate GI motility, supportive therapy.

Iron	Lethargy, nausea, vomiting, green or tarry stools, hypotension, weak rapid pulse, metabolic acidosis, shock, coma, hepatic necrosis, renal failure, local GI erosions	If immediately after ingestion and not already vomiting, give ipecac or lavage with saline solution; give deferoxamine mesylate I.V. at 15 mg/kg/hour in cases of severe poisoning (serum iron >350 µg/mL) until the urine color is normal, the patient is asymptomatic, or a maximum daily dose of 8 g is reached; urine output should be maintained >2 mL/kg/hour to avoid hypovolemic shock.
Isoniazid	Nausea, vomiting, blurred vision, CNS depression, intractable seizures, coma, metabolic acidosis	Control seizures with diazepam, give pyridoxine I.V. equal dose to the suspected overdose of isoniazid or up to 5 g empirically; give activated charcoal.
Nonsteroidal anti-inflammatory drugs	Dizziness, abdominal pain, sweating, apnea, nystagmus, cyanosis, hypotension, coma, seizures (rarely)	Induce emesis; give activated charcoal via NG tube; provide symptomatic and supportive care.
Opioids and morphine analogs	Respiratory depression, miosis, hypothermia, bradycardia, circulatory collapse, pulmonary edema, apnea	Establish airway and adequate ventilation; give naloxone 0.4 mg and titrate to a maximum of 10 mg; additional doses may be needed every 20-60 minutes. May need to institute continuous infusion, as duration of action of opiates can be longer than duration of action of naloxone.
Phenothiazines	Deep, unarousable sleep, anticholinergic symptoms, extrapyramidal signs, diaphoresis, rigidity, tachycardia, cardiac dysrhythmias, hypotension	Activated charcoal; do **not** dialyze; use I.V. benztropine mesylate 1-2 mg/dose slowly over 3-6 minutes for extrapyramidal signs; use I.V. fluids and norepinephrine to treat hypotension; avoid epinephrine which may cause hypotension due to phenothiazine-induced alpha-adrenergic blockade and unopposed epinephrine B_2 action; use benzodiazepines for seizure management and to decrease rigidity.
Salicylates	Nausea, vomiting, respiratory alkalosis, hyperthermia, dehydration, hyperapnea, tinnitus, headache, dizziness, metabolic acidosis, coma	Induce emesis or gastric lavage immediately; give several doses of activated charcoal, rehydrate, and use sodium bicarbonate to correct metabolic acidosis and enhance renal elimination by alkalinizing the urine; give supplemental potassium after renal function has been determined to be adequate. Monitor electrolytes; obtain stat serum salicylate level and follow.
Tricyclic antidepressants	Agitation, confusion, hallucinations, urinary retention, hypothermia, hypotension, tachycardia, arrhythmias, seizures	Give activated charcoal ± lavage; use sodium bicarbonate for QRS >0.1 msec; I.V. fluids and norepinephrine may be used for hypotension; benzodiazepines may be used for seizure management.

1093

OVERDOSE AND TOXICOLOGY INFORMATION *(Continued)*

Warfarin	Internal or external hemorrhage, hematuria	For moderate overdoses, give oral, S.C., or I.D., or slow I.V. (I.V. associated with anaphylactoid reactions) phytonadione; usual dose: 2.5-10 mg, adjust per prothrombin time; for severe hemorrhage, give fresh frozen plasma or whole blood.
Xanthine derivatives	Vomiting, abdominal pain, bloody diarrhea, tachycardia, extrasystoles, tachypnea, tonic/clonic seizures	Give activated charcoal orally; repeated oral doses of activated charcoal increase clearance; use 0.5-1 g/kg (30-60 g/dose) of activated charcoal every 1-4 hours (depending on the severity of ingestion) until nontoxic serum concentrations are obtained. Assure adequate GI motility, supportive therapy; charcoal hemoperfusion or hemodialysis can also be effective in decreasing serum concentrations and should be used if the serum concentration approaches 90-100 mcg/mL in acute overdoses.

ALLERGIC SKIN REACTIONS TO DRUGS

Skin eruptions are the most common clinically observed form of drug "allergy". Cutaneous manifestations of hypersensitivity may include pruritus, urticaria, and angioedema; maculopapular, morbilliform, or erythematous rashes; erythema multiforme; eczema; erythema nodosum; photosensitivity reactions; and fixed drug eruptions. The most severe drug-related reactions are exfoliative dermatitis and vesiculobullous eruptions such as the Stevens-Johnson syndrome and toxic epidermal necrolysis (Lyell's syndrome). This table lists the incidence of drugs associated with cutaneous manifestations reported in 22,227 consecutive medical inpatients in the Boston Collaborative Drug Surveillance Program.

Drug	Reaction per 1000 Recipients
Sulfamethoxazole and trimethoprim	59
Ampicillin	52
Semisynthetic penicillins	36
Blood, whole human	35
Corticotropin	28
Erythromycin	23
Sulfisoxazole	17
Penicillin G	16
Gentamicin sulfate	16
Practolol	16
Cephalosporins	13
Quinidine	13
Plasma protein fraction	12
Dipyrone	11
Mercurial diuretics	9.5
Nitrofurantoin	9.1
Packed RBCs	8.1
Heparin	7.7
Chloramphenicol	6.8
Trimethobenzamide	6.6
Phenazopyridine	6.5
Methenamine	6.4
Nitrazepam	6.3
Barbiturates	4.7
Glutethimide	4.5
Indomethacin	4.4
Chlordiazepoxide	4.2
Metoclopramide	4.0
Diazepam	3.8
Propoxyphene	3.4
Isoniazid	3.0
Guaifenesin and theophylline	2.9
Nystatin	2.9
Chlorothiazide	2.8
Furosemide	2.6
Isophane insulin suspension	1.3
Phenytoin	1.1
Phytonadione	0.9
Flurazepam	0.5
Chloral hydrate	0.2

Reference

Patterson R and Anderson J, "Allergic Reactions to Drugs and Biologic Agents", *JAMA*, 1982, 248:2637-45.

ANTACID DRUG INTERACTIONS

Drug	Antacid				
	Al Salts	Ca Salts	Mg Salts	NaHCO₃	Mg/Al
Allopurinol	↓				
Anorexiants				↑	
Atorvastatin	↓		↓		
Benzodiazepines	↑		↓	↓	↓
Calcitriol			x*		x*
Captopril					↓
Cimetidine	↓		↓		↓
Corticosteroids	↓		↓		↓
Digoxin	↓		↓		
Flecainide				↑	
Indomethacin	↓		↓		↓
Iron	↓	↓	↓	↓	↓
Isoniazid	↓				
Ketoconazole				↓	↓
Levodopa					↑
Lithium				↓	
Mycophenolate	↓		↓		
Naproxen	↑		↑	↓	↑
Nitrofurantoin			↓		
Penicillamine	↓		↓		↓
Phenothiazines	↓		↓		↓
Phenytoin		↓			↓
Quinidine		↑	↑		↑
Quinolones	↓	↓	↓		↓
Ranitidine	↓				↓
Salicylates				↓	↓
Sodium polystyrene sulfonate	x†		x†		x†
Sulfonylureas				↑	
Sympathomimetics				↑	
Tetracyclines	↓	↓	↓	↓	↓
Tolmetin				x‡	

Pharmacologic effect increased (↑) or decreased (↓) by antacids.

*Concomitant use in patients on chronic renal dialysis may lead to hypermagnesemia.

†Concomitant use may cause metabolic alkalosis in patients with renal failure.

‡Concomitant use not recommended by manufacturer.

ANTIDOTES

Antidote	Poison/Drug	Indications/Symptoms
Acetylcysteine	Acetaminophen	• Unknown quantity was ingested and <24 h have elapsed since the time of ingestion • >7.5 g ingested acutely • Serum acetaminophen >140 mcg/mL at 4 h postingestion • Ingested dose >140 mg/kg
Amyl nitrite, sodium nitrite, sodium thiosulfate	Cyanide	• Begin treatment at the first sign of toxicity if cyanide exposure is known or strongly suspected
Antivenin polyvalent	Pit viper bites (rattlesnake, cottonmouth, copperhead)	• History of envenomation by a pit viper and experiencing mild, moderate, or severe symptoms **Mild:** Local swelling (progressive), pain, no systemic systems **Moderate:** Ecchymosis and swelling beyond the bite site, some systemic symptoms, and/or lab changes **Severe:** Profound edema involving entire extremity, cyanosis, serious systemic involvement, significant lab changes
Atropine	Organophosphate and carbamate insecticides	• Myoclonic seizures, severe hallucinations, weakness, arrhythmias, excessive salivation, involuntary urination and defecation
Calcium EDTA (Versenate®)	Lead	• Symptomatic patients or asymptomatic children with blood levels >50 mcg/dL
Calcium gluconate	Hydrofluoric acid (HF)	• Calcium gluconate gel 2.5% for dermal exposure of HF <20% concentration •SC injections or intra-arterial administration of calcium gluconate for dermal exposures of concentrations >20% or failure to respond to gel
Deferoxamine (Desferal®)	Iron	• Serum iron >350 mcg/dL or unable to obtain SI in a reasonable time and patient has signs and symptoms consistent with iron toxicity
Digoxin immune Fab (Digibind®)	Digoxin	• Serious cardiac arrhythmias, progressive bradyarrhythmias, second or third degree heart block unresponsive to atropine, serum digoxin level >10 ng/mL or potassium levels >5 mEq/L
Dimercaprol (BAL in oil)	Arsenic	• Any symptoms of arsenic toxicity
	Lead	• All patients with symptoms, or asymptomatic children with blood levels 70 mcg/dL
	Mercury	• Serious, acute toxicity with inorganic mercury salts
Ethanol	Ethylene glycol or methanol	• Ethylene glycol or methanol blood levels >20 mg/dL or blood levels not readily available and suspected ingestion of toxic amounts, or any symptomatic patient with a history of ethylene glycol or methanol ingestion
Flumazenil (Mazicon®)	Benzodiazepines	• Complete or partial reversal of the sedative effects of benzodiazepines in cases where they were used in general anesthesia or for sedation for diagnostic or therapeutic procedures

ANTIDOTES *(Continued)*

Methylene blue (Methblue 65®) (Urolene Blue®)	Cyanide	• Begin treatment at the first sign of toxicity if cyanide poisoning is suspected or known
Naloxone	Opiates (heroin, morphine, etc)	• Respiratory depression ± coma from unknown cause, or from opioid overdose
Naltrexone	Opiates (heroin, morphine, etc)	• Respiratory depression ± coma from unknown cause, or from opioid overdose
Physostigmine (Antilirium®)	Atropine and anticholinergics	• Myoclonic seizures, hypertension, severe arrhythmias, hallucinations
Phytonadione (Vitamin K₁)	Warfarin	• Large acute ingestion of warfarin rodenticides or chronic exposure, or greater than normal prothrombin time
Pralidoxime (Protopam®)	Organophosphate insecticide	• An adjunct to atropine therapy for treatment of profound muscle weakness, respiratory depression, muscle twitching and cholinergic syndrome
Pyridoxine (Vitamin B₆)	Isoniazid	• Unknown overdose or ingested amount >80 mg/kg
Succimer (Chemet®)	Lead (unlabeled use: mercury, arsenic)	• Blood lead levels >45 mcg/dL • Symptoms of lead poisoning • Unlabeled: other heavy metal poisoning

ANXIOLYTIC/HYPNOTIC USE IN LONG-TERM CARE FACILITIES

One of the regulations regarding medication use in long-term care facilities concerns "unnecessary drugs." The regulation states, "Each resident's drug regimen must be free from unnecessary drugs." Recently, the Health Care Financing Administration (HCFA) issued the final interpretive guidelines on this regulation. The following is a summary of these guidelines as they pertain to anxiolytic/hypnotic agents.

A. **Long-Acting Benzodiazepines**

Long-acting benzodiazepine drugs should not be used in residents unless an attempt with a shorter-acting drug has failed. If they are used, the doses must be no higher than the listed dose, unless higher doses are necessary for maintenance or improvement in the resident's functional status. Daily use should be less then 4 continuous months unless an attempt at a gradual dose reduction is unsuccessful. Residents on diazepam for seizure disorders or for the treatment of tardive dyskinesia are exempt from this restriction. Residents on clonazepam for bipolar disorder, tardive dyskinesia, nocturnal myoclonus, or seizure disorder are also exempt. Residents on long-acting benzodiazepines should have a gradual dose reduction at least twice within 1 year before it can be concluded that the gradual dose reduction is "clinically contraindicated."

Long-Acting Benzodiazepines

Generic	Brand	Maximum Daily Geriatric Dose (mg)
Chlordiazepoxide	Librium®	20
Clonazepam	Klonopin™	1.5
Clorazepate	Tranxene®	15
Diazepam	Valium®	5
Flurazepam	Dalmane®	15
Halazepam	Paxipam®	40
Quazepam	Doral®	7.5

B. **Benzodiazepine or Other Anxiolytic/Sedative Drugs**

Anxiolytic/sedative drugs should be used for purposes other than sleep induction only when other possible causes of the resident's distress have been ruled out and the use results in maintenance or improvement in the resident's functional status. Daily use should not exceed 4 continuous months unless an attempt at gradual dose reduction has failed. Anxiolytics should only be used for generalized anxiety disorder, dementia with agitated states that either endangers the resident or others, or is a source of distress or dysfunction; panic disorder or symptomatic anxiety associated with other psychiatric disorders. The dose should not exceed those listed below unless a higher dose is needed as evidenced by the resident's response. Gradual dosage reductions should be attempted at least twice within 1 year before it can be concluded that a gradual dose reduction is "clinically contraindicated."

ANXIOLYTIC/HYPNOTIC USE IN LONG-TERM CARE FACILITIES (Continued)

Short-Acting Benzodiazepines

Generic	Brand	Maximum Daily Geriatric Dose (mg)
Alprazolam	Xanax®	0.75
Estazolam*	ProSom®	0.5
Lorazepam	Ativan®	2
Oxazepam	Serax®	30

*Primarily used as a hypnotic agent.

Other Anxiolytic and Sedative Drugs

Generic	Brand	Maximum Daily Geriatric Dose (mg)
Chloral hydrate	Noctec®, etc	750
Diphenhydramine	Benadryl®	50
Hydroxyzine	Atarax®, Vistaril®	50

Note: Chloral hydrate, diphenhydramine, and hydroxyzine are not necessarily drugs of choice for treatment of anxiety disorders. HCFA lists them only in the event of their possible use.

C. **Drugs Used for Sleep Induction**

Drugs for sleep induction should only be used when all possible reasons for insomnia have been ruled out (ie, pain, noise, caffeine). The use of the drug must result in the maintenance or improvement of the resident's functional status. Daily use of a hypnotic should not exceed 10 consecutive days unless an attempt at a gradual dose reduction is unsuccessful. The dose should not exceed those listed below unless a higher dose has been deemed necessary. Gradual dose reductions should be attempted at least three times within 6 months before it can be concluded that a gradual dose reduction is "clinically contraindicated."

Hypnotic Drugs

Generic	Brand	Daily Geriatric Dose (mg)
Alprazolam*	Xanax®	0.25
Chloral hydrate	Noctec®	500
Diphenhydramine	Benadryl®	25
Estazolam	ProSom™	0.5
Hydroxyzine	Atarax®, Vistaril®	50
Lorazepam*	Ativan®	1
Oxazepam*	Serax®	15
Temazepam	Restoril®	7.5
Triazolam	Halcion®	0.125
Zolpidem	Ambien®	5

*Not officially indicated as a hypnotic agent.

Note: Chloral hydrate, diphenhydramine, and hydroxyzine are not necessarily drugs of choice for sleep disorders. HCFA lists them only in the event of their possible use.

D. Miscellaneous Hypnotic/Sedative/Anxiolytic Drugs

The initiation of the following medications should not occur in any dose in any resident. Residents currently using these drugs or residents admitted to the facility while using these drugs should receive gradual dose reductions. Newly admitted residents should have a period of adjustment before attempting reduction. Dose reductions should be attempted at least twice within 1 year before it can be concluded that it is "clinically contraindicated."

Examples of Barbiturates

Generic	Brand
Amobarbital	Amytal®
Amobarbital/Secobarbital	Tuinal®
Butabarbital	Butisol Sodium®
Combinations	Fiorinal®, etc
Pentobarbital	Nembutal®
Secobarbital	Seconal™

Miscellaneous Hypnotic/Sedative/Anxiolytic Agents

Generic	Brand
Ethchlorvynol	Placidyl®
Glutethimide	Doriden®
Meprobamate	Equanil®, Miltown®
Methyprylon	Noludar®
Paraldehyde	Paral®

DEPRESSION SCALES

Short Form Geriatric Depression Scale*

NAME _____ AGE _____ SEX _____ DATE _____

WING _____ ROOM _____ PHYSICIAN _____

SCORING SYSTEM

Answers indicating depression are highlighted. Each BOLD-FACED answer counts one (1) point. Score greater than 5 indicates probable depression

1.	Are you basically satisfied with your life?	YES / **NO**
2.	Have you dropped any of your activities and interests?	**YES** / NO
3.	Do you feel that your life is empty?	**YES** / NO
4.	Do you often get bored?	**YES** / NO
5.	Are you in good spirits most of the time?	YES / **NO**
6.	Are you afraid that something bad is going to happen to you?	**YES** / NO
7.	Do you feel happy most of the time?	YES / **NO**
8.	Do you often feel helpless?	**YES** / NO
9.	Do you prefer to stay in your room/facility, rather than going out and doing new things?	**YES** / NO
10.	Do you feel you have more problems with memory than most?	**YES** / NO
11.	Do you think it is wonderful to be alive?	YES / **NO**
12.	Do you feel worthless the way you are now?	**YES** / NO
13.	Do you feel full of energy?	YES / **NO**
14.	Do you feel that your situation is hopeless?	**YES** / NO
15.	Do you think that most people are better off than you?	**YES** / NO

SCORE

NOTES / CURRENT MEDICATIONS:
ASSESSOR:

*This scale may be used when evaluating residents who do not have limited cognition.

Cornell Scale for Depression in Dementia*

NAME _____ AGE _____ SEX _____ DATE _____

WING _____ ROOM _____ PHYSICIAN _____

Ratings should be based on symptoms and signs occurring during the week before interview. No score should be given if symptoms result from physical disability or illness.

SCORING SYSTEM

a = Unable to evaluate   0 = Absent

1 = Mild to Intermittent   2 = Severe

> Score greater than 12 = Probable Depression

A. MOOD-RELATED SIGNS

	a	0	1	2
1. Anxiety; anxious expression, rumination, worrying				
2. Sadness; sad expression, sad voice, tearfulness				
3. Lack of reaction to pleasant events				
4. Irritability; annoyed, short tempered				

B. BEHAVIORAL DISTURBANCE

	a	0	1	2
5. Agitation; restlessness, hand wringing, hair pulling				
6. Retardation; slow movements, slow speech, slow reactions				
7. Multiple physical complaints (score 0 if gastrointestinal symptoms only)				
8. Loss of interest; less involved in usual activities (score only if change occurred acutely, i.e., in less than one month)				

C. PHYSICAL SIGNS

	a	0	1	2
9. Appetite loss; eating less than usual				
10. Weight loss (score 2 if greater than 5 pounds in one month)				
11. Lack of energy; fatigues easily, unable to sustain activities				

D. CYCLIC FUNCTIONS

	a	0	1	2
12. Diurnal variation of mood; symptoms worse in the morning				
13. Difficulty falling asleep; later than usual for this individual				
14. Multiple awakening during sleep				
15. Early morning awaking; earlier than usual for this individual				

E. IDEATIONAL DISTURBANCE

	a	0	1	2
16. Suicidal; feels life is not worth living				
17. Poor self-esteem; self-blame, self-depreciation, feelings of failure				
18. Pessimism; anticipation of the worst				
19. Mood congruent delusions; delusions of poverty, illness, or loss				

NOTES / CURRENT MEDICATIONS: SCORE

ASSESSOR:

*This scale may be used to evaluate residents with limited cognition.

FEVER DUE TO DRUGS

Allopurinol
Aminosalicylic acid
Antihistamines
Barbiturates
Cephalosporins

Iodides
Isoniazid
Methyldopa
Penicillins
Phenolphthalein

Phenytoin
Procainamide
Propylthiouracil
Quinidine
Sulfonamides

Reference
Abstracted from Harrison's *Principles of Internal Medicine*, 12th ed, Wilson JD, ed, New York, NY: McGraw-Hill Book Co, 1991 and Tabor PA, "Drug-Induced Fever," *Drug Intell Clin Pharm*, 1986, 20:413-20.

DISCOLORATION OF FECES DUE TO DRUGS

Black
Acetazolamide
Alcohols
Alkalies
Aluminum hydroxide
Aminophylline
Amphetamine
Amphotericin
Anticoagulants
Aspirin
Barium
Betamethasone
Bismuth
Charcoal
Chloramphenicol
Chlorpropamide
Clindamycin
Corticosteroids
Cortisone
Cyclophosphamide
Cytarabine
Dicumarol
Digitalis
Ethacrynic acid
Fenoprofen
Ferrous salts
Floxuridine
Fluorides
Fluorouracil
Halothane
Heparin
Hydralazine
Hydrocortisone
Ibuprofen
Indomethacin
Iodine drugs
Iron salts
Levarterenol
Levodopa
Manganese
Mefenamic Acid
Melphalan
Methylprednisolone

Methotrexate
Methylene blue
Nitrates
Oxyphenbutazone
Paraldehyde
Phenacetin
Phenolphthalein
Phenylbutazone
Phenylephrine
Phosphorous
Potassium salts
Prednisolone
Procarbazine
Pyrvinium
Reserpine
Salicylates
Sulfonamides
Tetracycline
Thallium
Theophylline
Thiotepa
Triamcinolone
Warfarin

Blue
Chloramphenicol
Methylene blue

Dark Brown
Dexamethasone

Gray
Colchicine

Green
Indomethacin
Iron
Medroxyprogesterone

Greenish Gray
Oral antibiotics
Oxyphenbutazone
Phenylbutazone

Light Brown

Anticoagulants

Orange-Red
Phenazopyridine
Rifampin

Pink
Anticoagulants
Aspirin
Heparin
Oxyphenbutazone
Phenylbutazone
Salicylates

Red
Anticoagulants
Aspirin
Heparin
Oxyphenbutazone
Phenolphthalein
Phenylbutazone
Pyrvinium
Salicylates
Tetracycline syrup

Red-Brown
Oxyphenbutazone
Phenylbutazone
Rifampin

Tarry
Ergot preparations
Ibuprofen
Salicylates
Warfarin

White/Speckling
Aluminum hydroxide
Antibiotics (oral)
Indocyanine green

Yellow
Senna

Yellow-Green
Senna

Reference
Adapted from Drugdex® — Drug Consults, Micromedex, vol 62, Rocky Mountain Drug Consultation Center, Denver, CO: January, 1995.

DISCOLORATION OF URINE DUE TO DRUGS

Black
Cascara
Ferrous salts
Iron dextran
Levodopa
Methocarbamol
Methyldopa
Naphthalene
Phenacetin
Phenols
Quinine
Sulfonamides

Blue
Anthraquinone
DeWitts pills
Indigo blue
Indigo carmine
Methocarbamol
Methylene blue
Nitrofurans
Resorcinol
Triamterene

Blue-Green
Amitriptyline
Anthraquinone
DeWitt's pills
Doan's® pills
Indigo blue
Indigo carmine
Methylene blue
Resoreinol

Brown
Anthraquinone dyes
Cascara
Chloroquine
Danthron
Furazolidone
Levodopa
Methocarbamol
Methyldopa
Metronidazole
Nitrofurans
Nitrofurantoin
Phenacetin
Phenols
Primaquine
Quinine
Rifampin
Senna
Sodium diatrizoate
Sulfonamides

Brown-Black
Methocarbamol
Methyldopa
Metronidazole
Nitrates
Nitrofurans
Phenacetin
Povidone iodine
Quinine
Senna

Dark
Aminosalicylic acid
Cascara
Furazolidone
Levodopa
Metronidazole
Nitrites
Phenacetin
Phenol
Primaquine
Quinine
Resorcinol
Riboflavin
Senna

Green
Amitriptyline
Anthraquinone
Chlorophyll, water soluble
DeWitt's pills
Indigo blue
Indigo carmine
Indomethacin
Methocarbamol
Methylene blue
Nitrofurans
Phenols
Resorcinol
Suprofen

Green-Yellow
DeWitt's pills
Methylene blue

Milky
Phosphates

Orange
Chlorzoxazone
Dihydroergotamine mesylate
Heparin sodium
Phenazopyridine
Phenindione
Rifampin
Sulfasalazine
Warfarin

Orange-Red
Chlorzoxazone
Doxidan
Phenazopyridine
Rifampin

Orange-Yellow
Fluorescein sodium
Rifampin
Sulfasalazine

Pink
Aminopyrine
Anthraquinone dyes
Cascara
Danthron
Deferoxamine
Merbromin
Methyldopa

Phenolphthalein
Phenothiazines
Phensuximide
Phenytoin
Salicylates
Senna

Purple
Phenophthalein

Red
Anthraquinone
Cascara
Daunorubicin
Deferoxamine
Dihydroergotamine mesylate
Dimethylsulfoxide
DMSO
Doxorubicin
Heparin
Ibuprofen
Methyldopa
Oxyphenbutazone
Phenacetin
Phenazopyridine
Phenolphthalein
Phenothiazines
Phensuximide
Phenylbutazone
Phenytoin
Rifampin
Senna

Red-Brown
Cascara
Deferoxamine
Methyldopa
Oxyphenbutazone
Phenacetin
Phenolphthalein
Phenothiazines
Phenylbutazone
Phenytoin
Quinine
Senna

Red-Purple
Chlorzoxazone
Ibuprofen
Phenacetin
Senna

Rust
Cascara
Chloroquine
Metronidazole
Nitrofurantoin
Phenacetin
Riboflavin
Senna
Sulfonamides

Yellow
Bismuth
Nitrofurantoin

Phenacetin
Riboflavin
Sulfasalazine

Yellow-Brown
Bismuth
Cascara
Chloroquine

DeWitt's pills
Methylene blue
Metronidazole
Nitrofurantoin
Primaquine
Quinacrine

Senna
Sulfonamides

Yellow-Pink
Cascara
Senna

Reference
Adapted from Drugdex® — Drug Consults, Micromedex, vol 62, Rocky Mountain Drug Consultation Center, Denver, CO: January, 1995.

HEMATOLOGIC ADVERSE EFFECTS

Hematologic Adverse Effects of Drugs

Drug	Red Cell Aplasia	Thrombo-cytopenia	Neutrope-nia	Pancyto-penia	Hemoly-sis
Acetazolamide		+	+	+	
Allopurinol			+		
Amiodarone	+				
Amphotericin B				+	
Amrinone		++			
Asparaginase		+++	+++	+++	++
Barbiturates		+		+	
Benzocaine					++
Captopril			++		+
Carbamazepine		++	+		
Cephalosporins			+		++
Chloramphenicol		+	++	+++	
Chlordiazepoxide			+	+	
Chloroquine		+			
Chlorothiazides		++			
Chlorpropamide	+	++	+	++	+
Chlortetracycline				+	
Chlorthalidone			+		
Cimetidine		+	++	+	
Codeine		+			
Colchicine				+	
Cyclophospha-mide		+++	+++	+++	+
Dapsone					+++
Desipramine		++			
Digitalis		+			
Digitoxin		++			
Erythromycin		+			
Estrogen		+		+	
Ethacrynic acid			+		
Fluorouracil		+++	+++	+++	+
Furosemide		+	+		
Gold salts	+	+++	+++	+++	
Heparin		++		+	
Ibuprofen			+		+
Imipramine			++	.	
Indomethacin		+	++	+	
Isoniazid		+		+	
Isosorbide dini-trate					+
Levodopa					++
Meperidine		+			
Meprobamate		+	+	+	
Methimazole			++		
Methyldopa		++			+++
Methotrexate		+++	+++	+++	++
Methylene blue					+
Metronidazole			+		
Nalidixic acid					+
Naproxen				+	
Nitrofurantoin			++		+
Nitroglycerine		+			
Penicillamine		++	+		

Hematologic Adverse Effects of Drugs (continued)

Drug	Red Cell Aplasia	Thrombo-cytopenia	Neutrope-nia	Pancyto-penia	Hemoly-sis
Penicillins		+	++	+	+++
Phenazopyridine					+++
Phenothiazines		+	++	+++	+
Phenylbutazone		+	++	+++	+
Phenytoin		++	++	++	+
Potassium iodide		+			
Prednisone		+			
Primaquine					+++
Procainamide			+		
Procarbazine		+	++	++	+
Propylthiouracil		+	++	+	+
Quinidine		+++	+		
Quinine		+++	+		
Reserpine		+			
Rifampicin		++	+		+++
Spironolactone			+		
Streptomycin		+		+	
Sulfamethoxazole with trimethoprim			+		
Sulfonamides	+	++	++	++	++
Sulindac	+	+	+	+	
Tetracyclines		+			+
Thioridazine			++		
Tolbutamide		++	+	++	
Triamterene					+
Valproate	+				
Vancomycin			+		

+ = rare or single reports.

++ = occasional reports.

+++ = substantial number of reports.

Adapted from D'Arcy PF and Griffin JP, eds, *Iatrogenic Diseases*, New York, NY: Oxford University Press, 1986, 128-30.

HEMODIALYSIS OF DRUGS

Dialyzable (50%-100%)

Acyclovir (Zovirax®)
Amdinocillin (Mecillinam®)
Amikacin (Amikin®)
Aspirin
Cefsulodin
Ceftazidime (Fortaz®)
Chloral hydrate (Noctec®)
Clavulanic acid
Ethanol
Fluconazole (Diflucan®)
Flucytosine (Ancobon®)

Gentamicin (Garamycin®)
Isoniazid (INH)
Kanamycin (Kantrex®)
Lithium (Lithobid®)
Methanol
Metronidazole (Flagyl®)
Minoxidil (Loniten®)
Neomycin
Netilmicin (Netromycin®)
Tobramycin (Nebcin®)

Moderately Dialyzable (20%-50%)

Acetaminophen (Tylenol®)
Acetazolamide (Diamox®)
Amoxicillin (Amoxil®)
Ampicillin (Omnipen®)
Atenolol (Tenormin®)
Azlocillin (Azlin®)
Aztreonam (Azactam®)
Bretylium (Bretylol®)
Captopril (Capoten®)
Carbenicillin (Geocillin®)
Cefaclor (Ceclor®)
Cefamandole (Mandol®)
Cefazolin (Kefzol®)
Ceforanide (Precef®)
Cefotaxime (Claforan®)
Cefoxitin (Mefoxin®)
Ceftizoxime (Cefizox®)
Cephalexin (Keflex®)
Cephalothin (Keflin®)

Cilastatin
Cyclophosphamide (Cytoxan®)
Enalapril (Vasotec®)
Ethosuximide (Zarontin®)
Fluconazole (Diflucan®)
Imipenem (Primaxin®)
Meprobamate (Equanil®)
Mezlocillin (Mezlin®)
Nadolol (Corgard®)
Penicillin G
Phenobarbital
Piperacillin (Pipracil®)
Primidone (Mysoline®)
Procainamide (Pronestyl®)
Sulfamethoxazole
Ticarcillin (Ticar®)
Tocainide (Tonocard®)
Trimethoprim (Trimpex®)

Slightly Dialyzable (5%-20%)

Amantadine (Symmetrel®)
Azathioprine (Imuran®)
Cefonicid (Monocid®)
Cefoperazone (Cefobid®)
Cefotetan (Cefotan®)
Chloramphenicol (Chloromycetin®)
Cimetidine (Tagamet®)
Erythromycin (E-Mycin®)
Ethambutol (Myambutol®)

Methaqualone (Quaalude®)
Methyldopa (Aldomet®)
Methylprednisolone (Solu-Medrol®)
Pentobarbital (Nembutal®)
Quinidine
Ranitidine (Zantac®)
Secobarbital (Seconal™)
Tetracycline (Achromycin®)

Not Dialyzable (0%-5%)

Ceftriaxone (Rocephin®)
Chlordiazepoxide (Librium®)
Clindamycin (Cleocin®)
Clonidine (Catapres®)
Cloxacillin (Tegopen®)
Colchicine
Diazepam (Valium®)
Dicloxacillin (Dynapen®)
Digitoxin
Digoxin (Lanoxin®)
Disopyramide (Norpace®)
Doxycycline (Vibramycin®)
Flecainide (Tambocor®)
Flurazepam (Dalmane®)
Itraconazole (Sporanox®)
Ketoconazole (Nizoral®)
Lidocaine (Xylocaine®)

Mebendazole (Vermox®)
Methicillin (Staphcillin®)
Methotrexate (Mexate®)
Metoclopramide (Reglan®)
Miconazole (Monistat®)
Minocycline (Minocin®)
Nafcillin (Unipen®)
Oxacillin (Prostaphlin®)
Oxazepam (Serax®)
Phenothiazines
Propoxyphene (Darvon®)
Propranolol (Inderal®)
Tolbutamide (Orinase®)
Valproate (Depakene®)
Vancomycin (Vancocin®)
Verapamil (Isoptin®)
Zidovudine (Retrovir®)

PRESSURE ULCER TREATMENT

Specific Treatment Options by Category	Description by Category	Advantages by Category	Disadvantages by Category
Surgical Debridement	Surgical excision of eschar by physician; may require concomitant treatment with systemic antimicrobials.	Repaid removal of necrotic tissue. Large wounds may be partially debrided reducing risk to resident.	May require hospitalization for procedure. Caution must be used with those who are immunosuppressed, debilitated, or have bleeding disorders. May leave some necrotic debris in place.
Autolytic Debriders Absorption Dressings Hydrocolloid Dressings Transparent Dressings	Use of occlusive dressings or dressings which impart moisture to soften and liquefy necrotic tissue.	Selective form of debridement (does not harm healing tissue). Effective alternative for debridement of small wounds. Readily available.	May lead to infection in large necrotic wounds. Not indicated for clinically infected wounds due to increased bacterial growth beneath dressing.
Enzymatic Debriders Accuzyme® Biozyme-C® Elase® Elase-Chloromycetin® Granulderm® Granulex Panafil® Panafil® White Santyl® Travase®	Enzyme topically applied to necrotic surface; usually covered with wet gauze and/or transparent dressing; applying a protectant (ie, moisture barrier cream) to surrounding tissue may be indicated; often requires concomitant treatment with topical or systemic antimicrobials; discontinue when wound is red and granulating or if it bleeds easily when cleansed.	Less traumatic than surgical debriding. Ease of application. Cost-effective debridement therapy.	Cross-hatching recommended if thick eschar is present. Some detergents and antiseptics may inactivate certain products. Effect on viable tissue varies by product. Takes longer than surgical debridement. May need barrier cream around wound to protect healthy skin. Requires secondary dressing.
Mechanical Debriders Wet-to-Dry Gauze Dressings Hydrotherapy	Removal of eschar using mechanical forces that pull off necrotic tissue; discontinue when wound is red and granulating or if it bleeds easily when cleansed.	Promotes softening and loosening of eschar. Potentially less traumatic than surgical debridement. Economical. Readily available.	Generally not as effective in severely necrotic wounds. Must monitor for signs of injury to healthy tissue.

PRESSURE ULCER TREATMENT (Continued)

Specific Treatment Options by Category	Description by Category	Advantages by Category	Disadvantages by Category
Cleansing Solutions Acetic Acid Cara-Klenz® Curasol® Dakins Hydrogen Peroxide Normal Saline Shur-Clens® Lactated Ringers	Cleansing solution that also hydrates; some products are bactericidal.	Cleanses wound. Maintains moist environment.	Can disturb granulation tissue. Can be cytotoxic if not diluted or used too vigorously.
Topical Antibiotics Silvadene® Betadine® Ointment Neosporin® Gentamicin	Antimicrobial solutions, ointments and creams; indicated for prophylaxis or for treatment of an infected wound.	Easy to apply. Water miscible creams easy to remove. Helps control bacterial growth until necrotic tissue can be debrided.	May have cytotoxic effects which may delay wound healing. Ointments are difficult to remove. Allergic reactions may occur. Bacteria may become resistant with prolonged use.
Absorption Dressings Bard® Comfeel® Envisan® Debrisan® DuoDERM® Hydragran® Intrasite® Iodoflex® Iodosorb® Kalostat® Sorbsan®	Includes granules, flakes, paste, and pads; placed directly into wound bed to absorb exudate; provides minor debriding action by retaining wound debris.	Absorbs wound exudate while maintaining wound moisture. Cleanses wound bed. Reduces wound odor.	Some dressings require irrigation to remove from wound. May increase time for dressing changes. May impair granulation and epithelialization by drying wound bed, if exudate is minimal. Permeable to fluids and bacteria. Contraindicated with tunneling. May sting upon application. Requires secondary dressing.
Gauze Dressings	Fine mesh gauze dressing used as vehicle for soaks, lubricants, or antimicrobials.	Economical. Readily available. Effective delivery of solution if kept moist. Cost-effective filler for large wounds.	May cause bleeding, pain, and remove healthy granulation tissue if allowed to dry. Requires increased nursing time to keep dressing moist.
Hydrocolloid Dressings DuoDERM® Restore® Comfeel® Tegasorb® Intact® Ultec®	Dressing that reacts with exudate to form a gel; creates a physical barrier and maintains a moist/acidic environment.	Totally occlusive; protects wound from physical injury and contamination. Maintains moist environment. Easy removal without adhesion to wound surface. May remain on wound for up to 5 days. Waterproof dressing allows resident to shower.	Difficult to observe wound. May promote development of infection in deep wounds. May accumulate excess fluid and macerate tissue. Dressing may soften, and wrinkles may increase pressure on wound base.
Nonadherent Dressings Telfa® Exu-Dry® Vaseline® Gauze Adaptic®	Nonocclusive, absorbent dressing; may be used with topical medications.	Easy to use. Inexpensive. Nontraumatic.	Nonocclusive. Does not physically protect wound site from injury. Less absorptive than plain gauze. Need secondary dressing.

Specific Treatment Options by Category	Description by Category	Advantages by Category	Disadvantages by Category
Transparent Dressings Op-Site® Tegaderm® Bioclusive® Acu-Derm® Blisterfilm® Uniflex®	Adhesive, transparent, thin film-type semipermeable dressing; semipermeable membrane allows moisture and oxygen exchange.	A barrier to contamination that also keeps wound moist. Allows for easy visual inspection. Good adhesive properties. Waterproof dressing allows resident to shower.Reduces pain. Time saving.	May lead to tissue maceration in extremely moist wounds. Some products are difficult to apply, and wrinkling may occur. May promote infection if necrotic tissue is present. Potential for adhesive injury. Expensive.
Hydrogels Carrington® Wound Gel Vigilon® Intrasite® Gel Elastogel®	Topicals with absorptive and moisturizing properties.	Nonadherent. May cool and/or soothe wound. Easy to apply. Comforms to wound bed.	Usually requires protective outer dressing. May require multiple daily dressing changes. May macerate surrounding tissue.

SERUM DRUG CONCENTRATIONS COMMONLY MONITORED: GUIDELINES

Drug	When to Sample	Therapeutic Concentration*	Usual Half-Life	Steady State (Ideal Sampling Time)	Potentially Toxic Concentration*
Antibiotics					
Gentamicin Tobramycin	30 min after 30 min infusion Trough: <0.5 h before next dose	Peak: 4-10 mcg/mL Trough: <2.0 mcg/mL	2 h	15 h	Peak: >12 mcg/mL Trough: >2 mcg/mL
Amikacin		Peak: 20-35 mcg/mL Trough: <8 mcg/mL	2 h	15 h	Peak: >35 mcg/mL Trough: >8 mcg/mL
Vancomycin	Peak: 1 h after 1 h infusion Trough: <0.5 h before next dose	Peak: 30-40 mcg/mL Trough: 5-10 mcg/mL	6-8 h	24 h	Peak: >80 mcg/mL Trough: >13 mcg/mL
Anticonvulsants					
Carbamazepine	Trough: Just before oral dose In combination with other anticonvulsants	4-12 mcg/mL 4-8 mcg/mL	15-20 h	7-12 d	>12 mcg/mL
Ethosuximide	Trough: Just before next oral dose	40-100 mcg/mL	30-60 h	10-13 d	>100 mcg/mL
Gabapentin					
Phenobarbital	Trough: Just before next dose	15-40 mcg/mL	40-120 h	20 d	>40 mcg/mL
Phenytoin Free phenytoin	Trough: Just before next dose Draw at same time as total level	10-20 mcg/mL 1-2 mcg/mL	Concentration dependent	5-14 d	>20 mcg/mL
Primidone	Trough: Just before next dose (**Note:** Primidone is metabolized to phenobarb, order levels separately)	5-12 mcg/mL	10-12 h	5 d	>12 mcg/mL
Valproic acid	Trough: Just before next dose	50-100 mcg/mL	5-20 h	4 d	>150 mcg/mL
Bronchodilators					
Aminophylline (I.V.)	18-24 h after starting or changing a maintenance dose given as a constant infusion	10-20 mcg/mL	Nonsmoking adult: 8 h Smoking adults: 4 h	2 d	>20 mcg/mL
Theophylline (P.O.)	Peak: Not recommended Trough: Just before next dose	10-20 mcg/mL	4-8 h	2 d	>20 mcg/mL
Cardiovascular Agents					
Digitoxin	Peak: Not necessary Trough: Prior to dose	20-35 ng/mL	7-8 days	5 wk	>45 ng/mL

(continued)

Drug	When to Sample	Therapeutic Concentration*	Usual Half-Life	Steady State (Ideal Sampling Time)	Potentially Toxic Concentration*
Digoxin	Trough: Just before next dose (levels drawn earlier than 6 h after a dose will be artificially elevated)	0.5–2 ng/mL	36 h	5 d	>2 ng/mL
Lidocaine	Steady-state levels are usually achieved after 6–12 h	1.2–5.0 mcg/mL	1.5 h	5–10 h	>6 mcg/mL
Procainamide	Trough: Just before next oral dose I.V.: 6–12 h after infusion started Combined procainamide plus NAPA	4–10 mcg/mL NAPA: 6–10 h 5–30 mcg/mL	Procain: 2.7–5 h >30 (NAPA + procain)	20 h	>10 mcg/mL
Quinidine	Trough: Just before next oral dose	2–5 mcg/mL	6 h	24 h	>10 mcg/mL
Other Agents					
Amitriptyline plus nortriptyline	Trough: Just before next dose	120–250 ng/mL	Amitriptyline: 9–25 h Nortriptyline: 28–31 h	4–8 d	>500 mcg/mL
Cyclosporine	Trough: Just before next dose or 12–18 h after oral dose	Months post-transplant: Plasma: 50–150 ng/mL Whole blood: 150–450 ng/mL	17–40 h	Variable 5 half-lives	>400 ng/mL
Desipramine	Trough: Just before next dose	125–160 ng/mL	12–54 h	3–11 d	>300 ng/mL
Imipramine plus desipramine	Trough: Just before next dose	150–300 ng/mL	9–24 h	2–5 d	
Lithium	12 hours after dose	0.6–1.2 mEq/mL (acute)	18–20 h	2–7 d	>3 mEq/mL
Nortriptyline	Trough: Just before next dose	50–140 ng/mL	28–31 h	4–19 d	>500 ng/mL
Trazadone	Trough: 30 min prior to next dose	0.5–2.5 mcg/mL	4–7.5 h	2 d	ND

*Due to methodology differences, reference ranges may vary from laboratory to laboratory; check with the laboratory service used for their appropriate levels.

SODIUM CONTENT OF SELECTED MEDICINALS

Name and Dosage Unit*	Sodium mg	mEq
Antibiotics		
Amikacin sulfate, 1 g	29.9	1.3
Aminosalicylate sodium, 1 g	109	4.7
Ampicillin, suspension 250 mg/5 mL, 5 mL	10	0.4
Ampicillin sodium, 1 g	66.7	3
Azlocillin sodium, 1 g	50	2.2
Carbenicillin indanyl sodium 382 mg (tablet)	22	1
Cefazolin sodium, 1 g	47	2
Cefotaxime sodium, 1 g	30.5	2.2
Cefoxitin sodium, 1 g	53	2.3
Ceftazidine, 1g	54	2.3
Ceftriaxone sodium, 1 g	83	3.6
Cefuroxime, 1 g	54.2	2.4
Chloramphenicol sodium succinate, 1 g	51.8	2.3
Dicloxacillin, 250 mg (capsule)	13	0.6
Dicloxacillin, suspension 65 mg/5 mL	27	1.2
Erythromycin ethyl succinate, susp 200 mg/5 mL	29	1.3
Erythromycin Base Filmtab®, 250 mg	70	3
Methicillin sodium, 1 g	66.7	2.9
Metronidazole, 500 mg I.V.	322	14
Mezlocillin sodium, 1 g	42.6	1.9
Nafcillin sodium, 1 g	66.7	2.9
Nitrofurantoin, suspension 25 mg/5 mL	7	0.3
Penicillin G potassium, 1,000,000 units I.V.	7.6	0.3
Penicillin G sodium, 1,000,000 units I.V.	46	2
Penicillin V potassium, suspension, 250 mg/5 mL	38	1.7
Piperacillin sodium, 1 g	42.6	1.8
Ticarcillin disodium, 1 g	119.6	5.2
Ticarcillin disodium/clavulanic acid, 1 g	109	4.75
Antacids, Liquid (content per 5 mL)		
Amphojel®	<2.3	<0.1
ALternaGEL®	2	0.1
Basaljel®	2.4	0.1
Extra Strength Maalox®-Plus	0.65	≅0.05
Gaviscon®	13	0.57
Maalox®	1.3	0.06
Tums E-X™	<4.8	<0.2
Sodium Content of Miscellaneous Medicinals		
Acetazolamide sodium, 500 mg	47.2	2.05
Chlorothiazide sodium, 500 mg	57.5	2
Cisplatin, 10 mg	35.4	1.54
Edetate calcium disodium, 1 g	122	5.3
Fleet® Enema, 4.5 oz	5000†	218
Fleet® Phospho®-Soda, 20 mL	2217	96.4
Hydrocortisone sodium succinate, 1 g	47.5	2.07
Hypaque® M 75%, injection, 20 mL	200	8.7
Hypaque® M 90%, injection, 20 mL	220	9.6
Metamucil® Instant Mix (orange)	6	0.27
Methotrexate sodium, 100 mg vial	20	0.86
Methotrexate sodium, 100 mg vial (low sodium)	15	0.65
Naproxen sodium, 250 mg (tablet)	23	1

Name and Dosage Unit*	Sodium	
	mg	mEq
Neutra-Phos®, capsule and 75 mL reconstituted solution	164	7.13
Oragrafin® (capsule)	19	0.8
Pentobarbital sodium, 50 mg/mL, 1 mL vial	5	0.2
Phenobarbital sodium, 65 mg, 1 mL vial	6	0.3
Phenytoin sodium, 1 g	88	3.8
Promethazine expectorant, 5 mL	53	2.3
Shohl's solution modified, 1 mL	23	1
Sodium ascorbate, 500 mg acid equivalent	65.3	2.84
Sodium bicarbonate, 50 mL 8.4%	1150	50
Sodium nitroprusside, 50 mg	7.8	0.34
Sodium polystyrene sulfonate, 1 g	94.3‡	4.1
Thiopental sodium, 1 g	86.8	3.8
Valproate sodium, 250 mg/5 mL, 5 mL	23	1

*Product formulations and hence sodium content are subject to change by the manufacturer.

†Average systemic absorption 250-300 mg.

‡Total sodium content. Only about 33% is liberated in clinical use.

TABLETS THAT CANNOT BE CRUSHED OR ALTERED

There are a variety of reasons for crushing tablets or capsule contents prior to administering to the patient. Patients may have nasogastric tubes which do not permit the administration of tablets or capsules; an oral solution for a particular medication may not be available from the manufacturer or readily prepared by pharmacy; patients may have difficulty swallowing capsules or tablets; or mixing of powdered medication with food or drink may make the drug more palatable.

Generally, medications which should not be crushed fall into one of the following categories.

- **Extended-Release Products.** The formulation of some tablets is specialized as to allow the medication within it to be slowly released into the body. This is sometimes accomplished by centering the drug within the core of the tablet, with a subsequent shedding of multiple layers around the core. Wax melts in the GI tract. Slow-K® is an example of this. Capsules may contain beads which have multiple layers which are slowly dissolved with time.

- **Medications Which Are Irritating to the Stomach.** Tablets which are irritating to the stomach may be enteric-coated which delays release of the drug until the time when it reaches the small intestine. Enteric-coated aspirin is an example of this.

- **Foul Tasting Medication.** Some drugs are quite unpleasant to taste so the manufacturer coats the tablet in a sugar coating to increase its palatability. By crushing the tablet, this sugar coating is lost and the patient tastes the unpleasant tasting medication.

- **Sublingual Medication.** Medication intended for use under the tongue should not be crushed. While it appears to be obvious, it is not always easy to determine if a medication is to be used sublingually. Sublingual medications should indicate on the package that they are intended for sublingual use.

- **Effervescent Tablets.** These are tablets which, when dropped into a liquid, quickly dissolve to yield a solution. Many effervescent tablets, when crushed, lose their ability to quickly dissolve.

Recommendations

1. It is not advisable to crush certain medications.

2. Consult individual monographs prior to crushing capsule or tablet.

3. If crushing a tablet or capsule is contraindicated, consult with your pharmacist to determine whether an oral solution exists or can be compounded.

Drug Product	Dosage Forms	Reasons/Comments
Accutane®	Capsule	Mucous membrane irritant
Acutrim®	Tablet	Slow release
Adalat® CC	Tablet	Slow release
Aerolate® SR, JR, III	Capsule	Slow release*†
Afrinol® Repetabs®	Tablet	Slow release
Anaplex SR	Capsule	Slow release
Ansaid®	Tablet	Taste††
Allerest® 12-Hour	Caplet	Slow release
Artane® Sequels®	Capsule	Slow release*†
Arthritis Bayer Time Release	Capsule	Slow release
Asacol®	Tablet	Slow release
ASA Enseals®	Tablet	Enteric-coated
Asbron G® Inlay	Tablet	Multiple compressed tablet†
Aspirin Delayed-Release	Tablet	Enteric-coated
Atrohist Plus	Tablet	Slow release*
Atrohist Sprinkle	Capsule	Slow release
Azulfidine® EN-tabs®	Tablet	Enteric-coated
Baros	Tablet	Effervescent tablet¶

Drug Product	Dosage Forms	Reasons/Comments
Betachron E-R	Capsule	Slow release
Betapen®-VK	Tablet	Taste††
Biphetamine	Capsule	Slow release
Bisacodyl	Tablet	Enteric-coated‡
Bisco-Lax®	Tablet	Enteric-coated‡
Bontril SR	Capsule	Slow release
Breonesin§	Capsule	Liquid filled§
Brexin® LA	Capsule	Slow release
Bromfed®	Capsule	Slow release†
Bromfed-PD®	Capsule	Slow release†
Calan® SR	Tablet	Slow release♦
Cama Arthritis Pain Reliever	Tablet	Multiple compressed tablet
Carbiset-TR®	Tablet	Slow release
Cardizem®	Tablet	Slow release
Cardizem® CD	Capsule	Slow release*
Cardizem® SR	Capsule	Slow release*
Carter's Little Pills®	Tablet	Enteric-coated
Cefal Filmtab®	Tablet	Enteric-coated
Charcoal Plus	Tablet	Enteric-coated
Chloral Hydrate	Capsule	**Note:** Product is in liquid form within a special capsule†
Chlorphedrine SR	Capsule	Slow release
Chlorpheniramine Maleate Time Release	Capsule	Slow release
Chlor-Trimeton® 12-Hour Allergy	Tablet	Slow release†
Choledyl® SA	Tablet	Slow release†
Chromagen®	Capsule	Taste††
Cipro™	Tablet	Taste††
Cleocin®	Capsule	Taste†††
Codimal-LA®	Capsule	Slow release
Codimal-LA® Half	Capsule	Slow release
Colace®	Capsule	Taste††
Comhist® LA	Capsule	Slow release*
Compazine® Spansule®	Capsule	Slow release†
Congess SR, JR	Capsule	Slow release
Contac®	Capsule	Slow release*
Cotazym-S®	Capsule	Enteric-coated*
Creon®	Capsule	Enteric-coated*
Creon® 10 Minimicrospheres	Capsule	Enteric-coated*
Creon® 25	Capsule	Enteric-coated*
Dallergy®	Capsule	Slow release†
Dallergy-D®	Capsule	Slow release
Dallergy-JR®	Capsule	Slow release
Deconamine® SR	Capsule	Slow release†
Deconsal® II	Tablet	Slow release
Deconsal® Sprinkle	Capsule	Slow release*
Demazin® Repetabs®	Tablet	Slow release†
Depakene®	Capsule	Slow-release-mucous membrane irritant†
Depakote®	Capsule	Enteric-coated
Desoxyn® Gradumets®	Tablet	Slow release
Desyrel®	Tablet	Taste††
Dexatrim® Max Strength	Tablet	Slow release
Dexedrine® Spansule®	Capsule	Slow release
Diamox® Sequels®	Capsule	Slow release
Dilacor™ XR	Capsule	Slow release

TABLETS THAT CANNOT BE CRUSHED OR ALTERED
(Continued)

Drug Product	Dosage Forms	Reasons/Comments
Dilatrate SR	Capsule	Slow release
Dimetane® Extentab®	Tablet	Slow release†
Disobrom®	Tablet	Slow release
Disophrol® Chronotab®	Tablet	Slow release
Dital	Capsule	Slow release
Docusate	Capsule	Liquid filled§
Docusate with Casanthranol	Capsule	Liquid filled§
Donnatal® Extentab®	Tablet	Slow release†
Donnazyme	Tablet	Enteric-coated
Doxidan® liquigels	Capsule	Liquid filled§
Drisdol®	Capsule	Liquid filled§
Drixoral®	Tablet	Slow release†
Drixoral® Sinus	Tablet	Slow release
Dulcolax®	Tablet	Enteric-coated‡
Dura-Vent®	Tablet	Slow release
Dura-Vent®/A	Capsule	Slow release
Dura-Vent®/DA	Tablet	Slow release
Dura-Tap/PD®	Capsule	Slow release
Duratuss	Tablet	Slow release♦
Easprin®	Tablet	Enteric-coated
Ecotrin®	Tablet	Enteric-coated
E.E.S.® 400	Tablet	Enteric-coated†
Efidac/24®	Tablet	Slow release
Elixophyllin® SR	Capsule	Slow release*†
E-Mycin®	Tablet	Enteric-coated
Endafed®	Capsule	Slow release
Entex® LA	Tablet	Slow release†
Entex® PSE	Tablet	Slow release†
Entozyme	Tablet	Enteric-coated
Equanil®	Tablet	Taste††
Ergostat®	Tablet	Sublingual form•
Eryc®	Capsule	Enteric-coated*
Ery-Tab®	Tablet	Enteric-coated
Erythrocin® Stearate	Tablet	Enteric-coated
Erythromycin Base	Tablet	Enteric-coated
Eskalith® CR	Tablet	Slow release
Fedahist® Timecaps®	Capsule	Slow release†
Feldene®	Capsule	Mucous membrane irritant
Fenesin™	Tablet	Slow release
Feocyte	Tablet	Slow release
Feosol®	Tablet	Enteric-coated†
Feosol® Spansule®	Capsule	Slow release*†
Ferrous Gluconate	Tablet	Film-coated
Feratab®	Tablet	Enteric-coated†
Fergon®	Tablet	May cause excessive GI upset
Fero-Grad 500® mg	Tablet	Slow release
Fero-Gradumet®	Tablet	Slow release
Ferralet® SR	Tablet	Slow release
Feverall™ Sprinkle Caps	Capsule	Taste* **Note:** Capsule contents intended to be placed in a teaspoonful of water or soft food.
Fumatinic	Capsule	Slow release

Drug Product	Dosage Forms	Reasons/Comments
Gastrocrom®	Capsule	**Note:** Contents should be dissolved in water for administration.
Geocillin®	Tablet	Taste
Gris-PEG®	Tablet	**Note:** Crushing may result in precipitation as larger particles.
Guaifed	Capsule	Slow release
Guaifed-PD	Capsule	Slow release
Guaimax-D	Tablet	Slow release
Halfprin	Tablet	Enteric coated
Humabid® DM	Tablet	Slow release
Humabid® DM Sprinkle	Capsule	Slow release*
Humabid® LA	Tablet	Slow release
Humabid® Sprinkle	Capsule	Slow release*
Hydergine® LC	Capsule	**Note:** Product is in liquid form within a special capsulet†
Hydergine® Sublingual	Tablet	Sublingual route†
Hytakerol®	Capsule	Liquid filled§†
Iberet®	Tablet	Slow release†
Iberet-500®	Tablet	Slow release†
Ilotycin®	Tablet	Enteric-coated
Imdur™	Tablet	Slow release♦
Inderal® LA	Capsule	Slow release
Inderide® LA	Capsule	Slow release
Indocin® SR	Capsule	Slow release*†
Ionamin®	Capsule	Slow release
Isoclor® Timesule®	Capsule	Slow release
Isoptin® SR	Tablet	Slow release
Isordil® Sublingual	Tablet	Sublingual form•
Isordil® Tembid®	Tablet	Slow release
Isosorbide Dinitrate Sublingual	Tablet	Sublingual form•
Isosorbide Dinitrate SR	Tablet	Slow release
Isuprel® Glossets®	Tablet	Sublingual form•
K+® 8	Tablet	Slow release†
K+® 10	Tablet	Slow release†
Kaon-Cl® 6.7 mEq	Tablet	Slow release†
Kaon-Cl® 10	Tablet	Slow release†
K + Care®	Tablet	Effervescent tablet†¶
K-Dur®	Tablet	Slow release♦
Klor-Con®	Tablet	Slow release†
Klor-Con®/EF	Tablet	Effervescent tablet†¶
Klorvess®	Tablet	Effervescent tablet†¶
Klotrix®	Tablet	Slow release†
K-Lyte®	Tablet	Effervescent tablet¶
K-Lyte/Cl®	Tablet	Effervescent tablet¶
K-Tab®	Tablet	Slow release†
Levsinex® Timecaps®	Capsule	Slow release
Macrobid®	Capsule	Slow release
Meprospan®	Capsule	Slow release*
Mestinon® Timespan®	Tablet	Slow release†
MI-Cebrin	Tablet	Enteric-coated
MI-Cebrin T	Tablet	Enteric-coated
Micro-K®	Capsule	Slow release*†
Motrin®	Tablet	Taste††
Motrin® IB	Tablet	Taste†††
Motrin® IB-sinus	Tablet	Taste†††

TABLETS THAT CANNOT BE CRUSHED OR ALTERED
(Continued)

Drug Product	Dosage Forms	Reasons/Comments
MS Contin®	Tablet	Slow release†
MSC Triaminic®	Tablet	Enteric-coated
Naldecon®	Tablet	Slow release†
Nasabid™	Capsule	Slow release
Nasatab LA	Tablet	Slow release
Nico 400	Capsule	Slow release
Nicobid®	Capsule	Slow release
Nitro-Bid®	Capsule	Slow release*
Nitrocine® Timecaps®	Capsule	Slow release
Nitroglyn®	Capsule	Slow release*
Nitrong®	Tablet	Slow release
Nitrostat®	Tablet	Sublingual route•
Nolamine®	Tablet	Slow release
Nolex® LA	Tablet	Slow release
Norflex®	Tablet	Slow release
Norpace® CR	Capsule	Slow release form within a special capsule
Novafed®	Capsule	Slow release
Novafed® A	Capsule	Slow release
Optilets-500® Filmtab®	Tablet	Enteric-coated
Optilets-M-500® Filmtab®	Tablet	Enteric-coated
Oragrafin®	Capsule	**Note:** Product is in liquid form within a special capsule
Ordrine® SR	Capsule	Slow release
Oramorph SR™	Tablet	Slow release†
Ornade® Spansule®	Capsule	Slow release
Oruvail®	Capsule	Slow release
Pabalate	Tablet	Enteric-coated
Pabalate SF	Tablet	Enteric-coated
Pancrease®	Capsule	Enteric-coated*
Pancrease® MT	Capsule	Enteric-coated*
Panmycin®	Capsule	Taste
Papaverine Sustained Action	Capsule	Slow release
Pathilon® Sequels®	Capsule	Slow release*
Pavabid® Plateau	Capsule	Slow release*
PBZ-SR®	Tablet	Slow release†
Pentasa®	Capsule	Slow release
Perdiem®	Granules	Wax coated
Peritrate® SA	Tablet	Slow release♦
Permitil® Chronotab®	Tablet	Slow release†
Phazyme®	Tablet	Slow release
Phazyme® 95	Tablet	Slow release
Phenergan®	Tablet	Taste†††
Phyllocontin®	Tablet	Slow release
Plendil®	Tablet	Slow release
Pneumonist®	Tablet	Slow release†
Polaramine® Repetabs®	Tablet	Slow release†
Prelu-2®	Capsule	Slow release
Prilosec™	Capsule	Slow release
Pro-Banthine®	Tablet	Taste
Procainamide HCl SR	Tablet	Slow release
Procan® SR	Tablet	Slow release
Procardia®	Capsule	Delays absorption§#
Procardia XL®	Tablet	Slow release **Note:** AUC is unaffected.

Drug Product	Dosage Forms	Reasons/Comments
Pronestyl-SR®	Tablet	Slow release
Proventil® Repetabs®	Tablet	Slow release†
Prozac®	Capsule	Slow release*
Quadra-Hist®	Tablet	Slow release
Quibron®-T SR	Tablet	Slow release†
Quinaglute® Dura-Tabs®	Tablet	Slow release
Quinalan® Lanatabs®	Tablet	Slow release
Quinalan® SR	Tablet	Slow release
Quinidex® Extentabs®	Tablet	Slow release
Respaire® SR	Capsule	Slow release
Respid®	Tablet	Slow release
Ritalin-SR®	Tablet	Slow release
Robimycin® Robitab®	Tablet	Enteric-coated
Rondec-TR®	Tablet	Slow release†
Roxanol SR™	Tablet	Slow release†
Ru-Tuss®	Tablet	Slow release
Ru-Tuss® DE	Tablet	Slow release
Seldane-D®	Tablet	Slow release
Sinemet® CR	Tablet	Slow release♦
Singlet®	Tablet	Slow release
Slo-bid™ Gyrocaps®	Capsule	Slow release*
Slo-Niacin®	Tablet	Slow release
Slo-Phyllin GG®	Capsule	Slow release†
Slo-Phyllin® Gyrocaps®	Capsule	Slow release*†
Slow FE®	Tablet	Slow release†
Slow-K®	Tablet	Slow release†
Slow-Mag®	Tablet	Slow release
Sorbitrate® SA	Tablet	Slow release
Sorbitrate® Sublingual	Tablet	Sublingual route
Sparine®	Tablet	Taste††
S-P-T	Capsule	**Note:** Liquid gelatin thyroid suspension.
Stamoist E	Tablet	Slow release
Stamoist LA	Tablet	Slow release
Sudafed® 12-Hour	Caplet	Slow release†
Surfak® Liquigels	Capsule	Liquid filled§
Tavist-D®	Tablet	Multiple compressed tablet
Teldrin®	Capsule	Slow release*
Temaril® Spansule®	Capsule	Slow release†
Tepanil® Tentab®	Tablet	Slow release
Tessalon® Perles	Capsule	Slow release
Theo-24®	Tablet	Slow release†
Theobid®	Capsule	Slow release*†
Theobid® Jr	Capsule	Slow release*†
Theoclear® L.A	Capsule	Slow release†
Theochron®	Tablet	Slow release
Theo-Dur®	Tablet	Slow release†♦
Theo-Dur® Sprinkle	Capsule	Slow release*†
Theo-Sav	Tablet	Slow release♦
Theolair™ SR	Tablet	Slow release†
Theovent®	Capsule	Slow release†
Theo-X®	Tablet	Slow release
Therapy Bayer	Caplet	Enteric-coated
Thorazine® Spansule®	Capsule	Slow release
Toprol XL®	Tablet	Slow release♦
Touro A&H®	Capsule	Slow release*
Touro EX®	Tablet	Slow release♦

TABLETS THAT CANNOT BE CRUSHED OR ALTERED
(Continued)

Drug Product	Dosage Forms	Reasons/Comments
Touro LA®	Tablet	Slow release♦
T-Phyl®	Tablet	Slow release
Trental®	Tablet	Slow release
Triaminic®	Tablet	Enteric-coated†
Triaminic-12®	Tablet†	Slow release†
Trilafon® Repetabs®	Tablet	Slow release†
Trinalin® Repetabs®	Tablet	Slow release
Tuss-LA®	Tablet	Slow release
Tuss-Ornade® Spansule®	Capsule	Slow release
ULR-LA®	Tablet	Slow release
Unicap®	Capsule	Liquid filled§
Uniphyl®	Tablet	Slow release
Valrelease®	Capsule	Slow release
Vanex® Forte	Caplet	Slow release
Vantin®	Tablet	Taste†††
Verelan®	Capsule	Slow release*
Volmax®	Tablet	Slow release†
Wyamycin® S	Tablet	Slow release
Wygesic®	Tablet	Taste
Zephrex LA®	Tablet	Slow release
ZORprin®	Tablet	Slow release
Zymase®	Capsule	Enteric-coated

Adapted from Mitchell JF and Pawlicki KS, "Oral Solid Dosage Forms That Should Not Be Crushed: 1996 Revision," *Hosp Pharm*, 1994, 29(7):666-75.

*Capsule may be opened and the contents taken without crushing or chewing; soft food such as applesauce or pudding may facilitate administration; contents may generally be administered via nasogastric tube using an appropriate fluid provided entire contents are washed down the tube.

†Liquid dosage forms of the product are available; however, dose, frequency of administration, and manufacturers may differ from that of the solid dosage form.

‡Antacids and/or milk may prematurely dissolve the coating of the tablet.

§Capsule may be opened and the liquid contents removed for administration.

††The taste of this product in a liquid form would likely be unacceptable to the patient; administration via nasogastric tube should be acceptable.

¶Effervescent tablets must be dissolved in the amount of diluent recommended by the manufacturer.

#If the liquid capsule is crushed or the contents expressed, the active ingredient will be, in part, absorbed sublingually.

•Tablets are made to disintegrate under the tongue.

♦Tablet is scored.

THERAPEUTIC CATEGORY INDEX

THERAPEUTIC CATEGORY INDEX

(Continued)

"Lexi-Comp's Clinical Reference Library™ (CRL) has established the new standard for quick reference information"

Lexi-Comp offers the Clinical Reference Library™ (CRL™), a series of clinical databases, as portable handbooks or integrated as part of a CD-ROM that also includes clinical decision support modules. CRL™ is delivered with a powerful search engine on a single CD-ROM and can be used with Microsoft® Windows™ release 3.1 or higher. In addition to our CD-ROM for Windows™, Lexi-Comp's databases can also be licensed for distribution on your Intranet, or used with your palmtop, Newton, or Windows™ CE device.

NEW titles targeted for release in print and on CD-ROM will include:

- **Drug Information Handbook for Nursing**
- **Drug Information Handbook for Cancer**
- **Drug Information Handbook for the Criminal Justice Professional**
- **Drug Information Handbook for Psychiatry**

Other titles offered by Lexi-Comp . . .

DRUG INFORMATION HANDBOOK 6th Edition 98/99

by Charles Lacy, PharmD; Lora L. Armstrong, BSPharm; Naomi Ingrim, PharmD; and Leonard L. Lance, BSPharm

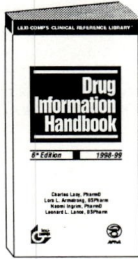

Specifically compiled and designed for the healthcare professional requiring quick access to concisely stated comprehensive data concerning clinical use of medications.

The Drug Information Handbook is an ideal portable drug information resource, containing 1100 drug monographs. Each monograph typically provides the reader with up to 29 key points of data concerning clinical use and dosing of the medication. Material provided in the Appendix section is recognized by many users to be, by itself, well worth the purchase of the handbook.

DRUG INFORMATION HANDBOOK POCKET 98/99

by Charles Lacy, PharmD; Lora L. Armstrong, BSPharm; Naomi Ingrim, PharmD; and Leonard L. Lance, BSPharm

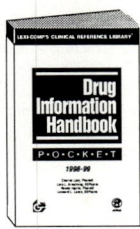

All medications found in the Drug Information Handbook, 6th Edition are included in this abridged pocket edition. It is specifically compiled and designed for the healthcare professional requiring quick access to concisely stated comprehensive data concerning clinical use of medications.

The outstanding cross-referencing allows the user to quickly locate the brand name, generic name, synonym, and related information found in the Appendix making this a useful quick reference for medical professionals at any level of training or experience.

ANESTHESIOLOGY & CRITICAL CARE DRUG HANDBOOK 98/99

by Andrew J. Donnelly, PharmD; Francesca E. Cunningham, PharmD; and Verna L. Baughman, MD

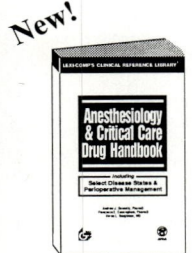

New!

Contains over 450 generic medications with up to 25 fields of information presented in each monograph. It also contains the following Special Issues and Topics: Allergic Reaction, Anesthesia for Cardiac Patients in Noncardiac Surgery, Anesthesia for Obstetric Patients in Nonobstetric Surgery, Anesthesia for Patients With Liver Disease, Chronic Pain Management, Chronic Renal Failure, Conscious Sedation, Perioperative Management of Patients on Antiseizure Medication, Substance Abuse and Anesthesia.

The Appendix contains over 140 pages of useful and valuable information including: Abbreviations & Measurements, Anesthesiology Information, Assessment of Liver & Renal Function, Comparative Drug Charts, Infectious Disease-Prophylaxis & Treatment, Laboratory Values, Therapy Recommendation, Toxicology, *and much more . . .*

PEDIATRIC DOSAGE HANDBOOK 5th Edition 98/99

by Carol K. Taketomo, PharmD; Jane Hurlburt Hodding, PharmD; and Donna M. Kraus, PharmD

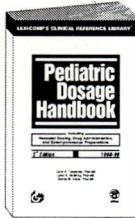

Special considerations must frequently be taken into account when dosing medications for the pediatric patient. This highly regarded quick reference handbook is a compilation of recommended pediatric doses based on current literature as well as the practical experience of the authors and their many colleagues who work every day in the pediatric clinical setting.

The Pediatric Dosage Handbook 5th Edition includes neonatal dosing, drug administration, and extemporaneous preparations for 619 medications used in pediatric medicine.

DRUG INFORMATION HANDBOOK FOR DENTISTRY 4th Edition 98/99

by Richard L. Wynn, BSPharm, PhD; Timothy F. Meiller, DDS, PhD; and Harold L. Crossley, DDS,

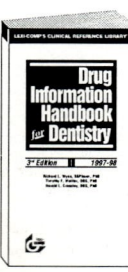

This handbook presents dental management and therapeutic considerations in medically compromised patients. Issues covered include oral manifestations of drugs, pertinent dental drug interactions, and dosing of drugs in dental treatment.

Selected oral medicine topics requiring therapeutic intervention include: managing the patient with acute or chronic pain including TMD, managing the patient with oral bacterial or fungal infections, current therapeutics in periodontal patients, managing the patient receiving chemotherapy or radiation for the treatment of cancer, managing the anxious patient, managing dental office emergencies, and treatment of common oral lesions.

DRUG INFORMATION HANDBOOK FOR THE ALLIED HEALTH PROFESSIONAL 5th Edition 98/99

by Leonard L. Lance, BSPharm; Charles Lacy, PharmD; and Morton P. Goldman, PharmD

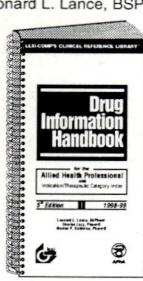

Working with clinical pharmacists, hospital pharmacy and therapeutics committees, and hospital drug information centers, the authors have assisted hundreds of hospitals in developing institution specific formulary reference documentation.

The most current basic drug and medication data from those clinical settings have been reviewed, coalesced, and cross-referenced to create this unique handbook. The handbook offers quick access to abbreviated monographs for 1441 generic drugs.

This is a great tool for physician assistants, medical records personnel, medical transcriptionists and secretaries, pharmacy technicians, and other allied health professionals.

INFECTIOUS DISEASES HANDBOOK 2nd Edition 97/98

by Carlos M. Isada MD; Bernard L. Kasten Jr. MD; Morton P. Goldman PharmD; Larry D. Gray PhD and Judith A. Aberg MD

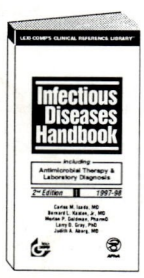

This four-in-one quick reference is concerned with the identification and treatment of infectious diseases. A unique feature of the handbook is that entries in each of the four sections of the book (164 disease syndromes, 143 organisms, 231 laboratory tests, and 222 antimicrobials) contain related information and cross-referencing to one or more of the other three sections.

The disease syndrome section provides straight-forward information on the clinical presentation, differential diagnosis, diagnostic tests, and drug therapy recommended for treatment of more common infectious diseases. The organism section presents discussion of the microbiology, epidemiology, diagnosis, and treatment of each organism. The laboratory diagnosis section describes performance of specific tests and procedures. The antimicrobial therapy section presents important facts and considerations regarding each drug recommended for specific diseases of organisms.

POISONING & TOXICOLOGY COMPENDIUM 98/99 (New 8½ x 11 Size!)
by Jerrold B. Leikin, MD and Frank P. Paloucek, PharmD

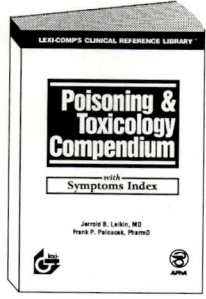

A six-in-one reference wherein each major entry contains information relative to one or more of the other sections. This handbook offers comprehensive concisely-stated monographs covering 645 medicinal agents, 256 nonmedicinal agents, 273 biological agents, 49 herbal agents, 254 laboratory tests, 79 antidotes, and 222 pages of exceptionally useful appendix material.

A truly unique reference that presents signs and symptoms of acute overdose along with considerations for overdose treatment. Ideal reference for emergency situations.

LABORATORY TEST HANDBOOK - CONCISE (New!)
by David S. Jacobs, MD, FACP, FCAP; Wayne R. DeMott, MD, FCAP; Harold J. Grady, PhD; Rebecca T. Horvat, PhD; Douglas W. Huestis, MD; Bernard L. Kasten Jr., MD, FCAP

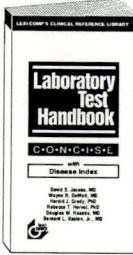

The authors of Lexi-Comp's highly regarded Laboratory Test Handbook have selected and extracted key information for presentation in this portable abridged version. It contains more than 800 test entries for quick reference and is ideal for residents, nurses, and medical students or technologists requiring information concerning patient preparation, specimen collection and handling, and test result interpretation.

LABORATORY TEST HANDBOOK 4th Edition 1996
by David S. Jacobs MD, FACP; Wayne R. DeMott, MD, FACP; Harold J. Grady, PhD; Rebecca T. Horvat, PhD; Douglas W. Huestis, MD; and Bernard L. Kasten Jr., MD, FACP

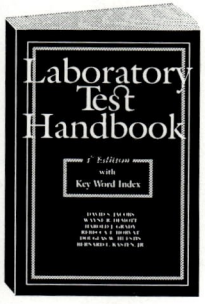

This is a single reference source that contains difficult to find general and interpretive information pertinent to the use of over 900 clinical laboratory tests.

Includes sections on Molecular Pathology and Trace Elements and each test entry in a section is complete in itself providing the user with the test name, synonyms, patient care recommendations, specimen requirements, reference ranges, methodology, footnotes, and references. Updated CPT and ICD-9 coding is also provided. This handbook delivers answers to many typical questions posed about laboratory tests. An extremely useful reference for practitioners and other healthcare professionals.

DIAGNOSTIC PROCEDURE HANDBOOK by Joseph A. Golish, MD

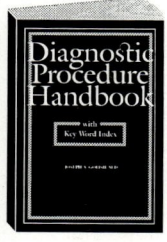

An ideal companion to the Laboratory Test Handbook this publication details 295 diagnostic procedures including: Allergy, Immunology/Rheumotology, Infectious Disease, Cardiology, Critical Care, Gastroenterology, Nephrology, Urology, Hematology, Neurology, Ophthalmology, Pulmonary Function, Pulmonary Medicine, Computed Tomography, Diagnostic Radiology, Invasive Radiology, Magnetic Resonance Imaging, Nuclear Medicine, and Ultrasound. A great reference handbook for healthcare professionals at any level of training and experience.